Lecture Notes in Computer Science   1679

Edited by G. Goos, J. Hartmanis and J. van Leeuwen

W0231962

Springer-Verlag Berlin Heidelberg GmbH

Chris Taylor   Alan Colchester (Eds.)

Medical
Image Computing
and Computer-Assisted
Intervention – MICCAI'99

Second International Conference
Cambridge, UK, September 19-22, 1999
Proceedings

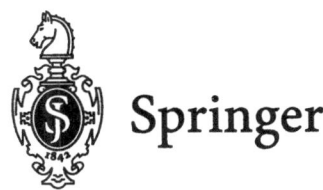 Springer

Series Editors

Gerhard Goos, Karlsruhe University, Germany
Juris Hartmanis, Cornell University, NY, USA
Jan van Leeuwen, Utrecht University, The Netherlands

Volume Editors

Chris Taylor
The University of Manchester
Oxford Road, Manchester M13 9PT, UK
E-mail: ctaylor@man.ac.uk

Alan Colchester
University of Kent
Canterbury, Kent CT2 7NT, UK
E-mail: a.colchester@ukc.ac.uk

Cataloging-in-Publication data applied for

Die Deutsche Bibliothek - CIP-Einheitsaufnahme

Medical image computing and computer assisted intervention : second
international conference ; proceedings / MICCAI '99, Cambridge, UK, September
19 - 22, 1999. Chris Taylor ; Alan Colchester (ed.). - Berlin ; Heidelberg ;
New York ; Barcelona ; Hong Kong ; London ; Milan ; Paris ; Singapore ; Tokyo :
Springer, 1999
(Lecture notes in computer science ; Vol. 1679)

CR Subject Classification (1998): I.5, I.3.5-8, I.2.9-10, I.4, J.3

ISSN 0302-9743

ISBN 978-3-540-66503-8   ISBN 978-3-540-48232-1 (eBook)
DOI 10.1007/978-3-540-48232-1

© Springer-Verlag Berlin Heidelberg 1999
Originally published by Springer-Verlag Berlin Heidelberg New York in 1999.
Typesetting: Camera-ready by author
SPIN: 10704282   06/3142 – 5 4 3 2 1 0   Printed on acid-free paper

Preface

This is the second MICCAI – the flagship international conference for medical image computing and computer-assisted intervention. MICCAI was created by merging three closely related and thriving conference series – VBC (Visualisation in Biomedical Computing), MRCAS (Medical Robotics and Computer Assisted Surgery) and CVRMed (Computer Vision, Virtual Reality and Robotics in Medicine) – to provide a single focus for the presentation of high-quality research in this important multi-disciplinary area. The first MICCAI was held in Boston, USA in October 1998. It attracted a large number of excellent submissions and was extremely well attended. The meeting went a long way towards meeting its ambitious objectives of bringing together the best theoretical and applied work in this rapidly emerging field, and encouraging constructive dialogue between computer scientists and clinicians.

We are delighted to report a similar level of interest in MICCAI'99. A total of 213 full-length papers were submitted, covering a broad range of topics. Of these, 133 were accepted for inclusion in the conference – 49 as oral presentations and 84 as posters. All the selected papers appear in these proceedings. Each paper was reviewed by four members of the Scientific Review Committee, selected for scientific or clinical expertise of relevance to the subject matter. Final decisions were made by the Programme Committee, following closely the advice of the reviewers. We are indebted to the members of the Scientific Review Committee for the time they devoted to the review process and for their well-informed and generally detailed feedback to authors.

The result is another volume of high-quality papers that we hope will contribute to the development of this important and exciting area. We are also indebted to the dedicated team of staff and students at Manchester who helped to put together the proceedings, particularly Angela Castledine, Alan Brett, Mike Rodgers, Danny Allen, Christine Beeston, Karen Davies, Tony Lacey, and Chris Wolstenholme. We were very pleased to welcome delegates to Cambridge and hope that you found MICCAI an enjoyable and stimulating experience. For readers unable to attend the conference, we hope that you will find this a valuable record of the scientific programme, and look forward to meeting you at MICCAI 2000, which will be held in Pittsburgh, USA.

September 1999   Chris Taylor and Alan Colchester

Conference Organising Committee

Second International Conference on
Medical Image Computing and Computer-Assisted Intervention
Cambridge, England
September 19–22, 1999

General Chair

Alan Colchester   University of Kent at Canterbury and Guy's
                                Hospital, London, UK

Co-chairs

Mike Brady   University of Oxford, UK
Jun-Ichiro Toriwaki   University of Nagoya, Japan

Programme Chair

Chris Taylor (Chair)   University of Manchester, UK

Programme Committee

Nicholas Ayache   INRIA Sophia Antipolis, France
Richard D Bucholz   St Louis University School of Medicine, USA
Brian Davies   Imperial College, UK
Tony DiGioia   Shadyside Hospital, Pittsburgh, USA
James Scott Duncan   Yale University, USA
Guido Gerig   University of North Carolina, USA
David Hawkes   Guy's Hospital, UK
Max A Viergever   Utrecht University, Netherlands

Clinical Advisory Committee Chair

Tony DiGioia   Shadyside Hospital, Pittsburgh, USA

Tutorials

Guido Gerig   University of North Carolina, USA

Industrial Liaison

Nicholas Ayache	INRIA Sophia Antipolis, France
Mike Brady	University of Oxford, UK
Bart ter Haar Romeny	University of Utrecht, Netherlands
Jocelyne Troccaz	University of Grenoble, France
Nigel John (Coordinator)	University of Manchester, UK

Local Organising Committee

Richard Prager	University of Cambridge, UK
Andrew Gee	University of Cambridge, UK

Scientific Review Committee

James Anderson	Johns Hopkins School of Medicine, USA
Takehide Asano	Chiba University School of Medicine, Japan
Gerard A Ateshian	Columbia University, USA
Nicholas Ayache	INRIA Sophia Antipolis, France
Isabelle Bloch	Ecole Nationale Superieure des Telecommunications, France
Fred Bookstein	University of Michigan, USA
Mike Brady	University of Oxford, UK
Richard D Bucholz	St Louis University School of Medicine, USA
Steve Charles	University of Tenessee, USA
Philippe Cinquin	Institut Albert Bonniot, France
Ela Claridge	University of Birmingham, UK
Court Cutting	New York University, USA
Paolo Dario	ARTS Lab, Italy
Brian Davies	Imperial College, UK
Scott Delp	Stanford University, USA
Tony DiGioia	Shadyside Hospital, Pittsburgh, USA
Takeyoshi Dohi	University of Tokyo, Japan
James Scott Duncan	Yale University, USA
Norberto Ezquerra	Universidad Politecnica de Catalunya, Spain
Elliot Fishman	The Johns Hopkins Hospital, USA
J Michael Fitzpatrick	Vanderbilt University, USA
Henry Fuchs	University of North Carolina, USA
Toshio Fukuda	Nagoya University, Japan
Guido Gerig	University of North Carolina, USA
Sarah Gibson	Mitsubishi Electric Research Lab, USA
Eric L Grimson	MIT AI Lab, USA
Blake Hannaford	University of Washington, USA
Dave Hawkes	Guy's Hospital, UK
Derek Hill	Guy's Hospital, UK

MICCAI Conference Series

MICCAI Board

Nicholas Ayache	INRIA Sofia Antipolis, France
Alan Colchester	University of Kent at Canterbury & Guy's Hospital, London, UK
Toni Digioia	Shadyside Hospital, Pittsburgh, USA
Takeyoshi Dohi	University of Tokyo, Japan
Jim Duncan	Yale University, USA
Eric Grimson	MIT Artificial Intelligence Laboratory, USA
Karl-Heinz Höhne	University of Hamburg, Germany
Ron Kikinis	Brigham and Women's Hospital, Boston, USA
Steve Pizer	University of North Carolina, USA
Richard Robb	Mayo Clinic, USA
Russ Taylor	Johns Hopkins Hospital, Baltimore, USA
Jocelyne Troccaz	University of Grenoble, France

Table of Contents

Data-Driven Segmentation

Segmentation Using Structural Models

Image Processing and Feature Detection

Surfaces and Shape

Measurement and Interpretation

Spatiotemporal and Diffusion Tensor Analysis

Registration and Fusion

Robotic Systems

Biomechanics and Simulation

Segmentation of Meningiomas and Low Grade Gliomas in MRI

M. R. Kaus[1,3], S. K. Warfield[1], A. Nabavi[1,2], E. Chatzidakis[1,2]
, P. M. Black[2], F. A. Jolesz[1], and R. Kikinis[1]

[1] Surgical Planning Laboratory, Department of Radiology,
[2] Department of Neurosurgery,
Brigham and Women's Hospital, Harvard Medical School,
75 Francis St., Boston, MA 02115
[3] Lehrstuhl Technische Elektronik, Universität Erlangen-Nürnberg,
D-91058 Erlangen, Germany
{kaus,warfield,arya,manos,jolesz,kikinis}@bwh.harvard.edu,
pmblack@bics.bwh.harvard.edu
http://splweb.bwh.harvard.edu:8000

Abstract. Computer assisted surgical planning and image guided technology have become increasingly used in neurosurgery. We have developed a system based on ATmC (Adaptive Template moderated Classification) for the automated segmentation of 3D MRI brain data sets of patients with brain tumors (meningiomas and low grade gliomas) into the skin, the brain, the ventricles and the tumor. In a validation study of 13 patients with brain tumors, the segmentation results of the automated method are compared to manual segmentations carried out by 4 independent trained human observers. It is shown that the automated method segments brain and tumor with accuracy comparable to the manual method and with improved reproducibility.

Keywords: Surgical planning, Image guided neurosurgery, Magnetic resonance (MR), segmentation, registration, brain, tumor

1 Introduction

Computer assisted surgical planning and image guided technology have become increasingly used in neurosurgery [1, 9, 15, 21]. 2D images accurately describe the size and location of anatomical objects. The process of generating 3D views to highlight structural information and spatial relationships of the anatomy, however, is a difficult task and usually carried out in the clinician's mind. Image processing tools can provide the surgeon with interactively displayed 3D visual information to facilitate the comprehension of the entire anatomy, and improve the spatial information about relationships of critical structures (e.g. motory and sensory cortex, vascular structures) and pathology [12].

Today commercially available systems usually provide the surgeon only with 2D cross-sections of the intensity value images and a 3D model of the skin. The main limiting factor for the routine use of 3D models of other important structures in clinical practice is the amount of time that an operator has to spend in the preparation of the data [7, 14]. The availability of automated methods will significantly reduce the time and is necessary to make such methods practical.

Conventional segmentation methods for tumor segmentation such as statistical classification or mathematical morphological operations may work well in some cases but may not differentiate between enhancing tumor, edema and normal tissue [8, 17, 18]. For the separation of these tissues, the acquisition of several tissue parameters alone has been shown to be insufficient [10]. A combination of statistical classification and anatomical information has been used for the segmentation of MRI images of the brain [3, 11, 20]. In a recent study, an anatomical knowledge guided fuzzy c-means method was used for automatic detection and segmentation of glioblastoma multiforme from a combination of T1-, T2- and Proton density (PD) MR images with promising results [2].

We have developed an automated segmentation method based on ATmC (Adaptive Template moderated Classification) [19] that combines statistical classification with anatomical knowledge from a digital atlas. The algorithm segments the skin surface, the brain, the ventricles and some of the most common tumor types, meningiomas and low grade gliomas. The purpose of the current study was to assess the accuracy and robustness of the algorithm by comparing the automated method to manual segmentation carried out by trained medical experts.

2   Materials and Methods

2.1   Patient Image Data

The MRI datasets consisted of a 3D sagittal spoiled gradient recalled (SPGR) acquisition (field of view (FOV): 240 mm; slice-thickness: 1.5 mm; 256× 256 × 124 matrix) after gadolinium-enhancement. 13 different patients with brain tumors of different size, shape and location were selected, i.e. 5 meningiomas (cases No. 1–3, 11, 12), and 8 low grade gliomas (cases No. 4–10, 13). A development database (cases No. 1–10) used for the design and validation of the automated segmentation method was extracted from a neurosurgical image database of approximately. 100 brain tumor cases that had been post-processed for image guided neurosurgery (manual outlining of the structures skin-surface, brain, ventricles, vessels and tumor). These cases provided a representative selection of meningioma and low grade glioma cases. Validation was also carried out on the datasets of 3 patients (cases No. 11-13) were image acquisition and processing took place after completion of the algorithm development.

2.2   Automated segmentation of brain and tumor

We adapted a general algorithm intended for the automated segmentation of anatomical objects in different locations in the human body [19]. The algorithm combines two approaches to image segmentation into an iterative process: statistical classification and segmentation by registration of an anatomical atlas

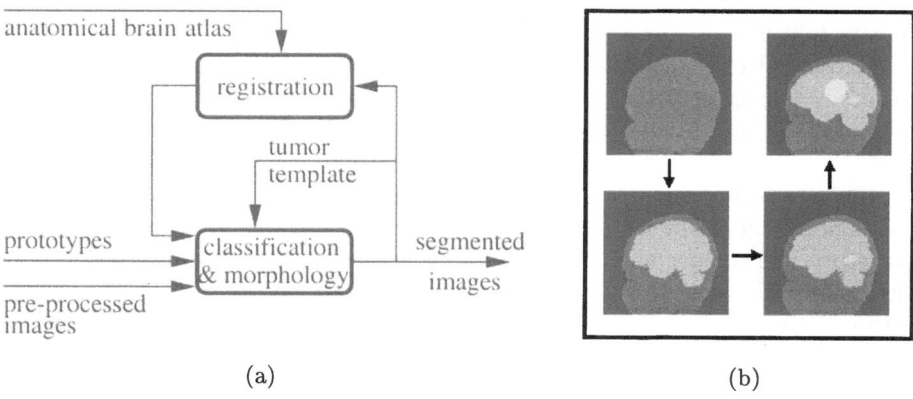

(a)   (b)

Fig. 1. ATmC (Adaptive Template moderated Classification) segmentation scheme (a) and brain tumor segmentation flow diagram (b).

(Fig. 1). We summarize here the concept of the segmentation framework and its application to brain tumor segmentation. For a mathematical description we refer to [19].

Image Segmentation Statistical classification (k-Nearest Neighbor rule) divides the image into different tissue classes based on the signal intensity value [5]. Overlap between signal intensity distributions of different tissue classes leads to mis-classifications. To resolve this problem, additional information is derived from a digital volumetric atlas of a normal brain that has been manually segmented into approximately. 250 different structures by medical experts [12]. By projecting anatomical templates from the atlas onto the individual patient data, different structures of interest in the patient dataset can be located according to their location in the atlas.

Comparing the images of two different brains requires non-linear registration for the projection of the atlas onto the patient data, capturing individual differences by allowing structures to shrink, grow, and twist, and to move or rotate locally and independently [4]. In our approach, the algorithm computes the spatial nonlinear transform on the basis of the segmented images, rather than the original signal intensity values, in order that the registration be less susceptible to image noise and intensity artifacts.

Instead of directly projecting anatomical templates onto the patient and thus having to rely on hard boundaries, a model of anatomical localization was formulated that reflects lower confidence in the localization towards the boundary of structures ("soft boundaries"). This was implemented by using Euclidian distance transforms computed from the templates as additional anatomical feature channels in the kNN classification. The approach has the advantage that a very precise registration is not necessary, because the method uses both the MR intensity information and the soft spatial location.

Statistical classification and registration of the anatomical brain atlas are iterated. The goal of the iteration is to improve the result of the registration by providing tentative image segmentations, and to improve the result of the classification by providing regions of interest.

Objects of interest are defined on the classified images, where every voxel was labeled according to the assigned tissue class. For the identification of each structure and removal of classification artifacts, a local segmentation strategy was used, consisting of a) a morphological erosion to "cut" classification artifacts such as thin connections between different objects, b) a connected-component algorithm to re-label every voxel as belonging to one object or another and c) a morphological dilation to restore previously eroded voxels on the object boundaries [16].

Application to tumor segmentation Five tissue classes were modeled: background, skin (fat/bone), brain, ventricles, and tumor. Due to the homogeneous tissue composition of meningiomas and low grade gliomas one tissue class was sufficient for the statistical model. A simple, hierarchical model of anatomy was used to define the order in which the different structures were segmented. By proceeding hierarchically from the outside to the inside of the head (Fig. 1), each segmented structure provided additional anatomical knowledge (i.e. a refined region of interest) for the next structure to be segmented. A standard normal brain atlas contains no tumor template. This has three consequences. First, anatomical templates from the atlas were derived only for the head, the ICC and the ventricles. Second, because the registration paradigm assumes correspondence between every structure in atlas and patient, a compound tissue class of the normal and pathologic brain structures was formed during ICC registration. The atlas brain was registered to the patient brain *and* pathology. Third, in a first tumor segmentation iteration, only atlas brain and ventricle templates were used. In a second iteration, the tumor segmentation from the first iteration was used as an anatomical template. Although this template was approximate, the additional information about the location of the tumor prevented the mis-classification of brain.

Initialization of the automated segmentation method Prior to the segmentation, the image data is preprocessed with an anisotropic diffusion filtering method to reduce the noise in the MR images while preserving edges [6]. The method requires the selection of 3–4 example points for each tissue class. For the 2D display of MR slices and the selection of example tissue points using a mouse a graphical user interface was developed. The program calculated a statistical model for the distribution of the grey values based on these manually selected tissue prototypes.

2.3   Validation

Since there is no "gold standard" to compare with, our definition of a segmentation "gold standard" is based upon the opinion of the medical expert, manifested in manual segmentations using interactive computer segmentation tools. However, manual segmentation is subject to inter-rater variability and human error. To minimize the influence of these factors while maintaining the means of measuring the segmentation accuracy of the individual raters, the standard was defined as the area of those voxels where at least 3 out of 4 experts agreed upon the identification. To determine inter- and intra-variability of the segmentation results, a fifth rater manually segmented each selected 2D slice 4 times over a period of one week, and the 4 experts carried out repeated initialization of the automated algorithm.

The experimental setup was the following: The automated algorithm was trained on a single MR slice containing the structures of interest and executed, resulting in a segmentation of the entire 3D dataset into the structures skin, brain, ventricles and tumor. A single 2D slice was randomly selected from the subset of MR slices containing the tumor. On those slices brain and tumor were manually segmented by 4 trained medical experts using an interactive segmentation tool (MRX, GE Medical Systems, Schenectady, NY). The structures were outlined slice-by-slice by pointing and clicking with a mouse. The program connected consecutive points with lines. An anatomical object was defined by a closed contour, and the program labeled every voxel of the enclosed volume.

Statistical analysis was carried out by comparing the volumes of the automatically with the manually segmented structures. Accuracy was defined as the percentage of correctly classified voxels with respect to the total number of voxels in the image. To measure the inter- and intra-rater variation, the coefficient of variation (CV% = 100*[(SD volume)/(mean volume)], SD: standard deviation) of the volume of the structure was calculated.

3   Results and Discussion

Examples for manual and automated segmentation (Fig. 2) for a meningioma (top row) and a low grade glioma (bottom row) illustrate high similarity between the two methods. Fig. 3 shows the accuracy for brain and tumor segmentation achieved by the automated and the manual method. The segmentation accuracy of the cases 11–13 is displayed in Tab. 1. The segmentation accuracy with the automated method is above 95 % for brain and above 99 % for tumor, and within or close (maximum difference 0.6 %) to the range of the minimum and maximum of the accuracy with the manual method. The errors of the automated brain segmentation are in part due to the over- and under-segmentation in the area of the tentorium cerebelli and the area of the lateral sulcus with abundant vessels. The algorithm tends to oversegment these areas, if voxels e.g. of the neck close to the cerebellum are mis-classified as brain and the template ICC derived from the atlas is mis-registered.

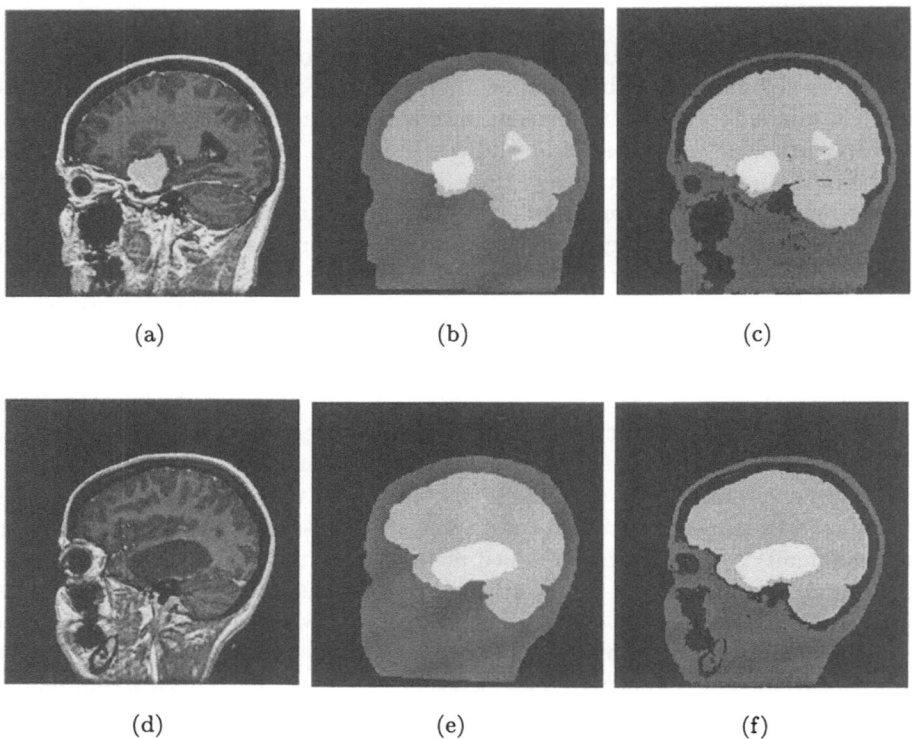

Fig. 2. Examples of manual and automated segmentation: Meningioma (SPGR image (a), manual (b), and automated segmentation (c)). Low Grade Glioma (SPGR image (d), manual (e), and automated segmentation (f).

The size of the structure affects the segmentation accuracy. Potentially, the boundaries are the areas of segmentation error. Since the comparison is based on measuring the number of correctly classified voxels (fore- and background), large objects tend to have a lower accuracy since there are more boundary voxels to mis-classify with respect to the entire image.

Fig. 4 and Fig. 5 show the inter- and intra-rater variability achieved by the manual and the automated methods. The horizontal lines mark the mean coefficient of variability over all 10 cases.

The inter- and intra-observer variability of both methods are lower for the brain than for the tumor. This is because the methods are consistent in labeling the "center" of an object, but vary in the determination of the boundaries. Since the brain is a larger structure than the tumor, the disagreement on the brain boundary with respect to the overall brain volume (not the entire image, as for the accuracy measurement) is less significant than for the tumor.

Table 1. Segmentation accuracy of the three cases 11-13, where image data was acquired and segmented after completion of the algorithm development.

Tumor Histology	Brain Accuracy [%]				Tumor Accuracy [%]			
	Manual			ATmC	Manual			ATmC
	min	max	mean		min	max	mean	
Meningioma	96.66	99.69	99.48	97.23	99.12	99.58	99.44	99.58
Meningioma	98.75	99.62	99.15	98.69	99.25	99.89	99.72	99.57
Low Grade Glioma	96.55	99.72	98.85	99.16	99.90	99.94	99.93	99.91

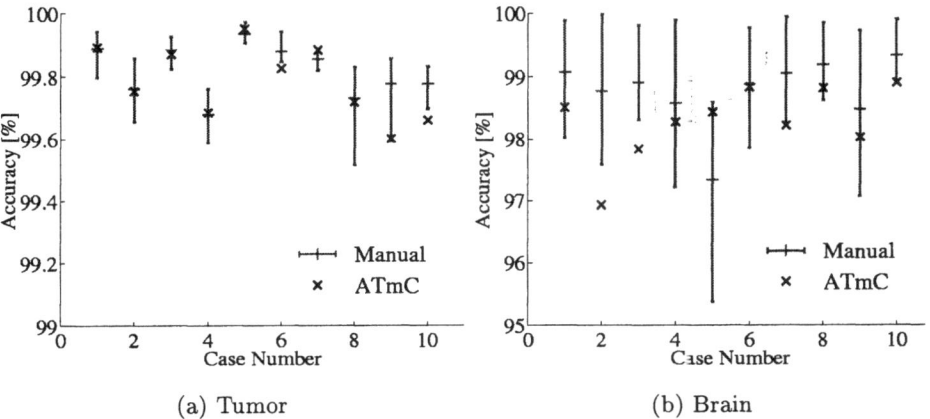

(a) Tumor   (b) Brain

Fig. 3. Segmentation accuracy of the manual (mean, minimum and maximum) and the automated method for each of the 10 brain tumor cases (1-3 Meningiomas), (7-10 Low Grade Gliomas).

The mean inter- and intra-observer variability of the automated method is lower than with manual outlining. While the inter-observer variability with the automated method is consistently lower than with the manual method, the intra-observer variability of the automated method is higher for most of the low grade glioma cases. This can be explained with the different grey value distributions of the meningioma and the low grade gliomas with respect to the brain. The meningioma tissue class partially overlaps with parts of the skin, fat in the neck and the straight and superior sagittal sinus. By restricting the region of interest (ROI) for the meningioma to the ICC, tissues that show signal intensity overlap with the meningioma are excluded and the meningioma can be successfully segmented. Low grade gliomas, however, are less distinguishable from brain tissue. Partial volume artifacts on the boundary of the brain and the tumor may cause signal intensity overlap between grey matter and tumor tissue, leading to mis-classifications, i.e. over- or under-segmentation of brain and tumor. Thus, the classifier is more sensitive to differences in the tissue prototype selection.

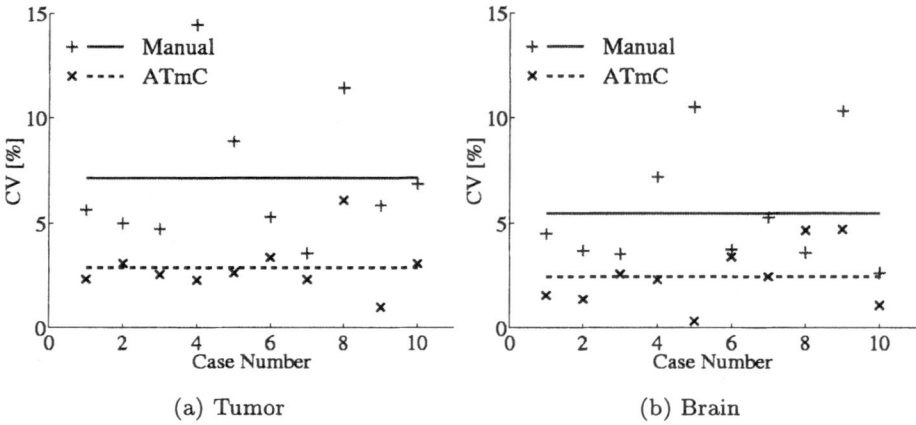

Fig. 4. Inter-observer variability of manual and automated method (coefficient of variation, CV). The horizontal line marks the mean of the CV values.

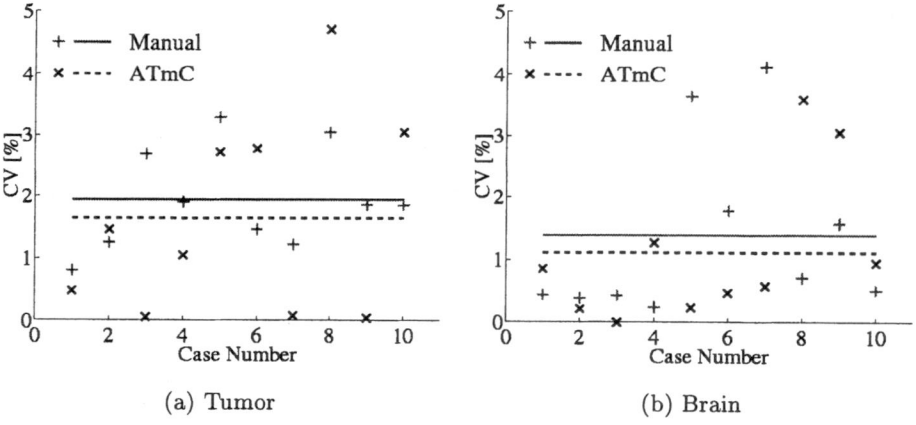

Fig. 5. Intra-observer variability of manual and automated method (coefficient of variation, CV). The horizontal line marks the mean of the CV values.

The mean computation time for the automated segmentation of the whole volume was 75 minutes on a Sun ES 6000 server with 20 CPUs and 5 GB of RAM (Sun Microsystems, Mountain View, CA). The overall operator time was approximately. 5–10 minutes for the selection of prototypes for each of the relevant tissue classes, while manual segmentation time for a neurosurgical case has been reported to be in the range of 180 minutes [14]. The reduction of operator time makes it practical to consider the integration of computerized segmentation into clinical routine.

3.1 Conclusion and Future Work

We have developed a method for the automated segmentation of meningiomas and low grade gliomas without edema. Accuracy and intra-observer variability of the automated method are comparable to the segmentation results from trained human observers, with improved inter-observer variability.

Further investigation is required to extend the algorithm to a broader range of brain tumors such as the glioblastoma multiforme or tumors with edema. Our algorithm is implemented on high performance computing hardware. However, through further algorithmic improvement and hardware speedups, we expect that this method will become practical in a clinical setting in the near future [13]. Currently, our tool is used in routine surgical planning to provide the basis for a clinical study based on a larger population to determine robustness and practical use in a clinical setting.

Acknowledgments

This work was supported (in part) by a grant from the Deutscher Akademischer Austauschdienst (DAAD). This investigation was supported (in part) by a Grant from the National Multiple Sclerosis Society (SW). This work was supported (in part) by NIH grants RO1 CA 46627-08, PO1 CA67165-01A1, PO1 AG04953-14, NSF grant BES 9631710 and Darpa grant F41624-96-2-0001. The authors thank Dr. Alexandra Chabrerie, Dr. Fatma Ozlen and Dr. Daniel Boll, Brigham and Women's Hospital, Boston for their help with the manual segmentations.

References

1. PM Black, T Moriarty, E Alexander, P Stieg, and EJ Woodward. Development and implementation of intraoperative magnetic resonance imaging and its neurosurgical applications. *Neurosurgery*, 41:831–845, 1997.
2. M Clark. *Knowledge Guided Processing of Magnetic Resonance Images of the Brain*. PhD thesis, University of South Florida, Tampa, Florida, 1998.
3. DL Collins, TM Peters, W Dai, and AC Evans. Model based segmentation of individual brain structures from MRI data. *SPIE Visualization in Biomedical Computing*, 1808:10–23, 1992.
4. J Dengler and M Schmidt. The dynamic pyramid - a model for motion analysis with controlled continuity. *International Journal of Pattern Analysis and Machine Intelligence*, 2(2):275–286, 1987.
5. RO Duda and PE Hart. *Pattern Classification and Scene Analysis*. John Wiley and Sons, New York, 1973.
6. G Gerig, R Kikinis, O Kübler, and FA Jolesz. Nonlinear anisotropic filtering of MRI data. *IEEE Transactions on Medical Imaging*, 11(2):221–232, 1992.

7. G Gerig, J Martin, R Kikinis, O Kübler, M Shenton, and FA Jolesz. Unsupervised tissue type segmentation of 3D dual-echo MR head data. *Image and Vision Computing*, 10(6):349–360, 1992.

8. P Gibbs, DL Buckley, SJ Blackband, and A Horsman. Tumor volume determination from MR images by morphological segmentation. *Physics in Medicine and Biology*, 41:2437–2446, 1996.

9. F Jolesz. Image-guided procedures and the operating room of the future. *Radiology*, 204:601–612, 1997.

10. M Just and M Thelen. Tissue characterization with T1, T2, and proton density values: Results in 160 patients with brain tumors. *Radiology*, 169:779–785, 1988.

11. M Kamber, R Shinghal, DL Collins, GS Francis, and AC Evans. Model-based 3-D segmentation of multiple sclerosis lesions in magnetic resonance brain images. *IEEE Transactions on Medical Imaging*, 14(3):442–453, 1995.

12. R Kikinis, PL Gleason, TM Moriarty, MR Moore, E Alexander III, PE Stieg, M Matsumae, WE Lorensen, HE Cline, PM Black, and FA Jolesz. Computer assisted interactive three-dimensional planning for neurosurgical procedures. *Neurosurgery*, 38(4):640–651, 1996.

13. R Kikinis, SK Warfield, and CF Westin. High performance computing (HPC) in medical image analysis (MIA) at the surgical planning laboratory (SPL). In *Proceedings of the 3rd High Performance Computing Asia Conference & Exhibition*, 1998.

14. S Nakajima, H Atsumi, A Bhalerao, FA Jolesz, R Kikinis, T Yoshimine, T Moriarty, and P Stieg. Computer-assisted surgical planning for cerebrovascular neurosurgery. *Neurosurgery*, 41:403–409, 1997.

15. DW Roberts, JW Strohbehn, JF Hatch, W Murray, and H Kettenberger. A frameless stereotaxic integration of computerized tomographic imaging and the operating microscope. *Journal of Neurosurgery*, 65:545–549, 1986.

16. J Serra. *Image analysis and mathematical morphology*. London Academic, London, 1982.

17. RP Velthuizen, LP Clarke, S Phuphanich, LO Hall, AM Bensaid, JA Arrington, HM Greenberg, and ML Silbinger. Unsupervised measurement of brain tumor volume on MR images. *JMRI*, 5:594–605, 1995.

18. S Vinitski, C Gonzalez, F Mohamed, T Iwanaga, RL Knobler, K Khalili, and J Mack. Improved intracranial lesion characterization by tissue segmentation based on a 3D feature map. *Magn Res Med*, 37:457–469, 1997.

19. SK Warfield, M Kaus, F Jolesz, and R Kikinis. Adaptive template moderated spatially varying statistical classification. In *Proceedings of the 1st International Conference on Medical Image Computing and Computer-Assisted Intervention*, pages 431–438, Boston, MA, 1998.

20. SK Warfield, J Dengler, J Zaers, CRG Guttmann, WM Wells, GJ Ettinger, J Hiller, and R Kikinis. Automatic identification of grey matter structures from MRI to improve the segmentation of white matter lesions. *Journal of Image Guided Surgery*, 1(6):326–338, 1995.

21. E Watanabe, T Watanabe, S Manaka, Y Mayanagi, and K Takakura. Three-dimensional digitizer (neuronavigator): new equipment for computed tomography-guided stereotaxic surgery. *Surgical Neurology*, 27(6):543–547, 1987.

Automated Segmentation of MS Lesions from Multi-channel MR Images

Koen Van Leemput[1], Frederik Maes[1], Fernando Bello[2], Dirk Vandermeulen[1], Alan Colchester[2], and Paul Suetens[1]

[1] Katholieke Universiteit Leuven, Medical Image Computing, Radiology-ESAT, UZ Gasthuisberg, Herestraat 49, B-3000 Leuven, Belgium
[2] Neurosciences Medical Image Analysis Group, Electronic Engineering Laboratory, University of Kent of Canterbury, Canterbury Kent CT2 7NT, UK
Koen.VanLeemput@uz.kuleuven.ac.be

Abstract. Quantitative analysis of MR images is becoming increasingly important as a surrogate marker in clinical trials in multiple sclerosis (MS). This paper describes a fully automated model-based method for segmentation of MS lesions from multi-channel MR images. The method simultaneously corrects for MR field inhomogeneities, estimates tissue class distribution parameters and classifies the image voxels. MS lesions are detected as voxels that are not well explained by the model. The results of the automated method are compared with the lesions delineated by human experts, showing a significant total lesion load correlation and an average overall spatial correspondence similar to that between the experts.

1 Introduction

The role of magnetic resonance (MR) imaging in assessing the progression of multiple sclerosis (MS) and in monitoring the effect of a drug therapy is of increasing importance. This is caused by the higher sensitivity and objectivity of an MR-based surrogate index compared to traditional clinical disability scales [1], in combination with the widespread availability of MR imaging.

In clinical trials, manual analysis of the MR images by human experts is too time-consuming because of the large amounts of data involved. Furthermore, the inter- and intra-observer variability associated with manual delineations complicates the analysis of the results. Finally, it is not clear how a human rater combines information obtained from the different channels when multi-spectral MR data are examined.

Therefore, considerable efforts have been made by the medical imaging community to come up with fast automated methods that produce more objective and reproducible results [2–4]. However, most of these techniques still require some human interaction and/or ad hoc processing steps, which can make the results not fully objective. Zijdenbos *et. al* [5,6] proposed and validated a fully automated pipeline for MS lesion segmentation from T1-, T2- and PD-weighted images. However, they used a fixed classifier that must be retrained in cases where different scanner types or pulse sequences produce contrast variations.

We present a fully automated technique for segmenting MS lesions from T1-, T2-, and PD-weighted MR images that automatically retrains the classifier. More specifically, a model-based iterative algorithm is used that simultaneously corrects for MR field inhomogeneities, estimates tissue class distribution parameters, and classifies the image voxels. The MS lesions are detected as voxels that are not well explained by the model.

The paper is organized as follows. The method is explained in section 2. Section 3 presents a validation of the automatic lesion segmentation by comparing it with the delineations of human experts. We discuss the results in section 4 and briefly formulate our conclusions in section 5.

2   Method

2.1   Model-based segmentation of normal MR images of the brain

Recently, we described a model-based method for fully automated classification of MR images of normal brains [7, 8]. Since we will build on this method in the rest of this paper, we briefly describe it here.

Suppose that there are J tissue types or so-called classes present in an MR image of the brain. Let the intensity of voxel i be denoted as y_i, then $y = \{y_1, \ldots, y_i, \ldots, y_N\}$ describes the observed intensities where N is the total number of voxels. An often-used simple model for the intensity distribution of a voxel i that belongs to class j is a normal distribution with parameters mean μ_j and variance σ_j^2, grouped in $\theta_j = \{\mu_j, \sigma_j^2\}$. MR images often suffer from an imaging artifact that introduces a spatially smoothly varying intensity inhomogeneity or so-called bias field in the images. We model the bias field in image y as a linear combination $\sum_k c_k \phi_k(x)$ of K smoothly varying basis functions $\phi_k(x)$, where x denotes the spatial position. With this model, the intensity distribution of a voxel i that belongs to class j is given by $p(y_i \mid \Gamma_i{=}j, \theta_j, C) = G_{\sigma_j}(y_i - \mu_j - \sum_k c_k \phi_k(x_i))$ where $G_\sigma()$ denotes a zero-mean normal distribution with variance σ^2, $\Gamma_i \in \{1, \ldots, j, \ldots, J\}$ denotes the class to which voxel i belongs, and $C = \{c_1, \ldots, c_K\}$ contains the bias field parameters. Assuming that the tissue types of the voxels are independently sampled from the J classes with some known probability $p(\Gamma_i{=}j)$, the overall model becomes $p(y \mid \theta, C) = \prod_i p(y_i \mid \theta, C)$ where

$$p(y_i \mid \theta, C) = \sum_j p(y_i \mid \Gamma_i{=}j, \theta_j, C)p(\Gamma_i{=}j) \tag{1}$$

and $\theta = \{\theta_1, \ldots, \theta_J\}$ denotes all the normal distribution parameters.

As shown in [7], assessing the maximum likelihood (ML) model parameters $\{\theta, C\}$ given the observed intensities y results in an iterative so-called Generalized Expectation-Maximization (GEM) algorithm that interleaves the following equations:

$$p(\Gamma_i{=}j \mid y_i, \theta, C) = \frac{p(y_i \mid \Gamma_i{=}j, \theta_j, C)p(\Gamma_i{=}j)}{\sum_j p(y_i \mid \Gamma_i{=}j, \theta_j, C)p(\Gamma_i{=}j)} \tag{2}$$

$$\mu_j = \frac{\sum_i p(\Gamma_i{=}j \mid y_i, \theta, C)(y_i - \sum_k c_k \phi_k(x_i))}{\sum_i p(\Gamma_i{=}j \mid y_i, \theta, C)} \tag{3}$$

$$\sigma_j^2 = \frac{\sum_i p(\Gamma_i = j \mid y_i, \theta, C)(y_i - \mu_j - \sum_k c_k \phi_k(x_i))^2}{\sum_i p(\Gamma_i = j \mid y_i, \theta, C)} \tag{4}$$

$$C = (A^T W A)^{-1} A^T W R \ , \ A_{ik} = \phi_k(x_i) \ , \ R_i = y_i - \tilde{y}_i \ , \ W = \mathrm{diag}(w_i) \tag{5}$$

$$\text{where} \quad \tilde{y}_i = \frac{\sum_j w_{ij} \mu_j}{\sum_j w_{ij}} \ , \ w_i = \sum_j w_{ij} \ , \ w_{ij} = \frac{p(\Gamma_i = j \mid y_i, \theta, C)}{\sigma_j^2}$$

This algorithm interleaves the following 3 steps until convergence: classification of the voxels (equation 2), estimation of the normal distribution parameters (equations 3 and 4), and estimation of the bias field (equation 5).

As described in [7], the method can be fully automated by introducing a digital brain atlas that contains spatially varying prior probabilities for gray matter, white matter and csf. After affine registration of the study image with a T1 template associated with the atlas, these prior probability maps can be used to initialize the algorithm, which makes the method fully automated. Additionally, the atlas spatially constrains the classification since it contains a spatially varying prior $p(\Gamma_i = j)$ that is used in equation 2.

Previously, we described the algorithm and its practical implementation in more detail. The interested reader is referred to [7,8]; suffice it here to say that the method is easily extended to multi-spectral MR images by substituting the normal distributions with multi-variate normal distributions with mean μ_j and covariance matrix Σ_j.

2.2   Adaptation for automated MS lesion segmentation

The simple mixture model described above works satisfactorily for MR images of normal brains. However, it does not include a model for MS lesions. Therefore, those lesions could be detected as voxels that are not well explained by the mixture model. We adopt the approach that was proposed by Guillemaud and Brady [9] for modeling non-brain tissues in MR images by adding a uniform intensity distribution to the mixture model, i.e. equation 1 is substituted by

$$p(y_i \mid \theta, C) = \sum_j p(y_i \mid \Gamma_i = j, \theta_j, C) p(\Gamma_i = j) + \lambda p(\Gamma_i = reject)$$

where λ is a small constant that is defined by the condition that the integral over all the intensities is unity.

Similar to the approach of Guillemaud and Brady, it can be shown that equations 2, 3 and 4 remain valid, provided that the new rejection class is added to equation 2. Voxels that are not well explained by the normal distributions, such as MS lesions, are pushed into the uniform rejection class. Also equation 5 for the bias estimation remains unchanged except that the weights w are now only calculated with respect to the normal distributions. That is, voxels that are rejected from the normal distributions have a zero weight for the estimation of the bias field.

Almost 95 % of the MS lesions are located inside white matter. This information can be added to the model by assigning the atlas prior probability map of white matter to $p(\Gamma_i{=}reject)$. Besides this spatial constraint, additional intensity constraints can be added. We use multi-spectral MR images that consist of T1-, T2- and PD-weighted images. MS lesions have an intensity between that of white matter and csf in T1, and appear hyper-intense in T2 and PD. We therefore exclude voxels with an intensity darker than the mean of csf in T1 or darker than the mean of gray matter in T2 and PD from the rejection class.

Upon convergence of the adapted GEM algorithm, a classification of the voxels is obtained along with an estimation of the parameters θ of the normal distributions and the bias field parameters C. The MS lesions can be expected to be found in the rejection class.

2.3   Post-processing

In practice, the rejection class does not contain the more subtle MS lesions, while on the other hand, non-lesion voxels that are not well explained by the normal distributions also end up in the rejection class. We therefore add a post-processing step in order to decrease the number of false positives and false negatives.

Final classification rule Given a single normal distribution with mean μ_j and variance σ_j^2, an intensity y_i can be said to be abnormal with respect to this distribution if its so-called mahalanobis-distance $d_j^i = (y_i - \mu_j)/\sigma_j$ exceeds a predefined threshold. In the case of a mixture of normal distributions, however, assessing the abnormality of an intensity y_i is more involved. Intuitively, an intensity is abnormal if the probability that it is generated by the mixture model is small, i.e. when the condition

$$\sum_j G_{\sigma_j}(y_i - \mu_j - \sum_k c_k \phi_k(x_i))p(\Gamma_i{=}j) \quad \leq \quad \kappa p(\Gamma_i{=}lesion)$$

holds with κ a small threshold. However, this would give bad results since a voxel that belongs to a class with a small variance is only detected as abnormal if its mahalanobis-distance is very large compared to a voxel belonging to a class with a large variance. The same rationale also explains the false positives and false negatives in the rejection class of the adapted GEM algorithm. Furthermore, it is not clear how κ should be chosen.

Instead, we weight each normal distribution with its variance, i.e. a voxel is labeled as MS lesion if the condition

$$\sum_j \sigma_j G_{\sigma_j}(y_i - \mu_j - \sum_k c_k \phi_k(x_i))p(\Gamma_i{=}j) \quad \leq \quad \kappa p(\Gamma_i{=}lesion) \qquad (6)$$

holds. The meaning of κ is now clear: it indirectly defines a mahalanobis-distance threshold above which a voxel is detected as abnormal, independent of the variance of the classes. This can be written more explicitly by $\kappa = 1/\sqrt{2\pi}exp(-0.5T^2)$ with T a mahalanobis threshold that we experimentally set to $\sqrt{3}$.

Given the parameters θ and C as calculated by the GEM algorithm, voxels where equation 6 holds, are classified as MS lesions. The other voxels are classified following equation 2.

Markov Random Fields Besides MS lesions, other voxels exist that are not well explained by the mixture model and, as a result, are misclassified as MS lesion. This is typically true for partial volume voxels along the sulci. Such misclassifications could be discarded by only withholding lesions at locations where the white matter a priori map exceeds a certain threshold (cf Zijdenbos et al. [5]), but this method is too crude in our experience.

Instead, we incorporate contextual information in the final segmentation process by making use of Markov-Random-Fields (MRF's). The segmentation Γ is assumed to be the realization of a random process where the probability that voxel i belongs to class j depends on the classification of its neighbors. The Hammersley-Clifford theorem states that the configurations of such a random field obey the distribution $p(\Gamma) = Z^{-1}exp(-U(\Gamma))$ where $U(\Gamma)$ is an energy function and Z is a normalization constant. We use the Potts model: $U(\Gamma) = \sum_i \sum_j \beta_{\Gamma_i,j} u_{i,j}$ where $u_{i,j}$ counts the number of neighbors of voxel i that belong to class j and $\beta_{l,j}, 1 \leq l, j \leq J$ are MRF parameters. We estimated these MRF parameters from an image that was manually labeled into grey matter, white matter, MS lesions, csf and non-brain tissues, using a histogramming technique [10]. Since the slice thickness in MRI can vary widely, we only use the 8 in-plane neighbors, although a full 3D neighborhood could also be used if a manual segmentation exists to estimate the appropriate 3D MRF parameters.

We incorporate contextual information in the final classification process by using the so-called Iterated-Conditional-Modes algorithm (ICM) [11]. More specifically, the prior probability that voxel i belongs to class j depends on the classification of its neighbors: $p(\Gamma_i=j) \sim exp(-\sum_j \beta_{\Gamma_i,j} u_{i,j})$ This prior replaces the atlas in the post-processing step, except for $p(\Gamma_i=lesion)$ where it is multiplied with the atlas prior probability for white matter. Starting from the segmentation obtained with the final classification rule as described above, we calculate $p(\Gamma_i=j)$ and re-apply the same rule with the updated prior. This is repeated until the classification stabilizes, for which 8 iterations are sufficient in our experience.

3   Results on BIOMORPH MS data

As part of the BIOMORPH project [12], we analyzed 12 serial scans from each of 20 MS patients, where each scan contained low-resolution T1-, T2- and PD-weighted images (24 axial 256x256 slices, voxel dimensions 0.9x0.9x5.5 mm^3). In addition to these time series, for each patient there was also at least one higher-resolution scan with the same modalities (52 axial 256x256 slices, voxel dimensions 0.9x0.9x2.5 mm^3). We processed these images after registering and resampling the T1-weighted images to the corresponding T2-weighted images using the affine multi-modality registration algorithm based on maximization of mutual information of Maes et al. [13]. The PD images were assumed to be perfectly aligned with the T2 images since they were acquired simultaneously. The images were then spatially normalized with the atlas by registering the T2-weighted images with the T1 template associated with the atlas using the same registration method.

3.1   Validation on low-resolution images

From 10 of the patients, 2 consecutive time points were manually analyzed by tracing MS lesions using only the T2-weighted images. We compared the delineation of the automatic algorithm with these expert segmentations by comparing the so-called total lesion load (TLL), measured as the number of voxels that were classified as MS lesion, on these 20 scans. Figure 1 shows the TLL of the expert segmentation along with the TLL of the automatic method. Also shown is the linear regression: the slope is unity, and the intercept is close to zero. The correlation coefficient between the automatically and manually detected lesion volumes is high: 0.96, $p < 10^{-10}$. However, a paired t-test reveals a significant difference between the TLL estimated by the expert and the TLL of the automated method (p = 0.029).

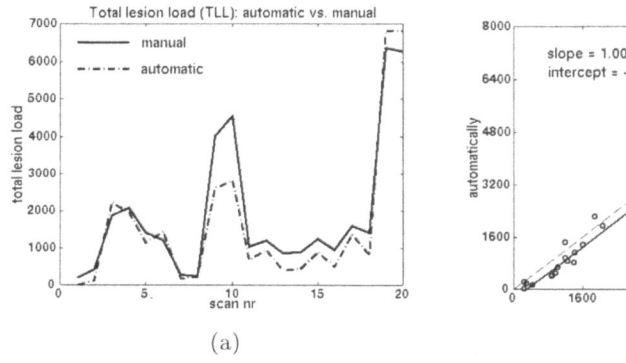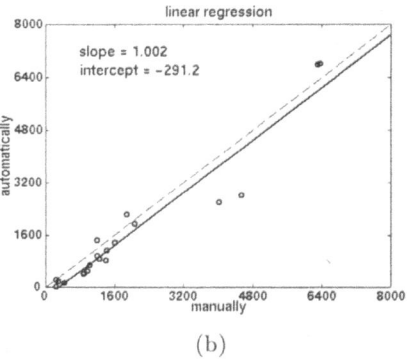

(a)   (b)

Fig. 1. Comparison between manual and automatic tracings of MS lesions on 20 low-resolution scans: total lesion load for each scan (a), and linear regression (b)

3.2   Results on high-resolution images

In addition to the manual expert segmentations on 20 low-resolution scans, 3 high-resolution (HR) scans from different patients were analyzed by 2 different human experts. Figure 2 shows a representative slice of the data with the lesion segmentation of the two experts and the automatic algorithm overlayed in bright color. The TLL of each of the experts and the TLL of the automatic algorithm are depicted in table 1. Expert 1 consistently found a larger lesion volume than expert 2, while the volume obtained by the automatic algorithm did not show a systematic relationship with that segmented by the human observers .

Comparing the TLL of two raters does not take into account any spatial correspondence of the segmented lesions [14]. We therefore calculated indices, the definition of which is given in table 2, which take account of the degree of correspondence between two segmentations: the similarity index which was previously used by Zijdenbos *et al.* [2], the overlap index, and the global spatial correspondence indices recently proposed by Bello and Colchester [14].

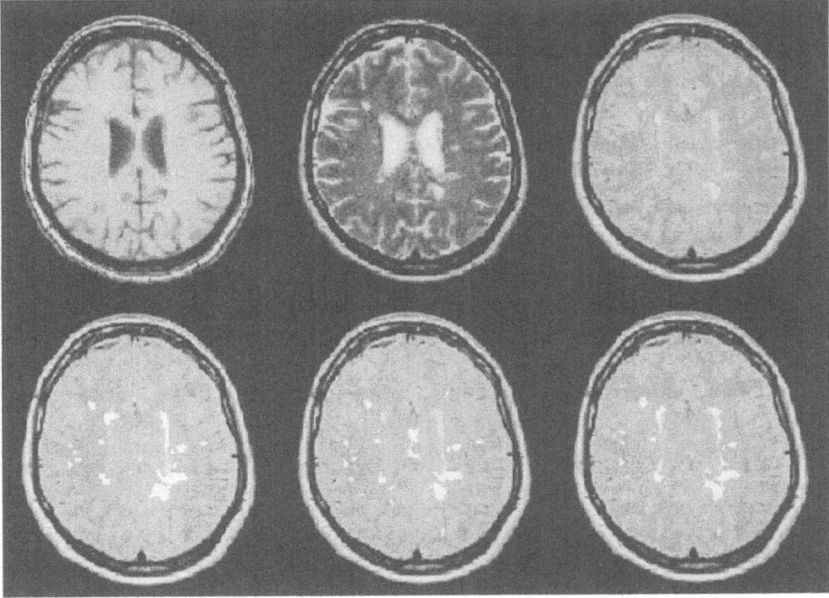

Fig. 2. Visual comparison of the MS lesion labeling by two experts and by the algorithm. Top: T1-, T2- and PD-weighted image. Bottom: MS lesions overlayed in bright color on the PD-weighted image. Left to right: expert 1, expert 2, automatic algorithm

The correspondence indices between expert 1, expert 2 and the automatic algorithm are depicted in table 3. We fused the segmentation maps of all 3 scans for each rater in order to have a single average index between each pair of raters. The non-symmetric nature of the global spatial correspondence indices is apparent in table 3 where the columns have been considered as the reference segmentation and the rows as the current observation. Thus, expert 1 has an average overall correspondence with expert 2 of 50.9 and expert 2 has an average overall correspondence of 43.8 with expert 1. This means that, on average, roughly half of the voxels labeled as lesion by expert 1 were also identified as lesion by expert 2, and that the common lesion voxels have a greater correspondence with the segmentations by expert 2 than with those by expert 1.

Regarding the automatic segmentation, the average similarity and overlap indices between the automatic method and the experts are smaller than between the experts, in particular for expert 1. The global spatial correspondence measures show the results of the automatic method to have an average overall correspondence of 33.4 with expert 1 and 39.8 with expert 2. At the same time, the segmentations done by expert 1 have an average overall correspondence of 39.9 with the automatic method, whereas those by expert 2 have an average overall correspondence of 40.8. These values indicate that the voxels identified as lesion by either of the experts and the automatic method in both cases had a slightly better correspondence with the automatic segmentation than with the manual segmentation. As expected from the definitions in table 2, the values of S are higher than those of O and C. However, all three measures show that the agreement between the experts is, on average, slightly better than between the automatic method and either of the experts, and that the automatic method has a better agreement with expert 2 than with expert 1.

Table 1. Total lesion load by two human experts and the automatic algorithm for 3 high-resolution data sets

TLL	scan 1	scan 2	scan 3
expert 1	5303	939	8172
expert 2	3772	598	6745
automatic	4609	228	8789

Table 2. Definition of spatial correspondence indices. V_1 and V_2 denote the total lesion volume of rater 1 and 2, and V_{12} denotes the volume of the voxels that both indicated as lesion. $I(\boldsymbol{X};\boldsymbol{Y})$ is the average total mutual information between rater 1 $(\boldsymbol{X})$ and rater 2 $(\boldsymbol{Y})$. $H(\boldsymbol{X})$ and $H(\boldsymbol{Y})$ denote the entropy of rater 1 and rater 2, respectively

symbol	name	definition
S	similarity index	$2V_{12}/(V_1 + V_2)$
O	overlap index	$V_{12}/(V_1 + V_2 - V_{12})$
C	global spatial correspondence	$I(\boldsymbol{X};\boldsymbol{Y}) \ / \ H(\boldsymbol{Y})$ and $I(\boldsymbol{X};\boldsymbol{Y}) \ / \ H(\boldsymbol{X})$

Table 3. Spatial correspondence indices between each pair of raters on the HR scans

		expert 1	expert 2	automatic
	expert 1	100	59.2	51.5
S (%)	expert 2	59.2	100	55
	automatic	51.5	55	100
	expert 1	100	42	34.7
O (%)	expert 2	42	100	38
	automatic	34.7	38	100
	expert 1	100	50.9	39.9
C (%)	expert 2	43.8	100	40.8
	automatic	33.4	39.8	100

4   Discussion

We validated the method by comparing the total lesion load (TLL) of automatically detected lesions on 20 scans with those detected by a human expert. A paired t-test revealed a significant difference between the TLL's of the automatic and the human rater. However, as pointed out in [1], the most important requirement for an automated method is that its measurements change in response to a treatment in a manner proportionate to manual measurements. We therefore performed a linear regression analysis, rather than concentrating on the absolute difference in TLL between the automated method and that of the manual segmentations. The regression analysis shows that the automatic segmentations indeed change proportionately to the manual segmentations.

Comparing the TLL of lesions detected by two different raters does not take into account the spatial correspondence between the two segmentations. If the automated method is used to study time correlations of lesion groups and lesion patterns in MS time series, it is important that the lesions are also spatially correctly detected. For 3 patients, we therefore calculated measures which assess this degree of correspondence between two human experts and between each of the experts with the automatic algorithm. Although the inter-observer variability for the experts was very large, the average overall agreement between the two experts was still better than the agreement between any of the experts and the automated algorithm. However, the average overall agreement between expert 2 and the automatic method was comparable to that between the experts.

The segmentation results were also analysed qualitatively. It was notable that the different segmentation methods (expert 1, expert 2 and automatic) showed certain differences which were consistent across patients. Expert 1 segmented many more brainstem and cerebellar lesions. Expert 2 generally segmented a larger number of lesions in the hemispheres. The automatic method tended to place the lesion boundary inside that chosen by the experts. Overall, very careful scrutiny of the segmentations did not reveal consistent failings in any of the methods. MS lesion segmentation is challenging for human observers and automated methods alike. Disagreement over *boundary placement* of specific lesions contributed only a small fraction of the total error. More important was disagreement over whether or not a lesion was present in a certain locality (*object identification*).

In this paper, the automatic method was validated by comparison of the segmentations with those of human experts. The automated algorithm uses multispectral data, while the manual segmentations used for validation were only based on T2-weighted images, which might have introduced errors in the manual tracings. Although the results presented in this paper look promising, a more thorough validation and assessment of intra- and inter-observer variability associated with manual delineation will require data of repeated manual tracings based on multi-spectral data by several human experts, as well as a study of the spatial correspondence between individual lesions and between group of lesions.

5   Summary and conclusions

This paper presented a fully automated model-based method for segmenting MS lesions from multi-channel MR images. The method simultaneously corrects for MR field inhomogeneities, estimates tissue class distribution parameters and classifies the image voxels. MS lesions are detected as voxels that are not well explained by the model. The results of the automated method were compared with the lesions delineated by human experts, showing a significant total lesion load correlation. When the degree of spatial correspondence between two segmentations was taken into account, considerable disagreement was revealed, both between the expert manual segmentations, and between expert and automatic methods. Qualitative evaluation of the results showed that the major source of disagreement lies in identification of lesions as opposed to boundary placement. There is no true gold standard available for evaluating methods, and correct identification of MS lesions remains a major challenge for human observers and automated methods alike.

Acknowledgments

This work was supported by the EC-funded BIOMORPH project 95-0845, a collaboration between the Universities of Kent and Oxford (UK), ETH Zürich (Switzerland), INRIA Sophia Antipolis (France) and KU Leuven (Belgium), by a grant for research specialization from the Flemish Institute for stimulation of the scientific-technological research in the industry (IWT), and by the Research Fund KU Leuven GOA/99/05 (Variability in Human Shape and Speech). The manual segmentations were performed by Dr. Basil Sharrack and Carla Rush.

References

1. A.C. Evans, J.A. Frank, J. Antel, and D.H. Miller. The role of MRI in clinical trials of multiple sclerosis: Comparison of image processing techniques. *Annals of Neurology*, 41(1):125–132, january 1997.
2. A.P. Zijdenbos, B.M. Dawant, R.A. Margolin, and A.C. Palmer. Morphometric analysis of white matter lesions in MR images: Method and validation. *IEEE Transactions on Medical Imaging*, 13(4):716–724, december 1994.
3. B. Johnston, M.S. Atkins, B. Mackiewich, and M. Anderson. Segmentation of multiple sclerosis lesions in intensity corrected multispectral MRI. *IEEE Transactions on Medical Imaging*, 15(2):154–169, april 1996.

4. J.K. Udupa, L. Wei, S. Samarasekera, Y. Miki, M.A. van Buchem, and F.I. Grossman. Multiple sclerosis lesion quantification using fuzzy-connectedness principles. *IEEE Transactions on Medical Imaging*, 16(5):598–609, october 1997.
5. A. Zijdenbos, A. Evans, F. Riahi, J. Sled, J. Chui, and V. Kollokian. Automatic quantification of multiple sclerosis lesion volume using stereotaxic space. In *Proceedings of Visualization in Biomedical Computing – VBC'96*, Lecture Notes in Computer Science, pages 439–448, 1996.
6. A. Zijdenbos, R. Forghani, and A. Evans. Automatic quantification of MS lesions in 3d MRI brain data sets: Validation of INSECT. In *Proceedings of Medical Image Computing and Computer-Assisted Intervention – MICCAI'98*, volume 1496 of *Lecture Notes in Computer Science*, pages 439–448. Springer, 1998.
7. K. Van Leemput, F. Maes, D. Vandermeulen, and P. Suetens. Automatic segmentation of brain tissues and MR bias field correction using a digital brain atlas. In *Proceedings of Medical Image Computing and Computer-Assisted Intervention – MICCAI'98*, volume 1496 of *Lecture Notes in Computer Science*, pages 1222–1229. Springer, 1998.
8. K. Van Leemput, F. Maes, D. Vandermeulen, and P. Suetens. Automated bias field correction and tissue classification of MR images of the brain using a digital atlas. *IEEE Transactions on Medical Imaging*, october 1999.
9. R. Guillemaud and M. Brady. Estimating the bias field of MR images. *IEEE Transactions on Medical Imaging*, 16(3):238–251, june 1997.
10. K. Van Leemput, F. Maes, D. Vandermeulen, and P. Suetens. Automated model-based tissue classification of MR images of the brain. *IEEE Transactions on Medical Imaging*, october 1999.
11. S.Z. Li. *Markov Random Field Modeling in Computer Vision*. Computer Science Workbench. Springer, 1995.
12. European project on brain morphometry (BIOMORPH, EU-BIOMED2 project nr. BMH4-CT96-0845, 1996–1998).
13. F. Maes, A. Collignon, D. Vandermeulen, G. Marchal, and P. Suetens. Multi-modality image registration by maximization of mutual information. *IEEE Transactions on Medical Imaging*, 16(2):187–198, April 1997.
14. F. Bello and A.C.F. Colchester. Measuring global and local spatial correspondence using information theory. In *Proceedings of Medical Image Computing and Computer-Assisted Intervention – MICCAI'98*, volume 1496 of *Lecture Notes in Computer Science*, pages 964–973. Springer, 1998.

Measurement of Infarct Volume in Stroke Patients Using Adaptive Segmentation of Diffusion Weighted MR Images

Anne L. Martel[1], Steven J. Allder[2], Gota S. Delay[3], Paul S. Morgan[3] and Alan R. Moody[3]

[1] Dept. Medical Physics, Queens Medical Centre, Nottingham, NG7 2UH, UK
[2] Dept. Clinical Neurology, University of Nottingham, NG7 2UH, UK
[3] Dept. of Academic Radiology, University of Nottingham, NG7 2UH, UK

Abstract. This paper describes a semi-automatic method of determining the infarct volume, an important parameter in the assessment of stroke patients, from MRI Diffusion Weighted Images (DWI). An adaptive thresholding algorithm incorporating a spatial constraint was used to segment the images. The relationship between adjacent pixels was modeled using a Markov Random Field (MRF) and the Iterative Conditional Modes (ICM) method was used to find a locally optimum solution. In order to improve the robustness of the ICM method, initial threshold levels were determined automatically using a non-spatial method. Preliminary results showed that the completely automatic technique failed if the infarct was too small or if the contrast was too low. The operator was therefore given a choice of modifying the initial threshold levels manually. It was also necessary to edit the final segmentation results in some cases as nerve tracts may also appear as bright regions on the images. Simulation studies were used to determine the accuracy of the technique. Reproducibility studies were carried out to determine the effect of inter and intra observer variability and patient positioning. The semi-automatic technique was quicker and more reproducible than manual segmentation and allowed the infarct volumes to be measured with a repeatability coefficient of < 6 cc.

1. Introduction

There has been considerable interest in the use of diffusion weighted imaging (DWI) to detect the site and size of ischaemic lesions in stroke patients [1, 2]. This information assists in classifying the stroke sub-type and may also be useful in predicting the clinical condition and eventual outcome [3]. Changes in infarct volumes over time have also been measured in a number of studies in an attempt to understand the natural history of stroke [4]. In future, measurements of infarct volume may have an important role to play in the assessment of stroke therapies in clinical trials.

In previous studies the DWI images have been segmented using manual region tracing methods in order to calculate infarct volumes [4, 5]. This is a laborious task and results are operator dependent. The aim of this work was to devise a method of segmenting the DWI images with a minimum of operator intervention that is quicker and more reproducible than existing methods.

We have used an adaptive segmentation technique [6] to automatically determine the brain and infarct volumes. This is based on the Iterative Conditional Modes (ICM) method [7] which allows the relationship between adjacent voxels to be taken into account during the segmentation. Since this method only converges to a local solution we have estimated the initial threshold values using an automatic technique [8]. In order to make the program completely robust it is designed to run under operator supervision. The operator is able to modify the initial threshold values if necessary and some editing of the final segmented image is also possible. The segmentation program was tested using simulation studies and inter and intra observer variability and inter-scan variability were determined using patient studies.

2. Theory

The contrast in a diffusion-weighted image is due to differences in mobility of water molecules in the tissue. If water is freely diffusible then the MRI signal is attenuated, if the movement of the water molecules is impeded in some way, for example along nerve bundles, then the MRI signal is larger. Acute cerebral ischaemia causes cell damage which results in edema due to the accumulation of intracellular water. This causes a restriction in the movement of water molecules therefore the infarct shows up as a region of increased signal intensity. The result is an image with three distinct regions: air, which has a signal intensity of close to zero; normal brain which has an intermediate grey scale value and infarcted tissue which has the highest signal intensity and is typically more heterogeneous than the other two regions. The problem is therefore to estimate the "true" image $X = \{x_s, s = 1...N\}$ (where N is the number of voxels in the image) with discrete values $x_s \in \{1,2,...K.\}$ (where K is the number of regions) from the noisy observed image $Y = \{y_s, s = 1...N\}$. $\mu(k)$ is the mean intensity of all pixels belonging to the k'th region and $\mu(1) < \mu(2) ... < \mu(K)$. From Bayes' Theorem $P(X|Y)$, the conditional probability of X given the observed image Y is given by

$$P(X|Y) \propto P(Y|X) \, P(X) \tag{1}$$

Where $P(Y|X)$ is the likelihood of observing the image Y given the true image X and $P(X)$ is the prior probability of X. The maximum *a posteriori* (MAP) estimate of the true image is the value of X which maximizes $P(X|Y)$. If we assume that the observed intensity values y_s are independently distributed with a mean x_s and variance σ^2 then $P(Y|X)$ is given by

$$P(Y|X) = \prod_{s=1}^{N} f(y_s | x_s) = \left(2\pi\sigma^2\right)^{-\frac{n}{2}} \exp\left\{\frac{-1}{2\sigma^2} \sum_{s=1}^{N} \{y_s - \mu(x_s)\}^2\right\} \tag{2}$$

If the probability of a pixel x_s having a particular value depends only on the pixel values in the neighborhood of s (η_s) then X corresponds to a Markov Random Field (MRF). We have used

$$P(x_s) \propto \exp\{\beta Z(x_s)\} \tag{3}$$

where $Z(x_s)$ is the number of pixels where $x_n = x_s$ for $n \in \eta_i$ and η_i is the 3-D, 2nd order neighborhood of i. The probability $P(X|Y)$ can be maximised using the method of iterated conditional modes (ICM) [7]. An initial estimate of the image X is generated and then each pixel s is updated in turn so that the new value of x_s is optimised for the current estimate of the true image, X_c. The function to be maximised is given by

$$p(x_s \mid Y, X_c) = p(x_s \mid y_s, x_n, n \in \eta_s) \propto \exp\left(\frac{-1}{2\sigma^2} \sum_{s=1}^{N} \{y_s - \mu(x_s)\}^2 + \beta Z(x_s)\right) \tag{4}$$

Several sweeps of the image are made until convergence is reached. This technique converges to a local rather than a global minimum but it is computationally simpler than alternative minimization schemes such as simulated annealing [9].

3. Methods

3.1 Adaptive Segmentation

Mardia and Hainsworth [6] describe an algorithm for adaptive thresholding based on ICM. From equation (4) it can be shown that the intensity level y for which $p(x_s=i|y_s, X_c)$ is equal to $p(x_s=j|y_s, X_c)$ is given by

$$y = \frac{1}{2}\{\mu(i) + \mu(j)\} + \beta\sigma^2\{Z(j) - Z(i)\}/\{\mu(i) - \mu(j)\} \tag{5}$$

where i,j = 1..K, i<j and $Z(i)$ is the number of pixels in the neighborhood of s with $x_n = i$. The decision variable is B defined as

$$B = y_s + \beta\sigma^2\{Z(j) - Z(i)\}/\{\mu(i) - \mu(j)\} \tag{6}$$

and the threshold level separating region i from region j is given by

$$t_{i,j} = \frac{1}{2}\{\mu(i) + \mu(j)\} \tag{7}$$

Using these definitions the algorithm is as follows:
1. Estimate the initial threshold values {$t_{i,j}$, i,j=1..K,i<j) and segment the image into K regions to obtain an initial estimate of X
2. Estimate the mean grey level $\mu(k)$ for each region.
3. For each region subtract the mean grey level $\mu(x_s)$ from the observed grey level y_s. and estimate the variance σ^2 from this modified data set.
4. Re-evaluate the threshold values, $t_{i,j} = \frac{1}{2}\{\mu(i) + \mu(j)\}$
5. For each pixel in the image do the following:

Set i=1
For j=2 to K do
   If $B > t_{i,j}$ set i=j: next j
Set $x_s = i$

6. Repeat steps 2-5 until the solution is stable. We have defined convergence as occurring when the percentage change in the number of pixels in the infarct region is < 0.1 %.

The ICM method finds a local rather than a global solution and the final segmentation may therefore be affected by the starting values [6]. The number of iterations required will also depend on how close the initial threshold values are to the final solution. For this reason we have used the iterative method described by Ridler and Calvard [8] to generate the initial threshold values. This method is equivalent to the adaptive segmentation algorithm described above for the special case when β=0. Since no spatial information is used the technique can be applied directly to the image histogram which makes it considerably faster to run than ICM which has to update each pixel in the image in turn. The algorithm used is as follows:

1. Generate the image histogram $h(v)$ from the observed image Y. $v = 0,... m$ and m is the maximum grey level in the image.
2. Estimate the initial threshold values by dividing the range of grey level values into K equal partitions so that $t_{i,j} = \{i \times m\}/K$ where $i < j = 1...K$
3. Calculate the mean intensity values for the regions defined by the threshold values.

$$\mu(k) = \frac{\sum\limits_{v=t_{k-1,k}}^{v<t_{k,k+1}} h(v) \times v}{\sum\limits_{v=t_{k-1,k}}^{v<t_{k,k+1}} v} \tag{8}$$

4. Calculate the new threshold values $t_{i,j} = \frac{1}{2}\{\mu(i) + \mu(j)\}$
5. Repeat steps 3-5 until the threshold values converge to a stable solution.
   This method always converges but the solution is dependent on starting points.

Figure 1 illustrates the whole segmentation process.

3.2 Semi-automatic Segmentation

The fully automatic technique described above worked well in most cases. However preliminary trials with patient data showed that in some images where the infarct was small and/or the contrast between the infarct and normal brain tissue was low the initial thresholding technique failed to separate normal brain from infarct. An example of this is shown in figure 2. The operator was therefore presented with a display showing the threshold contours superimposed on the DWI images, together with the intensity histogram. The thresholds could be modified manually by defining new threshold levels on the histogram.

Manual editing of the segmented images was also required in some cases. This was due to the presence of high intensity regions in the corpus callosum (due to the presence of nerve tissue) and in the base of the brain (due to susceptibility artifacts) which were incorrectly classified as infarct. A simple graphical user interface written in IDL (Boulder, CO) enabled the operator to reclassify these regions as normal brain.

3.3 Simulation Studies

The adaptive segmentation technique described in section 3.1 assumes that true image X is contaminated with white gaussian noise. This is a resonable assumption for the brain and infarct regions where the signal to noise ratio is high but in the low intensity background region where there is no signal the noise has a Rician distribution [10]. It is also assumed that the pixels in the true image X can only take one of three discrete values. This is only an approximation and in practice both the normal brain and the infarct regions will be heterogeneous.

The accuracy of the segmentation technique was assessed using simulation studies which attempt to model the true patient data. A patient scan with a moderate sized infarct (28 cc) was segmented manually into background, brain and infarct regions. The mean and standard deviation of pixel values within each region were calculated. Simulation studies were created by filling in the 3 regions with intensity values drawn from the appropriate distribution. 3 high contrast simulations were generated using $\mu=[0,130,430]$, $\sigma = [20,30,80]$. A second patient image with a much smaller, less distinct infarct was analyzed and the mean values from this were used to create 3 low contrast images ($\mu=[0,130,230]$, $\sigma = [20,35,40]$).

The effect of varying β between 0.5 and 2 and the effect of different initial threshold values on the segmentation results were investigated.

3.4 Image Acquisition

Patients diagnosed with a recent anterior circulation stroke were imaged on a 1.5 T Siemens Magnetom Vision using an echo planar DWI sequence. Imaging parameters were as follows: b value, 1100 s/mm^2; field of view, 250 mm; matrix size, 128x128 (sinc interpolated to 256x256); pixel size, 0.977 mm; slice thickness, 5 mm; number of slices, 25 (acquired interleaved with no slice gap); effective TE, 123 ms; total scan time, 7.044 s (for 25 slices).

A total of 63 patient studies were carried out with a median time between onset of stroke and acquisition of images of 26 hours. 10 of these studies were randomly selected for the inter- and intra- observer reproducibility studies (median time to scan: 11 hours). In a further 5 patients a second DWI image was acquired with different tilt angles and table positions to simulate the effect of changing the patients position in the scanner (median time to scan: 24 hours).

4. Results

4.1 Simulation Studies

The results in Table 1. give the mean values from 3 noisy simulations. The % miss-classification is the number of pixels incorrectly classified*100 / total number of pixels. The % error in the infarct volume is also given.

For the high contrast simulation the classification accuracy over the whole image was very good although the infarct volume was consistently underestimated. There was little difference between using the automatic and manually selected thresholds as starting values.

For the lower contrast simulations, the segmentation failed when $\beta<1$. The starting threshold levels selected by the automatic technique were clearly incorrect but despite this the ICM method converged to a reasonable solution. However this took an average of 11 iterations compared to 4 iterations needed for the manually selected thresholds (for $\beta = 1$)

There is little difference in the results for $\beta = 1$ and $\beta = 1.5$ but convergence occurred in fewer iterations when $\beta = 1$ so this value was selected for the patient studies.

Table 1. Summary of results for simulation studies.

		High Contrast		Low Contrast	
Initial Threshold	β	% Miss-classification (± 1SD)	% error in infarct volume (± 1SD)	% Miss-classification (± 1SD)	% error in infarct volume (± 1SD)
automatic	0	**0.60** (0.01)	**-3.2** (0.2)	**6.84** (0.02)	**1399.7** (0.1)
	0.5	**0.087** (0.002)	**-2.73** (0.08)	**0.301** (0.003)	**23.5** (0.7)
	1	**0.049** (0.001)	**-2.45** (0.03)	**0.104** (0.001)	**-1.0** (0.4)
	1.5	**0.049** (0.002)	**-2.13** (0.04)	**0.156** (0.008)	**1.4** (2.3)
manual	0.5	**0.081** (0.005)	**-2.6** (0.1)	**0.31** (0.01)	**18.0** (2.5)
	1	**0.045** (0.002)	**-2.24** (0.07)	**0.115** (0.003)	**-4.7** (0. 8)
	1.5	**0.048** (0.001)	**-1.89** (0.09)	**0.113** (0.006)	**-8.7** (1.9)

4.2 Patient Studies

The inter-observer, intra-observer and intra-scan reproducibility of the semi-automatic segmentation was assessed using the approach described in [11]. The difference between the repeated measures of infarct volume was calculated for each data set and the mean and standard deviation of these differences was calculated. The repeatability coefficient is defined as the 95% confidence interval, i.e. ±2SD.

The intra and inter observer variability for manual segmentation was also assessed. Manual segmentation was carried out using a graphical tool that provided access to a combination of thresholding, region growing and manual tracing techniques. The results show that the reproducibility is poor compared with the semi-automatic technique. The infarct volumes estimated by observer 1 were significantly higher than those estimated by observer 2 for the manual segmentation method. There was no significant bias with the semi-automatic technique.

The average time taken to segment both the normal brain and the infarct was 6 minutes for the semi-automatic technique and 15 minutes for the manual technique. Of the 6 minutes it took to carry out the semi-automatic segmentation, approximately 3 minutes were spent waiting for the ICM method to converge.

Table 2. Results of the reproducibility studies.

	Mean volume	Semi-Automatic		Manual	
		Mean difference	2SD	Mean difference	2SD
Intra-observer	94.0 cc (n=10)	0.9 cc	5.5 cc	1.8 cc	17.9 cc
Inter-observer	"	-0.5 cc	5.8 cc	11.0 cc	27.7 cc
Inter-scan	71.9 cc (n=6)	-0.2 cc	1.4 cc		

The median infarct volume for all 63 studies was 73cc. Automatic segmentation failed completely in 6 studies due to poor image quality. The initial thresholding step failed in a further 23 cases making it necessary to manually define the threshold level; the infarct size in this group was significantly lower than the remaining studies (11cc compared with 115cc).

The importance of the final manual editing step depended on the size of the infarct: in 27 cases the manual editing modified the infarct volume by < 1% (median infarct volume=125cc), in 12 cases the change was between 1-10% (median infarct volume=92cc) and in 18 cases the change was > 10% (median infarct volume=11cc). For all studies the median change in volume after manual editing was 1.2cc or 1.2% of infarct volume. There was no significant relationship between the time at which the scan was carried out and the quality of the segmentation.

Discussion

Previous studies have used manual segmentation techniques to determine the infarct volume from DWI images of the brain. The semi-automatic segmentation method described here is faster than the manual technique and has significantly improved reproducibility.

With the present technique the initial thresholding step tends to fail for small infarcts. The manual selection of a threshold level only takes seconds but in order to completely automate the process an alternative method is needed. One possibility would be to fit gaussian functions to the brain and background peaks in the intensity histogram and to derive the threshold values from the fitted parameters. Alternatively, if the b value and other acquisition parameters are kept the same for all images then the initial threshold levels could be based on intensity values obtained from training data. Improving the initial selection of the threshold would allow the segmentation to be carried out automatically. The initial results suggest that this would remove the need for any operator intervention at all for larger infarcts. For smaller infarcts the operator would only have to check the segmentation results and edit any miss-classified regions if necessary. We anticipate that this final editing step would only take 1-2 minutes depending on the quality of the initial segmentation. It may also be possible to predict the spatial distribution of the nerve tracts in order to exclude them automatically.

Previous studies have defined changes in infarct volumes of > 20% as significant [4]. If we assume a mean infarct volume of 35 cc [12] then this corresponds to an increase of 7 cc. Our results show that with the semi-automatic segmentation technique infarct volumes can be measured with a reproducibility of < 6 cc. Other groups [4, 5] have reported an inter-observer reproducibility of 5% using a manual region tracing technique. This is considerably better than our results and this may be due to better training of the observers or to differences in the manual region tracing method. It is difficult to compare results directly as details of how the reproducibility was measured are not given and the percentage error will depend on the infarct size.

Apparent diffusion coefficient (ADC) maps can be generated by acquiring DWI images with several different b values. ADC images provide quantitative information and may be of value in distinguishing between old and new lesions, however the contrast between infarcted and non-infarcted tissue is poor compared to the diffusion weighed images. We have therefore used the DWI images to estimate infarct volume. Some attempts have also been made to use multispectral segmentation techniques to segment the DWI images acquired with different b values [13, 14]. The disadvantage of this approach is that the multiple DWI images must be registered exactly so corrections must be made due to the presence of distortions in the image. It is also important that no patient movement occurs between images and this may be difficult to achieve when dealing with acute stroke patients.

References

[1] R. G. Gonzalez, P. W. Schaefer, F. S. Buonanno, L. H. Schwamm, R. F. Budzik, G. Rordorf, B. Wang, A. G. Sorensen, and W. J. Koroshetz,: Diffusion-weighted MR imaging: diagnostic accuracy in patients imaged within 6 hours of stroke symptom onset. Radiology **210** (1999) 155-62.

[2] K. O. Lovblad, H. J. Laubach, A. E. Baird, F. Curtin, G. Schlaug, R. R. Edelman, and S. Warach,: Clinical experience with diffusion-weighted MR

in patients with acute stroke [see comments]. AJNR Am J Neuroradiol **19** (1998) 1061-6.

[3]   K. O. Lovblad, A. E. Baird, G. Schlaug, A. Benfield, B. Siewert, B. Voetsch, A. Connor, C. Burzynski, R. R. Edelman, and S. Warach,: Ischemic lesion volumes in acute stroke by diffusion-weighted magnetic resonance imaging correlate with clinical outcome. Ann Neurol **42** (1997) 164-70.

[4]   A. E. Baird, A. Benfield, G. Schlaug, B. Siewert, K. O. Lovblad, R. R. Edelman, and S. Warach,: Enlargement of human cerebral ischemic lesion volumes measured by diffusion-weighted magnetic resonance imaging [see comments]. Ann Neurol **41** (1997) 581-9.

[5]   P. A. Barber, D. G. Darby, P. M. Desmond, Q. Yang, R. P. Gerraty, D. Jolley, G. A. Donnan, B. M. Tress, and S. M. Davis,: Prediction of stroke outcome with echoplanar perfusion- and diffusion- weighted MRI. Neurology **51** (1998) 418-26.

[6]   K. V. Mardia and T. J. Hainsworth,: Spatial thresholding method for image segmentation. IEEE Transactions on Pattern Analysis and Machine Intelligence **10** (1988) 919-927.

[7]   J. Besag,: On the statistical analysis of dirty pictures. J. R. Statist. Soc. B **48** (1986) 259-302.

[8]   T. W. Ridler and S. Calvard,: Picture Thresholding Using an Iterative Selection Method. IEEE Transactions on Systems, Man and Cybernetics **SMC-8** (1978) 630-632.

[9]   S. Geman and D. Geman,: Stochastic Relaxation, Gibbs Distributions, and the Bayesian Restoration of Images. IEEE Trans. Pattern Anal. Machine Intell. **PAMI-6** (1984) 721-741.

[10] H. Gudbjartsson and S. Patz,: The Rician distribution of noisy MRI data [published erratum appears in Magn Reson Med 1996 Aug;36(2):332]. Magn Reson Med **34** (1995) 910-4.

[11] J. M. Bland and D. G. Altman,: Statistical methods for assessing agreement between two methods of clinical measurement. Lancet **1** (1986) 307-10.

[12] K. J. van Everdingen, J. van der Grond, L. J. Kappelle, L. M. Ramos, and W. P. Mali,: Diffusion-weighted magnetic resonance imaging in acute stroke. Stroke **29** (1998) 1783-90.

[13] R. A. Carano, K. Takano, K. G. Helmer, T. Tatlisumak, K. Irie, J. D. Petruccelli, M. Fisher, and C. H. Sotak,: Determination of focal ischemic lesion volume in the rat brain using multispectral analysis. J Magn Reson Imaging **8** (1998) 1266-78.

[14] V. Nagesh, K. M. Welch, J. P. Windham, S. Patel, S. R. Levine, D. Hearshen, D. Peck, K. Robbins, L. D'Olhaberriague, H. Soltanian-Zadeh, and M. D. Boska,: Time course of ADCw changes in ischemic stroke: beyond the human eye! Stroke **29** (1998) 1778-82.

Fig. 1. Adaptive Segmentation. Top left: a slice taken from a DWI 3D image. Top right: the image histogram has a background, normal brain and infarct peak (the y axis has been clipped to show the infarct peak). The two automatically determined threshold levels (85 and 237) are displayed. Bottom left: the segmentation using the threshold levels cetermined using β=0. Bottom right: the segmentation with β=1.

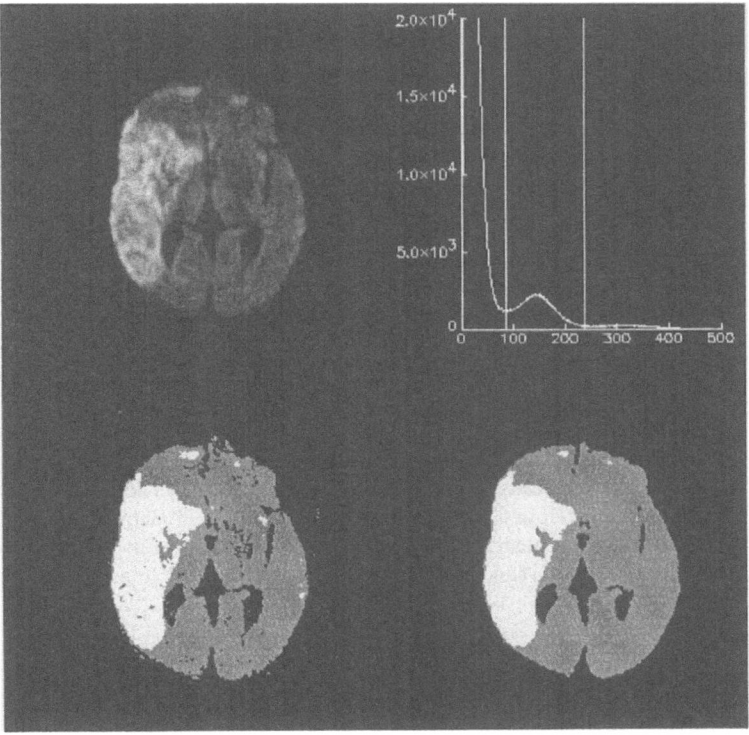

Fig. 2. In cases where the infarct is small (left) the image histogram only has two peaks (centre) and the automatically determined threshold values include normal brain (right)

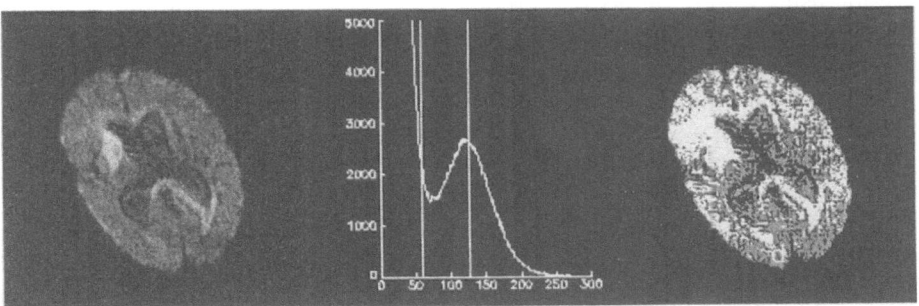

Quantitative Modelling of Microcalcification Detection in Digital Mammography

Andreas Rick , Serge Muller , Sylvie Bothorel , Michel Grimaud

GE Medical Systems
283 rue de la Minière
78533 Buc, France
Andreas.Rick@med.ge.com

Abstract. This article presents a simulation framework for the image acquisition on digital mammography systems. The framework is used to analyse the performance of a previously developed method for the detection of microcalcifications by a series of top-hat operators. The framework allows to determine the theoretical number of false positives and true positives for a given set of acquisition parameters and size of microcalcifications.

A minimal size of microcalcification that can be detected with sufficient certitude is analysed as a function of the pixel size of the detector and the acquisition conditions. An improved selection scheme for the detection threshold is developed which uses the model and the acquisition parameters to obtain a near-optimal detection for a wide range of acquisition conditions. Finally the model is evaluated on clinical images.

1 Introduction

Screening mammography is used today as the most important tool in the reduction of breast cancer mortality by early detection of the lesions. One of the early signs of breast cancer on mammography images are small depositions of radiologically very opaque materials like $Ca_3(PO_4)_2$, $CaCO_3$, $Mg_3(PO_4)_2$ which are called microcalcifications [9]. Many algorithms have been developed for their detection using a wide variety of methods like sub-band decomposition [1], fractals [2] or mathematical morphology [3][4]. When detecting microcalcifications we are facing the problem that their size has no lower limit and so their detection is always a compromise between detecting too much noise or missing very small calcifications. Some work has been done to estimate the noise level from the image itself [6], but this leads to an ambiguity of what is noise and what is image content. In our work we try to establish lower limits of the microcalcification detectability based on a model of the digital image chain. We use those limits for the selection of the local thresholds in our detection system for microcalcifications. In previous systems the selection of a threshold was often difficult as the noise is dependent on the image content. In this approach we can estimate the true and false positive rates as a function of the local thresholds and we can thereby optimise these thresholds to obtain the same compromise throughout the image. As the conditions of the image acquisition process are much more controlled for digital mammography system, as no film processing and scanning is required, high precision models can be used to perform a quantitative analysis of the breast tissue. Works have been done on mammography image normalisation [5] from digitalised films. Due to film processing and scanning process, the physical quantification is difficult but the results obtained are promising.

In section 2 we discuss the model of the image acquisition chain and include a brief description of the first stage of our previously published [3][4] detection system for microcalcifications.

In section 3 we analyse the systems performance for different sizes of microcalcifications, different pixel sizes and different doses.

In section 4 a new threshold selection method is derived from the model which allows an optimal distinction between microcalcifications and image noise for the whole range of acquisition parameters and tissue thicknesses.

Finally in section 5 we compare the theoretical detection rates with detection rates observed on clinical images acquired on a full-field digital mammography system.

2   Image Acquisition and Microcalcification Detection

A mammography image is obtained by a projection of X-rays through the breast. The X-rays are generated by the impact of electrons which are accelerated in a electric field ($\approx 30kV$) onto some anode material (Mo,Rh,W). The X-ray spectrum is a function of the anode material, the acceleration voltage and the angle of the rays relative to the anode.

The detector used for the mammograms analysed in this paper is a full-field digital mammography detector made of an amorphous silicon based photo-diode matrix which is covered with a CsI-scintillation screen which converts the X-rays to visible photons.

At any point in space the number $n(z, E)$ of direct X-rays of energy E arriving from the source can be calculated from the initial spectrum $n_0(E)$ generated at the anode by integrating the attenuation along the path of the ray for all energies.

$$n(z, E) = \frac{n_0(E)}{z^2} \cdot e^{-\int_{l=0}^{z} \mu(l, E) dl} dE \qquad (1)$$

2.1   Detector Model

Using the above model and the geometry of the acquisition, the number of photons $n(x, y, E)$ arriving on the surface of one pixel of the detector can be calculated:

$$n(x, y, E) = \frac{n_0(x, y, E)}{z^2} \cdot e^{-\int_{l=0}^{z} \mu(x, y, l, E) dl} dE \qquad (2)$$

A detector model which describes the conversion of the X-rays to visible photons in the scintillation material and the conversion of the photons to charges in the photo-diodes and finally the conversion from charges to pixel counts is used to link the number of X-ray-photons arriving at the entrance surface of a pixel $n(x, y, E)$ to the ideal pixel values $I_s(x, y)$.

$$I_s(x, y) = \int_0^{E_m} n(x, y, E) \cdot \eta(E) dE \qquad (3)$$

The detector model basically contains a conversion efficiency $\eta(E)$ between the X-ray energy and the pixel value. The modulation transfer function of the scintillator material can be taken into account by applying a spatial filter to the pixel values $I_s(x, y)$. The scattered photons are currently not taken into account in this model, as most of the scattered radiation can be eliminated using an anti scatter grid. One can use a deconvolution processing to estimate the scatter component (see [5] [7]).

2.2 Noise Model

The noise analysis of the detector has shown two principal noise sources, the quantum noise of the x-rays and the electronic readout noise. In total we can approximate the noise by a Gaussian noise with a standard deviation dependent on the signal and on a constant σ_e which represents the electronic noise.

$$\sigma_n(x, y) = \sqrt{\int n(x, y, E) dE + \sigma_e^2} \qquad (4)$$

2.3 Model of the Breast

We assume that the breast is composed of adipose and fibrous tissue and that its thickness l_b is know. Microcalcifications are modeled by a simple sphere of calcium inside the breast. To introduce this model in the detector model we replace the exponential term in equation 2 by a transmission term $t(x, y, E)$:

$$t(x, y, E) = e^{-\mu_b(E) \cdot l_b - (\mu_c(E) - \mu_b(E)) \cdot l_c(x,y)} \qquad (5)$$

where $\mu_b(E)$ and $\mu_c(E)$ are the attenuation coefficients of the breast tissue and of the calcification and l_b and l_c are the corresponding thicknesses. The $t(x, y, E)$ can be decomposed into two terms t_b and t_c, one for the breast tissue and one for the additional attenuation of the calcification:

$$t(x, y, E) = t_b(x, y, E) \cdot t_c(x, y, E) \qquad (6)$$
$$= e^{-\mu_b(E) \cdot l_b} \cdot e^{-(\mu_c(E) - \mu_b(E)) \cdot l_c(x,y)} \qquad (7)$$

In reality the breast tissue is not homogeneous but composed of different types of tissue. For a simulation any mixture of tissues can be considered, but in reality the only information about the tissue comes from the acquired image and therefore the exact decomposition into the different tissues is not possible. The decomposition becomes possible when only two different types of tissue are considered and the total thickness of the breast is known (see [5]).

2.4   Model of a Microcalcification

If we use a sphere with a radius r to model a microcalcification, we obtain:

$$t_c(x, y, E) = e^{-(\mu_c(E) - \mu_b(E)) \cdot \sqrt{r^2 - x^2 - y^2}} \tag{8}$$

It can be remarked that the position inside the breast in the direction of the x-rays has no influence on the microcalcification transmiss.on but due to the conic projection the calcifications closer to the tube are slightly magnified. The system we used for the evaluation has a tube to detector distance of 66cm. Under these conditions and with a maximum compressed breast thickness of 10cm the maximal magnification is 14% which should be taken into account during the detection process.

2.5   Detection System for Microcalcifications

We previously used the top-hat operator in a multi-scale scheme for microcalcification detection [4]. The top-hat operator, which combines the opening and subtraction of an image, is well adapted to the detection of structures like microcalcifications that have a small size and a hight contrast.

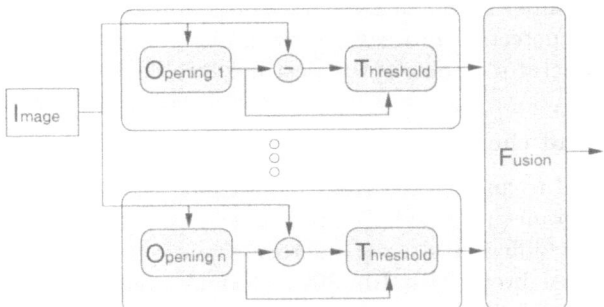

Fig. 1. Detection of microcalcifications using top-hat operators with different structuring element sizes

The opening removes all structures smaller than the structuring element from the image. The result of the subtraction from the original image gives only the small structures and a threshold is used to retain only the structures with a high contrast. As the sizes of the microcalcifications are not known in advance the top-hat operator is applied several times to the image using different sizes of structuring element and the result is combined (figure 1).

2.6   Overall Simulation Model

The simulation model shown in figure 2 can be constructed from the blocks described above. A number of parameters are fixed in each simulation, others

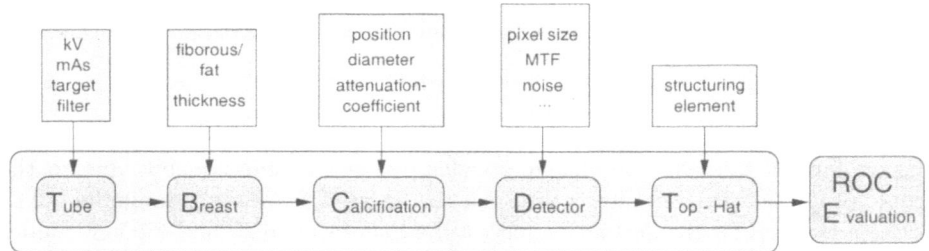

Fig. 2. Simulation model for the detection process

(position of the calcification, threshold, noise) are modified statistically and a Receiver Operating Characteristic curve is calculated. This model is used in the following to analyse the performance of each top-hat operator used in the detection system for microcalcifications.

3   Applications of the Simulation Model

Our goal in this paper is to calculate the limits of detectability of microcalcifications using the detection process described above and to adapt the threshold and the fusion operator to obtain the best possible detection rate.

3.1   Influence of the Pixel Size

The model is used to analyse the effect of changing the pixel size with all other factors being constant (e.g. dose). Figure 3 shows how the area A_z under the ROC curve changes for different sizes of microcalcifications. The conditions chosen are those of a dense breast (Rh/Rh, 30kV, 100mAs, 5cm). We observe that the detection quality globally increases with decreasing pixel size. At very high A_z values the lines for 50 and 100 μ come very close (see top of figure 3 left). A useful computer aided detection system must achieve very high detection rates with little false positives and therefore it must have a high A_z value. Under these constraints the smallest microcalcifications that can be detected are about 0.15 mm in dense regions of the breast. Reducing the pixel size below $100\mu m$ does not improve their detection.

For microcalcifications in adipose regions of the breast the detection performance A_z increases with decreasing pixel size. For the same high level of A_z the smallest microcalcifications that can be detected are about 70 to $100\mu m$ depending on the pixel size.

It is interesting to remark that the observer performance studies for the characterisation of malignant and benign microcalcification recently presented by Heang-Ping Chan [8] suggest the same optimum pixel size of either $70\mu m$ or $105\mu m$ and that $35\mu m$ pixel size gives worse results - even though they did not achieve sufficient statistical evidence in their study yet.

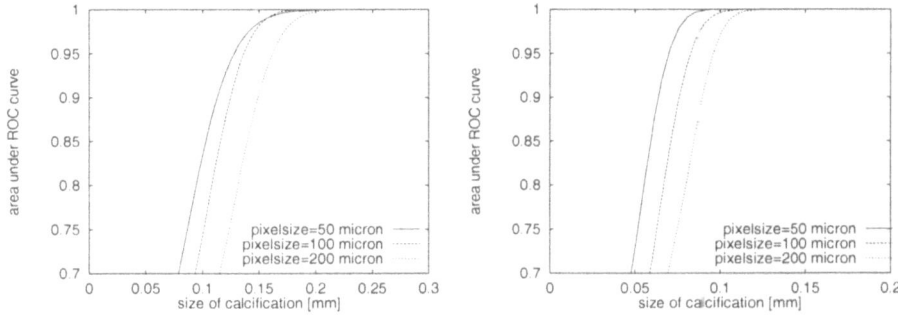

Fig. 3. Detection efficiency A_z as a function of calcification size and detector pixel size for a dense breast (left) and adipose breast (right)

3.2 Influence of Dose and Anode

The simulation model can also be used to calculate the influence of dose and anode/filter combination on the detectability of microcalcifications. We have chosen a dense breast and calculated the exposure (in mAs) necessary to obtain a detection performance given by an area under the ROC curve equal to 0.99 (figure 4). We can see that the Rh/Rh anode filter combination improves the

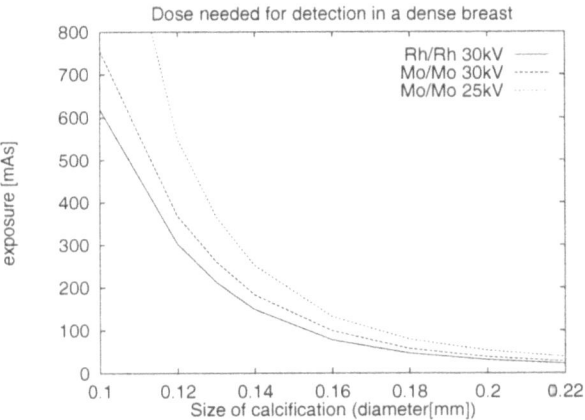

Fig. 4. Dose needed for detection of microcalcifications of different sizes using Mo or Rh anode with $A_z = 0.99$ in a dense breast

microcalcification detectability in dense breasts. In addition, we can see that the dose must increase dramatically as the size of microcalcification to be detected decreases.

4   Model Based Selection of Thresholds

The number of false positives obtained by using a given threshold t for the top-hat operator can be calculated using the noise model. For a Gaussian noise with standard deviation σ_n as given in equation 4 the probability $\tilde{p}_{fpr}$ of a pixel value to be higher than the threshold t for a given background value bg is expressed by the integrated normal distribution:

$$\tilde{p}_{fpr}(x,y) = \int_{t+bg(x,y)}^{\infty} \frac{1}{\sqrt{2\pi}\sigma_n(x,y)} e^{-\frac{1}{2}\left(\frac{g-bg(x,y)}{\sigma_n(x,y)}\right)^2} dg \tag{9}$$

For all the N pixels in the structuring element the probability of a false positive is given by:

$$p_{fpr}(x,y) = 1 - (1 - \tilde{p}_{fpr}(x,y))^N \tag{10}$$

The total number of false positives on a pixel basis is equal to the sum over all pixels of $p_{fpr}(x,y)$:

$$n_{fpr} = \sum_y \sum_x p_{fpr}(x,y) \tag{11}$$

The same reasoning can be applied for the calculation of the true positive rate for a spherical microcalcification of a given size.

Having calculated these detection rates we can choose an adapted detection strategy which represents a compromise between the true and false positives rates as a function of the microcalcification size and the image noise.

One strategy would be to select a constant true positive rate independent of the microcalcification size. Due to the higher image noise in the dense regions of the breast this leads to an unacceptably high false positive rate for small microcalcifications in these regions. The fusion stage which combines the results of the top-hats of different sizes must take into account this higher uncertainty for the small size top-hats.

A more interesting strategy is to give an a priori number of false positives coming from the combination of the top-hats and to select a number candidates from the top-hats until this selected number of false positive is reached. The block diagram for this approach is shown in figure 5.

For each size of the top hat operator, a number of false positives per pixel is estimated. For a given pixel, the threshold on the top-hat image which makes this pixel positive is used to estimate the number of false positives created by the noise corresponding to the local background value. The different false positive rates are then combined using the minimum operator. This operator allows to mark those microcalcification candidates for which the best adapted top-hat operator results in the lowest false positive rate. Finally a global threshold is used to choose the pixels with the lowest possible false positive rate.

This method has the advantage to combine the information from the different sizes of top-hat operators by taking into account their confidence values in a very intuitive way.

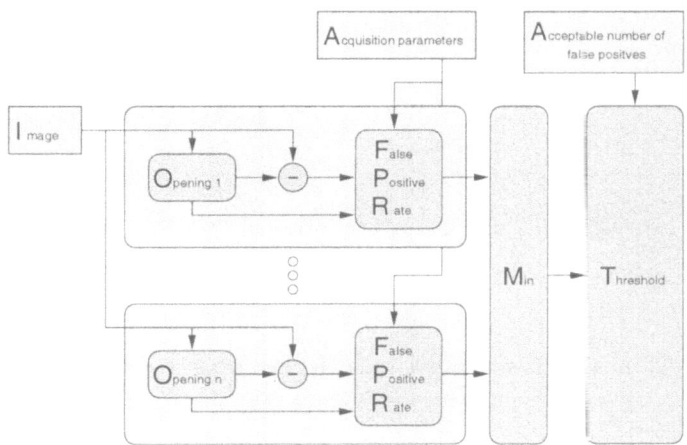

Fig. 5. Detection of microcalcifications using an estimated false positive rate per pixel

5   Evaluation on Clinical Images

An evaluation of this false positive rate estimation was performed on clinical images from the GE Full Field Digital Mammography (FFDM) [11] system from two different clinical sites.

5.1   Theoretical versus Measured False Positive Rate

Using the acquisition parameters selected to acquire an image on the FFDM system, the theoretical probability of false positives as function of the background grey-level and the threshold applied on the top-hats has been calculated (figure 6 left). The top-hat detector has been applied on a real image and the number of positives has been counted as a function of background and threshold (figure 6 right).

For regions with a low background value (regions with constant breast thickness) the correspondence between the predicted false positive rate and the measured detection rates on a real image is good. This confirms our hypothesis, that the detection problem inside the breast and especially for dense breasts is basically the problem of distinction from the image noise. For regions with high background values (breast border) the number of signal detected with higher thresholds is much higher than the predicted false positive rate due to noise. In these regions the dose arriving at the detector level is much bigger. It allows a much better distinction between breast structures and the noise is of lower importance. The detected structures are mostly fibrous structures and skin.

To distinguish fibrous structures from microcalcifications geometric or densitometric attributes can be used. Many algorithms about of false positives reduction have been published (e.g [10]). For illustration purpose, we show the

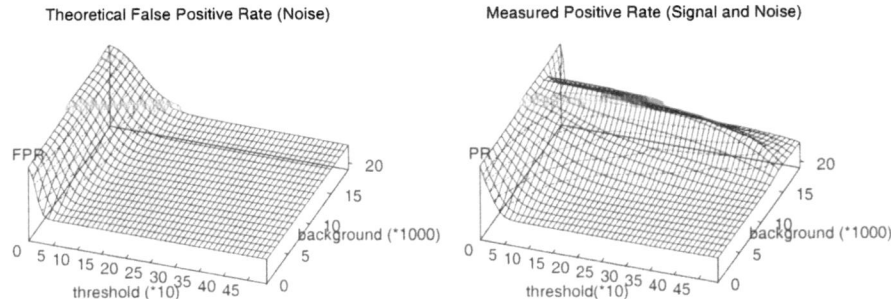

Fig. 6. Theoretical false positive rate(left) and measured positive rate (right)

effect of a densitometric constraint added to the detection process. The chosen constraint is a minimal attenuation coefficient for the detected structure which can be estimated from the size of the top-hat operator.

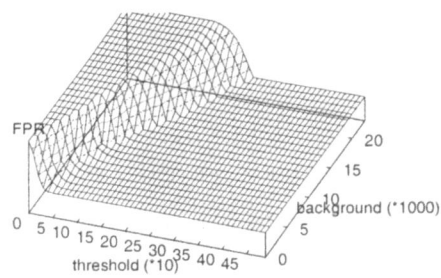

Fig. 7. Theoretical false positive rate including a densitometric constraint

The resulting theoretical false positive function shown in figure 7 is equal to the false positive function with noise only (figure 6) in dense regions (low background values) and exhibits a linear dependence between threshold and background values for higher background values. This allows to control the number of detected structures in the sub-cutaneous area.

6   Conclusions

In this paper we present a simulation system for the physics that underly the acquisition of images on digital mammography equipment. We use the model to calculate a minimal size of microcalcification that can be detected under given acquisition conditions and analyse the influence of pixel size and dose. The model is introduced in a detection system for microcalcifications to improve the detection performance across the different tissue thicknesses throughout the image. In addition, it becomes possible to calibrate the results relative to a theoretical false positive rate so that in order to obtain good detection results independently of the acquisition parameters. Finally we show that the correspondence between the theoretical false positive rate and the positive rate obtained on clinical images is good for regions inside the breast, where noise is the principal problem for the detection of calcifications.

References

1. M. Nafi Gurcan, Yasemin Yardimci, A. Enis Cetin, Rashid Ansari, *Automated Detection and Enhancement of Microcalcifications in Mammograms Using Nonlinear Subband Decomposition*, Proceedings of IEEE ICASSP97, International Conference on Acoustics, Speech, and Signal Processing, April 20-24, 1997, München, Germany.
2. François Lefebvre, Habib Benali, René Gilles, Edmond Kahn, Robert Di Paola *A fractal approach to the segmentation of microcalcifications in digital mammograms*, Medical Physics, Vol. 22, No.4, April 1995, pp.381 - 390
3. Sylvie Bothorel, *Analyse d'image par arbre de décision flcue - Application à la classification sémiologique des amas de microcalcifications en mammographie numérique*, Thèse de doctorat à l'université Paris 6, 1996
4. Michel Grimaud, *La géodesie numérique en morphologie mathématique. Application à la détéction automatique de microcalcifications en mammographie numérique*, Thèse de doctorat à l'Ecole Nationale Supérieure des Mines de Paris, 1991
5. Ralph Highnam, Michael Brady, Brasil Shepstone *A representation for mammographic image processing*, Medical Image Analysis, Vol. 1, No.1, 1996, pp. 1 - 18
6. Nico Karssemeijer, *Adaptive Noise Equalization and Recognition of Microcalcification Clusters in Mammograms*, in "State of the Art in Digital Mammographic Image Analysis", edited by K.W. Bowyer, S. Astley, World Scientific, 1994
7. J.M. Dinten, J.M. Volle, M. Darboux *Quantitative interpretation of mammogramms based on a physical model of the image formation process*, 4th International Workshop on Digital Mammography, Univerity of Nijmegen, The Netherlands, June 7-10, 1998
8. Heang-Ping Chan et.al. *Digital Mammography: Observer Performance Study of the Effect of Pixel Size on Radiologists Characterization of Malignant and Benign Microcalcifications*, SPIE Medical Imaging 99, International Conference on Acoustics, Speech, and Signal Processing, Feb. 20-26 1999, San-Diego, CA. USA.
9. Marton Lanyi, *Diagnosis and Differential Diagnosis of Breast Calcifications*, Springer Verlag 1986
10. Rufus H. Nagel, Robert M. Nishikawa, John Papaioanou, Kunio Doi, *Analysis of methods for reducing false positives in automated detection of clustered microcalcifications in mammograms*, Medical Physics, Vol. 25, No. 8, August 1998, pp. 1502 - 1506.
11. Serge Muller *Full-Field Digital Mammography designed as a complete system*, European Journal of Radiology, Invited Paper, to appear in 1999.

Interactive Direct Volume Rendering of Dural Arteriovenous Fistulae in MR–CISS Data

C. Rezk–Salama[1], P. Hastreiter[1], K. Eberhardt[2], B. Tomandl[2], and T. Ertl[1]

[1] Computer Graphics Group, University of Erlangen–Nuremberg,
Department of Computer Science , Am Weichselgarten 9, 91058 Erlangen, Germany
{rezk|hastreiter|ertl}@informatik.uni-erlangen.de
[2] Division of Neuroradiology, University of Erlangen–Nuremberg,
Department of Neurosurgery, Schwabachanlage 6, 91054 Erlangen, Germany

Abstract. Dural arteriovenous fistulae are the cause of various somatic diseases. For their analysis DSA is used in medical practice. However, the injection of contrast dye into the vertebral segmental arteries is a time–consuming and highly difficult procedure. Aiming at a reduction of the number of injections required for the detection and exact localization of the pathology, we introduce a new approach which provides meaningful visualization of MR–*CISS* volumes. Due to the limited spatial resolution of the image data an explicit segmentation of the small vascular structures is extremely difficult. Therefore, we propose a fast sequence of filtering operations and volume growing in order to separate the areas of background, spinal cord and cerebrospinal fluid. Consecutively, we suggest implicit segmentation within these sub–volumes. This is achieved by interactively adjusting transfer functions of pre–defined color lookup tables with a few manipulation operations. Thereby, the tiny target vessels contained within the area of cerebrospinal fluid are clearly delineated. Overall, the presented non–invasive approach ensures an optimal spatial understanding of vessel structures in relation to the surrounding anatomy and contributes significantly to reduce the number of injections during DSA examinations.

Keywords: Direct Volume Rendering, MR–*CISS*, Analysis of Dural Arteriovenous Fistulae, Surgery Planning

1 Introduction

Dural arteriovenous fistulae *(dAVF)* are pathologic connections between arterious and venous blood vessels within the vertebral column [1]. Such malformations cause a variety of somatic diseases, ranging from back pain to paraplegia and physical disabilities. Possible treatments are coagulation of the pathologic structure or excision of the whole abnormal area during a neurosurgical intervention.

The comprehensive analysis of dAVFs requires detailed knowledge of the related vascular structures in order to localize the malformation. Digital subtraction angiography *(DSA)* is still the method of choice to obtain a clear delineation of the vessels within the spinal column. However, a contrast medium has to be injected to differentiate the vessels from the surrounding tissue. This leads to projection images which contain no depth information. In order to determine the exact location of a fistula, multiple injections into the vertebral segmental arteries on both sides are necessary which is a time–consuming process. In order to accelerate the analysis and to reduce the risk of injuries to the spinal cord, it is desirable to minimize the number of injections.

With magnetic resonance *(MR)* it is possible to scan the vessels within the spinal column non–invasively, if a CISS *(Constructive Interference in the Steady State)* sequence [2] is applied. Revealing high contrast between the vascular structures and the cerebrospinal fluid *(CSF)* the slice images allow to substitute myelography since all the necessary information is available [3]. However, their two–dimensional *(2D)* representation is insufficient to track the course of the tiny vessels. This is mandatory to determine the location of a fistula allowing to perform DSA examinations more precisely and thereby to reduce the number of injections considerably. Therefore, an appropriate three–dimensional *(3D)* visualization of the MR–*CISS* data is required. This contributes considerably to understand the spatial relation of the involved structures producing meaningful images of spinal vascular structures with a diameter which is often below 1 mm.

After a short overview in section 2 explaining the representation of the target structures within MR–*CISS* slice images, the applied visualization technique based on 3D–texture mapping is discussed in section 3. Time–consuming explicit segmentation of the target vessels is avoided by using implicit delineation. This is conveniently obtained with transfer functions which are manipulated interactively to adjust pre–defined lookup tables for color an opacity values. As an advantage only a coarse separation of CSF and the spinal cord is required which is easily achieved with a sequence of fast and simple pre–processing steps, presented in section 4. Consequently, section 5 describes the pre–defined color lookup tables and the interactive process to adjust the transfer functions to a specific data set. Finally, section 6 presents several clinical examples demonstrating the value of the suggested approach.

2   MR–CISS Data

The flexibility of magnet resonance imaging (MRI) allows to differentiate a great variety of tissues non–invasively by using different sets of scanning parameters. The MR–*CISS* sequence provides image data with high signal of CSF and fat tissue, whereas vascular structures have low intensity. As can be seen in figure 1 the area between the spinal cord and the dura is filled with CSF which contains the target vessels. Further–on, the dura is surrounded by bone structures of low intensity and partly by epidural fat of high signal values. Since the spinal cord as well as the vascular and the bony structures are in the same range of data values it is impossible to apply a simple maximum intensity projection *(MIP)*. Contrary to that the explicit segmentation of the tiny vessels is a difficult and error–prone task since the resolution of the vessels is very limited and partial volume effects occur. However, using direct volume rendering semi–transparent views allow to delineate the vessels if an individual color lookup table is only locally applied to the area of CSF. An important prerequisite is the ability to manipulate the transfer functions interactively. This ensures accurate implicit segmentation within a very short time.

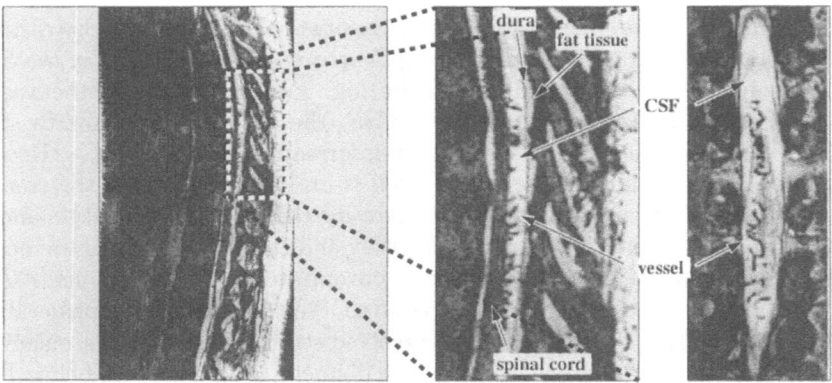

Fig. 1. MR–*CISS* with dAVF in the area of the thoracic spine: *(left)* Original saggital slice image — *(middle)* zoomed saggital view showing target vessels within CSF and *(right)* zoomed coronal view.

3   Visualization

In comparison to other approaches based on polygonal representations [4, 5], direct volume rendering has proved to be superior for the comprehensive and meaningful visualization of tomographic data [6, 7]. Additionally, the combination of interactive manipulation and resulting images of high quality are indispensable for clinical application [8, 9]. As presented previously [10] this is guaranteed with 3D texture mapping which provides hardware accelerated trilinear interpolation. According to the sampling theorem a 3D view of the volume is generated by drawing an adequate number of equidistant polygons parallel to the image plane with respect to the current viewing direction ("volume slicing"). During rasterization the respective polygons are textured with their corresponding image information directly obtained from the 3D–texture by trilinear interpolation. The final image is produced by successive blending of the textured polygons back–to–front onto the image plane. Due to the hardware accelerated interpolation and blending operations, the time consumed for rendering is negligible compared to software solutions.

During the rasterization process, transfer functions are applied to the 3D–texture, that specify color and opacity for each voxel value of the original data. The hardware integration allows to modify the lookup tables interactively providing direct visual feedback. Thereby, semi–transparent views lead to a fast and convenient implicit segmentation of the image data. This is most useful in pathologic cases with tiny and complex target structures. Moreover, it is the best way to deal with partial volume effects or noise inherent in the data which are usually very difficult to cope with using explicit segmentation.

For the interactive assignment of transfer functions, there are specific texture color tables of considerable depth on high–end graphics computers. They allow to apply the concept of "tagged volumes" which was previously presented in [11]. Using a voxel–based segmentation of the data, a unique tag number is assigned to every voxel in order to divide the data into disjoint subsets. According to the number of tags, the global lookup table is split into partitions. Thereby, individual transfer functions for color and opacity values are available for every sub–volume allowing to manipulate the 3D–representation locally.

In contrast to the described strategy based on 3D–texture mapping, approaches are currently gaining attention which avoid the computationally expensive trilinear interpolation by using 2D–textures and a shear–warp factorization of the viewing matrix [12]. However, they are less applicable for a detailed visualization during the analysis of tiny structures. Due to a fixed number of sampling points along the rays of sight and the spatially insufficient bilinear interpolation the resulting images might contain visual artifacts or appear blurred. This makes the clear delineation of small structures extremely difficult, especially if they are zoomed closely for a detailed inspection.

4   Segmentation

According to section 2 the slice images of MR–*CISS* data show high contrast between CSF and the spinal vessels. This is caused by the low intensity values of the vascular information and the high signal of CSF. However, both the surrounding tissue and the spinal cord are represented in the same range of intensity values as the target vessels. This prohibits an implicit delineation of the vascular structures if a lookup table is used which affects the volume data globally. Therefore, it is our strategy to isolate the region of CSF including the vascular structures and to apply transfer functions only locally. This approach is much faster and more convenient than an explicit segmentation of the vessels which might easily miss important features.

Subsequently, the sequence of pre–processing steps is explained which is used to separate the CSF including the spinal vessels, the spinal cord and the remaining part of the image data defined as background:

1. In most cases noise reduction is necessary as a first step to optimize the data for further pre–processing. Regions of higher homogeneity are obtained by anisotropic diffusion [13] while the exact object boundaries are preserved.
2. In order to segment the region of the CSF, containing the vascular structures, a morphologic 3D grey–value closing operation with a spherical filter kernel is applied to the voxel data. This operation removes the dark vascular structures within the region of CSF of high intensity, such that the whole region can be easily extracted by a simple threshold operation. For optimal

results the size of the spherical filter kernel must be greater than the largest
vessel diameter, but smaller than the diameter of the spinal cord.

3. Successively, the closed region of CSF is extracted by volume growing. Using
   bounding boxes to prevent volume off–shoots, the segmentation is computed
   stepwise starting at the top of the vertebral column.

4. Although this first segmentation already contains all the interesting structures, for an enhanced spatial understanding of the resulting images it is
   useful to additionally obtain a segmentation of the spinal cord. Again, this
   is easily achieved with volume growing of the closed image data, using the
   previous segmentation as a boundary.

5. Based on the segmentation results, the original image data is attributed
   using unique tag numbers for the CSF, the spinal cord and the surrounding
   dark tissue (see figure 2). Due to the immediate visual control and the low
   computational expense of the processing steps, the presented user–guided
   sequence leads to fast and robust segmentation results.

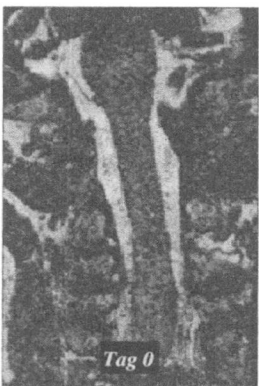 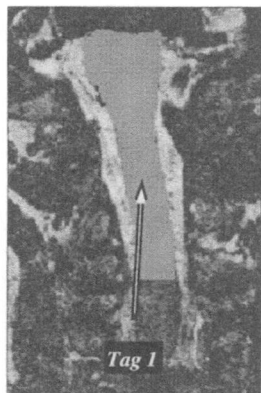 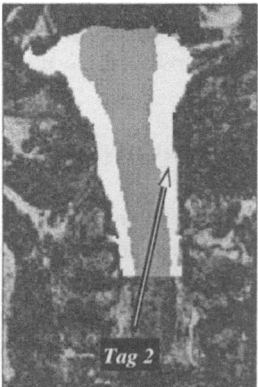

Fig. 2. Explicit segmentation of the significant regions represented by a tagged volume:
Background *(Tag 0)*, spinal cord *(Tag 1)*, CSF including target vessels *(Tag 2)*.

5   Transfer Functions

Using the coarse segmentation of the data described in the previous section,
a detailed implicit delineation is obtained directly during volume rendering by
interactively adjusting transfer functions. For every tagged sub–volume, four
separate curves are used describing the correlation between the original data
values and the displayed color components and opacity (RGBA).

Figure 3 shows the transfer functions which lead to the visualization presented in figure 5. As additional source of information the intensity histogram
of the volume data is displayed within the diagram. For the background region

(tag 0), the opacity is set to a constant low value and a linear ramp is specified for the color components. This results in a semi–transparent representation which supports the anatomical orientation. To reveal the small vessels within the CSF *(tag 2)*, the setting of the opacity function causes an implicit segmentation. Starting with high opacity for the low data values of the vascular structures, a slope must be adjusted to render the CSF of high intensity transparently. The red component is adjusted with a decay towards higher data values to enhance the impression of depth. The green and blue color components are completely switched off for this tag. Finally, the transfer functions of the spinal cord *(tag 1)* are set to full opacity and green color to additionally enhance the contrast.

To speed up the process of adjusting the transfer functions, pre–defined templates are used. These lookup tables look similar to those presented in figure 3. During the analysis of the image data the respective functions are either manipulated individually or as a combined set after grouping them arbitrarily. In order to find the optimal representation of every subregion only a few and simple operations are necessary. These comprise vertical and horizontal translations or simple movements of a handle in order to change the angle of a linear mapping.

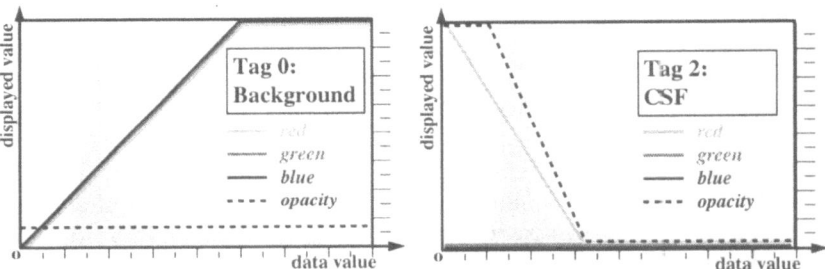

Fig. 3. Intensity histogram and transfer functions for the visualization shown in figure 5 *(e, f)*: *(left)* Setting for the semi–transparent background region — *(right)* Setting applied to delineate the vascular structures contained in the sub–volume of the CSF.

6   Results and Discussion

The presented approach was so far applied to the data of 12 patients with different locations of dAVFs. All MR–CISS volumes were acquired with a Siemens MR Vision 1.5 Tesla scanner which provides the necessary resolution to resolve the tiny vessel structures appropriately. In all cases volumes were used consisting of images with a 512^2 matrix and 40–70 slices. The size of the voxels was set to $0.5 \times 0.5 \times 0.7$ mm^3. In order to guarantee high frame rates the consecutive 3D–visualization was exclusively perform on a SGI Onyx2 (R10000, 195MHz) with BaseReality graphics hardware providing 64 Mbytes of texture memory.

To our experience direct volume rendering is the only visualization technique to produce meaningful 3D–representations of dAVFs contained in MR–CISS data. The following four cases demonstrate the clinical value of our strategy:

- Figure 4 comprises a DSA image of a dAVF and the 3D–visualization of MR–CISS data. This example shows the excellent correspondence between DSA and the 3D representation. The fully opaque spinal cord in green color enhances the spatial understanding. Additionally, clip planes are used to display the surrounding bone structures for the anatomical orientation.
- A highly complex vessel structure close to the medulla oblongata is presented in figure 5. While the spatial orientation is extremely difficult using DSA projections, this example clearly demonstrates the benefit of a 3D representation for the localization of the nidus of the fistula.
- The example in figure 6 shows a dAVF in the area of the lumbar spine. Although the vascular structure is surrounded by the roots of spinal nerves, the malformation is clearly delineated. In this case, the nidus of the fistula is located outside the area of CSF and thus cannot be visualized.
- Figure 7 displays a detailed 3D representation of a complex venous vessel in the area of the thoracic spine. Due to epidural fat tissue, the closing operation lead to segmentation artifacts (partly visible in *(b)*), which are successfully removed by interactive adjustment of independent clip planes.
- **Note: the color images can be found at**
  http://www9.informatik.uni-erlangen.de/eng/research/vis/dAVM/miccai.html

As demonstrated in these examples, the suggested approach based on non–invasively acquired image data assists tremendously to find the fistula and to define the related vertebrae. Finally, DSA is still applied since it represents a gold standard for the examination of dAVFs. However, knowing the exact location of the malformation the time–consuming process of multiple DSA projections is optimized by reducing the required number of injections to a minimum.

The size of the target structures and the spatial distribution of data values within MR–CISS data require a complex and time–consuming process to segment the vessels explicitly. Thus, for clinical application it is more appropriate to separate the whole area of CSF in a robust way. Overall the coarse pre–segmentation involving noise reduction, morphologic operations and volume growing takes approximately 10–15 minutes. For the meaningful and fast delineation of the vessel structures contained in the segmented subregion of the CSF the interactive adjustment of transfer functions is crucial, ensuring direct visual feedback. Using pre–defined color lookup tables, the adaptation of transfer functions to the individual data takes another 5 minutes. For interactive visualization 3D–texture mapping guarantees high frame rates and excellent image quality by using trilinear interpolation.

7   Conclusion

An approach was suggested for the interactive 3D–visualization of dural arteriovenous fistulae. Using MR–*CISS* data only the CSF and the spinal cord have to be segmented explicitly. The meaningful delineation of the target vessels is then performed implicitly by adjusting pre–defined color lookup tables for each separated area. Direct volume rendering based on 3D–texture mapping ensures the required interactivity and the necessary image quality to analyze the tiny vessels. The presented results demonstrate the value of our approach in practice which proved to effectively reduce the number of injections required for DSA examination. Therefore, our method assists pre–operative planning as a valuable approach for patients with dural arteriovenous fistulae.

References

1. M. Hamilton, J. Anson, and R. Spetzler. *The Practice of Neurosurgery*, chapter Spinal Vascular Malformations, pages 2272–2292. Williams & Wilkins, 1996.
2. M. Deimling and G. Laub. *Book of Abstracts*, chapter Constructive Interference in Steady State for Motion Sensitivity Reduction, page 842. Society of Magnetic Resonance in Medicine, 1989.
3. K. Eberhardt, I. Schäfer, M. Deimling, H.-P. Hollenbach, and F. Fellner. Diagnosis of Spinal Dural Arteriovenous Malformations Using a 3D–CISS Sequence. In *Proc. of Soc. of Magn. Res. in Med.*, volume 2, 1997.
4. S. Nakajima, H. Atsumi, A. Bhalerao, F. Jolesz, R. Kikinis, T. Yoshimine, T. Moriarty, and P. Stieg. Computer-assisted Surgical Planning for Cerebrovascular Neurosurgery. *Neurosurgery*, 41:403–409, 1997.
5. M.Melgar, L. Zamorano, Z. Jiang, M. Guthikonda, V. Gordon, and F. Diaz. Three–Dimensional Magnetic Resonance Angiography in the Planning of Aneurysm Surgery. *Comp. Aided Surgery*, 2:11–23, 1997.
6. B. Kuszyk, D. Heath, D. Ney, D. Bluemke, B. Urban, T. Chambers, and E. Fishman. CT Angiography with Volume Rendering : Imaging Findings. *American Jour. of Radiol. (AJR)*, pages 445–448, 1995.
7. G. Rubin, C. Beaulieu, V. Argiro, H. Ringl, A. Norbash, J. Feller, M. Dake, R. Jeffrey, and S. Napel. Perspective Volume Rendering of CT and MR Images: Applications for Endoscopic Viewing. *Radiology*, 199:321–330, 1996.
8. L. Serra, R. Kockro, C. Guan, N. Hern, E. Lee, Y. Lee, C. Chan and W. Nowinsky. Multimodal Volume–Based Tumor Nerurosurgery Planning in the Virtual Workbench. In *Proc. Med. Img. Comput. and Comp.–Assis. Interv. (MICCAI)*, volume 1496 of *Lec. Notes in Comp. Sc.*, pages 1007–1015. Springer, 1998.
9. P. Hastreiter, C. Rezk-Salama, , B. Tomandl, K. Eberhardt, and T. Ertl. Fast Analysis of Intracranial Aneurysms based on Interactive Direct Volume Rendering and CT–Angiography. In *Proc. Med. Img. Comput. and Comp.–Assis. Interv. (MICCAI)*, volume 1496 of *Lec. Notes in Comp. Sc.* Springer, 1998.
10. B. Cabral, N. Cam, and J. Foran. Accelerated Volume Rendering and Tomographic Reconstruction Using Texture Mapping Hardware. *ACM Symp. on Vol. Vis.*, pages 91–98, 1994.
11. P. Hastreiter, H. Çakmak, and T. Ertl. Intuitive and Interactive Manipulation of 3D Data Sets by Integrating Texture Mapping Based Volume Rendering into the OpenInventor Class Hierarchy. In *Worksh. Bildverarb. f.d. Med. (BVM)*, pages 149–154, 1996.
12. P. Lacroute and M. Levoy. Fast Volume Rendering Using a Shear–Warp Factorization of the Viewing Transform . *Comp. Graphics*, 28(4):451–458, 1994.
13. G. Gerig, O. Kübler, R. Kikinis, and F. Jolesz. Nonlinear Anisotropic Filtering of MRI Data. *IEEE Trans. on Med. Imag.*, 11(2):221–232, 1992.

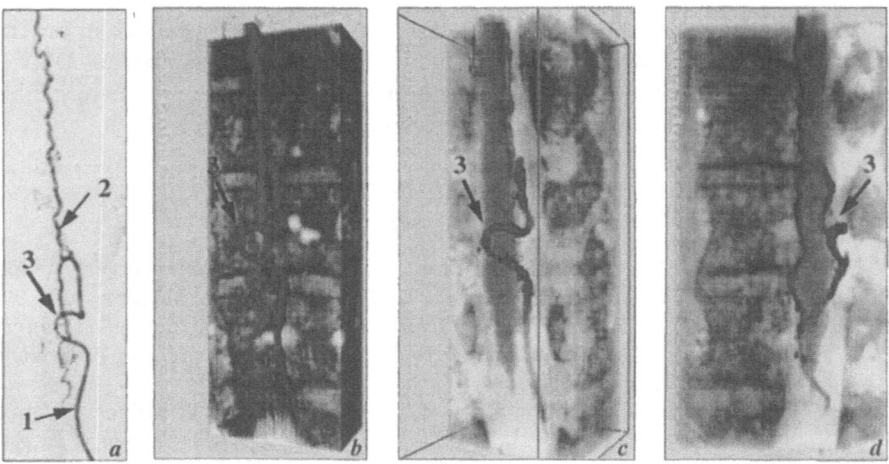

Fig. 4. Dural AV fistula in the area of the lower thoracic spine: *(a)* DSA shows the feeding artery (1 ⟶) and a perimedullary fistula (2 ⟶) — *(b)* Direct volume rending of MR–*CISS* shows optimal correspondence (3 ⟶) with the DSA — *(c, d)* The integration of the surrounding anatomy conveys the relation to the spinal cord (green) and the bone structures of the vertebral column.

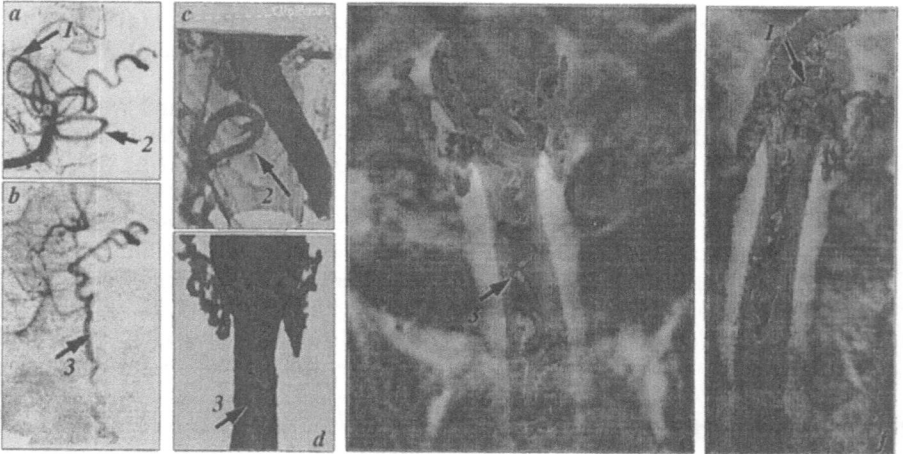

Fig. 5. Dural AV fistula in the area of the medulla oblongata: *(a,b)* DSA showing the vascular malformation — *(c-f)* Direct volume rendering leads to an excellent delineation showing the semi–transparent CSF and the opaque target vessels *(c)*, the opaque vessels and the opaque spinal cord *(d)*, and the relation to the surrounding anatomy *(e, f)*.

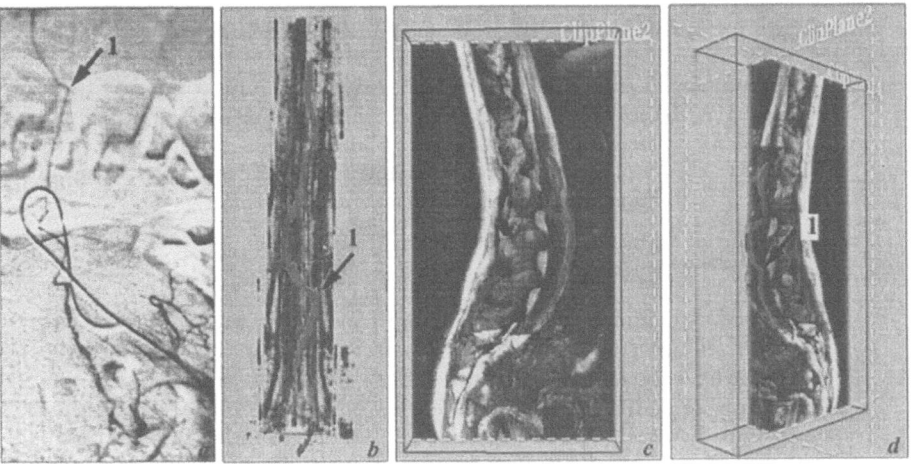

Fig. 6. Dural AV fistula in the area of the lumbar spine: *(a)* DSA shows a fistula (1 ⟶) coming from the right internal iliac artery. — *(b)* Volume rendering of the fistula and the roots of spinal nerves. *(c, d)* Lateral and frontal view of the malformation in relation to the surrounding anatomy.

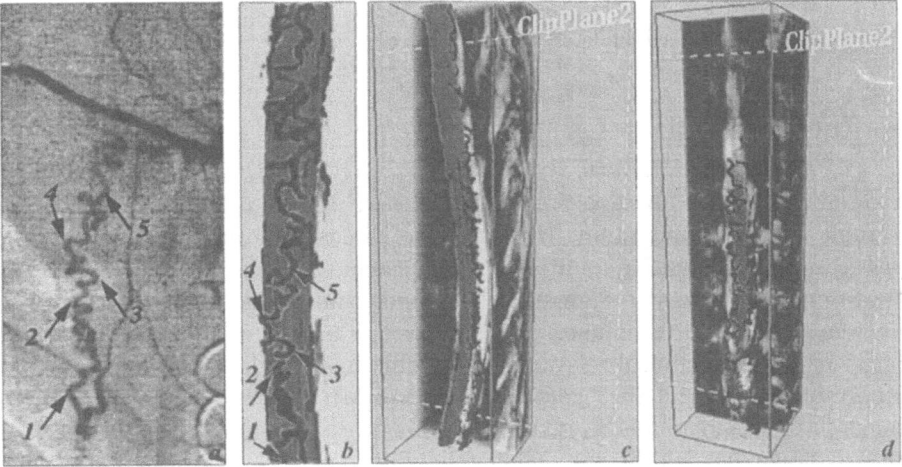

Fig. 7. Dural AV fistula in the area of the thoracic spine: Comparison of the complex vessel structure in a DSA projection image *(a)* and a corresponding 3D visualization of a MR–*CISS* volume *(b)* including a lateral *(c)* and a dorsal view *(d)*.

Segmentation of White Matter Lesions from Volumetric MR Images

S. A. Hojjatoleslami, F. Kruggel, and D. Y. von Cramon

Max-planck-institute of cognitive neuroscience
Stephanstraße 1A, D-04103 Leipzig, Germany

Abstract. Quantitative analysis of the changes to the brain's white matter is an important objective for a better understanding of pathological changes in various forms of degenerative brain diseases. To achieve an accurate quantification, an algorithm is proposed for automatic segmentation of white matter atrophies and lesions from T1-weighted 3D Magnetic Resonance (MR) images of the head. Firstly, white matter, gray matter and cerebrospinal fluid (CSF) compartments are segmented. Then, external and internal cisterns are separated by placing cutting planes relative to the position of the anterior and posterior commissure. Finally, a region growing method is applied to detect lesions inside the white matter. Since lesions may be adjacent to the gray matter, we use the external cisterns as a clue to prevent the algorithm from absorbing low gray level points in the gray matter.

The method is fully applied to detect the white matter lesions and relevant structures from a set of 41 MR images of normal and pathological subjects. Subjective assessment of the results demonstrates a high performance and reliability of this method.

1 Introduction

A number of brain diseases lead to focal and diffuse pathologic changes detectable by MR tomography. However, the clinical relevance of these findings with respect to cognitive abilities or impairments of a patient is often unclear. Traditionally, pathologic changes in MR tomograms are assessed visually or using semi-automatic techniques. These measures are compared with behavioral data to assess the clinical relevance of MR findings. While visual inspection and expert rating are still the "gold standard" in MR evaluation, it is hoped that image processing can assist and support this process and yield results which are rater-independent and have a higher reliability.

Extraction of such quantitative measures is concerned with computing a number of descriptors representing the properties of anatomical structures in the brain. The most important step in quantitative analysis is an accurate segmentation of tissues in MR images. The segmentation of tissues has received considerable attention in medical image processing community [1–4]. Although promising results on large sets of normal images is reported, validation of the

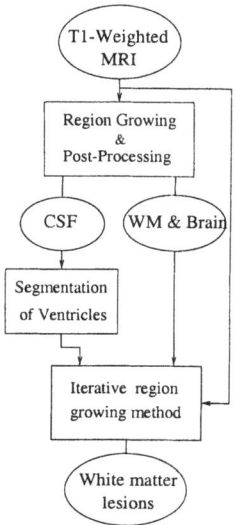

Fig. 1. Different processing steps for segmentation of white matter lesions in MR image.

techniques on pathological datasets remains a persistent problem. Not surprisingly, the problem of white matter lesion detection has also received a considerable interest in the literature where the use of various image analysis techniques including pyramidal approach [5], intensity based [6, 7] and model based [8] techniques, have been addressed. The reader is referred to good surveys on general purpose image segmentation techniques [9, 10] and those which are specifically designed or optimized for MRI segmentation purpose [1–4].

WM lesions are one of the main signs of various forms of degenerative brain diseases. In T1-weighted MR images, they appear as faint, dark, arbitrarily shaped blobs, which range from a few millimeters to several centimeters in size. A better understanding of the size, number and the spatial distribution of the lesions may give important clues to the mechanisms of the disease, provide a new tool for monitoring their change over time and allow drawing conclusions about the progression of a disease. A reliable detection of these lesions is difficult: fuzzy lesion boundaries, noise and non-uniformity in MR images produce a severe lack of definition of WM lesions. They may also lead to a reduction of the WM volume, which is also detected indirectly as an increase of the CSF compartment.

In this paper we aim to present a region based algorithm for the segmentation of the white matter, the internal and external CSF compartments and lesions from volumetric T1-weighted MR images of the head. As shown in Figure 1, we first segment the main tissues (WM, GM and CSF) from the MR data using a region growing method. The CSF compartment is split into internal and external cisterns using a heuristic technique. In the final step, the holes within the segmented WM are used as starting points for the region growing method to find the highest gradient boundary for every blob in the white matter. Since there are junctions between the lesions and the cortex, we use the external cisterns as clue to prevent the growing process from covering the low intensity points in the cortex.

This paper is organized as follows. Section2 presents a brief overview of the region growing method followed by a description of various processing steps applied to segment the white matter lesions from the brain. Section 3 considers the capability of the algorithm and evaluates its performance on a large set of normal and pathological datasets. The last section presents summary and conclusion of this study.

2   Methods

The method [11] starts from a seed point and absorbs the highest gray level point in its boundary to expand the region. During the growing process, it considers a discontinuity measure, called *peripheral contrast*, to choose from a set of regions evolved during the growing process, a region with the highest gradient boundary as the final output. The discontinuity measure computes the difference between the gray level average of internal boundary of the region and its current boundary. The "internal boundary" is the boundary produced by the set of connected outermost voxels of the current region and "current boundary" as the set of voxels adjacent to the current region. This algorithm is used in the first processing step to segment the scalp and other signal intense parts of the head.

A modified technique [12] which applies a new criterion is then employed to segment the white matter, gray matter and the CSF. Here, the segmented region in the previous step, called thereafter the mask, is used to prevent the growing process from joining the non-brain parts of the head. The criterion detects the point with the minimum gray level value in the current region which links the brain to the mask. These junctions are detected and blocked to allow the algorithm to consider the lower gray-level points in the local neighborhood without growing into the already segmented mask.

The criterion checks every new candidate point y_i with the set of points in the mask **S**. If the point is inside the mask, $y_\lambda \in \mathbf{S}$, the size of the region would reduce to k where $y_k = y_{min}$ is the last minimum gray level point joined to the region. The set of subsequently appended points, with index $i > k + 1$, will be labeled as the mask, and the growing process continues by absorbing a new point in the boundary. Such criterion can be formalized using:

$$y_i > y_k \quad for \quad i = k + 1, k + 2, ..., \lambda \tag{1}$$

where y_i is the sequence of pixels joining the region and y_λ belongs to the mask.

2.1   Segmentation of white matter, Gray matter and CSF

To demonstrate the capability of our algorithm for segmentation of white matter, gray matter and CSF, we consider the behavior of the algorithm applied to a 3D MR image shown in Figure 2-top. The mappings of gray level and peripheral contrast for the image for a starting point inside the brain stem is shown in Figure 2-bottom. The gray level mappings are shown for two conditions: (i) using the segmented scalp as a mask and, (2) using no mask and, therefore, ignoring the criterion (1). The mask is segmented using the algorithm when a point inside the scalp is used to start the growing process [11].

Let us consider the sequence of points absorbed by the growing process. If the algorithm is applied without the criterion (1), the region grows to include the white matter and then through bright junctions (i.e. optical nerves) joins the eyes and other signal intense parts of the head. The sharp increase in the gray level at index number $7.7e + 5$ is related to growing into the eyes and the scalp. When the mask is used, the mapping does not show any rise at this point. The criterion blocks the minimum point joining the scalp, and the current region continues to grow inside the brain. Comparing the two gray level mappings, it becomes evident that the gray level values of the new points are decreasing when the mask is used while fluctuations are observed when the mask is not applied. We, therefore, are interested to choose the locally highest gradient boundary by considering the peripheral contrast only when the mask and criterion (1) were used.

The peripheral contrast, see Figure 2-bottom, starts from low values and increases at the beginning of growing process. This rise is related to the relatively high gradient at the boundary of the white matter. The peripheral contrast changes slowly by the gradient inside the gray matter and shows a sharp increase when the gray matter is being covered. It then reduces when the growing process absorbs lower gray level values in the CSF. Because a low gradient inside the CSF is encountered, a clear peak for the brain compartment at index number $1.68e + 6$ is found. The third small peak at index number $2.3e + 6$ is related to the gradient at the boundary of CSF and the dura mater.

We use the three changes in the peripheral contrast as indicators for segmenting white matter, brain and CSF. For our pathological datasets, the white matter typically has a very fuzzy gradient boundary producing only a small change in the peripheral contrast measure. To increase the reliability of WM segmentation, we use the gradient of the peripheral contrast during the growing process and segment the region when a change in the gradient direction is observed. The global peak generated by the high gradient boundary of the brain is used as a reference for separating CSF and WM.

2.2   Post processing step

A post-processing step is applied to remove some thin structures, eg. parts of the optical nerves, veins and dura mater which connect the brain to its outer hulls. Typically, those junctions are very thin and, therefore, can be easily pruned

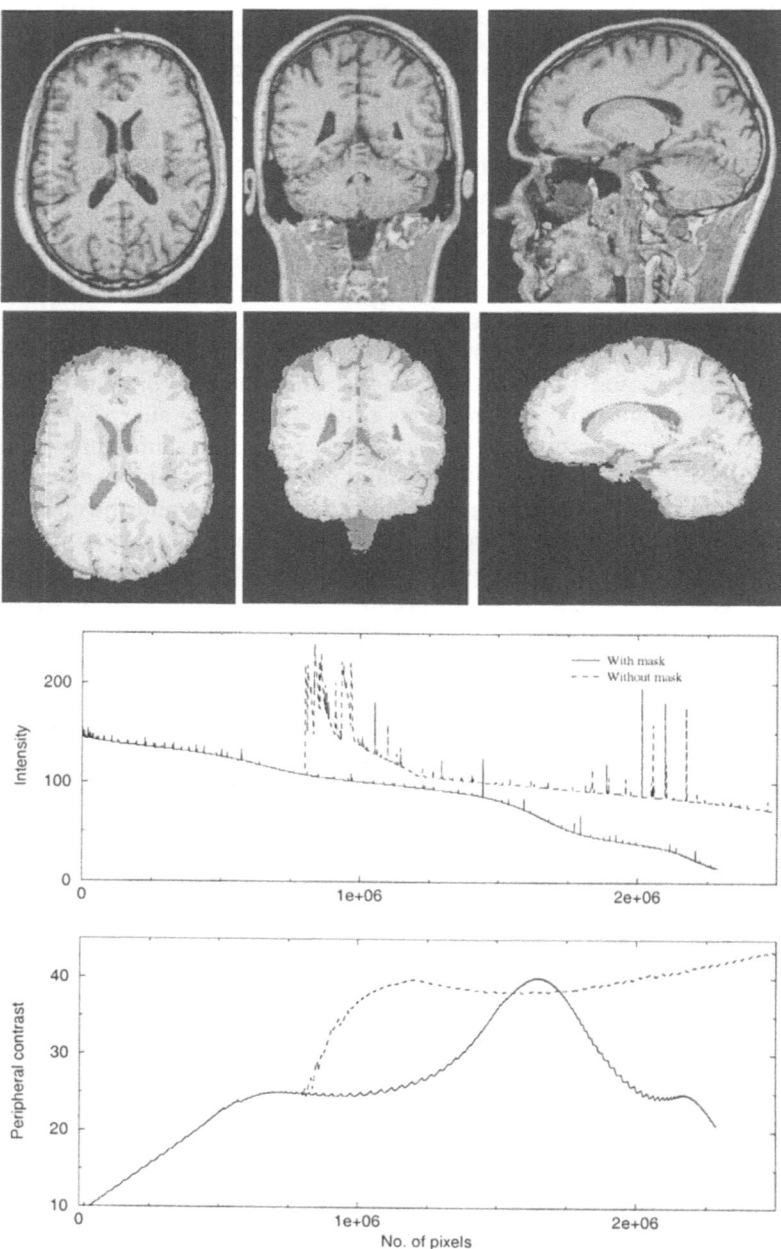

Fig. 2. First row: Orthogonal sections from a 3D brain dataset. **Second row:** The segmentation of tissues from the MR image (white: white matter, gray: gray matter and dark gray: CSF). The graph shows the gray level and peripheral contrast mappings for the two conditions during the growing process.

by applying morphological filters [13] with a small structuring element. This is performed using a closing filter followed by a dilation with spherical Structuring elements with diameters of 5 and 3 voxels, respectively.

2.3   Segmentation of ventricles

The inner cisterns mostly contain CSF and are surrounded by white matter. Only small connections exist which link the 3rd ventricle to the external cisterns. Cutting at this junction is expected to separate the external cisterns from the ventricles. The tiny membrane between the 3rd ventricle and the quadrigeminal cistern is often not fully connected due to the partial volume effect and thus leads to segmentation problems.

Because datasets are aligned with the stereotactical coordinate system, we can simply use the positions of the anterior (CA) and the posterior commissure (CP) to generate suitable cutting plains for separating inner and outer cisterns. The first cut is performed parallel to coronal plane with a thickness of 4mm, width of 16mm (centered at CP) starting from 1mm above CA down towards the neck. Two other cuts were performed with a reference from CP: one parallel to the axial plane starting from 8mm up and 7mm back of the head with the width of 18mm towards the neck. A small cut is also performed parallel to the sagittal plane, 3mm below CP with the width of 40mm connecting the two previous planes. However, this last cut was not necessary for most of the cases but useful for brains with extreme atrophies.

2.4   White matter lesion detection

To detect the small white matter lesions, we use the region growing method starting from the holes inside the segmented white matter. The growing process absorbs the low gray level points in its current boundary thus covering the lesion. The external cisterns are used as a mask to prevent the algorithm from growing into the gray matter or outside the brain. The peripheral contrast is then used to find the highest gradient boundary for each lesion.

An example of the gray level and peripheral contrast for two different lesions is shown in Figure 3. The peripheral contrast starts at a center point and reduces to a minimum value at index numbers 35 and 50. It then gradually approaches the zero level and increases sharply at the final stages of the growing process when most of boundary points are excluded based on criterion (1). This peak is related to very high gray level points (spikes) which will be absorbed at the end of process. The process is terminated when the number of boundary points are very low. The global minimum is used to segment the WM lesions. Limits for a minimum size of 5 voxels and a peripheral contrast of -6 are imposed to exclude false positive detections, which correspond to small and faint regions at resolution limits of the MR scanner.

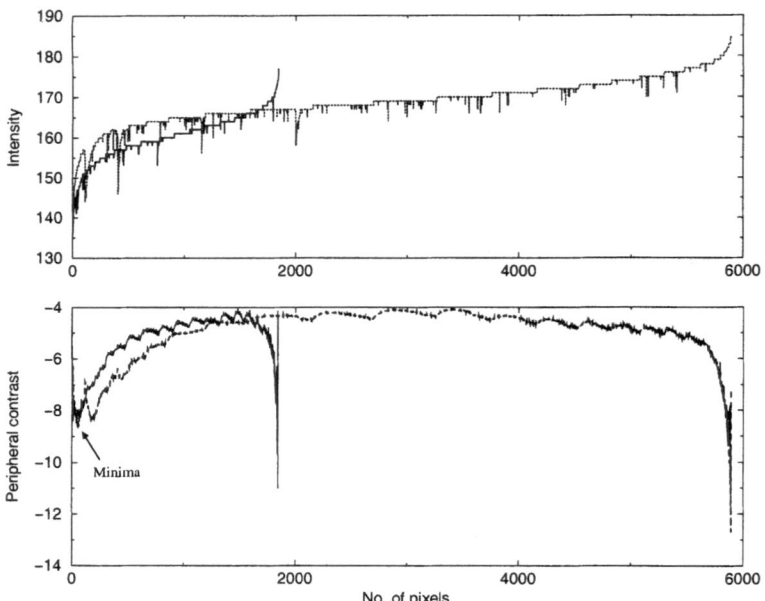

Fig. 3. Gray level and peripheral contrast mappings for two different white matter lesions.

3   Results

We used 41 T1-weighted MR images obtained by scanning persons suffering from brain atrophy (possible Alzheimer's disease), white matter disease, and lacunar infarcts. The images were obtained by a 1.5 Tesla clinical MR scanner at the university hospital Leipzig during a routine study of patients. All datasets were aligned with the stereotactical coordinate system before segmentation and their spatial resolution was interpolated to an isotropical resolution of 1mm.

The two starting points required for the segmentation algorithm were chosen inside the scalp and a bright part of the brain. Segmented tissues after the post-processing step are shown in Figure 4. WM lesions are shown in white overlayed on the original MR image (top row). Inner cisterns are shown in black, outer cisterns in gray (middle row) with respect to the segmented brain in white.

The results were assessed by a specialist in the field using visual inspection of cross-sections and 3D renderings of the segmented brains. Brain segmentation was very reliable and well in agreement with the specialist. White matter segmentation proved to be more difficult, partly due to the "routine" quality of the data, and partly due to the marked cortical atrophy in some cases. This problem also caused difficulty in detection of the relevant turning point from the peripheral contrast. The CSF and ventricles were segmented quite reliably. In some cases, the heuristic placement of the cutting planes clipped parts of the 3rd ventricle. However, the error induced hereby was less than 3% of the total ventricle volume in all cases.

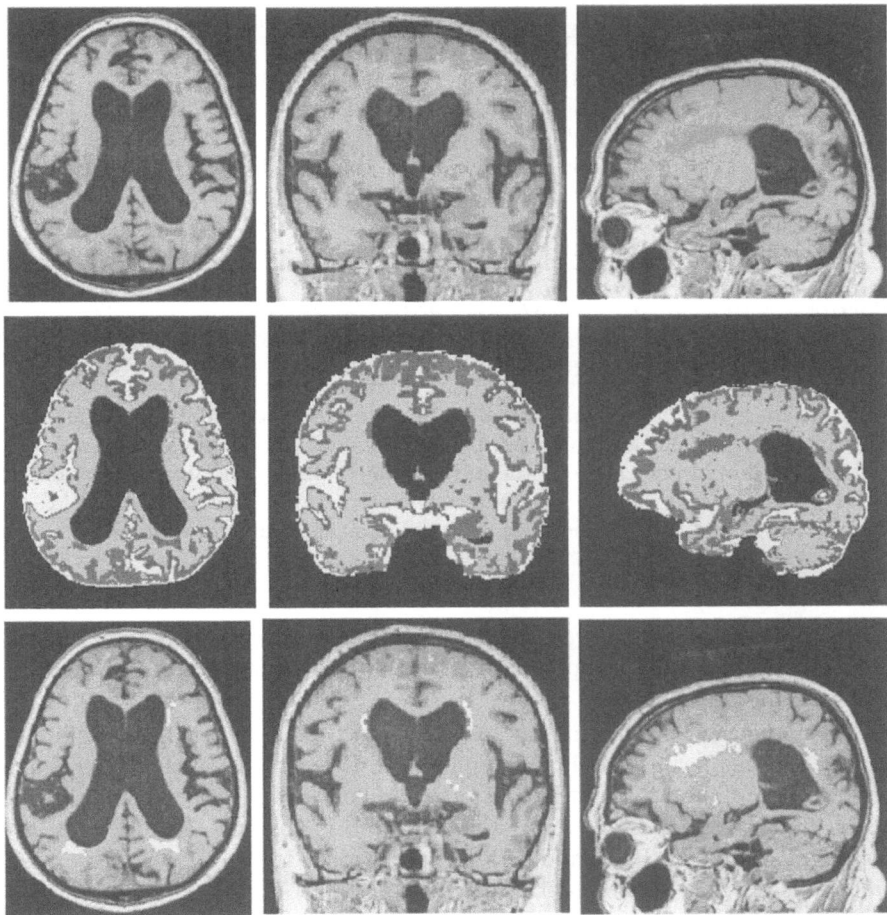

Fig. 4. Different structures segmented by our algorithm from a case of mixed dementia. **First row:** Original image. **Second row:** White matter (bright gray), Gray matter (dark gray), internal cisterns (black), external cisterns (white). **Third row:** White matter lesions (white) overlayed on the original image.

The validation of the white matter lesions is very difficult due to similarity and junctions of the lesions with gray matter. The performance as evaluated on the images were very well in agreement with an independently performed visual inspection by a specialist. Table 1 presents the size and number of white matter lesions for 3 normal subjects and 7 patients.

In comparison to normal subjects, all patients showed a reduction of the GM and the WM compartment (see Table 1), i.e. a global brain atrophy. In the first case, this atrophy led to a substantial increase of the inner cisterns, while in all other cases, only the outer cisterns were enlarged. A rough 1:1 ratio of the GM:

Diagnosis	Age	Sex	brain		EC		IC		WM		GM		LS	LN
			ml	%	ml	%	ml	%	ml	%	ml	%	ml	no
Mixed Dementia	81	m	1331	72	328	17.8	180	9.8	802	44	529	29	11.7	70
Mixed Dementia	82	f	1044	74	341	24.1	28	1.9	606	43	437	30	10.3	45
M. Alzheimer	84	m	1245	68	543	29.7	43	2.4	711	39	533	29	6.1	126
WM Disease	77	f	1036	70	395	26.8	44	3.0	518	35	517	35	8.8	63
WM Disease	75	m	1104	69	416	26.1	72	4.6	552	35	552	35	6.7	60
WM Disease	77	f	1298	74	437	24.9	22	1.2	649	37	649	37	9.5	90
WM Disease	77	f	1061	70	429	28.2	28	1.8	532	35	530	35	14.1	126
Control	32	m	1347	82	277	16.9	14	0.8	660	40	687	42	0	0
Control	25	m	1418	81	309	17.7	14	0.8	699	40	719	41	0	0
Control	24	m	1527	83	294	16.0	19	1.0	763	41	764	41	0	0

Table 1. Measures of intracranial compartments extracted from our segmentation algorithm for 7 pathological and 3 normal subjects. Volumes of the compartments are given in cm^3 and in percentage of the intracranial volume (CSF+brain) are tabulated for the brain, internal cisterns (IC), external cisterns (EC), white matter (WM), gray matter (GM), white matter lesion size (LS) and also the number of white matter lesions (LN).

WM compartment, which was found for the controls, was maintained for cases 4-7, indicating a global atrophy. For cases 1-3, a substantial atrophy of the GM compartment was detected.

We summarized our findings in Table 2 for patients suffering from Alzheimer's disease, a global brain atrophy in conjunction with a focus on the GM compartment was found, and the external cisterns were enlarged. Patients suffering from a WM disease retained the GM:WM ratio found in controls, although the brain volume was reduced. Both findings may overlap. It is still under study why in some cases only the inner cisterns are enlarged.

The main strength of the algorithm is that it needs only two starting points to segment the structures. The starting points were chosen automatically relative to CA and CP. Acceptable results were achieved on 36 out of 41 images without manual intervention. The starting points for other images were chosen manually.

4   Conclusion

We have proposed a new algorithm for segmentation of white matter lesions from T1-weighted volumetric images of the head. The algorithm applies a region growing algorithm to segment different tissues (WM, GM, CSF) based on changes in the discontinuity measure during the growing process. Inner and outer cisterns are separated by introducing cutting planes. Finally, small holes in the white matter are used as starting points to segment WM lesions. The external cisterns were used to prevent the region growing process from including gray matter in the lesions.

Diagnosis	Brain Volume	EC Comp.	IC Comp.	GM:WM Ratio
M. Alzheimer	↓	↑	=	↓
Mixed Dementia	↓	↑	=, ↑	↓
WM Disease	↓	↑	=	=

Table 2. Atrophy patterns for the subgroups of the patients.

The performance of the technique applied for white matter lesion segmentation from 41 datasets obtained by 1.5-Tesla scanner are very encouraging.

Acknowledgments

The authors are very grateful to Professor M.J. Gertz from Department of Psychiatry, University Clinic Leipzig, for providing the data.

References

1. M S Atkins and B T Mackiewich. Fully automatic segmentation of the brain in mri. *IEEE Trans Med Imag*, 17(1):98–107, 1998.
2. J C Bezdek, L O Hall, and L P Clarke. Review of mr image segmentation techniques using pattern recognition. *Med Phys*, 20(4):1033–1048, 1993.
3. L P Clarke, R P Velthuizen, M A Camacho, J J Heine, M Vaidyanathan, L O Hall, R W Thatcher, and M L Silbiger. Mri segmentation: Methods and applications. *Magn Reson Imag*, 13(3):343–368, 1995.
4. J C Rajapakse and F Kruggel. Segmentation of mr images with intensity inhomogeneities. *Image and Vision Computing*, 16:165–180, 1998.
5. C Pachai, Y M Zhu, J Grimaud, M Hermier, A Dromigny-Badin, A Boudraa, G Gimenez, C Confavreux, and J C Froment. A pyramidal approach for automatic segmentation of multiple sclerosis lesions in brain mri. *Computerized Med Imag and Graph*, 22:399–408, 1998.
6. B Johnston and MS Atkins. Segmentation of multiple sclerosis lesions in intensity corrected multispectral mri. *IEEE Trans Med Imag*, 15(2):154–167, 1996.
7. B Udupa, S Wei L Samarasekera, Y Miki, and M A Van Bucchem. Multiple sclerosis lesion quantification using fuzzy-connectness principles. *IEEE: Trans on Med Imag*, 16(5):598–609, 1997.
8. M Kamber, R Shinghal, L Collins, GS Francis, and A C Evans. Model based 3-d segmentation of multiple sclerosis lesions in magnetic resonance brain images. *IEEE Trans Med Imag*, 14(3):442–453, 1995.
9. R M Haralik and L G Shapiro. Survey: Image segmentation techniques. *Comput Vision, Graphics, Image Processing*, 29:100–132, 1985.
10. N R Pal and S K Pal. A review on image segmentation techniques. *Pattern Recognition*, 26:1277–1294, 1993.
11. S A Hojjatoleslami and J Kittler. Region growing: A new approach. *IEEE Trans Image Proc*, 7(7):1079–1084, 1998.
12. S A Hojjatoleslami, F Kruggel, and D Y von Cramon. A region based algorithm for brain segmentation in mri. *submitted*, 1999.
13. J Serra. *Image analysis and mathematical morphology: theoretical advances*, volume 2. Academic Press, New York, 1988.

Fractional Segmentation of White Matter

Simon K. Warfield[1], Carl-Fredrik Westin[1], Charles R. G. Guttmann[1], Marilyn Albert[2], Ferenc A. Jolesz[1], and Ron Kikinis[1]

[1] Surgical Planning Laboratory, Department of Radiology, Harvard Medical School and Brigham and Women's Hospital, 75 Francis St., Boston, MA 02115
{warfield,westin,guttmann,jolesz,kikinis}@bwh.harvard.edu
FAX: 617-732-7963   http://splweb.bwh.harvard.edu:8000
[2] Massachusetts General Hospital, Psychiatry/Gerontology (149-9124), Bldg. 149, 13th Street, Charlestown, MA, 02129

Abstract. Abnormalities in the white matter of the brain are common to subjects with multiple sclerosis and Alzheimer's disease. They also develop in normal, asymptomatic, subjects and appear more frequently with age. Clinically, it is interesting to be able to differentiate between different disease states and to find markers which allow early diagnosis. Conventional spin echo (CSE) magnetic resonance imaging (MRI) is sensitive to these white matter changes and has frequently been applied to their study.

Previous approaches to investigate white matter abnormalities have often been reported to have difficulty distinguishing between normal gray matter and abnormal white matter due to their similar appearance in MRI. Earlier methods have also often generated binary classifications, reporting white matter as either normal or abnormal.

We have developed a new approach which first identifies the region of white matter using a template moderated spatially varying classification, and then estimates the degree of white matter abnormality present at each voxel of the white matter. This fractional segmentation allows us to preserve the heterogeneous characteristics of white matter abnormalities and to investigate both focal and diffuse white matter damage. We compute, from the fractional segmentation, a white matter spectrum showing the different levels of white matter damage present in each subject.

We applied this automated image segmentation method to over 996 MRI scans of subjects affected by multiple sclerosis, 72 normal aging subjects and 29 scans of subjects with Alzheimer's disease. We investigated the ability to characterize these different subject groups based upon tissue volumes determined by spatially varying classification, and by the fractional segmentation of the white matter of each patient.

Keywords: automatic segmentation, brain, white matter, multiple sclerosis, Alzheimer's disease, normal aging.

1 Introduction

Abnormal white matter of the brain is common to patients with one of several different diseases (including multiple sclerosis (MS) and Alzheimer's disease (AD)) and also appears in normal (asymptomatic) aging (NA) subjects. Better characterization of the nature of these white matter changes can help to improve our understanding of the biological processes at work. Clinically, it is interesting to be able to differentiate between different disease states and to find markers which allow early diagnosis. Conventional spin echo magnetic resonance imaging is sensitive to these white matter changes. MRI studies of patients and volunteers have indicated that the patterns of brain change associated with these processes are different. An important goal is to be able to quantitatively study these differences.

Many automated and semi-automated segmentation algorithms for quantitatively assessing these brain changes have been developed and validated. Most of these algorithms have aimed at determining a binary characterization of each voxel as one of a group of possible tissue classes. This approach has been limited by two factors. First, abnormal white matter is often isointense with normal grey matter and previous studies have been limited by the inability to discriminate between some abnormal white matter and normal grey matter [1, 2]. Secondly, white matter damage appears as an heterogenous region of abnormal signal intensity but binarization of the segmentation treats all levels of signal intensity abnormality equally.

Segmentation methods for the assessment of white matter damage have in the past identified voxels in the region of white matter as either normal or as abnormal. This binarization of the state of white matter damage is at best a useful approximation to the actual underlying brain changes that cause the MRI signal intensity abnormalities.

Previous approaches for fractional segmentation of MRI have used geometric and probabilistic models. These methods have been developed in order to account for partial volume averaging to allow improved tissue volume estimates and to improve contrast between specific tissue types [3–6].

Often these methods attempt to assign to each voxel a fractional volume of each tissue class modelled (usually based on the relative probability of the signal intensity occuring for each of the classes proposed to be present in a voxel). Our work differs from these methods in two ways. First, we use an anatomical localization procedure to identify the region of white matter and grey matter, and then look for a fractional segmentation in the region of white matter. Secondly, empirical estimation of a probability density function for the signal intensity distribution of abnormal white matter has the following characteristics. The most commonly occuring abnormality dominates the probability distribution - regions of smaller and greater signal intersity are less probable. Consequently, a fractional segmentation based solely on the probability distribution of abnormal white matter signal intensity does not treat very bright regions differently from lower brightness regions (although they have different signal intensity characteristics, they can be equally probable). The use of relative weighting of the probability of white matter and abnormal white matter (a two class partial volume assignment) can also be problematic because typical estimation methods for white matter probability give very low (or zero) estimates in the region of typically abnormal white matter. This then leads to binarization of the region of abnormal signal intensity, which we would like to avoid.

Mitchell et al. [7] described a method for constructing a white matter - gray matter spectrum by projecting CSE MRI signal intensity onto the first principle component of the white matter (WM) and gray matter (GM) cluster. Intensity normalization was based on the CSF cluster but the inability to assign meaning to specific locations along the line of projection restricted the method to the use of arbitrary units. This method used manually determined ROIs to investigate the WM-GM spectrum of individual lesions. Spectrums were shown for a few time points of a few lesions in a few patients, and highlighted the possibility of such approaches for characterizing abnormal white matter.

We have developed a new automated image segmentation algorithm which is more sensitive and specific for white matter damage and which allows for the investigation of different levels of signal intensity abnormality. Our approach uses automated white matter segmentation, and so can characterize the entire white matter region, not just easily identifiable lesions. Our method is able to generate a calibrated scale for the degree of white matter damage present at each voxel in the white matter region. The goal of this new segmentation method is to allow improved measures of white matter damage to be developed and to allow quantification of damage suspected to be present in so-called normal-appearing white matter.

Our approach to the assessment of fractional white matter damage can be characterized as a geometric feature space model. Unlike earlier geometric models which relied upon more than two tissue classes, our use of automated segmentation of the white matter allows us to assess white matter damage without regard to other tissue classes (such as CSF). This makes our overall approach of first tissue segmentation and then fractional segmentation more robust than previously reported approaches for white matter characterization.

In the following sections, the image segmentation algorithm is presented, and several approaches to characterizing white matter damage are proposed. The algorithm and different white matter characterizations were applied to 72 MRI scans of normal aging subjects, 29 MRI scans of Alzheimer's disease subjects and 996 MRI scans involving 46 patients with multiple sclerosis.

2   Materials and Method

The image analysis is a two step process. First we generate a high sensitivity and specificity segmentation of the regions of white matter and grey matter. Then we generate a fractional segmentation of the region of white matter.

Nine hundred and ninety six MRI scans acquired during a previous study of the evolution of multiple sclerosis [8] were re-analyzed. Seventy two subjects participated in the study as part of a large study of normal aging [1]. There were 22 men and 50 women. All subjects provided informed consent consistent with the institutional IRB regulations.

Twenty nine subjects were included in the study with dementia of the Alzheimer type. The diagnosis of probable AD was made in concordance with NINCDS/ADRDA criteria. All patients had a history of a gradually progressive decline in cognition, demonstrated by difficulty in social or occupational function and impairments in memory and at least one other area of mental ability.

The conventional spin echo magnetic resonance images used in this study were prospectively acquired on a GE Signa 1.5T scanner. Each scan covered the entire brain with axial slices and each slice was acquired with an in-plane voxel size of 0.9375x0.9375 mm^2 and a slice thickness of 3.0 mm.

2.1   High Sensitivity and Specificity Tissue Class Segmentation

Recent review papers ([2, 9]) have highlighted the importance of developing new automated methods for segmentation in the presence of the overlapping intensity distributions of abnormal white matter and normal tissues.

The segmentation method we use involves a sequence of operations. First is intensity based classification with intensity correction using the EM algorithm [10]. This normalizes the intensities so that different scans acquired at different times are directly comparable. The intracranial cavity (ICC) is identified with a semi-automatic method that has previously been described and validated ([11]). The tissue classes identified inside the ICC which are segmented are CSF, white matter, gray matter and lesion. We then match a volumetric brain atlas to the subject with linear [12] and nonlinear registration [13], and resolve classification errors using anatomical context. We have previously described a general method for using anatomical context to resolve tissue class ambiguity due to overlapping intensity distributions [14]. The atlas is used to identify deep grey matter structures and to estimate the location of the cortical grey matter. It is then identified with region growing. The ability to segment cortical grey matter has previously been described and validated [15]. Our approach to the segmentation of deep gray matter structures has previously been described and validated [16].

We identify the white matter region by removing the gray matter structures and CSF tissue class from the ICC. The fractional segmentation described in the next section is then used to identify the level of white matter damage at every voxel in the white matter region.

2.2   Fractional Segmentation of the White Matter Region

The region of abnormal signal intensity associated with a focal lesion may contain areas of normal tissue as well as different histopathological components, such as edema, inflammation, gliosis, demyelination and axonal loss. Microscopic lesions of a size below the voxel resolution of the scanner occur in the normal-appearing white matter, and constitue an 'invisible' lesion load which a binary segmentation is unable to detect, because of the relatively small effect upon signal intensity these have. The inability to account for these factors (changes in normal-appearing white matter, different pathological factors of lesions) has been highlighted as a limitation of existing techniques for measurement of lesion burden [2] and recognized as an important goal for increasing the accuracy and efficacy of quantitative analysis of MS lesions from MRI [9]. However, it is also recognized that if a lesion burden measure is unbiased, reproducible and related to disease activity it can be used as a reliable indicator of disease progression, even if the measure does not fully reflect the underlying pathology [9].

Our work described here aims to investigate the potential for characterizing the variation in white matter signal intensity observed in conventional spin echo images (PDW and T2W images). The model we use is based on a simple observation of the signal intensity characteristics of normal and abnormal white matter in CSE images. Lesions appear relatively bright in both PDW scans and T2W scans. Normal white matter appears darker than grey matter in PDW and T2W scans. Focal white matter abnormalities are often the brightest region of the white matter and diffuse white matter abnormalities often appear as regions of slightly less intense white matter signal intensity increase.

We propose a projection of the signal intensity variation of white matter in this two dimensional MR intensity space onto a line joining the signal intensity characteristics of the darkest white matter and the most bright white matter. We hypothesise that the darkest white matter is the "healthiest" white matter and the brightest white matter is the "most damaged" white matter and we use this linearization to define a mapping beween two dimensional MR intensity space and our measure of white matter damage (0 is most healthy, 1 is most damaged). We can then characterize the dual channel signal intensity properties of the white matter regions in terms of its level of "white matter damage".

The observed voxel values are modelled as being due to a combination of the fraction of each tissue type present in the brain over the region from which the voxel value is measured and a white noise process. Of course, this is a simplification. For instance, even healthy individuals have some intrinsic signal intensity variation in the white matter which is related to the structure of the white matter rather than to disease processes (for example, regions of tight white matter bundles, such as the corpus callosum, appear darker). Let D be the voxel value that would be measured under ideal imaging conditions for a voxel containing maximum disease, and let H be the value measured for healthy tissue. In the presence of noise and imaging artifacts, the observed dual echo signal intensity of a voxel will be O', randomly perturbed away from the ideal position. Let O be the projection of an observed voxel O' onto the line joining D and H in the two channel feature space. We model the signal intensity at O as being due to fractions of diseased, fD, and healthy, $(1 - f)H$, tissues:

$$O = fD + (1 - f)H, \ f \in [0, 1]$$

This model includes the same information as a conventional binary classification (tissue classified as either healthy or diseased white matter) since a binary classification can be obtained from this model by thresholding at f = 0.5. Figure 1 is an illustration of the fractional segmentation of the white matter region of one image from a CSE MRI of the brain of one patient with multiple sclerosis.

2.3   Analyzing the Distribution of White Matter Damage

Once the white matter region has been identified and the fractional segmentation of the white matter region has been computed, we can study the distribution of the white matter damage as estimated by the fractional white matter segmentation, in order to gain a better understanding of the characteristics of white matter change.

One method for doing this is to compute a histogram of the fractional white matter segmentation. Normalizing this histogram generates a probability distribution function which gives the empirically determined probability that each level of white matter damage appears in the subject. We call this the white matter spectrum of the patient. It indicates the probability of different levels of white matter damage.

Computing a mean distribution (mean white matter spectrum) from the white matter fractional segmentation of a group of patients with AD gives an indication of the typical

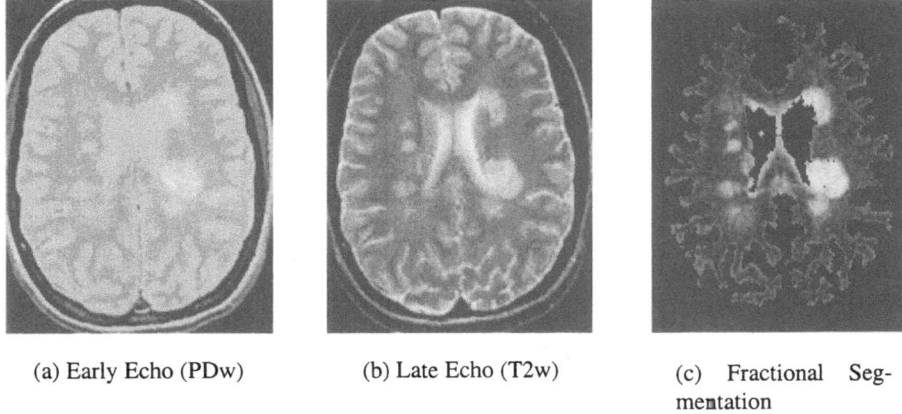

(a) Early Echo (PDw)   (b) Late Echo (T2w)   (c) Fractional Seg-
                                                            mentation

Fig. 1. This figure illustrates the fractional segmentation of the white matter region from one slice of a subject with multiple sclerosis. Intensity in image (c) is proportional to the fraction of white matter damage estimated to be present at the voxel. Note the preservation of the lesion heterogeneity and the easy visualization of the regions of diffuse white matter damage.

range of white matter abnormality present in patients with AD. Similarly, a mean white matter spectrum can be computed for normal subjects age matched to the AD subjects. Investigation of the differences between these distributions may indicate differences in the development of white matter abnormalities between these two groups.

3   Results

We first present conventional volumetric tissue measurements derived by spatially varying classification of MRI of normal aging (NA) and Alzheimer's disease (AD) subjects, and then show the white matter spectra of these and MS patients.

Figure 2 illustrates the differences between tissue volumes measured for normal aging and AD subjects. The AD subjects have lower relative white matter volume and higher relative lesion and CSF volumes than NA subjects and this effect is particularly pronounced with increasing age. The relationship of normal and abnormal white matter volume to ICC volume qualitatively reproduces that of an earlier study [1] which was carried out with a different image processing method, and so acts as a validation of the spatially varying classification technique used here.

Figure 3(a) shows the mean white matter spectrum computed from our databases of normal aging scans and AD scans, and the differences between these spectra in the region above the midpoint between healthy and diseased white matter (f = 0.5). Figure 3(b) shows the mean white matter spectrum of the normal aging subjects, the mean white matter spectrum derived from 996 scans of 46 MS patients, and the difference between these spectra in the region above the midpoint between healthy and diseased white matter (f = 0.5).

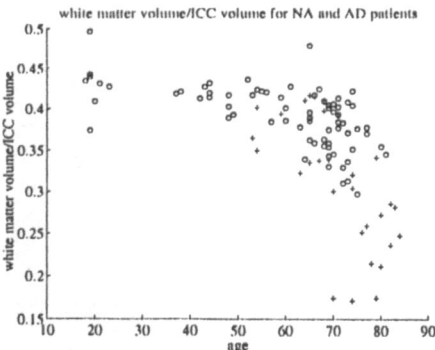

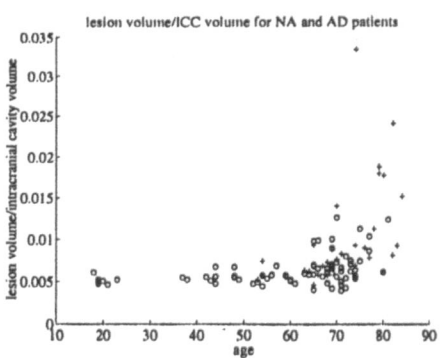

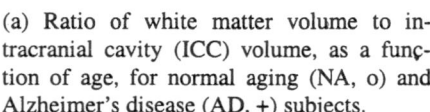

(a) Ratio of white matter volume to intracranial cavity (ICC) volume, as a function of age, for normal aging (NA, o) and Alzheimer's disease (AD, +) subjects.

(b) Ratio of abnormal white matter volume to intrancranial cavity volume, as a function of age, for normal aging (NA, o) and Alzheimer's disease (AD, +) subjects.

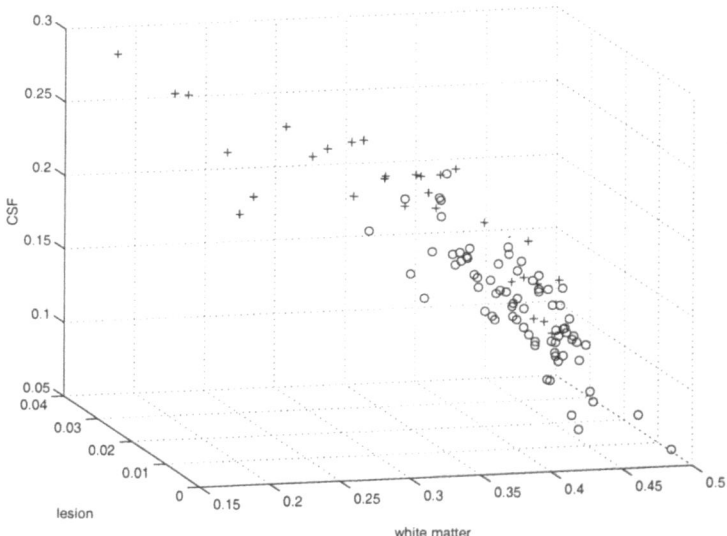

(c) Scatter plot of white matter, lesion and CSF tissue volume to ICC volume ratios for AD (+) and NA (o) subjects.

Fig. 2. Tissue volumes determined with spatially varying classification for normal aging and Alzheimer's disease subjects. The relationship of normal and abnormal white matter volume to ICC volume as a function of age qualitatively reproduces that of an earlier study carried out with a different image processing technique, and so acts as a validation of the spatially varying classification technique. It appears to be possible to distinguish many of the AD subjects from the NA subjects on the basis of the CSF/ICC, abnormal white matter/ICC and normal white matter/ICC ratios.

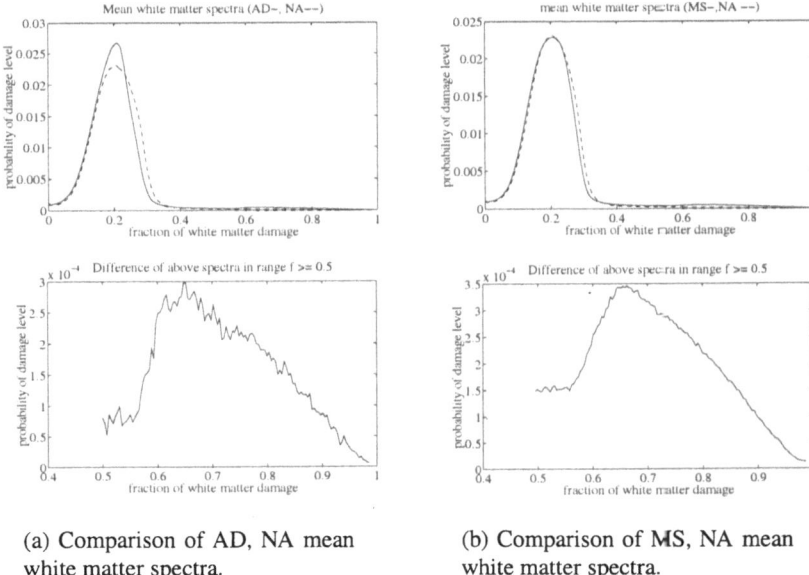

(a) Comparison of AD, NA mean
white matter spectra.

(b) Comparison of MS, NA mean
white matter spectra.

Fig. 3. Fractional segmentation of the white matter region from normal aging, Alzheimer's disease volunteers and multiple sclerosis patients was carried out. The mean white matter spectrum was calculated by averaging the normalized fractional segmentation histogram of each subject. The difference of the mean spectra is shown in detail for the damage level above 0.5. The nonzero differences raise the possibility that the white matter spectrum is indicative of different disease states.

For comparison with the fractional segmentation distributions, Figure 4 shows normalized histograms of the T2w intensity of the white matter and gray matter regions. The figure also shows the intensity distributions both before and after intensity normalization. Intensity normalization is achieved with the EM segmentation algorithm, which is a nonlinear, locally adaptive process. This figure shows that the intensity normalization process corrects for scanner and patient intensity variability, since the T2w distributions after intensity correction are quite similar. Note that while intensity normalization is necessary in order to derive the fractional segmentation and to allow comparison of intensities from different subjects, it does not distinguish between artifactual intensity inhomogeneity and disease related intensity inhomogeneity, so that, for example, if the T2w intensity of a disease process was uniformly brighter than a normal subject this difference would not be identified after intensity normalization. Although this does not appear to be a difficulty in practice, it is possible to consider intensity normalization schemes that attempt to separately identify artifactual intensity variations and intrinsic disease related intensity variations.

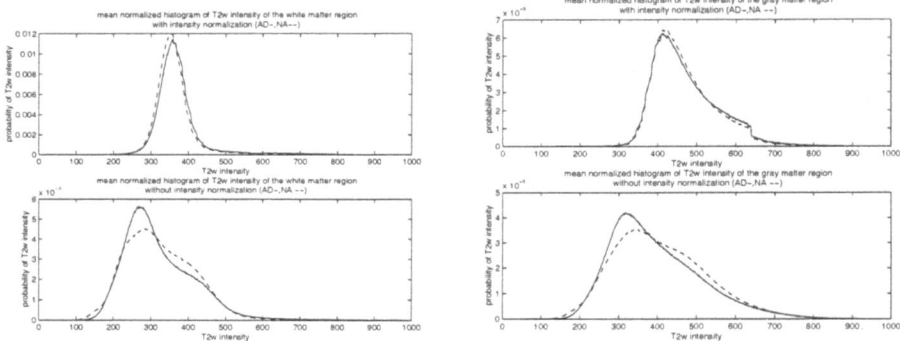

Fig. 4. This figure illustrates white matter and gray matter T2w MRI intensity distributions from the regions of white matter and gray matter of normal aging and Alzheimer's disease volunteers. This figure allows comparison of the T2w intensity distribution both before and after intensity normalization.

4   Discussion

The fractional segmentation of the white matter is a new descriptive mechanism for characterizing white matter change. It allows the visualization and quantification of both focal white matter lesions and diffuse white matter abnormality. Unlike binary classification, fractional segmentation preserves the inhomogeneity observed in the white matter. The fractional segmentation allows the construction of a white matter spectrum for each subject and for groups of subjects. Further analysis is necessary to determine if different diseases give rise to characteristic white matter spectra.

Tissue volumes determined by template moderated spatially varying classification indicate that a loss of normal white matter and an increase in CSF and abnormal white matter is characteristic of Alzheimer's disease. The relationship between age, CSF volume, and normal and abnormal white matter volume determined with this method (Figure 2) qualitatively reproduces earlier results [1]. This indicates that localization of the white matter region with spatially varying classification is a reasonable initial step prior to the computation of the fractional segmentation of this region.

We are currently investigating methods for differentiating between normal aging and Alzheimer's disease, and for identifying different sub-types of multiple sclerosis based on an analysis of the white matter spectra.

Acknowledgements

This investigation was supported (in part) by a grant from the National Multiple Sclerosis Society (SW) and by NIH grants P41 RR13218-01, R01 RR11747-01A, P01 CA67165-03 and P01 AG04953-14.

References

1. C. R. G. Guttmann, F. A. Jolesz, Ron Kikinis, R. J. Killiany, M. B. Moss, T. Sandor, and M. S. Albert, "White matter changes with normal aging", *Neurology*, vol. 50, pp. 972–978, 1998.

2. Robert I. Grossman and Joesph C. McGowan, "Perspectives on Multiple Sclerosis", *American Journal of Neuroradiology*, vol. 19, pp. 1251–1265, August 1998.

3. Hwan Soo Choi, David R. Haynor, and Yongmin Kim, "Partial Volume Tissue Classification of Multichannel Magnetic Resonance Images — A Mixel Model", *IEEE Transactions On Medical Imaging*, vol. 10, no. 3, pp. 395–407, 1991.

4. David C. Bonar, Kirt A. Schaper, Jon R. Anderson, David A. Rottenberg, and Stephen C. Strother, "Graphical Analysis of MR Feature Space for Measurement of CSF, Gray-Matter, and White-Matter Volumes", *Journal of Computer Assisted Tomography*, vol. 17, no. 3, pp. 461–470, 1993.

5. Yi-Hsuan Kao, James A. Sorenson, Mark M. Bahn, and Stefan S. Winkler, "Dual-Echo MRI Segmentation Using Vector Decomposition and Probability Techniques: A Two-Tissue Model", *Magnetic Resonance in Medicine*, vol. 32, no. 3, pp. 342–357, September 1994.

6. H. Donald Gage, Peter Santago, and Wesley E. Snyder, "Quantification of Brain Tissue Through Incorporation of Partial Volume Effects", in *SPIE Medical Imaging VI: Image Processing*, 1992, vol. 1652, pp. 84–96.

7. J. Ross Mitchell, Craig Jones, Stephen J. Karlik, Karen Kennedy, Donald H. Lee, Brian Rutt, and Aaron Fenster, "MR Multispectral Analysis of Multiple Sclerosis Lesions", *JMRI*, vol. 7, pp. 499–511, May/June 1997.

8. Charles R. G. Guttmann, Sungkee S. Ahn, Liangge Hsu, Ron Kikinis, and Ferenc A. Jolesz, "The Evolution of Multiple Sclerosis Lesions on Serial MR.", *AJNR*, vol. 16, pp. 1481–1491, 1995.

9. M. Filippi, M. A. Horsfield, P. S. Tofts, F. Barkhof, A. J. Thompson, and D. H. Miller, "Quantitative assessment of MRI lesion load in monitoring the evolution of multiple sclerosis", *Brain*, vol. 118, pp. 1601–1612, 1995.

10. W. M. Wells, R Kikinis, W. E. L. Grimson, and F. Jolesz, "Adaptive segmentation of MRI data", *IEEE Transactions On Medical Imaging*, vol. 15, pp. 429–442, 1996.

11. Ron Kikinis, Martha E Shenton, Guido Gerig, John Martin, Mark Anderson, David Metcalf, Charles R G Guttmann, Robert W McCarley, William E Lorenson, Harvey Cline, and Ferenc Jolesz, "Routine Quantitative Analysis of Brain and Cerebrospinal Fluid Spaces with MR Imaging", *Journal of Magnetic Resonance Imaging*, vol. 2, pp. 619–629, 1992.

12. Simon K. Warfield, Ferenc Jolesz, and Ron Kikinis, "A High Performance Computing Approach to the Registration of Medical Imaging Data", *Parallel Computing*, vol. 24, no. 9–10, pp. 1345–1368, September 1998.

13. Simon K. Warfield, Andre Robatino, Joachim Dengler, Ferenc A. Jolesz, and Ron Kikinis, *Nonlinear Registration and Template Driven Segmentation*, chapter 4, pp. 67–84, Progressive Publishing Alternatives, 1998.

14. Simon K. Warfield, Michael Kaus, Ferenc A. Jolesz, and Ron Kikinis, "Adaptive Template Moderated Spatially Varying Statistical Classification", in *MICCAI 98: First International Conference on Medical Image Computing and Computer-Assisted Intervention*. October 11–13 1998, pp. 231–238, Springer Verlag.

15. Simon Warfield, Joachim Dengler, Joachim Zaers, Charles R.G. Guttmann, William M. Wells III, Gil J. Ettinger, John Hiller, and Ron Kikinis, "Automatic identification of Grey Matter Structures from MRI to Improve the Segmentation of White Matter Lesions", *Journal of Image Guided Surgery*, vol. 1, no. 6, pp. 326–338, 1995.

16. Dan V. Iosifescu, Martha E. Shenton, Simon K. Warfield, Ron Kikinis, Joachim Dengler, Ferenc A. Jolesz, and Robert W. McCarley, "An Automated Registration Algorithm for Measuring MRI Subcortical Brain Structures", *NeuroImage*, vol. 6, pp 12–25, 1997.

A Modified Fuzzy C-Means Algorithm for MRI Bias Field Estimation and Adaptive Segmentation

M. N. Ahmed, S. M. Yamany, N. A. Mohamed, and A. A. Farag

Computer Vision and Image Processing Lab
Univ. of Louisville, E.E. Dept., Louisville, KY 40292 USA

Abstract. In this paper, we present a novel algorithm for adaptive fuzzy segmentation of MRI data and estimation of intensity inhomogeneities using fuzzy logic. MRI intensity inhomogeneities can be attributed to imperfections in the RF coils or some problems associated with the acquisition sequences. The result is a slowly-varying shading artifact over the image that can produce errors with conventional intensity-based classification. Our algorithm is formulated by modifying the objective function of the standard fuzzy c-means (FCM) algorithm to compensate for such inhomogeneities and to allow the labeling of a pixel (voxel) to be influenced by the labels in its immediate neighborhood. The neighborhood effect acts as a regularizer and biases the solution towards piecewise-homogeneous labeling. Such a regularization is useful in segmenting scans corrupted by salt and pepper noise. Experimental results on both synthetic images and MR data are given to demonstrate the effectiveness and efficiency of the proposed algorithm.

1 Introduction

Spatial intensity inhomogeneity induced by the radio frequency (RF) coil in magnetic resonance imaging (MRI) is a major problem in the computer analysis of MRI data. Such inhomogeneities have rendered conventional intensity-based classification of MR images very difficult, even with advanced techniques such as non-parametric, multichannel methods.[1, 2]. This is due to the fact that the intensity inhomogeneities appearing in MR images produce spatial changes in tissue statistics, i.e. mean and variance. In addition, the degradation on the images obstructs the physician's diagnoses because the physician has to ignore the inhomogeneity artifact in the corrupted images [3].

The removal of the spatial intensity inhomogeneity from MR images is difficult because the inhomogeneities could change with different MRI acquisition parameters from patient to patient and from slice to slice. Therefore, the correction of intensity inhomogeneities is usually required for each new image. In the last decade, a number of algorithms have been proposed for the intensity inhomogeneity correction. Meyer et al.[5] presented an edge-based segmentation scheme to find uniform regions in the image followed by a polynomial surface fit to those regions. The result of their correction is, however, very dependent on the quality of the segmentation step.

Several authors have reported methods based on the use of phantoms for intensity calibration. Wicks et al.[4] proposed methods based on the signal produced by a uniform phantom to correct for MRI images of any orientation. Similarly, Tincher et al.[6] modeled the inhomogeneity function by a second-order polynomial and fitted it to a uniform phantom-scanned MR image. These phantom approaches, however, have the drawback that the geometry relationship of the coils and the image data is typically not available with the image data. They also require the same acquisition parameters for the phantom scan and the patient. In addition, these approaches assume the intensity corruption effects are the same for different patients, an assumption which is not valid, in general [3].

The homomorphic filtering approach to remove the multiplicative effect of the inhomogeneity has been commonly used because of its easy and efficient implementation [2]. This method, however, is effective only on images with relatively low contrast. Some researchers [6, 7] reported undesirable artifacts.

Dawant et al.[7] used operator-selected reference points in the image to guide the construction of a thin-plate spline correction surface. The performance of this method substantially depends on the labeling of the reference points. Considerable user interactions are usually required to obtain good correction results. More recently, Gilles et al.[8] proposed an automatic and iterative B-spline fitting algorithm for the intensity inhomogeneity correction of breast MR images. The application of this algorithm is restricted to MR images with a single dominant tissue class, such as the breast MR images. Another polynomial surface fitting method [9] was proposed based on the assumption that the number of tissue classes, the true means, and standard deviations of all the tissue classes in the image are given. Unfortunately, the required statistical information is usually not available.

A different approach to segment images with intensity inhomogeneities is to simultaneously compensate for the shading effect while segmenting the image. This has the advantage of being able to use intermediate information from the segmentation while performing the correction. Recently, Wells et al.[1] developed a new statistical approach based on the EM algorithm to solve the bias field correction problem and the tissue classification problem altogether in an alternative fashion. Guillemaud and Brady [10] further refined this technique by introducing an extra class, "other". There are two main disadvantages of this EM approach. First, the the EM algorithm is extremely computationally intensive, especially for large problems. Second, the EM algorithm requires a good initial guess for either the bias field or for the classification estimate. Otherwise, the EM algorithm could be easily trapped in a local minimum, resulting in an unsatisfactory solution [3]. Xu et al.[11] followed Wells' approach and proposed a new adaptive fuzzy c-means technique to produce fuzzy segmentation while compensating for intensity inhomogeneities. Their method, however, is computationally intensive and is also very sensitive to noise.

In this paper, we present a different approach for adaptive fuzzy segmentation of MRI data. Our algorithm is formulated by modifying the objective function of the standard fuzzy c-means (FCM) algorithm to compensate for such inhomogeneities and to allow the labeling of a pixel (voxel) to be influenced by the labels in its immediate neighborhood. Taking into account the neighborhood effect acts as a regularizer and biases the solution towards piecewise-homogeneous labeling. Such a regularization is useful in segmenting scans corrupted by salt and pepper noise.

2   Background

The observed MRI signal is modeled as a product of the true signal generated by the underlying anatomy, and a spatially-varying factor called the gain field.

$$Y_k = X_k G_k \qquad \forall k \in \{1, 2, .., N\} \tag{1}$$

where X_k and Y_k are the corrected and observed intensities at the kth voxel, respectively, G_k is the gain field at the kth voxel, and N is the total number of voxels in the MRI volume. The application of a logarithmic transformation to the intensities allows the artifact to be modeled as an additive bias field [1]

$$y_k = x_k + \beta_k \qquad \forall k \in \{1, 2, .., N\} \tag{2}$$

where x_k and y_k are the corrected and observed log-transformed intensities at the kth voxel, respectively, and β_k is the bias field at the kth voxel. If the gain field is known, then it is relatively easy to estimate the tissue class by applying a conventional intensity-based segmentation to the corrected data. Similarly, if the tissue classes are known, then we can estimate the gain field. It may be problematic to estimate either without the knowledge of the other. We will show that by employing an iterative algorithm based on fuzzy logic, we can estimate both.

3   Modified Fuzzy C-means (MFCM) Objective Function

The standard FCM objective function for partitioning $\{x_k\}_{k=1}^N$ into c clusters is given by

$$J = \sum_{i=1}^{c} \sum_{k=1}^{N} u_{ik}^p \|x_k - v_i\|^2 \tag{3}$$

where $\{v_i\}_{i=1}^c$ are the prototypes of the clusters and the array $[u_{ik}] = U$ represents a partition matrix, $U \in \mathcal{U}$, namely

$$\mathcal{U}\{ u_{ik} \in [0, 1] \mid \sum_{i=1}^{c} u_{ik} = 1 \ \forall k \qquad and \qquad 0 < \sum_{k=1}^{N} u_{ik} < N \ \forall i\} \tag{4}$$

The parameter p is a weighting exponent on each fuzzy membership and determines the amount of fuzziness of the resulting classification. The FCM objective function is minimized when high membership values are assigned to voxels whose intensities are close to the centroid of its particular class, and low membership values are assigned when the voxel data is far from the centroid. We propose to modify Eq.(3) by introducing a term that allow the labeling of a pixel (voxel) to be influenced by the labels in its immediate neighborhood. As mentioned before, the neighborhood effect acts as a regularizer and biases the solution towards piecewise-homogeneous labeling. Such a regularization is useful in segmenting scans corrupted by salt and pepper noise. The modified objective function is given by

$$J_m = \sum_{i=1}^{c} \sum_{k=1}^{N} u_{ik}^p \|x_k - v_i\|^2 + \frac{\alpha}{N_R} \sum_{i=1}^{c} \sum_{k=1}^{N} u_{ik}^p \left(\sum_{x_r \in \mathcal{N}_k} \|x_r - v_i\|^2 \right) \quad (5)$$

where $\mathcal{N}_k$ stands for the set of neighbors of x_k and N_R is the cardinality of $\mathcal{N}_k$. The neighbors effect term is controlled by the parameter α. The relative importance of the regularizing term is inversely proportional to the signal to noise ratio (SNR) of MRI signal. Lower SNR would require higher value of the parameter α. Substituting Eq.(2) into Eq.(5), we have

$$J_m = \sum_{i=1}^{c} \sum_{k=1}^{N} u_{ik}^p \|y_k - \beta_k - v_i\|^2 + \frac{\alpha}{N_R} \sum_{i=1}^{c} \sum_{k=1}^{N} u_{ik}^p \left(\sum_{y_r \in \mathcal{N}_k} \|y_r - \beta_r - v_i\|^2 \right) \quad (6)$$

Formally, the optimization problem becomes

$$\min_{U,\ \{v_i\}_{i=1}^c,\ \{\beta_k\}_{k=1}^N} J_m \quad subject\ to \quad U \in \mathcal{U} \quad (7)$$

4   Parameter Estimation

The objective function J_m can be minimized in a fashion similar to the standard FCM algorithm. Taking the first derivatives of J_m with respect to u_{ik}, v_i, and β_k and setting them to zero results in three conditions for J_m to be at a minimum. In the following subsections, we will derive these three conditions.

4.1   Membership Evaluation

The constrained optimization in equation (7) will be solved using Lagrange multipliers

$$J_m = \sum_{i=1}^{c} \sum_{k=1}^{N} \left(u_{ik}^p D_{ik} + \frac{\alpha}{N_R} u_{ik}^p \gamma_i \right) + \lambda (1 - \sum_{i=1}^{c} u_{ik}) \quad (8)$$

where $D_{ik} = ||y_k - \beta_k - v_i||^2$ and $\gamma_i = \left(\sum_{y_r \in \mathcal{N}_k} ||y_r - \beta_r - v_i||^2 \right)$. Taking the derivative of J_m w.r.t. u_{ik} and setting the result to zero, we have

$$\left[\frac{\delta J_m}{\delta u_{ik}} = p u_{ik}^{p-1} D_{ik} + \frac{\alpha p}{N_R} u_{ik}^p \gamma_i - \lambda \right]_{u_{ik} = u_{ik}^*} = 0 \qquad (9)$$

Solving for u_{ik} we have

$$u_{ik}^* = \left(\frac{\lambda}{p(D_{ik} + \frac{\alpha}{N_R} \gamma_i)} \right)^{\frac{1}{p-1}} \qquad (10)$$

Since $\sum_{j=1}^c u_{jk} = 1 \quad \forall k$, then

$$\sum_{j=1}^c \left(\frac{\lambda}{p(D_{jk} + \frac{\alpha}{N_R} \gamma_j)} \right)^{\frac{1}{p-1}} = 1 \qquad (11)$$

or

$$\lambda = \frac{p}{\left(\sum_{j=1}^c \left(\frac{1}{(D_{jk} + \frac{\alpha}{N_R} \gamma_j)} \right)^{\frac{1}{p-1}} \right)^{p-1}} \qquad (12)$$

Substituting into equation (10), the zero-gradient condition for the membership estimator can be rewritten as,

$$u_{ik}^* = \frac{1}{\sum_{j=1}^c \left(\frac{D_{ik} + \frac{\alpha}{N_R} \gamma_i}{D_{jk} + \frac{\alpha}{N_R} \gamma_j} \right)^{\frac{1}{p-1}}} \qquad (13)$$

4.2   Cluster Prototype Updating

In the following derivation we use the standard Eucledian distance. Taking the derivative of J_m w.r.t. v_i and setting the result to zero we have;

$$\left[\sum_{k=1}^N u_{ik}^p (y_k - \beta_k - v_i) + \sum_{k=1}^N u_{ik}^p \frac{\alpha}{N_R} \sum_{y_r \in \mathcal{N}_k} (y_r - \beta_r - v_i) \right]_{v_i = v_i^*} = 0 \qquad (14)$$

Solving for v_i we have;

$$v_i^* = \frac{\sum_{k=1}^N u_{ik}^p \left((y_k - \beta_k) + \frac{\alpha}{N_R} \sum_{y_r \in \mathcal{N}_k} (y_r - \beta_r) \right)}{(1 + \alpha) \sum_{k=1}^N u_{ik}^p} \qquad (15)$$

4.3   Bias Field Estimation

In a similar fashion, taking the derivative of J_m w.r.t β_k and setting the result to zero we have

$$\left[\sum_{i=1}^{c} \frac{\partial}{\partial \beta_k} \sum_{k=1}^{N} u_{ik}^p (y_k - \beta_k - v_i)^2 \right]_{\beta_k = \beta_k^*} = 0 \qquad (16)$$

Since only the kth term in the second summation depends on β_k, we have

$$\left[\sum_{i=1}^{c} \frac{\partial}{\partial \beta_k} u_{ik}^p (y_k - \beta_k - v_i)^2 \right]_{\beta_k = \beta_k^*} = 0 \qquad (17)$$

Differentiating the distance expression, we obtain

$$\left[y_k \sum_{i=1}^{c} u_{ik}^p - \beta_k \sum_{i=1}^{c} u_{ik}^p - \sum_{i=1}^{c} u_{ik}^p v_i \right]_{\beta_k = \beta_k^*} = 0 \qquad (18)$$

Thus, the zero-gradient condition for the bias field estimator is expressed as

$$\beta_k^* = y_k - \frac{\sum_{i=1}^{c} u_{ik}^p v_i}{\sum_{i=1}^{c} u_{ik}^p} \qquad (19)$$

5   MFCM Algorithm

The MFCM algorithm for correcting the bias field and segmenting the image into different clusters can be summarized in the following steps:

Step 1 Select initial class prototypes $\{v_i\}_{i=1}^{c}$. Set $\{\beta_k\}_{k=1}^{N}$ to zero.

Step 2 Update the partition matrix using eq.13

Step 3 The prototypes of the clusters are obtained in the form of weighted averages of the patterns using Eq.15.

Step 4 Estimate the bias term using Eq.19.

Repeat steps 2-4 until convergence.

6   Results

In this section we describe the application of the adaptive segmentation on synthetic images corrupted with multiplicative gain and on brain MR images. All of the MR images shown in this section were obtained using a General Electric Signa 1.5 Tesla clinical MR imager. Results show that intensity variations across patients, scans, and equipment changes have been accommodated in the estimated bias field without the need for manual intervention. We implemented the MFCM algorithm on a Silicon Graphics Onyx Supercomputer. In all the examples, we set the parameter α (the neighbors effect) to be 0 7. Figure 1 shows

Fig. 1. Results of the MFCM on a two-class synthetic image corrupted by sinusoidal bias field. The original image is shown (left). The (Middle) presents the final results of the bias field and (right) the segmentation.

a synthetic test image. This image contains a two-class pattern corrupted by a sinusoidal gain field of higher spatial frequency. The test image is intended to represent two tissue classes, while the sinusoid represents an intensity inhomogeneity. This model was constructed so that it would be difficult to correct using homomorphic filtering or traditional FCM approaches. As shown in Figure 1, the MFCM has succeeded in correcting and classifying the data.

Figure 2 shows the results of applying the MFCM algorithm to segment an image of an axial-sectioned T1 MR brain. Strong inhomogeneities are apparent in the image. The MFCM algorithm segmented the image into three classes corresponding to background, gray matter, and white matter. The figure illustrates intensity profiles in the image before and after correction. These profiles correspond to the 128th column extract from the original bias field corrupted image and the corrected one using the MFCM algorithm. The figure demonstrates the ability of the MFCM algorithm to correct for the bias field. Figure 3 shows another example of T2 MR image where the MFCM was successful in recovering the bias field and segmenting the image. Figure 4 shows the results of applying the MFCM for the segmentation of a noisy brain image. The results of using the traditional FCM without considering the neighborhood field effect and the MFCM are presented. Notice that the segmentation of the MFCM, which uses the the neighborhood field effect, is much less fragmented compared to the traditional FCM approach. As mentioned before, the relative importance of the regularizing term is inversely proportional to the signal to noise ratio (SNR) of MRI signal. We compared our results with the Expectation-Maximization (EM) algorithm developed by Wells et al.[1]. The MFCM algorithm produces similar results as the EM algorithm with faster convergence and the added advantage that it requires no user interaction. Correct estimates of region statistics are crucial for the convergence of the EM algorithm while in the MFCM, approximate values for class centers are sufficient. In noisy images, the MFCM technique greatly outperforms the EM algorithm as it compensates for noise by including a regularization term. While only 2D results were presented in this summary, the MFCM can be easily extended to 3D segmentation and bias field correction.

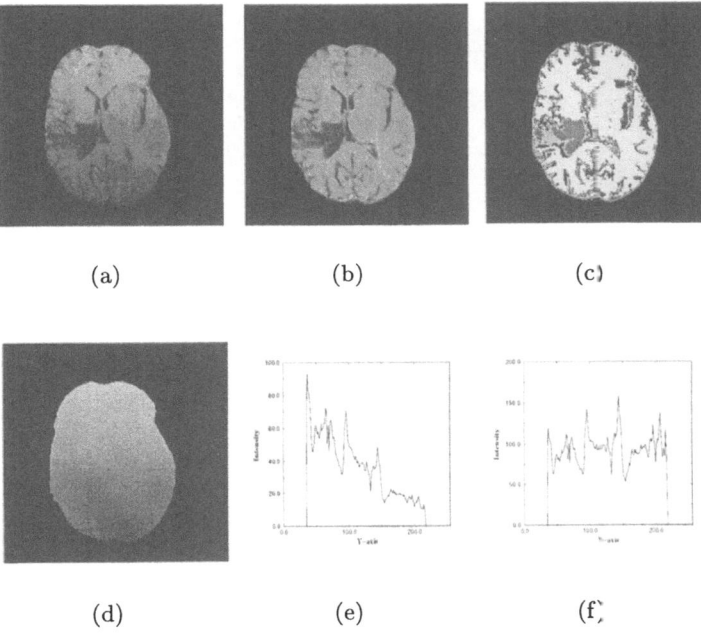

(a)   (b)   (c)

(d)   (e)   (f)

Fig. 2. Brain MRI example: (a) the original MR image corrupted with intensity in-homogeneities (b) the bias-field corrected image using the proposed algorithm. The segmented image is shown in (c) while the recovered bias field is displayed in (d). The cross section at the 128th column extract from (e) the original bias field corrupted image and (f) the corrected image using the MFCM algorithm. Intensity uniformity is clearly noticed in (f).

7   Conclusions

We have demonstrated a new modified fuzzy c-means (MFCM) algorithm for adaptive segmentation and intensity correction of MR images. The algorithm was formulated by modifying the objective function of the standard fuzzy c-means (FCM) algorithm to compensate for such inhomogeneities and to allow the labeling of a pixel (voxel) to be influenced by the labels in its immediate neighborhood. Taking into account the neighborhood effect acts as a regularizer and biases the solution towards piecewise-homogeneous labeling. Such a regu-larization is useful in segmenting scans corrupted by salt and pepper noise. The MFCM segmentation increases the robustness and level of automation available for the segmentation of MR images into tissue classes by correcting interscan intensity inhomogeneities. Via improved segmentation, this algorithm leads to an improvement in the quality of 3D reconstruction of brain structures, and for visualization, surgical planning, disease research, and for other purposes.

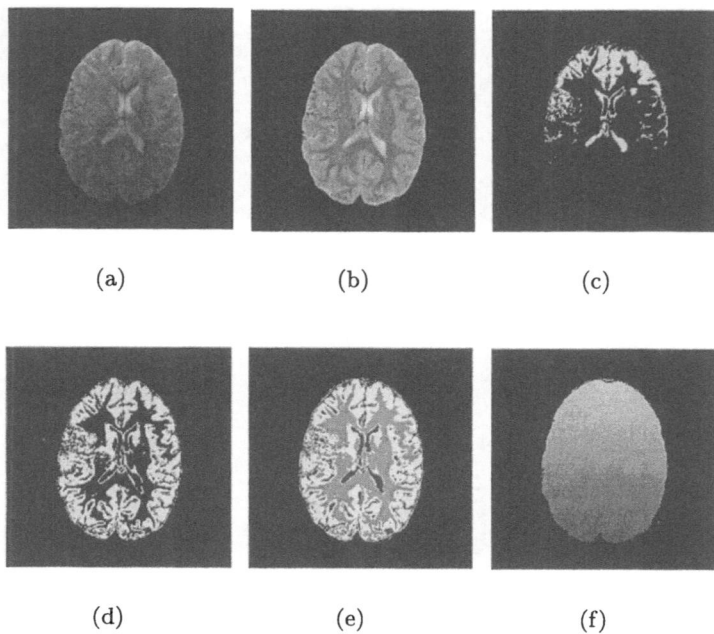

(a)   (b)   (c)

(d)   (e)   (f)

Fig. 3. Brain MRI example: (a) the original MR image corrupted with intensity inhomogeneities (b) the bias-field corrected image using the proposed MFCM algorithm. (c) Gray matter membership using traditional FCM. (d) Gray matter membership using MFCM. The segmented image using MFCM is shown in (e) while the recovered bias field is displayed in (f).

References

1. W.M. Wells, III, W.E.L. Grimson, R. Kikinis and F.A. Jolesz "Adaptive segmentation of MRI data," *IEEE Trans. Med. Imag.*, Vol. 15, pp. 429-442, 1996.

2. B. Johnston, M.S. Atkins, B. Mackiewich and M. Anderson, "Segmentation of multiple sclerosis lesions in intensity corrected multispectral MRI," *IEEE Trans. Medical Imaging*, Vol. 15, No.2, pp. 154-169, 1996.

3. S. Lai and M. Fang, "A new variational shape-from-orientation approach to correcting intensity inhomogeneities in MR images," *Workshop on Biomedical Image Analysis, CVPR98*, pp. 56-63, Sanata Barbara, California, 1998.

4. D.A.G. Wicks, G.J. Barker and P.S. Tofts, "Correction of intensity nonuniformity in MR images of any orientation," *Magnetic Resonance Imaging*, Vol. 11, pp. 183-196, 1993.

5. C.R. Meyer, P.H. Bland and J. Pipe, "Retrospective correction of intensity inhomogeneities in MRI," *IEEE Trans. Medical Imaging*, Vol. 14, No. 1, pp. 36-41, 1995.

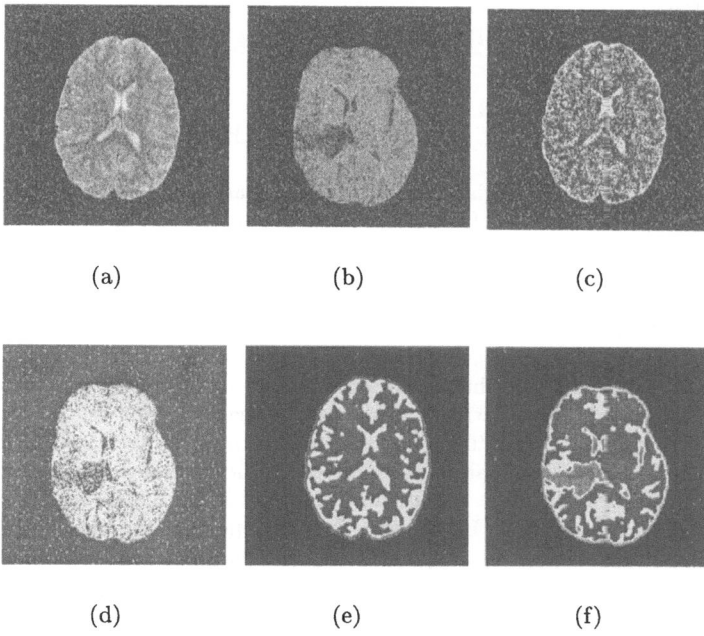

(a)   (b)   (c)

(d)   (e)   (f)

Fig. 4. Brain Tumor MRI examples corrupted with noise: The original MR images corrupted with salt and pepper noise are shown in (a) and (b). The segmented images using MFCM without any neighborhood consideration, are presented in (c) and (d). The segmented images using MFCM and neighborhood effect are presented in (e) and (f). See the text for a discussion on the results.

6. M. Tincher, C.R. Meyer, R. Gupta and D.M. Williams, "Polynomial modeling and reduction of RF body coil spatial inhomogeneity in MRI," *IEEE Trans. Medical Imaging*, Vol. 12, No. 2, pp. 361-365, 1993.
7. B. Dawant, A. Zijidenbos, and R Margolin "Correction of intensity variations in MR images for computer-aided tissue classification," *IEEE Trans. Med. Imag.*, Vol. 12, pp. 770-781 1993.
8. S. Gilles, M.Brady, J. Declerck, J.P. Thirion and N. Ayache, "Bias field correction of breast MR images," *Proceedings of the Fourth International Conf. on Visualization in Biomedical Computing*, pp. 153-158, Hamburg, Germany, Sep. 1996.
9. C. Brechbuhler, G. Gerig and G. Szekely, "Compensation of spatial inhomogeneity in MRI based on a parametric bias estimate," *Proceedings of the Fourth International Conference on Visualization in Biomedical Computing*, pp. 141,146, Hamburg, Germany, Sep. 1996.
10. R. Guillemaud and M. Brady, "Estimating the bias field of MR images," *IEEE Trans. Medical Imaging*, Vol. 16, No. 3, pp. 238-251, 1997.
11. C. Xu, D. Pham, and Jerry Prince "Finding the brain cortex using fuzzy segmentation, isosurfaces, and deformable surfaces," *Pro. of the XVth Int. Conf. on Information Processing in Medical Imaging (IPMI 97).*, pp. 399-404, 1997.

Statistical 3D Vessel Segmentation Using a Rician Distribution

Albert C. S. Chung and J. Alison Noble

Department of Engineering Science, Oxford University, Oxford, OX1 3PJ.
Email : {albert,noble}@robots.ox.ac.uk

Abstract. This paper presents an extended version of the fully automated 3D cerebral vessel reconstruction algorithm developed by Wilson
and Noble [11] which is applicable to time-of-flight (TOF) and phase
contrast (PC) magnetic resonance angiography (MRA) images. We introduce a Rician distribution for background noise modelling and use a
modified EM (Expectation-Maximization) algorithm for the parameter
estimation procedure. The proposed algorithm is applied to PC-MRA
images. It is shown that the estimated Rician distribution gives a better quality-of-fit to the observed background noise distribution than a
Gaussian distribution. In the experiments reported, the segmented 3D
vasculature is shown to be qualitatively comparable with the results obtained from higher resolution TOF MRA images.
Keywords : PC/TOF MRA, vessel segmentation, EM algorithm, endovascular treatment of aneurysms, neurology.

1 Introduction

Three dimensional vascular segmentation is an essential prior step for brain
aneurysm charaterization which has been shown, for example, to be extremely
useful for pre-GDC (Guglielmi detachable coil) treatment planning [12]. Pre-
treatment vessel examination is commonly performed using magnetic resonance
angiography (MRA) because the image intensity is flow related and MRA does
not require the use of contrast agent as for example X-ray analysis does. Two
typical and major groups of MRA techniques are phase contrast (PC) and time-
of-flight (TOF). The main advantage of PC-MRA over TOF-MRA is that it not
only gives information about vascular morphology but also provides, additionally, directional-flow images in each orthogonal direction. This work is entirely
driven by the growing need of PC-MRA image segmentation. This paper extends
the fully automated 3D cerebral vessel reconstruction algorithm developed by
Wilson and Noble [11] from TOF-MRA to PC-MRA. PC-MRA is employed for
capturing the flow rate (both magnitude and directions) information spatially
within a region of interest (ROI) at a particular time. Similar to TOF-MRA, the
voxel intensity is flow-encoded [8]. Intensity and flow rate are positively correlated in PC-MRA. However, unlike TOF-MRA, which shows detail anatomical
structures, a PC-MRA image displays two major and high contrast voxel types:
vessel and background. It is common to assume that the background intensities
are Gaussian distributed. However, in this paper, we adopt a Rician distribution
as the statistical representation of the background intensities because, theoretically, the background intensities follow a Rician distribution [4, 1, 9]. The experiments we present show that the Rician distribution gives a better quality-of-fit

than a Gaussian distribution. We present a method for estimating parameters based on modified EM (Expectation-Maximization) algorithm [2]. The proposed algorithm is tested on PC-MRA images and segmentation results are shown.

2 The Algorithm

This section briefly explains the statistical models of each voxel type based on the image formation process and physical characteristics of blood flow. These models are combined additively, and their parameters are estimated via a modified EM algorithm. Segmentation criteria are then described.

2.1 Derivation of the background noise and vessel models

We assume the following **background noise model** to describe the intensity characteristics of the voxels having approximately zero flow rate, i.e. air background or tissues with stationary flow rate. For PC-MRA, the flow-rate of each voxel is encoded separately in three orthogonal directions. The three orthogonal velocity components, v_x, v_y and v_z, are then combined to obtain the flow speed $v = \sqrt{v_x^2 + v_y^2 + v_z^2}$. These velocity components are complex numbers. Each component is computed by the difference between positive and negative gradient Fourier transformed images along the component direction [1,7]. We assume that the real and imaginary parts of these complex components are independently Gaussian distributed with different means μ_k, $k = 1 \ldots 6$, and the same variance σ^2. The probability density function (p.d.f.) of the flow v is then governed by a Rician distribution, which describes the distribution of the square root of the squared-sum of Gaussian random variables. Since the voxel intensity i and flow v are linearly related, the p.d.f. of the background voxel intensity $f_b(i)$ is also Rician distributed and given by,

$$f_b(i) = \frac{i}{\sigma^2} \left(\frac{i}{A} \right)^{\frac{N-2}{N}} e^{\frac{-(i^2 + A^2)}{2\sigma^2}} I_{\frac{N}{2}-1} \left(\frac{iA}{\sigma^2} \right) u(i), \tag{1}$$

where $A^2 = \sum_{k=1}^{N} \mu_k$, I is the modified Bessel function of real order, u is the unit step function and N is the number of independent Gaussian random variables. $N = 6$ for the rest of the paper. A plot of Rician distributions with difference Signal-to-Noise (SNR) ratios $\frac{A}{\sigma} = 0.001, 1, 2 \ldots 5$ and their corresponding skewness measures γ are shown in Figure 1a. It shows that a Rician distribution with small SNR tends to be positively skewed and that with large SNR it is symmetric and approximately Gaussian.

We assume a **vessel model**, in which the intensity characteristics of the vessel voxels are assumed to exhibit a laminar flow pattern. The velocity profile across the circular vessel cross-section is then parabolic [3], as shown in Figure 1b. Hence, the intensity profile is $i = C(1 - \frac{r^2}{R^2})$, where i is the intensity, C is a constant, R is the vessel radius and r is the distance from vessel centre to the boundary. The p.d.f. $f_v(i)$ for a vessel voxel that has intensity i is directly proportional to the area $a(x = i)$. $f_v(i)$ is calculated as the rate-of-change of area having intensity greater than or equal to i, i.e. $f_v(i) \propto |\frac{da(x \geq i)}{di}|$. The area $a(x \geq i)$ is given by $\pi R^2 (1 - \frac{i}{C})$. Therefore, the p.d.f. f_v is constant and can be

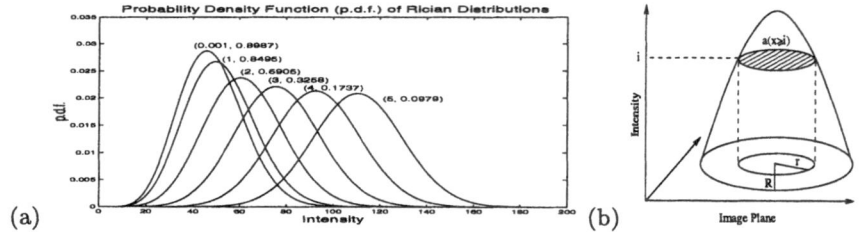

(a) (b)

Fig. 1. *(a) A plot of Rician distributions with different SNR and their corresponding skewness measures $(\frac{A}{\sigma}, \gamma)$. This shows that a Rician distribution with small SNR tends to be positively skewed and that with large SNR it is symmetric and approximately Gaussian. (b) A typical laminar flow pattern. $a(x \geq i)$ is the area having intensity x larger than i. The probability that a voxel has intensity equal to i is then given by $\left|\frac{da(x \geq i)}{di}\right|$.*

regarded as a uniform distribution, $f_v(i) = \frac{1}{i_{max}}$, where i_{max} is the maximum intensity in the frequency histogram. Although, in practice, the vessel voxel intensity mainly spreads over the high intensity region the number of vessel voxels is only a small proportion (1%) of the frequency histogram. Hence, for the sake of simplicity, we assume that the uniform distribution spreads over the entire intensity range $(0 \ldots i_{max})$.

The background noise and vessel models can be combined into a mixture model. The modified EM algorithm [2] can be used to estimate the parameters for the mixture $f(i) = w_b f_b(i|b) + w_v f_v(i|v)$, where $f_b(i|b)$ and $f_v(i|v)$ are the conditional probabilities that a voxel has intensity i given that it is a background noise and vessel voxel respectively, and w_b and w_v are the prior probabilities of a background noise and vessel voxel respectively. In other words, w_b and w_v are the weights of the background and vessel models respectively, and $w_b + w_v = 1$. A procedure for estimating the model parameters is outlined in the next subsection.

2.2   Parameter estimation procedure

This subsection concerns parameter estimation of a mixture density. Given a mixture model of a Rician and uniform distributions, there are four unknown parameters: w_b, w_v, A and σ^2 that need to be estimated. The modified EM algorithm is an iterative procedure that can be used to estimate the parameters which maximizes the log-likelihood of the mixture distribution in each iteration [2]. The iterative procedure terminates when the change in log-likelihood or the parameters is sufficiently small.

Let the log-likelihood function be $L = \sum_{i=0}^{i_{max}} h(i) \log f(i)$, where $h(i)$ is the frequency histogram of the observations and $f(i)$ is the mixture p.d.f.. The change in log-likelihood function is given by

$$L^{k+1} - L^k = \sum_{i=0}^{i_{max}} h(i) \log \left(\frac{f^{k+1}(i)}{f^k(i)} \right), \qquad (2)$$

where index k represents the kth iteration step. We aim to maximize the change of log-likelihood $L^{k+1} - L^k$ until the change is sufficiently small. Suppose that, given an intensity i, the posterior probabilities that a voxel belongs to the background noise and vessel are $p(b|i)$ and $p(v|i)$ respectively. Then $p(b|i) = w_b f_b(i|b)/f(i)$. The same applies to $p(v|i)$. Also $p(b|i) + p(v|i) = 1$. Equation (2) can be re-written as

$$L^{k+1} - L^k = \sum_{i=0}^{i_{max}} h(i) \log \left(p^k(b|i) \frac{w_b^{k+1} f_b^{k+1}(i|b)}{f^k(i)p^k(b|i)} + p^k(v|i) \frac{w_v^{k+1} f_v^{k+1}(i|v)}{f^k(i)p^k(v|i)} \right) \quad (3)$$

by expanding $f^{k+1}(i)$ and multiplying $p^k(b|i)$ and $p^k(v|i)$ to both numerator and denominator. By Jensen's inequality, $\log(\lambda_1 x_1 + \lambda_2 x_2) \geq \lambda_1 \log x_1 + \lambda_2 \log x_2$ and $\lambda_1 + \lambda_2 = 1$. Let $\lambda_1 = p^k(b|i)$ and $\lambda_2 = p^k(v|i)$. Then from Equation (3), we have

$$L^{k+1} - L^k \geq \sum_{i=0}^{i_{max}} h(i) \left(p^k(b|i) \log \frac{w_b^{k+1} f_b^{k+1}(i|b)}{f^k(i)p^k(b|i)} + p^k(v|i) \log \frac{w_v^{k+1} f_v^{k+1}(i|v)}{f^k(i)p^k(v|i)} \right) (4)$$

Therefore, maximizing the right-hand-size of the inequality in Equation (4) is equivalent to maximizing the change in log-likelihood until the log-likelihood converges to a stationary point.

Maximization with respect to w_b^{k+1} and w_v^{k+1} : the right-hand-side of Equation (4) can be rearranged to isolate the terms related to w_b^{k+1} and w_v^{k+1}. Let

$$Q_w = \sum_{i=0}^{i_{max}} h(i) \left(p^k(b|i) \log w_b^{k+1} + p^k(v|i) \log w_v^{k+1} \right). \quad (5)$$

Then we need to maximize Q_w under that constrain $w_b^{k+1} + w_v^{k+1} = 1$, i.e. maximize $Q_w + \lambda(1 - w_b^{k+1} - w_v^{k+1})$, where λ is the lagrange multiplier. Setting the derivatives with respect to w_b^{k+1} and w_v^{k+1} to zero gives,

$$\lambda w_b^{k+1} = \sum_{i=0}^{i_{max}} h(i)p^k(b|i) \quad and \quad \lambda w_v^{k+1} = \sum_{i=0}^{i_{max}} h(i)p^k(v|i) \quad (6)$$

Summing Equations (6) gives $\lambda = M$, which M is the total number of voxels. Hence, we obtain

$$w_b^{k+1} = \frac{1}{M} \sum_{i=0}^{i_{max}} h(i)p^k(b|i) \quad and \quad w_v^{k+1} = \frac{1}{M} \sum_{i=0}^{i_{max}} h(i)p^k(v|i). \quad (7)$$

The initial values of w_b^0 and w_v^0 we have used in our experiments are 0.99 and 0.01 respectively.

Maximization with respect to A_{k+1} and σ_{k+1}^2 : the right-hand-side of Equation (4) can be rearranged to isolate the terms related to A_{k+1} and σ_{k+1}^2.

$$Q_{A,\sigma^2} = \sum_{i=0}^{i_{max}} h(i)p^k(b|i) \log f_b^{k+1}(i|b). \quad (8)$$

Setting the derivatives of Q_{A,σ^2} with respect to A_{k+1} and σ_{k+1}^2 to zero gives

$$\frac{\partial Q_{A,\sigma^2}}{\partial A_{k+1}} = 0 \Rightarrow \sum_{i=0}^{i_{max}} h(i)p^k(b|i) \left[\left(1 - \frac{N}{2}\right) \frac{1}{A_{k+1}} - \frac{A_{k+1}}{\sigma_k^2} + \frac{I_v'}{I_v} \frac{i}{\sigma_k^2} \right] = 0, \quad (9)$$

$$\frac{\partial Q_{A,\sigma^2}}{\partial \sigma^2_{k+1}} = 0 \;\Rightarrow\; \sum_{i=0}^{i_{max}} h(i)p^k(b|i) \left[\frac{i^2 + A_k^2 - 2\sigma^2_{k+1}}{2\sigma^4_{k+1}} - \frac{I'_v}{I_v} \frac{iA_k}{\sigma^4_{k+1}} \right] = 0, \quad (10)$$

where $v = \frac{N}{2} - 1$, $I_v = I_v(y)$, $I'_v = \frac{dI_v}{dy}$. For Equation (9), $y = \frac{iA_{k+1}}{\sigma_k^2}$. For Equation (10), $y = \frac{iA_k}{\sigma^2_{k+1}}$.

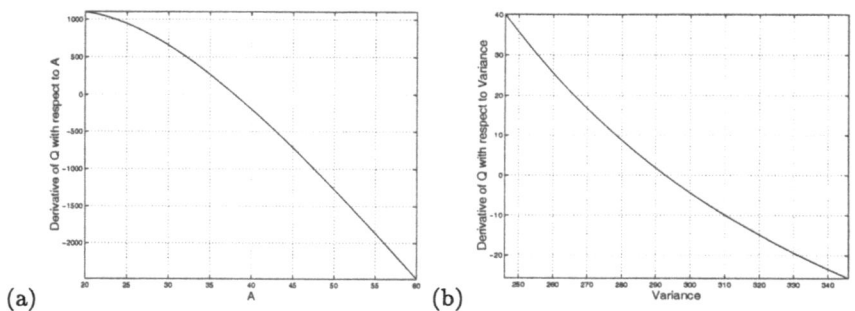

(a)   (b)

Fig. 2. *(a) and (b) show that the curves of derivatives versus A_{k+1} and σ^2_{k+1} are monotonic decreasing, which implies that the curves of Q_{A,σ^2} with varying A_{k+1} and σ^2_{k+1} are convex and have a unique maximum.*

Figures 2a and 2b show that the curves of derivatives of Q_{A,σ^2} with respect to A_{k+1} and σ^2_{k+1} versus A_{k+1} and σ^2_{k+1} are monotonic decreasing, which implies that the curves of Q_{A,σ^2} with varying A_{k+1} and σ^2_{k+1} are convex and have a unique maximum. Hence, the solutions A_{k+1} and σ^2_{k+1} of Equations (9) and (10) will maximize the value of Q_{A,σ^2}. Equations (9) and (10) can be solved numerically to find A_{k+1} and σ^2_{k+1} using, for example, the Newton-Raphson method. As shown in Figures 2a and 2b, both curves are approximately linear for a wide range of A_{k+1} and σ^2_{k+1}. Given the initial guesses of A_k and σ^2_k, the Newton-Raphson method converged after approximately 2 iterations in practice. The initial values of A_0 and σ_0^2 we have used in our experiments are $\sqrt{E[i^2] - N\sigma^2}$ and σ^2 the histogram variance respectively, where $E[i^2]$ is the expected value of i^2. The termination criterion for Newton-Raphson method was found empirically. The termination conditions in the Newton-Raphson method were set to be $|A_{k+1} - A_k| \le 0.1$ and $|\sigma^2_{k+1} - \sigma^2_k| \le 5$. These choices were found to keep the change in Q_{A,σ^2} approximately 0.5% per iteration of the EM algorithm. The EM algorithm applies the same termination criteria and converged after approximately 15 iterations.

2.3   Results

Figure 3a and 3b show a typical EM estimation result when the background voxel intensity f_b is assumed to be Rician and Gaussian respectively. Estimations were performed in each of the 64 slices of a PC-MRA volume. Figure 3c displays the absolute errors of the Rician (solid) and Gaussian (dashed) distributions versus slice number. Absolute error is defined as the absolute difference between the observed and estimated histograms $\sum_{i=0}^{i_{max}} \frac{1}{M} |h_{observed}(i) - h_{estimated}(i)| \times 100\%$.

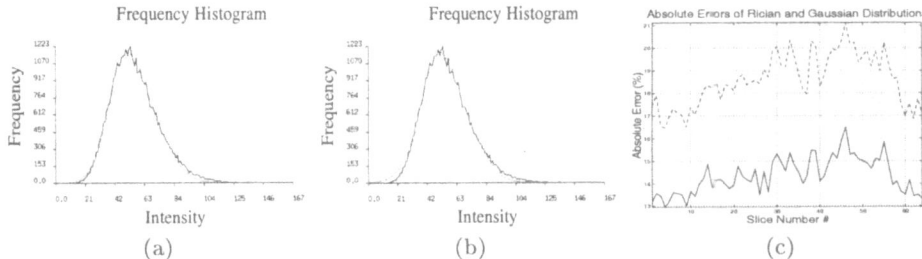

Fig. 3. *(a) and (b) show the estimation results when f_b is assumed to be Rician and Gaussian respectively. The solid line is the observed histogram and the dotted line is the estimated histogram. For 64 slices of a PC MRA volume, (c) shows the absolute errors (%) of the Rician (solid) and Gaussian (dashed) distributions versus the slice number. This shows that the Rician distribution gives a consistent better quality-of-fit for the background noise distribution than a Gaussian distribution*

Note that the Rician distribution consistently gives a better quality-of-fit (about 5%) for the background noise distribution than a Gaussian distribution. This is because of the low signal-to-noise ratio (SNR) of the background. Low SNR magnifies the contributions of Gaussian noise in each orthogonal component to the background signal. Therefore, the background distribution is corrupted from a Gaussian to a Rician distribution. A Gaussian distribution is still a good approximation when the SNR is significantly large ($\frac{A}{\sigma} \geq 3$) [4].

2.4 Segmentation Criteria

Given an estimated mixture model, a volume of PC-MRA can be segmented statistically on the basis of the MAP (Maximum-A-Posterior) criterion, which is conceptually different from the criteria of feature-based methods demanding the extraction of relevant spatial features, e.g. edge, curvature [5, 6] or intensity variance, or velocity coherence among neighbouring voxels [10], as the criteria for vessel segmentation. Using MAP, a voxel is classified as a vessel voxel when the vessel probability $w_v f_v(i|v)$ is greater than the background probability $w_b f_b(i|b)$. Therefore, a threshold i_t can be found by the intersection of the two probability distributions.

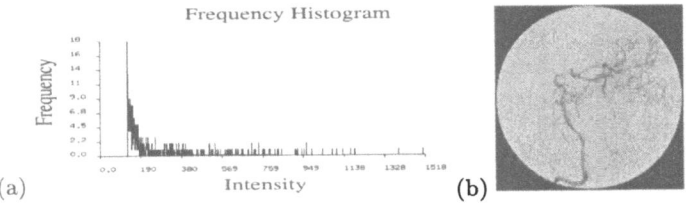

Fig. 4. *(a) shows that the histogram frequency increases as the intensity decreases. This is because the number of relatively slow flow (low intensity) small vessel voxels is greater than that of fast flow large vessel voxels. As shown in (b), which is an X-ray image of the same brain, most of the small subsidiary vessels lead from a single major vessel. The threshold is found by finding the point at the maximum planar curvature. In (a), the maximum curvature is at intensity value 198.*

The threshold i_t cuts the observed histogram into two portions. The high intensity portion describes the intensity distribution of the vessel voxels, as shown in Figure 4a. Note that the high intensity portion of the histogram follows the uniform distribution and is consistent with the vessel model. However, note also that the histogram frequency increases as the intensity decreases. This is because the number of relatively slow-flow (low intensity) small-vessel voxels is greater than that of fast-flow large-vessel voxels. As shown in Figure 4b, most of the small subsidiary vessels lead from the single major vessel. Therefore, when the intensity decreases, the number of voxels increases because of the increase in the number of low-intensity small vessels, which in turn causes an increase in the histogram frequency. This change in frequency can be found by finding the point i_t' at the maximum planar curvature of the smoothed curve. Curvature is defined as $\frac{d^2h(i)}{di^2}/[1 + (\frac{dh(i)}{di})^2]^{\frac{3}{2}}$. In Figure 4a, i_t and i_t' are approximately 120 and 198 respectively.

Figure 5a shows a sub-image from a PC-MRA slice. Figure 5b shows the segmentation results using the threshold i_t'. In this figure voxels with intensity greater than i_t' are labelled white. Figure 5c shows the segmentation results using the threshold i_t. Here voxels with intensity between i_t and i_t' are labelled white; those greater than i_t' labelled grey. This example illustrates that slow-flow small-vessel voxels are now detected and appear adjacent to the fast flow large vessel voxels. This means the estimated size of major vessels is larger without the correction.

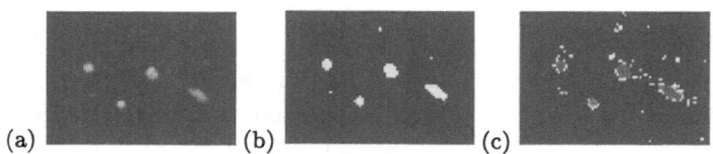

(a)   (b)   (c)

Fig. 5. *(a) shows a sub-image from a PC-MRA slice; (b) shows the segmented image using the corrected threshold I_t'; (c) shows the segmented image using the threshold I_t (found by MAP). Slow flow small vessel voxels are detected and appear adjacent to the fast flow large vessel voxels. This means the size of major vessels is overestimated without the correction.*

3 Results

Intracranial scans (both PC-MRA and TOF-MRA) of a volunteer (without an aneurysm) were performed using a 1.5 T Siemens Magnetom Vision MR scanner at the Radcliffe Infirmary, Oxford. The volume size was 192x256x48 voxels and voxel size 0.82mm x 0.78mm x 1.46mm. The segmentation algorithm was applied to the whole PC-MRA volume. The segmented 3D vasculature is shown in Figure 6a. A high resolution TOF-MRA image of the same volunteer was also acquired (voxel size 0.67mm x 0.39mm x 1.46mm and 225x512x48 voxels). The segmentation method [11] was applied to the data. The result is shown in Figure 6b. Observe that although PC-MRA is acquired at a lower scanning resolution, as compared with TOF-MRA, all the major vessels are clearly shown and reconstructed. To verify the aneurysm detection ability of the new algorithm, PC-MRA data from a patient with two small aneurysms was acquired at the same resolution and volume size. Figure 6c shows a 3D vascular segmentation of the data. The two aneurysms are clearly detected (pointed by the arrows). The computational time of the current implementation of the algorithm is approximately 10 seconds on a SGI 200MHz workstation.

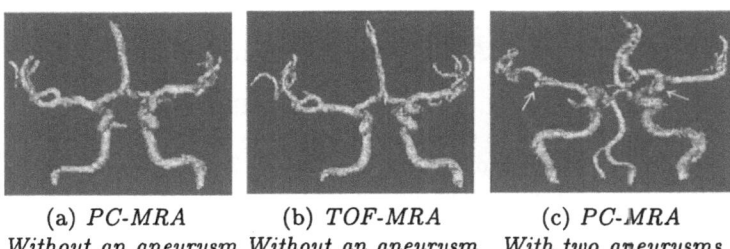

(a) *PC-MRA*   (b) *TOF-MRA*   (c) *PC-MRA*
Without an aneurysm Without an aneurysm   With two aneurysms
Fig. 6. *Segmentation Results*

4   Conclusion

We have presented an extended version of the fully automated 3D cerebral vessel segmentation algorithm [11] applicable to PC-MRA. Conceptually, the proposed algorithm falls into a probabilistic framework, in which the two major voxel types: background and vessel are statistically modelled. Statistical models were derived on the basis of the signal formation process and physical characteristics of the flow pattern. We show that a threshold found by the intersection of the two probabilistic distributions enables a good segmentation of the large major vessels to be performed. The results show that the estimated distribution well approximates the true (observed) background and vessel distributions. The main advantage of PC-MRA over TOF-MRA is that it gives additional directional flow images in the three orthogonal directions. Our next step is to perform directional velocity mapping on the segmented 3D vasculature such that the flow pattern around the region of aneurysm can be visualized and intensively studied.

Acknowledgements: We thank Dr. J. Byrne at the Department of Neuroradiology of the Radcliffe Infirmary, Oxford for providing data and helpful discussions. A. Chung is funded by a postgraduate scholarship award from the Croucher Foundation, Hong Kong.

References

1. A.H. Andersen and J.E. Kirsch. Analysis of noise in phase contrast MR imaging. *Med. Phy.*, 23(6):857–869,1996.
2. C. Bishop. *Neural Networks for Pattern Recognition.* Clarendon Press,1995.
3. C.G. Caro,T.J. Pedley et al. *The Mechanics of the Circulation.* O.U.P.,1978.
4. H. Gudbjartsson and S. Patz. The Rician distribution of noisy MRI data. *Mag. Reson. Med.*, 34:910–914,1995.
5. K. Krissian,G. Malandain and N. Ayache. Model-based multiscale detection and reconstruction of 3D vessels. *Tech. Report RR-3442*, INRIA,1998.
6. T.McInerney and D.Terzopoulos. Topologically Adaptable Snakes. *ICCV'95*, 840-5
7. N.J. Pelc,M.A. Bernstein et al. Encoding strategies for three-direction Phase Contrast MR imaging of flow. *J. Mag. Reson. Imag.*, 1:405–413,1991.
8. P.A. Rinck. *Magnetic Resonance in Medicine*, Blackwell,1993.
9. J. Sijbers,A.J. den Dekker,J.V. Audekerke,M. Verhoye and D. Van Dyck. Estimation of the noise in magnitude MR images. *Mag. Reson. Imag.*, 16(1):87–90,1998.
10. P. Summers,A. Bhalerao and D. Hawkes. Multi-resolution, Model-based segmentation of MR Angiograms. *J. Mag. Reson. Imag.*, 7(6):950-957,1997.
11. D. Wilson and J. Noble. Segmentation of cerebral vessels and aneurysms from MR angiography data. *IPMI*, 423–428,1997.
12. D.L. Wilson. *An Improved Planning Protocol for the Endovascular Treatment of Intracranial Aneurysms*, D.Phil.Thesis,U. of Oxford,1998.

Retinal Blood Vessel Segmentation by Means of Scale-Space Analysis and Region Growing

M. Elena Martínez-Pérez[1], Alun D. Hughes[2], Alice V. Stanton[2], Simon A. Thom[2], Anil A. Bharath[1], and Kim H. Parker[1]

[1] Department of Biological and Medical Systems.
Imperial College of Science, Technology and Medicine.
Prince Consort Road, London, SW7 2BY, UK
[2] Department of Clinical Pharmacology.
Imperial College of Science, School of Medicine at St. Mary's.
Paddington, London, W2 1NY, UK

Abstract. We present a method for retinal blood vessel segmentation based upon the scale-space analysis of the first and second derivative of the intensity image which gives information about its topology and overcomes the problem of variations in contrast inherent in these images. We use the local maxima over scales of the magnitude of the gradient and the maximum principal curvature as the two features used in a region growing procedure. In the first stage, the growth is constrained to regions of low gradient magnitude. In the final stage this constraint is relaxed to allow borders between regions to be defined. The algorithm is tested in both red-free and fluorescein retinal images.

1 Introduction

The eye is a window to the retinal vascular system which is uniquely accessible for the non-invasive, *in vivo* study of a complete vascular bed in humans. The detection and measurement of blood vessels can be used to quantify the severity of disease or as part of the process of automated diagnosis of disease. Retinal blood vessels can have measurable geometrical changes, in diameter, branching angles, lengths or tortuosity, as a result of a disease [4]. Thus a reliable method of vessel segmentation is needed for the early detection and characterisation of changes due to such diseases.

Different techniques are used to acquire images of retinal blood vessels. A relatively non-invasive technique, widely used clinically, is the retinal fundal photograph taken using a green filter. A more invasive technique is fluorescein angiography which involves an intravenous injection of dye which increases the contrast of the blood vessels against the background (Figure 3).

Previous studies have been carried out on the detection or enhancement of blood vessels in general and retinal blood vessels in particular [7]. Most of the work on segmentation of retinal images have been based in edge detectors or matched filters [1]. We have applied these two methods but because of the large regional variations in intensity inherent in these images and the very low contrast between vessels and the background, particularly in the red-free photographs, the results were disappointing. Techniques based on edge detectors lacked robustness in defining blood vessels without fragmentation and techniques based on matched filters were difficult to adapt to the variations of widths and orientation of blood vessels.

Multiscale analysis of the second derivative information was used to develop a vessel enhancement filter on X-ray images [3]. We present a method based on scale-space analysis from which we obtain retinal blood vessel width, size and orientation using two main geometrical features based upon the first and the second derivative of the intensity (edges and the maximum principal curvature) along the scale-space, that give information about the topology of the image. We then use a multiple pass region growing procedure which progressively segments the blood vessels using the feature information together with spatial information about the 8-neighbouring pixels.

2 Method

2.1 Scale-space representation

The idea behind scale-space representation is to separate out information at different scales. Any image can be embedded in one-parameter family of derived images $I(x, y; s)$ obtained by convolving the original image $I(x, y)$ with a Gaussian kernel $G(x, y; s)$ of variance s^2:

$$I(x, y; s) = I(x, y) \otimes G(x, y; s)$$

where s is a length scale factor. Figure 1(a) shows different scale-space representations of a portion of a red-free retinal image. Each scale slice is a version of the original after some amount of blurring, hence fine scale details disappear and images become more diffuse when scale parameter increases [5]. The use of Gaussian kernels to generate the scale-space information ensures that the objects in the images are *invariant* with respect to *translation, rotation* and *size* (scaling).

Under this framework, the derivative of an image $I(x, y)$ is defined as the linear convolution of the image with *scale-normalised derivative of Gaussian kernels.*

$$I_x = I(x, y) \otimes sG_x; \quad I_{xx} = I(x, y) \otimes s^2 G_{xx}$$
$$I_y = I(x, y) \otimes sG_y; \quad I_{xy} = I(x, y) \otimes s^2 G_{xy}$$
$$I_{yy} = I(x, y) \otimes s^2 G_{yy}$$

where subscripts indicate partial derivatives and

$$G(x, y; s) = \frac{1}{2\pi s^2} e^{-\frac{x^2 + y^2}{2s^2}}$$

$s = 2$ $s = 8$ $s = 14$ Maxima over scales

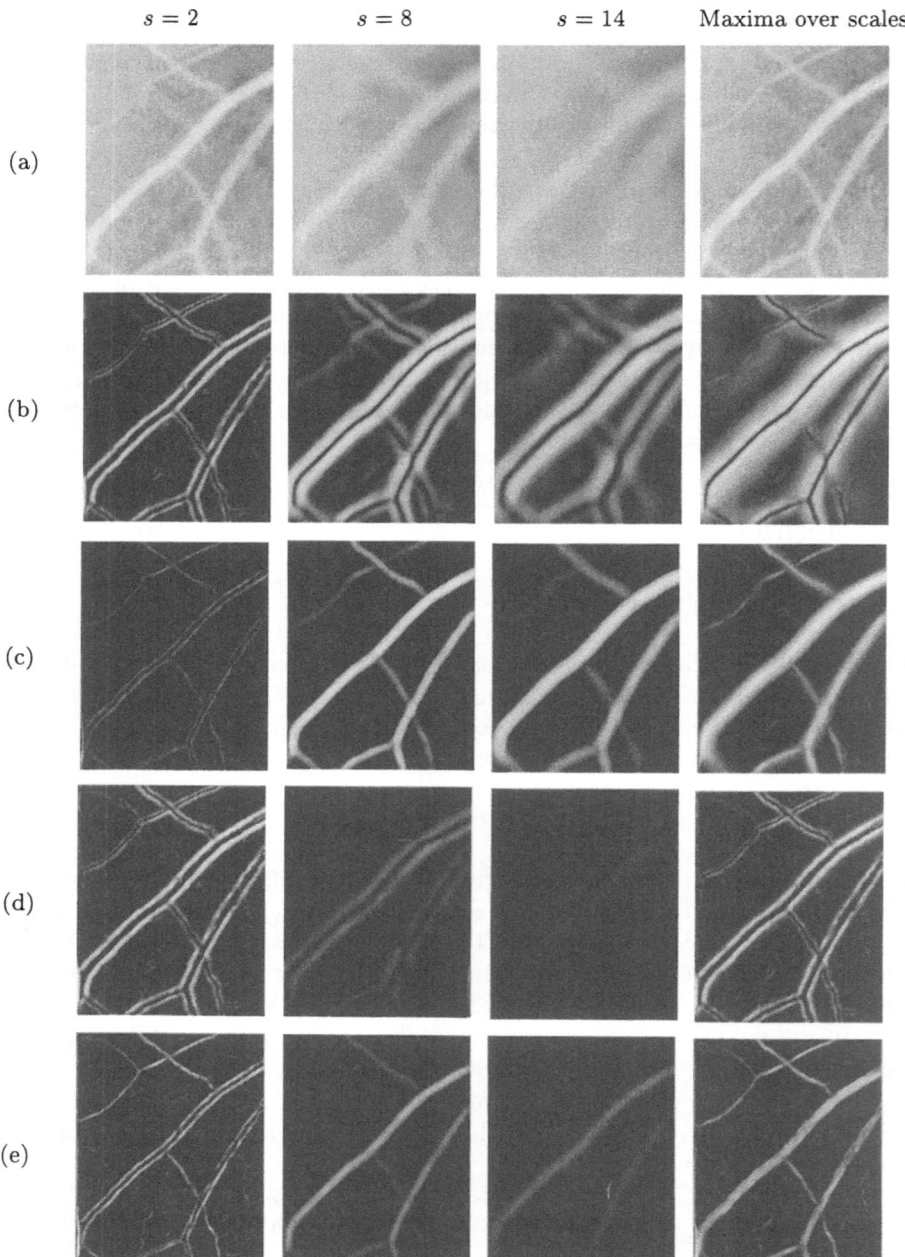

Fig. 1. Scale-space analysis for $s = 2$, 8 and 14 of a portion (360×290) of a red-free retinal image (1400×1200). (a) Original image, $I(s)$, (b) magnitude of the gradient, $|\nabla I(s)|$, (c) maximum principal curvature, $|\lambda_2(s)|$, (d) intensity scaled magnitude of the gradient, $|\nabla I(s)|/s$ and (e), intensity scaled maximum principal curvature, $|\lambda_2(s)|/s$. The last column in the first row is the original image and in the other rows is the maxima over scales.

2.2   Feature extraction

The measurements of feature strength that we used to characterise blood vessels are edges and maximum principal curvatures (ridges).

Edge strength. An edge point is weighted by the magnitude of the gradient of the image. The gradient is a vector function which represents the changes in intensity in the coordinate directions, and its magnitude is equal to the value of the slope, which is high at the edges and low at uniform regions:

$$|\nabla I| = \sqrt{I_x^2 + I_y^2}$$

Ridge strength. A ridge point is a point for which the intensity image has a local maximum in the direction for which the gradient of the image undergoes the largest change (largest concavity) [2]. The second derivative information can be derived from the Hessian of the intensity image $I(x,y)$:

$$H = \begin{pmatrix} I_{xx} & I_{xy} \\ I_{yx} & I_{yy} \end{pmatrix}$$

Since $I_{xy} = I_{yx}$ the Hessian matrix is symmetrical with real eigenvalues and orthogonal eigenvectors which are rotation invariant. The eigenvalues of the Hessian, λ_1 and λ_2, where we take $|\lambda_1| \leq |\lambda_2|$, measure convexity and concavity in the corresponding eigendirections. The maximum eigenvalue ($|\lambda_2|$) will correspond to the *maximum principal curvature*. Thus, a pixel belonging to a vessel region will be weighted as a ridge pixel if $|\lambda_2| \gg 1$, for both red-free and fluorescein images (Figures 1(b) and (c)).

Intensity scaling. From last column of Figures 1(b) and (c), it is noticeable that the local maxima response is much higher for large blood vessels than for small ones. This might be expected since the vessels are approximately cylindrical so that the total amount of blood in the light path corresponding to each pixel is larger in large vessels. Thus, there will be more absorption of non-red light in the red-free images and increased fluorescence in fluorescein images in the larger vessels.

To account for this effect, we introduce an *intensity scale* factor which is related to the size of the blood vessels. Because the parameter s is related to the width of the vessels, we normalise each feature with this factor over the scale-space and then keep the local maxima:

$$\gamma = \max_s \left[\frac{|\nabla I(s)|}{s} \right] \quad ; \quad \kappa = \max_s \left[\frac{|\lambda_2(s)|}{s} \right]$$

Figures 1(d) and (e) show these two new scale-space representations with the local maxima over scales in the last column.

2.3   Using the scale-space information

We calculate the scale-space information in intervals $s_{min} \leq s \leq s_{max}$ where s_{min} and s_{max} are fixed according to the sizes of the smallest and largest vessels to be detected in the image. In this case we use $2 \leq s \leq 20$ with steps of 1.

The approach we use to extract information across the scales is to keep the local maxima over scales for both measurements of feature strength. These values, the local maxima of the intensity scaled gradient magnitude, γ, and the local maxima of the intensity scaled maximum principal curvature, κ, are then used as the two features to classify pixels in the image into two region classes, *background* and *vessel*, using a multiple pass region growing procedure.

2.4 Region growing

The labelling algorithm is designed using information from the histograms of both features $h(\gamma)$ and $h(\kappa)$ and spatial information from the 8-neighbouring pixels. In the first stage the growing for both classes is restricted to regions with low gradients, allowing rapid growth of regions outside of the boundaries, and allowing vessels to grow where the values of κ lie within a wide interval.

For $h(\gamma)$ only one class is used: *low gradient*, which is defined as $\gamma < \mu_g + \sigma_g$ for the complete histogram (Figure 2(a)). $h(\kappa)$ is divided into two classes using the Otsu threshold algorithm [6], and their means and standard deviations are calculated: *background*, for $\kappa/\kappa_{max} \in [0, t]$ with mean μ_b and variance σ_b^2 ; and *vessel*, for $\kappa/\kappa_{max} \in (t, 1]$ with mean μ_v and variance σ_v^2, where t is the threshold (Figure 2(b)).

The algorithm begins by planting seeds for each region: background seeds are pixels for which $\kappa \leq \mu_b$, whereas vessel seeds are defined as $\kappa \geq \mu_v$. Region growing is by an iterative process: An unlabelled pixel is classified as belonging to class i if it fulfils a specific condition with initial parameters $a_i{=}1$. Growing is repeated until no more pixels are classified. The constraints are relaxed by incrementing the parameters a_i by 0.5 and the growing is repeated.

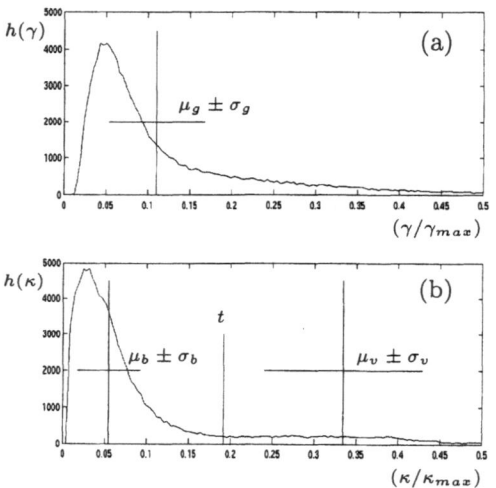

Fig. 2. Parameters used in the region growing algorithm. (a) Histogram of the local maxima of the edge strength, γ. One class: *low gradient*, $\gamma < \mu_g + \sigma_g$. (b) Histogram of the local maxima of the ridge strength, κ, where t is the threshold. Two classes: *background*, $\kappa/\kappa_{max} \in [0, t]$ and *vessel*, $\kappa/\kappa_{max} \in (t, 1]$.

For the first stage, the condition for class *vessel* is:

$$(\mu_v - a_v\sigma_v) \leq \kappa \ \ AND \ \ \gamma \leq (\mu_g + a_g\sigma_g) \ \ AND \ \ N_v \geq 1$$

whereas the condition for class *background* is:

$$\kappa \leq (\mu_b + a_b\sigma_b) \ \ AND \ \ \gamma \leq \mu_g \ \ AND \ \ N_b \geq 1$$

where N_i is the number of neighbours already labelled as class i.

After alternating these two procedures until no further classifications are found, the final stage of the algorithm grows vessel and background classes simultaneously without the gradient restriction. Now the condition for class i is:

$$(\mu_i - a\sigma_i) \le \kappa \le (\mu_i + a\sigma_i) \ AND \ N_i \ge 1$$

and again the condition is relaxed by increasing the value of a until all pixels are classified. With this final stage, borders between classes are defined. The complete procedure was applied to both red-free and a fluorescein images. Results are shown in Figure 3.

3   Results and Conclusion

From these results it can be seen that despite the much poorer contrast, the red-free image segmentation is nearly as good as that of the fluorescein image. We also find that the segmentation is relatively insensitive to the wide variations in intensity that are inherent in these images. Note in the fluorescein image, for example, the similar detail in the segmented image in the much brighter region just below the darker optic disk in the upper centre of the image.

It should be pointed out that although the idea of the intensity scale factor applied to the scale-space information is empirical, it can be justified by a simple model in which the intensity of the image is proportional to the amount of blood in the light path corresponding to that pixel. In any case, the method seems to work well in detecting retinal blood vessels over a large range of widths.

We have presented an algorithm which combines: 1) the scale-space representation that gives information about width, length and orientation of blood vessels, 2) two important geometrical properties of tube-like structures based on the first and second derivative information which give weights to pixels with a high probability of belonging to vessels, and 3) a multiple pass region growing procedure. The region growing algorithm is relatively fast because in the initial stage growth is restricted to regions with low gradients, allowing vessels to grow where the values of the maximum principal curvature lie within a wide interval. This allows rapid growth of regions outside the boundaries. In the final stage when the borders between classes are defined, the algorithm grows vessel and background classes simultaneously without the gradient restriction.

The appearance of the retinal blood vessels can be an important diagnostic indicator of various disorders of the eye and the body. From the segmented images, the morphology of retinal blood vessels can be measured in order to study changes resulting from disease: geometrical factors such as diameters, branching angles, lengths, tortuosity, etc. and network properties such as connectivity, branch ordering and, if appropriate, fractal properties. We are currently applying this segmentation algorithm to analyse these properties using clinical fundus photographs from normal subjects and hypertensive patients.

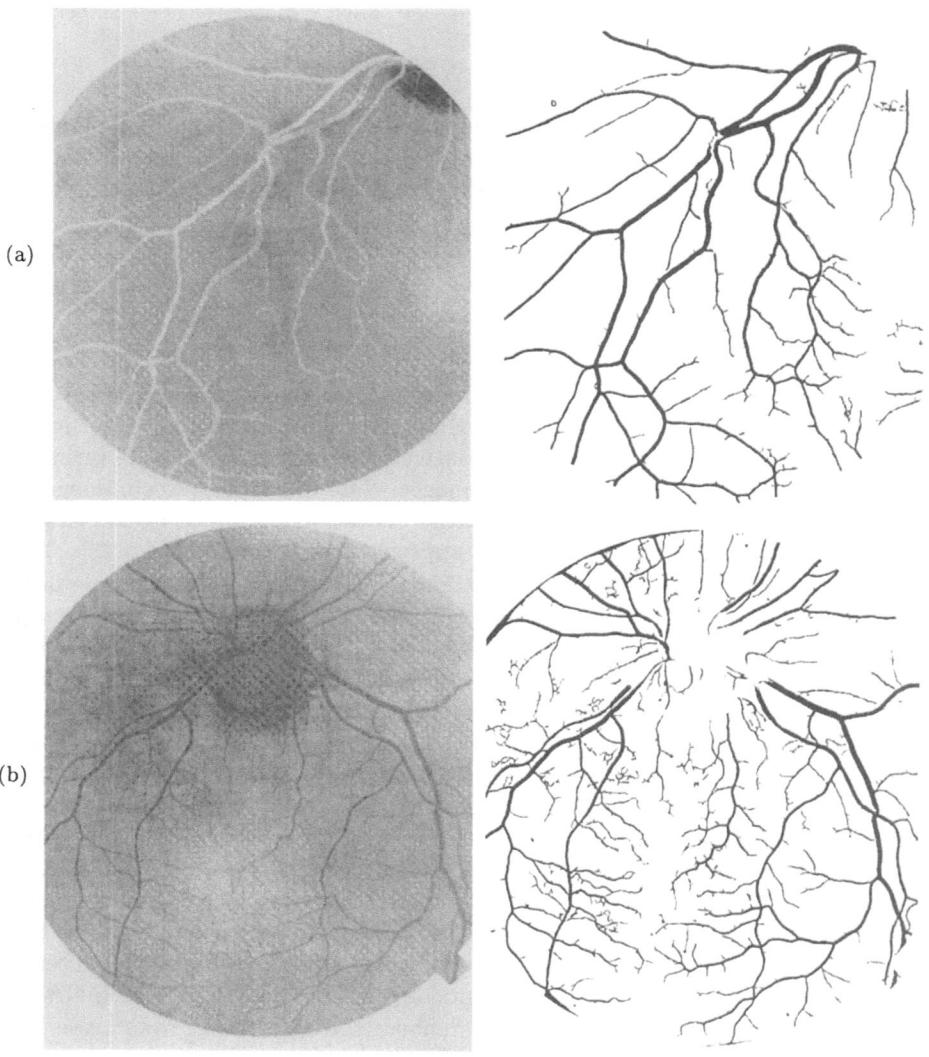

Fig. 3. Application of scale-space analysis and region growing segmentation to (a) red-free and (b) fluorescein fundal retinal images. The first column shows the original images. The second column shows the segmented vessels. Both images were photographed with the same resolution (size 1400×1200 pixels), the images correspond to the scanned negatives.

References

1. S. Chaudhuri, S. Chatterjee, N Katz, M. Nelson, and M. Goldbaum. Detection of blood vessels in retinal images using two-dimensional matched filters. *IEEE Trans. Med. Imag.*, 8:263–269, 1989.
2. D. Eberly. *Ridges in Image and Data Analysis*. Computational Imaging and Vision. Kluwer Academic Publishers, Netherlands, 1996.
3. A.F. Frangi, W.J. Niessen, K.L. Vincken, and M.A. Viergever. Multiscale vessel enhancement filtering. In W.M. Wells, A. Colchester, and S. Delp, editors, *Medical Image Computing and Computer-Assisted Intervantion- MICCAI'98*, number 1496 in Lecture Notes in Computer Science, pages 130–137, Berlin, 1998. Springer.
4. L.A. King, A.V. Stanton, P.S. Sever, S. Thom, and A.D. Hughes. Arteriolar length-diameter (l:d) ratio: A geometric parameter of the retinal vasculature diagnostic of hypertension. *J. of Hum. Hypertens.*, 10:417–418, 1996.
5. T. Lindeberg and B.M. ter Haar Romeny. Linear scale-space. In B.M. ter Haar Romeny, editor, *Geometry-Driven Diffusion in Computer Vision*, Computational Imaging and Vision, pages 1–72. Kluwer Academic Publishers, Dordrecht, 1994.
6. N. Otsu. A threshold selection method from gray-level histograms. *IEEE Trans. Syst., Man, Cybern.*, SMC-9:62–66, Jan 1979.
7. S.A. Thom, X. Gao, A.V. Stanton, J.N. Chapman, A. Bharath, and A.D. Hughes. A computer system for automated retinal microvascular architecture quantification. *J. Hypertens.*, 16(S2):1421, 1998.

Liver Blood Vessels Extraction by a 3-D Topological Approach

Petr Dokládal, Christophe Lohou, Laurent Perroton, and Gilles Bertrand

ESIEE Cité Descartes, B.P. 99, 93 162 Noisy-le-Grand Cedex, France
{dokladap, lohouc, perrotol, bertrang}@esiee.fr

Abstract. We propose in this paper a new approach to segmentation of 3-D tomography of liver vessel system. The approach is based on a point-wise reconstruction with restriction to simple points manipulation to preserve the homotopy. We propose and compare two dual methods of the vessel system extraction. The efficiency of these methods is demonstrated on a raw X-ray tomography image. The desired level of detail in the vein ramification system is obtained by adjusting one parameter controlling the admitted level of light intensity.

The paper is organized as follows: In the introductory section we present the main principles of the approach using simple points. We explain the algorithm as well as the aspects of efficient computer implementation. Experimental results for different parameter values are given together with discussion and conclusions.

Keywords: Segmentation, simple point, homotopy.

1 Introduction

The proposed segmentation technique is based on a priori knowledge of the processed images. The category of images that we consider in this paper is an X-ray tomography scan of liver. Closer examination of such an image gives a rough idea of the topology, morphology and geometry which is analogous for every human being and varies only in minor changes for each patient. The blood vessel circuitry is composed of bright-textured areas surrounded by darker regions which are also non-uniformly textured. The morphology of the image is due to the used contrasting substance. The substance is most concentrated in the portal vein being therefore the region of the highest luminosity in the image. The healthy part of liver, fairly flooded with the contrasting substance appears somewhat darker. The non-flooded liver lesions appear in the image as dark areas.

The vessel system flooded with the contrasting substance is composed of one voluminous portal vein which develops into thinner ramifications. The vessel circuitry forms a system without cycles [Sol98]. The conclusions on the topology are immediate: the vessel system is a simply connected object without cavities and holes and forms itself a cavity in respect to its complement.

The principle of the segmentation techniques proposed in this paper is based on the hypothesis that the resulting object is simply connected, contains no holes and no cavities. The resulting object is reconstructed by iterative adding simple points which ensures preservation of topology. During the reconstruction procedure we process the points in the order determined by their luminosity. The advantages of our methods is the ability to give a result that is thin, rich in detail and topologically correct. The methods complete in one phase and do not require any pre-treatment nor any subsequent correction

The paper is organized as follows: In the introductory section we present the main principles of the approach using simple points. We explain the algorithm and also give the aspects of efficient computer implementation. Experimental results for different parameter values are given together with discussion and conclusions.

The segmentation techniques presented in this paper are new and have not yet been published.

2 Basic notions

We present some basic notions of 3-D topology needed to outline the principles of the algorithm, see also [MR80], [BM94].

A 3-D *grey-scale image* is an application $\mathbb{Z}^3 \to \mathbb{N}$. A point $x \in \mathbb{Z}^3$ is defined by (x_1, x_2, x_3) with $x_i \in \mathbb{Z}$. We use the following neighborhoods: $N_6(x) = \{y \mid \sum_{i=1,2,3} |x_i - y_i| = 1\}$, $N_{26}(x) = \{y \mid \max_{i=1,2,3}(|x_i - y_i|) = 1\}$. The points x, y are said to be *n-adjacent* (or *neighbors*) for $n = 6, 26$ if $x \neq y$ and $x \in N_n(y)$. We use 26-adjacency and 6-adjacency for the object and the background, respectively, see also [KR89].

Let $X \subset \mathbb{Z}^3$. An *n-path* γ, $\gamma \subset X$ is a sequence of points $x_0, \ldots, x_k$, where $x_i \in X$, $\forall i = 0, \ldots k$ and x_i is *n*-adjacent to x_{i+1}, for $i = 0, \ldots, k-1$. We say that a path is closed if $x_0 = x_k$.

To introduce the notions of hole and simply connected object we need to outline the notion of path deformation. For exhaustive definition see Bertrand and Malandain [BM94]. Let γ and γ' be two paths. We will consider γ' an *elementary deformation* of γ if γ and γ' are identical with the exception of a little neighborhood. This neighborhood depends on the used connectivity. A non-elementary deformation of a path is obtained by successive applications of elementary deformations.

An object $X \subset \mathbb{Z}^3$ is said to be *n-connected* if for any two points $x, y \in X$ there is an *n*-path γ, $\gamma \subset X$ from x to y. An object X is said to be *simply connected* if every possible path γ, $\gamma \subset X$ can be reduced by successive deformations to a single point. We say that there is a *hole* in X, if there is a closed path contained in X that cannot be deformed in X to a single point.

A *cavity* in X is a finite and isolated connected component of $\overline{X}$.

A *simple point* $x \in X$ is a point the deletion of which doesn't change the topology of the object X. Bertrand and Malandain [BM94] have proposed a characterization of simple point based on calculation of connected components in the neighborhood of the point. A point of a cubic grid is simple if in the neighborhood of the point there is exactly one connected component of the

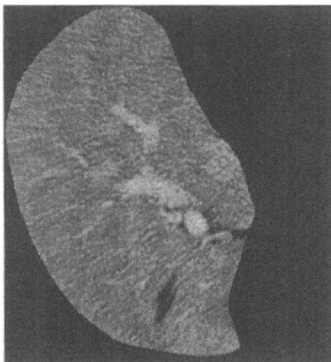

Fig. 1. 2-D slice cut from a 3-D tomography scan of liver. The vessels appear as bright areas whereas the liver lesions as dark ones.

object and exactly one connected component of the complement. Recall that different connectivities must be used for the object and for the complement.

The test whether a particular point is simple or non-simple is implemented using a fast algorithm based on binary decision diagrams [RM96]. This algorithm decomposes the neighborhood of the point to a decision tree. The complexity of this algorithm is constant in time and requires 26 tests (26 neighbors of the point) in the worst case.

3 Principle of the segmentation algorithm

The principle is analogous to the 3-D hole closing algorithm by Aktouf *et al.* [ABP96] and is based on iterative point-wise growing restricted exclusively to simple points. The growing is done preferentially with the points of the same or resembling luminosity. If the object is bright, surrounded with darker background then the growing proceeds with the bright points first.

The constraint of processing exclusively only simple-points ensures the homotopy. However, during the iterations of the object growing some points having once been classified as non-simple may become simple later on. This happens due to modifications in the neighborhood. The algorithm is conceived in the way that the points having once been refused for non-simplicity may be revisited later.

Firstly we present the notion of hierarchical-priority lists needed to explain the algorithm.

3.1 Priority lists

The hierarchical priority lists is an ordered group of FIFO lists. Each list is assigned a priority value corresponding to a certain value of luminosity. The higher the luminosity, the higher the priority of the particular list.

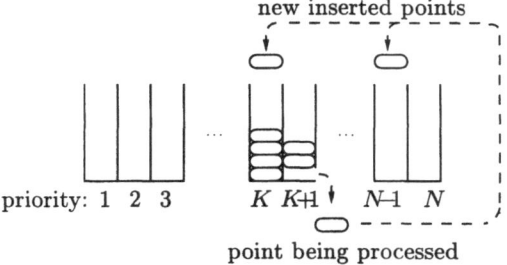

Fig. 2. Hierarchical waiting lists. $K+1$ is the current value of priority for retrieval of a point.

The maximum length each list can grow up to is known and can be decided from the picture. It equals the number of points of the corresponding grey level.

The principle is outlined in Fig. 2. The lists are accessed for insertion of new points randomly since the arriving points are of random level of grey. Retrieval of a point is done always on the non-empty list of the highest priority. The conditions on which some points are inserted in the waiting lists are explained below. It is possible that one of the arriving points has higher priority than the one of the list being processed at this moment. The list containing the new point then becomes the list of the highest priority. The lists once emptied may again be accessed for point insertion and therefore cannot be freed from memory.

See the Figure 2. The current priority of the list being read is $K+1$. The new-arriving points are inserted in the corresponding lists. The next point to be processed in the forthcoming iteration is the one being inserted into the list $N-1$.

3.2 Principle of the reconstruction

The procedure reconstructs an object according to a given stop criterion K. Initially the object is the empty set. The waiting lists are also empty with exception of one or more points inserted in to seed the growing. Iteratively, from the highest-priority non-empty list, a point x_i is retrieved to be processed. If this point is simple then it will make part of the output object. Whether the point is simple or not its neighbors are inserted into the respective waiting lists if their level of grey is superior or equal to K. The iteration is repeated as long as there are any points in the lists the priority of which is superior to K.

See the illustration given by Fig. 3. Let's suppose the object in form of a disc constituted by the points superior to 100. The background of the image is formed by the points inferior to this value. Let's suppose the point 120 is a marker to start the object growing.

The object growth proceeds in two directions on the boundary of the disc with the points $119, \ldots, 115$ being classified as simple. The points already inserted in the object at this moment are typeset in boldface. When the growing procedure

1		3	2	1	1	3	2
2		1	**118**	**117**	**116**	0	1
1	**119**	113	112	111	**115**	2	
0	120	113	112	111	114	1	
1	**119**	113	112	111	**115**	0	
3		2	**118**	**117**	**116**	1	1
1		2	3	1	1	2	4

Fig. 3. The object is formed by points superior to 100. The point 114 once classified as non-simple is revisited for insertion.

inserts the two points of 115 then the point 114 becomes non simple. It cannot be inserted at this stage since its insertion would create a hole by disconnecting the interior from the exterior of the "C"-like object. The growing then continues with the points 113, . . . , 111 filling the interior. Once the disc filled in, the point 114 is revisited. At this moment it is classified as simple and is inserted to the object.

The algorithm of reconstruction can be used in two dual modifications: *segmentation by reconstruction of the object* and *segmentation by reconstruction of the background*. We will see that these modifications are dual but not symmetric.

Segmentation by reconstruction of the object A marker must be given to start the object growing. It can be found manually by an expert or it may be the result of another forthcoming image analysis. A stop criterion K has to be provided to stop the growing procedure.

Segmentation by reconstruction of the background This method works on the grey-scale complement of the input image. The reconstruction algorithm starts with the border of the image and iteratively reconstructs the background. The points are iteratively added the bright (originally dark) points first until there are no simple points of luminosity superior to K.

The reconstructed object is free of ruptures and is reconstructed till the very extremities of the blood vessels. There is no need of marker since the object is being extracted as the complement of the background and the reconstruction is seeded with the image border.

The maximum calculation complexity is equivalent for the two variants. It is almost (because of the waiting list) a liner function of the size of the image. The execution time of the two methods may however differ as it depends of the dimensions of the object. If the volume of the object is considerably smaller than the volume of the background then the reconstruction of the object is significantly faster.

4   Experimental results

Segmentation by reconstruction of the object Let's see the segmentation results obtained by the object reconstruction method given by Fig. 5 a) and c). The result a) comprises a few principal branching of the portal artery. Lowering the threshold value however results both in rendering the result richer in the circuitry structure as well as in thickening of the arteries, cf. Fig. 5 c). It is not possible, whatever the value of the stop criterion, to obtain identical results for the two methods.

The object is topologically correct, i.e. it doesn't contain any holes or cavities in either of the two modifications. It is evident from the principle of the method that the resulting object is a simply connected 3-D object.

The disadvantage of this method is its sensitivity to noise. The growing of very thin structures deteriorated with noise can be prematurately stopped. Points which level of grey is inferior to the stop criterion will cause ruptures in the vein circuitry. See the illustration given by Figure 4. The ruptures are due to the texture-like nature of the vessels. The points which luminosity is inferior to the stop criterion are not inserted. This is the mechanism how in the worst case the cracks prevent the vessel extremities from reconstruction. This effect is quite frequent since the image is heavily noised. The segmentation by reconstruction of the background alleviates this annoying effect.

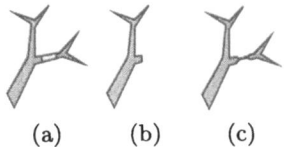

(a)   (b)   (c)

Fig. 4. The two methods give different results, a) a blood vessel with a region of faint contrast in center, b) segmentation by reconstruction of the object, c) reconstruction of the background.

Segmentation by reconstruction of the background The advantage of this method is that ruptures present in the vessels do not stop the reconstruction, see Fig. 4. The segmentation by reconstruction of the background, Fig. 4 c), is more appropriate) since the restriction to simple points prevents from creating unconnected objects.

Let's now examine the results of the background reconstruction method given by Fig. 5 b) and d).

You can see that the results of segmentation by reconstruction of the background are considerably thinner than those obtained by reconstruction of the object. Fine threshold modifications enable simple means of controlling the detail level in the resulting object. The richness of the vessel structure is quite sensitive to the parameter.

The background reconstruction method may suffer from the effect dual to the cracks in the result by reconstruction of the object. If the stop criterion is too high, this method creates thin fake vessels. This effect is caused by a noise present in the image. Bright (in the original image) points that do not belong to the object are linked with the vessel structure due to the condition of homotopy preservation.

5 Conclusion

Visual appraisal of the results of two segmentation methods approves the ability of the latter to produce richer and thinner result. The results of the segmentation by object reconstruction are either rather undersegmented when compared visually with the original image or too voluminous to be of practical use. The sensitivity to the stop criterion has proven better for the second method.

Further modifications and extensions : Alleviating the annoying effects of the noise doesn't seem impossible. Erroneous ramifications might be eliminated by hysteresis applied to the grey level of the branches. Employing the distance transform at the same time may give priority to filter rather the branch extremities while preserving the central artery.

The principle of the latter of the two methods enables to obtain also the skeleton of the vessel system instead of its segmentation, see [DLPB99]. To obtain the skeleton, the algorithm proceeds until unity diameter. When the current luminosity level overruns the K criterion then another condition is supplied to protect the vessel extremities from shortening. This condition is needed since the contraction of vessel extremities is a homotopic operations.

References

[ABP96] Z. Aktouf, G. Bertrand, and L. Perroton. A 3d holes closing algorithm. In *6th workshop on Discrete Geometry for Computer Imagery*, November 1996.

[BM94] G. Bertrand and G. Malandain. A new characterization of three-dimensional simple points. *Pattern Recognition Letters*, (15):1003–1011, 1994.

[DLPB99] P. Dokládal, C. Lohou, L. Perroton, and G. Bertrand. A new thinning algorithm and its application to extraction of blood vessels. In *BioMedSim'99*, ESIEE Noisy-le-Grand, France, pages 32-37, 1999.

[KR89] T. Y. Kong and A. Rozenfeld. Digital topology: introduction and survey. *Comp. Vision Graphics and Image Processing*, (48):357–393, 1989.

[MR80] D.G. Morgenthaler and A. Rozenfeld. Three dimensional topology: the genus. Technical Report TR-980, Computer Science Center, University of Maryland, College Park, 1980.

[RM96] Luc Robert and Gregoire Malandain. Fast binary image processing using binary decision diagrams. Technical Report 3001, INRIA Sophia-Antipolis, 1996.

[Sol98] Luc Soler. *Une nouvelle méthode de segmentation des structures anatomiques et pathologiques: application aux angioscanners 3D du foie pour la planification chirurgicale*. PhD thesis, INRIA Sophia-Antipolis, 1998.

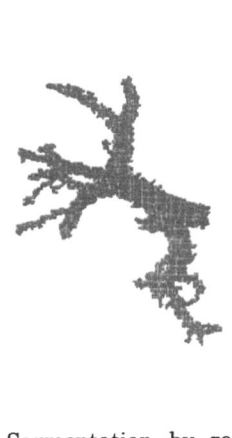

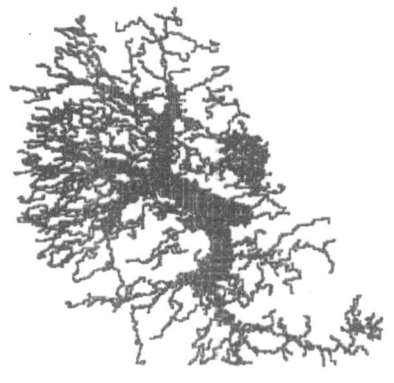

(a) Segmentation by reconstruction of the object $K = 166$

(b) Segmentation by reconstruction of the background $K = 80$

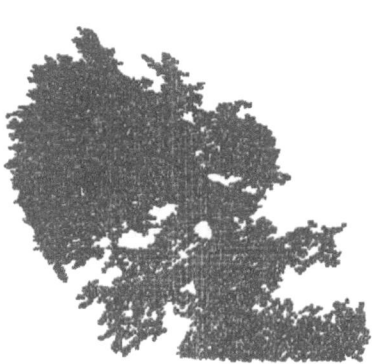

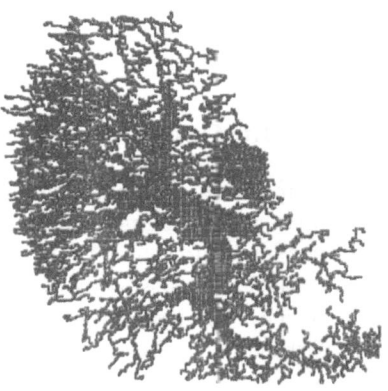

(c) Segmentation by reconstruction of the object $K = 140$

(d) Segmentation by reconstruction of the background $K = 90$

Fig. 5. Results of the liver blood vessel extraction by two dual approaches for different values of the stop criterion. (2-D rendering of 3-D objects)

Tamed Snake: A Particle System for Robust Semi-automatic Segmentation

Johannes Hug, Christian Brechbühler, and Gábor Székely

Swiss Federal Institute of Technology, ETH Zentrum
CH-8092 Zürich, Switzerland
[jhug | brech | szekely]@vision.ee.ethz.ch

Abstract. Semi-automatic segmentation approaches tend to overlook the problems caused by missing or incomplete image information. In such situations, powerful control mechanisms and intuitive modelling metaphors should be provided in order to make the methods practically applicable. Taking this problem into account, the usage of subdivision curves in combination with the simulation of edge attracted mass points is proposed as a novel way towards a more robust interactive segmentation methodology. Subdivision curves provide a hierarchical and smooth representation of a shape which can be modified on coarse and on fine scales as well. Furthermore, local adaptive subdivision gives the required flexibility when dealing with a discrete curve representation. In order to incorporate image information, the control vertices of a curve are considered mass points, attracted by edges in the local neighbourhood of the image. This so-called Tamed Snake framework is illustrated by means of the segmentation of two medical data sets and the results are compared with those achieved by traditional Snakes.

1   Introduction

Fully automatic and manual segmentation methods represent two extremes of a wide spectrum of segmentation algorithms. Between these, a whole family of interactive semi-automatic tools [2, 5, 10, 11] has been developed, promising to combine the advantages of computational support, resulting in precise border detection, with the benefits from manual manipulation possibilities. The application of these algorithms to the segmentation of medical imagery supports the human operator considerably in the case of clear and sharp organ outlines. But whenever edge information at organ boundaries is disturbed or missing, as is often the case in rather demanding tasks, such as the model-making of an abdominal cavity [12], manual outlining based on interpolating B-splines proved superior in every respect to the semi-automatic approaches. In particular, the controllability of geometric shapes is very poor in interactive operation mode. The generic gap-closing mechanism provided by these algorithms between clear border segments seems to be unsuited and not sufficiently under control of the operator.

Most existing segmentation tools lack an intuitive manipulation semantic, especially on coarse scales, and sometimes on finer scales as well. Hence the geometric representation must be chosen in order to alleviate the interaction difficulties arising when the human operator is required to intervene during the segmentation process. Fortunately, the computer graphics community supplies us with a large number of animation and modelling techniques well suited to overcome the aforementioned inadequacies. In particular, hierarchical multiresolution representations are promising candidates regarding the necessary interactive modelling capabilities and the suitability for numerical simulations.

The work presented in this paper is a first step towards combining traditional computer vision approaches with intuitive modelling semantics in order to provide a truly operational interactive segmentation system. At first, we will review selected representatives of the class of interactive segmentation algorithms which have been developed during the last twenty years. Having taken a quick glance at recent advances in geometric modelling, Sect. 2 presents a novel combination of edge attracted mass points with subdivision curves, adopting both automatic boundary detection and interactive modelling. Finally, Sect. 3 compares this new framework with traditional Snakes on the basis of two medical data sets.

1.1   Earlier Interactive Segmentation Approaches

The first class of algorithms we would like to mention considers the image I as a discrete neighbourhood graph, where each pixel corresponds to a node in the graph. A cost function $P(I)$ assigns a value to each node in the graph. For edge tracking purposes, the cost function is usually based on the magnitude of the gradient of the low-pass filtered image. A very popular cost function for minimisation algorithms is therefore

$$P(I) = 1 - \frac{||\nabla(\text{Gauss} \otimes I)||}{\max(||\nabla(\text{Gauss} \otimes I)||)} . \tag{1}$$

With such a cost function, edge tracking can be considered as a minimal cost path search problem between two points in the image graph. Fischler, Tenenbaum and Wolf [2] used the well known $F^\star$ algorithm to solve this minimisation problem in a semi-automatic framework for road detection; Barrett and Mortensen [10] applied the very similar $A^\star$ algorithm for the interactive segmentation of medical imagery. Interaction possibilities are limited to the choice of start and end points of the path. Subsequent modifications of the shape can only be accomplished by moving each single polygonal vertex.

In order to link polygonal vertices together, whilst abandoning the discrete working domain, Kass, Witkin and Terzopoulos [5] introduced Snakes: A Snake is the simulation of a physical system consisting of an elastically deformable mass-spring object living in a potential field, $P(I)$, as defined above. Unfortunately, the shape regularisation provided by the elasticity and rigidity terms is only available during automatic evolution, wherefore manual editing still remains very cumbersome. Several extensions, such as Ziplock Snakes [11], have been developed, but the basic problem with the underlying geometry was not addressed until the invention of B-spline Snakes [6, 7] using dynamic knot insertion. Despite manual modifications on coarse scales being possible with B-Snakes, fine scale editing results in a proliferation of control points, destroying the coarse scale manipulation semantic.

1.2   Hierarchical Modelling

Hierarchical modelling is composed of two very general key components: Iterative refinement of the geometry which defines a hierarchy of representations with increasing degrees of freedom; and local detail encoding which represents the details of a finer level with respect to the next coarser one. These two building blocks enable a natural editing semantic on coarse and on fine scales, as required for a practically useful segmentation tool. This concept has been introduced by Forsey and Bartels [3] for B-spline curves and surfaces, and has led to several experimental and industrial modelling systems [13, 4].

Subdivision curves and surfaces are well suited for hierarchical modelling since their representation implicitly comprises a hierarchy of refined shapes. Furthermore, local detail encoding is only a simple extension in the context of subdivision schemes. The favourable properties of this geometric description have already been used among others for finite element based shape recovery [9], and for feature based indirect volume rendering [8].

2   Tamed Snakes

In order to take advantage of the benefits from both the Snake-like edge tracking and hierarchical modelling, we present a new combination of the two underlying components. In the following paragraphs, we will give a detailed description of the components establishing the core of the Tamed Snake framework.

2.1   Subdivision Curves

Univariate subdivision schemes are usually defined as the iterative application of an operator which maps a given polygon $\mathcal{P}_k = [\mathbf{p}_i^{(k)}]$ to a refined polygon $\mathcal{P}_{k+1} = [\mathbf{p}_i^{(k+1)}]$. Such an operator is given by two rules for computing the new so-called even vertices $\mathcal{P}_{k+1}^{\natural} = \{\mathbf{p}_{2i}^{(k+1)}\}$ and the new odd vertices $\mathcal{P}_{k+1}^{\sharp} = \{\mathbf{p}_{2i+1}^{(k+1)}\}$. For interpolatory refinement, the rule for even points is always $\mathbf{p}_{2i}^{(k+1)} = \mathbf{p}_i^{(k)}$.

In our Tamed Snake implementation, the first smooth interpolating subdivision scheme from Dyn, Levin and Gregory [1] is employed. The subdivision rules, which are also known as DLG-subdivision scheme, are given by

$$\mathbf{p}_{2i}^{(k+1)} = \mathbf{p}_i^{(k)}, \qquad \mathbf{p}_{2i+1}^{(k+1)} = (\frac{1}{2} + \omega)(\mathbf{p}_i^{(k)} + \mathbf{p}_{i+1}^{(k)}) - \omega(\mathbf{p}_{i-1}^{(k)} + \mathbf{p}_{i+2}^{(k)}) \ . \quad (2)$$

If the magnitude of the free tension parameter ω is chosen inside the interval $(0, \frac{1}{4})$, the limit curve will be continuous, and for $0 < \omega < \frac{1}{8}$, the limit curve has a continuous tangent vector given by the following equation:

$$\mathbf{p}_i' = \frac{1}{1 - 4\omega} \left[\frac{1}{2}(\mathbf{p}_{i+1} - \mathbf{p}_{i-1}) - \omega(\mathbf{p}_{i+2} - \mathbf{p}_{i-2}) \right] \tag{3}$$

An example depicting three refinement steps carried out with this 4-point subdivision stencil is displayed in Fig. 1.

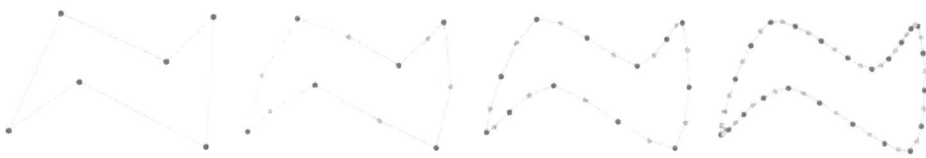

Fig. 1. Interpolatory refinement: The iterative application of the DLG-subdivision operator transforms an initial control polygon $\mathcal{P}_0$ (left) into a finer polygon $\mathcal{P}_3$ (right). Black vertices represent even points, and grey vertices denote odd points.

Local detail encoding is achieved by establishing a local coordinate system $f_i^{(k)}$ in each vertex $\mathbf{p}_i^{(k)}$ and by representing details with respect to this local frame (see Fig. 2). A very natural choice for $f_i^{(k)}$ is the normalised tangent $\frac{\mathbf{p}_i'}{\|\mathbf{p}_i'\|}$ together with the normal vector counterclockwise perpendicular to the tangent in each vertex.

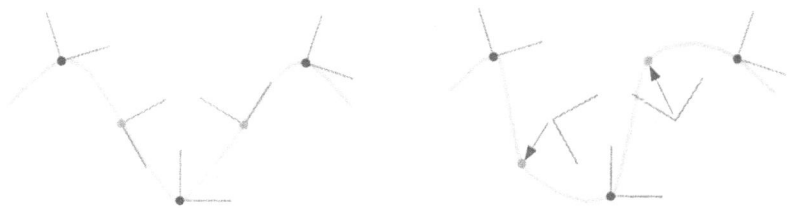

Fig. 2. Local coordinate frames for detail encoding. The two odd points of the left curve are modified by adding local detail coefficients (right).

2.2 Local Adaptive Subdivision

In order to have efficient data structures and fast algorithms at hand, we can exploit the hierarchical, tree-like structure of a subdivision curve as well as the local support of the refinement operator. As illustrated in Fig. 3, a flexible representation of the hierarchy of vertices is a combination of a doubly linked list with a collection of binary trees. In the following, we will refer to such a structure as a *listed tree*. Each point $\mathbf{p}_i^{(k)}$ is represented by a node on level k in a tree. The links between two nodes can be interpreted as the polygonal segments in between two points $\mathbf{p}_i^{(k)}$ and $\mathbf{p}_{i+1}^{(k)}$. Please notice that the nodes are also connected across tree boundaries, admitting of fast navigation in different resolution levels. In order to save memory, it is advantageous to separate the real vertex data from the tree nodes and to keep it in a dynamic array, since that way even points must only be stored once.

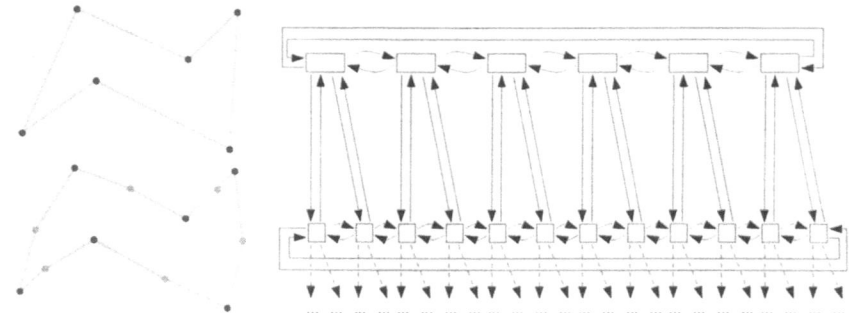

Fig. 3. A *listed tree* as a data structure for efficient and adaptive subdivision. The corresponding polygons $\mathcal{P}_0$ and $\mathcal{P}_1$ are displayed on the left of the nodes representing the points $\mathbf{p}_i^{(0)}$ and $\mathbf{p}_i^{(1)}$.

The main reason for choosing such a sophisticated data structure is the fact that flat regions of a curve need only a small number of subdivision steps, while segments with high curvature or with fine details require more degrees of freedom. Therefore the refinement operator is only applied to those parts of the curve that have additional details or where the local flatness is still too small. Figure 4 shows the effect of such an adaptive synthesis of a curve using a discrete curvature estimator as a flatness oracle.

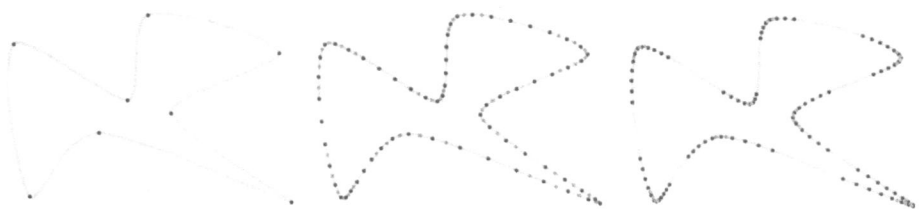

Fig. 4. Adaptively subdivided curve with vertices of level 0 (left), level 4 (middle), and level 5 (right). A discrete curvature estimator served as a flatness criterion. Regions with high curvature are subdivided, while flat regions remain unrefined.

Applying adaptive synthesis interactively produces very dynamic data structures. The resulting listed trees may become pretty unbalanced when flat regions and highly detailed segments occur in the same curve. Nevertheless, adaptive synthesis is well suited for interactive segmentation since it always assures an appropriate sampling of the shape.

As a consequence of the local support of the DLG-subdivision operator, the modification of a point $\mathbf{p}_i^{(k)}$ does not enforce the recalculation of the whole curve, but only a small part of it, depending on $\mathbf{p}_i^{(k)}$. Figure 5 shows these dependencies between two successive subdivision levels. The refinement of level k triggered by the modification of the point $\mathbf{p}_i^{(k)}$ can be sketched as follows: Firstly, the invalidated positions of the dependent vertices $\mathbf{p}_{2i-3}^{k+1}$, $\mathbf{p}_{2i-1}^{k+1}$, $\mathbf{p}_{2i+1}^{k+1}$, and $\mathbf{p}_{2i+3}^{k+1}$ must be recalculated using (2). Secondly, all affected local frames in level $k+1$ are updated using (3), and lastly, detail coefficients are added. For the refinement of the next level $k+1$, only those of the altered vertices — those not passing the flatness test — are regarded as modified. This procedure is applied iteratively until no further segments need refinement.

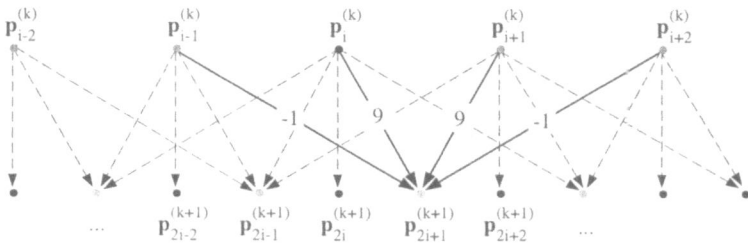

Fig. 5. Local support of the points in level k; weights according to $\omega = \frac{1}{16}$ for the recalculation of the point $\mathbf{p}_{2i+1}^{(k+1)}$.

2.3   Particle Systems for Interactive Segmentation

The hierarchical structure of subdivision curves suggests starting the segmentation process with a reasonably coarse model and then to iteratively adjust and refine the control vertices of the resulting curve. Since we apply an interpolating subdivision scheme, all odd points of the current working level must be moved to a correct boundary position, before proceeding to the next finer resolution. If this holds for all vertices on coarser levels, the prediction of the refinement operator improves continuously with respect to the vertex positions on the next finer level and converges to the correct boundary position.

In order to combine such a coarse-to-fine strategy with Snake-like edge tracking, we must modify the traditional Snake energy to be optimised (see [5, 11]). Since the regularisation term provided by the elastic rod model is useless on a coarse scale, we drop it in favour of a spring energy originating from springs attached to each odd control point (see Fig. 6). A spring allows for a snapping of the attached control vertex $\mathbf{p}_i$ into the correct boundary position, within the vicinity of its starting position $\mathbf{p}_i(0) = \mathbf{p}_i \mid_{t=0}$. The imposed restriction on the search space to the local neighbourhood is reasonable under the assumption of working with a good initialisation. Additionally, since the error of the refinement operator's prediction tends to decrease with each subdivision step, we can increase the spring constant $\delta^{(k)}$ in order to restrict the search area accordingly. Hence, the energy originating from all springs on refinement level k is given by:

$$E_S = -\frac{1}{2} \sum_{\mathbf{p}_i \in \mathcal{P}_k^\sharp} \delta_i^{(k)} \|\mathbf{p}_i(t) - \mathbf{p}_i(0)\|^2 \qquad (4)$$

Besides the spring energy, Tamed Snakes incorporate a kinetic energy E_{kin} depending on the mass μ, and an image energy E_I originating from the potential function defined in (1). The full energy term $E_{\text{TS}} = E_{\text{kin}} + E_{\text{pot}}$, is therefore as follows:

$$E_I = - \sum_{\mathbf{p}_i \in \mathcal{P}_k^\sharp} P(I) \mid_{\mathbf{p}_i(t)}, \quad E_{\text{kin}} = \frac{1}{2} \sum_{\mathbf{p}_i \in \mathcal{P}_k^\sharp} \mu_i \left| \frac{\partial \mathbf{p}_i(t)}{\partial t} \right|^2, \quad E_{\text{pot}} = E_S + E_I$$

$$E_{\text{TS}} = \frac{1}{2} \sum_{\mathbf{p}_i \in \mathcal{P}_k^\sharp} \left[\mu_i \left| \frac{\partial \mathbf{p}_i(t)}{\partial t} \right|^2 - \delta_i^{(k)} \|\mathbf{p}_i(t) - \mathbf{p}_i(0)\|^2 - 2P(I) \mid_{\mathbf{p}_i(t)} \right] \qquad (5)$$

Since a Tamed Snake defined by (5) can be regarded as an energy conserving physical system, we introduce as usual the Rayleigh dissipation functional depending on the viscosity γ in order to stabilise the numerical simulation. Using variational calculus for the derivation of the Euler-Lagrange equations of motion, we end up with (6) describing the motion of all mass points $\mathbf{p}_i$ at the time t:

$$\forall \, \mathbf{p}_i \in \mathcal{P}_k^\sharp : \ \mu_i \frac{\partial^2 \mathbf{p}_i(t)}{\partial t^2} + \gamma_i \frac{\partial \mathbf{p}_i(t)}{\partial t} + \delta_i^{(k)} (\mathbf{p}_i(t) - \mathbf{p}_i(0)) = -\nabla_\perp P(I) \mid_{\mathbf{p}_i(t)} \qquad (6)$$

In order to prevent the control vertices from drifting along the boundary, the gradient of the potential is projected in normal direction of the curve. This operation has been denoted by $\nabla_\perp$ in (6).

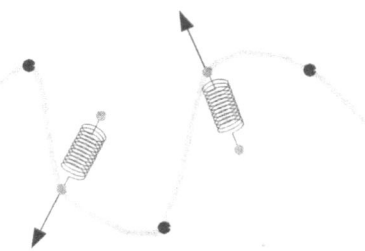

Fig. 6. Springs are attached to all odd vertices $\mathbf{p}_i \in \mathcal{P}_k^\sharp$.

Since we dropped the regularisation term in the energy functional, there are no longer derivatives with respect to a parameterisation along the curve. The odd points of the curve are therefore not correlated during energy minimisation and, as a direct consequence, the physical system degrades to an uncorrelated particle system. For this reason, the governing differential equation (6) is only an ordinary second order differential equation which can be solved for each vertex $\mathbf{p}_i$ separately. Using backward differences and resolving for $\mathbf{p}_i^{[t]}$, a simple discretisation results for numerical simulation, as illustrated in (7), where the symbol p_i represents either the x- or y-component of $\mathbf{p}_i$:

$$p_i^{[t]} = \frac{1}{(\mu_i + \gamma_i + \delta_i^{(k)})} \left[\mu_i(2p_i^{[t-1]} - p_i^{[t-2]}) + \gamma_i p_i^{[t-1]} + \delta_i^{(k)} p_i^{[0]} - \nabla_\perp P(I) \mid_{\mathbf{p}_i^{[t-1]}} \right]$$

(7)

Note, the equations for x- and y-components are semi-linear since they are coupled by the image term $P(I)$ and by the spring term. Fortunately, the latter can be decoupled by replacing the spring with two orthogonal springs in x- and y-direction, respectively.

3   Segmentation Results

Without any prior knowledge of the structure to be segmented, a Tamed Snake must be initialised by a small number of points defining a very rough outline of the shape. The (upper) left images in Fig. 7 and Fig. 8 depict possible initialisations for the segmentation of a bladder and a corpus callosum, respectively. The more points are provided by the human operator, the closer the vertices of the subsequently refined curves are to their correct boundary position. Although the number and position of the initial points are not decisive for the quality of the resulting segmentation, the initialisation has a strong impact on the additional manual editing required for achieving good results. This can be illustrated by the second and third image in Fig. 8, where the initial position of the vertices in the Splenium and the Genu of the corpus callosum must be adjusted manually to bring them into the local neighbourhood of their correct position.

The segmentation itself is a quick interplay between automatic edge tracking and manual manipulation. The optimisation of the boundary position for all odd vertices in the current working level stops as soon as the simulated physical system has reached a stable state. Afterwards, the operator can intervene manually if necessary or proceed to the next finer representation. This iterative refinement of the segmentation is illustrated in Fig. 7 and Fig. 8. The first five images depict the shapes with increasing refinement after edge optimisation and occasional manual corrections where necessary.

Good results can be achieved applying an exponential weighting function to the spring constants $\delta^{(k)} := \delta^{(0)} e^k$. Although the working range for automatic edge tracking consequently becomes very restricted on finer levels, it proved to be necessary to use such a strong weighting function in order to conserve a regular sampling of the curve. Nevertheless, since the prediction of the subdivision scheme is sufficiently precise on fine scales, the exponential weighting is not a restricting limitation of the framework.

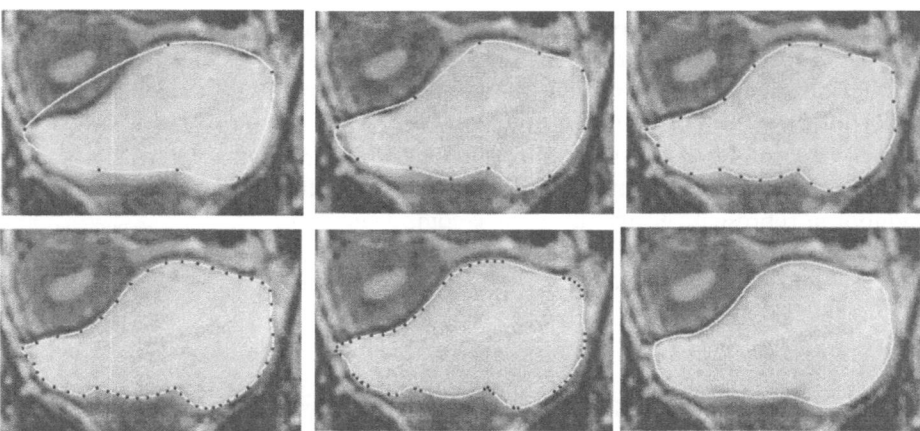

Fig. 7. Segmentation of a bladder with a Tamed Snake. The upper row and the two lower left images depict a Tamed Snake with increasing refinement after edge optimisation and occasional manual modifications. The lower right picture shows the best possible solution with a traditional Snake.

In order to compare the results with traditional approaches, the lower right image in Fig. 7 and the rightmost image in Fig. 8 show the segmentation results achieved with a traditional Snake. While the result for the bladder is, on a coarse scale, of equal quality as the Tamed Snake segmentation, the original Snake is shown to partially fail in the case of the corpus callosum. Although manual editing of the resulting polygonal shape is theoretically possible, it would be a tedious and time consuming task to adjust all the misdirected vertices. Equally time consuming is the manual modification of the bladder-Snake required to capture the intricate details obtained by the Tamed Snake at its finest scale.

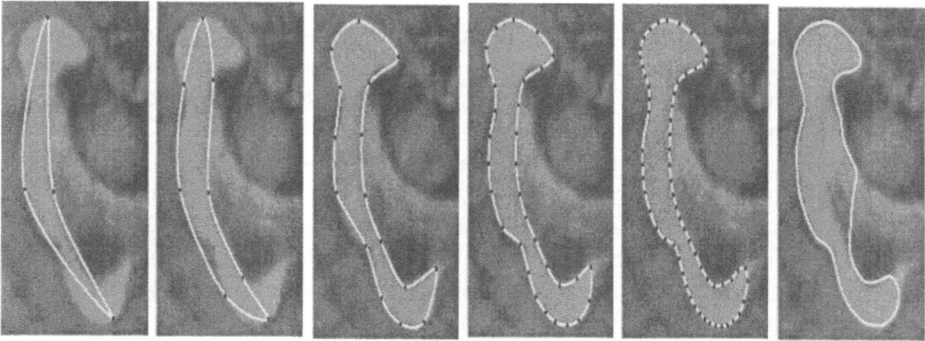

Fig. 8. Segmentation of a corpus callosum with a Tamed Snake. The rightmost picture shows the partial failure of a traditional Snake, in spite of a good manual curve initialisation.

4 Conclusion and Future Research

Tamed Snakes combine powerful editing semantics with traditional edge tracking methods so as to provide a robust segmentation tool. Although Tamed Snakes are, in the case of clear boundaries, not as fast and elegant as traditional Snakes, the advantages of better controllability and stronger editing semantics are, given all considerations, superior to all interactive segmentation algorithms we have tested up to the present day.

Further research has to be carried out in the field of model-based initialisations in order to reduce the necessary initial user interaction. Additionally, we plan to extend Tamed Snakes for the segmentation of three-dimensional medical datasets, where controllability of the shape is even more important than in the two-dimensional case.

References

1. Nira Dyn, David Levin, and John A. Gregory. A 4-point interpolatory subdivision scheme for curve design. *Computer Aided Geometric Design*, 4(4):257–268, 1987.
2. M. A. Fischler, J. M. Tenenbaum, and H. C. Wolf. Detection of roads and linear structures in low-resolution aerial imagery using a multisource knowledge integration technique. *Computer Graphics and Image Processing*, 15:201–233, 1981.
3. David R. Forsey and Richard H. Bartels. Hierarchical B-spline refinement. In *Computer Graphics Proceedings 1988*, pages 205–212. ACM SIGGRAPH, 1988.
4. Steven J. Gortler and Michael F. Cohen. Hierarchical and variational geometric modeling with wavelets. In *1995 Symposium on interactive 3D Graphics*, pages 35–42, April 1995.
5. Michael Kass, Andrew Witkin, and Demetri Terzopoulos. Snakes: Active contour models. *International Journal of Computer Vision*, 1(4):321–331, 1988.
6. F. Leitner, I. Marque, S. Lavallée, and P. Cinquin. Dynamic segmentation: Finding the edge with Snake splines. In *Curves and Surfaces*, pages 279–284, 1991.
7. Haihong Li. *Semi-automatic Road Extraction from Satellite and Aerial Images*. PhD thesis, Swiss Federal Institute of Technology Zürich, Switzerland, 1997.
8. C. Lürig, L. Kobbelt, and T. Ertl. Deformable surfaces for feature based indirect volume rendering. In *Proceedings of CGI98*, pages 752–760, June 1998.
9. Chhandomay Mandal, Baba C. Vemuri, and Hong Qin. A new dynamic FEM-based subdivision surface model for shape recovery and tracking in medical images. In *Proceedings of MICCAI98*, pages 753–760. Springer, October 1998.
10. E. N Mortensen and W. A. Barret. Fast, accurate, and reproducible live-wire boundary extraction. *Proceedings of VBC96*, pages 183–192, September 1996.
11. Walter M. Neuenschwander. *Elastic Deformable Contour and Surface Models for 2-D and 3-D Image Segmentation*. PhD thesis, Swiss Federal Institute of Technology Zürich, Switzerland, 1996.
12. G. Székely, M. Bajka, J. Hug, M. Manestar, P. Groscurth, and U. Haller. Anatomical model generation for laparoscopic surgery simulation. In *The Second Visible Human Project Conference Proceedings*, October 1998.
13. Denis Zorin, Peter Schröder, and Wim Sweldens. Interactive multiresolution mesh editing. In *Computer Graphics Proceedings 1997*, pages 259–268, Los Angeles, August 1997. ACM SIGGRAPH.

Interactive Medical Image Segmentation with United Snakes

Jianming Liang[1,2], Tim McInerney[2,3], and Demetri Terzopoulos[2]

[1] Turku Centre for Computer Science, DataCity, Lemminkäisenkatu 14 A, 20520 Turku, Finland
[2] Department of Computer Science, University of Toronto, 6 King's College Road, Toronto, ON M5S 3H5, Canada
[3] Department of Math, Physics and Computer Science, Ryerson Polytechnic University, Toronto, ON M5B 2K3, Canada

Abstract. Snakes have become a standard image analysis technique with several variants now in common use. We have developed a software package called "United Snakes". It unifies the most important snake variants, including finite difference, B-spline, and Hermite polynomial snakes, within the framework of a general finite element formulation with a choice of shape functions. Furthermore, we have incorporated into united snakes a recently proposed snake-like technique known as "livewire", via a method for imposing hard constraints on snakes. Here, we demonstrate that the combination of techniques in united snakes yields generality, accuracy, ease of use, and robustness in several medical image analysis applications, including the segmentation of neuronal dendrites in EM images, dynamic chest image analysis, and the quantification of growth plates.

1 Introduction

Snakes (active contour models) [8] have met the challenge of extracting clinically useful information from medical images in numerous applications to a wide range of medical image analysis tasks, including segmentation, registration, tracking, and shape analysis [14, 18]. Extensive research activity worldwide over the past decade has resulted in a host of snake variants (e.g., finite element snakes [5], B-snakes [15, 3], Fourier snakes [19]) as well as snake-like "livewire" techniques [16, 2, 17, 6]. The result is a confusing array of choices for the user.

There exists a need for definitive software which unites the best features of the various snake(-like) techniques in a portable, reusable package. To this end, we have developed *United Snakes* [11] in Java as a JavaBean (reusable Java software component). United snakes unify the most important snakes variants, including finite difference, B-spline, and Hermite polynomial snakes, in a comprehensive finite element framework, where any particular type of snake can be chosen by simply changing the finite element shape functions. Furthermore, united snakes combine snakes and livewire via a simple yet effective method for imposing constraints.

Hence, we offer a general purpose tool for interactive medical image analysis that provides more flexible control than its component techniques alone while reducing the need for user interaction. In the remainder of the paper, we will describe united snakes and demonstrate their generality, accuracy, ease of use, and robustness using clinical images from several different medical image analysis projects.

2   United Snakes

This section presents a non-mathematical description of united snakes. The relevant mathematical formulations are found in [11]).

2.1   Snakes

A snake is a dynamical system taking the form of a parametric contour in the image plane, whose shape is dictated by a potential energy comprising a contour deformation term and an image term. The final shape of the snake results when the dynamical system reaches equilibrium, corresponding to a minimum of the potential energy. Traditionally, a snake is initialized manually by the user or automatically through image processing operators with a rough approximation to an image feature of interest (edge, boundary, etc.). If the snake has been initialized appropriately, it will accurately localize and conform to the image feature. With a dynamic snake it is natural to incorporate user guidance via constraints in order to drive the snake out of one local energy minimum into another, and it is also possible to track moving objects in image sequences.

2.2   Finite Element Framework

Several variants of the original finite difference formulation [8] have been proposed in an effort to improve its performance in some respect (e.g. to decrease initialization sensitivity, increase the range of object shapes that can be modeled, decrease noise susceptibility, improve segmentation reproducibility for a class of objects, etc.). Finite element snakes [5, 13], B-snakes [15, 3], and Fourier descriptor snakes [19] are representative examples of these variants.

We have unified several snake variants within a finite element framework with different shape functions: Hermitian, B-spline, NURBS [20], Catmull-Rom, Bézier, Fourier, and Dirac delta. The shape functions generate different stiffness matrices and, in turn, yield different snake behaviors suitable for different tasks. For example, snakes that use B-spline shape functions are typically characterized by a low number of degrees of freedom, typically use polynomial basis functions of degree 2 or higher, and are inherently very smooth. Therefore, these "B-snakes" [15, 3] can be effective in segmentation or tracking tasks involving noisy images and where the target object boundaries may exhibit significant gaps in the images. Alternatively, object boundaries with many fine details or rapid curvature variations may best be segmented by a snake that uses simpler shape functions and many degrees of freedom such as the finite difference snake [8]. The unification of different shape functions in a single framework enhances the range of object modeling capabilities.

2.3   Initialization

An accurate initialization is generally needed in order for the snake to lock onto the image features. Therefore, researchers have been actively investigating techniques to mitigate the sensitivity of snakes to their initialization. Among these techniques is the use of an inflation force [5], the use of a chamfer distance map [5] and gradient vector flow [21]. These techniques can work well if the image feature map is relatively clean. However, most clinical images are noisy, contain many uninteresting edges, or texture is present. Hence, these more automatic techniques do not work as expected. For this reason, we are exploring an alternative direction—instead of attempting to automatically remove or decrease initialization sensitivity, we seek to increase the efficiency of interactive initialization. In particular, we enable the user to initialize snakes quickly and with minimal effort by exploiting the strengths of the livewire technique.

2.4 Livewire

Livewire is a recently proposed interactive boundary tracing technique [16, 2, 17, 6]. Although it shares some similarities with snakes—it was originally developed as an interactive 2-D extension to previous stage-wise optimal boundary tracking methods— it is generally considered in the literature as a competing technique to snakes. Like snakes, the idea behind the livewire technique is to allow image segmentation to occur with minimal user interaction, while at the same time allowing the user to exercise control over the segmentation process. However, livewire realizes the idea differently from snakes.

In livewire, the user places an initial *seed* point near the boundary of the object of interest to begin the segmentation process. As the cursor, or *free* point is moved around, the current calculated boundary, the *livewire* or *trace*, is interactively displayed from the seed point to the free point. If the displayed trace is acceptable, the free point may be collected as an additional seed point, and the trace between the two adjacent seed points is frozen (locked). Each trace given by the livewire is the path with minimal cost between the two seed points resulting from the application of two-dimensional dynamic programming [6] or Dijkstra's graph search algorithm [17] with a local cost function. The local cost function assigns a lower cost to image features, such as edges, and consequently the livewire tends to stick to the object boundary guided with the seed points from the user. The resulting livewire boundaries are piecewise optimal (*i.e.* optimal between seed points), while the snake gives a global optimal solution over the entire contour.

2.5 Union of Snakes and Livewire

With livewire, the user has no control of the traces between seed points other than by backtracking. When the shape of the object boundary is complex, or when it is near other strong but uninteresting object boundaries, many seed points are needed in order to generate an acceptable result. Furthermore, when a section of the desired object boundary has a weak edge relative to a nearby strong edge, the livewire snaps to the strong edge rather than the desired weaker boundary. A method called *on-the-fly training* has been proposed to mitigate this problem [17]. However, the method relies on the assumption that the edge property is relatively consistent along the object boundary.

Livewire is fundamentally image-based. Thus, it cannot effectively bridge gaps where the desired object boundaries are missing, and the smoothness of the traces cannot be guaranteed. Therefore, it is desirable to allow the user to exercise control over the livewire traces between seed points, impose smoothness on livewire traces, and bridge gaps along object boundaries. This is what snakes are very good at doing. Snakes adhere to edges with sub-pixel accuracy and they may also be adjusted interactively as parametric curves with intuitively familiar physical behaviors. Moreover, unlike livewire, snakes have the power to track moving objects.

In most cases, however, livewire can quickly give much better results than casual manual tracing. Hence, the resulting livewire boundary can serve to quickly and effectively initialize a snake. The livewire seed points carry the user's prior knowledge of the object boundary. They can therefore serve as either hard or soft point constraints for the snake, depending on the user's confidence in the accuracies of the livewire seed points.

Because a livewire-traced initial object boundary is usually more accurate than a hand-drawn boundary, the incorporation of the seed points provided by the livewire trace as snake constraints results in a snake that very quickly locks onto the desired object boundary. If necessary, the user may correct errors inherited from the livewire-generated boundary, by applying mouse-controlled spring forces to the snake. Because the user still has the opportunity to correct the errors on the traces as the snake is deforming, the number of seed points needed to generate the initial livewire object boundary can be further reduced.

The combination of snakes and livewire relies on an efficient constraint mechanism. A constraint on a snake may be either soft or hard. Hard constraints generally compel the snake to pass through certain positions or take certain shapes [7, 1], while soft constraints merely encourage a snake to do so. Two kinds of soft constraints, springs and volcanos, were described in the original finite difference snakes paper [8] and they are incorporated into our finite element formulation. A simple yet efficient way to impose hard constraints on snakes for the integration of snakes and livewire is to properly update the stiffness matrix and encode constraint values in the system force vector. This approach maintains the symmetry of the stiffness matrix for economical skyline storage and efficient computation via a single factorization [11]. Since they are encoded in the system force vector, the constraint values may be updated and other hard (or soft) constraints may be added as the snake is deforming. Therefore, the user may dynamically adjust the constraints to refine the object boundary during snake deformation.

2.6 Summary

To summarize, the united snakes software unites several snake variants with livewire to provide a general purpose tool for interactive medical image segmentation which amplifies the efficiency, flexibility, and reproducibility of the component techniques. United snakes offer more control for relatively less user interaction. As it quickly locks onto the image features of interest with reasonable tolerance to errors in the livewire, the snake fully exploits the user guidance and expert prior knowledge reflected captured by the initial livewire trace.

As an initial demonstration that united snakes improves upon the robustness and accuracy of its component techniques, Fig. 1 shows a synthetic image of a known curve degraded with strong Gaussian white noise (variance 0.25). Given its image-based nature, the livewire is sensitive to noise as shown in Fig. 1(a). A snake initialized with the livewire gives a better result (Fig. 1(b)). Fig. 1(c) shows that the united snakes result

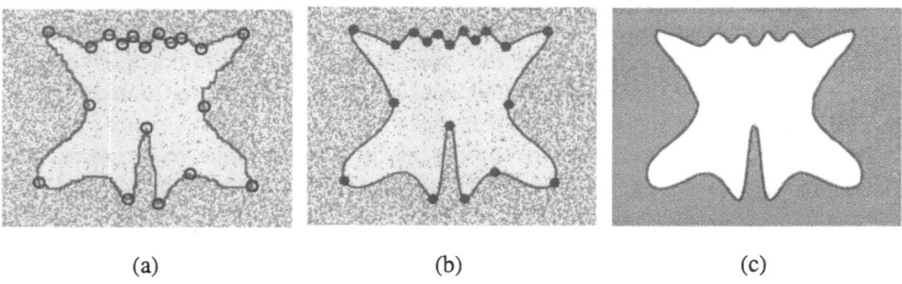

(a)   (b)   (c)

Fig. 1. Performance of united snakes demonstrated using a synthetic image with strong Gaussian white noise (variance 0.25). (a) A livewire is sensitive to noise (the required seed points are shown). (b) The united snake is robust to noise and accurately conforms to the boundary. (c) The united snake segmentation is close to the ideal boundary. The superior performance is a consequence of the imposed hard constraints (indicated by asterisks in (b)), without which the snake would slip away from high curvature points.

is very close to the boundary in the ideal image, despite the strong noise. This performance is a consequence of the imposed hard constraints, without which the snake would slip away from high curvature points.

3 Applications

In this section, we demonstrate the potential of the united snakes technique in a series of experiments with medical images.

3.1 Segmenting Neuronal Dendrites in EM Images

A neuronal dendrite is the receiving unit of a nerve cell. The area of contact between the dendrites of different cells is called a synapse and is located on the dendritic spines. In humans, changes in dendritic spines are seen with aging and with diseases that affect the nervous system, such as dementia, brain tumors and epilepsy [4]. Detailed anatomical models of dendritic spines and their synapses will provide new insights into their function, thus providing better opportunities to understand the underlying causes and effects of these diseases. To build such models, the dendrite must be segmented from the surrounding tissue in positive electron micrography (see [4] for a detailed description of how snakes are used in reconstruction of 3D nerve cell models from serial microscopy). Here, we are interested in localizing nerve cell membranes, which appear dark in positive micrography.

In the United Snakes system, the user begins an image segmentation task using a livewire. An initial seed point is placed near the boundary of the object of interest. As the cursor, or free point, is moved around, the livewire, or trace, is interactively displayed from the seed point to the free point. If the displayed trace is acceptable, the free point is collected as an additional seed point.

We can capture an approximate cell boundary in Fig. 2(a) with just three seeds. The livewire tends to stick to the object boundary using the seed points as a guide. The trace between the two adjacent seeds is frozen. The user has no further control over these traces other than backtracking. In order to generate a more accurate result in the area indicated by a rectangle, more seed points may be placed as in Fig. 2(b). Although the livewire boundary is somewhat jagged and exhibits some small errors, it is in general as accurate as manual tracing, but more efficient and reproducible.

Next, we instantiate a snake using the livewire-generated boundary to initialize the snake and using the seed points to constrain it. The user may select a shape function for the snake which is suitable for the object boundary. In our cell segmentation example, if the livewire result with five seed points is used to construct a finite difference snake, it is able to tolerate the livewire errors and very quickly and accurately lock onto the cell boundary without any need for further user interaction (Fig. 2(c)). Using the livewire result with three seed points, the snake becomes "stuck" in the problematic area (Fig. 2(d)) due to the livewire-generated boundary errors. However, this situation can be easily remedied using the mouse spring (Fig. 2(e)). Furthermore, as the snake is deforming, the hard constraints may be adjusted to refine the snake boundary. In Fig. 2(f) for example, constraint point 2 is moved to illustrate this snake boundary adjustment capability. By contrast, it is not nearly as easy to adjust a seed point in the livewire algorithm.

We refer to this form of livewire-snake integration as *static* integration—once the livewire result is used to initialize a snake, the segmentation process continues using only the constrained, user-controlled snake. The user may also set the united snake system to a more *dynamic* integration "mode"—once the livewire trace between the last seed point and the free point is formed, a corresponding open snake with constraints at the seed point and the free point is constructed and automatically set in motion for deformation. When the free point is collected as a seed point, this open snake is merged with the snake constructed from the previous livewire traces (if they exist). All seed points are automatically applied as constraints. Fig. 3 illustrates this process where "+" indicates the current free point. The livewire and snake results are shown separately in 3(a) and (b) respectively. Since the snake is automatically set in motion, the user may use the mouse spring to correct it in any problematic areas along the snake (Fig. 3(c)).

3.2 Dynamic Chest Image Analysis

The aim of the dynamic chest image analysis project is to show focal and general abnormalities of lung ventilation and perfusion based on a sequence of digital chest fluoroscopy frames collected over a short time period (typically about 4 seconds) [10, 12, 9]. The project uses only plain X-ray fluoroscopy (with and without breathing) for the ventilation and perfusion studies. Consequently, the radiation dose to patients is low and, unlike a nuclear medicine scan, no preparation is required before the examination and radioactive isotopes are unnecessary. The information gleaned from these images is helpful in several aspects of cardiothoracic radiology. Diseases directly related to the parameters being measured include pulmonary embolism, pulmonary emphysema, cardiac failure, congenital heart disease and other diseases (tumors, obstructive lesions or infections) which may change pulmonary ventilation and/or perfusion. An essential

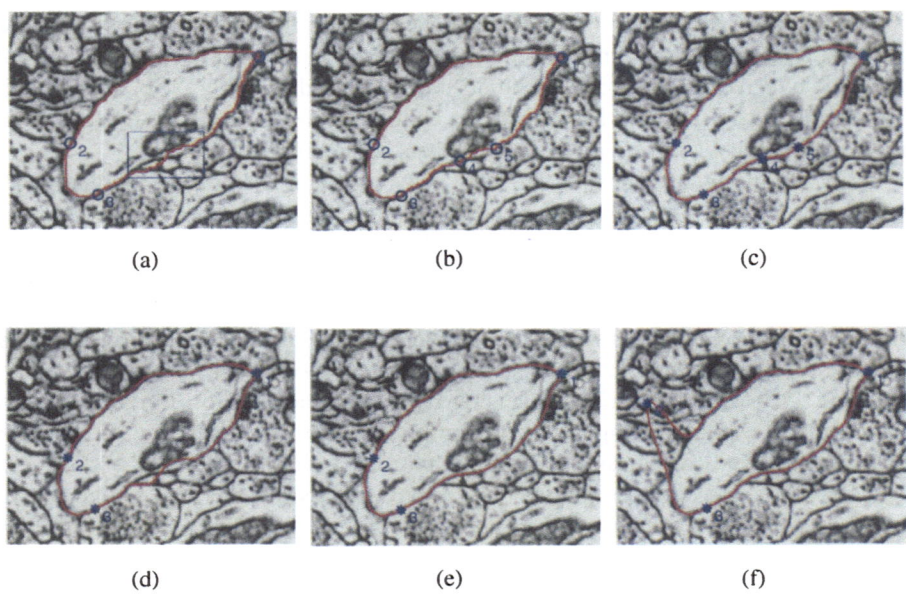

Fig. 2. Using united snakes in static mode to segment neuronal EM images. (a) Approximate livewire boundary using just 3 seeds (blue rectangle indicates a problem area). (b) Additional seed points can improve livewire's accuracy. (c) Initialized from the livewire in (b), the snake tolerates livewire errors and locks on cell boundary without further user interaction. (d) Initialized from the livewire in (a), the snake "sticks" in the problem area, but it is easily adjusted (e) using the mouse. (f) Snake adjustment capability illustrated by moving constraint point 2.

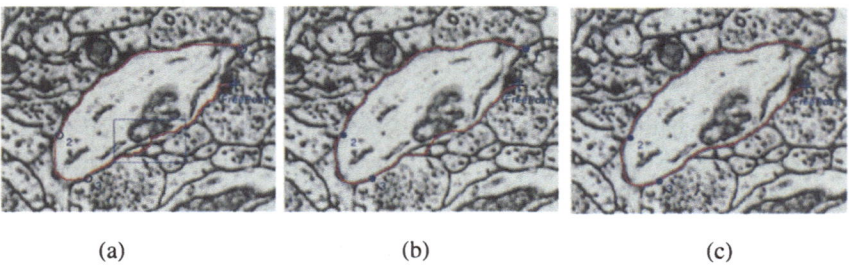

Fig. 3. Using united snakes in dynamic mode to segment neuronal EM images. (a) Livewire boundary showing 3 seeds and free point (blue rectangle indicates a problem area). (b) Open snakes dynamically generated from the livewire trace and constrained by seed and free points. (c) Third snake corrected in the problem area using the mouse.

first step for ventilation and perfusion analysis is the delineation of the lungs and the heart from each frame in a chest image sequence. The united snakes system is used to perform the delineation. Typically most of the user interactions to initialize and edit the snake are applied to the first image of the sequence only. The resulting snake is then propagated and deformed through the remaining frames of the image sequence.

As the chest image (Fig. 4(a)) shows, some segments of the lung boundary have strong edges and some segments are rather weak. The elliptical viewport generates very strong edges, consequently, part of the livewire between seed point 4 and seed point 1 snaps to the strong viewpoint edges rather than the desired lung boundary (Fig. 4(b)). On-the-fly training is not effective since the lung boundary does not exhibit consistent edge properties. Thus, the livewire alone requires much backtracking and many seed points (Fig. 4(c)) to generate an accurate lung boundary.

We construct a Hermite snake from the livewire traces in Fig. 4(b) and the first seed is used as a hard constraint on the snake since the edge information there is very weak. The snake can easily be pulled out of the strong edge and locked onto the lung boundary (as shown in Fig. 4(d)) without the use of on-the-fly training. Thanks to this hard constraint, it can firmly stick to the lung apex and follow the lung motion throughout the entire chest image sequence with minimal user interaction, by propagating the result from one frame to next frame. The first image contains the largest lung boundary in the sequence while the smallest lung boundary is shown in Fig. 4(e). Fig. 4(f) shows an additional example.

In the case of the heart, Fig. 5(a) illustrates that part of the livewire trace from seed point 1 to seed point 2 is a straight line where the cardiac boundary is missing. Furthermore, at the bottom of the image, the livewire technique does not generate an acceptable cardiac boundary (i.e. from seed point 3 to seed point 1), so we have manually drawn a rough curve between the points. A least squares approximation to the initial livewire curve with a cubic B-spline with 5 knots (shown in Fig. 5(b)) can be used as an initialization to a B-snake. A hard constraint may be further imposed on control polygon node 3 to effectively bridge the gap along the heart boundary. The result is shown in Fig. 5(c) after only a few iterations. The B-snake then is used to track the heart motion through the image sequence.

3.3 Quantifying Growth Plates in MR images

The aim of the growth plate project is to determine the right time for surgery for patients with abnormal growth of the legs. To this end, the four tiny (essentially horizontal) lines in the image (Fig. 6(a)) must be detected to quantify the growth plate.

In this scenario, it is difficult for the user to manually trace an initial contour for a snake because of the small size of the lines and the small distance between each pair of lines. However, livewires can be used to quickly generate an acceptable snake initialization with just two or three seed points as shown in Fig. 6(b). In the final results shown in Fig. 6(c), two hard boundary conditions are applied on each of four finite difference snakes.

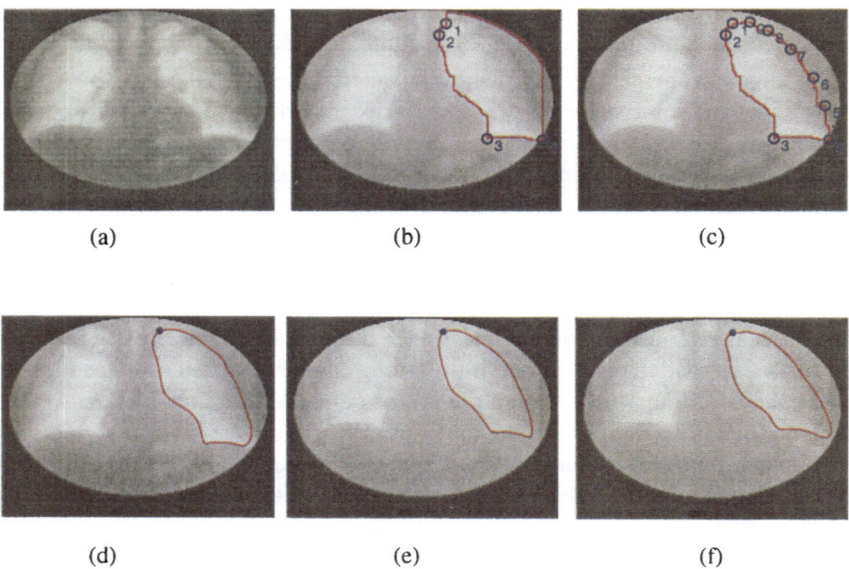

Fig. 4. Lung delineation in X-ray fluoroscopy image sequence. (a) First image in sequence. (b) Livewire generated boundary. (c) Livewire trace requires backtracking and additional seed points to correct boundary delineation. (d) Hermite snake constructed from livewire trace in (b) and constrained by seed point 1. (e–f) Segmentation of other images in the sequence.

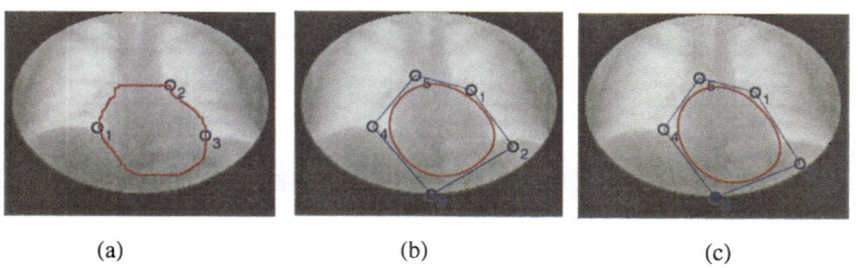

Fig. 5. Heart delineation in X-ray fluoroscopy image sequence. (a) Initial livewire generated boundary. (b) Initial B-spline snake (red) and control polygon (blue) constructed from livewire trace. Control point 3 is used as a hard constraint. (c) Resulting segmentation.

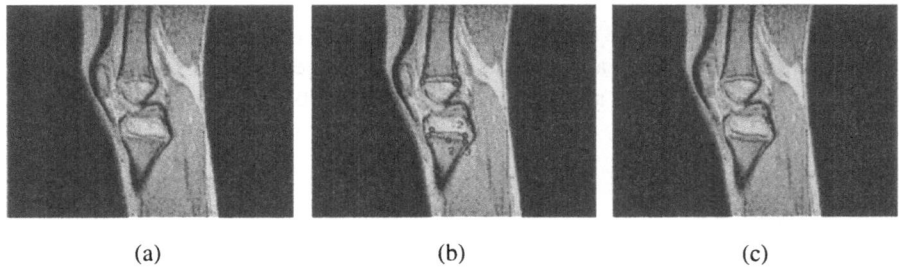

Fig. 6. Quantifying growth plates in MR images. (a) An MR growth plate image. (b) The livewire results. (c) The united snakes results.

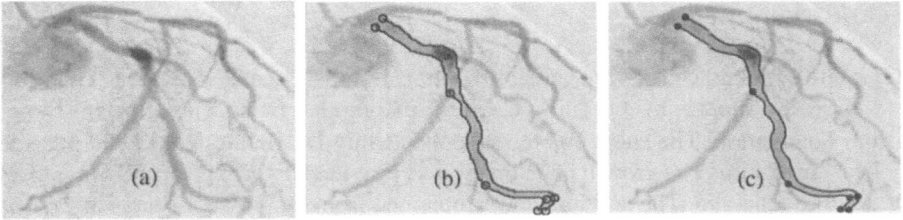

Fig. 7. Segmenting a vessel in an angiogram. (a) The image used in [17]. (b) Livewire segmentation. (c) United snake generates boundaries comparable to *ideal* boundaries in [17].

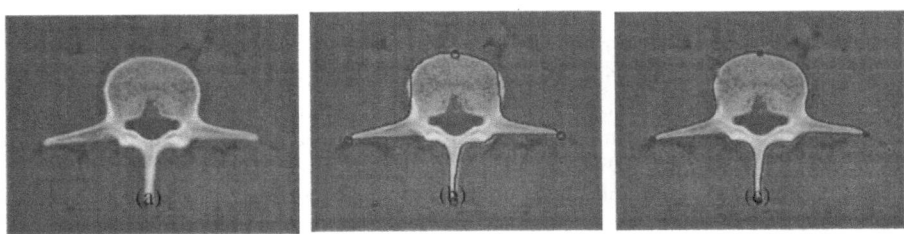

Fig. 8. Segmenting the outer boundary of a vertebra. (a) The image used in [17]. (b) Livewire segmentation. (c) United snake boundary is comparable to the *ideal* boundary in [17].

3.4   Other Segmentation Examples

We have applied united snakes to two other medical images, an angiogram (Fig. 7) and a vertebra image (Fig. 8), to which Mortensen and Barrett applied their livewire algorithm in [17]. With only a few seeds, united snakes generate the boundaries shown in Figs. 7(c) and 8(c), which are comparable to the ideal boundaries used as references in [17].

4   Conclusion

We have developed a software package called "United Snakes" which unites several snake variants with livewire to offer a general purpose tool for interactive medical image segmentation and tracking. The union of these techniques provides more flexible control than the individual techniques while reducing user interaction. We have demonstrated the generality, accuracy and robustness of united snakes in applications to the segmentation of neuronal dendrites in EM images, to dynamic chest image analysis, and to the quantification of growth plates, among other segmentation examples. It appears that united snakes are in several ways superior to livewire or snakes alone.

Acknowledgments

JL gratefully acknowledges the valuable comments and suggestions of Prof. Timo Järvi as well as the support of the Turku Centre for Computer Science and the Instrumentarium Foundation. The chest image was collected by Dr. Raimo Virkki and provided by Dr. Aaro Kiuru. The growth plate image was provided by Prof. Martti Kormano and Dr. Matti Sauna-aho. The cell image was obtained from Dr. Kristen Harris of the Harvard Medical School. The angiogram and spine images were provided courtesy Eric Mortensen of Brigham Young University.

References

1. A. Amini, T. Weymouth, and R. Jain. Using dynamic programming for solving variational problems in vision. *IEEE Trans. on Pattern Analysis and Machine Intelligence*, 12(9):855–867, 1990.
2. W. Barrett and E. Mortensen. Interactive live-wire boundary extraction. *Medical Image Analysis*, 1(4):331–341, 1997.
3. A. Blake and M. Isard. *Active Contours*. Springer-Verlag, 1998.
4. I. Carlbom, D. Terzopoulos, and K. Harris. Computer-assisted registration, segmentation, and 3D reconstruction from images of neuronal tissue sections. *IEEE Trans. on Medical Imaging*, 13(2):351–362, 1994.
5. L. Cohen and I. Cohen. Finite element methods for active contour models and balloons for 2D and 3D images. *IEEE Trans. on Pattern Analysis and Machine Intelligence*, 15(11):1131–1147, 1993.
6. A. X. Falão, J. K. Udupa, S. Samarasekera, and S. Sharma. User-steered image segmentation paradigms: Live wire and live lane. *Graphical Models and Image Processing*, 60:233–260, 1998.

7. P. Fua and C. Brechbühler. Imposing hard constraints on deformable models through optimization in orthogonal subspaces. *Computer Vision and Image Understanding*, 65:148–162, 1997.

8. M. Kass, A. Witkin, and D. Terzopoulos. Snakes: Active contour models. *International Journal of Computer Vision*, 1(4):321–331, 1988.

9. J. Liang, A. Haapanen, T. Järvi, A. Kiuru, M. Kormano, E. Svedström, and R. Virkki. Dynamic chest image analysis: Model-based pulmonary perfusion analysis with pyramid images. In E. A. Hoffman, editor, *Medical Imaging 1998: Physiology and Function from Multidimensional Images*, pages 63–72, San Diego, CA, 1998.

10. J. Liang, T. Järvi, A. Kiuru, M. Kormano, E. Svedström, and R. Virkki. Dynamic chest image analysis: Model-based ventilation study with pyramid images. In E. A. Hoffman, editor, *Medical Imaging 1997: Physiology and Function from Multidimensional Images*, pages 81–92, Newport Beach, CA, 1997.

11. J. Liang, T. McInerney, and D. Terzopoulos. United snakes. In *Proc. Seventh International Conf. on Computer Vision (ICCV'99)*, Kerkyra (Corfu), Greece, September 1999. IEEE Computer Society Press.

12. J. Liang, R. Virkki, T. Järvi, A. Kiuru, M. Kormano, and E. Svedström. Dynamic chest image analysis: Evaluation of model-based ventilation study with pyramid images. In R. Zurawski and Z.-Q. Liu, editors, *IEEE First International Conference on Intelligent Processing Systems*, pages 989–993, Beijing, China, 1997.

13. T. McInerney and D. Terzopoulos. A dynamic finite element surface model for segmentation and tracking in multidimensional medical images with application to cardiac 4D image analysis. *Computerized Medical Imaging and Graphics*, 19(1):69–83, 1995.

14. T. McInerney and D. Terzopoulos. Deformable models in medical image analysis: A survey. *Medical Image Analysis*, 1(2):91–108, 1996.

15. S. Menet, P. Saint-Marc, and G. Medioni. B-snakes: Implementation and application to stereo. In *Proceedings DARPA*, pages 720–726, 1990.

16. E. N. Mortensen and W. A. Barrett. Intelligent scissors for image composition. In *Proceedings of Computer Graphics (SIGGRAPH'95)*, pages 191–198, Los Angeles, CA, August 1995.

17. E. N. Mortensen and W. A. Barrett. Interactive segmentation with intelligent scissors. *Graphical Models and Image Processing*, 60:349–384, 1998.

18. A. Singh, D. Goldgof, and D. Terzopoulos, editors. *Deformable Models in Medical Image Analysis*. IEEE Computer Society Press, 1998.

19. L. Staib and J. Duncan. Boundary finding with parametrically deformable models. *IEEE Trans. on Pattern Analysis and Machine Intelligence*, 14(11):1061–1075, 1992.

20. D. Terzopoulos and H. Qin. Dynamic NURBS with geometric constraints for interactive sculpting. *ACM Transactions on Graphics*, 13(2):103–136, 1994.

21. C. Xu and J. L. Prince. Snakes, shapes, and gradient vector flow. *IEEE Transactions on Image Processing*, 7(3):359–369, 1998.

Active Shape Model-Based Segmentation of Digital X-ray Images

G. Behiels[1], D. Vandermeulen[1], F. Maes[1], P. Suetens[1], and P. Dewaele[2]

[1] Medical Image Computing, Katholieke Universiteit Leuven, Leuven, Belgium
[2] Agfa-Gevaert NV, Mortsel, Belgium

Abstract. We propose an improved search procedure for Active Shape Model (ASM) based delineation of anatomical structures in digital X-ray images. Whereas the original ASM search method [1] iteratively improves the current estimate of the location of boundary points by a limited least squares adjustment of the pose and shape parameters, our method additionally requires the subsequent changes in shape during the search to be smooth, which is achieved by using a minimum cost path search algorithm. We compare the two methods on a database of more than 400 manual segmentations of digital X-ray images of the femur, humerus and calcaneus. We evaluate the accuracy and robustness of both methods using a cross-validation procedure.

1 Introduction

Accurate detection and segmentation of anatomical structures is an essential component in many biomedical image analysis procedures. Delineation of bone structures, for instance in digital X-ray (DRX) images, is a prerequisite in many orthopaedic examinations. Since manual delineation of these anatomical structures is very tedious and time consuming, fast and accurate computer-aided segmentation methods are required.

Cootes et al. [1] represent objects as sets of labeled points and examine the statistics of their coordinates over a number of training examples. The characteristic pattern of a shape class is described by the average shape vector and a linear combination of eigenvectors of the variations around the average shape. These representations are called Point Distribution Models (PDM). During image search, new target points, e.g. edges, are searched in a region of the image around each model point and the model is updated to best fit these new target points. This update consists of two steps. First, the pose parameters (rotation, translation, scaling) are determined, and second, the remaining residuals are projected onto the eigenvector basis. The resulting shape parameters are limited to ensure that the current shape remains similar to the training set. In the context of locating object boundaries in images using an iterative search algorithm to fit the statistical object model to the image data, Point Distribution Models are coined Active Shape Models (ASM).

A shortcoming of this search method, however, is the independent estimation of each point to a new target position by a local search along the normal direction toward the strongest image edges. Inaccuracies in this estimation, e.g. edges corresponding to a different object, cannot be accommodated for appropriately by the pose and shape parameters, even when using a different criterion for positioning new target points like maximum similarity of grey level profiles [2].

We therefore propose to estimate the position of new target points while incorporating a regularisation term imposing smoothness of shape changes. New target point positions are determined using a minimum cost path search algorithm before the adjustment of pose and shape parameters.

2   Point Distribution Model: Capturing Shape Statistics

Point Distribution Models represent each object boundary as a vector s of boundary point coordinates: $s = (x_0 \ y_0 \ x_1 \ y_1 \ \ldots \ x_n \ y_n)^T$. These boundary points correspond to expert-labeled landmark points on examples of objects belonging to the same shape class. To eliminate changes in scale, rotation and translation, shapes in the training set are aligned by minimizing a weighted sum of squared distances between corresponding points on the different examples of the training set for a single shape class [4]. The average or mean shape $\bar{s}$ and the covariance matrix C_{tr} of variations about the mean are computed. The eigenvectors p_k of the covariance matrix represent an orthogonal basis of linear deformation modes that describe how landmark points tend to move together as the shape varies. The eigenvalue λ_k associated to each eigenvector p_k is equal to the variance explained by each linear deformation mode. Each shape s of the training set can then be represented as a weighted sum of the eigenvectors p_k and the mean $\bar{s}$, $s = \bar{s} + Pb$, wherein $P = (p_1 \ p_2 \ \ldots \ p_{2n})$ is a matrix with the eigenvectors as its columns, and $b = (b_1 \ b_2 \ \ldots \ b_{2n})$ the vector of weights or the shape coefficients of the shape in our the model-space $(\bar{s}, P)$. Suitable limits for the shape parameters are, for example, $-3\sqrt{\lambda_k} \leq b_k \leq 3\sqrt{\lambda_k}$. Because most of the variance is explained by the eigenvectors with the largest eigenvalue, the number of eigenvectors can be limited to $t < 2n$, defined e.g. as the smallest number of modes such that the sum $\sum_{i=1}^{t} \lambda_i$ of variance explained, is a sufficiently large proportion of the total variance, $\lambda_T = \sum_{i=1}^{2n} \lambda_i$. In our experiments we choose t to be the smallest number satisfying the following condition

$$\frac{\sum_{i=1}^{t} \lambda_i}{\lambda_T} > 0.9$$

thus explaining more than 90% of the variance of the training set.

Each PDM for a particular shape class is built using a bootstrap-procedure. The first image is presented to a trained expert who carefully delineates the object. For the next three images, the first delineation can be interactively transformed and the shape boundary points are manually adjusted to the correct object boundary. After these four manual segmentations, a shape model is computed and used to automatically segment the other images. Each presented solution can be edited before it is in turn added to the shape model.

3   Image Model: Capturing Image Appearance

Given a shape model and an image containing an example of the modelled shape class, detection or segmentation of the object involves searching for the model parameters that best fit the model to the image. The image model defines which image feature and/or which similarity function to use for measuring the quality of the fit of the model to the image data. During optimization, new target point positions that best fit the image model are searched for in a local neighborhood. In the original ASM implementation, these points were defined to have the highest image gradient magnitude within a search window, along a line normal to the current estimate of the contour.

Similarly to [2] where different image models on photographic images of a human face are compared, we observed that searching for the highest gradient point is not the most reliable measure to define the boundary. We performed an extensive test on a database of over 400 digital X-rays of 6 different bone structures such as the femur, humerus, etc. By way of example we show the results pictorially for the femur. In Fig. 1, one image of the training set is shown together with the manual delineation as a solid line. For each of the 104 examples of femur images, we virtually displaced each contour point to the point with the largest gradient magnitude within a local search interval of 20 pixels along the normal to the contour. The mean displacement over all images for each contour point is displayed as a circle in Fig. 1 together with the corresponding standard deviation as a bar through these circles. We observe that there is a strong bias and variance for those contour points in areas of weak contrast and vice versa for contour points on strong edges.

Alternative image appearance models define a similarity measure on image feature values along one-dimensional profiles normal to the contour. Similarly to the boundary point coordinates, these profiles can be modelled during a learning phase as follows. Each profile g of the training set can be represented by the mean profile $\bar{g}$ and a number of modes of variation P_g

$$g = \bar{g} + P_g b_g$$

A suitable similarity measure defining the fit of a new input profile x with n_p points to the model profile is given by the Mahalanobis distance M

$$M = \sum_{j=1}^{n_p} \frac{b_{gj}}{\lambda_j} \tag{1}$$

wherein b_{gj} is the projection of the input pattern x onto the j-the eigenvector p_{gj}. If we only use a limited number of eigenvectors t_g, Equation (1) can be approximated by (see [2])

$$F = \sum_{j=1}^{t_g} \frac{b_{gj}^2}{\lambda_j} + \frac{2\epsilon^2}{\lambda_{t_g}} \tag{2}$$

wherein ϵ^2 is the sum of squares of differences between the input pattern x and the reconstruction of this pattern $\bar{g} + P_g b_g$.

We compared four different image features g (intensity, normalized intensity, gradient, normalized gradient) on the database. We graphically show the results for the femur in Fig. 1 and summarize the results for the other structures in Table 1. From these experiments, we conclude that normalized intensities are the better image features in combination with the Mahalanobis distance similarity measure.

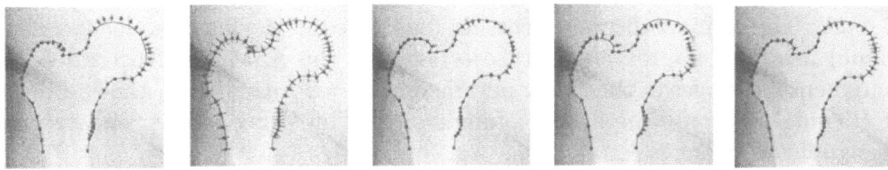

Fig. 1. Mean error (*circle*) and standard deviation (*bars*) for a local search along the normals using the gradient-magnitude or (2). The first image displays the results for a local search to the image points with the largest magnitude of the gradient. The second image displays the results for intensity profiles, the third represents normalized intensity and the fourth and fifth respectively gradient and normalized gradient profiles.

Table 1. Mean error and standard deviation when searching for the maximum gradient (Δ) and for profile matching using intensity (I), normalized intensity ($\tilde{I}$), gradient (G) and normalized gradient ($\tilde{G}$) profiles.

	Δ	I	$\tilde{I}$	G	$\tilde{G}$
calcaneus	1.81 ± 2.59	5.73 ± 6.96	1.46 ± 2.36	1.95 ± 2.87	1.61 ± 2.50
femur(de,lv)	1.74 ± 2.73	5.56 ± 6.67	1.26 ± 2.14	1.77 ± 2.88	1.46 ± 2.30
femur(pe,vv)	2.19 ± 2.63	6.14 ± 7.24	1.20 ± 2.16	2.48 ± 2.96	1.96 ± 2.68
femur(de,vv)	1.54 ± 2.46	5.91 ± 7.01	1.17 ± 1.94	1.56 ± 2.69	1.17 ± 2.10
tibia	2.01 ± 2.75	5.11 ± 6.25	1.30 ± 1.98	2.25 ± 2.91	1.79 ± 2.55
humerus	0.99 ± 1.83	5.35 ± 7.71	0.89 ± 1.74	1.16 ± 2.00	0.99 ± 1.75

4   Search Algorithms

Given the statistical shape and image appearance models for a particular structure in a particular imaging modality, our aim is to use them to segment these structures into new images by searching for the shape parameters $b = (b_1 \; b_2 \; \dots \; b_t)^T$ and pose parameters (scale s, rotation θ and translation t_x and t_y) that best fit the model to the data. In Sect. 4.1, we explain the original search algorithm used by Cootes et al. [3] and in Sect. 4.2 we explain the modifications we propose to constrain the search procedure.

4.1   Iterative Search

Given an initial estimate of the pose and shape parameters of an instance of the object in the image, a region of the image around each boundary point is examined to determine a displacement required to move that point to a better image position. In our implementation we search along the normal to the curve for that point with the smallest Mahalanobis distance (or its approximation given by (2)) between the model profile and the image feature profile centered at that point. The pose and shape parameters are then adjusted to move the boundary points as close as possible to the suggested target points, while still satisfying the model shape constraints. The original method suggested by Cootes et al. [2] first calculates the pose parameters (scale, translation, rotation) that best fit (in a least squares sense) the current estimate X to the suggested set of points $X + dX$. The residual displacements dx (expressed in the local model coordinate frame) are then approximated (projected onto the ASM eigenvectors) by the incremental changes in the shape parameters $db = P_t^T dx$ with P_t the sub-matrix of P containing only the first t columns of P. This procedure is repeated until no significant changes result.

4.2   Regularized Iterative Search using Dynamic Programming

At each update step in the previous search algorithm, pose and shape parameters are adjusted using a least squares approximation procedure. This least squares fit criterion is known to be sensitive to outliers occasionally suggested by the imperfect image model. (Fig. 2). Indeed, suppose we start from an initialized shape model X and take the target points with the smallest Mahalanobis distance, we might end up with a shape like the dotted line in Fig. 2. Here, model point p_2 is attracted to an outlier position. Adjusting the shape and pose parameters then leads to a biased boundary estimate that cannot be corrected during further iterations. We propose to correct the suggested movements dX before adjusting pose and shape parameters in the following way.

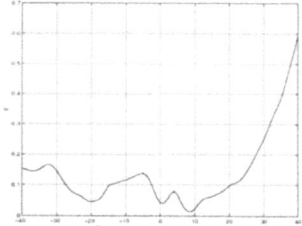 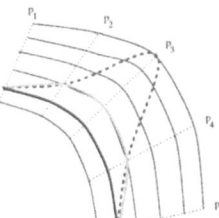

Fig. 2. Left:Mahalanobis distance calculated using (2) with normalized intensity profiles. The values are computed for a given boundary point along a path normal to the curve. Right:Starting from an initialized shape model (bold line), displacements to target points p_i with the smallest Mahalanobis distance can result in an outlier configuration (dashed line). Instead, a regularized target point configuration (grey line) is more appropriate.

We construct a "cost-matrix" K with dimensions $n \times l$ (n being the number of boundary points), containing the associated Mahalanobis distance values along the one-dimensional search profiles (length l pixels) normal to the curve. We then incorporate a regularization constraint penalizing outlier configurations by minimizing the function f

$$f(X) = K_{1,x_1} + \sum_{i=2}^{n} (K_{i,x_i} + \alpha \, |x_i - x_{i-1}|) \tag{3}$$

wherein α is a weight factor. We minimize f for X where X are the displacements in pixels along the normal to the curve: $X = (x_1 \; x_2 \ldots x_n), -\frac{l}{2} \leq x_i \leq \frac{l}{2}$. The last term in (3) indeed penalizes local outlier positions. This function can be minimized using dynamic programming. The corrected displacements are then used for updating the shape and pose parameters as in the previous search procedure.

5   Results

In this section we describe experiments designed (1) to test how well Point Distribution Models can model manual delineations of bone structures, (2) to test how well the image model can model the expected appearances of these structures in DRX, (3) to compare the results of the original iterative ASM search procedure and the proposed improved MCP search procedure.

These tests are based on a cross-validation or jack-knifing (leave-one-out) procedure. For each training set of a particular anatomical structure, we iteratively leave one example out and compute a shape and image model based on the remaining examples. This model is then used to segment the one image left out, and the average and maximal correspondence error and boundary error between the solution and the manual segmentation are computed. The correspondence error E_c of each point is the distance of the point to its corresponding point of the manual segmentation. The average and maximal error of the correspondence (over all boundary points of all examples) are denoted by E_{ca} and E_{cm}, respectively. The boundary error E_b of a point is the distance between this point and the closest boundary point of a spline computed through the manual segmentation. The average and maximal boundary error are denoted by $E_{ba} \leq E_{ca}$ and $E_{bm} \leq E_{cm}$.

Each test is performed on a database of more than 400 segmentations with the following subdivision: femur 104 (proximal end, ventral view), humerus 65 (proximal end, ventral view), calcaneus 91 (lateral view), femur 92 (distal end, lateral view), femur 56 (distal end, ventral view), tibia 17 (proximal end, ventral view).

The first experiment is designed to test how well the contours drawn manually by an expert can be modelled by the Point Distribution Models. Since we iteratively left one example out of the training set and since we also use a limited number of eigenvectors and limit the shape parameters between $-3\sqrt{\lambda_k} \leq b_k \leq 3\sqrt{\lambda_k}$, we cannot expect the PDM based on the remaining examples to model the one example perfectly. The average as well as maximal correspondence and boundary errors are given in Table 2. These values represent lower limits on the errors obtained in the other experiments.

In the second test we compare both search algorithms, the iterative search algorithm (ASM)and the Minimal Cost Path-based (MCP) search algorithm,

Table 2. Error measure for modelling the shape of the objects: E_{ca} is the average correspondence error; E_{ba} is the average boundary error; E_{cm} is the maximum correspondence error. E_{bm} is the maximum boundary error.

	E_{ca}	E_{ba}	E_{cm}	E_{bm}
calcaneus	1.93	1.32	12.49	8.20
femur (de,lv)	1.51	1.13	12.79	9.35
femur (pe,vv)	1.55	1.00	9.78	6.79
femur (de,vv)	1.83	1.41	8.28	7.10
tibia	2.14	1.43	8.80	6.46
humerus	1.08	0.82	7.04	4.21

with respect to their capability of finding the object boundary if the initial position is optimal w.r.t. the shape model (the solutions of the first test are given as initial positions). In both cases we use as image-model fit measure the Mahalanobis distance on the normalized grey-level profiles. We stop the search algorithm after 1 iteration and compute the errors (see Table 3). These errors reflect the stability of both search algorithms around the optimal shape. Corresponding errors after convergence are also listed in Table 3.

Table 3. Error measure for stability of the search algorithm near the correct solution. The values given in the left section of the table are the average correspondence (E_{ca}) and boundary (E_{ba}) errors, and maximal correspondence (E_{cm}) and boundary (E_{bm}) errors for both the original ASM search method and the improved MCP method after one iteration. The values in the right section of the table are the errors compiled after convergence of the algorithm.

		E_{ca}	E_{ba}	E_{cm}	E_{bm}	E_{ca}	E_{ba}	E_{cm}	E_{bm}
calcaneus	Asm	2.45	1.65	21.48	14.09	5.89	2.56	46.24	26.13
	Mcp	2.16	1.58	19.61	12.48	2.61	1.53	21.49	21.09
femur (de,lv)	Asm	2.15	1.69	14.81	11.58	3.87	2.33	31.20	31.00
	Mcp	1.95	1.51	14.56	11.79	2.68	1.78	32.05	27.85
femur (pe,vv)	Asm	1.90	1.26	11.16	7.24	3.25	1.76	29.84	20.75
	Mcp	1.69	1.02	10.77	7.94	1.91	1.03	13.80	9.63
femur (de,vv)	Asm	2.41	1.81	13.10	12.28	5.33	3.19	60.74	52.51
	Mcp	2.02	1.45	10.56	10.00	2.46	1.57	18.27	16.34
tibia	Asm	2.51	1.70	15.45	12.54	4.51	2.65	24.37	18.43
	Mcp	2.32	1.49	12.35	7.33	2.78	1.61	17.83	12.93
humerus	Asm	1.53	1.18	9.31	8.90	2.77	1.75	22.88	21.58
	Mcp	1.23	0.91	7.40	6.38	1.36	0.93	8.85	8.39

The third test compares the accuracy of both algorithms when starting from the registered mean shape with each manual segmentation. This experiment evaluates the stability of both search methods given that the pose parameters are already optimal. The results of this test are found in Table 4. Examples of segmentations with the worst correspondence are given in Fig. 3.

The last experiment examines the robustness of both search algorithms w.r.t. changes in the initial pose parameters. After registration of the mean shape with the manual segmentation, one of the pose parameters is varied and the model is

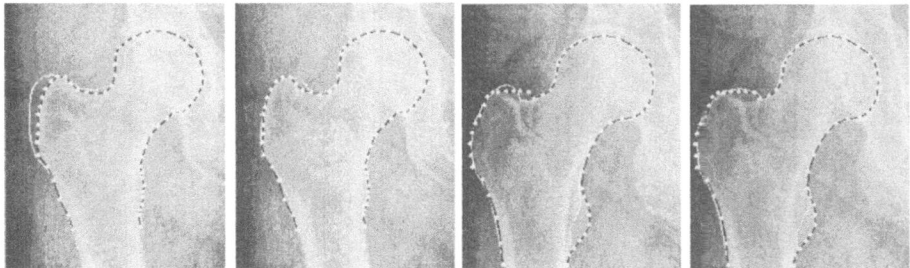

Fig. 3. Segmentation of the femur with the worst correspondence error (ASM: first, MCP: last image) computed after registering the average shape model with the manual segmentation. Corresponding segmentation obtained with the other method (MCP: second, ASM: third image). The manual segmentation is given by the dotted line.

Table 4. Error measures for segmentation after registering the mean shape with the manual segmentation using the ASM and MCP search technique.

		E_{ca}	E_{ba}	E_{cm}	E_{bm}
calcaneus	Asm	7.61	2.96	64.95	44.96
	Mcp	4.10	1.70	39.45	24.35
femur (de,lv)	Asm	5.84	2.72	46.34	28.28
	Mcp	4.19	2.27	27.84	26.25
femur (pe,vv)	Asm	4.95	2.43	36.71	36.71
	Mcp	3.10	1.34	23.75	18.03
femur (de,vv)	Asm	7.66	4.47	68.07	50.15
	Mcp	3.49	1.87	24.73	21.03
tibia	Asm	5.15	2.99	35.73	31.44
	Mcp	3.33′	1.75	17.92	13.42
humerus	Asm	4.09	2.12	28.18	22.63
	Mcp	2.24	1.09	18.05	14.27

fitted to the image. To make the search-algorithms more robust, we adaptively increase the number of eigenvectors for the shape during the search. In Table 4 the average correspondence errors for both search algorithms are displayed.

To evaluate the speed of both search algorithms, we measured the total calculation time on a search of a shape containing 25 points over 56 images after registration of the mean with the manual segmentation. The test was done on an Intel Pentium 300MHZ processor using Linux. The average calculation times till convergence for one shape are 0.2 s for the original search method and 0.18 s for the MCP-algorithm.

6   Discussion

We compared the original ASM iterative search method to the regularized MCP search method using a cross-validation procedure with expert manual segmentations as the standard. Tables 1 and 2 represent independent lower limits on the obtainable accuracy because of limitations in the shape model and limitations

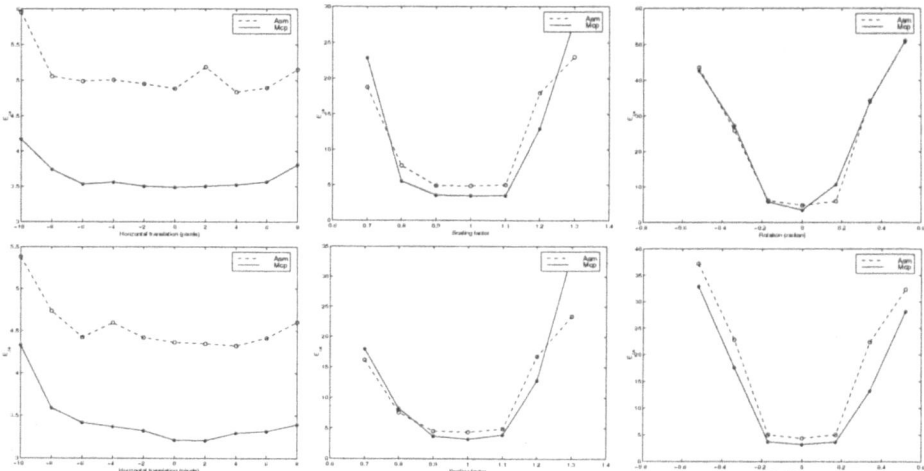

Fig. 4. Sensitivity to initial parameters experiment for the tibia (first row) and the femur (pe,vv,second row). These values are computed using a scheme which increases the number of eigenvectors used during the search.

and imperfections in the image model resp. which prevents both search methods from perfectly recovering the manual segmentations.

Comparing the results of the stability test (one iteration starting from the shape fitted to the manual segmentation) of both algorithms (Table 3) to these lower limits indicates that the one iteration of the MCP method consistently outperforms the ASM method but still occasionally fails to correct for outliers suggested by the image fit model. These errors are not recovered during remaining iterations as shown in Table 3.

When starting from the mean shape after registration with the manual segmentation, the MCP method again performs better according to all error measures (Table 4). Figure 3 shows two examples of worst results for both algorithms as well as the corresponding solution by the other algorithm. From this figure we observe that ASM worst case delineations tend to be associated more with gross overall misalignments. This can be attributed to the fact that outliers in ASM are inevitably propagated to pose and gross shape parameters, whereas the MCP algorithm regularizes these outliers and generates delineations with only local deviations.

Figure 4 illustrates that both search algorithms are relatively robust for initial mismatches in model translation, but degrade abruptly for slight changes in both scale and rotation. Overall the MCP algorithm performs more robustly. However, in general, we can conclude that both automatic delineation methods require that the initial pose parameters (translation, rotation, scaling) be fairly close to their final values. This sensitivity to mismatches of the initial model position can be reduced to some extent by using global optimization search algorithms such as

Genetic Algorithm search [6] or by a multi-resolution search (which includes a multi-resolution shape and image model as well) [5].

Despite the added algorithmic complexity of the minimum cost path search algorithm, the MCP algorithm is still, but only marginally, faster than the original ASM algorithm. Each iteration of the MCP algorithm indeed takes more time than the ASM algorithm, but far less iterations are needed for convergence.

7   Conclusions

This work presents a new search technique for delineation of anatomical structures in DRX using statistical Point Distribution Models. The image-model fit function that performs best for these examples is shown to be the Mahalanobis distance similarity function on normalized grey-level profiles. In order to minimize the sensitivity of the original iterative search procedure [1] to outliers, we incorporate a regularization constraint penalizing outlier configurations that we minimize using a dynamic programming algorithm. Extensive cross-validation experiments comparing both search procedures indicate that although the search procedure proposed in this paper consistently outperforms the original procedure for similar execution times, it still occasionally diverges to incorrect solutions because of limitations in both the shape and image model. Current work focuses on improving both components and rephrasing the procedure by optimizing a Bayesian Maximum a Posteriori (MAP) objective function [7]

Acknowledgements

This work was supported by a grant of Agfa-Gevaert NV, by a grant for research specialization from the Flemish Institute for stimulation of the scientific-technological research in the industry (IWT), and by the Research Fund KU Leuven GOA/99/05 (Variability in Human Shape and Speech). The manual segmentations were performed by Dr. Tom De Jaegere.

References

1. T. F. Cootes and C. J. Taylor. Active shape models - "smart snakes". In *BMVC*, pages 256–275, 1992.
2. T. F. Cootes and C. J. Taylor. Active shape model search using local grey-level models: A quantitative evaluation. In *BMVC*, pages 339–348, Sept. 1993.
3. T. F. Cootes, C. J. Taylor, D. H. Cooper, and J. Graham. Training models of shape from sets of examples. In *BMVC*, pages 9–18, 1992.
4. T. F. Cootes, C. J. Taylor, D. H. Cooper, and J. Graham. Active shape models - their training and application. *Computer Vision and Image Understanding*, 61(1):38–59, January 1995.
5. T. F. Cootes, C. J. Taylor, and A. Lanitis. Active shape models : Evaluation of a multi-resolution method for improving image search. In *BMVC*, pages 327–336, 1994.
6. A. Hill, C. J. Taylor, and T. Cootes. Object recognition by flexible template matching using genetic algorithms. In *2nd European Conference on Computer Vision*, pages 852–856, May 1992.
7. Y. Wang and L. H. Staib. Boundary finding with correspondence using statistical shape models. In *Proc. IEEE Conf. Computer Vision and Pattern Recognition*, pages 338–345, 1998.

Nonrigid 3-D/2-D Registration of Images Using Statistical Models

M. Fleute[1] and S. Lavallée[2]

[1] TIMC Laboratory, University Joseph Fourier, Grenoble, France
[2] PRAXIM, 4 Av. Obiou, 38 700 La Tronche, France

Abstract. This paper presents a new algorithm for reconstruction of 3D shapes using a few x-ray views and a statistical model. In many applications of surgery such as orthopedics, it is desirable to define a surgical planning on 3-D images and then to execute the plan using standard registration techniques and image-guided surgery systems. But the cost, time and x-ray dose associated with standard pre-operative Computed Tomography makes it difficult to use this methodology for rather standard interventions. Instead, we propose to use a few x-ray images generated from a C-Arm and to build the 3-D shape of the patient bones or organs intra-operatively, by deforming a statistical 3-D model to the contours segmented on the x-ray views. In this paper, we concentrate on the application of our method to bone reconstruction. The algorithm starts from segmented contours of the bone on the x-ray images and an initial estimate of the pose of the 3-D model in the common coordinate system of the set of x-ray projections. The statistical model is made of a few principal modes that are sufficient to represent the normal anatomy. Those modes are built by using a generalization of the Cootes and Taylor method to 3-D surface models, previously published in MICCAI'98 by the authors. Fitting the model to the contours is achieved by using a generalization of the Iterative Closest Point Algorithm to nonrigid 3D/2D registration. For pathological shapes, the statistical model is not valid and subsequent local refinement is necessary. First results are presented for a 3-D statistical model of the distal part of the femur.

1 Introduction

X-ray images are the dominating image modality in the operating room. Due to his anatomical knowledge the surgeon is used to mentally fuse 2D images taken from different view points. However for many applications this mental registration is not sufficient to obtain all necessary information about the anatomical situation to properly perform the surgery. Therefore, since the introduction of Computed Tomography many surgical interventions are preceded by the construction of a CT-based 3D model of the object of interest to provide the surgeon with spatial information which is leaking when using only 2D images. To combine preoperative acquired CT data with intra-operatively acquired X-ray images, marker based or surface based registration methods are usually applied.

But the CT data acquisition process is associated with several drawbacks: First, the total X-ray dose for the patient raises considerably. Further it significantly increases the overall intervention costs as well as its duration. Therefore it is desirable to infer 3D-information from the 2D X-ray images to facilitate the navigation within the patient and thus allowing to abandon CT data acquisition at least for many standard surgical applications.

In [Hof97] for instance, authors propose to acquire several images using a classical C-arm equipped with an image intensifier and to track the position and orientation of the surgical tools, the image intensifier and a patient's reference with an optical localizer, thus allowing to compute relative movements of the patient or the surgical tools with respect to each acquired image during the intervention. Although this system is a considerable improvement, real 3D information is still missing.

The objective of this paper therefore is to recover the surface of an object using a very limited number (2 - 6) of calibrated X-ray images. We concentrate here on bone reconstruction but the proposed method is also applicable to other anatomical structures.

Image intensifiers are subject to geometric distortions due to non planar shape of the image intensifier and external magnetic fields. Calibration techniques such as the NPBS method [CLSC92] for instance can be used to correct these distortions as well as to compute a pseudo focal point of the source. This calibration is not further addressed in this paper. However full digital X-ray detectors without any geometric distortion [CCD98] begin to appear on the market and are likely to replace the image intensifiers in the future.

The remainder of this paper is organized as follows: In section 2 we give a brief overview about related work and introduce the statistical shape model of Cootes and Taylor. Section 3 presents a generalization of the Iterative Closest Point algorithm [BM92] for contour based 3D/2D registration. Section 4 shows how to efficiently compute matched point pairs by computing the model's contour generators. Section 5 shows how to fit the model to the projection data. Section 6 provides results obtained with simulated data and in Section 7 we draw a short conclusion.

2   Related Work

First considering the simpler case of recovering only the pose parameters of a 3D model from its 2D projections (rigid 2D/3D registration), one can distinguish two different concepts: One type of algorithm is based on contours and requires prior segmentation of the object in the 3D-image as well as in the 2D-image [LS95,FAB94] although in [HSLC95] authors propose a cooperative approach between registration and 2D segmentation. The other concept does not need segmentation and compares the grey value distribution of the 2D-image with the distribution obtained when projecting the 3D-image under current registration parameters [LFK94]. Due to the high computational cost for projecting the 3D image this method is rather slow although in [Wee99] authors recently proposed a promising technique for considerable acceleration by using the shear-warp factorization.

Much less work has been done in the field of nonrigid 3D/2D registration: In [PV97] for instance, authors aim to recover shape from one single X-ray image by exploiting both, geometric and densitometric constraints while making two assumptions: the density of the structure to be recovered is approximately constant and the surface of each structure is smooth. This approach shares ideas from the work of [TWK88]. In [Nik96] authors reconstruct femurs from 2 orthogonal X-ray images. They separate the femur into 3 subparts each of them assumed to be round. They fit cubic parametric surface patches to the subparts and then assemble them to a complete model. For a general overview about image registration techniques see for instance [MV98].

We propose to formulate the shape recovery problem as a nonrigid registration between a deformable shape model and the contour data extracted from the X-ray views. As we aim to recover the shape from very few projections it is necessary to incorporate a priori knowledge. One possibility is to consider models such as deformable superquadrics [MT93], however those models are appropriate to capture shapes defined by many data (the superquadrics convey information about the global shape but this part of the model is not accurate enough for our applications). Similarly, using volumetric deformations with regularization constraints such as octree-splines [SL96] can be expected to preserve the shape of an anatomical structure, but this will be true only in the neighborhood of the available data. The result of those methods is not guaranteed to be a shape that respects the anatomy.

Another approach is to to consider statistically based shape models in order to infer the anatomical information. One well known approach is to use statistical models based on Fourier representations, such as [SD92,SkBG96]. Another method is based on extracting features such as crest-lines and to perform modal analysis on these features [STA96]. A third approach is to consider a statistical model with modal representation based on principal component analysis directly applied to the nodal representation of a mean contour.

Cootes and Taylor [CTCG95] have proposed to use Point Distribution Models (PDM). A PDM is a deformable model built from the statistical analysis of examples of the object being modeled. Given a collection of N 3D training shapes of an object, the Cartesian coordinates of M landmark points are recorded for each image. Each training example is represented by a vector $\mathbf{m} = (x_1, y_1, z_1, ..., x_M, y_M, z_M)$.

After aligning of the training shapes the pointwise mean shape

$$\bar{\mathbf{m}} = \frac{1}{N} \sum_{i=1}^{N} \mathbf{m}_i \tag{1}$$

is then calculated. Modes of variation are found using Principal Component Analysis (PCA) on the deviations of examples from the mean. These modes are represented by $3M$ orthonormal eigenvectors $\mathbf{e}_i$. A new instance of the shape is generated by adding linear combinations of the t most significant variation vectors to the mean shape:

$$\mathbf{m} = \bar{\mathbf{m}} + \sum_{i=1}^{t} w_i \mathbf{e}_i \qquad (2)$$

where w_i is the weighting factor for the ith variation vector. By ensuring $t < 3M$, only the important deformations are extracted, discarding training data noise, and thus object shape and variation can be captured compactly.

A key requirement for building such a model is the collection of several sets with corresponding landmarks from training images. Doing this manually for a 3D model is impractical due to the considerable effort required for image-model registration. In [FL98] the authors present a method which performs an automatic landmark point generation using a template triangle mesh while ensuring point correspondence between the training shapes.

Fig.1 shows the effect of applying ±3 standard deviations of the first two modes to the mean shape of a model constructed of 10 dry femurs.

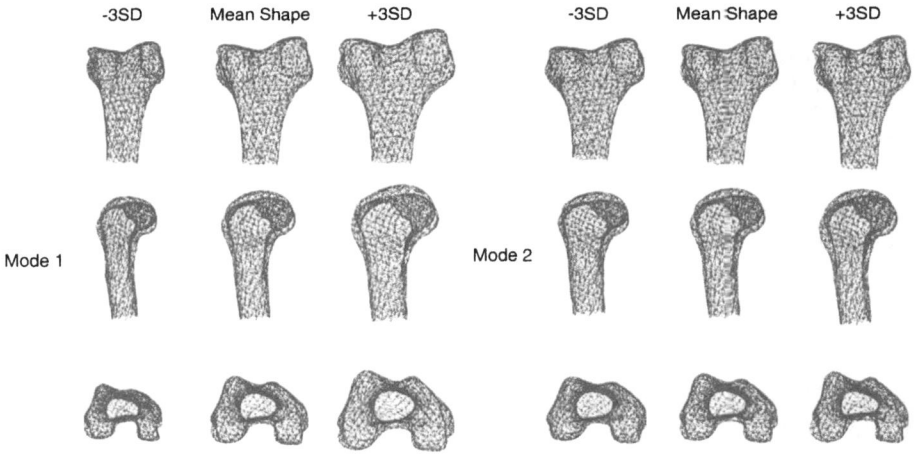

Fig. 1. Applying 3 standard deviations of the first and second deformation modes on the mean shape

3 Using the ICP algorithm for 2D/3D registration

A well known method for rigid registration of a 3D data point set with a 3D model point set is the Iterative Closest Point algorithm introduced in [BM92]. Each iteration of the ICP algorithm is divided into two steps. Step 1 establishes

142   M. Fleute and S. Lavallée

point to point correspondence between the data set and the model set. Step 2 calculates a rigid transformation by a direct method using quaternions such that the sum of the squared distances between the corresponding points becomes minimal. To be able to use the ICP algorithm for 3D/2D registration we have to define the correspondence between the model and each projection ray $\mathbf{p}_{i,i=1...P}$ of the X-ray images defined by the coordinates of the contour points x_i, y_i in the image plane and the focal point $\mathbf{f}$ of the source. We associate the endpoints of that line segment originating on the projection ray and ending on the model surface such that their distance to each other is minimal. Note that at each iteration step new points on both, the model and the projection rays may be selected, while in the 3D/3D case the points in the data set remains the same throughout all iterations. In [WH96] authors describe this approach for rigid 2D/3D registration of CAD models to video camera images but do not address the problem of quickly finding those points on the projection ray and the model having the smallest distance to each other. This is a key step for applicability within intra-operative applications. We address this problem in the next section.

4   Efficient matched point pair building

To efficiently find the above defined correspondence we use the approach described in [Gue98] by first computing the actual contour generators $\mathbf{g}_{i,i=1...G}$ of the model. Contour generators are those object features constituting the (inner and outer) contours of the object in image space with respect to the current projection parameters. As we use a triangle mesh for presentation of our model, the contour generators are a subset of all triangle edges. Thus establishing correspondence results in the simple computation of shortest lines between two 3D line segments. When the model is perfectly aligned with the projection rays, the latter intersect those triangle edges previously found to be contour generators. In [Gue98] authors call the contour generators 'apparent contours' and use them for a rigid registration algorithm to match a CT model with fluoroscopic images. We define the triangles in the mesh by pointers to an edge list. Each edge in the edge list points to the two vertices in a vertex list defining the edge. This representation enables us to efficiently compute the contour generators using the following criterion: For each triangle the viewing direction is defined as the vector originating from the center of projection to the triangle centroid. If the triangle normal, defined by the cross product of ordered orientated triangle edges constitutes an obtuse angle with the viewing direction, the triangle is said to be visible and invisible otherwise. An edge is a contour generator if the triangle on one side of the edge is visible and the triangle on the other side of the edge is invisible. We store all edges meeting this criterion in a list and rather than performing brutal force search within the complete edge list of the model we only have to search within this subset to find matched point pairs. For our model, consisting of about 5000 edges there are only about 300 contour generators for each perspective projection. Fig 2 shows the correspondence between one projection ray and the current contour generators of the model.

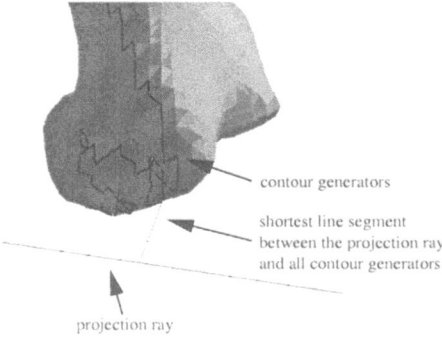

contour generators

shortest line segment
between the projection ray
and all contour generators

projection ray

Fig. 2. Correspondence between one projection ray and the current contour generators of the model

5   Model Fitting

To recover the shape from the projection rays it is necessary to find the rigid transformation (rotation $\mathbf{R}$, translation $\mathbf{T}$) between the matched point pairs and the decomposition of the t preserved eigenvectors in such a way that the distances between them are minimized. The objective function to be minimized is defined as follows:

$$E(\mathbf{R}, \mathbf{T}, w_1...w_t) = \sum_{j=1}^{P} \min_{1 \leq k \leq G} \|\mathbf{p}_j - (\mathbf{R}\mathbf{g}_k(w_1...w_t) + \mathbf{T})\|^2 \qquad (3)$$

In theory, we could simultaneously optimize the rigid and the nonrigid parameters. However, in practise we have found it more efficient to adjust them sequentially. Given an estimate for the pose parameters $\mathbf{R}, \mathbf{T}$ by applying the generalized ICP algorithm we adjust the deformation parameters $w_1...w_t$ using the Down Hill Simplex Algorithm. Bounds to the deformation parameters are applied to force the model to deform only in an anatomical reasonable range.

6   Results

Experiments with simulated data have been established using a simulator tool allowing to interactively rotate and translate a 3D model of the distal part of a femur, to project its contour generators onto an image plane and to record the image together with the projection parameters (Fig. 3 a). Fig 3 (b) shows 4 simulated X-ray shots taken from different view points around the object. The experiments were performed using an image plane / focal point distance of 1000mm thus roughly approximating real conditions when using a C-arm. Fig 4 shows the shape model before registration (a), after rigid (b) and after nonrigid

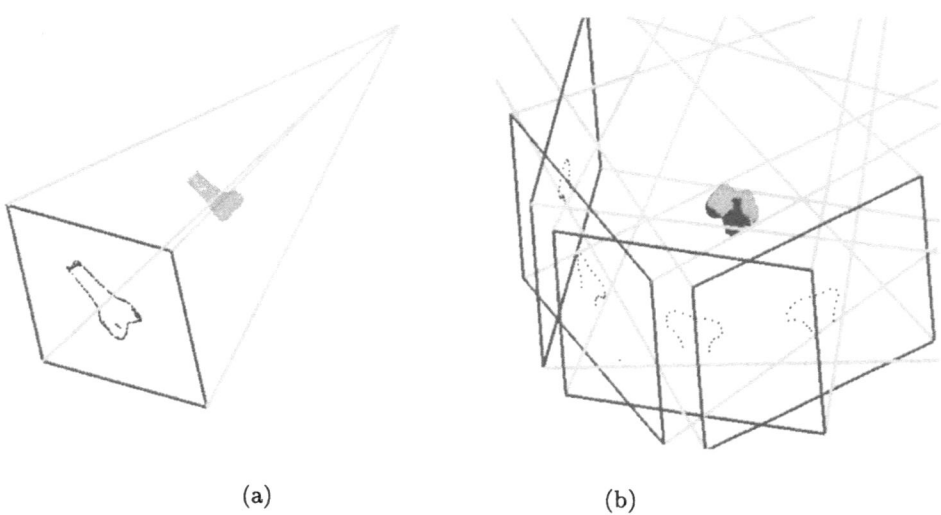

(a)   (b)

Fig. 3. (a) Interactive X-ray simulation to compute contours under known perspective projection parameters. (b) Four simulated X-ray shots taken around the object

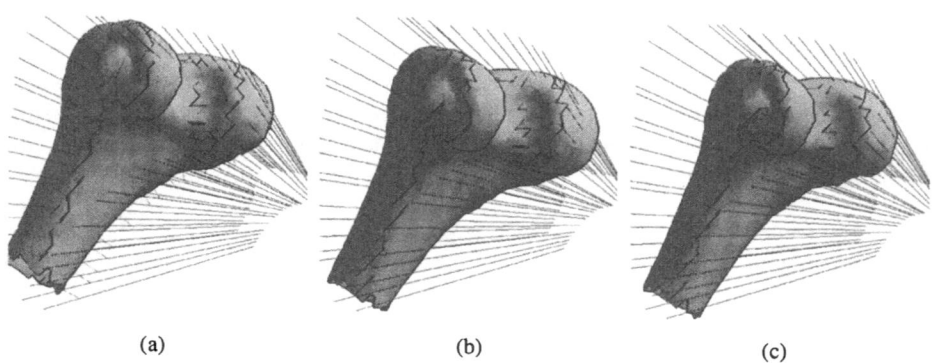

(a)   (b)   (c)

Fig. 4. Surface model of the distal part of the femur: (a) before registration, (b) after initial rigid registration, (c) after nonrigid registration

(c) registration. One recognizes that the projection rays are tangential to the object surface after the nonrigid registration.

Experiments using different numbers of X-ray images and varying numbers of deformation modes show that within the current implementation two orthogonal views and 4 deformation modes establish the best compromise between accuracy and computation time. Table 1 shows registration results for different numbers of calculated projection rays per X-ray image. In this experiment we used 2 orthogonal X-ray views and 4 deformation modes. We calculated the RMS between the projection rays and the model and the RMS between the surface model of the shape to be recovered (reference) and the deformed model.

	RMS (mm)	
rays	rays-model	reference-model
10	0.34	1.3
20	0.52	1.2
50	0.49	1.13
100	0.55	1.05
200	0.77	0.99

Table 1. RMS for different number of projection rays per view

We also compared the accuracy of our 2D/3D matching algorithm with the 3D/3D registration algorithm presented on MICCAI'98. Approximately 500 points randomly distributed on the surface of the shape to be recovered were first registered rigidly with the mean shape, resulting in a RMS of 2.44mm. The nonrigid registration between the 3D data set of the test femur and the deformable model using 4 deformation modes results in a final RMS of 0.85mm. Using 2 (orthogonal) views, each with about 200 projection rays results in a final RMS between the deformed model and the shape to be recovered of 0.99mm.

7   Conclusion

Statistical shape models have been proven to be effective for different tasks in the field of computer vision such as segmentation of 2D, 3D images or nonrigid 3D/3D registration. This paper has presented a new approach to perform nonrigid 3D/2D registration between such a model and relatively few segmented contour points from calibrated X-ray images. Contour based registration algorithms suffer from the potential drawback that their accuracy directly depends on the correct segmentation of the objects contour in the image. Our approach is robust with respect to this problem in such a way that good matching results are obtained even when considerable parts of the objects contour cannot reliably be segmented. Computation time of the current implementation directly depends on the number of used projection rays and is less than one minute on a standard workstation when using a total number of 400 projection rays and 4 deformation modes. When dealing with pathological shape deformations which are not covered by the statistical model, local refinements of the model are necessary to obtain a sufficient good fit between the model and the projective data. Experiments with real data acquired with a new distortion free digital X-ray detector (Pixium 4600, Trixell, France) are in progress and will be presented soon.

Acknowledgments

Authors wish to thank the Anatomy Department of Grenoble University (Pr. JP Chirossel) for providing the specimen of femurs. This research is financially supported by the Region Rhone-Alpes.

References

[BM92] P.J. Besl and N.D. McKay. A method for registration of 3-D shapes. *IEEE Transactions on Pattern Analysis and Machine Intelligence*, 14(2):239–256, 1992.

[CCD98] C. Chaussat, J. Chabbal, T. Ducourant, V. Spinnler, and G. Vieux. New superior detectivity csi/a-si 43cm x 43cm x-ray flat panel detector for general radiography provides immediate direct digital output and easy interfacing to digital radiographic systems. In H.U. Lemke, editor, *CAR*, 1998.

[CLSC92] G. Champleboux, S. Lavallee, P. Sautot, and P. Cinquin. Accurate calibration of cameras and range imaging sensors, the NPBS method. In *IEEE Int. Conf. on Robotics and Automation*, pages 1552–1558, Nice France, May 1992.

[CTCG95] T.F. Cootes, C.J. Taylor, D.H. Cooper, and J. Graham. Active shape models - Their training and application. *Computer Vision and Image Understanding*, 61(1):38–59, 1995.

[FAB94] J. Feldmar, N. Ayache, and F. Betting. 3D-2D projective registration of free-form curves and surfaces. Technical Report 2434, INRIA, France, 1994.

[FL98] M. Fleute and Stephane Lavallee. Building a Complete Surface Model from Sparse Data Using Statistical Shape Models: Application to Computer Assisted Knee Surgery. In W. M. Wells, A. Colchester, and S. Delp, editors, *Medical Image Computing and Computer-Assisted Intervention-MICCAI'98*, pages 880–887. Springer Verlag, October 1998.

[Gue98] A. Gueziec. Anatomy-based registration of ct-scan and intraoperative x-ray images for guiding a surgical robot. *IEEE Transactions on Medical Imaging*, 17(5):715–728, October 1998.

[Hof97] R. Hofstetter. Fluoroscopy based surgical navigation-concept and clinical applications. In H.U. Lemke, editor, *CAR*, 1997.

[HSLC95] A. Hamadeh, P. Sautot, S. Lavallee, and P. Cinquin. Towards automatic registration between CT and X-ray images : cooperation between 3D/2D registration and 2D edge detection. In *Second Symposium on Medical Robotics and Computer Assisted Surgery Proc. (MRCAS'95)*, pages 39–46, Baltimore, MA, nov. 1995. Wiley.

[LFK94] L. Lemieux, D.R. Fish, and N.D. Kitchen. A patient-to-computed-tomography image registration method based on digitally reconstructed radiographs. *Medical Physics*, november 1994.

[LS95] S. Lavallee and R. Szeliski. Recovering the position and orientation of free-form objects from image contours using 3-D distance maps. *IEEE PAMI (Pattern Analysis and Machine Intelligence)*, 17(4):378–390, 1995.

[MT93] D. Metaxas and D. Terzopoulos. Shape and nonrigid motion estimation through physics-based synthesis. *IEEE Trans PAMI*, 15(6):580–591, 1993.

[MV98] A. Maintz and M. Viergever. A survey of medical image registration. *Medical Image Analysis*, 2(1):1–36, 1998.

[Nik96] B. Nikkhahe. 3d reconstruction of the femoral bone using two x-ray images from orthogonal views. In H.U. Lemke, editor, *CAR*, 1996.

[PV97] R. Poli and G. Valli. Shape from radiological density. *Computer Vision and Image Understanding*, 65(3):361–381, March 1997.

[SD92] L.H. Staib and J.S. Duncan. Boundary finding with parametrically deformable models. *IEEE Trans. on PAMI*, 17(11):1061–1075, 1992.

[SkBG96] R. Szekely, A. kelemen, C. Brechbuler, and G. Gerig. Segmentation of 2D and 3D objects from MRI volume data using constrained elastic deformations of flexible Fourier surface models. *Medical Image Analysis*, 1(1):19–34, 1996.

[SL96] R. Szeliski and S. Lavallee. Matching 3-D anatomical surfaces with non-rigid deformations using octree-splines. *Int. J. of Computer Vision (IJCV)*, (18)(2):171–186, 1996.

[STA96] G. Subsol, J.P. Thirion, and N. Ayache. Application of an automatically built 3D morphometric brain atlas: study of cerebral ventricle shape. In K.H. Hohne and R. Kikinis, editors, *Visualization in Biomedical Computing (VBC'96) Proc. LNCS 1131*, pages 373–382, Berlin, 1996. Springer-Verlag.

[TWK88] D. Terzopoulos, A. Witkin, and M. Kass. Constraints on deformable models: Recovering 3D shape and nonrigid motion. *Artificial Intelligence*, 36:91–123, 1988.

[Wee99] J. Weese. Fast voxel-based 2d/3d registration algorthm using a volume rendering method based on the shear-warp factorization. In *SPIE*, 1999.

[WH96] P. Wunsch and G. Hirzinger. Registration of cad-models to images by iterative inverse perspective matching. In *International Conference on Pattern Recognition*, 1996.

A New Approach to 3D Sulcal Ribbon Finding from MR Images

X.Zeng[1], L.H.Staib[1], R.T.Schultz[2], H.Tagare[1], L.Win[2], and J.S.Duncan[1]

[1] Departments of Electrical Engineering and Diagnostic Radiology,
[2] Child Study Center,   Yale University, New Haven, CT, 06520-8042

Abstract. Sulcal medial surfaces are 3D thin convoluted ribbons embedded in cortical sulci, and they provide distinctive anatomical features of the brain. Here we propose a new approach to automatic intrasulcal ribbon finding, following our work on cortex segmentation with coupled surfaces via level set methods, where the outer cortical surface is embedded as the zero level set of a high-dimensional distance function. Through the utilization of this distance function, we are able to formulate the sulcal ribbon finding problem as one of surface deformation, thus avoiding possible control problems in other work using sliding contour models. Using dynamic programming and deformable surface models, our method requires little manual intervention and results parameterized sulcal ribbon surfaces in nearly real-time. Though a natural follow up to our earlier segmentation work, we describe how it can be applied with general segmentation methods. We also present quantitative results on 15 MR brain images.

1   Introduction

A great amount of recent anatomical MRI studies of the human brain have been focused on the cerebral cortex, which is characterized by its convoluted cortical surface. The narrow groove separating adjacent cortical convolutions is called a sulcus, and the intrasulcal medial surface can be modeled as a 3D thin ribbon embedded in the cortical fold. The deepest part of a sulcus is called the fundus, and it often demarcates the boundary between cortical regions with observable differences in their cytoarchitecture (the packing density and laminar distribution of different neuron types) and function [14].

Because of the importance of sulcal ribbons in brain structural and functional analysis, a number of recent efforts have begun to deal with the automatic extraction of sulci [15, 8], the probabilistic study of sulcal geometry and configuration [9], and automatic sulcal labeling [11].

Of all the work cited above, ours is most closely related to that of Vaillant and Davatzikos [15]. The aim is to automatically extract a sulcal ribbon surface and provide a parametric representation, thereby further facilitating quantitative shape analysis and cortical-constrained brain matching and warping. Vaillant and Davatzikos start by initializing an active contour at the exterior part of a sulcus (see Figure 1). A parametric representation of the sulcal medial surface is obtained as the active contour slide down toward the deep sulcal bottom under the influence of weighted external forces, such as the center-of-mass force and the inward force which is a combination based on surface normal, curve sliding speed and sliding acceleration. This deformable model uses characteristics of the cortical shape, and has been successfully applied to MR brain images to extract sulcal ribbons. However, the manual placement of the initializing curve is a limitation, and so could be the tuning of the weights on the external forces.

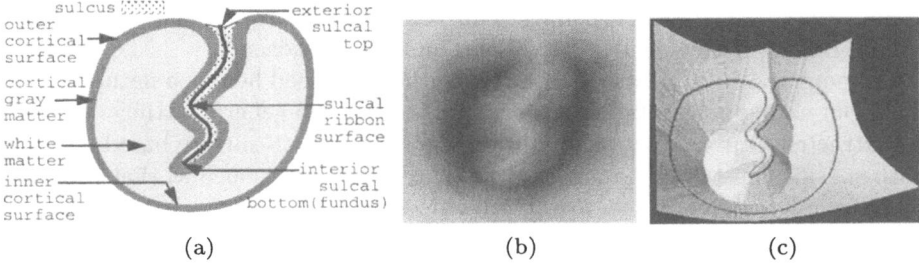

(a)   (b)   (c)

Fig. 1. (a): 2D schematic representation of a sulcus; Gray scale view (b) and surface view (c) of the signed distance function corresponding to the outer cortical boundary shown in (a).

2   Our Method

Following our earlier work on cortex segmentation with coupled surfaces using a level set implementation [19], we propose a new approach to automatic sulcal ribbon finding. Through the utilization of the distance function in which the outer cortical surface is embedded as its zero level set, we are able to formulate the sulcal ribbon finding problem as one of surface deformation, avoiding possible control problems of tuning weights on external forces in the sliding contour method. Our sulcal ribbon finding algorithm starts from the outer cortical surface and its associated level function, and takes three steps as shown in Figure 2.

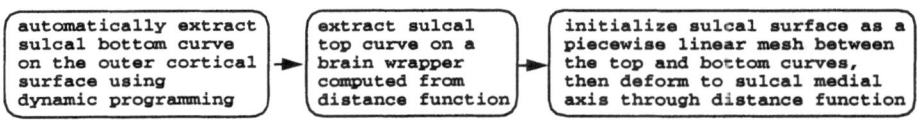

Fig. 2. Diagram of our algorithm.

2.1   Brain Segmentation

We first perform segmentation of brain images using our coupled surfaces propagation algorithm with a level set implementation [19]. Starting from concentric spheres, the outer and inner surfaces propagate out, looking for image features of CSF/gray boundary (outer cortical surface) and gray/white boundary (inner cortical surface) respectively, while maintaining a nearly constant thickness in between. When the propagation ends, we have two level functions Ψ_{out} and Ψ_{in} in which the outer and inner cortical surfaces S_{out} and S_{in} are embedded as zero level sets respectively.

Because of the level set implementation, our segmentation algorithm has the advantage of handling highly convoluted structures. As a result, S_{out} captures the deep sulcal folds and gets down to the interior sulcal bottom (see Figure 1 and Figure 5) rather than staying at the exterior sulcal top. Therefore, we can use this surface to extract a sulcal bottom curve at the fundus, which greatly facilitates the sulcal ribbon finding. This is an important difference of our sulcal ribbon finding from that due to Vallaint and Davatzikos.

Though the sulcal ribbon finding algorithm proposed here is a natural follow up to our earlier segmentation work, it easily applies in general settings. S_{out} can be extracted from any segmented brain volume using iso-surface based methods with specific constraints to preserve high curvature areas, such as that proposed by Gibson [7]. Ψ_{out} can then be calculated as the signed distance function:

$$\Psi_{out}(x) = \begin{array}{ll} -dist(x, S_{out}) & if \ x \in brainvolume, \\ dist(x, S_{out}) & else. \end{array}$$

where $dist$ is the Euclidean distance from position x on 3D image grid to S_{out}. Narrow band techniques [20] can be used here to limit the calculation of Ψ_{out} to positions close to S_{out} for computational efficiency.

2.2   Automatic Tracing of Sulcal Curves on Outer Cortical Surface

Our first step in sulcal ribbon finding is to define the interior sulcal bottom curve at the fundus. Based on the fact that crest curves consist of points corresponding to local maxima of maximum principal curvature, defining sulcal bottom curves becomes a problem of finding curves that pass through regions of high maximum principal curvature while confined to the outer cortical surface. In the continuous case, this can be posed as a problem of finding curvature-weighted minimal geodesic curves. On our discretized outer cortical surface net, the goal is to find paths that go through surface vertices corresponding to maximal curvature values. The maximum principal curvature on each vertex $Curv(v_i)$ on S_{out} is calculated directly from Ψ_{out} as described in [19]. Figure 3 shows an example of high maximum principal curvature points on an outer cortical surface.

We introduce the following notation for the description of our automatic curve extraction method.

- $V = \{v_i \mid 0 \leq i < M\}$: the set of all vertices on the surface net, where M is the number of vertices;
- $T = \{t_j\}$: the set of all triangles on the surface net;
- $E = \{e_{i,j}\}$: the set of all edges on the surface net, where $e_{i,j}$ is an edge if for some triangle $t \in T$, v_i, v_j are vertices of t. $e_{i,j}$ is a degenerate edge if $i = j$.
- $N(v_i) = \{v_j \mid e_{i,j} \in E\}$: the set of neighbors of vertex v_i;
- $Cost(e_{i,j}) = cost(Curv(v_i), Curv(v_j)) \cdot dist(v_i, v_j)$: the cost of stepping through edge $e_{i,j}$, where function $cost(,)$ penalizes small maximum principal curvatures,

and $dist(v_i, v_j)$ gives the Euclidean distance between vertices v_i and v_j. Function $cost(Curv(v_i), Curv(v_j))$ can take on forms such as $Curv_{max} - \frac{Curv(v_i)+Curv(v_j)}{2}$, where $Curv_{max}$ is the largest maximum principal curvature of all surface vertices.

- $P_{i_0,i_1,...,i_K}$: a path from v_{i_0} to v_{i_K}, consisting of a sequence of edges e_{i_0,i_1}, e_{i_1,i_2}, ..., e_{i_{K-1},i_K} (degenerate edges are allowed), where K is the number of steps.

We now formulate the problem of finding a sulcal curve given the starting point v_{start} and the ending point v_{end}, to be finding the optimal path:

$$P^* = \arg \min_{P_{i_0,i_2,...,i_K}} \Sigma_{k=0}^{K-1} Cost(e_{i_k,i_{k+1}})$$

where $v_{i_0} = v_{start}, v_{i_K} = v_{end}$, and K is the number of steps taken.

Dynamic programming ([2,3])is a technique suited for such an optimization problem. Similar application can be found in [10]. The basic idea is as follows. Suppose there are M vertices on the surface net, then the optimal path P^* takes no more than M steps, i.e. $K \leq M$. If we can find an optimal path of step $K-1$ to the neighbors of v_{end}, then P^* is just the optimal path to one particular neighbor of v_{end}, plus the edge from that particular neighbor to v_{end}.

The algorithm works in the following fashion. Initialize a *pathvalue* for v_{end} to be 0, and $+\infty$ for the rest of the vertices. Let PV_t denote the set of possible vertices at the end of step $t (0 \leq t \leq K - 1)$. Since v_{end} is the end of step K, it is obvious that $PV_{K-1} = N(v_{end})$. So for each $v_i \in PV_{K-1}$, we store *pathvalue* to be $Cost(e_{end,i})$, and assign v_{end} to be the *successor* of such a v_i. By similar reasoning, we have $PV_t = \{N(v_i) \mid v_i \in PV_{t+1}\}$. Now for $t = K - 1$ down to 0, for each $v_i \in PV_t$, we compare $Pathvalue(v_j) + Cost(e_{ji})$ where $v_j \in N(v_i)$, to find the optimal *pathvalue* for v_i and assign its corresponding *successor*. When the operation is done for $t = 0$, starting from v_{start}, we trace back from the *successor* all the way to v_{end}, which gives us the optimal path.

Note that such an optimal path is only an approximation of the weighted geodesic curve on the continuous surface. However, since our triangulation of the surface is done at the level of voxel size (each cortical surface net has about 500,000 triangles), we have found the discrete path to be a fine enough approximation, as verified by expert inspection. In our implementation, the starting and ending points of a particular sulcus are specified by the user to allow flexibility, which only takes two mouse clicks on a surface rendering. The step number K is usually set to be 300 (large enough for the possible steps for each sulcus) to provide real-time operation. Example automatic traces are shown in Figure 4.

2.3 Brain Wrapper and Exterior Sulcal Top Curves

After extracting the interior sulcal bottom curve, we then define the exterior sulcal top. One simple way is to use the signed distance level function Ψ_{out}. While the outer cortical surface S_{out} is the zero level set of Ψ_{out}, a positive value ϵ can be chosen so that the ϵ level set of Ψ_{out} provides a brain wrapper – a surface that wraps around the brain volume, while following indentations at exterior sulcal tops. In our implementation, ϵ is chosen to be $3mm$, which results in a consistent brain wrapper suitable for subsequent sulcal ribbon extraction. After the brain wrapper surface is extracted, sulcal top curves are automatically traced out on the brain wrapper surface in the same fashion that sulcal bottom curves are on the cortical surface (see Figure 5).

2.4   Sulcal Ribbon Surface Extraction

The sulcal ribbon surface corresponds to the medial axis of a particular sulcus. There are different ways of extracting the medial axis of 3D structures, such as those using Voronoi diagrams [4, 13, 12]. The drawbacks of 3D Voronoi methods lie in their algorithmic difficulties caused by sampling problems and pruning procedures. Moreover, a parametric representation of the sulcal ribbon does not follow immediately from these methods.

From the level function Ψ_{out} and the sulcal bottom and top curves traced out automatically, we have a simple and natural way of defining the entire sulcal ribbon. Our method is based on the fact that the medial axis of a sulcus corresponds to directional local maximum of the signed distance function Ψ_{out}. This is illustrated by the 2D schematic drawing in Figure 1. Figure 1 (b) and (c) show the image and surface view of the signed distance function of the outer cortical boundary in Figure 1(a). The ridge curve in the sulcal region shown in Figure 1(c) is the medial axis of the sulcus, and has the property of being located at a local maximum of the distance function along its normal direction. The 3D case is similar, only differing in that the medial axial ridge curve becomes a surface that has a local maximum of Ψ_{out} along its normal direction. Our goal now is to capture such a surface through Ψ_{out}.

We will define a sulcal surface mesh $R(u, v)$ on the domain $[0, 1] \times [0, 1]$, so that parameter u runs in the direction parallel to the sulcal top and bottom curves, while parameter v runs across the sulcal depth. Figure 7 helps in illustrating this process. To start, we map $R(u, 0)$ to be the interior sulcal bottom curve, and $R(u, 1)$ to be the exterior sulcal top curve. We reparameterize $R(u, 1)$ in u so that it has the same u parametric speed as $R(u, 0)$. In this way, we set up a correspondence between the points on the sulcal top and bottom curves, which helps to offer a reasonable concept of sulcal depth discussed later in Section 3.1.

We then realize a piece-wise linear triangulation between the sulcal bottom and top curves to generate the entire mesh as an initialization of the sulcal ribbon surface: $R(u, v) = (1 - v)R(u, 0) + vR(u, 1)$.   The number of v iso-parametric curves is chosen to be 20 in our implementation, so that the triangulation of sulcal ribbon surfaces are fine enough to be on the order of a voxel or less. Figure 7(a,b) shows such an initialization of a central sulcal surface and a superior frontal sulcal surface.

We then deform the surface according to the following equation while fixing the sulcal bottom curve $R(u, 0)$:

$$\frac{\partial R(u, v)}{\partial t} = F_{smooth} + F_{image}$$

$$= a(R_{uu} + R_{vv}) + (\nabla \Psi_{out} \cdot N_R(u, v))N_R(u, v), \quad (u, v) \in [0, 1] \times (0, 1]$$

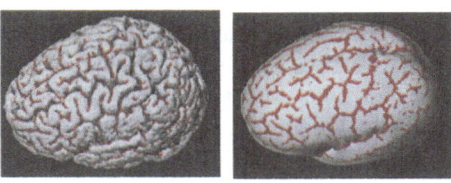

Fig. 3. Left: An outer cortical surface with high maximum principal curvature points shown in red. Right: Flattening makes more high curvature points visible.

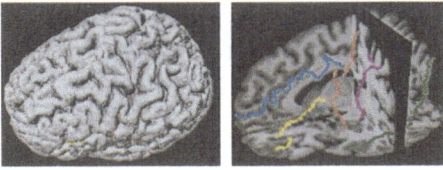

Fig. 4. Automatically traced sulci shown with cortical surface and orthogonal image cards are central (magenta), superior (blue) and inferior (yellow) frontal, superior temporal (green) and pre-central (tan) sulci.

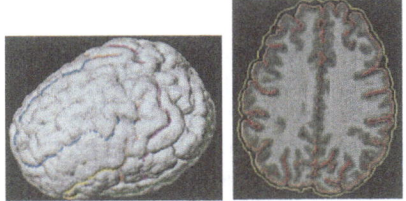

Fig. 5. Left: Corresponding sulcal top curves (also see Figure 4) on brain wrapper. Right: Cut view of brain wrapper (yellow) and cortical surface (red) on axial slice.

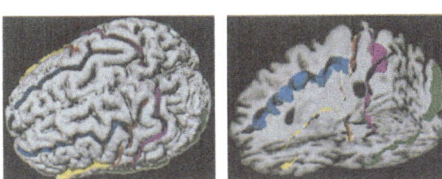

Fig. 6. Sulcal ribbon surfaces corresponding to sulcal curves in Figure 4 shown on cortical surface and orthogonal image cards.

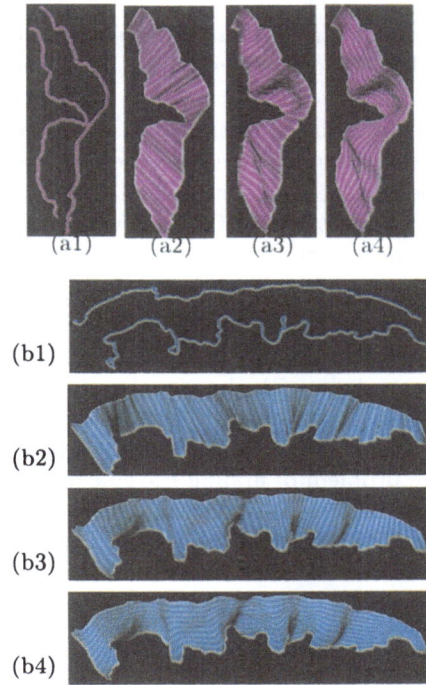

(a1)   (a2)   (a3)   (a4)

(b1)

(b2)

(b3)

(b4)

Fig. 7. Deformation of (a): central and (b): superior frontal sulcal ribbons. (1): Sulcal top and bottom curves traced automatically. (2): Piece-wise linear mesh as initialization. Sulcal ribbons with isoparametric (3):u and (4):v curves superimposed.

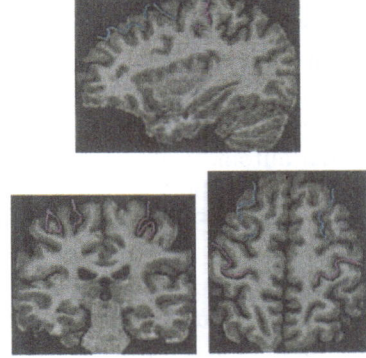

Fig. 8. Central (magenta) and superior frontal (blue) sulcal ribbons shown on sagittal, coronal and axial image slices.

where $N_R(u, v)$ denotes the unit normal of the sulcal ribbon surface. The first term on the right hand side of the equation guarantees the smoothness of the sulcal ribbon surface, while the second force drives the sulcal surface in its normal direction towards the local maximum of Ψ_{out} which corresponds to the sulcal medial axis. Thus, the surface deforms to the sulcal medial axis while maintaining a certain smoothness decided by parameter a. This equation is discretized on the surface mesh and solved iteratively. The iteration stops when the increase of $\int\int_{R(u,v)} \Psi_{out} du dv$ falls below a certain threshold, which is set to be 0.05.

Figure 7(c,d) shows the captured central and superior frontal sulcal surfaces with their iso-parametric u and v curves superimposed. The iso-u parametric curves show the correspondence between the points on sulcal top and bottom curves which is used in the sulcal depth measurement, and the iso-v parametric curves help with the visualization of the convolution across the sulcal depth.

The advantage of our approach is that the information defining the sulcal medial axis is implicit in the signed distance function Ψ_{out}, and by using Ψ_{out}, the problem of finding the sulcal ribbon becomes explicitly one of surface deformation. This formulation avoids the difficulty in tuning the weights of multiple inward force components in the sliding contour model.

3   Applications

In this section, we present results of our sulcal ribbon finding algorithm on high resolution MR images (1.5 T GE scanner, SPGR, $1.2 \times 1.2 \times 1.2 mm^3$ voxel size), and discuss how they can be used for structural and functional analysis of sulci.

We first ran our coupled surfaces algorithm to segment cortical gray matter from white matter and non-brain tissues, which resulted in the outer cortical surface S_{out} and its level function Ψ_{out}. The segmented cortical gray matter volume was then inspected by an expert, and corrections were made. Accordingly, S_{out} and Ψ_{out} were modified locally at the places of correction. This completed the pre-processing step of the sulcal ribbon finding algorithm.

As described in section 2.3, a brain wrapper surface S_{wrap} was extracted based on Ψ_{out}, and maximum principal curvature was calculated on both S_{out} and S_{wrap}. Our expert then dropped starting and ending points of sulcal top and bottom curves on S_{wrap} and S_{out} respectively. After the sulcal curves were extracted automatically, sulcal ribbon surface was initialized and deformed as described in section 2.4. Software written in C++/Open Inventor was used for these steps on a SGI Octane machine with a 255MHz R10000 processor. The automatic tracing of sulcal curves is done in real-time, and the deformation of each ribbon surface takes about $3 - 5$ seconds.

Shown in Figure 6 are the ribbon surfaces of central (magenta), superior frontal (blue), inferior frontal (yellow), superior temporal (green) and pre-central (tan) sulci with the outer cortical surface and orthogonal image cards. The cut views of central and superior frontal sulcal ribbon on orthogonal image slices shown in Figure 8 demonstrate the complexity of 3D sulcal convolution captured by our algorithm.

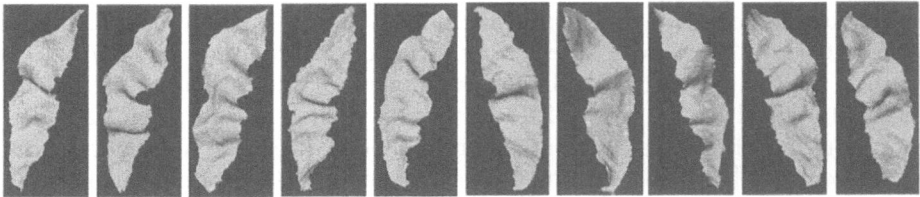

Fig. 9. Corresponding left (left 5) and right (right 5) central sulcal ribbons of 5 normal subjects extracted from MR images using our algorithm.

3.1   Quantitative Measurement of Central Sulcal Ribbons

Once the sulcal ribbons are captured in their parametric form, we can make quantitative measurements such as surface area, sulcal depth and sulcal curvature etc. Sulcal ribbon surface area is calculated as the sum of the area of all the triangles used to compose the surface. A reasonable and consistent way to measure sulcal depth is to measure the geodesics to sulcal fundus along the top curve, in other words, the geodesics between $R(u, 1)$ to $R(u, 0)$ for all $u \in [0, 1]$. The geodesics are computed using the dynamic programming technique described in Section 2.2, with the cost function set to be simply the length of a step, i.e. $dist(v_{i_k}, v_{i_{k+1}})$. Our experiments suggest that most of time the geodesic from $R(u_0, 1)$ to $R(u_0, 0)$ for a particular u_0 coincides with the iso-u curve $R(u_0)$.

We measured the depth and intrasulcal ribbon surface area of the complete course of the central sulcus in both hemispheres across 15 right handed subjects to demonstrate our methods in an area of interest to neuroscientists. The fundus of the central sulcus is the dividing point for the primary motor region (Brodmann area 4) on the anterior bank and the primary somatosensory strip (Brodmann area 3b) on the posterior bank of the sulcus. In addition to serving as boundaries, the depth of sulci and the total intrasulcal surface area may bear some relationship to the functional capacity of that region. There is a somatotopic mapping of the body on the primary motor and somatosensory regions, such that different regions of these cortical strips process information from different regions of the body. Recent work has suggested that anatomic asymmetry in the depth and surface area of the region of the central sulcus which maps to the hand and arm may be associated with asymmetry in motor function; right handers have a deeper central sulcus in this region in the left hemisphere, while the opposite is true in left handers [18, 1, 17].

Figure 9 shows the central sulcal ribbons of 5 of the subjects to demonstrate the sulcal variability captured by our algorithm. Although not presented here, ongoing work in our lab is comparing regional measurements corresponding to the representation of the hand in this group and a matched comparison group of left handers, in order to test for structure function relationships. Results for the total central sulcus in this group of 15 neurologically healthy young adults of normal general intelligence (IQ mean $\pm SD = 108 \pm 15$) including 7 males and 8 females between the ages 9 and 41 years are as follows. Average sulcal depth of the complete central sulcal ribbon was $18.12(\pm1.66)mm$ on the left and $18.08(\pm1.67)mm$ on the right, with no significant right-left difference. Total surface area of the cortical ribbon (corresponding to surface area of one bank, not both sulcal banks) was $1724(\pm202)mm^2$ on the left and $1764(\pm205)mm^2$ on the right. These measurements are roughly commensurate with postmortem measurements [17] and prior in vivo morphometry [1], especially considering the differences in measurement procedure (the cited methods were based on interpolation between traces on 2D slices).

3.2   Brain Matching With Cortical Constraints

Another potential use of the extracted sulcal surfaces lies in non-rigid brain warping and cortical atlas building. As distinctive features of the brain, sulcal surfaces can be used as geometric guidelines in shape transformation methodologies. There has already been work toward this direction [16, 6, 5], and our method offers an alternative to getting a starting point.

4   Discussion

We have presented a new approach to automatic 3D sulcal ribbon finding. Dynamic programming is used to automatically extract interior sulcal bottom curves on the outer cortical surface, and exterior sulcal top curves on a brain wrapper computed from the distance function Ψ_{out} associated with the outer cortical surface. A sulcal ribbon surface is then initialized through a piecewise linear triangulation between the sulcal top and bottom curves, and deformed to sulcal medial axis through the distance function Ψ_{out}. The use of Ψ_{out} makes the information defining sulcal medial axis implicit, and the resulting surface deformation formulation is simpler without multiple forces to tune. Though a natural follow up to our segmentation method, our sulcal ribbon finding algorithm can be adapted to follow other segmentation procedures. By allowing the user to define a sulcal ribbon with a few mouse clicks, our method offers automation, flexibility and real-time operation.

All the sulcal ribbon surfaces captured by our algorithm are evaluated slice by slice on axial image slices by an expert. The positions of the ribbon surfaces are always within one voxel's distance from the sulcal medial axis by visual inspection. However, since any type of expert tracing of the sulcal ribbon suffers from its limitation in capturing the 3D nature of sulci, we feel the best way to do full quantitative analysis of our algorithm is to create a phantom with known convolutions, and experiment on its images.

Our method for extracting the brain wrapper has potential for further improvement. There are no well defined methods to locate the exterior top edge of a sulcus. Although our way of extracting a fixed ϵ level set surface is consistent in it own right, ideally different values of ϵ need to be chosen for different sulci in order to obtain a more geometry-specific definition. Other directions of future research include localized sulcal measurement and shape analysis, and the study of structure and function relationships in the sulcal region.

Acknowledgements

This work was supported in part by NIH grant NINDS R01 NS35193, NSF grant IRI-9530768, and NIH grant NICHD 5 P01 HDIDC 35482.

References

1. K. Amunts et al. Asymmetry in the human motor cortex and handedness. *Neuroimage*, 4(3 Pt 1):216-22, Dec 1996.
2. D.H. Ballard and C.M. Brown. *Computer Vision*, chapter 4. Prentice-Hall Inc., New Jersey, 1982.
3. R. Bellman and R. Kalaba. *Dynamic Programming and Modern Control Theory*. Academic Press Inc, 1965.
4. H. Blum. *Models for the Perception of Speech and Visual Form*. MIT Press, 1967.
5. H. Chui, J. Rambo, R. Schultz, J. Duncan, and A. Rangarajan. Registration of cortical anatomical structures via robust 3D point matching. In *Proc. IPMI*, 1999.
6. D.L. Collins, G.L. Goualher, and A.C. Evans. Non-linear cerebral registration with sulcal constraints. In *Proc. MICCAI*, pp.974-984, MIT, 1998.
7. S. Gibson. Constrained elastic surface nets: Generating smooth surfaces from binary segmented data. In *Proc. MICCAI*, pp.888-898, MIT, 1998.
8. G.L. Goualher, C. Barillot, and Y.Bizais. Modeling cortical sulci using active ribbons. *Int. Journal of PRAI*, 11(8):1295-1315, 1997.
9. G.L. Goualher, D.L. Collins, C. Barillot, and A.C. Evans. Automatic identification of cortical sulci using a 3D probabilistic atlas. In *Proc. MICCAI*, pp.509-518, 1998.
10. N. Khaneja, M.I. Miller, and U. Grenander. Dynamic programming generation of curves on brain surfaces. *IEEE Trans. PAMI*, 20(11):1260-1265, 1998.
11. J. Mangin, J. Regis, I. Bloch, V. Frouin, Y. Samson, and J. LopezKrahe. A MRF based random graph modeling the human cortical topography. In *Proc. CVRMed*, pp.177-183, Nice, 1995.
12. L.R. Nackman and S.M. Pizer. Three-Dimensional shape description using the symmetric axis transformation I: Theory. *IEEE Trans. PAMI*, 7(2):187-202, 1985.
13. M. Naf, O. Kubler, R. Kikinis, M.E. Shenton, and G. Szekely. Characterization and recognition of 3d organ shape in medical image analysis using skeletonization. In *Proc. MMBIA*, pp.139-150, 1996.
14. J. Rademacher, V.S. Caviness Jr, H. Steinmetz, and A.M. Galaburda. Topographical variation of the human primary cortices: implications for neuroimaging, brain mapping, and neurobiology.. *Cerebral Cortex*, 3(4):313-329, 1993.
15. M. Vaillant and C. Davatzikos. Finding parametric representations of cortical sulci using an active contour model. *Medical Image Analysis*, pp.295-315, Sep 1997.
16. M. Vaillant and C. Davatzikos. Mapping the cerebral sulci: Application to morphological analysis of cortex and to non-rigid registration. In *Proc. IPMI*, pp.141-154, 1997.
17. L.E. White, T.J. Andrews, C. Hulette, A. Richards, M. Groelle, J. Paydarfar, and D. Purves. Structure of the human sensorimotor system. II: Lateral symmetry. *Cerebral Cortex*, 7(1):31-47, 1997.
18. L.E. White, G. Lucas, A. Richards, and D. Purves. Cerebral asymmetry and handedness. *Nature*, 368(6468):197-8, 1994.
19. X. Zeng, L.H. Staib, R.T. Schultz, and J.S. Duncan. Segmentation and measurement of the cortex from 3D MR images. In *Proc. MICCAI*, pp 519-530, 1998.
20. X. Zeng, L.H. Staib, R.T. Schultz, and J.S. Duncan. Volumetric layer segmentation using coupled surfaces propagation. In *Proc. CVPR*, pp.708-715, 1998.

Automated Segmentation of Sulcal Regions

Maryam E. Rettmann[1], Chenyang Xu[2] , Dzung L. Pham[2,4], and
Jerry L. Prince[1,2,3]

[1] Biomedical Engineering, [2] Electrical and Computer Engineering, [3] Radiology,
The Johns Hopkins University, Baltimore MD 21218, USA.
[4] Laboratory of Personality & Cognition, GRC/NIH, Baltimore, MD 21224, USA.

Abstract. Automatic segmentation and identification of cortical sulci play an important role in the study of brain structure and function. In this work, a method is presented for the automatic segmentation of sulcal regions of cortex. Unlike previous methods that extract the sulcal spaces within the cortex, the proposed method extracts actual regions of the cortical surface that surround sulci. Sulcal regions are segmented from the medial surface as well as the lateral and inferior surfaces. The method first generates a depth map on the surface, computed by measuring the distance between the cortex and an outer "shrink-wrap" surface. Sulcal regions are then extracted using a hierarchical algorithm that alternates between thresholding and region growing operations. To visualize the buried regions of the segmented cortical surface, an efficient technique for mapping the surface to a sphere is proposed. Preliminary results are presented on the geometric analysis of sulcal regions for automated identification.

1 Introduction

With the advancement of magnetic resonance (MR) imaging techniques, high-resolution, high contrast three-dimensional images of the brain can now be routinely acquired in vivo. Techniques for modeling and automatically extracting information from such images have therefore emerged as a crucial component in furthering the understanding of brain structure and function. In particular, a topic that has recently received increased attention is the segmentation and identification of sulci [1–6]. Sulci identified on the cortex can then be used in applications such as localizing activation sites in functional imaging and deformable atlas registration algorithms. In addition, the geometric analysis of sulci will lead to a better understanding of normal versus diseased cortical geometry and the morphological changes that occur with disease.

Most previous work in the segmentation of sulci has focused on either fitting a surface [1–3] or finding a set of points [5] in between the sulcal banks. In this work, we present a method that segments the actual cortical regions surrounding sulci as opposed to extracting the sulcal spaces. The advantage of segmenting the actual surface is that a direct mapping of the cortical geometry is obtained.

This work was partially supported by the NSF Presidential Faculty Fellow Award MIP93-50336, NIH R01NS37747 and a Whitaker Foundation graduate fellowship.

For ease of terminology, we refer to our segmented regions as "sulcal regions", meaning precisely the buried regions of cortex surrounding the sulcal spaces. Another advantage of the proposed method is that it segments sulcal regions on the medial surface as well as the lateral and inferior surfaces. Also, this segmentation method is completely automated except for picking a seed point on the reconstructed cortical surface.

The segmentation is accomplished by reconstructing two surfaces for each hemisphere— the true cortical surface and an outer "shrink-wrap" surface. Sulcal regions on the true cortical surface are then segmented by their distance to the shrink-wrap surface. Because the sulcal regions are buried beneath the cortical folds, we briefly describe a fast method for generating a spherical representation of the cortical surface that facilitates their visualization. After the sulcal regions have been segmented, the next step is to anatomically identify each region as corresponding to a particular sulcus. We present some preliminary results on evaluating the characteristics of segmented sulcal regions that have potential for automatic sulcal identification.

2   Methods

Initial Data and Model   Although our method is generally applicable to any reconstructed cortical surface [7–12], in this work, we use surfaces reconstructed from MR images generated by the technique described in [13]. This technique combines fuzzy segmentation, isosurfaces and deformable surface models to reconstruct the layer of cortex lying in the geometric center, which is approximately cytoarchitectonic layer 4. MR data was obtained from the Baltimore Longitudinal Study on Aging [14]. The reconstruction method is composed of three major steps. First, a three-class fuzzy segmentation of the MR data is computed corresponding to gray matter, white matter and cerebrospinal fluid. Second, an initialization for the deformable surface model is created by generating a smoothed isosurface from the white matter membership function obtained from the segmentation. The result of the isosurface algorithm is a mesh that is a discrete representation of the continuous isosurface. Finally, a deformable surface model is used to refine the initial surface to the central layer of the gray matter. The cortex reconstruction method requires a minimal amount of manual interaction and is capable of fully resolving deep convoluted folds.

To allow visualization of the buried sulcal regions, a spherical representation of the reconstructed cortical surface is generated that maintains a one-to-one mapping with the original reconstructed surface. This "spherical map" is generated by reducing the number of vertices in the cortical surface mesh to a few points and then rebuilding the mesh to a sphere in conjunction with a multi-resolution relaxation process. The mesh is reduced by a progressive mesh decimation originally described in [15] and subsequently in [16]. In a progressive mesh decimation, a complex mesh is reduced to a simplified base mesh while storing the information necessary to rebuild the original mesh. In the spherical map generation, we first decimate the cortical surface mesh and then use the resulting base mesh and stored information to rebuild the mesh to a sphere. This is accomplished by initially projecting each vertex of the base mesh to a sphere. As each vertex is subsequently added back to the mesh, it is placed on the sphere while maintaining the correct neighbor topology. At various stages in the rebuilding process the vertices on the sphere are allowed to undergo elastic relaxation in order to avoid anomalous topologies. Compared to methods based purely on elastic deformations, this iterative rebuilding and multi-resolution smoothing process is typically six times faster, requiring only about one hour on an Silicon Graphics O2 R10000 workstation.

Segmentation.   In this section, we describe the method for automatically segmenting the sulcal regions from a reconstructed cortical surface. The basic principle of the segmentation method is that regions of cortex that are not part of the outer, gyral surface are considered to lie in sulci. This outer surface, which we call a "shrink-wrap", tightly surrounds the reconstructed cortical surface, but does not enter into the cortical folds. Sulcal regions are then defined based on distances between the cortical surface and the shrink-wrap surface. In order to segment the sulcal regions on the medial surfaces as well as the lateral and inferior surfaces, a shrink-wrap surface must be generated for each hemisphere separately. To this end, the reconstructed cortical surface is divided into two separate hemispheres by applying a cut through the corpus callosum. This step requires a user-defined seed point at the center of the corpus callosum, the only manual interaction required during the entire segmentation procedure.

The shrink-wrap surface is generated for each hemisphere using a deformable surface model. Focusing on one hemisphere, a deformable surface is initialized as an ellipsoidal mesh and allowed to deform to the outer cortical surface according to external and internal forces. The external forces drive the deformable surface model toward the cortical surface using standard gradient based potential forces [17] derived from an edge map. The edge map, shown in Fig. 1(a), is generated by discretizing one hemisphere of the reconstructed cortical surface. High internal forces are used to force the deformable surface to have a high tension, thus reducing its ability to enter into the cortical folds. The use of high internal forces, however, can sometimes cause the deformable surface to break through the gyri as shown in Fig. 1(b). To avoid this, an additional external force is introduced into the model. This force, which we call a barrier force, prevents the deformable surface from moving into parts of the image marked as barrier regions. A barrier region that prevents the deformable surface from shrinking into the gyri is created by applying a unidirectional inward dilation to the edge map. Additionally, the hole introduced at the corpus callosum is filled by adding points along the path originally used to introduce the cut. The resulting barrier region, shown in Fig. 1(c), allows for high tension on the deformable surface while preventing it from shrinking into the cortical surface. Fig. 1(d) is a coronal cross-section showing a contour of the final shrink-wrap surface in gray and the reconstructed cortical surface in white. Parameter values required for the deformable surface algorithm were determined empirically from one data set and held fixed for subsequent data sets.

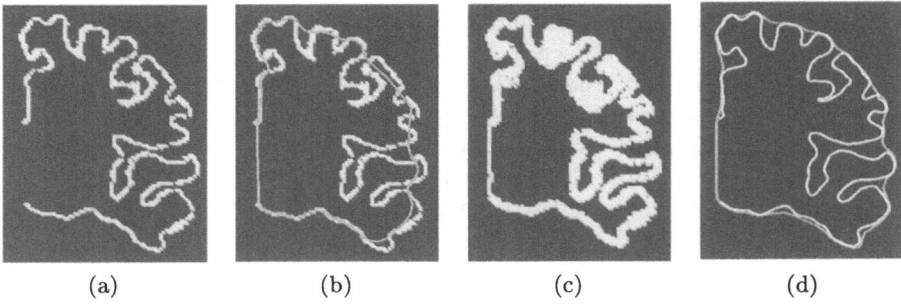

(a)   (b)   (c)   (d)

Fig. 1. Cross-sectional view of (a) the edge map generated from the cortical surface, (b) the deformable surface breaking through gyral regions, (c) the barrier region, and (d) the shrink-wrap surface superimposed on the cortical surface.

In the next step, the deep sulcal regions are discriminated from outer, gyral regions by computing the three-dimensional Euclidean distance from each vertex on the cortical surface to the nearest vertex on the corresponding shrink-wrap surface. Fig. 3(a)[1] shows a resulting depth map plotted on a lateral view of the spherical map, where larger depths are plotted in red and gray and smaller depths are plotted in blue. The corresponding lateral view of the convoluted cortical surface is shown in Fig. 3(b). This figure illustrates that buried sulcal regions can be identified by their greater distances to the outer shrink-wrap surface. For example, the largest gray region towards the bottom of the spherical map is the insular cortex and the vertical region above the insula with a slight posterior to anterior orientation is the cortical region surrounding the Central sulcus.

In order to obtain separate parametric surface segments for each sulcal region, points within a sulcal region must be connected. A simple approach would be to apply a single thresholding operation to the depth map, followed by a region growing algorithm that connects clustered regions to form sulcal segments. The shortcoming of this approach is that, because of the complex cortical geometry, there is no single threshold that can simultaneously extract the full extent of each sulcal region while preventing separate sulcal regions from joining together. This is because a high depth threshold segments only the deepest portions of a sulcal region, while a low depth threshold results in the joining of distinct sulcal regions. Thus, a hierarchical approach is applied that initially sets the threshold to a large value and relationships between regions are defined as the threshold is gradually decreased. This allows for sulci to be defined as distinct at the deeper regions of the cortex where they are believed to be more stable.

First, an initial sulcal segmentation map is computed from the depth map using a threshold of 10 pixels, where a pixel is .9375 millimeters. Vertices on the cortical surface with a depth greater than the initial threshold are considered to lie in sulcal regions. Clustered vertices are then joined to form parametric sulcal

---

[1] Figures are referenced out of order because color figures appear at end of text.

segments and each region is assigned a distinct but arbitrary numerical label. The resulting sulcal map, shown in Fig. 5(a) extracts the most buried portions of the deeper sulci. Next, the depth threshold is slightly decreased. Clustered vertices that have a depth between the previous threshold and the new threshold are joined to form new regions. These new regions are assigned numerical labels according to a set of rules designed to expand previously extracted regions while preventing separate regions from joining together. These rules are given as follows:

1. If a region is not adjacent to any previously labeled regions, it is assigned a new numerical label.
2. If a region is adjacent to a single previously labeled region, it is assigned the numerical label of the adjacent region.
3. If a region is adjacent to two or more previously labeled regions, it is labeled as a bridge region.
4. If a region is adjacent to a bridge, this region is also labeled as a bridge (this rule applies only to subsequent hierarchical levels).

After the region growing is complete, non-bridge regions with areas below a specified size are removed. This process is repeated for each thresholding level. Fig. 5 shows the sulcal map at various thresholding levels where the bridges are shown in black. This figure demonstrates how this hierarchical thresholding and region growing algorithm segments the full extent of the sulcal regions, but prevents separate sulcal regions from connecting together. After the final iteration of the above process, all bridges are relabeled as gyral regions.

3   Segmentation Results and Discussion

The sulcal segmentation method was applied to three reconstructed cortical surfaces with a typical result shown in Fig. 6. In each image of Fig. 6, the segmented regions are superimposed on either a translucent cortical reconstruction or its spherical map. Once segmented, each sulcal region can be manually identified as the region of cortex surrounding a specific sulcus. For example, on the right lateral surface are the regions corresponding to the Superior Temporal sulcus (green), Sylvian fissure (magenta) and Central sulcus (blue). On the medial surface, the Parieto-Occipital (orange), and Calcarine (purple) sulcal regions are segmented as well as the Cingulate sulcal region which is composed of several segments arcing from anterior to posterior. Sulcal regions segmented from the medial surface are also visible in the top view of the spherical map. Several other sulcal regions, such as the right Superior Frontal seen at the bottom left of Figs. 6(b) and (e), are segmented as several pieces. The fragmented segmentation of sulci that are interrupted or pseudo-interrupted (meaning the interruption occurs within the sulcal fold [18]) has both advantages and disadvantages. The disadvantage is that fragmented regions need to be identified as belonging to a single sulcal region. The advantage is that these fragments can be used to quantitatively analyze the characteristics of interrupted sulci. Another complexity of cortical geometry is that two distinct sulci may be joined, meaning there is no gyral ridge separating them, even at the sulcal fundi. In this segmentation method, a single sulcal region will be extracted for two sulci that are joined.

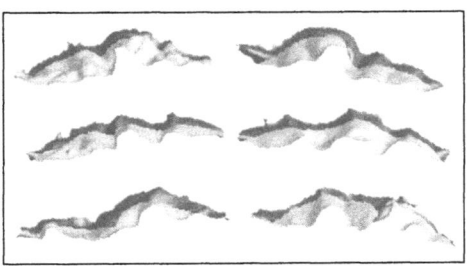

Fig. 2. Region of cortex surrounding the Central sulcus segmented from six hemispheres.

The segmented regions corresponding to the Central sulcus from the six hemispheres are shown in Fig. 2. To aid in visualization, the side of the surface closer to the white matter is colored light gray, while the side closer to the cerebral spinal fluid is colored dark gray. This figure illustrates that although variability exists across subjects, these sulcal regions share some characteristic geometric features.

4   Geometric Analysis of Segmented Sulcal Regions

In this section, we investigate the potential for using geometric quantities computed for each sulcal region to automatically identify their anatomical designation. Three geometric features are computed for each segmented sulcal region and evaluated on the basis of whether the sulci might be distinguishable based on these features. The features used in this preliminary study are area, center of mass in Talairach coordinates and orientation.

For the area computation, the surface area in mm^2 is computed for each polygonal face in the region and these areas are summed. In order to compute the center of mass of each segment in Talairach coordinates, the surface is transformed into the standard three-dimensional Talairach space [19] and then computed as follows:

$$\mu = \frac{1}{N}\sum_{i=1}^{N} v_i \qquad (1)$$

where N is the number of vertices in the extracted sulcal segment and v_i is the location of each vertex in three-dimensional space. The orientation of each segmented region in the standard three-dimensional Talairach coordinate space is characterized by an orientation vector. This vector is computed by first computing the covariance matrix,

$$\Sigma = \frac{1}{N-1}\sum_{i=1}^{N}(v_i - \mu)(v_i - \mu)^T. \qquad (2)$$

The eigenvector associated with the maximum eigenvalue of Σ yields the orientation of the segmented region. The eigenvectors are restricted to point in the positive Z direction guaranteeing uniqueness.

The surface areas computed for each segmented region of three cortical surfaces are shown in Fig. 4(a). The x-axis is the identification number of each segmented region and the y-axis is the surface area in mm^2. The regions of cortex corresponding to the right and left Sylvian fissures are easily identified as having the two largest area measurements in each plot. Fig. 4(b) shows the Talairach centers of mass for a few selected sulcal regions from six hemispheres where regions corresponding to a particular sulcus are colored the same. The color scheme is as follows: Central sulcus (yellow), Sylvian fissure (green), Parieto-Occipital sulcus (blue) and Calcarine sulcus (red). In one of the hemispheres, the Parieto-Occipital and Calcarine sulci were connected resulting in a single segmented region corresponding to both sulci. This region is colored in cyan. This figure illustrates that the centers of mass for these sulcal regions in all six hemispheres cluster quite well in three-dimensional space, especially for regions corresponding to the Central sulcus and Sylvian fissure. Fig. 4(c) shows the orientation vectors computed for each segmented region from one cortical surface superimposed on the segments themselves. The origin of each orientation vector is the center of mass of its corresponding segment. This figure illustrates that the orientation vector describes the directionality of each segmented region. The orientation vectors of a few selected regions from six hemispheres are plotted in Fig. 4(d) with each vector centered at the origin. The color scheme used is the same as in Fig. 4(b). This plot illustrates the strong y orientation of the Calcarine sulcal region as opposed to the strong z orientation of the Parieto-Occipital sulcal region, indicating that this quantity could be used to discriminate these two regions that have similar locations in three-dimensional space. The three geometric quantities computed can be combined to form a high-dimensional geometric feature vector that characterizes the geometry of each segmented region. Used alone, these geometric features may not be sufficient to automatically identify sulcal regions. But from the results of our preliminary analysis, automatic identification may be possible when the various geometric features are combined.

5   Conclusions and Future Work

We have described an automated method that segments the full extent of sulcal regions while maintaining separate regions as distinct. Geometric quantities computed for each sulcal segment show promise for the automatic identification of their anatomic designation. We are currently working to apply our segmentation method and geometric analysis on additional data sets. This will allow us to test our hypothesis of automated labeling based on high-dimensional geometric feature vectors.

Acknowledgments

The authors are grateful to Swen Campagna and Hans Peter Seidel for allowing use of their progressive mesh software.

References

1. P. M. Thompson, C. Schwartz, and A. W. Toga. High-resolution random mesh algorithms for creating a probabilistic 3D surface atlas of the human brain. *Neuroimage*, 3:19–34, 1996.
2. M. Vaillant and C. Davatzikos. Finding parametric representations of the cortical sulci using an active contour model. *Medical Image Analysis*, 1(4):295–315, 1997.
3. G. Le Goualher, C. Barillot, and Y. Bizais. Modeling cortical sulci with active ribbons. *IJPRAI*, 11(8):1295–1315, 1997.
4. G. Le Goualher, D. L. Collins, C. Barillot, and A. C. Evans. Automatic identification of cortical sulci using a 3D probabilistic atlas. In *Proc. of (MICCAI)*, pages 509–517, 1998.
5. J.F. Mangin, V. Frouin, I. Bloch, J. Regis, and J. Lopez-Krahe. From 3D magnetic resonance images to structural representations of the cortex topography using topology preserving deformations. *Math. Imag. and Vision.*, 5:297–318, 1995.
6. J.F. Mangin, J. Regis, I. Bloch, V. Frouin, Y. Samson, and J. Lopez-Krahe. A MRF based random graph modelling the human cortical topography. In *Lecture Notes in Computer Science*, pages 177–183, Nice, France, 1995. CVRMed'95.
7. A. M. Dale, B. Fischl, and M. I. Sereno. Cortical surface-based analysis I. Segmentation and surface reconstruction. *Neuroimage*, 9:179–194, 1999.
8. D. MacDonald, D. Avis, and A. C. Evans. Multiple surface identification and matching in magnetic resonance images. In *SPIE Proc. VBC '94*, volume 2359, pages 160–169, 1994.
9. H.A. Drury, D.C. Van Essen, C.H. Anderson, C.W. Lee, T.A. Coogan, and J.W. Lewis. Computerized mappings of the cerebral cortex: A multiresolution flattening method and a surface-based coordinate system. *J. Cogn. Neuro.*, 8(1):1–28, 1996.
10. C. Davatzikos and R. N. Bryan. Using a deformable surface model to obtain a shape representation of the cortex. *IEEE Trans. Med. Imag.*, 15:785–795, December 1996.
11. S. Sandor and R. Leahy. Surface-based labeling of cortical anatomy using a deformable atlas. *IEEE Trans. Med. Imag.*, 16(1):41–54, 1997.
12. C. Xu, D. L. Pham, and J. L. Prince. Finding the brain cortex using fuzzy segmentation, isosurfaces, and deformable surface models. In *the XVth Int. Conf. Inf. Proc. Med. Imag. (IPMI)*, pages 399–404. Springer-Verlag, 1997.
13. C. Xu, D. L. Pham, J. L. Prince, M. E. Etemad, and D. N. Yu. Reconstruction of the central layer of the human cerebral cortex from MR images. In *Proc. of (MICCAI)*, pages 481–488. Springer-Verlag, 1998.
14. N. W. Shock, R. C. Greulich, R. Andres, D. Arenberg, P. T. Costa Jr., E. Lakatta, and J. D. Tobin. Normal human aging: The Baltimore longitudinal study of aging. U.S. Governement Printing Office, Washington, D.C., 1984.
15. Hughes Hoppe. Progressive meshes. In *Computer Graphics (SIGGRAPH '96 Proceedings)*, pages 99–108, 1996.
16. S. Campagna and H.-P. Seidel. Generating and displaying progressive meshes. In H.-P. Seidel, B. Girod, and H. Niemann, editors, *3D Image Analysis and Synthesis '97*, pages 35–42, 1997.
17. M. Kass, A. Witkin, and D. Terzopoulos. Snakes: Active contour models. *International Journal of Computer Vision*, 1(4):321–331, 1987.
18. M. Ono, S. Kubick, and C. D. Abernathey. *Atlas of the cerebral sulci*. Thieme, New York, 1990.
19. J. Talairach and P. Tournoux. *Co-Planar Stereotaxic Atlas of the Human Brain. 3-Dimensional Proportional System: An Approach to Cerebral Imaging*. Thieme Medical Publisher, Inc., Stuttgart, New York, 1988.

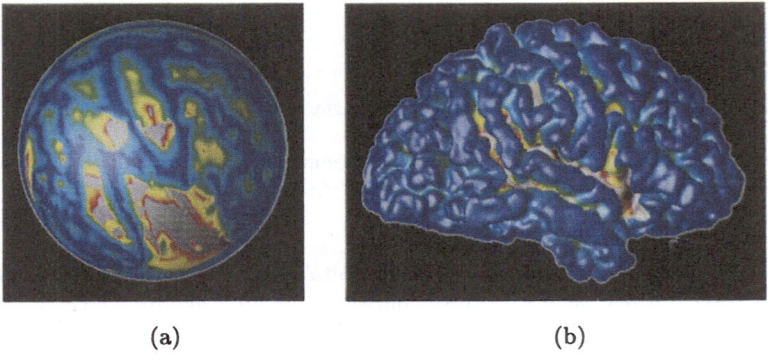

Fig. 3. Computed depths displayed on a lateral view of (a) the spherical map and (b) the convoluted cortical surface.

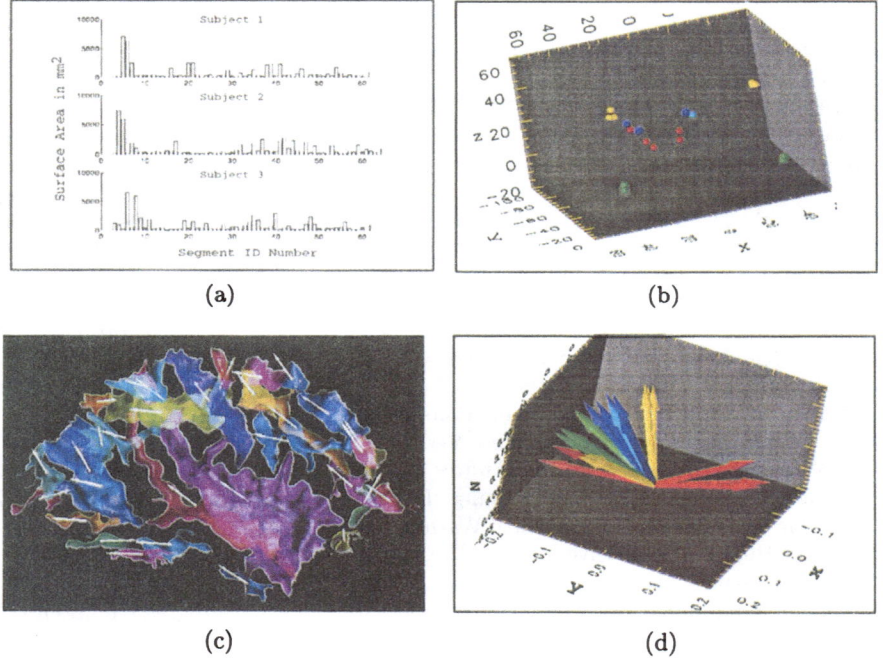

Fig. 4. Geometrical features: (a) surface areas of all segmented sulcal regions from three cortical surfaces, (b) Talairach centers of mass of selected sulcal regions from three cortical surfaces, (c) orientation vectors of all segmented regions from one cortical surface and (d) orientation vectors of selected sulcal regions from three cortical surfaces.

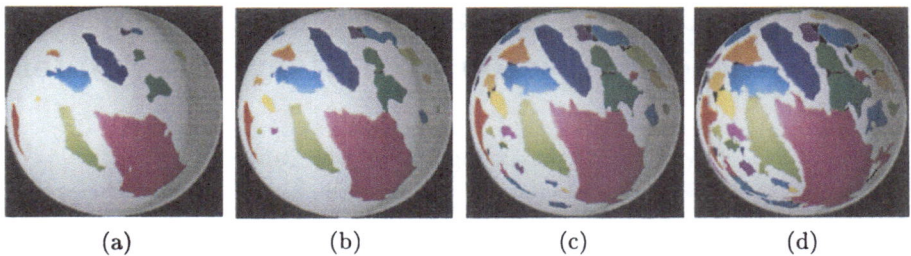

Fig. 5. Sulcal map shown at a threshold of (a) 10 (b) 7 (c) 4 and (d) 2 pixels, where a pixel is .9375 mm.

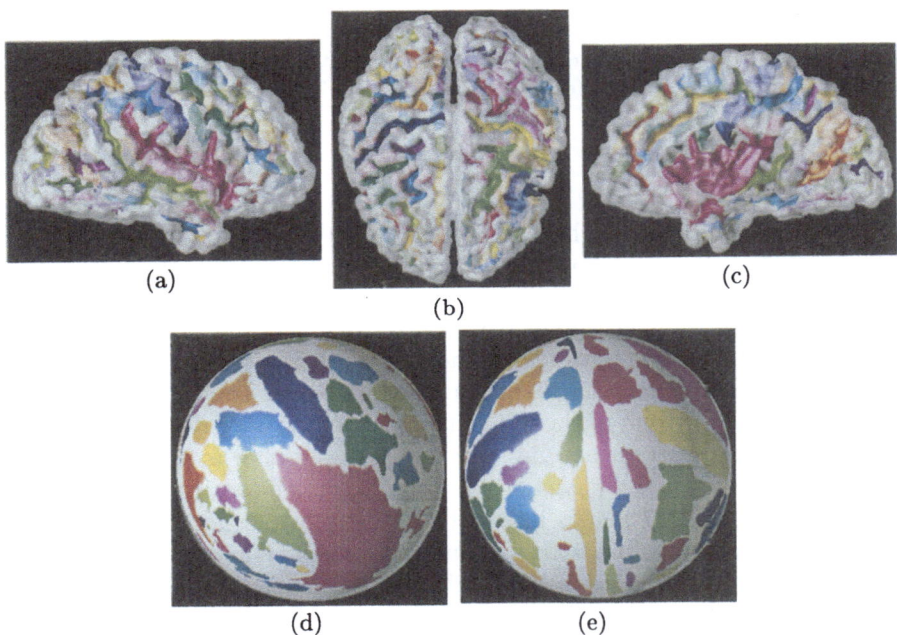

Fig. 6. Resulting sulcal segmentation superimposed on (a) lateral (b) top and (c) medial views of the reconstructed cortical surface and (d) lateral and (e) top views of the spherical map.

Cylindrical Echocardiographic Image Segmentation Based on 3D Deformable Models

J. Montagnat, H. Delingette, and G. Malandain

INRIA Sophia, Epidaure project, BP 93
2004 route des Lucioles, 06902 Sophia-Antipolis Cedex France
http://www-sop.inria.fr/epidaure/

Abstract. This paper presents a 3D echocardiographic image segmentation procedure based on deformable surfaces. We first propose to adapt filtering techniques to the cylindrical geometry of several 3D ultrasound image devices. Then we compare the effect of different external forces on a surface template deformation inside volumetric echocardiographic images. An original method involving region grey-level analysis along the model normal directions is described. We rely on an *a priori* knowledge of the cardiac left ventricle shape and on region grey-level values to perform a robust segmentation. During the deformation process the allowable surface deformation is modified. Finally, we show experimental results on very challenging sparse and noisy images and quantitative measurements of the left ventricle volume.

1 Introduction

Since its introduction over the past few years, 3D ultrasound imagery has been very promising due to its low cost and non-invasive nature. Furthermore, the development of real-time 3D ultrasound probes reveals numerous applications for the diagnosis and therapy of patients. Cardiac left ventricle modeling permits a quantitative computation of the ventricle ejection fraction which is of major importance in detecting heart pathologies. In this paper, we propose a 3D reconstruction algorithm of the left ventricle based on 3D deformable models.

In many cases, 3D ultrasound systems are based on a mobile 2D probe acquiring along non-aligned planes [13]. In this paper, we consider rotative probes producing a set of 2D planes intersecting each other along a revolution axis. These images are acquired with a cylindrical geometry implying that the density of information decreases as a function of the distance to the axis (figure 1).

Previous work of Winterfeldt [14] and Jacob [6] have mainly considered 2D image segmentation and tracking approaches without any spatial coherence between slices. Statistical information (mainly principal component analysis) has also been used to restrain the allowable deformations of a model [6, ?]. Several authors proposed to reduce speckle level by spatial compounding [11] or to detect boundaries in US images by modeling speckle noise [1].

In this paper, we propose to use "naive" image processing techniques based on rough approximations of the image speckle and noise. The introduction of

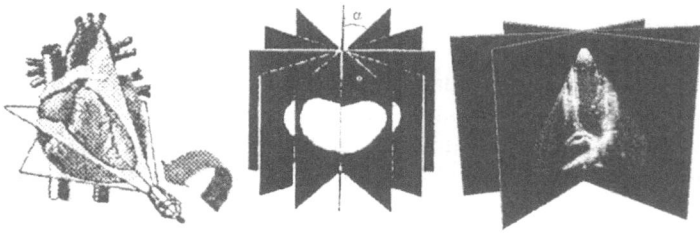

Fig. 1. The rotative probe and the resulting US images with cylindrical symmetry.

3D deformation and some basic *a priori* knowledge about the data's reliability compensate for the presence of outliers and increase the robustness of the image segmentation. The main contributions of our approach are to consider the full 3D problem with 3D model deformations inside a volumetric image, to adapt image filtering techniques to the ultrasound images cylindrical geometry, and to use a region-based approach for finding the boundaries of the left ventricle.

2 Simplex Meshes

A 2-simplex mesh is a discrete non-parametric representation of a surface in $\mathbb{R}^3$ defined by a set of vertices $\{\mathbf{V}_i\}_i$ and their connectivity. It is a regular 3-connected mesh, its topology is dual to a triangulation, and it can represent surfaces of any topology. The geometry of simplex meshes allows one to define discrete quantities such as mean curvature at each vertex (see [2] for details). All vertices follow a Newtonian law of motion. Three kinds of forces are computed at each vertex $\mathbf{V}_i$. The internal force f_i^{int} enforces some regularization behavior (such as C^2 continuity). The external force f_i^{ext} pulls the model towards the ventricle boundaries. The global displacement force f_i^{global} is computed from a global transformation with few degrees of freedom designed to constrain all the vertices displacements. The law of motion is discretized using finite differences and an explicit iterative scheme:

$$\mathbf{V}_i^{t+1} = \mathbf{V}_i^t + (1-\gamma)(\mathbf{V}_i^t - \mathbf{V}_i^{t-1}) + \alpha f_i^{int} + \beta(\lambda f_i^{ext} + (1-\lambda)f_i^{global}),$$

where $\mathbf{V}_i^t$ denotes the position of vertex $\mathbf{V}_i$ at time t, γ is a damping coefficient, α and β are the internal and external force weights, and λ is a locality weight. The time step is hidden in the α, β and γ coefficients. We use a refinement approach, limiting model deformation capabilities by setting λ to zero at the beginning of the deformation process, then letting it gradually increase to allow more deformations. The α coefficient value is set to 1 thus having β variations weight the respective influence of the internal and the external forces. The β coefficient varies from 1 to 0.1 as λ increases. The damping value γ is fixed to 0.35 based on some empirical results. An automatic algorithm for governing λ evolution was proposed in [10].

3   Gradient Computation in Cylindrical Geometry

In 3D images based on a regular lattice (Cartesian images), the computation of gradient vectors is mostly based on separable filters (*e.g.*, Sobel operators) or recursive filtering (*e.g.*, Canny-Deriche filters [9]). When considering images of cylindrical geometry, classical approaches can be used in each slice, computing 2D gradients and neglecting the tangential component. It is also possible to interpolate the image on a regular lattice before applying 3D operators. Unfortunately, this approach is hopeless due to the important angular resolution and the low signal-to-noise ratio. Instead, we compute a 3D gradient vector for each image voxel in the cylindrical geometry (see [5] for a similar approach in 2D). Let M_0 be a point in Euclidean space with Cartesian coordinates (x_0, y_0, z_0) and cylindrical coordinates (r_0, θ_0, z_0) (see figure 2 left). Let I be the cylindrical image defined as $I : B \subset \mathbb{R}^3 \rightarrow \mathbb{R}$, where B is the discrete cylindrical grid over which the grey-level values are known. The convolution of a 3D signal S by a filter f at point M_0 is defined in Cartesian space as:

$$(S \otimes f)(M_0) = \int_{-\infty}^{\infty} \int_{-\infty}^{\infty} \int_{-\infty}^{\infty} S(x_0 - x, y_0 - y, z_0 - z) f(x, y, z) dx dy dz. \quad (1)$$

To express this equation in cylindrical space we use the coordinate transformation $x = r \cos(\theta)$, $y = r \sin(\theta)$, and $z = z$. Let J be the Jacobian matrix corresponding to this transformation. A variable change in equation 1 leads to:

$$(S \otimes f)(M_0) = \int_{-\infty}^{\infty} \int_{0}^{2\pi} \int_{0}^{\infty} S(x_0 - r\cos(\theta), y_0 - r\sin(\theta), z_0 - z) f(x, y, z) |J| dr d\theta dz. \quad (2)$$

Since image I is a discrete signal, we discretize equation 2. Let δr, $\delta\theta$, and δz be the dimensions of the discrete filter to apply to I, the filtered value of I at point $M_0 \in B$, knowing that $|J| = r$, is:

$$(I \otimes f)(M_0) = \sum_{z=z_0-\delta z}^{z_0+\delta z} \sum_{\theta=\theta_0-\delta\theta}^{\theta_0+\delta\theta} \sum_{r=r_0-\delta r}^{r_0+\delta r} -I(r, \theta, z) r f(x_0 - r\cos(\theta), y_0 - r\sin(\theta), z_0 - z).$$

We use Deriche filters [3] to perform gradient computation in cylindrical geometry. Let D_d and S_d be the mono-dimensional Deriche derivative and smoothing filters respectively, in dimension $d \in \{x, y, z\}$: $D_d(u) = ue^{-\alpha|u|}$ and $S_d(u) = (\alpha|u| + 1)e^{-\alpha|u|}$. The directional gradient operators are defined as $G_x(u) = D_x(u)S_y(u)S_z(u)$, $G_y(u) = S_x(u)D_y(u)S_z(u)$, and $G_z(u) = S_x(u)S_y(u)D_z(u)$. The discrete masks are computed by sampling G_x, G_y, and G_z values then normalizing mask coefficients such that the sum of positive coefficients equals 1 and the sum of negative coefficients equals -1. This ensures that the derivative mask coefficients sum is nul.

Figure 2 (center) illustrates the filter response on a slice of a synthetic cube image for a 3^3 (top) and a 7^3 (bottom) filter. Figure 2 (right) compares the output of the 2D Sobel filters (left) and a 3D cylindrical operator (right) in one image plane. The cylindrical operator improves significantly the edge detection and reduces the speckle effect by filtering along the axial direction, especially close to the rotation axis where dense data is available.

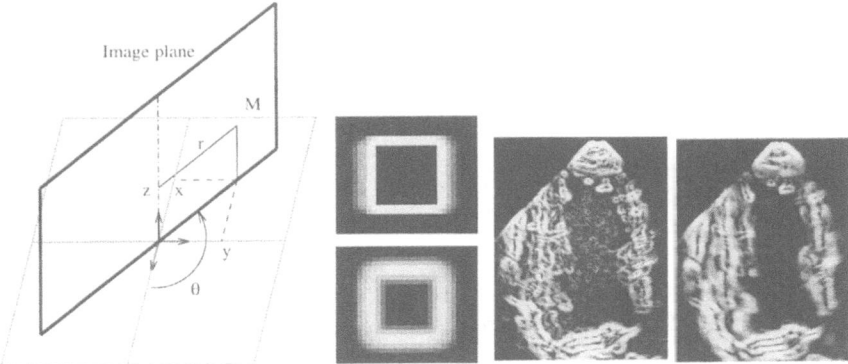

Fig. 2. (left) Cylindrical geometry; (center) cylindrical gradient filter response on a cube; (right) comparison of Sobel operators and the cylindrical gradient filter.

4 External Forces for 3D US Image Segmentation

Our deformable simplex mesh relies on external forces for segmenting the left ventricle in 3D US images. These forces should attract each model vertex towards the closest left ventricle boundary voxel. In echocardiographic images several difficulties arise for finding object boundaries. The *speckle*, inherent to the image formation of US imagery, and the image *noise* mainly originating from the digitalization process, are responsible for causing false contour detections (false positives). The *variable information density*, due to the cylindrical geometry of the image, and the *missing information*, due to the low energy of the ultrasound beam reflected at the organ interfaces and the rib occlusions, make the ventricle contours hard to detect (false negatives). We rely on the model regularizing behavior and the robust force expressions proposed below to deal with the false positives and the false negatives.

4.1 Scan-Line Algorithm

The force expressions are computed for each vertex by scanning along the model normal direction until a boundary voxel is reached. Indeed, it has been shown in [8] that the class of surface deformations is not restricted by only considering displacement along each vertex normal. Thus, we restrict the search for boundary points along the normal direction $\mathbf{n}_i$ of each vertex $\mathbf{V}_i$.

We proceed by scanning all the cylindrical voxels which intersect with the normal line $(\mathbf{V}_i, \mathbf{n}_i)$ in the volumetric image within a fixed range centered on each vertex (see figure 3 left). The image intensity $I(\mathbf{P})$ at any normal line point $\mathbf{P}$ is tri-linearly interpolated from the eight closest image voxel intensities I_0 to I_7 (see figure 3 center). This algorithm outputs a list of voxels for which we store their interpolated intensity value and their Euclidian distance from $\mathbf{V}_i$. The scan-line range is fixed as a percentage of the image size. We used a ten-voxel length scan-line in our experiments.

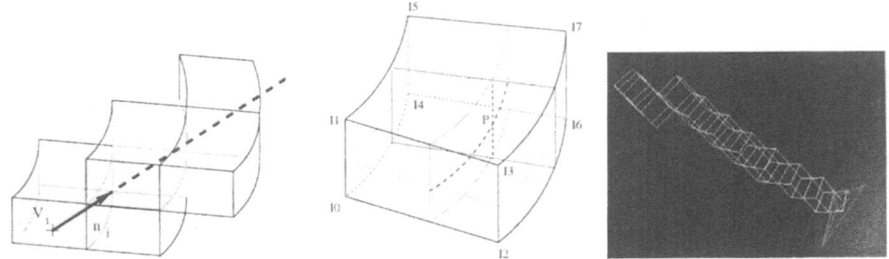

Fig. 3. Normal line and the scanned voxels; Tri-linear interpolation on a cylindrical voxel; 3D display of the scanned voxels.

4.2   Gradient Norm Extremum

We first use the extracted scan line in order to find the extremum of the gradient norm along the normal direction. In practice, the normal direction at a gradient vertex quickly converges towards the direction of the gradient vector in presence of a strong boundary. In order to improve this external force computation, we propose to add two additional constraints for a voxel to be considered as the closest boundary voxel. Since the cavity of left ventricle is surrounded by structures that appear brighter, we use a *gradient orientation constraint* to retain only boundaries whose gradient vector direction is roughly the same that normal direction. We constrain the boundary voxel to belong to a given *interval of intensity* in order to eliminate spurious boundary information.

4.3   Region-Based Algorithm

The previous algorithm may still fail due to the presence of strong edges in the ventricle boundaries vicinity, if such a neighboring edge has a higher gradient than the ventricle edge, and if it meets the two additional constraints listed above. In order to improve the discrimination of the boundary search algorithm, we propose to use both the notion of region and boundary. Region-based image segmentation has been proposed in [12] and has proven to be more powerful than gradient-based approaches. We first extract the intensity profile of a vertex and filter the intensity values to decrease the speckle effect (both Gaussian and Median smoothing have been implemented). The smoothed profile is scanned from the inside to the outside to find a set of consecutive voxels within a given intensity range and of length greater than a minimum threshold. Once the beginning of a region has been found, we search for the first voxel value that does not belong to the region intensity range thus corresponding to the end of the region. Given that such a voxel has been found we then look for a voxel whose gradient norm is above a given threshold in the vicinity of the region end. This algorithm requires to set the region intensity range and the gradient norm threshold parameters depending on the segmented images. The minimum region length is a trade-off between computation time and the algorithm accuracy. We used a four-voxel length in our experiments.

5   Experimental Results

We first study the effects of the image angular resolution on the model deformation process. A set of synthetic cylindrical slice images was generated by
intersecting the geometric face model shown in figure 4 (left) with planes sampled every 20, 10, 5, and 3 degrees. We then deform a spherical model in the
3D cylindrical images produced. The results are shown in the rest of figure 4.
Unsurprisingly, the retrieved surface shape improves as the angular resolution
increases. For low resolution images the model has to be more constrained so
that it correctly interpolates sparse data. Forces computed from higher resolution images are more reliable and the *a priori* model information is less critical
in that case.

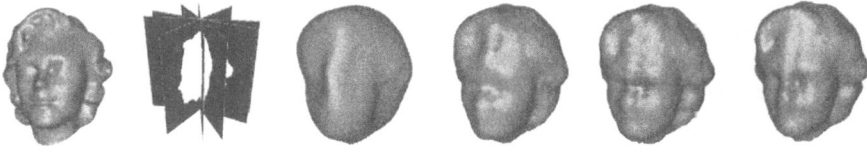

Fig. 4. Face model; Sampled planes; Deformed models for an angular resolution of 20,
10, 5, and 3 degrees of an arc.

The next experiment compares the cardiac left ventricle reconstruction from
a 3D echocardiographic image using a gradient of the gradient norm guiding force
as introduced by Kass *et al* [7] and the forces introduced in section 4. The model
is initialized as an ellipsoïde roughly centered inside the ventricle. Figure 5 shows
the reconstructed surfaces and the intersection of each surface with one of the
image planes. The template image quality is high (4 degrees of arc resolution) and
gradients are compute using a 7^3 cylindrical filter. The gradient of the gradient
norm is not reliable enough due to the large amount of speckle which introduces
too many false positives. The scan-line algorithm provides better results for both
the gradient extremum and the inner dark regions search. The region approach
better smoothes the boundary and is more accurate as can be clearly seen in the
mitral valve area.

Finally, we show the temporal evolution of the cardiac left ventricle extracted
from a series of eight 3D echocardiographic images. Due to the images'poor
quality (20 degrees of arc resolution and a very high noise level due to video signal
digitization) we prefer the more robust region based approach. The model built
in the previous experiment is used as a template for the first image segmentation
and at each time step, the model is initialized from its position at the previous
time instant. Figure 6 shows one out of two reconstructed models from end
diastole to end systole (left to right). The intersection of each surface model
with three image planes at 20 (second row), 80 (third row), and 140 (fourth row)
degrees of arc is shown. The surface model allows for an accurate computation

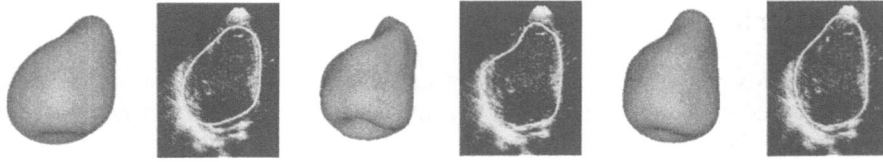

Fig. 5. gradient of the gradient norm (left), gradient extremum (center), and region based (right) reconstruction.

of the ventricle volume variation through the cardiac cycle (figure 6 top, left), and therefore, of the ejection fraction (here we found 38%).

6   Conclusion

In this paper we demonstrate the ability of 3D deformable models to segment cylindrical echocardiographic images. The model provides enough intrinsic (shape) and extrinsic (grey-level range) *a priori* knowledge to constrain the deformations properly even in the presence of very sparse and noisy data. Due to its simplicity, the proposed method is efficient (about 5 minutes to generate the 8 surface models shown in figure 6 on a Digital PWS500). The 3D approach allows an accurate computation of the left ventricle ejection fraction, yet, this model does not take advantage of the time continuity that could be used since the computations are performed off-line. We also plan to improve the region matching algorithm by introducing more accurate knowledge of image grey-level distributions.

Acknowledgments

We are grateful to Gary Schwartz from ATL Ultrasound, a Philips Medical Systems Company, Marie-Odile Berger from ISA research, Loria, and Dr Lethor, CHU Brabois, for providing the 3D ultrasound images used in this paper.

References

1. R. N. Czerwinski. Line and boundary detection in speckle images. *IEEE Transactions on Image Processing*, 7(12):1700–1714, 1998.
2. H. Delingette. General object reconstruction based on simplex meshes. to appear in *International Journal of Computer Vision*, 1999.
3. R. Deriche. Using Canny's criteria to derive a recursively implemented optimal edge detector. *International Journal of Computer Vision*, 1(2), 1987.
4. A. Giachetti. On-line analysis of echocardiographic image sequences. *Medical Image Analysis*, 2(3):261–284, 1999.
5. I. Herlin and N. Ayache. Feature extraction and analysis methods for sequences of ultrasound images. In *Proceedings of the European Conference in Computer Vision (ECCV'92)*, pages 43–57, 1992.

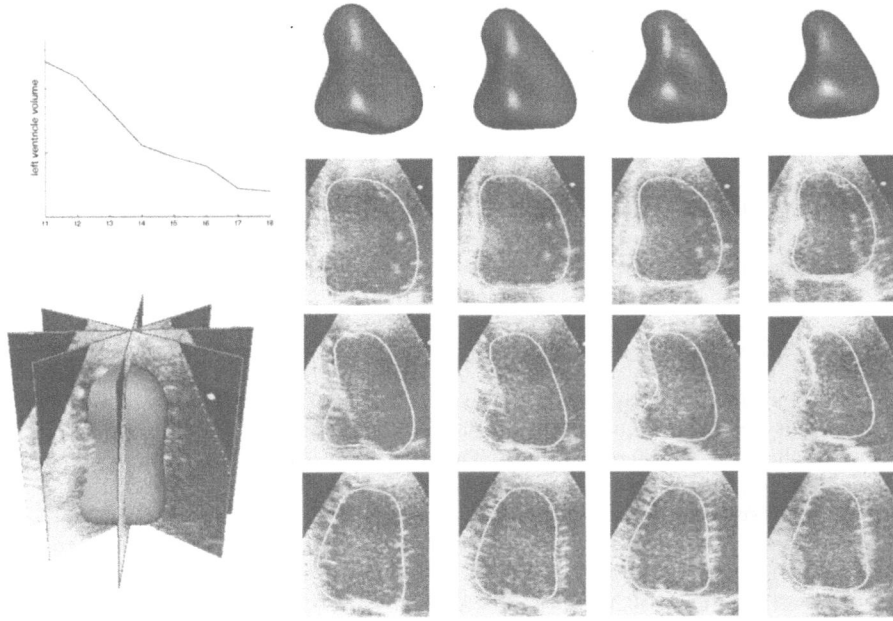

Fig. 6. Four out of the eight instants reconstructed from a 4D echocardiographic image.

6. G. Jacob, A. Noble, M. Mulet-Parada, and A. Blake. Evaluating a robust contour tracker on echocardiographic sequences. *Medical Image Analysis*, 3(1):63–75, 1999.
7. M. Kass, A. Witkin, and D. Terzopoulos. Snakes: Active Contour Models. *International Journal of Computer Vision*, 1:321–331, 1988.
8. B. Kimia, A. Tannenbaum, and S. Zucker. On the evolution of curves via a function of curvature i. the classical case. *Journal of Mathematical Analysis and Applications*, 163:438–458, 1992.
9. O. Monga, R. Deriche, G. Malandain, and J.-P. Cocquerez. Recursive filtering and edge tracking: two primary tools for 3-D edge detection. *Image and Vision Computing*, 9(4):203–214, August 1991.
10. J. Montagnat and H. Delingette. Globally constrained deformable models for 3D object reconstruction. *Signal Processing*, 71(2):173–186, December 1998.
11. R. Rohling, A. Gee, and L. Berman. Three-dimensional spatial compounding of ultrasound images. *Medical Image Analysis*, 1(3):177–193, 1997.
12. R. Ronfard. Region-based strategies for active contour models. *International Journal of Computer Vision*, 13(2):229–251, 1994.
13. G. Treece, R. Prager, A. Gee, and L. Berman. Fast surface and volume estimation from non-parallel cross-sections, for freehand 3-d ultrasound. Technical Report 326, Cambridge University Engineering Department, july 1998.
14. G. Winterfeldt, MO. Berger, JP. Lethor, and M. Handschuhmacher. Expert Model Based 3D Reconstruction of the left Ventricle Using Transthorasic Echographic Images. In *Computers in Cardiology*, sept 1997.

Active Model Based Carotid Ultrasonic Data Segmentation

Alexandre Moreau-Gaudry*, Philippe Cinquin* and Jean-Philippe Baguet+

[1] TIMC-IMAG, Institut Albert Bonniot, 38706 La Tronche cedex, FRANCE
{Alexandre.Moreau-Gaudry, Philippe.Cinquin}@imag.fr
[2] Department of Internal Medicine and Cardiology, Hôpital Michallon, CHU
Grenoble, FRANCE

Abstract. To diagnose cardiovascular diseases, the most significant mortality causes in industrialized countries, the study of the carotid artery wall plays a preferential part. This paper presents a three dimensional active model based carotid ultrasonic data segmentation. A C1 continuous surface, defined by a deformable skeleton and envelope, includes the Y-shape topology and gray level as a priori knowledge. It is automatically fitted to a sequence of 2.5D ultrasonic branching data by an iterative quadratic method. The quality of the fit is illustrated by figures. Result of this 3D fitting can be used as initial position for quantification of the intima-media thickness.

1   Introduction

Among cardiovascular diseases, coronary diseases represent the most important part in terms of frequency, morbidity and mortality. Lesions of the carotid artery wall (infraclinic atherosclerosis) reflect their effects. With the introduction of 2.5D ultrasound imaging (2D ultrasonic data located in 3D space), 3D analysis of the whole artery appears to be feasible. To initialize this study, a global branching model fits ultrasonic slices in an automatic way. It is made possible by the use of a priori knowledge : the **Y**-shape topology of the model and gray level modelling. This defines an absolute reference system. Tissular modifications (intima plus media thickness) and clinical parameters (degree of stenosis, plaque volume), evaluated from the result fitting, can be followed in this reference system, improving so the reproducibility.

2   An active branching model

In [1], we mention the particularity of the branching topology and explain why we don't use deformable models or reconstruction methods like [7, 4]. Recently, in [5], a branching reconstruction was performed from two dimensional carotid CT images. Contrary to these, ultrasonic images are often of poor quality. The maximum of a priori knowledge has to be used to compensate the lack of informations. A natural and powerful a priori knowledge is the particular **Y-shape** of the branching. This knowledge is introduced by the use of ε global branching model. Although topologically adaptive deformable models quoted in [6] have been shown to be promising in segmenting vascular structures in 2D and 3D images, we develop in [1] an explicit C1 continuous surface based on a deformable skeleton and envelope (see figure 1). It is totally defined by 24 model parameters. Thanks to the add of gray level a priori knowledge, a rough fully automatic carotid ultrasonic data segmentation will be realized.

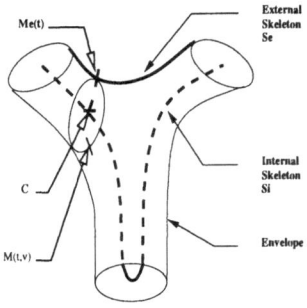

Fig. 1. Surface Description

S_e, the external skeleton, represents the upper branching convexity. It is a planar curve parameterized by $t, t \in [-1..1]$.

S_i, the internal skeleton, is the set of centers C of planar curves, continuously built on S_e. Each planar curve (superquadric [3]) are parameterized by $\iota, v \in [-\pi..\pi]$. The envelope of S_i defines the branching surface. By a one-to-one mapping between S_e and S_i, an explicit equation $M(t, v)$ of the surface is obtained, which was a main point for the numerical efficiency. For complementary explanations, see [1].

3 Data collection

Data are obtained with collaboration of the Department of Internal Medicine and Cardiology at the Grenoble University Hospital. Echographic images are acquired by a HP SONOS (Hewlett-Packard, Santa Clara, California, USA) ultrasonic system at a frequency of 50Hz. Figure 2 explains how to compute 2.5D data from these 2D data.

Because of the high frequency of acquisition, we are in front of an huge amount of information, which requires an automatic treatment. This will be possible thanks to the a priori knowledge contained in the branching shape. In a first approach, only cross-sectional data acquired during one cardiac cycle along the carotid artery are treated.

4 Methods

Let $X = (X_j, j = 1..24)$ be the vector of 24 model parameters, dX, an elementary shifting in the space of model parameters; $M(t, v; X)$, a point of current parameters (t,v) on the surface of parameter X, $dM(t, v; X)$, the elementary movement of a point $M(t, v; X)$ in the real 3D space.

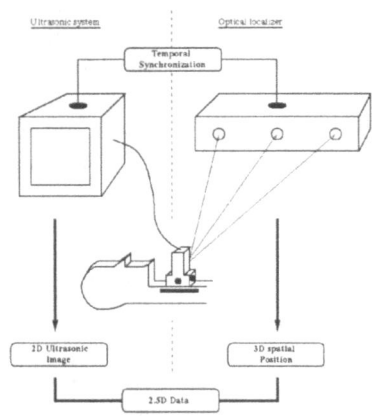

Fig. 2. Acquisition of 2.5D ultrasonic data.

2D images are acquired on a HP ultrasonic system at a frequency of 50 Hz. During the medical exploration, the ultrasonic system is connected to an optical localizer (Optotrak Northern Digital Inc.).

To collect 2.5D data, a six degrees-of-freedom optical tracking device attached to the ultrasound probe is used. The optical tracking system works with infrared diodes put on the probe which are then located by three fixed CCD cameras (Optotrak Northern Digital Inc.) at a frequency of 100Hz. Position and orientation of the echographic planes are thus obtained during all the exploration.

Thanks to a temporal synchronization between echographic and spatial data, 3D spatial coordinates for each 2D points of echographic plane can be computed.

4.1   Initialization

Shape initialization Thanks to the particular shape of the model, it is made easy. We choose manually four points on the 2.5D data, corresponding roughly to the top of the bifurcation position (the lowest point of the external skeleton) and the three branching extremities (the bottom, the right and the left extremities of the Y). A initial set $X0$ of parameter is then automatically computed from positions and distances between these different points. $X0$ is chosen so that the initial branching surface is in the lumen of the vessel.

Gray level initialization From this initial position, the intersections of the surface (see 4.2) with the ultrasonic planes are computed (closed curves). For each point of the curves, a gray level profile (10 pixel) is extracted towards the inside. We model the inside by a gaussian of mean μ and of variance σ.

4.2   Calculating a suggested movement

Intersection computing To determine surface intersection with ultrasonic planes, we compute first their intersections with three plane curves $Ci, i = 1..3$ judiciously chosen on the surface (see Figure 3). Two half spaces are defined by each ultrasonic plane. By determining the change of sign of the signed distance function, the exact intersections of planes with Ci are calculated by a Brent's method ([9]). From these points or germs, we compute, by a similar process, step by step, points $M_i(t_i, v_i; X)$ on the surface intersection, taking into account of the provenance direction.

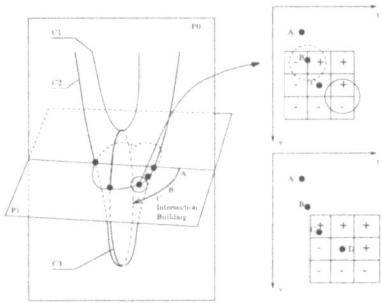

Fig. 3. Intersection computing: an overview.

Left: from germ A, intersection between the ultrasonic plane P1 and C2, we build step by step the intersection: points A,B,C.
Right: at the current point C, the signed distance map in its neighborhood is computed. After having identified the two changes of signs (circle with solid and dashed line), the point which maximizes the sum of distances with the three last points A,B,C is chosen and computed. This makes the process to go forward by choosing D (circle with solid line). The process is then iterated.

Suggested movement dM_i Let $\overrightarrow{n_i}$ be the projection in the current plane of the normal $\overrightarrow{N_i}$ of the surface in M_i. For each point M_i, the elementary movement dM_i in the 2D plane along $\overrightarrow{n_i}$ according to the gaussian gray model is computed: shifting from the inside (-10 pixels) of the branching intersection to the outside (+5 pixels), we go on until pixel intensity I at current point along the profile does not verify gaussian threshold: $\left(\frac{I-\mu}{\sigma}\right)^2 > 1$. If $M_i + dM_i$ is outside, a weight α_i of 1 is associated to it. On the contrary, if $M_i + dM_i$ is inside, to retract the surface, a weight proportional to $\|dM_i\|^2$ is chosen. By this asymmetry of balancing, a controlled inflating strategy is created, which prevents to go through the border of the vessel. dM_i computed, the movement along $\overrightarrow{N_i}$ is inferred from it.

4.3   Suggested shifting dX

Computing dX from n elementary movements dM_i, weighted by $\alpha_i, i = 1..n$, was a main point to establish a relation between the space parameter and the real 3D space. Each point $M_i(t_i, v_i; X) \equiv M_i(X)$ is seen as a function from $\Re^{24}$ to $\Re^3$: it associates to the vector X, the 3D point $M_i(X)$ on the surface of parameter X. With an approximation at the first order, the following relation is achieved: $dM_i(X) = J_{M_i}(t_i, v_i; X)(dX)$, where $J_{M_i}(X) \equiv J_{M_i}(t_i, v_i; X)$ is the jacobian matrix of function M_i. Because we have an *explicit* definition of the surface, an explicit expression of $J_{M_i}(X)$ is computed with Maple software (Maple V Release 4). To determine the shifting dX from $dM_i, i = 1..n$, we choose to minimize in $\Re^{24}$ the quadratic problem Q (1), which comes down to resolve a linear system in $\Re^{24}$.

$$Q = \sum_{i=1}^{n} \alpha_i \|dM_i(t_i, v_i; X) - J_{M_i}(t_i, v_i; X)dX\|^2 . \tag{1}$$

4.4   Algorithm

The natural process consists then to iterate the last three steps. To stop the process, we define a cost function, sum of 2D elementary movements in each plane along the outline: each movement is counted positive when it goes outside the surface, and negative in the other case. Process is stopped when the cost function is minimal.

4.5   Modelling a gray level appearance according to the incidence of ultrasonic rays

Because ultrasonic images are often of poor quality, to model the relation between the incidence of ultrasonic rays and the gray levels in the image is a precious a priori knowledge: we have indeed to remember that the wall of the vessel is particularly well identifiable if ultrasonic rays are normal to its surface, and vice versa.

Let $\vec{d}$ be the incidence direction of ultrasounds. At first approximation, the border of the vessel is circular on cross-sections. A polar angle θ of nil value in the direction $\vec{d}$ (see figure 4) is then naturally introduced. This angle is *the parameter* which gives us informations on the expected quality of gray levels. A new a priori knowledge is injected under the form of a statistical gray level modelling coming from [10], and *function* of θ. This model is applied on the result of the precedent step, to determine in an more acute way the limit of the vessel: we indeed have *to be close* to the vessel wall to compute a realistic angle with the incidence direction of ultrasounds.

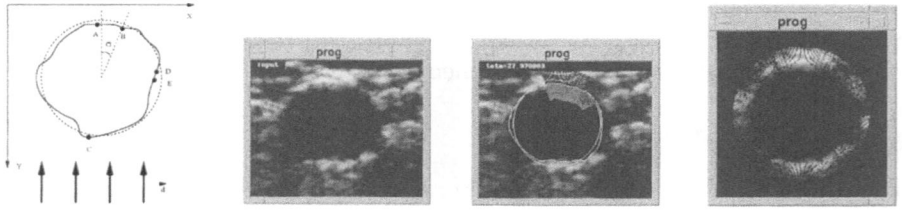

Fig. 4. A parameter which gives informations on the expected quality of gray levels : θ.
Left: $\vec{d}$ is the incidence direction of ultrasonic rays. For θ values close to zero or π, (*points A,B,C*), the ultrasonic echo is of good quality and this part of the image is meaningful. For θ values close to $\frac{pi}{2}, -\frac{pi}{2}$, (*points D,E*), we have a lack of information.
Middle left: Example of image on which gray level extraction will be applied.
Middle right: Extraction in course; the best circle fitting the border of the vessel, manually determined, can be seen.
Right: Result of the gray level profile extraction in each point of the border.

Model Building The statistical model is built from m ultrasonic images of the vessel ($m = 6$). Each image $im_j, j = 1..m$ is manually segmented. To extract gray level profiles according to the incidence angle of the ultrasonic rays, we fit, according to [13], the best circle on the border. A scaling transform is applied on each image to align circles with respect to each other, so that the images represent the same informations. Using a tri-linear interpolation, for each image im_j, for each degree $\theta, \theta = 1..360$, a gray level profile $p_{j,\theta}$ of 20 pixel centered on the border is extracted (see figure 4). Following [10, 8], a Principal Components Analysis on gray level profiles of identical angle $p_{j,\theta=cst}, j = 1..m$ is performed, in order to recover the principal components of the wall: we thus obtain, for each θ, the mean m_θ, and keep the eigenvectors $p_{\theta,k}$ corresponding to 95 percent of gray level information (four or five eigenvectors: $k = 1..4, 5$). Thus, 360 gray level profiles along the border of the vessel are defined.

Model fitting Let M_i be a current point of the vessel wall. To fit the gray level model with informations contained in the image in M_i to calculate a more accurate displacement, we compute the angle θ between $\vec{d}$ and $\vec{n_i}$, the previously defined direction of profile extraction. 20 gray level profiles along $\vec{n_i}$ are then extracted. For each profile, its Mahalanobis distance ([7]) from the mean m_θ, which is a measure of how well it fits the model, is computed. The point, for which this distance is minimum, is the new $M_i + dM_i$.

5   Results

After a manual initialization, the model modifies its shape by an active process to fit the border of the vessel. Figure 5 shows different intersections of the surface with ultrasonic planes. One can clearly notice a visual improvement with regard to the border of the vessel, particularly in the critical region of the bifurcation (plane 21). Furthermore, it appears that the model is not enough inflated. Improvements concerning the stop measure or the displacement of points have to be done.

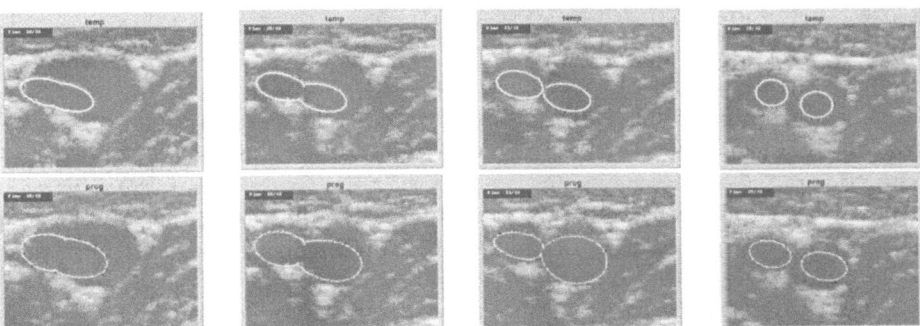

Fig. 5. Result.
Line 1: Intersection of the initial surface with ultrasonic planes.
Line 2: Intersection of the final surface with the same ultrasonic planes as for line 1.

6   Discussion and conclusion

6.1   Advantages and pitfalls

Advantages Because ultrasonic images are renowned for their poor quality, a priori knowledge is required to deal with them. In our case, the intrinsic information carried by our model is its shape. It makes possible an easy 3D and gray model initialization, which makes feasible the autonomous active search of the border of the vessel. A priori shape modelling is an active research topic ([10]). Only few methods are able to automatically describe the division of one artery in two branches [4, 2]: to our knowledge, no *explicit continuous active deformable* branching model incorporating *the **Y-shape topology** as an a priori information* had been developed. Furthermore, the compactness of the branching description, totally defined by 24 parameters, has to be underlined. The relatively small number of parameters results in a certain stiffness of deformation. This is the cost to pay for compactness. It would be possible to improve it by the use of deformable superquadrics with local and global deformations [11], or by other methods [12]. We don't adopt this strategy principally for two reasons: the implementation is heavy, and the result that we obtain is sufficient for the next step of the vessel study (quantification of the thickness of the wall). Our result provides a mean position of the carotid during the cardiac cycle, position from which we're going to start to study more precisely the wall of the vessel in other slices, at different time of the cardiac cycle.

Pitfalls It's necessary to evaluate the impact of the initial position for the model fitting, especially with regard to the spatial initialization (near or away from the bifurcation). The fitting is relatively slow on a HP A 9000/715 workstation. The calcul of intersections of the surface with ultrasonic planes represents the blocking step. A C (and not C++) or a parallel implementation could be certainly more efficient.

6.2   Perspectives

Given this initial position, the addition of the statistical gray level a priori information (build but not totally tested) will be useful for a more acute wall study. The addition of ultrasonic acquisitions of the same vessel under different incidences will be interesting to rebuilt more precisely the vessel: the next natural step will be the introduction of longitudinal slices. Our geometric model is the first step to an accurate quantification (quantification of the variations of the wall thickness during a cardiac cycle). It will be a measurement tool to evaluate new medical therapeutics tested to slow down atherosclerosis evolution. It could be an element in medical decision making, in order to optimize the cost/benefit equation.

Our data collection corresponds to a cross sectional study. We need some longitudinal information to test the reproducibility and the parameters sensibility of our model. This tool is promising. It could be used for all the branching vessels acquired by ultrasonic system (femoral, renal, popliteal divisions). It is known that ultrasonic slices are very noisy. Investigations by CT scan or MRN could be interesting. The use of our model could be extended, particularly to cerebral, coronary or hepatic branching vessels.

At last, in physiological medical research, our model which creates a virtual branching surface from 3D real data could be included in hemodynamic vascular model to test the local repercussion of turbulence on the atherosclerosis outcome.

Acknowledgments: This work was supported by Hewlett-Packard and Medasys Digital Systems.

References

1. A. Moreau-Gaudry, J.P. Baguet, and P. CINQUIN A New Branching Model: Application to Carotid Ultrasonic Data. *Medical Image Computing and Computer-Assisted Intervention-MICCAI'98-LNCS*, pages 1049–1056, 1998.
2. D.Attali E.Ferley, M.P.Cani-Gascuel. Skeletal Reconstruction of Branching Shapes. *The Eurographics Association*, 1997.
3. F.Solina and R.Bajcsy. Recovery of parametric models from range images:The case for superquadrics with global deformations. *IEEE Transactions on Pattern Analysis and Machine Intelligence*, 12(2):131–147, February 1990.
4. V.Juhan B.Nazarian K.Malkani R.Bulot J.M.Bartoli and J.Secueira. Geometrical modeling of abdominal aortic aneurysms. *CVRED-MRCAS*, pages 243–252, 1996.
5. G.Abdoulaev, S.Cadeddu, G.Delussu, M.Dinizelli, L.Formaggia, A.Giachetti, E.Gobbetti, A.Leone, C.Manzi, A.Scheinine, M.Tuveri, A.Varone, A.Veneziani, G.Zanetti and A.Zorcolo. ViVa: The Virtual Vascular Project. *IEEE Transactions on Infromation Technology in Biomedecine*, 2:268–273, December 1998.
6. T. McInerney and D. Terzopoulos. Deformable models in medical image analysis: a survey. *Medical Image Analysis*, 1(2):91–108, 1996.
7. S. Benayoun C.Nastar N.Ayache. Dense non-rigid motion estimation in sequence of 3d images using differential constraints. *CVRMed*, 1995.
8. C. Nastar B. Moghaddam A. Pentland. Generalized matching for recognition and retrieval in an image database. *Proceedings of the Third International Conference: Communicating by Image and Multimedia*, May 1996.
9. W.H.Press W.T.Vetterling S.A.Teukolsky and B.P.Flannery. Numerical recipies in c:Second edition.
10. T.F.Cootes A.Hill C.J.Taylor and J.Haslam. The use of active shape models for locating structures in medical images. *Image and Vision Computing*, 12(6):355–366, July 1994.
11. D. Terzopoulos and D. Metaxas. Dynamic 3D models with local and global deformations: Deformable superquadrics. *IEEE Transactions on Pattern Analysis and Machine Intelligence*, 13(7):703–714, July 1991.
12. D. Terzopoulos and M. Vasilescu. Sampling and reconstruction with adaptive meshes. In *IEEE Computer Society Conference on Computer Vision and Pattern Recognition (CVPR'91)*, pages 70–75, Maui, Hawaii, June 1991.
13. A.Bjorck. *Numerical Methods for Least Squares Problems*. SIAM, 1996.

Automatic Segmentation of Lung Fields in Chest Radiographs

Bram van Ginneken and Bart M. ter Haar Romeny

Image Sciences Institute, Utrecht University, The Netherlands.
E-mail: bram@isi.uu.nl, URL: http://www.isi.uu.nl/

Abstract. We present algorithms for the automatic delineation of lung fields in chest radiographs. We first develop a rule-based scheme that detects lung contours using a general framework for the detection of oriented edges and ridges. This algorithm is compared to several pixel classifiers using different combinations of features. We propose a hybrid system that combines both approaches. The performance of each system is compared with interobserver variability and results available from the literature. Our hybrid scheme turns out to be accurate and robust; the accuracy is 0.969 ± 0.00803, and above 94% for all 115 test images.

1 Introduction

Chest radiographs make up 40 percent of all conventional diagnostic radiographic procedures in general hospitals [1]. The advent of digital thorax units makes it in principle possible to use computerized methods for the analysis of chest radiographs on a routine basis. Our particular interest is the development of tools for computer assistance in mass chest screening against tuberculosis.

We focus on segmentation of lung fields in standard PA chest radiographs. Automatic segmentation is a mandatory pre-processing step for computer analysis of thorax images and has received considerable attention in recent literature. The two main approaches are rule-based reasoning and pixel classification with neural networks. Rule-based schemes have been proposed by Xu et al. [2,3], Duryea and Boone [4], and Carrascal et al. [5]. Lung segmentation by pixel classification has been investigated by McNitt-Gray [6,7], Hasegawa et al. [8], Tsujii et al. [9], and Vittitoe et al. [10].

We consider both a rule-based system and pixel classification with several sets of features. The rule-based scheme we present is new and employs a general and flexible framework for detection of subdimensional structures. Furthermore, we propose a new hybrid segmentation scheme that combines the rule-based approach with pixel classification. We show that this system compares favourably with literature results and approaches the accuracy of segmentation by hand. Such direct comparisons between segmentation methods have not been made before.

2   Materials and methods

Our database consists of standard PA chest radiographs from a tuberculosis screening program for people seeking political asylum in The Netherlands. We randomly selected normal and abnormal cases of adult subjects. Images were taken with a mobile Electrodelca (Oldelft BV, Delft, The Netherlands), a system commonly used in mass chest screening. Tube voltage was 117 kV and the images were printed on 10 by 10 cm. film. The films were digitized with a Lumisys 100 scanner (Lumisys, Inc., Sunnyvale, CA) to 996 by 996 pixels with 10 bit intensity, and subsampled to 256 by 256 pixels, which is sufficient for our purposes. Images were randomly divided in a test set and a training set, each containing 115 images. We indicate the coordinate of the upper left corner of the image with (0,0) and the lower right with (1,1) and express scales accordingly.

All software for displaying and drawing the digitized radiographs and the segmentation algorithms presented here was written by the first author in C++ using Borland C++ Builder (Borland International Inc.) and runs on a PC with Windows NT 4.0. The lung fields were traced with a mouse by each author independently, under supervision of an experienced radiologist.

3   Lung segmentation algorithms

3.1   Rule-based detection of lung contours

Starting point of our rule-based approach is the observation that the borders between anatomical structures in chest radiographs largely coincide with edges and ridges in the image. A difficulty is that these structures are highly connected and correspond only partly to the borders between anatomical regions. It is not straightforward to pick out the "correct" structures or parts of structures. We propose to use directional derivatives to overcome this problem.

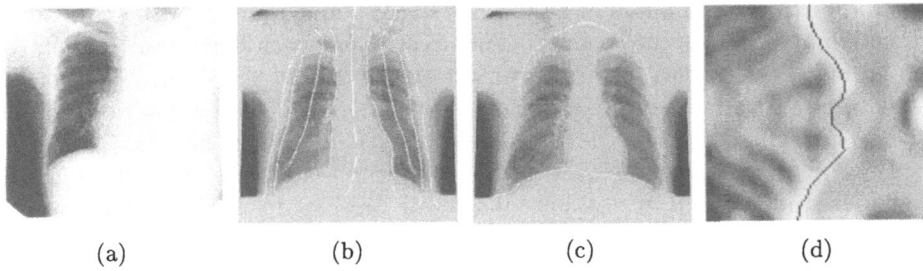

(a)   (b)   (c)   (d)

Fig. 1. (a) Example of an image that is rejected because no thorax center line is found; (b) Typical result of detection of vertical structures (thorax center line, mediastinum edges, lung edges, rib cage); (c) Typical result of detected diaphragm and lung top detected; (d) Polar transformation of a hemicircle of the image used in the detection of the lung top. The horizontal axis is the radius, the vertical is the polar angle; the center of the circle is at half height on the left of the image.

Edges are usually defined as those points in an image where the gradient magnitude is maximum in the gradient direction. Ridges are commonly defined as extrema in the direction of the largest curvature. Instead of these definitions, we consider structures defined by extrema in a *fixed* direction α, for derivatives of a certain order in that same direction. In this way, we obtain structures that cannot cross, because in the direction α consecutive points cannot both be extremal. The order of derivative n and the choice for minima and maxima determines the nature of the detected structures. Using order $n = 0$, one detects axes of bright and dark blobs; $n = 1$ yields edges from dark to bright regions, or vice versa; $n = 2$ gives bright and dark line structures, all in the direction perpendicular to α. The problem of connected structures is much reduced in this way. To solve the problem of selecting the proper structures, we use a straightforward voting technique. For the detection of diaphragm and lung top, voting mechanisms may fail to detect the correct structure. Since the lung top and diaphragm are generally the strongest lines and edges, we used dynamic programming to detect them. Putting this all together, estimates of the diaphragm, the border between lung fields and mediastinum, the boundaries of the rib cage and the lung tops are obtained. Figure 1 shows representative results. We now give a detailed description of the algorithm.

System 1. Rule-based reasoning
1. Detection of thorax center line. ROI is a rectangle defined by $0.3 < x < 0.7$ and $0.2 < y < 0.6$. This y-range is also used in steps 2-5. The 0th order derivative is computed at scale 0.05. Pixels which are maximal in the horizontal direction are detected and grouped into 8-connected structures. For each horizontal line in the ROI, the structure closest to the vertical centerline of the ROI is voted for. The structure that receives most votes is selected. Other structures are added, in order of received votes, as long as they don't overlap in their y-coordinates. If no center line is detected, the image is rejected.
2. Detection of the right/left edge of mediastinum. ROI is bounded on the right/left by the thorax center line and has 0.4 width. The 1st derivative in the x-direction is computed at a scale of 0.03. Maxima/minima in the horizontal direction are grouped into connected structures. For each horizontal line, starting from the center line, the first structure encountered is voted for. Again, other structures are added, in order of received votes, as long as they don't overlap in their y-coordinates. The same voting procedure is used in steps 3 to 5.
3. Detection of lung center lines. The mediastinum edges are the right and left boundaries of the ROI, which has a 0.3 width. We look for horizontal minima of the 0th order derivative at a scale of 0.03.
4. Detection of right/left lung edges. The lung center lines are the right and left boundaries of the ROI which has a 0.4 width. We look for horizontal minima/maxima of the 1st order derivative in the x-direction at a scale of 0.03.
5. Detection of right/left rib cage. The lung edges are the right/left boundaries of the ROI which has a 0.2 width. We look for horizontal maxima of the 2nd order derivative at a scale of 0.02.

6. Detection of diaphragm. The right and left diaphragm are determined with dynamic programming to find a line from left to right in a rectangular ROI. The ROI contains the 1st derivative in the y-direction of the image computed at a scale of 0.02. The line is allowed to have a slope between -1 and 1. The right diaphragm is detected first, because it is visible more clearly, owing to the absence of heart and stomach bubbles. The x-range of the ROI is from the lowest x-coordinate of the rib cage to the lowest x-coordinate of the thorax center line. We find a point on the right diaphragm by taking the right lung center at $y = 0.40$, moving down from this point to a maximum in the 1st derivative. The y-range of the diaphragm is 0.4, centred around this point. After the right diaphragm detection, crossings with the right rib cage and mediastinum edge are determined. These landmark points are added to the right diaphragm starting point. The y-range of the ROI for the left diaphragm is given by the smallest y-coordinate of these points minus 0.2 and the lowest y-coordinate plus 0.2. The x-range is from the highest x-coordinate of the thorax center line to the highest x-coordinate of the left rib cage.

7. Detection of lung tops. We use the fact that the top is a bright line structure, just like the rib cage. It is more or less circular, so we make a polar transformation of a hemicircle in the image. As center point we take the thorax center line at $y = 0.40$. The radius of the hemicircle is estimated to be half the distance between the right and left rib cage at this height. Minimum and maximum radius are set at 0.7 and 1.3 times this radius. We take the 2nd derivative along the circle radius and find a maximum path with dynamic programming. In this path, we allow deviations from a circular path of at most 45°.

8. Lung contours from a reference image with 15 control points along each contour are moved in horizontal or vertical direction until they coincide with the detected mediastinum, lung top, rib cage or diaphragm respectively. The contour interpolated based on the displacements of control points is taken as final lung contour.

System 2-7. Pixel classifiers

Segmentation can also be treated as a pixel classification problem by calculating a feature vector for each pixel in the input image. Output is the anatomical class the pixel belongs to. Although different types of classifiers will obviously lead to different results, the performance of these segmentation algorithms will depend mostly on the features of the input vector. As features we use *pixel location*, *pixel intensity*, *entropy*, and the *corrected location* computed from a scaling and translation computed from the rule based scheme. The entropy measure is motivated by the fact that the lung fields contain overlying ribs and lung vasculature and are therefore less homogeneous than areas outside the lungs. It is computed by subtracting a slightly blurred version of the image from the original, taking the absolute value of this image and blurring this slightly.

We use k-nearest-neighbour classification with $k = 31$. This setting of k was determined as optimal in several pilot experiments. We used 1024 points from each image in the training set (32 by 32). In all systems, scaling factors were

Method	Accuracy	Sensitivity	Specificity
Interobserver variability	0.984 ± 0.00475	0.957 ± 0.0174	0.993 ± 0.00306
Classification correction (8)	0.969 ± 0.00803	0.943 ± 0.0330	0.978 ± 0.0106
Rule-based (1)	0.961 ± 0.0116	0.940 ± 0.0389	0.969 ± 0.0153
PC int., entropy, corr. location (7)	0.956 ± 0.0157	0.912 ± 0.0617	0.972 ± 0.0248
PC int., corrected location (6)	0.953 ± 0.0177	0.906 ± 0.0649	0.970 ± 0.0288
PC int. and location (5)	0.933 ± 0.0219	0.854 ± 0.0771	0.966 ± 0.0309
PC location (3)	0.898 ± 0.0382	0.784 ± 0.0984	0.947 ± 0.0339
PC int. (4)	0.847 ± 0.0356	0.727 ± 0.122	0.891 ± 0.0447
All negative (2)	0.736 ± 0.0551	0 ± 0	1 ± 0
Duryea's rule-based method [4]	0.959 ± 0.054	0.863 ± 0.11	0.987 ± 0.044
Vittitoe's MRF [10]	0.948 ± 0.016	0.907 ± 0.044	0.972 ± 0.020
McNitt-Gray's 59 features [7]	0.932	0.949	0.922
Tsujii's PC corr. int., location [9]	0.923		
McNitt-Gray's 8 features [7]	0.918	0.903	0.930
Vittitoe's PC int. 3x3 [10]	0.893 ± 0.027	0.846 ± 0.057	0.925 ± 0.038
Vittitoe's PC location [10]	0.880 ± 0.035	0.820 ± 0.08	0.920 ± 0.044
Duryea's classifying location [4]	0.879 ± 0.063	0.785 ± 0.10	0.934 ± 0.063
Vittitoe's fixed thresholding [10]	0.806 ± 0.071	0.860 ± 0.058	0.781 ± 0.112
Duryea's all negative [4]	0.751 ± 0.063	0 ± 0	1 ± 0

Table 1. Accuracy, sensitivity and specificity of all 8 systems on the complete test set. PC stands for pixel classification. The number in parentheses denotes the system number. The systems are sorted according to accuracy. Below the line are results from literature for which the same performance measures could be found or calculated. Note that the test sets in these studies are different.

calculated to obtain zero mean and unit standard deviation for each feature over the whole training set. These scaling factors were also applied to the features of pixels in the test images.

System 2 uses no features and thus classifies each pixel using the most likely class, i.e. the background. *System 3* uses pixel location, *System 4* uses intensity (a multiple threshold), *System 5* uses location and intensity, *System 6* uses intensity and corrected location, *System 7* uses all features.

System 8. Rule-based reasoning and correction using pixel classification
This system reclassifies those pixels in the image for which systems 1 and 6 yield different classes. There are 2 possibilities, pixels can be classified as lung by system 1 and as non-lung by system 6, or vice versa. For each case, we determine a training set consisting of all the pixels in the training set for which this situation occurs. We use corrected location as feature.

4   Results and discussion

Table 1 lists the results of our schemes together with results reported in the literature, in terms of accuracy, sensitivity and specificity. We found no significant

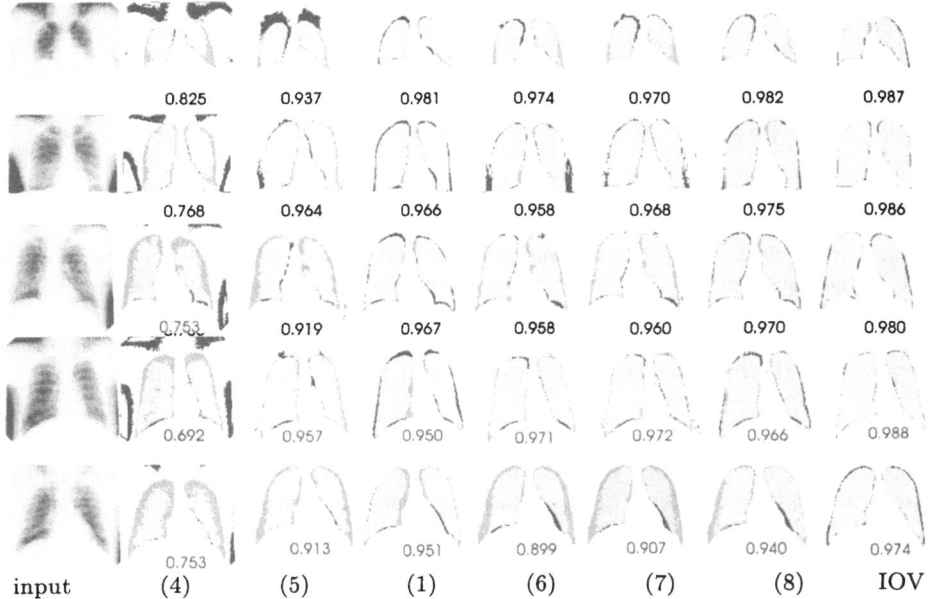

0.825	0.937	0.981	0.974	0.970	0.982	0.987
0.768	0.964	0.966	0.958	0.968	0.975	0.986
0.753	0.919	0.967	0.958	0.960	0.970	0.980
0.692	0.957	0.950	0.971	0.972	0.966	0.988
0.753	0.913	0.951	0.899	0.907	0.940	0.974
input	(4)	(5)	(1)	(6)	(7)	(8)	IOV

Fig. 2. Segmentation results for 5 radiographs of the test set for which system 8 gave respectively, best, good, average, poor and worst results. Systems are indicated in parentheses under each column. The right column shows the interobserver variability (a comparison of the segmentations of the first and second author). True negative pixels are shown white, true positive light gray, false positive pixels are dark gray and false negative pixels are shown in black.

differences in segmentation accuracy for normal versus abnormal radiographs. Key result is the accuracy of 96.9% of system 8, which approaches the interobserver variability. Figure 2 shows results of several systems for 5 images. The images were chosen to range from best to worst performance for System 8, the overall most accurate system.

Using only intensity as feature, which can be seen as using an optimal multiple threshold, yields an accuracy 84.7%. Vittitoe determined a single optimal threshold for his dataset, which scored 80.6%. Using a neural network classifier with the intensities of a 3 by 3 neighbourhood (with the images subsampled to 64 by 64 pixels) of each pixel as input vector, he achieved 89.3% correct classification. The fact that our result with intensity as a single feature scores half-way between indicates that the performance increase of the 3 by 3 intensity classification versus fixed thresholding is partly due to the fact that a classifier determines multiple thresholds and partly due to the textural context information obtained from the pixel neighbourhood.

The interobserver variability, an accuracy of 98.4%, provides a theoretical upper bound for the performance of any algorithm. This variability is mainly due to the difficulty in assessing the exact borders of mediastinum. Given the

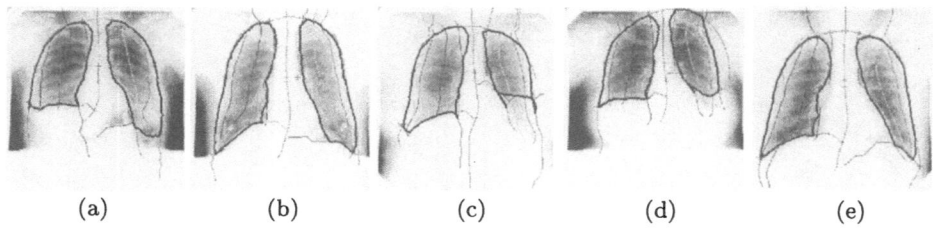

| (a) | (b) | (c) | (d) | (e) |

Fig. 3. Overview of occasional failures of the rule-based segmentation scheme. (a)-(b) Largely and slightly incorrect detection of left diaphragm due to the presence of stomach gasses (occurred in 18 of 115 cases). (c) Incorrect detection of left diaphragm due to a dense low left lung field. (d) Incorrect detection of the lung top. (e) Incorrect detection of the right mediastinum edge due to a pronounced right hilus.

performance of "simple" systems and the interobserver variability, a segmentation scheme for lung fields in chest radiographs will in practice have an accuracy between 90% and 98%.

It is surprising that a classifier using intensity and the location of pixels as feature (system 5) already gives an accuracy of 93.3%, especially if this is compared with the results of McNitt-Gray [7] who obtained 93.2% using 59 features and spatial information. It might be partly explained by the difference in database. However, it may also indicate that, apart from spatial information, the use of many more local features than (raw) intensity, can hardly improve the discriminating power of pixel classifiers in segmenting lung fields.

The rule-based system is accurate and robust, but there is still room for improvements. We distinguish *structural* and *occasional* errors. The detected edge of left lung and mediastinum in the upper lung part is structurally too much to the right. Another example is the outer rib cage, which is detected as a line structure and located on the center of the overlapping ribs. The lung fields end slightly more medial. Because of the coarse scales used to detect the lung edges, their location has shifted. Figure 3 gives an overview of occasional errors. The most important is failure to correctly detect the left diaphragm. Indications for failure are differences between the average height of right and left diaphragm and the presence of diaphragm-like structures above/below the detected diaphragm (in case of unexpectedly low/high left diaphragms). Adding rules is the obvious way to extend a rule-based system and this has prompted Xu [3] to develop tests to classify thoraxes into several categories based on stomach gasses appearance.

The remaining pixel classifiers use the corrected location as feature. This is not sufficient to outperform the rule-based method. Therefore we attempted to combine the strengths of both methods in a system that reclassified those pixels for which rule-based segmentation and pixel classification with corrected location and intensity gave different results. This (system 8) increased the accuracy from 0.961 to 0.969. This improvement may seem small, but in fact it bridges 35% of the gap between the rule-based scheme (96.1%) and the maximally achievable interobserver variability of 98.4%, and therefore may be considered a significant amelioration. Even more important is the increase of robustness. Reclassification is a means to correct those cases where the rule-based systems makes an occasional gross failure. If we consider the 10% of images that scored worst with the rule-based scheme, the average accuracy is 93.7%. For the corrected scheme this percentage is 95.2%. Note that these are different images, so for the 10 worst cases for the rule-based method, the performance gain is even larger. The worst case of all 115 images using the rule-based system scored 90.1%, for the corrected scheme the worst result was 94.0%.

Segmentation requires about 10 seconds for the hybrid scheme using a standard 350 MHz PC. Our implementation is not optimized for speed. We expect that an improved implementation can segment a radiograph, even at the resolution used in clinical practice, within a second.

Acknowledgements The authors are indebted to the radiologists Wallid Haddad, Ad van Gils, Erik Beek, and Paul van Waes. This work is supported by the IOP Image Processing, funded by the Dutch Ministry of Economic Affairs.

References

1. R. E. Bunge and C. L. Herman. Use of diagnostic imaging procedures: a nationwide hospital study. *Radiology*, 163:569–573, 1987.
2. X.W. Xu and K. Doi. Image feature analysis for computer-aided diagnosis: Accurate determination of ribcage boundary in chest radiographs. *Medical Physics*, 22(5):617–626, 1995.
3. X.W. Xu and K. Doi. Image feature analysis for computer-aided diagnosis: Detection of right and left hemidiaphragm edges and delineation of lung field in chest radiographs. *Medical Physics*, 23(9):1613–1624, 1996.
4. J. Duryea and J.M. Boone. A fully automatic algorithm for the segmentation of lung fields on digital chest radiographic images. *Medical Physics*, 22(2):183–191, 1995.
5. F.M. Carrascal, J. Carreira, M. Souto, P.G. Tahoces, L. Gomez, and J.J. Vidal. Automatic calculation of total lung capacity from automatically traced lung boundaries in postero-anterior and lateral digital chest radiographs. *Medical Physics*, 25(7):1118–1131, 1998.
6. M.F. McNitt-Gray, J.W. Sayre, H.K. Huang, and M. Razavi. A pattern classification approach to segmentation of chest radiographs. *Proc. SPIE*, 1898:160–170, 1993.
7. M.F. McNitt-Gray, H.K. Huang, and J.W. Sayre. Feature selection in the pattern classification problem of digital chest radiograph segmentation. *IEEE Transactions on Medical Imaging*, 14(3):537–547, 1995.
8. A. Hasegawa, B. Lo. Shih-Chung, M. T. Freedman, and S. K. Mun. Convolution neural network based detection of lung structures. *Proc. SPIE*, 2167:654–662, 1994.
9. O. Tsuji, M. Freedman, and K.M. Seong. Automated segmentation of anatomic regions in chest radiographs using an adaptive-sized hybrid neural network. *Medical Physics*, 25(6):998–1007, 1998.
10. N.F. Vittitoe, R. Vargas-Voracek, and E.F. Jr. Carey. Identification of lung regions in chest radiographs using markov random fiel modeling *Medical Physics*, 25(6):976–985, 1998.

Automatic Reconstruction of 3D Geometry Using Projections and a Geometric Prior Model

J. Lötjönen[1,2,3], I. E. Magnin[2], L. Reinhardt[1,3], J. Nenonen[1,3], and T. Katila[1,3]

[1] Laboratory of Biomedical Engineering, Helsinki University of Technology, P.O.B. 2200, FIN-02015 HUT, Finland
{Jyrki.Lotjonen, Lutz.Reinhardt, Jukka.Nenonen, Toivo.Katila}@hut.fi
[2] Creatis, INSA 502, 69621 Villeurbanne Cedex, France
Isabelle.Magnin@creatis.insa-lyon.fr
[3] BioMag Laboratory, Helsinki University Central Hospital, P.O.B. 503, FIN-00029 HYKS, Finland

Abstract. A method has been developed to reconstruct 3D surfaces from two orthogonal X-ray projections. A 3D geometrical prior model, composed of triangulated surfaces, is deformed according to contours segmented from projection images. The contours are segmented by a new method based on free-form deformation. First, virtual X-ray images of the prior model are constructed by simulating real X-ray imaging. Thereafter, the contours segmented from the virtual projections are elastically matched with patient data. Next, the produced 2D vectors are back-projected onto the surface of the prior model and the prior model is deformed using the back-projected vectors with shape-based interpolation. The accuracy of the method is validated by a data set containing 20 cases. The method is applied to reconstruct thorax and lung surfaces. The average matching error is about 1.2 voxels, corresponding to 5 mm.

1 Introduction

Modern medical imaging devices produce detailed 3D volume images. However, these imaging modalities are not always available. Hence, a method to reconstruct individualized 3D information using only two approximately orthogonal X-ray projections was developed. In this paper, the method is demonstrated with two applications: creation of patient specific thorax models and reconstruction of lung volumes from the X-ray projections. Patient-specific thorax models are needed in magnetocardiographic (MCG) and electrocardiographic (ECG) forward and inverse problems [1].

Terzopoulos *et al.* [2] presented a method to recover the 3D shape from 2D profiles of an object using a deformable tube coupled to a deformable spine. The deformation was controlled by physically based intrinsic and extrinsic forces. Bardinet *et al.* [3] proposed a method to match a parametric deformable model to unstructured 3D data. First, they matched a superquadric model to a given point set. Second, the generated superquadric model was deformed locally by a free-form deformation (FFD) [4] using a 3D deformation grid. Because of the parametric model and the regularization, the method can be used to model sparse data. Several other methods exist to create a 3D surface from a set of 3D points [5, 6]. However, the application of these methods to projection images has not been reported. Laurentini has discussed theoretical limitations of surface reconstruction from 2D silhouettes [7].

Our method differs considerably from the methods referred above. In general, the detailed 3D reconstruction of the geometry is not possible using only information from two orthogonal projections. We introduce a method based on 3D elastic deformation of a geometric prior model. First, the contours, created from the prior model by simulating real X-ray imaging conditions, are elastically matched with the contours extracted from real projections. The segmentation method proposed in this paper produces elastic matching between the contours automatically. Second, the generated 2D-vector field is back-projected onto the 3D surface of the model. Finally, the deformation of the prior model is accomplished by shape-based interpolation utilizing the back-projected 3D vectors.

2   Segmentation

The segmentation is based on our previous work [8]. The most important difference is the definition of the prior model. Compared to magnetic resonance (MR) images, edges are smoother and more difficult to define in X-ray projections. Therefore, distance maps, calculated from binarized edges in MR data and used to attract the prior model surfaces in 3D or contours in 2D, can not be easily utilized with X-ray images. In this paper, the prior model is an X-ray image similar to the one to be segmented but taken from a different patient (Fig. 1). The prior model is a representative of mean anatomy. The model is matched with the input image using the FFD in such a way that the similarity between two images is maximized. Since the model is pre-segmented, the segmentation of the input image is automatically produced. Therefore, even very weak edges can be correctly localized because they appear in same positions both in the input image and in the prior model. In practice, we matched the gradient images calculated by the Canny-operator (Fig. 1) [9] because they are less sensitive to the contrast and brightness differences than the original X-ray images. The matching error E_{data} between the model and data is defined by

$$E_{data} = \frac{1}{N_G} \sum_{i=1}^{N_G} \|\mathbf{G}^D(x_i, y_i) - \mathbf{G}_i^M\|^2, \qquad (1)$$

where the function $\mathbf{G}^D(x, y)$ is the gradient image of input data, $\mathbf{G}_i^M$ is a gradient vector from the gradient image of the prior model, and N_G is the total number of these vectors. The function $\mathbf{G}^D(x, y)$ is evaluated at the position (x_i, y_i) of the gradient $\mathbf{G}_i^M$. The symbol $\| \; \|$ denotes vector norm. It is worth noting that the function $\mathbf{G}^D(x, y)$ and the gradients $\mathbf{G}_i^M$ remain constant during deformation. Only the position (x_i, y_i) of each model gradient is varying.

The minimization of E_{data} does not guarantee that the prior knowledge of the model shape is preserved. Therefore, deformation is regularized. The changes in

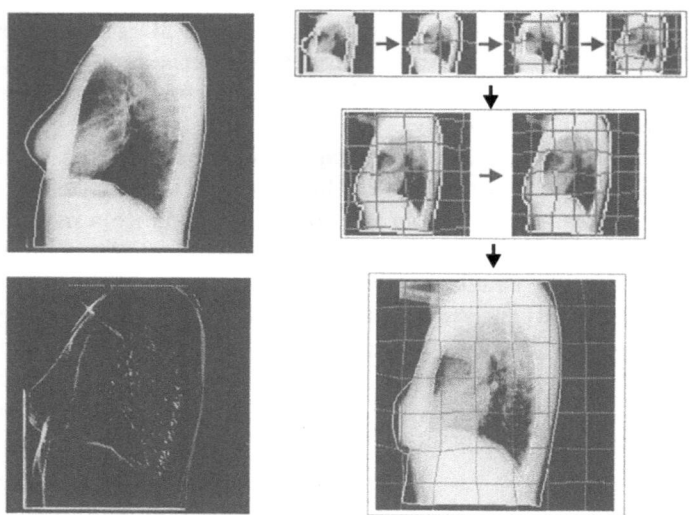

Fig. 1. *On the left: The prior model (up) and corresponding gradient image (bottom), showing only the magnitude of the gradient. On the right: the multiresolution and the global-to-local approach. The deformed prior model contour and a deformation grid are superimposed onto the input data.*

the normal directions of the contour points, defined by the pre-segmented model, are restricted. The energy E_{model} is calculated as follows

$$E_{model} = \frac{1}{N_C} \sum_{l=1}^{N_C} (1.0 - \mathbf{n}_l \cdot \mathbf{n}_l^*), \tag{2}$$

where N_C is the total number of contour points in the model, $\mathbf{n}_l$ and $\mathbf{n}_l^*$ are the deformed and the original normals of the contour point l, respectively, and $\cdot$ stands for the dot product. Other regularization terms, such as curvature based measures, could be also used [8].

The total energy E_{total} is defined by

$$E_{total} = E_{data} + \gamma E_{model}, \tag{3}$$

where γ is a parameter to control the balance between the two energy components.

The FFD is controlled by a deformation grid. The relation between the displacements of the grid points and the points of the prior model were defined by bilinear interpolation.

Since distance maps are not used, the minimization process is more sensitive to local minima. Two different methods were chosen to improve robustness:

1. The multiresolution approach is used, i.e. the matching is started at a low resolution level and followed by increasing resolution during the process. The

method is a trade off between computation time and convergence towards the global minimum. The multiresolution approach is visualized by vertical arrows in Fig. 1.

2. The *global-to-local* approach is used, i.e. more degrees of freedom are added to the model during deformation. First, input data and the prior model are coarsely registered. In this paper, this is accomplished by matching the centers of mass when the mass of each pixel is the magnitude of the gradient (the first image on the right side of Fig.1). Next, the prior model is deformed by a grid size of 3×3. When a minimum is found, the number of grid points is increased. In practice, only one grid point is added in both directions at each step until the specified grid size is reached. The highest grid size used depends on the geometric details needed. A grid size of 10×10 is usually large enough for thorax images. After reaching the highest grid size the resolution level is changed. The global-to-local approach is demonstrated by horizontal arrows in Fig. 1.

Local rigidity constraints can be easily added to the prior model. One coefficient can be attached to each prior model vector in Eq. 1. Similar effects with lower computation time can be achieved by locally reducing the number of prior model gradients (Eq. 1). Local rigidity is increased at areas where the model does not represent data well. Moreover, rigidity can be set higher at areas where the gradients are nearly constant in order to reduce computation time.

3   Reconstruction of the 3D geometry

3.1   Prior model

The prior model should be a good representation of the object to be modeled. Cootes *et al.* [10] and Székely *et al.* [11] propose 3D models which represent mean shapes in a statistical sense. Moreover, the models are deformed using deformation modes, which are statistically defined using a training set. In our approach, a prior model library was constructed from MR data of ten different subjects. The geometric prior models (Fig. 2a) were built by triangulating the segmented MR volumes [12].

The matching between real data and the prior model can not be accomplished straightforwardly, because the X-ray projections are in 2D and the model in 3D. Therefore, virtual projections are produced from the model by simulating X-ray imaging conditions, i.e. the orthogonal side and frontal views are generated. The distances from the film to the X-ray source and to a patient correspond to the values used in clinical practice. The X-ray source is regarded as a point because the blurring effect is less than one millimeter. Noise is added to the signal. The imaging process has been simplified in two ways: 1) The radiation is monochromatic, 2) The bone structures were excluded because CT images covering the whole thorax were not available for this study. Despite these simplifications, the virtual X-ray images correspond visually well to real images (Fig. 2b). Since the surfaces of the body and lungs are to be reconstructed, the effect of the excluded ribs is not important.

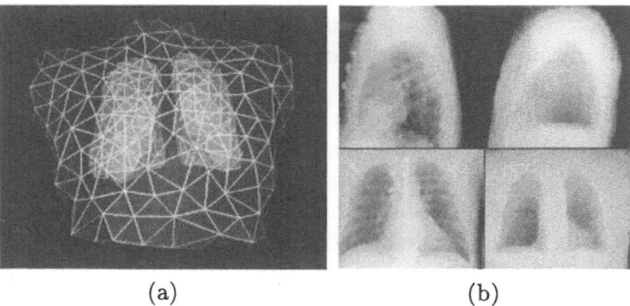

(a)   (b)

Fig. 2. *a) The prior model. b) Real (left) and virtual (right) X-ray projections.*

3.2 Sparse vector field

The contours extracted from real and virtual X-ray projections are matched elastically. The segmentation method automatically gives a 2D displacement vector $\mathbf{V}_k$ for each contour point of the virtual X-ray image (Fig. 3a).

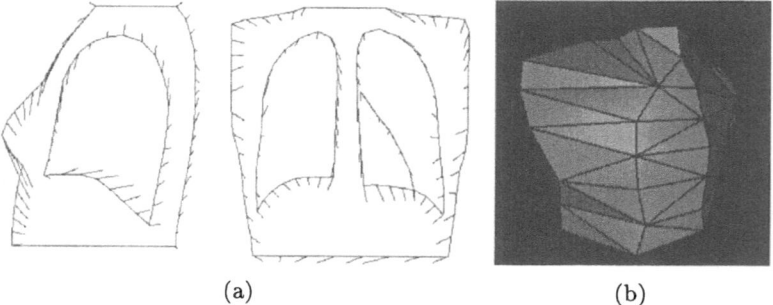

(a)   (b)

Fig. 3. *a) Displacement vectors of the contour points produced by segmentation. b) The positions of the back-projected contour points on the surface of the 3D prior model.*

Thereafter, each vector is back-projected onto the surface of the 3D prior model. A ray is cast from each contour point towards the X-ray source. The closest surface points, to which the ray is tangential, are selected and denoted by $\mathbf{p}_k$. Because of parallax effect, the symmetry of the thorax has to be taken into account separately. Next, the vector $\mathbf{V}_k$ is back-projected onto the plane, which is orthogonal to the ray going through the point $\mathbf{p}_k$ and which contains the point $\mathbf{p}_k$. The end-points of the vector $\mathbf{V}_k$ are projected separately. The projection is accomplished by the ray from the point to be projected to the X-ray source. The effect of parallax effect to the length of the projected vector is automatically considered. Back-projection leads to a sparse 3D vector field. In Fig. 3b, the apex points of the triangles represent the positions $\mathbf{p}_k$.

3.3   Dense vector field

To deform the prior model, the displacement vectors have to be defined for each node of the model $\mathbf{p}_l^*$ (Fig. 2a). Each displacement vector $\mathbf{v}_l^*$ is a weighted sum of the back-projected vectors $\mathbf{v}_k$. Only the vectors $\mathbf{v}_k$ located close to the node $\mathbf{p}_l^*$ affect the vector $\mathbf{v}_l^*$. We consider a geodesic distance between the points, computed on the model surface. This is similar to the so-called natural neighbor coordinate used in the computational geometry and geological modeling. The geodesic closeness is defined using the Voronoi areas on the surface for the all points $\mathbf{p}_k$ and each prior model node $\mathbf{p}_l^*$ separately [12]. The weights s_k for each vector $\mathbf{v}_k$ are calculated as follows:

$$ s_k = \frac{1/d_k}{\sum_{m=1}^{N_{nb}} 1/d_m}, \tag{4} $$

where d_k is the geodesic distance from $\mathbf{p}_k$ to $\mathbf{p}_l^*$ on the model surface, and N_{nb} is the number of neighboring Voronoi areas. For non-neighboring Voronoi areas weights s_k are zero. The benefit in using geodesic distances is that in some geometries the model nodes may be close to each others according to Euclidean measures, although they are on different sides of the surface.

Linear interpolation gives optimal results if the surface between the back-projected vectors is well represented by a plane. However, this approximation is not valid for some large triangles in Fig. 3b. Therefore, a heuristic interpolation method was developed tending to preserve the normal direction of the prior model surface. A 2D example of shape based interpolation is shown in Fig. 4a. The thick black line describes the known model surface; $\mathbf{v}_k$ and $\mathbf{v}_{k+1}$ are back-projected vectors. A displacement vector on the dashed line is defined as follows. 1) Search a point $\mathbf{p}_l^S$ in such a way that the angle between the lines, defined by points $\mathbf{p}_l^S$ and $\mathbf{p}_k$, and $\mathbf{p}_l^S$ and $\mathbf{p}_{k+1}$, is $\pi/2$. 2) These lines are moved according to the displacement vectors $\mathbf{v}_k$ and $\mathbf{v}_{k+1}$. The cross-section point of the displaced lines is calculated resulting in the vector $\mathbf{v}_l^S$. 3) The displacement vector for the point $\mathbf{p}_l^L$ is calculated by linear interpolation between the vectors $\mathbf{v}_k$ and $\mathbf{v}_{k+1}$. 4) The displacement vector between the points $\mathbf{p}_l^S$ and $\mathbf{p}_l^L$ is defined by linear interpolation with the corresponding vectors, otherwise the vector $\mathbf{v}_l^S$ is used.

In general, the prior shape can not be preserved in 3D but an approximation is used (Fig. 4b). The lines in 2D correspond to planes in 3D. The definition of the planes to define the vector $\mathbf{v}_l^S$ can not be directly transformed to 3D. Instead, the orientation of the plane is defined in 3D by the following two vectors: 1) the vector from the point $\mathbf{p}_k + \mathbf{v}_k$ to the point $\mathbf{p}_{k+1} + \mathbf{v}_{k+1}$ and 2) the vector from the point $(\mathbf{p}_k + \mathbf{p}_{k+1})/2$ to the point $\mathbf{p}_l^S$.

4   Results

4.1   Segmentation

Segmented thorax X-ray images are shown in Fig. 5. The γ factor was 1000 and the lowest resolution 32×32. Overall, the results are visually good. Usually,

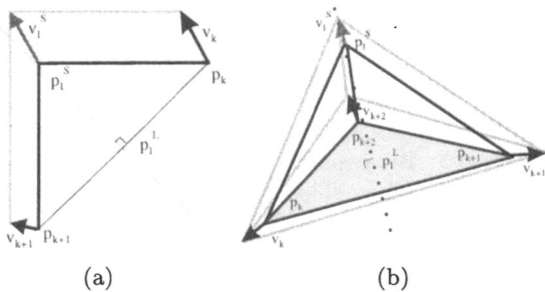

(a)   (b)

Fig. 4. *Shape-based interpolation in 2D and in 3D.*

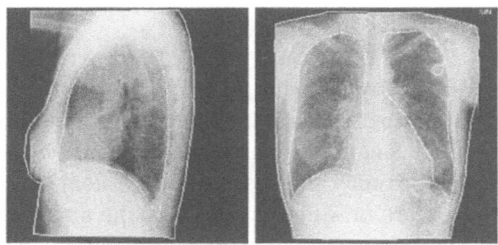

Fig. 5. *A segmentation result of thorax images.*

only small interactive corrections are needed. The computation time was about 10 seconds using a Sun Ultra10 workstation.

4.2   Extraction of 3D surfaces

The accuracy of the reconstruction method was tested by a simulation. Virtual X-ray projections were created from 20 segmented MR volumes. The resulting X-ray images were segmented and the prior model was deformed. The results were compared to the original volumes. The size of the volumes was about 128x128x100 voxels with a voxel size 3.9 mm. The matching error is defined as the shortest Euclidean distance from each model node to the surface in the MR volume.

Ten different prior models were tested. The model that produced the smallest average error was selected out of 20 patients. The results are shown in Table 1a. The error corresponds to about 5 mm. If linear interpolation was used instead of shape based interpolation, the error would be about 5% higher. Fig. 6 shows the deformed model superimposed onto the segmented MR volume in the best case (patient 20, T=1.03, LL=0.93, LR=0.90 voxels) and in the worst case (patient 15, T=1.25,LL=1.8, LR=1.21 voxels). The overall match is good, except for the left lung in Fig. 6b. In general, the highest matching error is concentrated on the areas where the distance to the nearest back-projected vector is high. The time to create the deformed model from the contours is less than one second with a Sun Ultra10 workstation.

Two simple matching methods were used for comparison: 1) The centers of mass of the contours were matched, 2) The contours were affine registered. The results using these simple matching methods and the elastic deformation method presented in this paper are represented in Table 1b. The column 'Mean' is the mean error for the thorax and lungs of all 20 patients (20 patients and 3 objects leading to 60 measures). The columns 'Min' and 'Max' represent the lowest and the highest value out of 60 matching errors.

Object	Error	Stdev	Max
T	1.22	0.91	5.4
LL	1.19	0.91	4.8
LR	1.21	0.90	4.6

Method	Mean	Min	Max
Mass	2.81	1.47	6.60
Affine	1.61	0.96	3.01
Elastic	1.21	0.85	1.80

Table 1. *a) Mean error (N=20), standard deviation and maximum error (in voxels) for thorax (T), left lung (LL) and right lung (LR). b) Mean, minimum and maximum matching errors of 20 patients using different matching methods.*

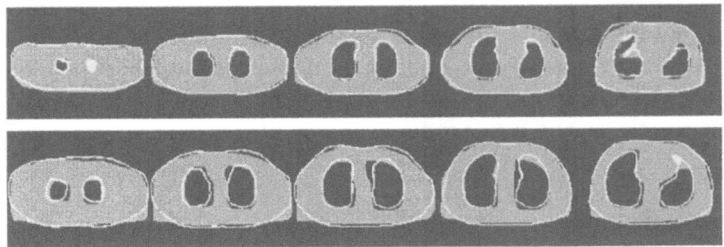

Fig. 6. *A deformed model superimposed onto MR images in the best case (top) and in the worst case (bottom).*

The effect of the error in imaging geometry was tested. An error of 3 cm in the position of the X-ray source increased the matching error maximally by 10%.

4.3 Extraction of 3D volume

The same simulation data set was used as in the previous section to define the volume of lungs from projections. The model producing the lowest error was chosen. The average error for right and left lungs were 5% and 7%, respectively. The maximum error was 14% and the minimum error less than 1%.

4.4 Thorax library

A method was developed and tested to choose the best model from the prior model library to be used with each separate patient. The idea was to test if the shape of 2D contours in X-ray images has a relation to the 3D shape of the areas far from the back-projected vectors. For example, if a model library contains two models, a cube and a ball, and the 2D contours are circles, the ball-shaped model should be chosen better.

Altogether 90 parameters were calculated from the contours in both directions. These parameters include harmonic coefficients up to the 10th order, different moments, lengths and the area of the object. The differences between the parameters of each model and patient data were calculated. Moreover, several other parameters were defined, such as an error after affine registration. Each model was matched with a data set of 15 different patients and the error was calculated. Thereafter, a linear regression analysis was applied to find out the best linear model to calculate the matching error between a model and a patient using the parameters defined from X-ray images. The best prior model for a patient is the one which gives the lowest matching error using the linear model. The goodness of the model was tested with the data set of 15 patients, and also with a set of 5 patients who were not included in the regression analysis.

If the model giving the lowest error was correctly chosen, the average error in 3D surface reconstruction for thorax, left lung and right lung would be 1.10 voxels. The corresponding value for the model producing the lowest average error was 1.21, as reported above. This means that the error would be about 10% lower in the optimal case. When the linear model was applied, the results for a data set used to create the model was about 2% lower and for the whole data set 1% higher than with the lowest average error model. Thereby, the statistical model is not able to choose the best model from the library with given contours.

5   Discussion

A method was proposed to deform a 3D geometric prior model based on X-ray projections of a patient. The 3D model generated does not describe the anatomy of the patient as well as a model extracted, for example, from MR images, but is a good trade off between accuracy and cost. The accuracy of the elastic matching is superior to affine registration tested. The absolute value of the error was 1.21 voxels using $128 \times 128 \times 100$ volumes. So far, it is not known what is the correlation between the geometric error of the model and the accuracy of MCG/ECG source localization.

The segmentation method developed is robust and fast. Moreover, the construction of the prior model is easy because only one X-ray image with segmented contours is needed. So far, we have applied the method to thorax images. However, to validate the method, it should also be tested with other types of X-ray images.

The pose, the size and the orientation of the prior model should approximately correspond to the patient data. Otherwise, the model has to be coarsely registered with the patient data. If the variability of the shape in the patient data is large, the coarse registration does not solve the problem. Therefore, we used a thorax library to select the best model. However, the shape parameters of the 2D contours did not contain enough information to choose the best model from the library. The analysis should be continued by using intensity information of X-ray images with the shape parameters. Another approach would be to use a statistical mean model and to deform it using statistically defined deformation modes. After deformation the model should follow the positicns defined by the back-projected vectors.

The accuracy of the 3D reconstruction method could be improved by using more than two X-ray projections. However, the improvement of the geometric accuracy compared to the extra dose captured by a patient should be validated. Moreover, a calibration system to produce X-ray images in specific angles should be used.

Besides of the described applications, the method can be used to create patient specific 3D heart models from fluoroscopic images. These models can be fused to the body surface potential mapping system used in a catheterization laboratory. The method could be also applied in registration of 3D images with 2D projections or as an initialization in model based segmentation.

Acknowledgements

The authors express thanks to The Department of Radiology, Helsinki University Central Hospital, Finland and Oy IMIX Ab, Tampere, Finland for providing MR volumes and X-ray images for the study

References

1. J. Nenonen. Solving the inverse problem in magnetocardiography. *IEEE Eng. Med. Biol.*, 13:487–496,1994.
2. D. Terzopoulos, A. Witkin and M. Kass. Constraints on Deformable Models: Recovering 3D Shape and Nonrigid Motion. *Artificial Intelligence* 36:91–123,1988.
3. E. Bardinet, L. Cohen and N. Ayache. A Parametric Deformable Model to Fit Unstructured 3D Data. *CVGIP: Image Understanding*, 71(1):39–54,1998.
4. T. Sederberg and S. Parry. Free-form deformation of solid geometrical models. *SIGGRAPH*, 20:151–160,1986.
5. H. Hoppe, T. DeRose, T. Duchamp, J. McDonaldand and W. Stuetzle. Surface Reconstruction from Unorganized Points. *Computer Graphics*, 26(2):71–78,1992.
6. R. Poli, G. Coppini and G. Valli. Recovery of 3D Closed Surface from Sparse Data. *CVGIP: Image Understanding*, 60(1):1–25,1994.
7. A. Laurentini. How Far 3D Shapes Can Be Understood from 2D Silhouettes. *IEEE PAMI*, 17(2):188–195,1995.
8. J. Lötjönen, P-J. Reissman, I. E. Magnin and T. Katila. Model Extraction from Magnetic Resonance Volume Data Using the Deformable Pyramid. *Medical Image Analysis*, 1999, in press.
9. J. Canny. A computational approach to edge detection. *IEEE Trans. PAMI*, 8:679-698,1986.
10. T. F. Cootes, C. J. Taylor, D. H. Cooper and J. Graham. Active shapes models–their training and application. *Computer Vision and Image Understanding*, 61(1):38–58,1995.
11. G. Székely, G. Kelemen, C. Brechbühler and G. Gerig. Segmentation of 2-D and 3-D objects from MRI volume data using constrained elastic deformations of flexible Fourier contour and surface models. *Medical Image Analysis*, 1:19–34,1996.
12. J. Lötjönen, P-J. Reissman, I. E. Magnin, J. Nenonen, and T. Katila. A Triangulation Method of an Arbitrary Point Set for Biomagnetic Problems. *IEEE Trans. Magn.*, 34(4):2228–2233,1998.

3D Image Matching Using a Finite Element Based Elastic Deformation Model

Matthieu Ferrant[1,2], Simon K. Warfield[1], Charles R.G. Guttmann[1],
Robert V. Mulkern[1,3], Ferenc A. Jolesz[1], and Ron Kikinis[1]

[1] Radiology, Brigham and Womens Hospital, Harvard Medical School, Boston, USA.
[2] Telecommunications Laboratory, Université catholique de Louvain, Belgium.
[3] Radiology, Children's Hospital, Boston, USA.
{ferrant,warfield,guttmann,jolesz,kikinis}@bwh.harvard.edu

Abstract. We present a new approach for the computation of the deformation field between three dimensional (3D) images. The deformation field minimizes the sum of the squared differences between the images to be matched and is constrained by the physical properties of the different objects represented by the image. The objects are modeled as elastic bodies. Compared to optical flow methods, this approach distinguishes itself by three main characteristics: it can account for the actual physical properties of the objects to be deformed, it can provide us with physical properties of the deformed objects (i.e. stress tensors), and computes a global solution to the deformation instead of a set of local solutions. This latter characteristic is achieved through a finite-element based scheme. The finite element approach requires the different objects in the images to be meshed. Therefore, a tetrahedral mesh generator using a pre-computed case table and specifically suited for segmented images has been developed. Preliminary experiments on simulated data as well as on medical data have been carried out successfully. Tested medical applications included muscle exercise imaging and ventricular deformation in multiple sclerosis.

1 Introduction

During the last decade, physically realistic models for surgical planning and image registration have gained increased attention in the medical imaging community. The reason for this is that purely image-based statistical methods do not take into account the physical properties of the objects depicted in the image and often cannot predict any changes in the image. Different imaged objects have very different properties and react in a way defined by their material characteristics (e.g. bone and soft tissues have very different behaviors when submitted to equivalent stresses). Therefore, we believe that using a model incorporating the object's physical characteristics can improve the accuracy of a deformable model significantly.

The discretization of deformation problems using the Finite Element (FE) Method and elastic bodies is becoming more and more popular for various applications such as surgical simulation and surgical planning [1–3]. This method, in conjunction with an elastic deformation model, is often chosen for its reliable behavior and accuracy as compared to simpler analogies such as mass-spring models and others [4, 5].

Previous work for recovering image deformation is mainly based on local image structure [6, 7]. These methods compute a deformation field between images simultaneously minimizing a local similarity measure and satisfying some kind of arbitrarily chosen smoothness constraint. They are often referred to as optical flow (OF) methods. Later, the image registration community proposed physical deformation models to constrain the deformation field using elastic [8, 9] or even viscous fluid deformation models [10, 11] . It is only recently that biomechanical models have been explicitly proposed to constrain the deformation of images [12, 13]. Currently, the drawback of the latter methods is that they either require user intervention, or another means to compute the forces applied to the model. Another drawback is that these methods have only been applied to 2D images thereby limiting the clinical utility and the possibility to efficiently assess the accuracy of the method.

We propose a new integrated approach that implicitly computes the forces applied to the 3D model by constraining the deformation field to satisfy both the elasticity model and the local image similarity criterion. This is achieved by embedding an image similarity constraint on the deformation field into the minimization scheme that leads to the constitutive equations of the deformation model. The equations are discretized using the finite element method.

We apply this method to synthetic 3D images as well as to sequences of arm exercise and enlarging ventricles in 3D brain MRI. In these applications, the deformations happen over time and are, at least in part, intrinsically due to small biomechanical deformations for which our elastic model is very well suited.

2 Theory

2.1 Mathematical formulation of the problem

We formulate the elastic matching of two images as an energy minimization procedure, where the energy comprises a term modeling the physical behavior of the object to be deformed and another term driving the model so as to match both images. The matching criterion between both images is modeled as the minimization of the sum of the squared differences between both images.

Assuming a linear elastic continuum with no initial stresses or strains, the potential energy of an elastic body submitted to externally applied forces can be expressed as [14]:

$$E = \int_{\Omega} \sigma^t \epsilon \, d\Omega + \int_{\Omega} Fu \, d\Omega \qquad (1)$$

where F is the vector representing the forces applied to the elastic body (forces per unit volume, surface forces or forces concentrated at the nodes), u the displacement vector, and Ω the body on which one is working. ϵ is the strain vector, defined as

$$\epsilon = \left(\frac{\partial u}{\partial x}, \frac{\partial u}{\partial y}, \frac{\partial u}{\partial z}, \frac{\partial u}{\partial x} + \frac{\partial u}{\partial y}, \frac{\partial u}{\partial y} + \frac{\partial u}{\partial z}, \frac{\partial u}{\partial x} + \frac{\partial u}{\partial z} \right)^t = Lu \qquad (2)$$

and σ the stress vector, linked to the strain vector by the material's constitutive equations. In the case of linear elasticity, with no initial stresses or strains, this relation is described as

$$\sigma = \left(\sigma_x, \sigma_y, \sigma_z, \tau_{xy}, \tau_{yz}, \tau_{xz} \right)^t = D\epsilon \qquad (3)$$

where D is the elasticity matrix characterizing the material's properties [14].

The external forces F can be computed as a classical optical flow field between the images to be matched , providing us with a semi-implicit method where the optical flow field would be an initial estimate of the deformation field being regularized by the elastic model. The estimates can then be iteratively refined until an equilibrium is reached.

To avoid the separate computation of the forces F, the elastic deformation, and the matching criterion, we propose to directly compute a deformation field that readily satisfies both the elasticity constraint and a local image similarity constraint between the images to be matched (I_1 and I_2). Hence, the total energy to be minimized is expressed as:

$$E = \int_\Omega \sigma^t \epsilon \, d\Omega + \int_\Omega \left(I_1(x + u(x)) - I_2(x) \right)^2 d\Omega \qquad (4)$$

Assuming that the deformation field is small and the variation of I_1 smooth, the first order Taylor expansion of $I_1(x + u(x))$ can be expressed as

$$I_1(x + u(x)) \cong I_1(x) + \langle \nabla I_1(x), u(x) \rangle \qquad (5)$$

Using the material's constitutive equation (3) and (5), equation (4) becomes (the dependencies to x are omitted in further developments to clarify the equations) :

$$E = \int_\Omega \epsilon^t D \epsilon \, d\Omega + \int_\Omega \left(I_1 - I_2 \right)^2 - 2\left(I_1 - I_2 \right) \nabla I_1 u + u^t \nabla I_1^t \nabla I_1 u \, d\Omega \qquad (6)$$

Within a finite element discretization framework, an elastic body can be approximated as an assemblage of discrete finite elements interconnected at nodal points on the element boundaries. The displacements are a function of the displacement at the element's nodal points weighted by the element's shape functions $N_i^{el}(x)$ (7).

$$u(x) = \sum_{i=1}^{4} N_i^{el}(x) u_i^{el}(x) \qquad (7)$$

The elements we use are tetrahedra, with linear interpolation of the displacement field. Hence, the shape function of node i of tetrahedron el is defined as follows:

$$N_i^{el} = \frac{1}{6V^{el}} \left(a_i^{el} + b_i^{el} x + c_i^{el} y + d_i^{el} z \right) \qquad (8)$$

The computation of the volume of the element V^{el} and the other constants is detailed in [14]. For every node i of each element el, we define the matrix $B_i^{el} = L_i N_i^{el}$. The function to be minimized at every node i of each element el can thus be expressed as :

$$E(u_{ij}^{el}) = \int_\Omega \sum_{j=1}^{4} u_i^{el^t} B_i^{el^t} D B_j^{el} u_j^{el} \, d\Omega$$

$$+ \int_\Omega \left(I_1 - I_2 \right)^2 - 2\left(I_1 - I_2 \right) \nabla I_1 N_i^{el} u_i^{el} \, d\Omega$$

$$+ \int_\Omega \sum_{j=1}^{4} u_i^{el^t} N_i^{el} \nabla I_1^t \nabla I_1 N_j^{el} u_j^{el} \, d\Omega \qquad (9)$$

We seek the minimum of this function by solving for $\frac{dE(u_i^{el})}{du_i^{el}} = C$. Equation (9) then becomes :

$$\int_\Omega \sum_{j=1}^{4} \left(B_i^{el\,t} D B_j^{el} + N_i^{el} \nabla I_1^t \nabla I_1 N_j^{el} \right) u_j^{el}\, d\Omega = \int_\Omega (I_1 - I_2) \nabla I_1 N_i^{el}\, d\Omega \quad (10)$$

This last expression can be written as a matrix system for each finite element:

$$\left(K^{el} + G^{el} \right) u^{el} = F^{el} \tag{11}$$

Matrices K^{el}, G^{el} and F^{el} are defined as follows: $K_{i,j}^{el} = \int_\Omega B_i^{el\,t} D B_j^{el}\, d\Omega$, $G_{i,j}^{el} = \int_\Omega N_i^{el} \nabla I_1^t \nabla I_1 N_j^{el}\, d\Omega$, $F_j^{el} = \int_\Omega (I_1 - I_2) \nabla I_1 N_i^{el}\, d\Omega$; where every element i, j refers to pairs of nodes of the element el (i and j range from 1 to 4). $K_{i,j}^{el}$ and $G_{i,j}^{el}$ are 3 by 3 matrices, F_j^{el} is a 3 by 1 vector. The 12 by 12 matrices K^{el} and G^{el}, and the vector F^{el} are computed for each element and are then assembled in a global system the solution of which will provide us with the deformation field corresponding to the global minimum of the total energy.

2.2 Tetrahedral mesh generation

Within the finite element framework, objects need to be meshed, i.e. divided into finite elements. We have chosen tetrahedral elements for their simplicity in terms of shape functions and data structure. Most available packages do not allow meshing of multiple objects [17],[19], and are often designed for regular objects, which is not the case for labeled medical data. Therefore, we have developed our own tetrahedral mesh generator, specifically suited for labeled 3D volumes.

The labeled 3D image is first divided into cubes of a given size, which are further divided into 5 tetrahedra with an alternating pattern so as to avoid diagonal crossings on the shared quadrilateral faces of neighboring cubes. For each tetrahedron, the image labels at its nodes are checked. A case table draws the elements to be added to the mesh. If all 4 nodes have non-object labels, no tetrahedron is added to the mesh. If all nodes have an object label, the tetrahedron is added to the mesh as is. If the tetrahedron lies across two objects (i.e. all nodes do not have the same label), the subdivision of the original tetrahedron is looked up in the case table. Figure 1 shows the 5 basic

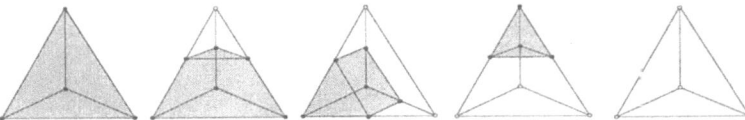

Fig. 1. Different tetrahedral cases depicted from left to right. Case 1: all nodes belong to structure; case 2: 3 nodes belong to structure; case 3: 2 nodes belong to structure; case 4: 1 node belongs to structure; case 5: no nodes belong to structure.

cases. There are actually 16 cases, but the remaining cases are symmetric to cases 2, 3 and 4. The resolution of the mesh can easily be adapted by varying the tetrahedra's sizes. The resulting prisms are divided into tetrahedra using Nielson's index connexion rule [15] so as to avoid edge crossings on the quadrilateral faces shared by neighboring prisms. The mesh structure is built such that for images containing multiple objects, a

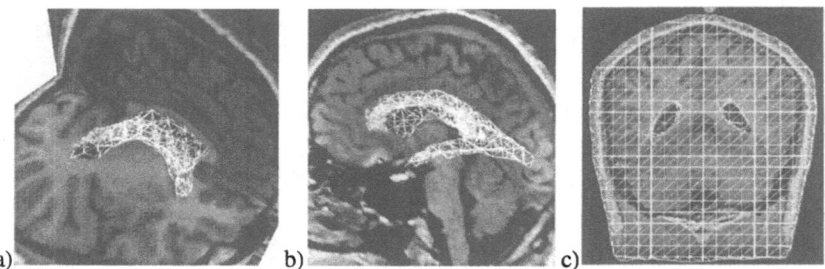

a)   b)   c)

Fig. 2. a) and b) 3D rendering of the wireframe tetrahedral mesh of lateral ventricles. c) coronal cut through tetrahedral mesh of head and lateral ventricles.

fully connected and consistent tetrahedral mesh is obtained with for every cell, a given label corresponding to the object the cell belongs to. Therefore, different biomechanical properties can easily be assigned to the different cells or objects composing the mesh.

2.3   Material properties

An isotropic linear elastic material is characterized by two parameters: Young's elasticity modulus E and Poisson's ratio ν [14]. They determine the elastic behavior of the object to be deformed and are related to the Lamé constants λ and μ by the following relations :

$$E = \frac{\mu(2\mu + 3\lambda)}{\mu + \lambda} \qquad \nu = \frac{\lambda}{2(\lambda + \mu)} \qquad (12)$$

where E relates tension in the object and its stretch in the longitudinal direction, and ν is the ratio of the lateral contraction to longitudinal stretch.

The choice of these values is of course critical to the reliability of a physics based deformation model. Their determination has not been addressed very consistently in the literature as the coefficients used often differ significantly from study to study and do not always include the physical units of the values. Recently, Hagemann et. al. [13] published a comparative study of brain elasticity coefficients proposed by different authors, and came to the conclusion that for their application, the only comparable and meaningful values presented by other authors are the ratios of the coefficients. This has also been our choice for all the presented experiments.

3   Experiments

We have implemented our own FE algorithm. The assembly and solving of the linear matrix system has been parallelized using the PETSc library [16]. The matching algorithm, using a mesh with approximately hundred thousand tetrahedra, only takes a few minutes on a parallel machine with 20 Ultra Sparc II 250Mhz CPUs. The size of the edges of the tetrahedra was approximately 5 mm, so as to have a good compromise between capture range and local precision. The 3D visualization module has been programmed using The Visualization Toolkit library [17].

An experiment with a synthetic image was carried out to verify the plausibility of our model and to show the advantage, for medical imaging applications, of our matching using an elastic model instead of just considering local image structure with a smoothness constraint (Optical Flow methods). To demonstrate the applicability of our method, we also chose two experiments with medical data.

3.1 Growing sphere experiment

We have applied the algorithm to a synthetic sequence of two spheres (gray regions) centered at the same location with a radius of 15 and 17 pixels. On figure 3, one can observe that the deformation field yielded by OF is located only at the voxels where the difference between both images is non-zero, while the FE elastic deformation algorithm propagates the deformation all along the surrounding elastic body (which in this experiment was stiffer and had a larger Young modulus than the sphere itself).

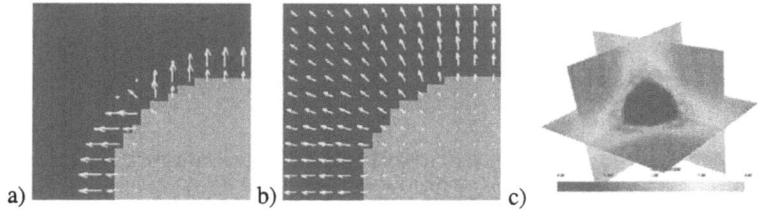

a)   b)   c)

Fig. 3. Growing sphere. a) and b): close-ups of 2D cuts through 3D image with a) classical OF, and b) FE matching deformation fields overlayed, c) and 3D orthogonal cuts through the FE mesh with intensity coding of the displacement field. The displacement field is mainly located at the boundaries of the sphere and is propagated through the surrounding elastic medium.

3.2 Arm data

The next example studies the deformation occurring when a muscle of the arm is exercised by a two finger flexion [18]. Exercise causes a muscle on the left part of the image to expand. The aim of this exercise related muscle deformation experiment was to characterize the physical change happening during exercise, by comparing both images when they are aligned together.

In this experiment, the Young modulus of the tissue has been set to 2 kPa (and ν to 0.3), and was constant over the whole arm volume. Future enhancements will include different coefficients for the bones and the skin. The results of Figure 4 confirm that the muscular exercise manifests itself essentially on the left part in the image, where the displacement field is the most important.

3.3 Ventricular matching

In this experiment, the ventricles and the intra-cranial cavity of an MS patient have been segmented at two different time points (approx. 3 years apart) from 3D T2 weighted

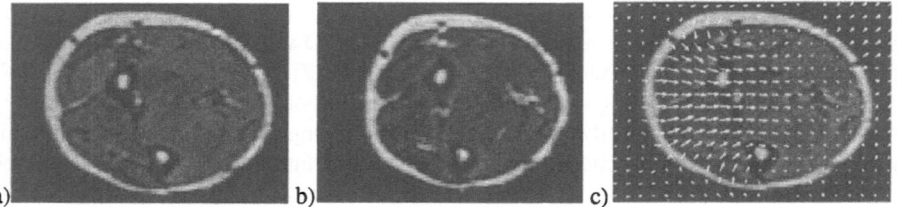

Fig. 4. Arm exercise. Slice of 3D MR dataset a) at exercise, b) at rest, c) deformation field over-layed on exercise slice

MR images. During that period, significant enlargement of the ventricles occurred. The matching of these time points allows us to observe the change in shape of the brain and ventricles ($E = 3kPa, \nu = 0.4$).

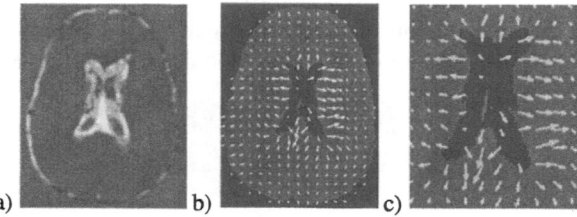

Fig. 5. Enlarging ventricles.a) slice of difference between segmented images at both time points (gray means no difference), b)deformation field superimposed on same image at the first time point. c) close-up

4   Conclusions and perspectives

We have presented a new, physics-based deformable model for tracking physical deformations using image matching. The model results from the minimization of a deformation field simultaneously satisfying the constraints of an elastic body and a local image similarity measure. The model provides us with a physically realistic deformation field and also allows us to inspect the characteristics of the deformed objects. This can be very useful for the inspection of stresses induced by the deformation of certain objects on their surroundings. For example, the model could be used to predict deformations consequent to the growth of a tumor, to predict brain shift during neurosurgy, etc.

In the experiments we presented, the objects were considered to be homogeneous elastic bodies. Further improvements of the algorithm include the assignment of different elasticities to the different objects represented in the image. This will require a preliminary segmentation of the objects to be deformed so as to be able to set appropriate elasticity coefficients to every cell of the mesh. Also, the anisotropy of certain tissues could be included into the model by modifying the elasticity matrix D appropriately.

Acknowledgements

M. Ferrant is working towards a Ph.D. degree with a grant from the Belgian FRIA. This investigation was also supported in part by a grant from the National Multiple Sclerosis Society (SW)

and by the Neuroimage Analysis Center (NIH P41 RR132118-01), Core Segmentation Tools for Computer Assisted Surgery (NIH R01 RR11747-01A), and MR Guided Therapy (NIH P01 CA67165-03). The authors would also like to thank Dr. Xingchang Wei for providing us with the segmented images for the ventricular matching experiment.

References

1. H. Delinguette. Toward Realistic Soft-tissue Modeling in Medical Simulation. *Proceedings of the IEEE*, 86(3):512–523, march 1998.
2. D.D. Paulsen, M.I. Miga, F.E. Kennedy, P.J. Hoopes, A. Hartov, and D.W. Roberts. A Computational Model for Tracking Subsurface Tissue Deformation During Stereotactic Neurosurgery. *IEEE Transactions on Biomedical Engineering*, 46(2):213–225, february 1999.
3. O. Skrinjar, D. Spenser, and J. Duncan. Brain Shift Modeling for use in Neurosurgery. In *MICCAI '98*, pages 641–649, 1998.
4. S.F. Gibson. 3D Chainmail : a Fast Algorithm for Deforming Volumetric Objects. In *Symposium on Interactive 3D Graphics, ACM SIGGRAPH*, pages 149–154, 1997.
5. M. Bro-Nielsen. Modeling Elasticity in Solids using Active Cubes: Application to Simulated Operations. In *Computer Vision, Virtual Reality and Robotics in Medicine*, pages 535–541, 1995.
6. S. Bauchemin and J.L. Barron. The Computation of Optical Flow. *ACM computing surveys*, 27(3), 1995.
7. J. Dengler and M. Schmidt. The Dynamic Pyramid - a Model for Motion Analysis with Controlled Continuity. *International Journal of Pattern Recognition and Artificial Intelligence*, 2:275–288, 1988.
8. R. Bajcsy and S. Kovacic. Multi Resolution Elastic Matching. *Computer Vision, Graphics and Image Processing*, 46:1–21, 1989.
9. C. Davatzikos. Spatial Transformation and Registration of Brain Images using Elastically Deformable Models. *Computer Vision and Image Understanding*, 66(2):207–222, may 1997.
10. G.E. Christensen, S.C. Joshi, and M.I. Miller. Volumetric Transformation of Brain Anatomy. *IEEE Transactions on Medical Imaging*, 16(6):864–877, december 1997.
11. M. Bro-Nielsen and C. Gramkow. Fast Fluid Registration of Medical Images. In *Visualization in Biomedical Computing (VBC '96)*, pages 267–276, 1996.
12. D.K. Kyriacou and C. Davatzikos. A Biomechanical Model of Soft Tissue Deformation with Applications to Non-rigid Registration of Brain Images with Tumor Pathology. In *MICCAI '98*, pages 531–538, 1998.
13. A. Hagemann, Rohr K., H.S. Stiel, U. Spetzger, and Gilsbach J.M. Non-Rigid Matching of Tomographic Images Based on a Biomechanical Model of the Human Head. In *SPIE Medical Imaging '99*, 1999.
14. O.C. Zienkewickz and R.L. Taylor. *The Finite Element Method*. McGraw Hill Book Co., 1987.
15. G.M. Nielson and J. Sung. Interval Volume Tetrahedrization. In *Visualization '97*, pages 221–228, 1997.
16. S. Balay, W.D. Gropp, L. Curfman McInnes, and B.F. Smith. PETSc 2.0 for MPI - Portable, Extensible Toolkit for Scientific Computations. http://www.mcs.anl.gov/petsc, 1998.
17. Will Schroeder, Ken Martin, and Bill Lorensen. *The Visualization Toolkit: An Object-Oriented Approach to 3D Graphics*. Prentice Hall PTR, New Jersey, 1996.
18. J.L. Fleckenstein, J.V. Crues III, and C.D. Reimers. *Muscle Imaging in Health and Disease*. Springer, 1996.
19. B. Geiger. *Three Dimensional Modeling of Human Organs and its application to diagnosis and surgical planning*. Report 2105, INRIA Sophia-Antipolis France, 1993.

Quantitative Comparison of Sinc-Approximating Kernels for Medical Image Interpolation

Erik H. W. Meijering, Wiro J. Niessen, Josien P. W. Pluim, Max A. Viergever

Image Sciences Institute, Utrecht University
Heidelberglaan 100, 3584 CX Utrecht, The Netherlands
URL: http://www.isi.uu.nl E-mail: {erik,wiro,josien,max}@isi.uu.nl

Abstract. Interpolation is required in many medical image processing operations. From sampling theory, it follows that the ideal interpolation kernel is the sinc function, which is of infinite extent. In the attempt to obtain practical and computationally efficient image processing algorithms, many sinc-approximating interpolation kernels have been devised. In this paper we present the results of a quantitative comparison of 84 different sinc-approximating kernels, with spatial extents ranging from 2 to 10 grid points in each dimension. The evaluation involves the application of geometrical transformations to medical images from different modalities (CT, MR, and PET), using the different kernels. The results show very clearly that, of all kernels with a spatial extent of 2 grid points, the linear interpolation kernel performs best. Of all kernels with an extent of 4 grid points, the cubic convolution kernel is the best (28% - 75% reduction of the errors as compared to linear interpolation). Even better results (44% - 95% reduction) are obtained with kernels of larger extent, notably the Welch, Cosine, Lanczos, and Kaiser windowed sinc kernels. In general, the truncated sinc kernel is one of the worst performing kernels.

1 Introduction

Interpolation of sampled data is required in a variety of medical image processing operations, such as rotation, translation, deformation, or magnification, which are frequently applied for registration or visualization purposes. In many applications, it is of paramount importance to limit as much as possible the grey-value errors introduced by interpolation. For example, in image registration, interpolation errors may introduce artifacts in the optimization cost function, which may lead to registration errors [1]. Furthermore, it has been pointed out that, especially in the case of functional images, interpolation errors may affect the interpretation of longitudinal studies [2]. It has also been shown that the errors made by interpolation kernels influence the results of measurements carried out in maximum intensity projection images [3].

Whereas from sampling theory it follows that the ideal interpolation kernel is the sinc function, it is not the ideal kernel from an implementational point of view, since this function is of infinite extent and has a very low rate of decay. In the attempt to obtain practical and computationally efficient image processing algorithms, many sinc-approximating interpolation kernels have been devised. However, an extensive quantitative comparison of the performance of these kernels when using them to apply geometrical transformations to medical images, has never been described. The purpose of this paper is to present the results of such a comparison.

2   Sinc-Approximating Kernels

In this section we briefly present the sinc-approximating kernels most frequently encountered in the literature. These can be divided into piecewise polynomial kernels and windowed sinc kernels.

2.1   Piecewise Polynomial Kernels

A frequently used approach to obtain a sinc-approximating kernel is to model the shape of the sinc kernel by piecewise polynomials. The simplest approach in this respect is to use zeroth order polynomials, resulting in the so-called nearest neighbor kernel:

$$h_{NN}(x) = \begin{cases} 1 \,, -\frac{1}{2} \leqslant x < \frac{1}{2} \\ 0 \,, x < -\frac{1}{2} \ \vee \ x \geqslant \frac{1}{2} \end{cases} \tag{1}$$

Higher order piecewise polynomial kernels can be written in the form [4]:

$$h(x) = \begin{cases} a_{0j} + a_{1j}|x| + \ldots + a_{nj}|x|^n \,, j \leqslant |x| < j+1 \\ 0 \qquad\qquad\qquad\qquad\qquad ,\, m \leqslant |x| \end{cases} \tag{2}$$

where n is the order of the polynomials, $j = 0, 1, \ldots, m - 1$, the parameter $m \in \mathbb{N}_{\backslash\{0\}}$ determines the extent of the kernel, and n and m are related by $n = 2m - 1$. The $(n + 1)m$ coefficients a_{ij} can be solved by imposing constraints on the polynomials, derived from the shape of the sinc kernel [4].

For $n = 1$, Eq. (2) boils down to the linear interpolation kernel, h_{Lin}. The resulting kernels for $n > 1$ can be shown to be functions of a free parameter, α. In order to obtain a unique value for α, one additional constraint needs to be imposed. In the literature on cubic convolution ($n = 3$), several constraints have been proposed [5]: (i) The slope constraint, which implies that α is chosen such that the slope of the kernel equals the slope of the sinc function at $x = 1$. This value is denoted α_ς. (ii) The continuity constraint. For $n > 1$, the piecewise polynomial kernels are elements of C^{n-2}. The continuity constraint implies that α is chosen such that the $(n - 1)$th-order derivative of the kernel is continuous at $x = 1$. The resulting value is denoted $\alpha_\sim$. (iii) The flatness constraint, which implies that α is chosen such that the Fourier spectrum of the kernel, $\tilde{H}(f)$, is flat at $f = 0$. This value of α is denoted $\alpha_\flat$. These three constraints can also be applied to the higher order schemes. The resulting values of α for the cubic (h_{Cub}), quintic (h_{Qui}), septic (h_{Sep}), and nonic (h_{Non}) piecewise polynomial interpolation kernels, are presented in Table 1.

Kernel	α_ς	$\alpha_\sim$	α_b
h_{Cub}	-1	$-\frac{3}{4}$	$-\frac{1}{2}$
h_{Qui}	$\frac{11}{96}$	$\frac{1}{13}$	$\frac{3}{64}$
h_{Sep}	$-\frac{1027}{452574}$	$-\frac{3133}{2275008}$	$-\frac{71}{83232}$
h_{Non}	$\frac{34814699}{2509872453120}$	$\frac{17671607}{2324998440576}$	$\frac{3829}{788235264}$

Table 1. Values of the free parameter α for the cubic (h_{Cub}), quintic (h_{Qui}), septic (h_{Sep}), and nonic (h_{Non}) piecewise polynomial interpolation kernels, resulting from the slope constraint (α_ς), continuity constraint ($\alpha_\sim$), and flatness constraint (α_b).

2.2 Windowed Sinc Kernels

Another approach to obtain a sinc-approximating kernel is to multiply the sinc function with a window function of limited extent:

$$h(x) = \omega(x)\mathrm{sinc}(x) , \quad \text{with} \quad \omega(x) = \begin{cases} w(x) , 0 \leqslant |x| < m \\ 0 \qquad , m \leqslant |x| \end{cases} \tag{3}$$

where $\omega : \mathbb{R} \to \mathbb{R}$ is the window function, and $w : \mathbb{R} \to \mathbb{R}$ determines the shape of the window in the interval $(-m, m)$, with $m \in \mathbb{N}_{\backslash\{0\}}$. The window functions which were used in the quantitative comparison described in the next section are listed in Table 2.

3 Quantitative Comparison

The sinc-approximating kernels presented in the previous section were quantitatively compared by using them to apply several geometrical transformations to a number of medical images, and by analyzing the resulting interpolation errors in the transformed images. In this section we present the evaluation strategy and the results.

3.1 Evaluation Strategy

Medical images were obtained from a collection of 3-D brain datasets from three different modalities, *viz.*, computed tomography (CT), magnetic resonance imaging (MR; T1-weighted), and positron emission tomography (PET). From every subset (modality), we selected five images. The five CT images were of size 512×512 times 28, 29, 33, 30, and 28 voxels, respectively, all with a voxel size of $0.654 \times 0.654 \times 4.0$ mm^3. The five T1-weighted MR images were all of size $256 \times 256 \times 26$ voxels, with a voxel size of $1.25 \times 1.25 \times 4.0$ mm^3. The five PET images were of size $128 \times 128 \times 15$ voxels, one with a voxel size of $1.94 \times 1.94 \times 8.0$ mm^3, and the others with a voxel size of $2.59 \times 2.59 \times 8.0$ mm^3.

Window	Definition
Bartlett	$w_{Bar} \triangleq 1 - \frac{|x|}{m}$
Blackman	$w_{Bla} \triangleq 0.42 + 0.50 \cos\left(\frac{\pi x}{m}\right) + 0.08 \cos\left(\frac{2\pi x}{m}\right)$
Blackman-Harris	$w_{BHa} \triangleq 0.42323 + 0.49755 \cos\left(\frac{\pi x}{m}\right) + 0.07922 \cos\left(\frac{2\pi x}{m}\right)$
Bohman	$w_{Boh} \triangleq \left(1 - \frac{|x|}{m}\right) \cos\left(\frac{\pi x}{m}\right) + \frac{1}{\pi} \sin\left(\frac{\pi |x|}{m}\right)$
Cosine	$w_{Cos} \triangleq \cos\left(\frac{\pi x}{2m}\right)$
Hamming	$w_{Ham} \triangleq 0.54 + 0.46 \cos\left(\frac{\pi x}{m}\right)$
Hann	$w_{Han} \triangleq 0.5 + 0.5 \cos\left(\frac{\pi x}{m}\right)$
Kaiser	$w_{Kai} \triangleq \frac{I_0(\beta)}{I_0(\alpha)}, \ \beta = \alpha\sqrt{1 - \left(\frac{x}{m}\right)^2}$
Lanczos	$w_{Lan} \triangleq \operatorname{sinc}\left(\frac{\pi x}{m}\right)$
Rectangular	$w_{Rec} \triangleq 1$
Welch	$w_{Wel} \triangleq 1 - \frac{x^2}{m^2}$

Table 2. Window functions and their definitions. Throughout this paper, the corresponding kernels are given the same subscript. In the definition of the Kaiser window, $\alpha \in \mathbb{R}^+$ is a free parameter, for which we used values of 5.0, 6.0, 7.0, and 8.0. I_0 is the zeroth order modified Bessel function of the first kind, which can accurately be approximated by using its series expansion. For details, see Harris [6] or Wolberg [5].

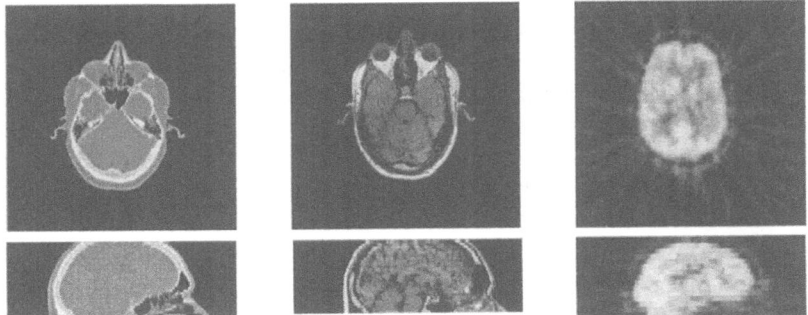

Fig. 1. Examples of the medical test-images used in the experiments. Top row (left-to-right): a transversal slice of a 3-D CT, MR-T1, and PET dataset, respectively. Bottom row: sagittal slices of the same datasets. Note that for display purposes, the images of the sagittal slices shown in this figure were scaled, thus correcting for the voxel anisotropy. Nearest neighbor interpolation was used for this purpose.

In order to be able to study the performance of the interpolation kernels in different slice directions, we selected, for each of the 3-D images, one transversal and one sagittal slice. This resulted in a total of 30 different 2-D test-images (see Fig. 1 for examples).

The test-images were subjected to several geometrical transformations, including rotations and subpixel translations, as these are frequently required in (multimodality) registration. In the rotation experiments, the test-images were successively rotated over 0.7°, 3.2°, 6.5°, 9.3°, 12.1°, 15.2°, 18.4°, 21.3°, 23.7°, 26.6°, 29.8°, 32.9°, 35.7°, 38.5°, 41.8°, and 44.3°, which adds up to a total of 360°. In the subpixel translation experiments, the images were successively shifted over 0.01, 0.04, 0.07, 0.11, 0.15, 0.18, 0.21, 0.24, 0.26, 0.29, 0.32, 0.35, 0.39, 0.43, 0.46, and 0.49 pixels, which adds up to a total of 4.0 pixels. For every test-image, both experiments were carried out for all interpolation kernels. Of the two families described in Section 2, we used all kernels for which $m \leqslant 5$, which amounts to a total of 84 kernels. In order to avoid border problems, the test-images were mirrored around the borders in each dimension.

For every combination of test-image, experiment (rotation or translation), and interpolation kernel, the root-mean-square error (RMSE) of the grey-values in the processed image was computed. Since in these experiments the grid points of the processed images coincide with those of the original images, a gold standard is available: for the rotation experiments, the references images are simply the original images, and for the translation experiments, the reference images are obtained by translating the original image by four pixels (which requires no interpolation). In order to avoid quantization errors, all computations were carried out with double precision floating-point numbers (12 significant decimals).

3.2   Results

As can be concluded from the literature, the linear interpolation kernel, h_{Lin}, is by far the most frequently used kernel [7]. Therefore, in this study, our main interest was to investigate the performance of alternative kernels compared to h_{Lin}. To this end, we computed for every test-image and type of experiment, the percentile RMSE of every interpolation kernel compared to h_{Lin}. Since, in all cases, the percentile errors of the five images from a given combination of modality and slice direction were very similar, they were averaged. The results of the translation experiments are presented in Table 3, and those of the rotation experiments in Table 4. For every modality, type of experiment, and kernel extent, only the top-3 best kernels are shown.

4   Discussion

The performance of interpolation kernels may be assessed by subjective visual inspection of image quality, after having used the kernels to perform certain resampling operations [8, 5]. An alternative evaluation approach is to compare the spectral characteristics of the kernels to those of the ideal sinc kernel [9, 10], or to compare their abilities to reconstruct certain mathematical test-functions [11]. In the evaluation described in this paper, we have chosen to use a more pragmatic approach, in which the different interpolation kernels are used to apply actual geometrical transformations, which are frequently required in *e.g.*

Mod	Slc	Extent				
		$m=1$	$m=2$	$m=3$	$m=4$	$m=5$
CT	Tr	h_{Lin} 100.0	$h_{Cub}^{\alpha b}$ 33.4	$h_{Kai}^{\alpha=5}$ 12.3	$h_{Kai}^{\alpha=6}$ 6.3	$h_{Kai}^{\alpha=7}$ 4.7
		h_{NN} 497.1	$h_{Kai}^{\alpha=6}$ 63.6	h_{BH3} 26.7	h_{BH3} 10.4	h_{BH3} 5.6
		h_{Wel} 805.4	h_{Ham} 163.0	h_{Bla} 28.3	h_{Bla} 16.6	h_{BH4} 8.6
	Sa	h_{Lin} 100.0	$h_{Cub}^{\alpha b}$ 70.1	$h_{Kai}^{\alpha=5}$ 52.0	h_{Lan} 42.7	h_{Lan} 37.5
		h_{Wel} 193.9	$h_{Kai}^{\alpha=5}$ 76.2	h_{Lan} 54.0	h_{Cos} 42.9	h_{Cos} 37.9
		h_{NN} 281.1	h_{Ham} 79.2	h_{Cos} 54.1	$h_{Kai}^{\alpha=5}$ 43.8	$h_{Kai}^{\alpha=5}$ 39.0
MR	Tr	h_{Lin} 100.0	$h_{Cub}^{\alpha b}$ 66.9	$h_{Kai}^{\alpha=5}$ 47.1	h_{Lan} 37.8	h_{Lan} 31.5
		h_{Wel} 211.2	$h_{Kai}^{\alpha=5}$ 74.5	h_{Ham} 49.9	$h_{Kai}^{\alpha=5}$ 38.4	h_{Cos} 31.9
		h_{NN} 310.0	h_{Ham} 78.2	h_{Lan} 50.9	h_{Cos} 38.5	$h_{Kai}^{\alpha=5}$ 33.3
	Sa	h_{Lin} 100.0	$h_{Cub}^{\alpha \sim}$ 71.7	h_{Cos} 55.9	h_{Cos} 46.4	h_{Lan} 41.6
		h_{Wel} 162.3	$h_{Kai}^{\alpha=5}$ 79.3	h_{Lan} 56.1	h_{Lan} 46.4	h_{Cos} 41.7
		h_{Cos} 230.6	h_{Wel} 79.8	$h_{Kai}^{\alpha=5}$ 56.3	h_{Wel} 47.8	h_{Wel} 42.8
PET	Tr	h_{Lin} 100.0	$h_{Cub}^{\alpha b}$ 36.5	$h_{Kai}^{\alpha=5}$ 21.2	$h_{Kai}^{\alpha=6}$ 16.9	$h_{Kai}^{\alpha=6}$ 15.3
		h_{Wel} 448.6	$h_{Kai}^{\alpha=6}$ 62.5	h_{BH3} 31.4	h_{BH3} 19.8	h_{BH3} 16.4
		h_{NN} 542.7	h_{Ham} 90.9	h_{Bla} 31.8	h_{Bla} 20.9	h_{Bla} 17.0
	Sa	h_{Lin} 100.0	$h_{Cub}^{\alpha b}$ 66.5	$h_{Kai}^{\alpha=5}$ 47.9	h_{Lan} 39.2	h_{Lan} 34.6
		h_{Wel} 173.3	$h_{Kai}^{\alpha=5}$ 72.0	h_{Lan} 48.7	h_{Cos} 39.5	h_{Cos} 34.7
		h_{Cos} 247.6	h_{Ham} 74.9	h_{Cos} 49.0	$h_{Kai}^{\alpha=5}$ 40.4	h_{Wel} 35.8

Table 3. The percentile root mean square errors (RMSEs) resulting from the different interpolation kernels in the translation experiments, relative to the RMSEs of the linear interpolation kernel, h_{Lin}. For every extent (m), modality (Mod), and slice direction (Slc), either transversal (Tr) or sagittal (Sa), only the top-3 best kernels are shown.

medical image registration problems. The design of the evaluation was such that true gold standards were available, *viz.*, the original images.

The results of the evaluation allow us to draw some important conclusions. For $m=1$, *i.e.*, a spatial extent of 2 grid points, the best interpolation kernel is the linear interpolation kernel. For $m=2$, *i.e.*, a spatial extent of 4 grid points, the best approach is to use a cubic convolution kernel, although the optimal value for the free parameter, α, may differ for different types of images. For the test-images used in this study, cubic convolution resulted in a considerable (28% - 75%) reduction of interpolation errors, as compared to linear interpolation. Even better results (44% - 95% reduction) were obtained with kernels of larger extent. These latter results showed that, for $m \geqslant 3$, most windowed sinc kernels give better results than piecewise polynomial kernels, although one must be very careful in choosing a window function. Of the window functions incorporated in this study, the Welch, Cosine, Lanczos, and Kaiser windows appeared to be the best. It was also concluded that a truncated sinc kernel (resulting from applying a rectangular window), was one of the worst performing kernels. Finally, we notice that due to the anisotropic nature of 3-D medical datasets, the through-

Mod	Slc	Extent				
		$m=1$	$m=2$	$m=3$	$m=4$	$m=5$
CT	Tr	h_{Lin} 100.0	$h_{Cub}^{\alpha b}$ 24.7	$h_{Kai}^{\alpha=5}$ 10.8	$h_{Kai}^{\alpha=6}$ 5.7	$h_{Kai}^{\alpha=7}$ 5.1
		h_{NN} 173.6	$h_{Kai}^{\alpha=6}$ 56.2	h_{BH3} 21.7	h_{BH3} 9.9	h_{BH3} 5.5
		h_{Wel} 997.5	h_{Ham} 247.6	$h_{Qui}^{\alpha b}$ 22.5	h_{BH4} 14.0	h_{BH4} 7.0
	Sa	h_{Lin} 100.0	$h_{Cub}^{\alpha \sim}$ 58.9	$h_{Kai}^{\alpha=5}$ 45.1	h_{Wel} 35.4	h_{Wel} 30.2
		h_{NN} 143.1	$h_{Kai}^{\alpha=6}$ 76.0	h_{Wel} 46.0	h_{Cos} 36.5	h_{Cos} 30.8
		h_{Wel} 240.7	h_{Ham} 83.4	h_{Cos} 48.0	$h_{Kai}^{\alpha=5}$ 38.6	h_{Lan} 32.1
MR	Tr	h_{Lin} 100.0	$h_{Cub}^{\alpha \sim}$ 59.2	$h_{Kai}^{\alpha=5}$ 43.7	h_{Wel} 35.2	h_{Wel} 30.3
		h_{NN} 153.2	$h_{Kai}^{\alpha=6}$ 74.1	h_{Wel} 46.1	h_{Cos} 36.3	h_{Cos} 30.8
		h_{Wel} 250.8	h_{Ham} 83.4	h_{Cos} 50.4	$h_{Kai}^{\alpha=5}$ 37.8	h_{Lan} 32.0
	Sa	h_{Lin} 100.0	$h_{Cub}^{\alpha \sim}$ 62.3	h_{Wel} 49.4	h_{Wel} 40.5	h_{Wel} 36.3
		h_{NN} 139.3	$h_{Kai}^{\alpha=5}$ 76.5	$h_{Kai}^{\alpha=5}$ 50.2	h_{Cos} 41.2	h_{Cos} 36.7
		h_{Wel} 201.0	h_{Ham} 80.8	h_{Cos} 51.7	h_{Lan} 42.9	h_{Lan} 37.9
PET	Tr	h_{Lin} 100.0	$h_{Cub}^{\alpha b}$ 30.1	$h_{Kai}^{\alpha=5}$ 18.3	$h_{Kai}^{\alpha=6}$ 15.7	$h_{Kai}^{\alpha=7}$ 14.7
		h_{NN} 177.1	$h_{Kai}^{\alpha=6}$ 54.2	h_{BH3} 27.6	h_{BH3} 18.2	h_{BH3} 15.5
		h_{Wel} 515.7	h_{Ham} 123.3	$h_{Qui}^{\alpha b}$ 28.5	h_{Bla} 20.7	h_{Bla} 16.8
	Sa	h_{Lin} 100.0	$h_{Cub}^{\alpha b}$ 57.1	$h_{Kai}^{\alpha=5}$ 42.1	h_{Wel} 33.5	h_{Wel} 29.1
		h_{NN} 135.5	$h_{Kai}^{\alpha=6}$ 72.6	h_{Wel} 44.3	h_{Cos} 34.8	h_{Cos} 29.7
		h_{Wel} 231.5	h_{Ham} 79.8	h_{Cos} 48.1	$h_{Kai}^{\alpha=5}$ 36.5	h_{Lan} 30.9

Table 4. The percentile root mean square errors (RMSEs) resulting from the different interpolation kernels in the rotation experiments, relative to the RMSEs of the linear interpolation kernel, h_{Lin}. For every extent (m), modality (Mod), and slice direction (Slc), either transversal (Tr) or sagittal (Sa), only the top-3 best kernels are shown.

plane interpolation errors were considerably larger than the in-plane errors. This implies that through-plane interpolation usually requires larger kernels in order for the errors to be comparable to in-plane linear interpolation errors.

5   Conclusions

In this paper we have presented the results of a quantitative comparison of sinc-approximating kernels for medical image interpolation. The evaluation involved the application of several geometrical transformations (rotations and subpixel translations) to a number of medical images from different modalities (CT, MR, and PET), using the different interpolation kernels, and by comparing the resulting grey-value errors to those resulting from linear interpolation. A total of 84 different kernels were evaluated, with spatial extents ranging from 2 to 10 grid points in each dimension.

The results of the evaluation show very clearly that, of the kernels with a spatial extent of 2 grid points, the linear interpolation kernel is the best. Of the kernels with an extent of 4 grid points, the cubic convolution kernel is the best (28% - 75% reduction of the errors as compared to linear interpolation). Even better results (44% - 95% reduction) were obtained with kernels of larger extent, notably the Welch, Cosine, Lanczos, and Kaiser windowed sinc kernels. The truncated sinc kernel was one of the worst performing kernels.

Acknowledgment

The images used in the experiments described in this paper were obtained from Vanderbilt University, and were originally used in the project "Evaluation of Retrospective Image Registration", National Institutes of Health, Project Number: 1 R01 NS33926-01, Principal Investigator: Prof. Dr. J. Michael Fitzpatrick, Vanderbilt University, Nashville, TN, USA.

References

1. J. P. W. Pluim, J. B. A. Maintz, & M. A. Viergever, "Interpolation artefacts in mutual information based image registration", *Computer Vision and Image Understanding*, 1999. In Press.
2. J. L. Ostuni, A. K. S. Santha, V. S. Mattay, D. R. Weinberger, R. L. Levin, & J. A. Frank, "Analysis of interpolation effects in the reslicing of functional MR images", *Journal of Computer Assisted Tomography*, vol. 21, no. 5, pp. 803–810, 1997.
3. S. Schreiner, C. B. Paschal, & R. L. Galloway, "Comparison of projection algorithms used for the construction of maximum intensity projection images", *Journal of Computer Assisted Tomography*, vol. 20, no. 1, pp. 56–67, 1996.
4. E. H. W. Meijering, K. J. Zuiderveld, & M. A. Viergever, "Image reconstruction by convolution with symmetrical piecewise nth-order polynomial kernels", *IEEE Transactions on Image Processing*, vol. 8, no. 2, pp. 192–201, 1999.
5. G. Wolberg, *Digital Image Warping*, IEEE Computer Society Press, Washington, USA, 1990.
6. F. J. Harris, "On the use of windows for harmonic analysis with the discrete Fourier transform", *Proceedings of the IEEE*, vol. 66, no. 1, pp. 51–83, 1978.
7. G. J. Grevera & J. K. Udupa, "An objective comparison of 3-D image interpolation methods", *IEEE Transactions on Medical Imaging*, vol. 17, no. 4, pp. 642–652, 1998.
8. J. A. Parker, R. V. Kenyon, & D. E. Troxel, "Comparison of interpolating methods for image resampling", *IEEE Transactions on Medical Imaging*, vol. 2, no. 1, pp. 31–39, 1983.
9. S. K. Park & R. A. Schowengerdt, "Image reconstruction by parametric cubic convolution", *Computer Vision, Graphics and Image Processing*, vol. 23, no. 3, pp. 258–272, 1983.
10. E. Maeland, "On the comparison of interpolation methods", *IEEE Transactions on Medical Imaging*, vol. 7, no. 3, pp. 213–217, 1988.
11. R. G. Keys, "Cubic convolution interpolation for digital image processing", *IEEE Transactions on Acoustics, Speech, and Signal Processing*, vol. 29, no. 6, pp. 1153–1160, 1981.

A Post-processing Technique to Suppress Fluid Signal and Increase Contrast in Multispectral MR Exams of MS Patients

J.R. Mitchell[1,2,3], P. Gareau[1], S. Karlik[1,2,3], B. Rutt[1,2,3]

Imaging Research Laboratories, John P. Robarts Research Institute[1]; Department of Diagnostic Radiology and Nuclear Medicine, University of Western Ontario[2], and, The London Health Sciences Center[3], London Ontario, Canada N6A 5A5

Abstract. We present a new method to extract data from multispectral MR exams of patients with Multiple Sclerosis. Our technique produces images of "spectral phase" relative to cerebro-spinal fluid (CSF-SP images). It provides a convenient way of reducing multispectral MR exams to a single, intuitive image with contrast characteristics similar to anatomical photographs. Our new images provide better tissue contrast than that found in any of the MR images. Contrast between CSF and white matter (WM) was increased from a maximum of 19.5 in the T1w MR image to 56 in the CSF-SP image (+187%). Contrast between CSF and gray matter (GM) increased from a maximum of 14.5 in the T1w image to 35.2 in the CSF-SP image (+143%). Finally, contrast between WM and GM increased from a maximum of 7.5 in the T2w image to 11.5 in the CSF-SP image (+53%). The additional contrast in CSF-SP images may aid the quantification and analysis of lesion activity in MR exams of MS patients.

1 Introduction

MRI provides very sensitive detection of the lesions of Multiple Sclerosis (MS)[1]. We are developing new techniques to provide information about temporal changes in MS lesion intensity composition from sequential multispectral MR exams of MS patients[2]. Our methods are based upon analysis of the multispectral "feature space" distributions of tissue and lesion intensities[3]. However, as the number of images in each exam increases the feature space dimension also increases making feature space visualization and analysis more difficult.

In this paper we present a new method to extract data from multidimensional feature spaces while minimizing the loss of information. Our new technique provides images of "spectral phase" (SP) relative to a reference tissue. SP images have a number of important advantages: a) they are largely insensitive to intensity inhomogeneities in the multispectral MR exam; b) they allow retrospective suppression of reference tissue signals; c) they provide information about the underlying MR characteristics of lesions and other tissues while retaining high spatial resolution; and, d) they can provide tissue contrast much greater than any of the MR images. In this paper we describe the construction of spectral phase images relative to cerebro-spinal fluid (CSF) and show their application to MR exams of five MS patients selected from a clinical trial underway at our institute.

2   Methods

Multispectral analysis was performed on MR exams of five MS patients selected at random from a clinical trial underway at our institute. Patients were imaged on a 1.5T Signa scanner (General Electric Systems). Four MR contrasts at each of 24 slices covering the head were acquired from each patient using spin echo imaging: proton density weighted (PDw); T2 weighted (T2w); T1 weighted (T1w); and, T1 weighted after administration of gadolinium-DTPA contrast agent (GAD). Imaging parameters were as follows: FOV = 22 x 16.5 cm.; slice thickness = 5 mm. with no gap; matrix = 256 x 192; flow compensation was enabled. For the proton density/T2 weighted images, TR/TE1/TE2 = 5000/30/80 msec; BW1/BW2 = 15.6/7.81 khz; 1 nex. Total scan time was 10 minutes 24 seconds. For the T1 weighted images TR = 550 msec; TE = 13 msec; BW = 16 khz; 2 nex. Total scan time was 5 minutes 23 seconds. After the initial T1 acquisition 0.1 mmol per kg gadolinium-DTPA was injected intravenously, without disturbing the patient setup. After 5 minutes a second gadolinium enhanced T1 weighted sequence was acquired with the same parameters as above. A standard patient setup and exam slice orientation procedure was used to minimize patient motion between the PD/T2w and T1w scans and provide slice positioning which varied less than 1 mm over the entire patient volume.

Images were transferred to a SUN Ultrasparc 10 workstation (Sun Microsystems, Mountainview, California) for preprocessing. Initially, intensity non-uniformity in each multispectral exam was corrected using the non-parametric, non-uniform intensity normalization algorithm developed by Sled et. al[4]. Next, a non-linear anisotropic diffusion based filter was applied to improve the signal-to-noise ratio within the images. The filter is based on one reported by Perona and Malik[5] but extended to incorporate information from an arbitrary number of spectral bands when calculating the diffusion coefficient. This filter requires two input parameters: the number of iterations; and, an estimate of image noise. We selected three iterations as suggested by Gerig et al[6]. Image noise was estimated using twice the standard deviation measured in a large region of interest (ROI) placed in air. Although signal in air typically follows a Rician distribution, it can be used to predict the Gaussian distribution of signals in tissues[7]. Finally, in each exam four slices covering the lateral ventricles were selected for processing. A single 4-D feature space was constructed for each patient from the four MR exam intensities in the selected slices.

The 4-D feature spaces were used to calculate spectral phase images relative to cerebro-spinal fluid (CSF). CSF was selected as a reference signal since it is easily identifiable, allows definition of large homogenous ROI's and has stable MR image signal through disease progression. ROI's were placed were placed within the lateral ventricles of each patient. ROI's were placed well away from the ventricle edges to reduce any partial volume effects between slices. For each patient 'p' a CSF reference intensity vector was formed as follows:

220 J. R. Mitchell et al.

$$\vec{CSF}_p = \left[\bar{R}_{PDw,p} \quad \bar{R}_{T2w,p} \quad \bar{R}_{T1w,p} \quad \bar{R}_{GAD,p} \right]^T \tag{1}$$

where

$$\bar{R}_{b,p} = \frac{\sum_{ij} I_{bijp}}{n_p}, \, ij \in ROI, \, b \in \{PDw, T2w, T1w, GAD\} \tag{2}$$

given that: I_{bijp} is the voxel value from spectral band 'b' in voxel 'ij' within patient 'p'; and, n_p is the number of voxels in the CSF ROI. Here 'i,j' were restricted to indicate voxels within the CSF ROI.

Spectral phase images for each patient were then constructed by determining the CSF-relative spectral phase at every exam location 'xy':

$$CSF - SP_{xyp} = \vec{CSF}_p \cdot \vec{V}_{xyp} \tag{3}$$

where

$$\vec{V}_{xyp} = [I_{bxyp}]^T, b \in \{PDw, T2w, T1w, GAD\} \tag{4}$$

given that: I_{bxyp} is the voxel value from spectral band 'b' in voxel 'xy' within patient 'p'. With this algorithm tissues which are spectrally "close" to CSF have small values in the output image, while those that are "far" from CSF have high values.

Contrast in the original MR and CSF-SP images was determined from the signal difference to noise ratio (dSNR) between: CSF and normal-appearing white matter (NAWM); CSF and gray-matter (GM); and NAWM and GM. dSNR between pairs of tissues was calculated using the following equation:

$$dSNR = \frac{|\bar{x}_1 - \bar{x}_2|}{\sqrt{\frac{(n_1 - 1) \cdot s_1^2 + (n_2 - 1) \cdot s_2^2}{n_1 + n_2 - 2}}} \tag{5}$$

where: $\bar{x}_i$ is the mean signal measured within each tissue ROI; s_i^2 is the variance within each tissue ROI; and n_i is the number of voxels within each ROI. Note that this is similar to a two-sample unpaired t-test under the assumption of equal variances[8]. The mean and standard deviation of the dSNR measurements across the 5 patients were then plotted and compared.

3   Results

Figure 1 shows PDw, T2w, T1w and contrast enhanced T1w images from a single slice in Patient 1. The lesion burden in this patient is very small with only one prominent lesion on the anterior horn of the left lateral ventricle. This lesion is not readily visible in the T1 weighted image nor in the gadolinium enhanced image. These images are typical of those for patients in the early stages of disease.

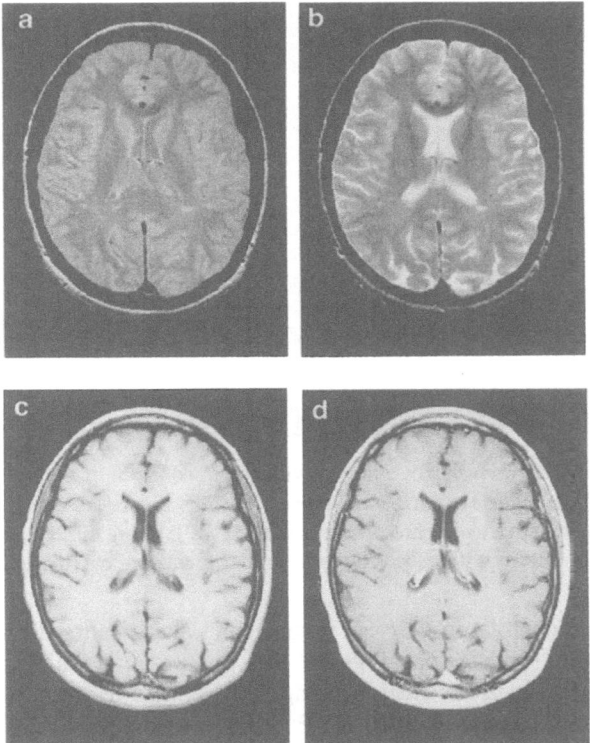

FIG. 1. *a)* through *d)* are respectively spin-echo PDw, T2w, T1w, and T1w after administration of gadolinium-DTPA contrast agent. This patient has one lesion near the anterior horn of the left lateral ventricle. However, this lesion does not enhance after administration of contrast agent. These images are typical of those analyzed in these experiments

Figure 2 shows the CSF-SP image calculated at the same slice as the images in Figure 1. The image has high contrast, with an overall appearance similar to anatomical images. Indeed, some white-matter tracks are visible. Figure 3 shows tissue contrasts measured between CSF and NAWM; CSF and GM; and, NAWM and GM, in the MR and CSF-SP images from the 5 MS patient exams. The CSF-SP images provided higher tissue contrast than any of the MR images. Part of the increased contrast resulted from application of the anisotropic diffusion filter algorithm which reduced the standard deviation within tissues by 33% on average. In turn, this increased dSNR between tissues by 33% on average. However, calculation of CSF-SP images increased tissue contrast further: CSF-NAWM contrast was increased from a maximum of 19.5 in the T1w image to 56 in the CSF-SP image (+187%). CSF-GM contrast increased from a maximum of 14.5 in the T1w image to 35.2 in the CSF-SP image (+143%). Finally, NAWM-GM contrast increased from a maximum of 7.5 in the T2w image to 11.5 in the CSF-SP image (+53%).

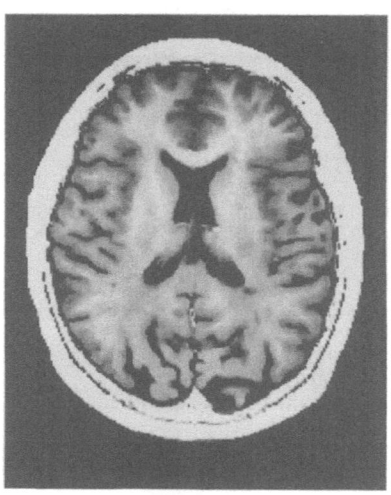

FIG. 2. Spectral phase images not only provide high contrast, but also allow selective suppression of tissue signals during post-processing.This figure shows a cross-sectional spectral phase image relative to cerebro-spinal fluid (CSF-SP). Using this technique to suppress fluid signal produces images with tissue contrasts similar to anatomical images

The increased contrast in CSF-SP images may allow better visualization of the heterogeneity within some lesions. Figure 4 shows close-up views of a single periventricular lesion in Patient 2.The CSF-SP image reveals heterogeneity within the lesion region which is not apparent in either the PDw or T2w images. Much of the lesion is not visible in the T1w images. Visualization of subtle changes in contrast within and around the lesion region in CSF-SP images may provide a sensitive indication of change, and thus disease activity.

4   Discussion

A number of authors have shown that analysis of multi-dimensional feature spaces can aid the identification and detection of various pathologies. For example Vinitski et al have shown that cluster classification in a 3-dimension feature space improves tissue segmentation compared to classification in a 2-dimensional feature space[9]. They have also shown that utilization of a 3-dimensional feature space allows identification of additional tissues within tumor regions which correlate with histologic samples[10].

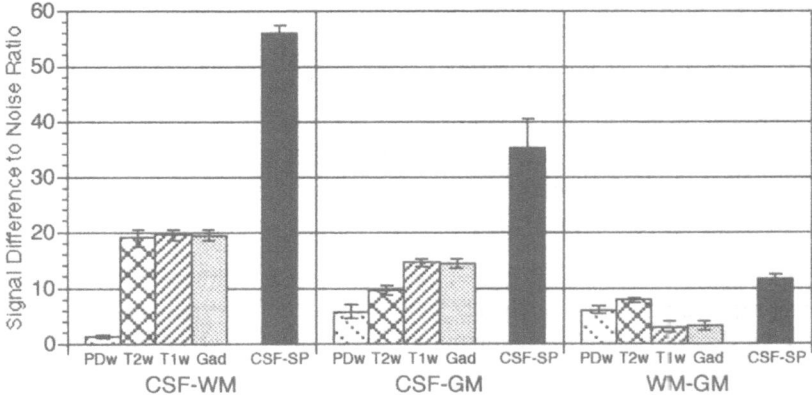

FIG. 3. The mean signal-difference to noise ratios (dSNR) measured between tissues in MR and CSF-SP images from 5 MS patients. The error bars indicate one standard error about each mean. CSF spectral phase images provide better dSNR between CSF, normal-appearing white matter (WM) and gray matter (GM) than any of the MR images. The mean dSNR between CSF and WM in CSF-SP images is 56, while it is only 20 at most the MR images. The improved contrast may aid detection of subtle changes in lesions over time

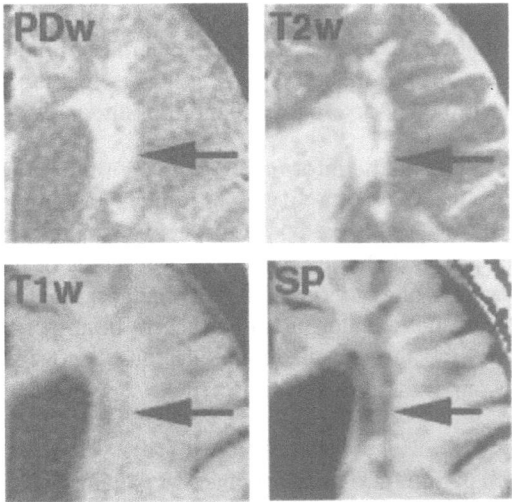

FIG. 4. Increased contrast in CSF spectral phase images may aid the visualization of lesion heterogeneity. The images are close-up views of a large lesion in the original proton-density weighted *(PDw)*, T2 weighted *(T2w)*, T1 weighted *(T1w)* and spectral phase relative to cerebro-spinal fluid *(SP)* images. The lesion *(arrow)* is barely visible in the T1w image, and appears relatively homogenous in the PDw and T2w images. The CSF-SP image reveals structure within the lesion region. Notice also the good suppression of CSF signal in the SP image

They speculate that analysis of additional contrast (i.e. analysis of higher dimensional feature spaces) may improve segmentation further.

However visualization and analysis of feature spaces becomes more difficult as their dimension increases. One solution is to use tissue class information to construct a transformation from a higher dimensional feature space down to a 2-D or 3-D feature space. Zadeh et. al. have shown one such transformation which has the added benefit of increasing class separability[11],[12].

Brunetti et. al. describe a different technique which combines multi-spectral MRI data into a quantitative color image[13]. They found that this new color image helped improve the detectability of white matter lesions in multiple sclerosis. It also improved the agreement and reduced the variability between radiologists compared to conventional spin echo studies. However their technique incorporates information from exactly three MR images and is therefore incapable of incorporating information from additional contrast.

In this paper we have presented a new technique to extract information from multi-dimensional feature spaces constructed from MR images of patients with multiple sclerosis. Our new technique provides images of spectral phase relative to CSF. CSF was selected as the reference signal since it is easily identifiable and maintains intensity characteristics through disease progression. However, alternative reference signals could be selected from other tissues, or phantom materials within the exam volume and may provide even better discrimination of lesions and normal tissues. A more extensive study needs to be performed to determine the merit of alternative reference signals.

CSF-SP images can combine information from an arbitrary number of MR image contrasts. This may be useful for simplifying or reducing a complex data set down to a single image. CSF-SP images also allow retrospective suppression of reference tissue signals. This may be useful if the reference tissue obscures or has contrast similar to another tissue of interest in one or more of the MR images. Finally, CSF-SP images can provide tissue contrast much greater than that present in any of the MR images. This increased contrast may aid the visualization of lesion heterogeneity and improve the detection of subtle changes in lesions over time.

Figure 5 shows CSF-SP images calculated from MR exams acquired every 4 weeks over a 5 month period from an additional MS patient. Each image was produced within the same 3mm thick slice. Although registration between exams is not perfect, this slice was selected for analysis since all lesions visible in this slice were also visible in the slices immediately superior and inferior to this slice. A number of diffuse abnormalities are visible in this image sequence which are not apparent in the original MR images. For example, a dark, diffuse region appears around a prominent lesion in the left anterior region on Day 26. Monitoring of subtle changes in CSF-SP images may provide a more sensitive indication of disease activity than analysis of standard MR exams of MS patients. However, an ROC analysis comparing the detectability of MS lesions in conventional and CSF-SP images must be performed to demonstrate this point conclusively.

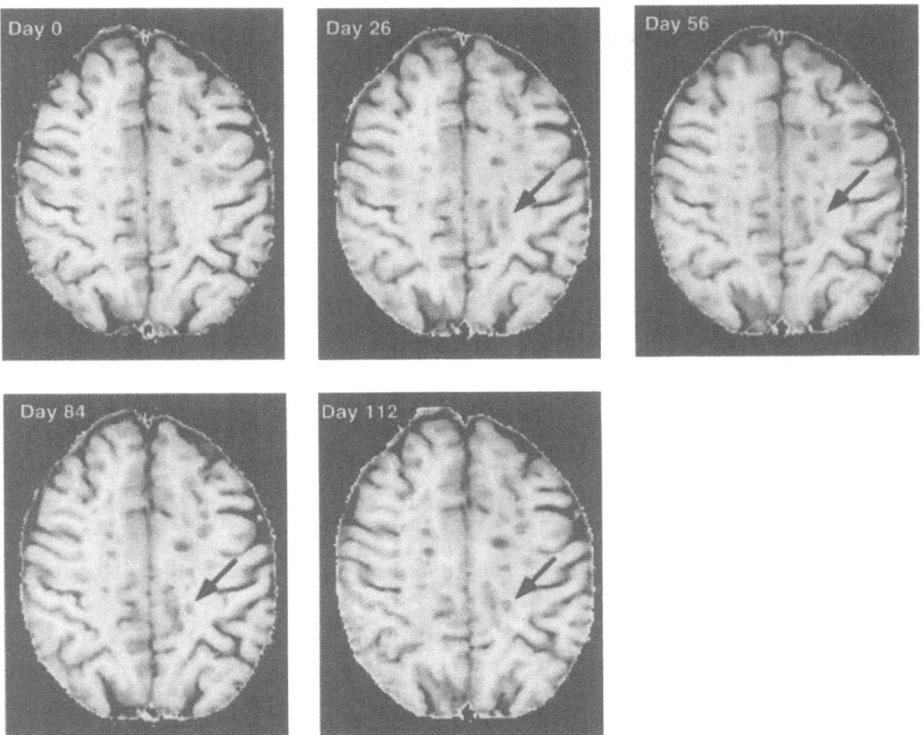

FIG. 5. Spectral phase images may indicate subtle changes in MR exam intensities over time. These are CSF-SP images derived from MR exams acquired over 5 months within the same 3mm thick axial cross-section from an additional MS patient. Note, for example, the growth of a diffuse abnormality in the lower right quadrant by Day 26 *(arrow)*. This abnormality recedes by Day 84 leaving two small focal lesions

5   Conclusions

A new technique has been developed to calculate "spectral phase" images from multispectral MR exams of MS patients. The technique provides a convenient way of reducing multispectral MR exams to a single image. Spectral phase images relative to CSF provide better tissue contrast than that found in any of the MR images. The increased contrast may aid the quantification and analysis of lesion activity in MR exams of MS patients.

226   J. R. Mitchell et al.

Acknowledgments and References

This work was supported by the Canadian Multiple Sclerosis Society.

1   Evans AC, Frank JA, Antel J, Miller DH "The role of MRI in clinical trials of multiple sclerosis: comparison of image processing techniques". Ann. Neurol., 41(1), 125-132 (1997).

2   M.W. Vannier et. al, "Multispectral analysis of magnetic resonance images". Radiology, 154:221-224, (1985).

3   Mitchell JR, Jones C, Karlik SJ, Kennedy K, Lee DH, Rutt B and Fenster A. "MR multispectral analysis of multiple sclerosis lesions." Journal of Magnetic Resonance Imaging; 7:499-511 (1997).

4   Sled JG, Zijdenbos AP and Evans AC. "A nonparticipant method for automatic correction of intensity nonuniformity in MRI data". IEEE Transactions on Medical Imaging; 17(1):87-97 (1998).

5   Perona P, Malik J. "Scale-space and edge detection using anisotropic diffusion." IEEE Transactions on Pattern Analysis and Machine Intelligence 12(7):629-639 (1990)

6   Gerig G., Kubler O, Kikinis R, Jolesz FA, "Nonlinear anisotropic filtering of MRI data." IEEE Transactions on Medical Imaging, 11 (2), 221-232, (1992).

7   Gudbjartsson H, Patz S. "The Rician distribution of noisy MRI data" Magnetic Resonance in Medicine; 34(6):910-914 (1995).

8   Armitage P, Berry G. Statistical methods in medical research. 2nd edition. Oxford: Blackwell Scientific Publications. (1990)

9   Vinitski S, Gonzalez C, Andrews D, Knobler R, Curtis M, Mohamed F, Gordon J and Khalili K. "In vivo validation of tissue segmentation based on a 3D feature map using both a hamster brain tumor model and stereotactically guided biopsy of brain tumors in man". Journal of Magnetic Resonance Imaging; 8(4):814-819 (1998).

10   Viniski S, Gonzalez, Mohamed P, Iwanga T, Knobler R, Khalili K and Mack J. "Improved intracranial lesion characterization by tissue segmentation based on a 3D feature map". Magnetic Resonance in Medicine; 37(3):457-469 (1997).

11   Soltanian-Zadeh H, IEEE Member, Windham JP and Peck DJ. "Optimal linear transformation for MRI feature extraction". IEEE Transactions on Medical Imaging; 15(6):749-767 (1996).

12   Soltanian-Zadeh H, Peck DJ, Windham JP and Mikkelsen T. "Brain tumor segmentation and characterization by pattern analysis of multispectral NMR images". Nuclear Magnetic Resonance in Biomedicine; 11:201-208 (1998).

13   Brunetti A, Tedeschi G, Di Costanzo A, Covelli EM, Aloj L, Bonavita S, Ciarmiello A, Alfano B and Salvatore M. "White matter lesion detection in multiple sclerosis: improved interobserver concordance with multispectral MRI display." Journal of Neurology; 244:586-590 (1997).

De-noising h_{int} Surfaces: A Physics-Based Approach

Margaret Yam, Ralph Highnam, and Michael Brady

Medical Vision Laboratory, Engineering Science, Oxford University,
Oxford OX1 3PJ, UK.
Email : {margaret,rph,jmb}@robots.ox.ac.uk

Abstract. The h_{int} representation is a normalised, quantitative version of a mammogram which has substantial quantum noise components because of the way in which it is computed. This paper presents a physics-based approach to de-noising the h_{int} representation of a mammogram. We investigate the major contributions to noise and the steps in the h_{int} generation that amplify noise, such as removal of intensifying screen glare. Estimating the radiographic noise components using parameters derived from physics models, we filter the original mammographic images with an adaptive wiener filter, W. Generating the h_{int} representation from the filtered images yields a de-noised version which has substantially improved signal-to-noise ratio, and which is far better to use for further-processing, such as microcalcification detection. The accuracy of the de-noised h_{int} representation is verified using experimental results on phantom images and mammograms with microcalcifications.
Keywords: mammography, radiographic mottle, de-noising, physics-based

1 Introduction

X-ray mammography plays an important role, and remains the primary imaging modality, in breast cancer screening. However, the quality of mammograms is always subject to variations in the imaging conditions; this makes robust and reliable mammographic analysis difficult, for human observers and machines alike. Acknowledging this fact, Highnam and Brady [3, 4] developed a normalised mammographic representation, the h_{int} representation, by modeling the X-ray imaging process and removing a number of image degrading factors, including scattered radiation, extra-focal radiation and intensifying screen glare. Every pixel value in the original image is converted into a floating point number which quantifies the amount of "interesting" (or non-fat) tissue present in the cone of breast above that pixel. However, removal of blur greatly amplifies the effects of high frequency noise componenets such as those due to radiographic mottle. Figure 3(a) and 4(a) show examples of noisy h_{int} surfaces. The reduced signal-to-noise ratio (SNR) of the noise-corrupted h_{int} surface greatly hinders potential applications of it. The work presented in this paper is aimed at de-noising the h_{int} surfaces by taking radiographic mottle into account. The correctness of the de-noised h_{int} surface is verified experimentally using both phantom images and mammograms with microcalcifications.

2 Image Degrading Factors in the Mammographic Process

Various image degrading factors exist in different parts of the mammographic imaging process. Some of the most important ones are:

- scattered radiation in the X-ray path through the breast;
- glare from the intensifying screen to the film; and
- radiographic mottle from the stochastic nature of the imaging process.

Scatter and glare result in low-frequency "noise" components and have been taken into account in the current h_{int} model [3]. In this paper, we deal with the effect of radiographic mottle which introduces a high-frequency noise component. Some of the image degrading sources are depicted schematically in Figure 1.

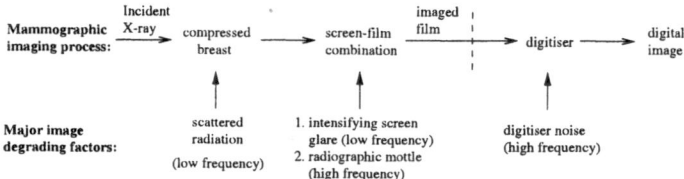

Fig. 1. A schematic representation of some of the major image degrading factors along the chain of mammographic imaging process.

Radiographic mottle is the spatial fluctuation of film density due to noise intrinsic to the screen-film combination, and comprises three primary components, namely quantum mottle, film granularity and structure mottle [1]. Quantum mottle ($\sigma_q(D)$) is caused by the spatial fluctuations in the number of X-ray photons absorbed per unit area of the intensifying screen; film granularity ($\sigma_g(D)$) is due to fluctuations in the number of silver halide grains per unit area of the film emulsion; and structure mottle ($\sigma_s(D)$) arises from random inhomogeneities in the phosphor coating of the intensifying screen. Since these three components are independent random processes, the total radiographic mottle, $\sigma(D)$, can be formulated as:

$$\sigma(D) = (\sigma_q^2(D) + \sigma_g^2(D) + \sigma_s^2(D))^{\frac{1}{2}} \quad (1)$$

where $\sigma(D)$ is the standard deviation of the film density, D. Amongst these three components, quantum mottle and film granularity contribute more significantly to the total radiographic noise while structure mottle makes up only 10% of it typically [7]. It is therefore reasonable to ignore for the present work the effect of structure mottle and approximate $\sigma(D)$ as:

$$\sigma(D) = (\sigma_q^2(D) + \sigma_g^2(D))^{\frac{1}{2}} \quad (2)$$

Incorporating fluctuations in the energy absorbed per interacting photon and those in the number of light photons emitted per unit energy absorbed, Barnes [1] formulates $\sigma_q(D)$ as:

$$\sigma_q(D) = \frac{0.434G}{(n_x A_e)^{\frac{1}{2}}} \left[1 + \frac{\langle \Delta E^2 \rangle}{\langle E \rangle^2} \right]^{\frac{1}{2}} \left[1 + \frac{\langle \Delta w^2 \rangle}{\langle w \rangle^2} \right]^{\frac{1}{2}} \quad (3)$$

where G is the gradient of the film screen curve at density D; n_z is the average X-ray photon fluence absorbed in the intensifying screen; A_e is the effective noise sampling aperture; $\langle E \rangle$ and $\langle \Delta E^2 \rangle$ are the mean and variance of the energy imparted in the screen per interacting photon; $\langle w \rangle$ and $\langle \Delta w^2 \rangle$ are the mean and variance of the light photon yield per absorbed energy.

Film density fluctuation due to film granularity $(\sigma_g(D))$ is given by:

$$\sigma_g(D) = \left(\frac{0.434 a_g}{A} \right)^2 [\langle D \rangle]^{\frac{1}{3}} \tag{4}$$

where a_g is the average grain area, A the sampling area, and $\langle D \rangle$ is the average film density.

Both fluctuations in the number of absorbed X-ray photons and those in the number of film grains follow a Poisson distribution, but can be effectively modeled as Gaussian noise [2].

3   The De-noising Algorithm

The essence of our de-noising algorithm is to first filter radiographic mottle from the film density surface of the original mammogram and then generate the h_{int} representation using the smoothed film density surface. We identify that the pronounced noise resulting in the h_{int} representation, generated from intensity images, is due to amplification of the effect of quantum noise after removing the effects of blur due to glare from the intensifying screen. Glare arises from the isotropic emission of light by the phosphor in the intensifying screen to the film, which results in a small blurred exposure to the film. Its removal, therefore, increases image sharpness, but at the same time amplifies high frequency noise due to radiographic mottle. This is evident from the fact that the SNR of h_{int} surfaces with glare removed is significantly smaller than those without glare removed (Table 2).

From Equations 3 and 4, it is obvious that the amplitudes of the noise components are signal-dependent. In the case of quantum mottle, $\sigma_c(D)$ is dependent on the photon fluence, n_x, which is in turn related to the film density via the film screen curve. For film grain noise, its standard deviation, $\sigma_g(D)$, is proportional to the cube root of the local average density. Modeling radiographic noise as being Gaussian distributed (which will be justified experimentally in Section 4.1), we filter the original film density surface using an adaptive wiener filter, W, [5], which is a spatially-variant filter taking local statistics into consideration. Given the original noisy signal h, elements of the filtered signal, $f(x, y)$, is:

$$f(x, y) = m_s(x, y) + \frac{\sigma_s^2(x, y)}{\sigma_s^2(x, y) + \sigma_n^2(x, y)} (h(x, y) - m_s(x, y)) \tag{5}$$

where $m_s(x, y)$ and $\sigma_s^2(x, y)$ are the signal mean and variance of a local neighbourhood around (x, y) respectively; and $\sigma_n^2(x, y)$ is the local noise estimate computed using Equations 2, 3 and 4.

The de-noised h_{int} surface is then obtained by generating the h_{int} representation using methods described in [3] but having the original film densities replaced by the filtered version.

230   M. Yam et al.

4   Experimental Results

4.1   Radiographic Noise Analysis Using a Step Wedge Phantom

We investigate the statistical properties of the radiographic noise using a 12-step lucite wedge phantom image. Experiments are performed on the middle 5 steps, the film densities of which lie in the linear region of the film-screen curve and correspond to the film density range within the breast area in mammograms. From the film density image of each step, we extract 24 smaller squares, each of 32×32 pixels, pair them off and obtain 12 difference images of film density by subtracting each image pair. The mean, variance, skew and kurtosis are computed for each difference image of each step. The plots are shown in Figure 2 and the average values for each step are presented in Table 1. The skew and kurtosis values shown in Table 1 reflect that it is reasonable to approximate its distribution as Gaussian which has skew and kurtosis of 0 and 3 respectively.

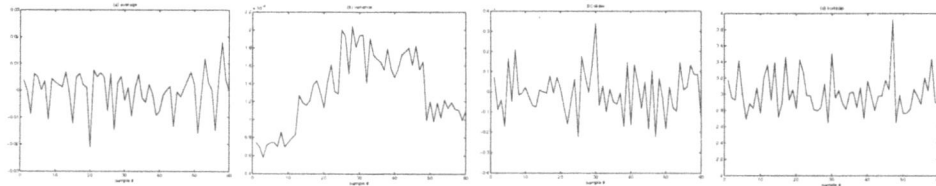

Fig. 2. Plots of (a) average, (b) variance, (c) skew, and (d) kurtosis of the difference images of film density. The x-axis refers to the label of individual samples. The line plots are solely for clearer presentation; no connectivity between records is implied.

step number	average film density	difference image average	variance	skew	kurtosis
4	0.54	0.0008	0.0007	0.0001	3.0235
5	0.83	0.0010	0.0013	-0.0109	3.0720
6	1.30	-0.0018	0.0018	0.0228	2.9541
7	1.76	-0.0024	0.0017	-0.0243	3.0265
8	2.19	0.0015	0.0011	-0.0020	2.9753

Table 1. Statistics of radiographic noise for different steps of the step wedge phantom

4.2   De-noising h_{int} Surfaces of Step Wedge Images

We run our de-noising algorithm on the same 5 steps of the wedge as used in section 4.1. The images are digitised to a resolution of $50\mu m$ per pixel. Film-screen gradient G is set to 3.6, corresponding to the gradient of the linear region of our film-screen curve. Sampling area, A, is set to the pixel area, which is $0.0025mm^2$. We adopt the values of a couple of physical parameters as quoted in [1] ($A_e = 0.79mm^2$; $a_g = 5.31\mu m^2$). Assuming the variance of energy absorbed per interacting photon, ΔE^2, and that of light photon yield per absorbed energy, Δw^2, to be negligible, $\left[1 + \langle \Delta E^2 \rangle / \langle E \rangle^2\right]^{1/2} \approx 1$ and $\left[1 + \langle \Delta w^2 \rangle / \langle w \rangle^2\right]^{1/2} \approx 1$. n_x is computed from the energy imparted values. A mask size of 5×5 pixels is used to define the local neighbourhood in the filtering.

A comparison of the average, variance and signal-to-noise ratio (SNR) of the original h_{int}, the h_{int} plus glare (i.e. the h_{int} surface generated without glare removed), and the de-noised h_{int} is given in Table 2. Since the h_{int} surface of the step wedge should have constant height over each individual step, we define its SNR to be $\frac{\mu(h_{int})}{\sigma(h_{int})}$, where $\mu(h_{int})$ and $\sigma(h_{int})$ are the mean and standard deviation of h_{int} values.

step	lucite thickness	original h_{int}			h_{int} plus glare			de-noised h_{int}		
		ave	var	SNR	ave	var	SNR	ave	var	SNR
4	4.40	2.15	0.168	5.23	2.11	0.00313	37.8	2.11	0.00565	28.0
5	3.96	2.02	0.143	5.34	1.99	0.00296	36.7	1.99	0.00512	27.8
6	3.52	1.81	0.121	5.20	1.79	0.00238	36.7	1.79	0.00437	27.0
7	3.08	1.69	0.092	5.58	1.68	0.00142	44.6	1.67	0.00261	32.7
8	2.64	1.57	0.081	5.51	1.56	0.00128	43.5	1.55	0.00254	30.7

Table 2. Comparison of average (ave), variance (var) and SNR of the original h_{int}, h_{int} plus glare and de-noised h_{int} surfaces of different steps of the step wedge phantom.

It is interesting to note, from Table 2, that the average h_{int} for the three versions of h_{int} surface are very similar and are about 50% of the total lucite thickness, which agrees well to the fact that lucite approximates 50/50 interesting tissue/fat [3]. The increasing trend of variance with increasing lucite thickness of the steps reflects that as the thickness increases, the number of X-ray photons incident on the screen reduces hence increasing quantum noise.

The SNR of the de-noised h_{int} surface is above 5 times larger than that of the original h_{int}, but is about 1.4 times less than that of the h_{int} plus glare. This shows that the de-noised h_{int} suppresses the noise power by a significant amount as compared to the original one. However, due to approximations made in the radiographic noise estimation, such as the omission of structure mottle, the SNR of the de-noised h_{int} is slightly smaller than that of h_{int} plus glare. The highest SNR of the h_{int} plus glare also highlights the smoothing effect of glare on the h_{int} surface. In the next section, we show that this blurring effect imposed by glare decreases image sharpness and affects the accuracy of the h_{int} values.

Figure 3 shows the surface plots of the original h_{int}, the h_{int} plus glare and the de-noised h_{int} of one of the steps of the wedge, and their 1-D profiles along $y = 100$.

4.3   De-noising h_{int} Surfaces of Microcalcification Images

The experiment is performed on a set of 20 isolated microcalcifcations in 15 image samples, each of 230×180 pixels. All image samples are digitised to a resolution of $50\mu m$ per pixel. The de-noising procedure and parameters used are identical to that on the step wedge phantom given in Section 4.2. Figure 4(a)–(c) show the surface plots of the original h_{int}, the h_{int} plus glare and the de-noised h_{int} of one of the image samples with a microcalcifications about (120, 74). Figure 4(d) and (e) compare the 1-D profiles, across the microcalcification at $y = 74$, of the de-noised h_{int} with that of the original h_{int} and the h_{int} plus glare respectively. It can be seen from the plots that whilst removing much of the noise from the original h_{int} surface, the de-noised h_{int} retains image contrast

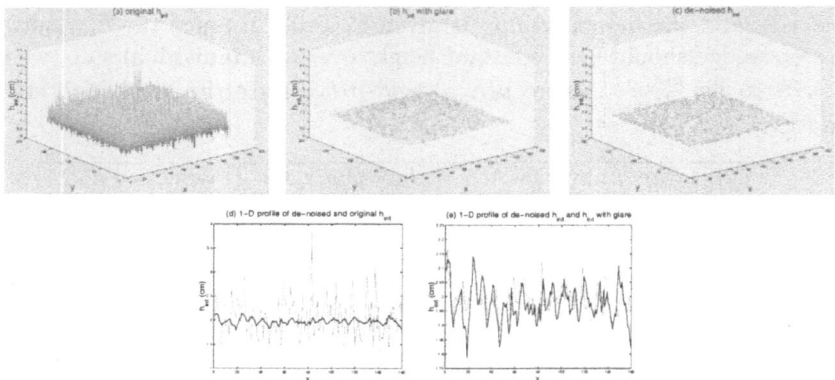

Fig. 3. (a)–(c): surface plots of the original h_{int}, the h_{int} plus glare, and the de-noised h_{int} of a step of the step wedge; (d): comparison of the 1-D profile of the original h_{int} (dotted line) and the de-noised h_{int} (solid line) along $y = 100$; (e): comparison of the 1-D profile of the h_{int} plus glare (dotted line) and the de-noised h_{int} (solid line) along $y = 100$.

and sharpness without inducing a blurring effect on the microcalcification as in the case of the h_{int} plus glare.

Using a physics-based model [3], we simulate the X-ray mammographic imaging process and obtain simulated image samples from the original h_{int}, the h_{int} plus glare and the de-noised h_{int} representation. Figure 5 show their respective appearances along with the original mammogram image sample. The better image quality of the de-noised h_{int} over the original h_{int}, and the improved image contrast and sharpness of the de-noised version over the one with glare and the original image are apparent.

To evaluate the accuracy of the de-noised h_{int} model, we use it to quantify microcalcifications by means of their volume ratios to their corresponding estimated 3-D volumes based on an ellipsoid model. The method is similar to that described in [8]. The segmentation uses iso-contours and an area constraint on the de-noised h_{int} surface to pick out regions which correspond to candidate calcifications. The actual calcification thickness, h_{calc}, is related to the h_{int} values by (from [3]): $h_{calc}(x,y) \approx 0.018 \times (h_{int}(x,y) - h_{int}^{surr})$, where h_{int}^{surr} is the average h_{int} thickness of the surrounding tissue obtained by performing a morphological dilation of the extracted region. Then we compute the ratio of the microcalcification volume to its estimated 3-D volume (the computation of both quantities is described in [8]), v_{calc}^{ratio}, which has a theoretical value of 1.

The computed v_{calc}^{ratio}s of the 20 microcalcifications, using the three versions of h_{int}, are given in figure 6(a). The values obtained using the de-noised h_{int} approximate the theoretical value of 1, while those using the original h_{int} are greater than 1 due to the inclusion of quantum noise and those using h_{int} with glare are less than 1 due to the excessive smoothing that lowers the h_{int} values. The rms error of the v_{calc}^{ratio} from 1 is 0.062, 0.511 and 0.415 for the de-noised h_{int}, the original h_{int} and the h_{int} plus glare respectively.

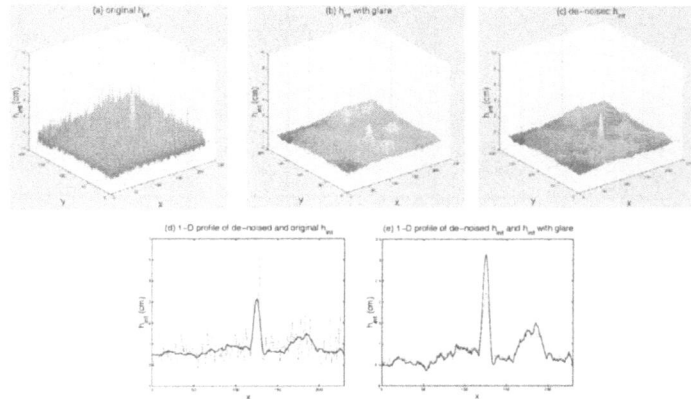

Fig. 4. (a)–(c): surface plots of the original h_{int}, the h_{int} plus glare, and the de-noised h_{int} of a mammogram sample with a microcalfication about (120,74); (d): comparison of the 1-D profile of the original h_{int} (dotted line) and the de-nosied h_{int} (solid line) along $y = 74$; (e): comparison of the 1-D profile of the h_{int} plus glare (dotted line) and the de-noised h_{int} (solid line) along $y = 74$.

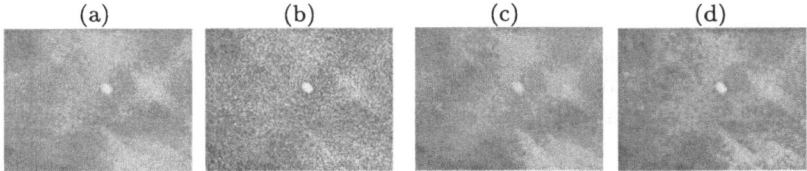

Fig. 5. (a): original mammogram sample; simulated X-ray mammograms using (b): the original h_{int}, (c): the h_{int} plus glare, and (d): the de-noised h_{int} respectively.

This physical quantity, v_{calc}^{ratio}, can be used in a quantitative approach for microcalcification detection. Previous work using volume to characterise calcifications can be found in [6]. In an initial trial, the 20 microcalcifications are all successfully detected with no false positives using a v_{calc}^{ratio} threshold of 0.8. Using Receiver Operating Characteristics (ROC) analysis, we show that our results are better than those obtained using a grey level contrast measure and thresholding (Figure 6(b)).

5   Discussion and Conclusions

We have presented a physics-based approach to de-noising h_{int} surfaces. The reliability of our restoration scheme is related to the underlying physics model of radiographic mottle in terms of a number of physically-defined parameters, hence eliminating the need to fine-tune variables in a heuristic manner.

The accuracy of our de-noised h_{int} model was verified experimentally using a step wedge phantom image and mammograms with microcalcifciations. The computed h_{int} thickness of steps of the phantom approximates the theoretical value, which is half of the lucite thickness of the corresponding step. On microcalcifications, we quantify them by means of the physical quantity, v_{calc}^{ratio}, which

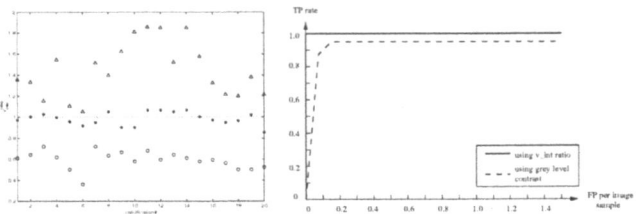

Fig. 6. *Left:* A scatter plot showing the computed v_{calc}^{ratio} of 20 microcalcifications using the original h_{int} (triangle), the h_{int} plus glare (circle), and the de-noised h_{int} (star); *Right:* Comparison of microcalcification detection results using our method and using grey level contrast thresholding.

is the ratio of the computed volume of a microcalcification to its estimated 3-D volume. We have shown that v_{calc}^{ratio}s computed on the de-noised h_{int} surface have smallest deviations from the theoretical value of 1 as compared with those obtained from the original h_{int} and the h_{int} plus glare.

In essence, our de-noising algorithm is capable of rescuing the h_{int} from the amplified effect of quantum noise without inducing a blurring effect on the h_{int} signal. The de-noising algorithm also makes feasible applications concerning analysis of the h_{int} surface, such as the detection of calcifications by means of quantitative volume analysis. Future work will employ the de-noised h_{int} representation on microcalcification detection and evaluate its performance using a larger data set.

Acknowledgements

Margaret Yam is supported by a postgraduate scholarship from the Croucher Foundation (Hong Kong) and an Overseas Research Student Award (UK). Ralph Highnam and Michael Brady's work in mammography is supported by a grant from the Engineering and Physical Sciences Research Council (UK).

References

1. G. T. Barnes. Radiographic mottle: A comprehenive theory. *Medical Physics*, 9(5):656–667, 1982.
2. K. R. Castleman. *Digital Image Processing*, Prentice Hall, 1996.
3. R. P. Highnam, and J. M. Brady. *Mammographic Image Processing*, Kluwer Academic Publishing, 1999.
4. R. P. Highnam, M. Brady, and B. J. Shepstone. A representation for mammographic image processing. *Medical Image Analysis*, 1:1–19, 1996.
5. J. S. Lee Digital image enhancement and noise filtering by use of local statistics. *IEEE Transaction on Pattern Analysis and Machine Intelligence*, 2:165–168, 1980.
6. R. M. Nishikawa, Y. Jiang, M. L. Giger, C. L. Vyborny, R. A. Schmidt, and U. Bick. Characterization of the mammographic appearance of microcalcifications: applications in computer-aided diagnosis. *SPIE vol.1898 Imag. Proc.* 422–29, 1993.
7. S. Webb. *The Physics of Medical Imaging*, Institute of Physics Publishing, 1988.
8. M. Yam, J. M. Brady, R. P. Highnam, and R. English. Detecting calcifications using the h_{int} representation. *The 13th International Congress on Computer Assisted Radiology and Surgery*, Paris, June 1999.

ERS Transform for the Detection of Bronchi on CT of the Lungs

François Chabat, David M. Hansell, and Guang-Zhong Yang

Imaging Department, Royal Brompton Hospital. Sydney Street,
London SW3 6NP. UK
f.chabat@rbh.nthames.nhs.uk

Abstract. The identification of bronchi on Computed Tomography (CT) images of the lungs provides valuable clinical information for the assessment of patients with suspected bronchiectasis, emphysema, or constrictive obliterative bronchiolitis. The automated recognition of the airways is an important part of a diagnosis-aid system. It resolves potential ambiguities associated with intensity-based feature extractors. On CT images, cross-sections of bronchi normally appear as elliptical rings and this paper presents a novel technique for their recognition. The proposed method, the ERS transform, is based on the analysis of the distribution of edges in local polar co-ordinates. Pixels are ranked according to local edge (E) strength, radial (R) uniformity, and local symmetry (S). A discrete implementation of the technique is provided which reduces the computational cost of the ERS transform by using a geometric approximation of the intensity patterns. The method compares favourably to other methods such as template matching or Hough transform. Noise-sensitivity of the technique was evaluated on a set of synthetic images and patient study was undertaken with a set of 27 cross-sectional images showing different lung pathologies. Agreement with an experienced radiologist was reached in 76 out of 136 bronchi (agreement rate: 57 %). which suggests satisfactory statistical significance for using the ERS transform as part of a computerised diagnosis aid system.

1 Introduction

Computed Tomography (CT) is a valuable imaging modality for assessing lung diseases such as bronchiectasis, emphysema, or constrictive obliterative bronchiolitis. From a set of cross-sectional images of the lungs, experienced radiologists achieve differential diagnosis by taking into account CT findings such as the density differences of the lung parenchyma, the size and distribution of the pulmonary vessels, and the state of the bronchi. For the detection of small airways disease, the most important finding is the identification of areas of decreased attenuation in the lung parenchyma. Based on global intensity distribution, we have developed several methods for the quantification of the extent of under-attenuated areas of the lungs [1][2][3]. The inherent problem with these methods is that the contextual information is not taken into account. Indeed, dark patches in the lung parenchyma cannot be confidently labelled as abnormal without ancillary findings, such as the morphology of the pulmonary vessels and the airways. Several low level feature extractors need to be combined in a high-level system incorporating *a priori* knowledge to achieve computerised diagnosis aid. Within this framework, essential clinical information can be derived from the morphology of the airways by measuring bronchial dilation and wall thickening. As an example, the presence of intensity differences in the lung parenchyma (known as mosaic attenuation pattern) can be caused by different pathologies: interstitial lung disease, vascular abnormalities, or airway disease. The identification of bronchial wall dilation on inspiratory scans suggests an airway disease rather than a vascular cause. This example stresses that there are ambiguities associated with the sole consideration of intensity differences. To resolve them and derive clinically meaningful conclusions, an algorithm for the automated detection of bronchi is necessary.

On cross-sectional images, bronchi running near perpendicular to the image plane appear as bright elliptical rings. This paper presents a novel technique for the recognition of elliptical rings, based on their geometric properties. An Edge-Radius-Symmetry (ERS) transform is used for the analysis of gradient maxima and minima in local polar co-ordinates. Based on the intensity (measured by function E), radial distribution (measured by function R), and symmetry (measured by function S) of these maxima and minima, the pixels are ranked to provide a sorted list of the most likely positions of all dominant elliptical rings. The algorithm was evaluated on synthetic and patient data showing different lung pathologies.

2   Background

Along a short distance, bronchi can be assimilated to cylindrical structures. They are filled with air and thus the luminal CT density is of the value of -1000 Hounsfield Units (H.U.). The bronchial wall consists of tissues of higher density (typically 100 H.U.). On CT images, perpendicular cross-sections of bronchi therefore appear as circular bright rings superimposed on the lung parenchyma, which has a low average CT density (typically –900 H.U.). When the plane of acquisition is not precisely

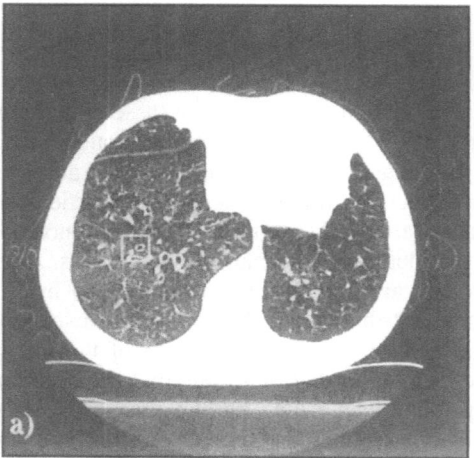
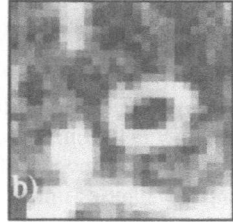

Fig. 1. *a)* Example of an HRCT scan of the lungs (window settings: level = -800 H.U. / width = 1000 H.U.). Bronchi perpendicular to the plane of acquisition appear as bright rings. The white square highlights the position of a major bronchus. *b)* Magnified view of the major bronchus highlighted in Figure (1b).

perpendicular to the main axis of a bronchus, the bronchial wall appears as an elliptical ring. Figure (1) provides an example of High-Resolution Computed Tomography (HRCT) scan of the lungs, with the conspicuous near-perpendicular cross-section of a major airway, which can be identified as a bright elliptical ring. Because of partial volume effect and the limits in image resolution, small bronchi may be partially hidden and difficult to detect.

There is little work reported in the literature for the automated identification of bronchi on CT images of the lungs, but semi-automated techniques requiring user interaction have been described [4]. This may be due to the difficulty for automated methods to match the subjective assessment made by experienced radiologists. Indeed, it has been demonstrated that inter-observer agreement for the detection of bronchial wall thickening, for instance, is consistent (kappa value $\kappa = 0.6$) [5]. Still, to incorporate contextual information into a diagnosis aid system based firstly on the analysis of intensity differences [1], it is necessary to design an automated technique for the detection of bronchi. The transform presented in this paper is a necessary tool meant to be used in conjunction with other features extractors, combined in a high-level framework to resolve local ambiguities.

3 Automated pattern identification

Template matching and Hough transform are common for the detection of circular patterns. Although they are suitable for the current application of detecting bronchial wall, they can be computationally expensive due to the high number of parameters required to define a ring-shaped structure. These parameters include position, size, orientation, ratio of the short and long axes, and width of the ring. The five parameters involved for detecting an ellipse, for instance, can make a standard Hough transform impractical in terms of computational and memory demands and even adaptive and two-pass methods remain time consuming [6].

3.1 ERS Transform

The ERS transform introduced in this paper is based on the analysis of the distribution of gradient maxima and minima in the neighbourhood of each pixel. Ellipses and rings are patterns symmetrical relatively to their centroids. In polar co-ordinates, the expression of the intensity and spatial distribution of the most significant edges has characteristic properties of symmetry and uniformity. The ERS transform is based on the analysis of edge distribution in local polar co-ordinates. In the case of CT images, given the CT densities of air, bronchial wall, and lung parenchyma, the intensity gradient should show local maxima and minima at the points on the inner border (i.e. at the interface between airway and bronchial wall) and outer border (i.e. at the interface between bronchial wall and lung parenchyma) of a bronchus respectively.

Let $I(x, y)$ be the original image, we consider the local polar co-ordinates (r, θ) centred at (x_o, y_o), and a neighbourhood Ω of radius r_o. The maximum of the intensity gradient within Ω along direction θ is defined as $e_I(\theta)$:

$$e_1(\theta) = \max_{0 < r < r_0}\left(\frac{\partial I}{\partial r}(r,\theta)\right) \tag{1}$$

with its corresponding radius defined as $r_1(\theta)$. The size r_0 of the neighbourhood Ω is to be defined according to the resolution of the image and the typical size of the patterns to identify. Similarly, the minimum of the intensity gradient along direction θ within the neighbourhood Ω is defined as $e_2(\theta)$:

$$e_2(\theta) = \min_{0 < r < r_0}\left(\frac{\partial I}{\partial r}(r,\theta)\right) \tag{2}$$

and its radius is denoted as $r_2(\theta)$. This generates four functions in relation to θ: $e_1(\theta)$, $e_2(\theta)$, $r_1(\theta)$, and $r_2(\theta)$ which describe the radial distribution of edges around point (x_o, y_o). Figure (2) gives a schematic representation of the definition of $e_1(\theta)$, $e_2(\theta)$, $r_1(\theta)$, and $r_2(\theta)$ for a pixel (x_o, y_o) located inside an elliptical ring, shown in Figure (2a). By searching along direction d_θ, the gradient maximum $e_1(\theta)$, shown in the gradient profile in Figure (2b), is found at the inner border of the ring. Similarly, the gradient minimum $e_2(\theta)$ is found at the outer border of the ring. The positions $r_1(\theta)$ and $r_2(\theta)$ of these maximum and minimum, relatively to (x_o, y_o), provide the intersection points of the ring along direction d_θ.

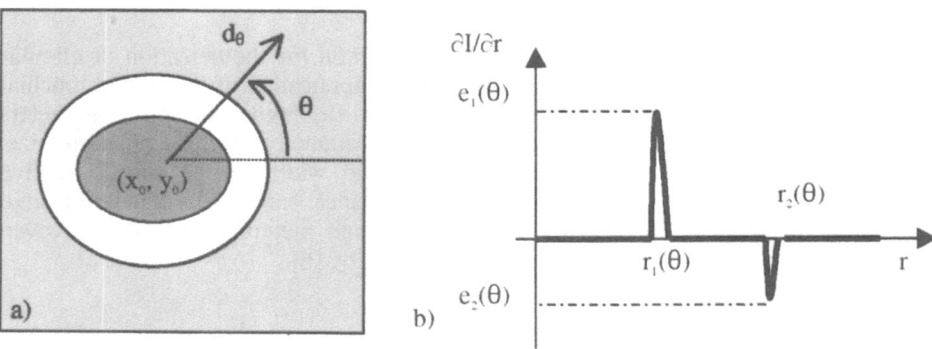

Fig. 2. *a)* Schematic representation of the function $I(x, y)$ for an elliptical ring. The darkest areas represent the lowest intensities. At pixel (x_o, y_o), the maximum and minimum of the intensity gradient are searched along each direction d_θ. *b)* The profile of the intensity gradient along direction d_θ. The distance to the pixel (x_o, y_o) is denoted r, and $\partial I/\partial r$ measures the intensity gradient. At the inner border of the ring, a sharp intensity increase results in a maximum peak $e_1(\theta)$ at a distance $r_1(\theta)$. Further, at the outer border of the ring, a sharp intensity decrease results in a minimum peak $e_2(\theta)$ at a distance $r_2(\theta)$.

At every pixel (x, y), three quantities E, R, and S are then derived from the functions $e_1(\theta)$, $e_2(\theta)$, $r_1(\theta)$, and $r_2(\theta)$.

- The value $E(x, y)$ measures the strength of the edges found in the neighbourhood of (x, y). It is defined as:

$$E(x, y) = \frac{1}{\underset{0 \le \theta < 2\pi}{mean} \left(\left|e_1(\theta)\right|\right) + \underset{0 \le \theta < 2\pi}{mean} \left(\left|e_2(\theta)\right|\right)} \tag{3}$$

For a well-defined ring with sharp edges, the values of $e_1(\theta)$ are highly positive and the values of $e_2(\theta)$ are highly negative, making $E(x, y)$ small.

- The value $R(x, y)$ measures the uniformity of the radial distribution of the edges. It can be computed as:

$$R(x, y) = \sigma(r_1(\theta)) + \sigma(r_2(\theta)) \tag{4}$$

where $\sigma(f(\theta))$ is the average deviation of $f(\theta)$.
For a perfectly circular ring centred at (x, y), the values of $r_1(\theta)$ are all identical, and so are the values of $r_2(\theta)$, yielding to a minimal value of $R(x, y)$ of zero.

- The value $S(x, y)$ measures the symmetry of the strength of the edges. It is defined as:

$$S(x, y) = \underset{0 \le \theta < 2\pi}{mean}(\delta_1(\theta)) + \underset{0 \le \theta < 2\pi}{mean}(\delta_2(\theta)) \tag{5}$$

where:

$$\delta_j(\theta) = \frac{\max(e_j(\theta), e_j(\theta + \pi))}{\min(e_j(\theta), e_j(\theta + \pi))} - 1 \tag{6}$$

The value of $\delta_j(\theta)$ measures the difference of contrast between two opposing edges relatively to (x, y). For a pattern that is perfectly symmetrical in relation to (x, y), the function $\delta_j(\theta)$ is always nil, yielding to a minimum value $S(x, y)$ of zero.

If (x, y) denotes the location of a well-defined elliptical ring, the values $E(x, y)$, $R(x, y)$ and $S(x, y)$ should therefore be small. The ERS transform is performed by combining numerically these three measures. Each pixel is given a rank n_E reflecting its position in the list of pixels sorted according to $E(x, y)$. The pixel with rank $n_E = 1$ represents the location with the lowest value of $E(x, y)$ (i.e. the sharpest edges) found on the image. Similarly, each pixel is given a rank n_R and a rank n_S according to its value of $R(x, y)$ and $S(x, y)$ respectively. The three ranks are then combined to provide a list of pixels sorted according to the value of n defined as:

$$n = n_E + n_R + n_S \tag{7}$$

The pixel with the highest rank n represents the position of the most dominant elliptical ring within the image. This ranking mechanism ensures that there is no need to normalise and weight the three quantities $E(x, y)$, $R(x, y)$ and $S(x, y)$. Since pixels are sorted according to each of the criteria independently, the final ranking does not depend on how rapidly the numerical expressions of E, R, and S increase.

3.2   Discrete approximation

Since the typical size of the elliptical patterns to be identified is less than 12 pixels, it is possible to derive a precise approximation of them by considering only 8 points, taken along 8 principal directions, rather than considering all points of an ellipse. The 8 directions $\{d_i\}_{1 \leq i \leq 8}$ are taken along the horizontal, vertical and principal diagonal axes, and are indexed clockwise consecutively. Edge information is derived from the original image by pre-computing the gradient along directions d_1, d_2, d_3, and d_4. The intensity gradient maxima and minima along directions $\{d_i\}_{1 \leq i \leq 8}$ are represented by 8-dimensional vectors $e_1 = (e_{1,i})_{1 \leq i \leq 8}$ and $e_2 = (e_{2,i})_{1 \leq i \leq 8}$ respectively, whereas the radial distribution of the edges are represented by vectors $r_1 = (r_{1,i})_{1 \leq i \leq 8}$ and $r_2 = (r_{2,i})_{1 \leq i \leq 8}$. The definitions of $E(x, y)$, $R(x, y)$ and $S(x, y)$ are the discrete equivalent of those given in equations and **(3)** , **(4)** and **(5)**.

In the discrete implementation of the ERS transform, the ranking procedure involved is done using the quicksort algorithm. On average, the computational cost of the discrete implementation of the ERS transform is $O(N \log N, r_0)$, with N being the number of pixels, and r_0 being the radius of the neighbourhood searched at each point.

As an example, Figure (3) demonstrates the pixels ranked according to E, R, and S for a synthetic image. Figure (3a) represents an image with elliptical rings and non-elliptical patterns with different sizes. The arrow highlights incomplete rings and partly occluded patterns. The SNR of this image is 44 dB, which is close to that of a typical HRCT scan. The locations surrounded by significant edges have high ranks n_E as shown in Figure (3b), signified by the brightness of the pixels. The results for $R(x, y)$ (uniformity) and $S(x, y)$ (symmetry) are illustrated in Figures (3c) and (3d) respectively. The incomplete patterns highlighted by the arrow on Figure (3a) are penalised by low ranks n_S, as shown in Figure (3d).

4   Results

4.1   Noise sensitivity

Since the proposed method is effectively based on the analysis of local maxima and minima of the first derivatives of the image intensity, it is necessary to evaluate its sensitivity to noise. A synthetic image, shown in Figure (3a), displaying various elliptical rings with different sizes was created to evaluate the noise-sensitivity of the edge-based technique. The intensity of the patterns is typical of the structures seen on HRCT scans of the lungs. The added Gaussian noise is similar to the noise inherent to the imaging modality. In the first 100 locations found by the algorithm, no false positive was detected, and all rings were identified.

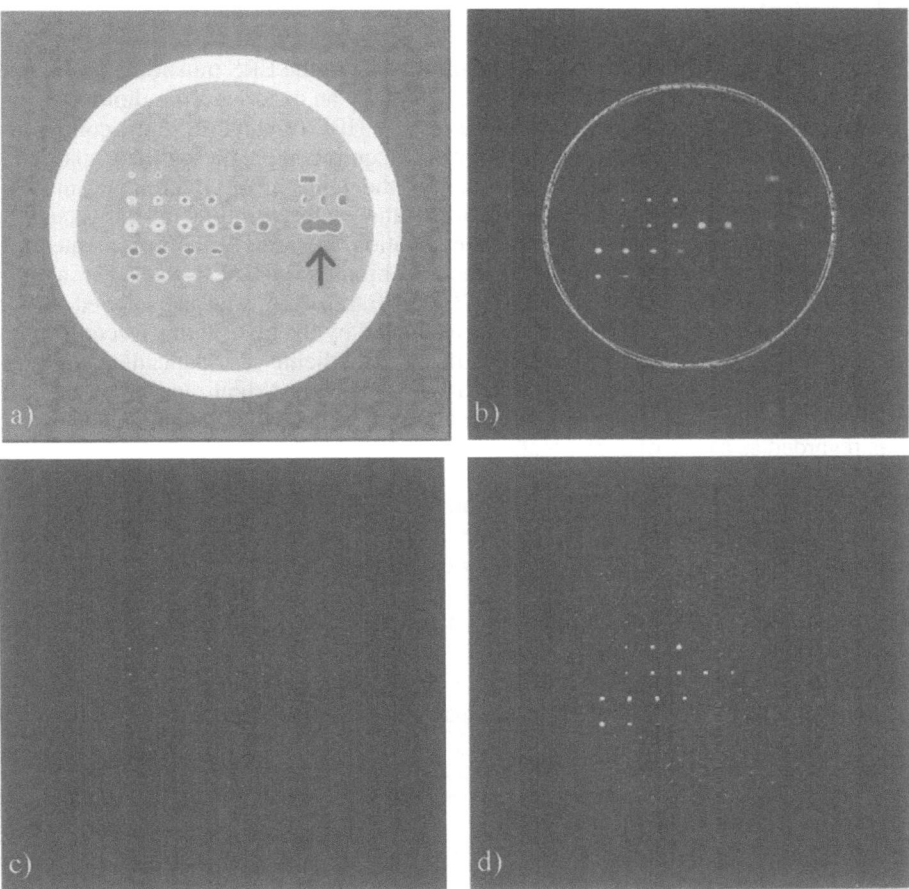

Fig. 3. *a)* Original synthetic image showing various elliptical and non-elliptical patterns with different sizes. The arrow highlights incomplete and partly occluded patterns. Gaussian noise was superimposed to the image (SNR=44dB). *b)* Ranks n_E derived from $E(x, y)$ (displayed only in the large inner circle). Pixels surrounded by strong edges have high ranks n_E and appear brighter. *c)* Ranks n_R derived from $R(x, y)$. The centres of the elliptical patterns are highlighted. *d)* Ranks n_S derived from $S(x, y)$. The partly occluded patterns have poor edge strength symmetry and appear darker.

Measuring how the method copes with added Gaussian noise of higher variance shows that, for a signal-to-noise ratio (SNR) equal to or lower than 14 dB, no false positive is found amongst the first 100 results. With an SNR equal to 12 dB, 3 % of false negatives and 4 % of false positive can be found in the first 100 results.

4.2   Patient studies

To assess the value of the method in a clinical context, the ERS transform was applied to CT scans of the lungs, which were also scored by an experienced radiologist. For 9 patients presenting suspected airways disease, 3 HRCT scans (1.5 mm collimation, sharp kernel reconstruction algorithm) were acquired at 3 pre-defined anatomical level in the upper, mid and lower zones of the lungs respectively. A radiologist identified on each of these 27 cross-sectional images the positions of the bronchi he regarded as most significant in a clinical evaluation. Because of the documented high inter-observer agreement for the assessment of bronchi on HRCT scans [5], a single human observer was considered reliable. The ERS transform was also applied and, for each scan, the list of the N first positions estimated by the algorithm was compared to the N positions determined by the human observer (N being case-dependent, and fixed for each case by the radiologist). Each location found both in the N-long list established by the radiologist and the N-long list established by the automated method was regarded as a case of agreement.

On a set of 27 cross-sectional images, the radiologist found 136 significant bronchi. Agreement with the ERS transform was reached in 76 instances, giving a rate of agreement of 57 %. Figure (4) shows an example of the compared results found by the human observer, as displayed by the crosses on Figure (4a), and the proposed algorithm, as displayed by the crosses on Figure (4b). In this case, agreement was reached in 9 out of 10 instances.

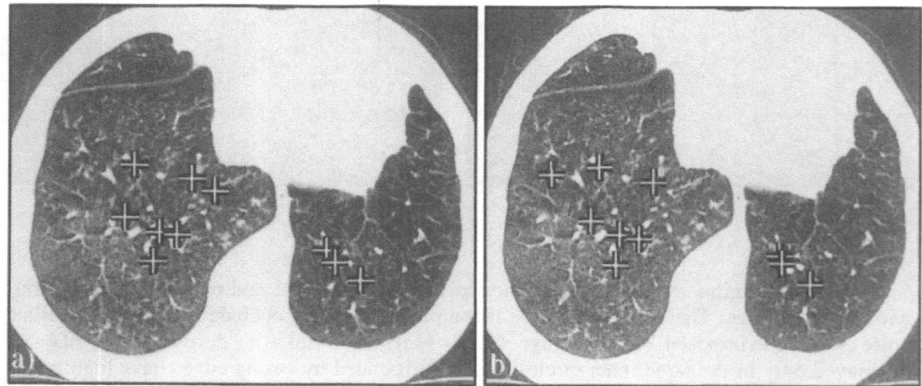

Fig. 4. *a)* HRCT scan of the lower zone of the lungs. The most significant bronchi, as identified by an experienced radiologist, are marked with a cross. *b)* Bronchi found by the ERS transform on the same image. The automated method matches the results of the human observer in 9 out of 10 instances.

Figure (5) shows an example of HRCT scan yielding to strong disagreement between the human observer and the automated method. The bronchi that the radiologist highlights for their clinical value, shown on Figure (5a), may not have the most clearly defined contours. Therefore, agreement with ERS transform cannot be reached, as shown in Figure (5b). However, by reading Figure (5b) retrospectively, it appears that the patterns identified by the ERS transform are indeed elliptical rings, in accordance with the expected behaviour of the algorithm.

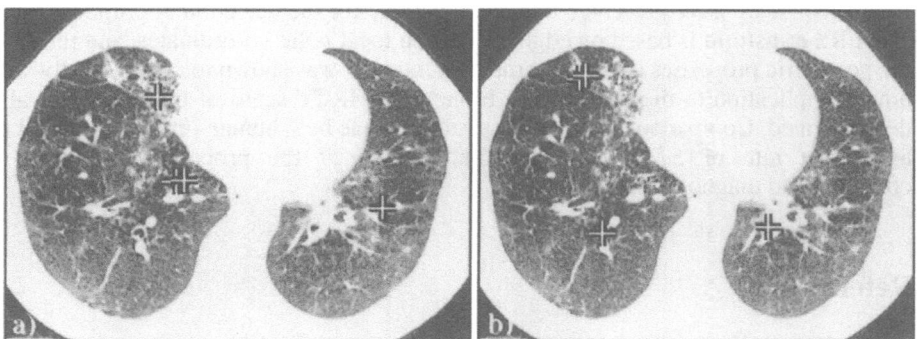

Fig. 5. Example of an HRCT scan with strong disagreement between the human and automated assessment. *a)* Airways identified by the human observer. The bronchi retained for the clinical information they provide are not necessarily the best-defined patterns with the strongest edges. *b)* ERS transform. Elliptical rings are detected but they were not selected by the radiologist for their clinical value.

5   Discussion

The elliptical rings to identify being defined by 6 parameters, the computational cost of methods like template matching and Hough transform (complexity $O(N^{6})$) is considerable [7]. The implementation of the ERS transform compares favourably with these techniques.

The agreement rate of 57 % is satisfactory for a low-level feature extractor such as the ERS transform. The patient study showed that the bronchi identified by the algorithm presented the expected geometric properties. When the human observer did not primarily choose them, it was due to high-level clinical knowledge. For example, the structures identified within consolidated lung or at a level near bifurcation, as shown in Figure (5b), are indeed bronchi, but are discarded by an experienced observer because the reliable interpretation of airways in these situations is problematic. This radiological expertise is out of the scope of the proposed algorithm. However, using the ERS transform, detection of bronchi is still possible. In a computerised diagnosis-aid system, multiple feature extractors are used. Their outputs are combined in a statistical high-level framework incorporating *a priori* knowledge in order to reach valid clinical conclusions. In that context, the agreement rate of 57 % between the proposed method and a human observer suggests satisfactory statistical significance.

6   Conclusion

In this paper, we have presented a novel technique for the detection of elliptical rings. The ERS transform is based on edge analysis in local polar co-ordinates, and relies on the geometric properties of the patterns to identify. It was shown to cope robustly with noise. Application to the detection of bronchi on HRCT scans of the lungs was also demonstrated. Comparison with the assessment made by a human observer showed an agreement rate of 57 %, allowing for the use of the proposed method in a computerised diagnosis aid system.

References

[1] Chabat F, Hansell DM, Yang GZ. CT Lung image classification with correction for perfusion gradient. *in* Proceedings of the Seventh IEE Conference on Image Processing and Applications; 1999. *In press.*

[2] Yang GZ, Chabat F, Hansell DM. Enhancement of subtle intensity differences of the lung parenchyma on CT. British Journal of Radiology; 1998, 71(846):686-90.

[3] Yang GZ, Hansell DM. CT Image enhancement with wavelet analysis for the detection of small airways disease. IEEE Transactions on Medical Imaging; 1997, 6(16):953-961.

[4] Senéterre E, Paganin F, Bruel JM, Michel FB, Bousquet J. Measurement of the internal size of bronchi using high resolution computed tomography (HRCT). Eur Respir J; 1994, 7: 596-600.

[5] Reiff DB, Wells AU, Carr DH, Cole PJ, Hansell DM. CT Findings in bronchiectasis: limited value in distinguishing between idiopathic and specific types. AJR; 1995, 165:261-267.

[6] Yuen HK, Illingworth J, Kittler J. Detecting partially occluded ellipses using the Hough transform, Image and Vision Computing; 1989, vol. 7, 1:31-37.

[7] Haralick RM, Shapiro LG. Computer and Robot Vision, Volume 1. Addison-Wesley publishing company, 1992.

Detection of Pulmonary Nodules on CT and Volumetric Assessment of Change over Time

Margrit Betke[1] and Jane P. Ko[2]

[1] Computer Science Department,
Boston College, Chestnut Hill MA 02167, USA,
betke@oak.bc.edu
http://oak.bc.edu/~betke
[2] Department of Radiology, Massachusetts General Hospital,
Harvard Medical School, Boston, MA 02114, USA

Abstract. We present a computer vision system that automatically detects pulmonary nodules in computed tomography (CT) scans of oncology patients, performs size analysis and assesses for change in volume over time.

Thresholding, backtracking, and smoothing algorithms have been developed to recognize the thorax and trace the lung border. The regions within the lung that potentially contain nodules are evaluated for their shape, size, and position. These candidate regions are then characterized as nodules versus other structures by comparing consecutive CT slices in the same study. A preliminary system for the registration of studies has also been developed. It estimates nodule volume in each study and evaluates the volumetric change over time.

Our system has been tested on initial and follow-up studies of four patients. Preliminary results were detection of 284 nodules ranging between 1 and 32 mm at various locations and assessment of their volumetric change over time.

Our techniques have future applications for determining disease progression, remission, and stability in oncologic patients in addition to coregistration of different modalities within the thorax.

1 Introduction

Chest computer tomography (CT) is used to diagnose pulmonary metastasis and evaluate for progression in cancer patients. CTs are obtained at intervals determined by treatment regimens, protocols, and acute clinical issues. The radiologist searches the CT images for pulmonary nodules and compares the results with neighboring images in the same study and corresponding images on preceding studies. The radiologist then determines if a given nodule is stable, increased, decreased or resolved from prior studies.

The radiologist typically uses bidimensional measurements in the axial plane to estimate volumetric change in nodule size. However, in general, volumetric change is not accurately quantified.

The process of systematically evaluating several CT studies of the same patient is very time consuming for the radiologist. If a study contains $n = 30$ images, there are $3(n - 2) = 84$ triplet images that are compared with each other, the image and its neighbors above and below. If two studies are evaluated, each image in one study is compared to approximately three images in the second study to register corresponding nodules, so a total of $9(n - 2) = 252$ comparisons are made.

Our work addresses both issues. We developed a computer vision system that detects nodules in CT images, analyzes the size of the nodules and then assesses for any change on subsequent studies. The system quantitatively evaluates whether a nodule has changed in size. This estimate helps evaluate for disease response or progression.

Kanazawa et al. [4] and Giger et al. [2] have described preliminary diagnostic systems which have high sensitivities for detecting nodules of diameters > 4 mm and 3 – 18 mm, respectively. Work has also been done in nodule detection on chest radiographs [1, 5]. Our work complements the previous work in nodule detection and focuses on volumetric quantization and comparison of consecutive studies.

2   Algorithms

Our computer vision system processes each CT image separately to obtain a set of regions in the lung that contain potential nodules. The properties of candidate regions on sequential slices are then compared. The results of the comparisons are used to classify candidate regions as nodules and to estimate their volumes.

2.1   Analysis of Individual CT Images

Thorax and Lung Border Detection. The patient's thorax is detected in the CT image by analyzing vertical and horizontal profiles of pixel grey levels. Since the surrounding soft tissues and bones are denser than the air-filled lung, they are visible as bright grey values, while the lung is dark. To find the border of the lung, the CT image is thresholded to create a binary image that is then analyzed to find the lung border. We developed a recursive backtracking algorithm that is similar to well-known maze algorithms [6] to trace along the border. Backtracking is used to detect narrow channels that could be due to vessels or artifacts. Since such channels are not considered to be border-forming structures, the tracing algorithm bridges them. The cropped center of a typical chest CT image and its traced lung border is shown in Figure 1 d.

Lung Border Correction and Lung Interior Detection. Our system addresses the problem of misinterpreting nodules that abut the border. Nodules in this location can be falsely excluded from the lung. Therefore the computed curve along the lung border is corrected. The locations of such nodules are detected by comparing the slopes of the points on the curve. A rapid change in slope indicates a nodule, large vessel, or bronchus. Pixels that are enclosed within the adjusted border curve are then labeled as belonging to the lung parenchyma. Figure 1 shows how the border curve is adjusted so that two large nodules are included in the lung.

The "main centroid" and the centroid of each individual lung are calculated using these pixels. The "main centroid" is computed using pixels of both lungs. Figures 1 d and 2 show the centroids as white crosses.

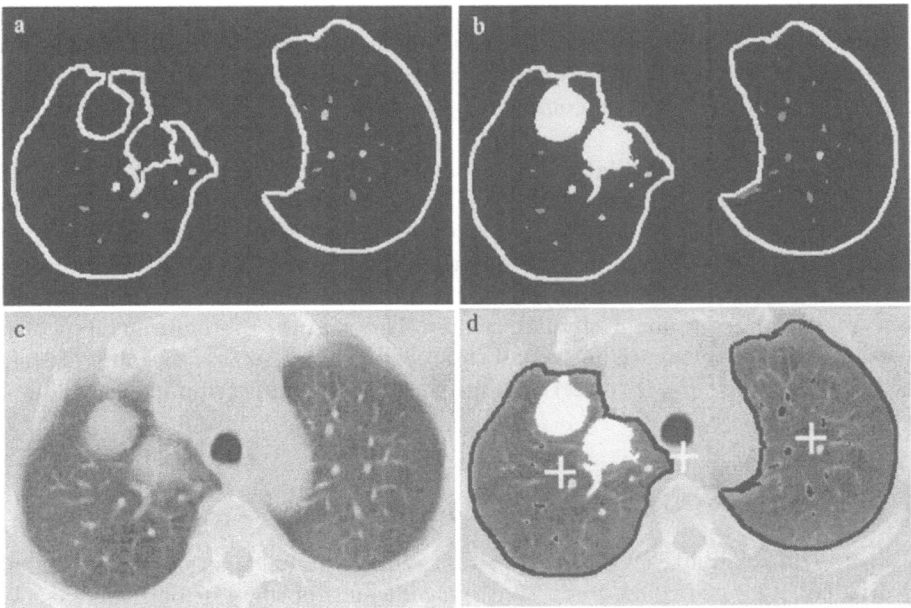

Fig. 1. The border curve in **1 a** is adjusted so that the two large nodules are included in the lung (**1 b**). **1 c** and **d** show a crop of the original CT image and the result of the processing. Detected nodules and centroids are shown in white, potential nodules in grey.

Determining Candidate Regions. Once the set of pixels belonging to the lung parenchyma has been determined, pixels can be divided into lighter and darker subsets. The lung parenchyma is dark on a CT image, except where there are normal vessels and bronchi, or nodules and other pathology. These would be lighter regions. The grey value at a pixel is a density average that describes the underlying volume (voxel). Therefore, lighter structures that fill the whole slice thickness appear bright. Structures that are smaller than the slice thickness are averaged with their surrounding air and appear fainter. Therefore, we use several grey-level thresholds to create binary images of the lung parenchyma that contain different candidate regions (Fig. 2). We then use the sequential labeling algorithm described by Horn [3] to distinguish and label candidate regions uniquely.

Computing Properties of Candidate Regions. For each candidate region, the number of pixels within the region is computed as a first estimate of the *2D axial area* of the region. This estimate is then used to compute the region's centroid and its *distance* to the lung centroids and to the lung border. Large candidate regions close to the border of the lung are likely to be nodules.

The *shape* of a candidate region is important for classification of the region. Nodules are typically spherical. Therefore circular regions on 2D CT images may be spherical nodules, but they also could be vessels in cross section. Elongated regions indicate vessels. A combination of two methods is used to determine shape.

First, for each candidate region, we find the line of pixels for which the sum E_{min} of the square of the distance to points in the region is a minimum. This line is the axis of least second moment or the "major axis" of the region. Maximizing the sum E_{max} of the square of the distance to points in the region yields the minor axis of the region. The ratio E_{min}/E_{max} is zero for a straight-line region and one for a circular region. The ratio is therefore an important measure for how elongated or round the region is. Our second measure of shape is the percentage P_{csc} of pixels within the circle circumscribing the candidate region.

2.2   Analysis of Consecutive CT Slices

To compare consecutive CT slices, we first register global positions which include individual lung centroids, main centroid and lung borders in both images. We then compare local nodule positions in both images and determine correspondences.

Nodules that appear in only one CT image have a diameter that is smaller than the slice thickness, so their diameter can be upper bounded by this thickness. They can be lower bounded by the 2D diameter of the disk visible in the CT image.

Similarly, we can estimate the diameter of a nodule that appears in more than one CT image by bounding its diameter from above by the number of slices times their thickness. We then determine the 3D center of the nodule. We use the axial image on which the nodule appears brightest along with the 2D center of the nodule on this image. We use the diameter of the nodule cross section as a lower bound on the nodule's diameter.

2.3   Time Analysis

Identifying corresponding nodules in separate studies is considerably more difficult than identifying corresponding nodules in consecutive images within the

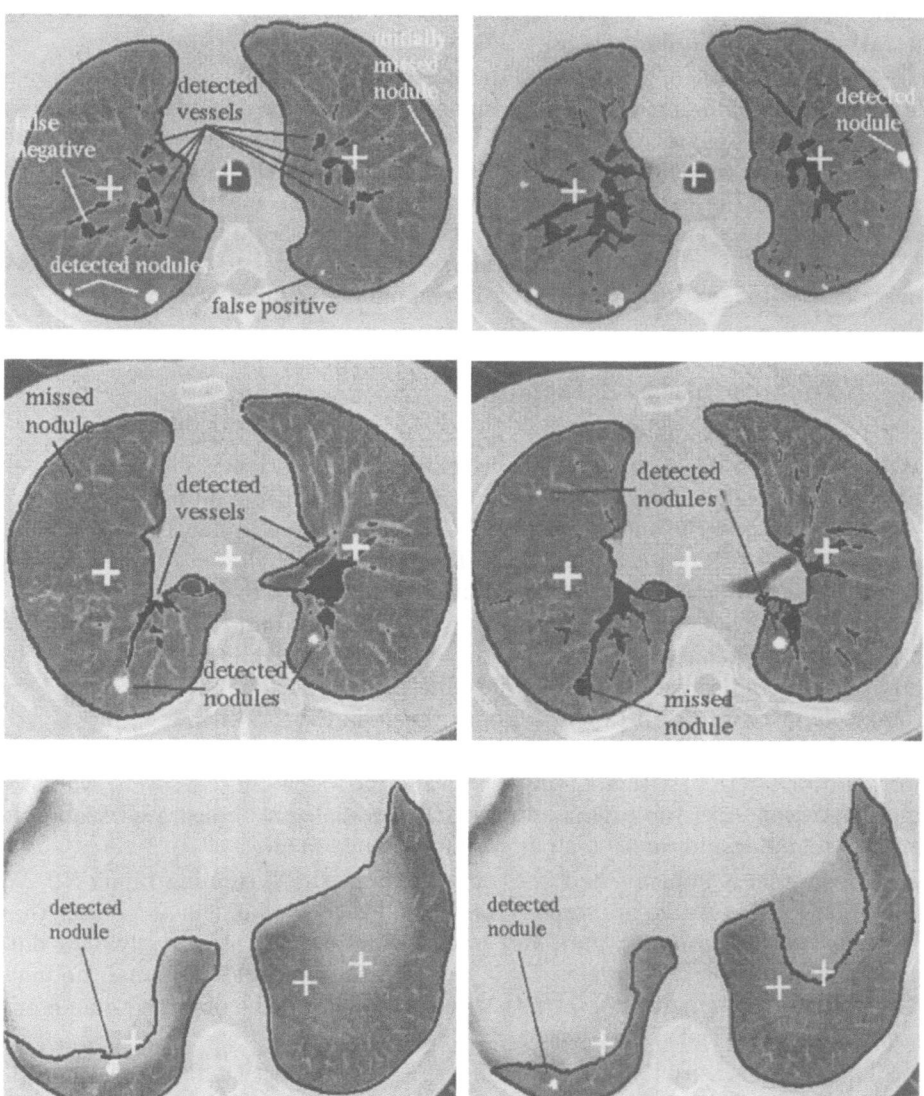

Fig. 2. On the left, each row shows the detection results for a CT image processed with a high grey-level threshold. On the right, the same CT image is shown processed with a lower threshold. Nodules initially missed using a high threshold can be detected using a low threshold and vice versa.

same study. Differences in patient position and inspiration complicates the registration between studies.

Given a CT image, we first need to find the closest CT image on a subsequent study. In our preliminary system, we identify CT slices by hand in both studies that show the apex of the lung. With the initial registration of apex images, we simplify the search for corresponding CT images in the rest of the lung. For each image in the earlier study we identify a possible matching image in the subsequent study and examine the two surrounding slices. Once corresponding CT images are identified, the images are registered similar to the 3D registration described above, and the volumes of corresponding nodules are compared.

3   Experiments and Results

We evaluated an initial and a follow-up study for four patients. The patients were identified through a database of reports as having multiple pulmonary nodules. The patients had melanoma, renal carcinoma, and rectal cancer. The studies were obtained 1, 2 or 6 months apart. The studies were chosen to reflect a wide variety of nodule number, size, distribution, and change over time.

The helical thoracic CT scans were obtained at 10 mm increments from the apices to the adrenal glands with 5 mm increments through the hila. On average 30 images were processed per CT study, which gives a total of 240 images. Each image contains a 512×512 matrix, each pixel is quantized using 16 bits.

A thoracic radiologist evaluated the scans using a clinical IMPAX PACS workstation (AGFA) with a 12-bit display and the follow-up scans were evaluated in comparison with the original studies. The radiologist interpreted sequential studies together and made comparisons for change in size.

The system is implemented in C on a Pentium II PC running Linux 5.2. We define nodules to be *large, medium,* and *small* if their diameter is greater than 1 cm, between 1 cm and 5 mm, and smaller than 5 mm, respectively. Our data contains a total of 323 nodules, 52 large, 108 medium, and 163 small nodules. The volume V of a nodule can be easily computed from the obtained diameter d assuming a spherical shape, $V = 4/3\pi(d/2)^3$.

The overall sensitivity of the system was 88% for detecting all nodules in eight studies. The individual study sensitivities are 84% (A1), 84% (A2), 100% (B1), 100% (B2), 85% (C1), 100% (C2), 84% (D1), and 92% (D2). Table 1 summarizes our nodule detection results.

Nodule sizes range between 1 mm – 4 cm, 2.5 mm – 1.6 cm, 2 mm – 1 cm, and 1.9 mm – 2.5 cm for patients A, B, C, and D, respectively. Size analysis results are shown in Table 2. Of the 39 missed nodules, 29 are small, 8 are medium, and 2 are large. The missed nodules either abut a lung border (20) or vessel (13), or are too small and faint (6).

The radiologist detected a total of 156 nodules changed and 44 remained stable, while the computer demonstrated change in 175 nodules with 25 nodules remaining stable (Table 3).

Table 1. Nodule Detection: Class 1 = Detected Extremely Likely Nodule, Class 2 = Detected Likely Nodule, Class 3 = Missed Nodule. Total = Total Number of Nodules Identified by Radiologist

Class	Study 1				Study 2			
	1	2	3	total	1	2	3	total
Patient								
A	26	36	12	74	26	38	12	76
B	6	4	0	10	7	3	0	10
C	10	1	2	13	9	3	0	12
D	16	16	6	38	59	24	7	90

Table 2. Volumetric Analysis of Detected Nodules: Detected nodules are separated into size categories. Large nodules: > 1cm, medium-sized nodules: between 5mm and 1cm, and small nodules: < 5mm.

Patient	Nodule	Number of Nodules and Average Sizes in mm							
		Study 1				Study 2			
		l	m	s	total	l	m	s	total
A	number	5	13	44	62	5	12	47	64
A	av. size	24.7	6.3	3.3	5.6	25.1	7.0	3.1	5.1
B	number	1	4	5	10	3	3	4	10
B	av. size	15	7.3	3.1	6.0	14.4	7.8	3.5	8.1
C	number	1	8	2	11	1	8	3	12
C	av. size	10.0	6.4	3.3	6.2	10.5	6.7	3.5	6.2
D	number	5	18	9	32	29	34	20	83
D	av. size	13.7	7.1	3.7	7.2	13.8	6.6	3.5	8.4

Table 3. Change in Volume: Disease progression: decrease (d), no change $(=)$ and increase (i) in nodule size.

Studies Compared	Change in Size of Nodules					
	Radiologist			Computer		
	d	$=$	i	d	$=$	i
A1 – A2	37	20	13	38	9	23
B1 – B2	2	4	6	3	3	6
C1 – C2	1	12	0	1	11	1
D1 – D2	15	8	82	17	2	86

4   Conclusions

We presented a computer vision system for pulmonary nodule detection, automated quantification of volume, and assessment for change in volume over time. The system detects nodules of a wide range in diameter (1 – 32 mm), and location, for example, abutting the lung border or a vessel. The system uses thresholding, backtracking, and smoothing techniques and 3D registration techniques. Registration of thoracic CT between studies is challenging because of differences in patient position and respiration. We presented a preliminary registration technique for comparing the same nodules on sequential studies. These techniques have future applications for determining disease progression, remission, and stability in oncologic patients in addition to coregistration of different modalities within the thorax.

Acknowledgements

The authors thank Gordon Harris, Robert Lewis, and Steven Hodge, Computer-Aided Diagnostics Laboratory at Massachusetts General Hospital, for data transfer and Nicholas Makris, Massachusetts Institute of Technology, for computer facilities.

References

1. Carreira, M., Diego, C. Penendo, M. Mosquera, A.: Computer-Aided Diagnosis: Automatic Detection of Lung Nodules. Med. Phys. **25**:10 (1998) 1998–2006.
2. Giger, M., Bae, K., MacMahon, H.: Computerized Detection of Pulmonary Nodules in Computed Tomography Images. Invest Radiol. **28** (1994) 459–465.
3. Horn, B. K. P.: Robot Vision. MIT Press, 1986.
4. Kanazawa, K., Kawata, Y., Niki, N., Satoh, H., Ohmatsu, H., Kakinuma, R., Kaneko, M., Eguchi, K., Moriyama, N.: Computer-Aided Diagnostic System for Pulmonary Nodules Using CT Images. Proc. Medical Image Computing and Computer-Assisted Intervention, 1998, 449–456.
5. Matsumoto, T., Yoshimura, H., Giger, M. Doi, K., MacMahon H. Montner, S. Nakanishi, T.: Potential Usefulness of Computerized Nodule Detection in Screening Programs for Lung Cancer. Invest Radiol. **27** (1992) 472–475.
6. Wirth, N. Algorithmen und Datenstrukturen. B. G. Teubner, 1983.

Improving the Detection Performance in Semi-automatic Landmark Extraction

Sönke Frantz, Karl Rohr, and H. Siegfried Stiehl

Universität Hamburg, Fachbereich Informatik, Arbeitsbereich Kognitive Systeme
Vogt-Kölln-Str. 30, D-22527 Hamburg, Germany
{frantz,rohr,stiehl}@informatik.uni-hamburg.de
http://kogs-www.informatik.uni-hamburg.de/PROJECTS/imagine/Imagine.html

Abstract. Manually extracting 3D anatomical point landmarks from tomographic images is generally tedious and time-consuming. A semi-automatic procedure for landmark extraction, which allows for interactive control, offers the possibility to improve on this. The detection performance is decisive for the applicability of such a procedure. However, existing computational approaches to landmark detection often suffer from a larger number of false detections. A considerable number of false detections is caused by neighboring anatomical structures that are captured by the region-of-interest (ROI) at a landmark. In this paper, we present two different approaches to reducing false detections caused by neighboring structures. First, we present a statistical, differential approach to automatically selecting a suitable size for the 3D ROI. Second, we present a differential approach that incorporates additional prior knowledge of the intensity structure at a landmark. Combining both approaches with a robust 3D differential operator for landmark detection, we develop a new algorithm for landmark detection. In estimating the partial derivatives of the intensity function, we can cope with anisotropic voxel sizes using a scheme based on B-spline image interpolation. The new algorithm is applied within a semi-automatic procedure to extract anatomical point landmarks from 3D MR and CT images of the human head.

1 Introduction

Anatomical landmarks are useful features for a wide spectrum of applications in medical image analysis. If selected suitably, such landmarks may represent substantial image information very concisely, which is important in medical applications considering the vast amount of data one has to deal with. Among the different types of landmarks, we are particularly interested in 3D anatomical point landmarks of the human head. The driving application is landmark-based 3D image registration. One advantage of using point landmarks is efficiency, e.g., in establishing correspondences. Also, point landmarks are well suited for interactive control, which we consider crucial in clinical practice. However, manual landmark extraction from images is generally tedious and time-consuming. A (semi-)automatic procedure offers the possibility to improve on this.

Only a few computational approaches to extracting 3D anatomical point landmarks exist (e.g., [1],[2],[3]). In these approaches, 3D differential operators are used to detect different types of landmarks. The complexity of these operators ranges from those using only first order partial derivatives of the intensity function [2] to those using derivatives up to the second or even the third order [3],[1]. In our case, we apply operators within a semi-automatic procedure, which has the advantage that the user can control the results. Semi-automatic means that (i) the user interactively determines the position of a landmark coarsely, (ii) a differential operator is applied within a region-of-interest (ROI) to detect landmark candidates, and (iii) the user selects one candidate. However, a general problem with differential operators is that often a larger number of false detections occurs (see [4] for a study of the detection performance of 3D differential operators for landmark detection). A large number of false detections not only affects the selection of the correct candidate but also the confidence in the results, which in turn would reduce the acceptance of such a procedure. One reason for false detections is that only local intensity information is used, which makes the operators sensitive to noise and small intensity variations. Operators that use high order derivatives are particularly affected by this. Second, a considerable number of false detections is caused by neighboring anatomical structures that are captured by the ROI.

In this paper, we introduce two different approaches to reducing false detections caused by neighboring structures. First, we address the problem of selecting a suitable 3D ROI at a landmark. We present a statistical, differential approach to automatically selecting an optimal ROI size (Sect. 2). Second, we take advantage of prior knowledge of the intensity structure at a landmark to impose additional constraints on the detected candidates. Based on the curvature of the isointensity surfaces at the detected positions, we automatically reject those candidates where the present intensity structure is inconsistent with the prior knowledge of the landmark at hand (Sect. 3). Combining both approaches with a robust 3D differential operator for landmark detection, which uses only first order derivatives, we present a new algorithm for landmark detection. In image derivative estimation, we can cope with the typical case of anisotropic voxel sizes using a scheme based on B-spline image interpolation (Sect. 4). The new algorithm is applied within a semi-automatic procedure to extract anatomical point landmarks from 3D MR and CT images of the human head (Sect. 5).

2   Automatically Selecting a Suitable 3D ROI Size

Within our semi-automatic procedure, the user interactively determines the position of the landmark at hand coarsely. At this position, a 3D ROI is placed in which a differential operator is applied to detect landmark candidates. In previous work [2],[5], we used a fixed ROI size. Because of this, however, neighboring anatomical structures were often captured by the ROI, which gave rise to additional detections. Here, we present a statistical approach to automatically selecting a suitable ROI size based on a 3D differential edge intersection approach, which was previously used for refined landmark localization [6]. In the edge intersection approach, tangent planes are computed to locally approximate the surface at a landmark. The landmark position is estimated by intersecting the tangent planes using the least-squares method. This approach can be used for ROI size selection by taking the statistical uncertainty of the position estimate as a criterion for isolating an anatomical landmark (e.g., a tip) within the ROI. First results based on a 2D version of this approach were presented in [7].

Consider a cubic ROI of width w centered at the interactively determined position. Let $\hat{x}_w$ denote the position estimate resulting from the 3D edge intersection approach [6]. The statistical uncertainty of $\hat{x}_w$ is given by the covariance matrix,

$$\Sigma_w = \sigma_\varepsilon^2 \left(\sum_i \nabla g(\mathbf{x}_i) \nabla g(\mathbf{x}_i)^T \right)^{-1},$$

where σ_ε^2 is a data-dependent noise term and $\nabla g(\mathbf{x}_i)$ is the intensity gradient at $\mathbf{x}_i$; the sum index i addresses all voxels within the ROI. The matrix Σ_w reflects the consistency of the observed data with the assumed polyhedral model of the surface at the landmark. A scalar measure for the uncertainty is the determinant of the covariance matrix, $U_w = det(\Sigma_w)$ (generalized variance). The idea behind ROI size selection is to vary the ROI size and then to select the optimal ROI size based on minimal uncertainty.

The procedure for ROI size selection is as follows: We start with a user-specified minimal ROI size (e.g., $w_{min} = 7$ voxels). When the ROI does not capture sufficient intensity information to reliably estimate the landmark position, U_w is large. Hence, taking more image information into account by enlarging the ROI, U_w can be expected to decrease. However, when neighboring structures are captured by the ROI, U_w significantly increases, which suggests that further enlargement of the ROI is not useful. In our implementation, we detect such a change of U_w at $w_{increase}$, say, by requiring that (a) U_w increases and (b) the relative spatial variation of the position estimate exceeds a threshold t_V. Additionally, a maximal ROI size w_{max} is prescribed. Finally, the optimal ROI size w_{opt} is selected in between, i.e., $w_{opt} = \arg\min U_w$, $w_{min} \leq w \leq \min\{w_{increase}, w_{max}\}$.

3   Incorporating Prior Knowledge of the Landmark

We take advantage of prior knowledge of the intensity structure at a landmark to impose additional constraints on the detected candidates. In general, the user knows the landmark type (e.g., a tip or a saddle point) as well as the used modality and the imaging parameters. Here, we distinguish between tips and saddle points. Additionally, we distinguish between dark and bright tips w.r.t. the background. To classify these structures, we exploit curvature properties of the isointensity surfaces at the detected positions.

Suppose we have detected a point $\mathbf{x}_d$ on the surface of an anatomical structure. Let K denote the Gaussian curvature and H the mean curvature of the isointensity surface at $\mathbf{x}_d$, which is implicitly defined by $g(\mathbf{x}) - g(\mathbf{x}_d) = 0$ (for details on computing differential measures of isointensity surfaces, see, e.g., [8],[1]). Using the sign of K, we distinguish between tips ($K > 0$) and saddle points ($K < 0$). Using the sign of H, we further distinguish between dark ($H < 0$) and bright ($H > 0$) tips w.r.t. the background. The candidate is rejected if the classification of the present intensity structure is inconsistent with the expected intensity structure.

4   Improved Algorithm for Landmark Detection

In sum, our new algorithm for landmark detection comprises three constituents:

(1) A cubic ROI is centered at the interactively determined position, and then an optimal size for the ROI is automatically selected (Sect. 2).
(2) Landmark candidates are detected by applying a computationally efficient 3D differential operator [2]. The operator is applicable to different types of landmarks and is relatively robust w.r.t. noise since only first order derivatives are used (cf. [4]). The operator reads $Op3 = det(\mathbf{C})/trace(\mathbf{C})$, where $\mathbf{C}$ denotes the averaged dyadic product of the intensity gradient, $\mathbf{C} = \overline{\nabla g \nabla g^T}$.
(3) Detected candidates with an intensity structure being inconsistent with the prior knowledge of the landmark at hand are automatically rejected (Sect. 3).

In addition, in estimating the partial derivatives of the intensity function, we can cope with anisotropic voxel sizes. Based on [9], we implemented a scheme using cubic B-spline image interpolation and Gaussian smoothing. The derivatives are calculated based on the reconstructed continuous signal, taking anisotropic image resolution into account. In contrast, in the previous algorithm for landmark detection (e.g., [2],[5]) the detection operator $Op3$ was applied within a ROI of fixed size. Reduction of false detections by incorporating additional prior knowledge of the landmark was not considered.

5   Experimental Results Using 3D MR and CT Images

5.1   Experimental setting

Data. We used five T1-weighted MR/CT image pairs from different patients: one (*C06*) acquired at Utrecht University Hospital and four (*V101, V104, V107,* and *V109*) acquired at Vanderbilt University. The voxel sizes of the *C06* data are $0.86 \times 0.86 \times 1.2\text{mm}^3$ (MR) and $0.63 \times 0.63 \times 1.0\text{mm}^3$ (CT). The voxel sizes of the remaining original data are $0.85 \times 0.85 \times 3.0\text{mm}^3$ (MR) and $0.42 \times 0.42 \times 3.0\text{mm}^3$ (CT). Instead of the original data in the latter case, we used up-sampled images with a slice thickness of 1.0mm based on cubic B-spline interpolation [9].

Landmarks. We considered visually salient features located on the skull and within the brain: the saddle points at the zygomatic bones (MC15), the tip of the external occipital protuberance (MC5e), the topmost concavity of the fourth

ventricle (MC2), the junction at the upper end of pons (MC18), and the tips of
the frontal (MC6) and occipital ventricular horns (MC7) (see Fig. 1). A suffix
added to the landmark symbols indicates the respective hemisphere, e.g., MC15l
refers to the saddle point at the left zygomatic bone.

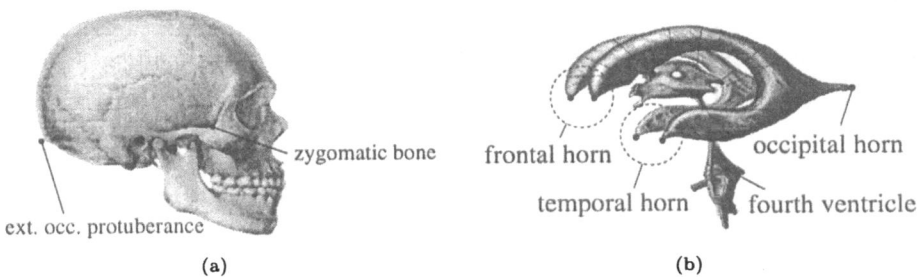

(a)   (b)

Fig. 1. Anatomical point landmarks located (a) on the skull (adapted from [10]) and
(b) on the ventricular system (adapted from [11]).

Parameters. The minimal and maximal width of the cubic ROI was set to
$w_{min} = 7$ voxels and $w_{max} = 21$ voxels, resp. The threshold for the spatial
variation of the position estimate was set to $t_V = 0.5$mm. In the experiments
with the previous algorithm for landmark detection, we used a fixed ROI width
of $w = w_{max} = 21$ voxels. In estimating the derivatives, we used two different
scales for the Gaussian filters, depending on the scale of the respective landmark:
$\sigma = 1.0$mm for MC15 as well as MC18 and $\sigma = 1.5$mm for MC5e, MC2, MC6,
and MC7 (note that these scales were automatically adapted according to the
actual voxel size). Averaging the intensity gradient (matrix $C = \overline{\nabla g \nabla g^T}$) was
done within a $5 \times 5 \times 5$ window. Local maxima of the operator responses were
determined in $3 \times 3 \times 3$ neighborhoods.

5.2   Evaluation of the Detection Performance

To evaluate the detection performance, we use a certain type of performance
visualization as well as a scalar quantity measuring the detection capability [12].
Additionally, we consider the number of detections. The operator responses at
the detected candidates are plotted as a function of the distance to the ROI
center. Thus, in these plots the spatial scatter of the detected positions within
the ROI, the number of detections, as well as the significance of the different
detections (in terms of the strength of the operator response) are reflected. To
quantitatively evaluate the detection performance, we use a measure that takes
into account both the number of detections as well as the significance of the
different detections. Suppose we have obtained n detections for a landmark. Let
$R_i > 0$, $i = 1, \ldots, n$, denote the operator responses at the detected positions

and let R_{max} denote the maximum of these values. We consider the measure

$$\psi = \begin{cases} 0 & n = 0, \\ \sum_{i=1}^{n} \frac{R_i}{R_{max}} & n \geq 1. \end{cases}$$

If we obtain only one correct detection, we have $\psi = 1$. Additional false detections with small operator responses give $\psi \approx 1$. In this case, the correct detection can clearly be distinguished. On the other hand, if there are detections with operator responses similar to the maximal operator response, ψ is much larger than 1. Thus, the closer ψ is to 1, the better the detection performance.

5.3   Analysis of the Efficacy in Reducing False Detections

Exemplarily, we consider six landmarks located within the mid-sagittal plane and within the left hemisphere. We compare the detection performance of the new algorithm for landmark detection with that of the previous algorithm (see Sect. 4). Here, we present in detail the results obtained for the *V109* MR/CT image pair. In the experiments, the ROI centers are the positions resulting from best manual landmark localization (in agreement of two persons). Using this 'ground truth', we can also study the impact of our approaches on the localization performance. No thresholds were applied to the operator responses. In Fig. 2 (MR) and Fig. 3 (CT), the detection performance is visualized as described in Sect. 5.2. Thick bars indicate the detections obtained with the new algorithm for landmark detection. Narrow bars indicate those detections that would additionally be obtained with the previous algorithm. Note that the new algorithm always yields a subset of those candidates obtained with the previous algorithm. Additionally, the number of detections n obtained with both algorithms as well as the detection performance measure ψ are given.

For both modalities, the new algorithm showed a significantly better detection performance than the previous algorithm. A larger number of false detections with significant operator responses were suppressed, e.g., in MR in the case of the occipital protuberance and the fourth ventricle (Figs. 2b,c) and in CT in the case of the fourth ventricle, the top of pons, and the left occipital horn (Figs. 3c,d,f). Note that in MR in the case of the fourth ventricle (Fig. 2c) and in CT in the case of the fourth ventricle and the top of pons (Figs. 3c,d) the previous algorithm yielded a number of false detections with larger operator responses than those candidates with minimal distance to the manual positions. These detections were rejected with the new algorithm. In almost all cases, the localization performance was not affected, i.e., the detections with minimal distance to the manual positions were retained. The fact that the detections obtained with the new algorithm are better distinguishable w.r.t. the operator response is also reflected by smaller values of ψ. Both approaches to reducing false detections complementarily improve the performance. For example, in MR in the case of the fourth ventricle (Fig. 2c) ROI size selection alone yielded two detections, while incorporation of prior knowledge of the landmark yielded four detections. The combination of both approaches yielded only one detection. For the other four MR/CT image pairs, we obtained similar results.

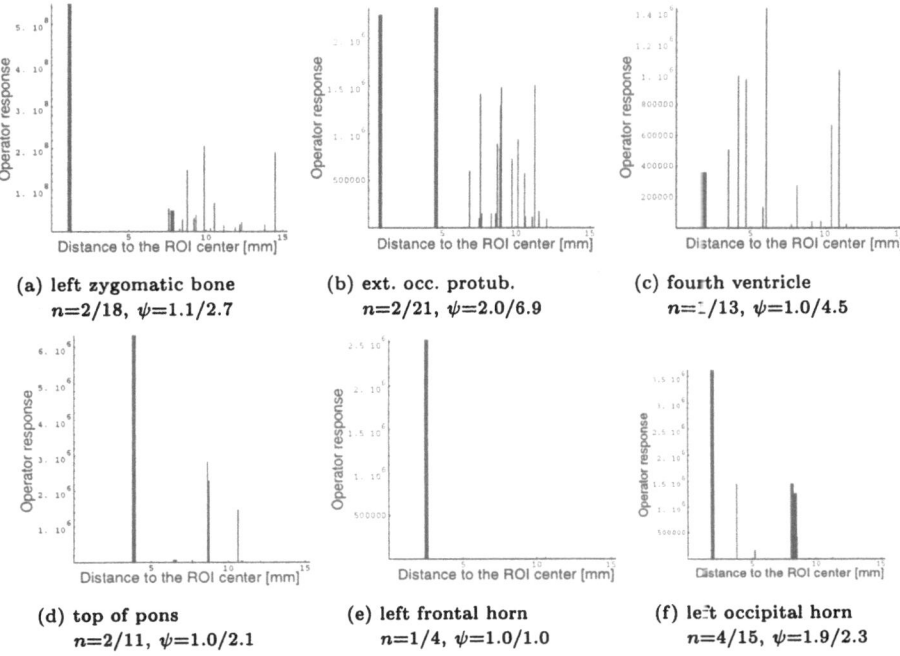

(a) left zygomatic bone
$n=2/18$, $\psi=1.1/2.7$

(b) ext. occ. protub.
$n=2/21$, $\psi=2.0/6.9$

(c) fourth ventricle
$n=1/13$, $\psi=1.0/4.5$

(d) top of pons
$n=2/11$, $\psi=1.0/2.1$

(e) left frontal horn
$n=1/4$, $\psi=1.0/1.0$

(f) left occipital horn
$n=4/15$, $\psi=1.9/2.3$

Fig. 2. Comparison of the detection performance of the new algorithm with that of the previous algorithm (*V109* MR image). The operator responses at the detected positions are drawn as a function of the distance to the ROI center. Thick bars indicate the remaining detections within the selected ROI obtained with the new algorithm. Narrow bars indicate those detections that would additionally be obtained with the previous algorithm. For both algorithms, the number of detections n as well as the detection performance measure ψ are given. For example, in (a) $n = 2/18$ means two detections for the new algorithm and 18 detections for the previous algorithm.

5.4   Application to Five MR/CT Image Pairs

We applied our new algorithm to extract landmarks from all five different MR/CT image pairs specified in Sect. 5.1. Depending on the field-of-view, the image quality, and lesions, we selected for each image pair 7–9 landmarks, which were simultaneously extracted from both modalities using the semi-automatic procedure. In the experiments, we applied a dynamic threshold to the operator responses to suppress insignificant detections (10% of the maximal operator response). The user inputs (e.g., the interactively determined positions and the selected candidates) were automatically recorded by the computer system. In Tables 1 and 2, the detection performance of the new algorithm is documented. Table 1 shows the results obtained for the five MR images, and Table 2 shows the results obtained for the five CT images (see Sect. 5.1 for the landmark symbols used for abbreviation). We compare the detection performance with that of the previous algorithm, which we applied at the same positions. For each landmark,

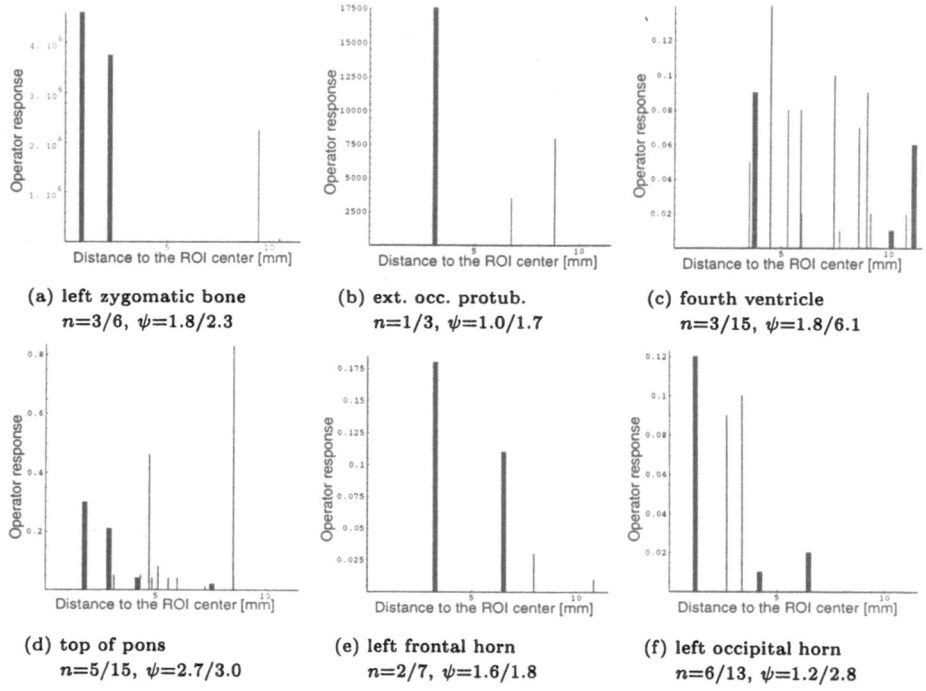

Fig. 3. Same as Fig. 2 but for the *V109* CT image.

we consider the mean $\bar{n}$ and the maximal number n_{max} of detections, the relative difference $\Delta\bar{n}$ between these mean values, as well as the mean $\bar{\psi}$ and the maximum ψ_{max} of the detection performance measure ψ.

For all landmarks, the mean number of detections was reduced using the new algorithm. In most cases, we obtained significantly fewer detections. The values of ψ are significantly smaller, which indicates that the remaining detections are better distinguishable w.r.t. the operator responses. In MR, especially for the saddle points at the zygomatic bones (MC15), the occipital protuberance (MC5e), the fourth ventricle (MC2), and the top of pons (MC18) the results were significantly improved. In CT, for MC2 and MC18 we obtained significantly better results. In general, the detection performance was better for the CT images, i.e., the number of detections were smaller and ψ was smaller. In most cases, we obtained only 1–2 detections with the improved algorithm (in MR in 72% of all cases and in CT in 83% of all cases). In either case, we obtained not more than five detections for a landmark, while the previous algorithm yielded 15 detections in the worst case. Using the improved algorithm, in most cases the candidate with the maximal operator response was selected (in MR in 89% of all cases and in CT in 78% of all cases).

Recently, we also validated our improved algorithm for landmark detection within an application study in which five different observers participated [13].

Table 1. Comparison of the detection performance of the new algorithm with that of the previous algorithm (for five MR images). For each landmark, the mean $\bar{n}$ and the maximal n_{max} number of detections, the relative difference $\Delta\bar{n}$ between these mean values, as well as the mean $\bar{\psi}$ and the maximum ψ_{max} of the detection performance measure ψ are given. For example, for MC15l $\bar{n} = 2.0/4.8$ denotes 2.0 detections in the mean for the new algorithm and 4.8 detections for the previous algorithm.

	MC15l	MC15r	MC5e	MC2	MC18	MC6l	MC6r	MC7l	MC7r
$\bar{n}$	2.0/4.8	3.3/8.3	1.8/8.3	1.0/12.0	1.0/5.0	2.5/3.0	2.4/3.4	1.8/2.8	2.0/3.4
n_{max}	3/8	5/12	2/13	1/15	1/7	3/4	3/5	3/4	3/5
$\Delta\bar{n}$	59%	61%	79%	92%	80%	17%	30%	36%	42%
$\bar{\psi}$	1.5/2.6	1.8/3.6	1.5/4.0	1.0/4.9	1.0/2.6	1.7/1.8	1.7/2.2	1.3/1.5	1.4/1.8
ψ_{max}	2.1/4.5	2.8/4.9	2.0/6.0	1.0/4.9	1.0/3.5	2.3/2.7	2.4/3.6	1.9/2.0	1.6/2.5

Table 2. Same as Table 1 but for five CT images.

	MC15l	MC15r	MC5e	MC2	MC18	MC6l	MC6r	MC7l	MC7r
$\bar{n}$	1.6/2.6	1.8/3.0	1.5/2.3	1.0/8.0	3.0/6.0	1.3/2.0	2.8/3.6	1.6/3.8	2.0/3.8
n_{max}	2/3	2/4	2/4	1/10	5/7	2/2	5/6	2/7	3/7
$\Delta\bar{n}$	39%	40%	35%	88%	50%	35%	23%	58%	48%
$\bar{\psi}$	1.3/1.9	1.6/2.1	1.2/1.4	1.0/3.5	1.7/2.7	1.0/1.2	1.9/2.2	1.3/2.1	1.5/2.0
ψ_{max}	1.8/2.3	2.0/2.8	1.5/2.0	1.0/3.9	2.6/3.3	1.2/1.2	3.6/3.9	1.9/2.6	1.8/2.9

The aim of this study was to evaluate the performance of the semi-automatic procedure in extracting landmarks from MR/CT images in comparison to a manual procedure (e.g., in terms of the elapsed time spent for landmark extraction as well as the registration results using a rigid transformation). The main findings were that (a) the elapsed time spent for landmark extraction can significantly be reduced with the semi-automatic procedure (the mean relative reduction of the elapsed time compared to a manual procedure was 38%) and (b) the registration results of both procedures generally showed similar quality.

6 Conclusion

Existing computational approaches to extracting 3D anatomical point landmarks from medical images often suffer from false detections, which may seriously affect the applicability and the acceptance of such an approach. A considerable number of these false detections is caused by neighboring anatomical structures. In this paper, we introduced two different approaches to reducing false detections caused by neighboring structures. Combining both approaches with a robust 3D differential operator for landmark detection, we presented an improved algorithm for landmark detection. In estimating the partial derivatives of the intensity function, we can cope with the typical case of anisotropic voxel sizes. We applied our new algorithm within a semi-automatic procedure to extract anatomical point landmarks from 3D MR and CT images of the human head. Experimental results showed that both automatically selecting the ROI size as well as incorporating additional prior knowledge of the landmark are very effective in reducing the number of false detections. Results of applying our novel semi-automatic procedure for landmark extraction to five MR/CT image pairs demonstrated the applicability of our procedure.

Acknowledgments

Support of Philips Research Hamburg, project IMAGINE (IMage- and Atlas-Guided Interventions in NEurosurgery), is gratefully acknowledged. Images were provided as part of the E.U. AIM project COVIRA and as part of the project "Evaluation of Retrospective Image Registration", National Institutes of Health, Project Number 1 R01 NS33926-01, Principal Investigator, Dr. J. Michael Fitzpatrick, Vanderbilt University, Nashville, TN.

References

1. J.-P. Thirion. Extremal Points: Definition and Application to 3D Image Registration. In *Proc. CVPR'94*, pp. 587–592. IEEE Computer Society Press, 1994.
2. K. Rohr. On 3D differential operators for detecting point landmarks. *Image and Vision Computing*, 15(3):219–233, 1997.
3. W. Beil, K. Rohr, and H.S. Stiehl. Investigation of Approaches for the Localization of Anatomical Landmarks in 3D Medical Images. In *Proc. CAR'97*, pp. 265–270. Elsevier Science, 1997.
4. T. Hartkens, K. Rohr, and H.S. Stiehl. Performance of 3D differential operators for the detection of anatomical point landmarks in MR and CT images. In *Proc. SPIE's Medical Imaging 1999: Image Processing.* vol. 3661, pp. 32–43. SPIE, 1999.
5. K. Rohr. Image Registration Based on Thin-Plate Splines and Local Estimates of Anisotropic Landmark Localization Uncertainties. In *Proc. MICCAI'98*, LNCS 1496, pp. 1174–1183. Springer-Verlag, 1998.
6. S. Frantz, K. Rohr, and H.S. Stiehl. Refined Localization of Three-Dimensional Anatomical Point Landmarks Using Multi-Step Differential Approaches. In *Proc. SPIE's Medical Imaging 1998: Image Processing*, vol. 3338, pp. 28–38. SPIE, 1998.
7. S. Frantz, K. Rohr, and H.S. Stiehl. Multi-step Procedures for the Localization of 2D and 3D Point Landmarks and Automatic ROI Size Selection. In *Proc. ECCV'98*, vol. I, LNCS 1406, pp. 687–703. Springer-Verlag, 1998.
8. L.M.J. Florack, B.M. ter Romeny, J.J. Koenderink, and M.A. Viergever. General Intensity Transformations and Differential Invariants. *Journal of Mathematical Imaging and Vision*, 4:171–187, 1994.
9. M. Unser, A. Aldroubi, and M. Eden. B-Spline Signal Processing: Part I—Theory. *IEEE Trans. on Signal Processing*, 41(2):821–833, 1993.
10. R. Bertolini and G. Leutert. *Atlas der Anatomie des Menschen*, volume 3: Kopf und Hals, Gehirn, Rückenmark und Sinnesorgane. Springer-Verlag, 1982.
11. J. Sobotta. *Atlas der Anatomie des Menschen*, volume 1: Kopf, Hals, obere Extremität, Haut. Urban & Schwarzenberg, 19th edition, 1988.
12. K. Rohr. Extraction of 3d anatomical point landmarks based on invariance principles. *Pattern Recognition*, 32(1):3–15, 1999.
13. S. Frantz, K. Rohr, H.S. Stiehl, S.-I. Kim, and J. Weese. Validating Point-based MR/CT Registration Based on Semi-automatic Landmark Extraction. In *Proc. CARS'99*. Elsevier Science, to appear.

Automatic Classification of Linear Structures in Mammographic Images

Reyer Zwiggelaar[1]*, Christopher J. Taylor[2], and Caroline R. M. Boggis[3]

[1] Division of Computer Science, University of Portsmouth, Portsmouth, UK
[2] Wolfson Image Analysis Unit, University of Manchester, Manchester, UK
[3] Greater Manchester Breast Screening Service, Withington Hospital, Manchester, UK

Abstract. Certain kinds of abnormalities in x-ray mammograms are associated with specific anatomical structures - in particular, linear structures. This association can, in principle, be exploited to improve the specificity and sensitivity with which the abnormalities can be detected. We compare annotated and the automatic detection of the scale and orientation associated with linear structure in mammograms. We investigate methods of classifying the detected structures into anatomical classes (spicules, vessel, duct, fibrous tissue etc) from their cross-sectional profiles. Automatic (linear and non-linear) classification results are compared with expert annotations using receiver operating characteristic analysis. We show that useful discrimination between anatomical classes is achieved. Some of this relies on simple attributes such as the width and contrast of the profile, but there is also important information carried by the shape of the profile.

1 Introduction

The UK Breast Screening Programme alone generates 1.5 million mammograms per annum. Potential malignancies can be detected from subtle abnormalities in radiographic appearance but it is known that radiologists fail to detect a significant proportion of these abnormalities. It has been shown that their performance would improve if they were prompted with the possible locations of abnormalities [1–5]. The abnormalities of interest include microcalcification clusters, masses, spiculated lesions, asymmetry and architectual distortions [6]. Normal mammograms also contain a variety of linear structures: vessels, ducts, fibrous tissue, skinfolds, edges and others that are difficult to classify anatomically. In abnormal mammograms linear structures called 'spicules' may also be present. Abnormalities are non-accidentally associated with these linear structures. For example, microcalcifications are more likely to imply malignancy if they are located in ducts [7] and spicules are always associated with lesions (called spiculated lesions). Each type of linear structure has a characteristic appearance which we hypothesize should be reflected in the cross-sectional intensity profiles.

Spiculated lesions can be detected from the characteristic arrangement of linear structures (the spicules) in a radial pattern [1, 4, 5]. This is, however, less than perfect because other linear structures can be accidentally arranged in similar patterns in normal

---

* email: reyer.zwiggelaar@port.ac.uk

mammograms. We suggest that these methods could be made more specific by applying them to just those linear structures that have a high probability of being spicules.
Linear structures can be detected using various approaches [8]. Here we investigate the
ability to classify detected structures into anatomical classes using their cross-sectional
intensity profiles, with particular emphasis on detecting spicules. Anatomical classification has been developed and tested using real screening mammograms, annotated by
an expert radiologist. Raw intensity profiles are extracted and normalised for intensity
and scale. The dimensionality of the observations is reduced using principal component
analysis (PCA) and both linear and non-linear classification are investigated.

2   Mammographic Data

We will be giving a comparison between the width and orientation as obtained from
the Line Operator approach [8] and those same parameters as provided by a radiologist
based on real mammographic data (in [8] the comparison was based on synthetic data).

2.1   Anatomical Annotations

The Line Operator was applied to 29 mammograms from the MIAS database [9]. Once
the linear structures were detected, a selection was labelled by an expert radiologist into
anatomically distinct classes: *ducts*, *edges*, *fibrous tissue*, *skin folds*, *spicules*, *vessels*
and *others*. Linear structures were randomly selected, taking the detected line strength
into account, so that for each class the total number of profiles obtained approximately
represented their prevalence in mammograms. In addition to providing the anatomical
annotation, the radiologist also gave an indication for the width of the linear structures.

2.2   Profile Width

A comparison between the width as provided by the Line Operator and that as provided
by the radiologist can be found in Fig. 1. Large deviations are possible and the distributions tend to be skewed to the negative side (indicating that the width provided by the
radiologist tended to be larger than the width derived from the Line Operator).

Instead of using the raw scale from the Line Operator it is also possible to obtain
a scale distribution for each linear structure and derive a more robust width. We have
used the median width from the distribution for each structure. The reason we assume
this to be more robust is indicated in Fig. 1, which also shows the deviation between
the annotated widths and those derived from the median scale as provided by the Line
Operator for linear structures. These results indicate that the distribution becomes closer
to that given by the radiologists.

2.3   Profile Orientation

A comparison between the orientation as provided by the Line Operator and that as
provided by the annotations can be found in Fig. 2. As for the width of the linear structures (see previous section) there is a wide distribution. These direct results from the
Line Operator can be compared with the median orientation as obtained for the linear
structures. Improvements in the orientation are not as clear as for the width.

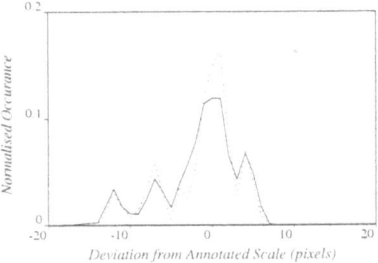

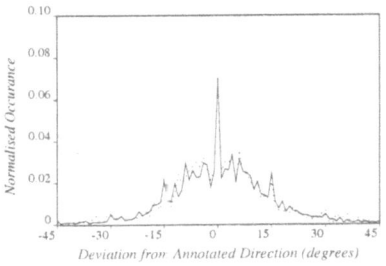

Fig. 1. Deviation between the annotated widths (range 2 to 30 pixels) and those derived from the scale as provided by the Line Operator for individual profiles (continuous lines) and those derived from the median scale as provided by the Line Operator for linear structures (dashed lines).

Fig. 2. Deviation between the annotated orientation and those derived from the orientation as provided by the Line Operator for individual profiles (continuous lines) and those derived from the median orientation as provided by the Line Operator for linear structures (dashed lines).

2.4   Extracting Profiles

Cross-sectional profiles were obtained by taking the normal to the orientation found by the line operator and bilinear interpolation was used to sample grey-level values from the original mammograms. The cross-sectional length of the profiles was taken to be three times the width of the linear structure. To use these variable length profiles for statistical analysis, each profile was re-scaled to a constant number of pixels, 30 in this case, allowing each observation to be represented by an equal number of elements.

2.5   Profile Preprocessing

Instead of using the profiles directly it is also possible to use information derived from them. The motivation for such an approach is that a raw grey-level profile provides not only shape information but also describes the local background grey-level and contrast.

The grey-level values from the original mammogram were represented on a logarithmic scale (to represent tissue thickness). If a local background grey-level gradient existed this was removed by subtracting the gradient as obtained by a simple linear fit to the raw profile. In addition to remove the remaining effects of the grey-level background the mean grey-level was subtracted. To remove grey-level variations within the profiles normalisation with respect to the standard deviation of the grey-level was used. After this preprocessing the resulting profile should contain only the shape information.

2.6   Profile versus Linear Structure Classification

Using statistical modelling we obtain a class probability for every profile. However, we are in general interested in the classification of the linear structures. This can be obtained by a simple summation of the probabilities of the profiles (multiplication is more appropriate but resulted in probabilities equal to zero for the majority of structures).

3   Results for Annotated Profiles

Models were trained on a dataset comprising 318 linear structures (47,812 profiles). To avoid bias the modelling was applied using a three-way split of the dataset (on an image basis). In addition, to avoid bias between left and right mammograms all profiles were included twice for the modelling, once in the original format, but also in reverse order.

As we are interested in the detection of the linear structures that are associated with spiculated lesions we will restrict the classification results to the anatomical class of spicules. This means that for the classification results presented the spicules are regarded as the targets and will indicate the true positives and false negatives, while the other classes are regarded as the non-targets and will indicate the false positives and true negatives. Similar results could be presented for the other anatomical classes.

We have investigated two variations on the input information from the profiles that was used to obtain the classification results; classification based on the full profile and classification based on the PCA data derived from the profiles (using those principal components that covered 99% of the data variance). Two different artificial neural networks were used. The first network used 30 input nodes to represent the elements of the profiles. The second network used a lower number of input nodes, the exact value being determined by the PCA modelling. At the output level (i.e. the classification level) we used two nodes representing the class and non-class options.

3.1   Principal Component Analysis

For models based on the raw profiles the cumulative variance associated with the first five principal components are respectively: 85.5%, 95.3%, 98.8%, 99.4% and 99.6%. Fig. 3 shows the mean profile and the first three principal components of a PCA model based on raw profiles. The first principal component indicates a basic change in the mean grey-level of the profiles. The second principal component shows changes in the gradient of the background grey-level on which the profile is situated. The higher principal components capture changes in the shape of the profiles.

For models build using the normalised profiles the cumulative variance associated with the first five principal components are respectively 19.1%, 35.0%, 49.4%, 58.2% and 65.0%. The effect of the first three principal components and the mean profile are shown in Fig. 4. All the three principal components indicate variations in the shape of the profiles, without any of the effects of the background present. The first principal component seems to be an indication of the overall shift of the profile from left to right. The second and third principal components indicate changes in the width and multi-modal effects of the profiles.

3.2   Classification

ROC curves for linear and non-linear classification of the linear structures based on the original profiles are shown in Fig. 5. The classification shows a significant improvement for the non-linear classification of the linear structures.

ROC curves for linear and non-linear classification based on the normalised profiles are shown in Fig. 6. This indicates an improvement when the non-linear modelling is

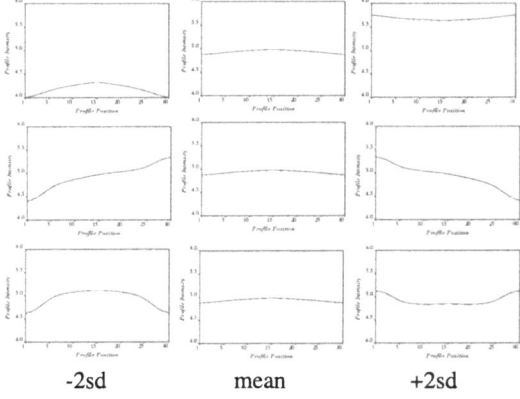

-2sd   mean   +2sd

Fig. 3. Annotated Profiles: The mean (centre column) and first three (from top to bottom) principal components (±2 standard deviations) of the PCA model based on the raw profiles.

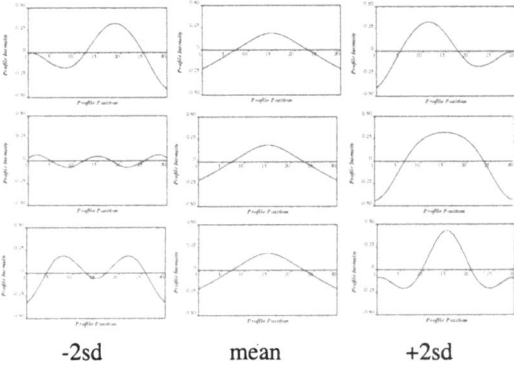

-2sd   mean   +2sd

Fig. 4. Annotated Profiles: The mean (centre column) and first three (from top to bottom) principal components (±2 standard deviations) of the PCA model based on the normalised profiles.

used. In saying this it has to be kept in mind that the improvements are small and that this preprocessing of the profiles does not result in large discrimination effects.

These results indicate that the shape of the profile on its own might not be sufficient for the classification of anatomical linear structures. But when the raw profiles are used the results look very promising, with optimum ROC results of 80% True Positives at the cost of 35% False Positives. The differences between the classification based on the raw and normalised profiles are an implicit indication of the classification potential of the width, mean grey-level and standard deviation of the profiles.

4   Results for Automaticly Extracted Profiles

For an automatic system the width and orientation of the linear structures has to be determined by a computer vision approach. In this section we present results obtained

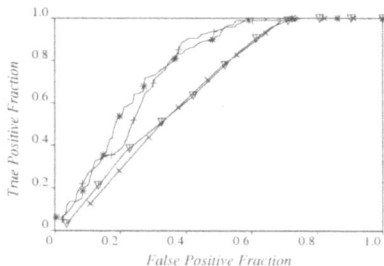

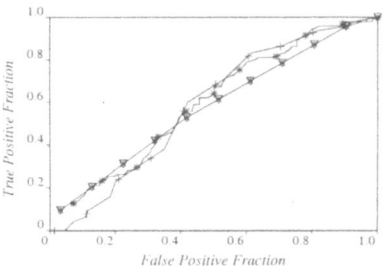

Fig. 5. Annotated Profiles: ROC linear structure classification based on the original profiles for spicule/non-spicule classification. Where ▽: linear classification based on the full profile, ×: linear classification based on the PCA data, ∗: non-linear classification based on the full profile, and +: non-linear classification based on the PCA data.

Fig. 6. Annotated Profiles: ROC linear structure classification based on preprocessed profiles for spicule/non-spicule classification. Where ▽: linear classification based on the full profile, ×: linear classification based on the PCA data, ∗: non-linear classification based on the full profile, and +: non-linear classification based on the PCA data.

using the scale and orientation provided by the Line Operator [8]. The median scale for each structure is used (see Section 2.2). The preprocessing of the profiles is identical to those described in Section 2.5.

4.1 Principal Component Analysis

For the PCA model based on the raw profiles the cumulative variance associated with the first five principal components are respectively: 95.0%, 98.3%, 98.9%, 99.2% and 99.5%. The mean profile and the principal components of a PCA model based on the raw profiles are very similar to those presented using the annotated width and orientation as presented in Fig. 3.

For models build using the normalised profiles the cumulative variance associated with the first five principal components are respectively 19.5%, 37.0%, 48.9%, 57.1% and 63.4%. Again, the resulting PCA models are very similar to those presented for the profiles extracted using the annotated width (see Fig. 4), except for the change-over of the first two principal components (both of them covering about 19% of the variation in the profile data).

4.2 Classification

ROC curves for linear and non-linear classification based on the original profiles is shown in Fig. 7. This shows a small improvement for the non-linear classification of the linear structures.

ROC curves for linear and non-linear classification based on the normalised profiles is shown in Fig. 8. Classification into class/non-class indicates no improvement when the non-linear method is used.

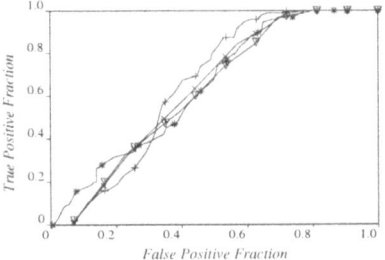

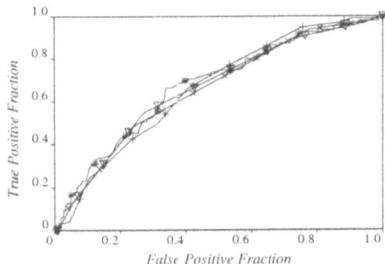

Fig. 7. Median Line Operator Profiles: ROC linear structure classification based on the original profiles for spicule/non-spicule classification. Where ▽: linear classification based on the full profile, ×: linear classification based on the PCA data, ∗: non-linear classification based on the full profile, and +: non-linear classification based on the PCA data.

Fig. 8. Median Line Operator Profiles: ROC linear structure classification based on preprocessed profiles for spicule/non-spicule classification. Where ▽: linear classification based on the full profile, ×: linear classification based on the PCA data, ∗: non-linear classification based on the full profile, and +: non-linear classification based on the PCA data.

The comparison between the results presented in this section and those presented in Section 3.2 indicate large differences with an overall degradation of the classification results. The only difference between the two approaches has been a change in the width and orientation of the profiles that were extracted. It seems that the width as selected by the radiologists results in profiles which are easier to classify.

5   Discussion and Conclusions

An automated technique for detecting specific anatomical types of linear structures in digital mammograms has been described. We have demonstrated how principal component analysis can be used to successfully model the shape of the cross-sectional intensity profiles of the anatomically different linear structures. In addition non-linear aspects of profile classification have been investigated.

A three-way split classification experiment demonstrated anatomical classification with a significantly better than random correct classification for the spicule profiles. A correct classification rate of 80% for spicules/non-spicules could be achieved (at a false positive percentage of ∼35%), which will clearly be useful for the verification of potential spiculated lesions and architectural distortions. In similar experiments, good classification results have also been obtained for vessels and ducts. The potential of this technique for discriminating between ducts and vessels to reduce the number of false positives generated by automated micro-calcification detection algorithms is clear [7]. The detection and classification of ducts is likely to provide useful information for automated techniques attempting to locate the nipple.

However, it does not seem to be the shape of the profile that contributes most significantly to the classification of the linear structures. The width, mean grey-level and standard deviation of the profiles are implicated as being good parameters for classification of the profiles. As soon as these factors have been removed from the profiles the classification potential is reduced, but still better than random, indicating some useful classification potential for the shape of the profiles.

Large classification differences occurred when automaticly determined width and orientation were used when compared with the results obtained when these parameters were derived from the annotations provided by the radiologist. This indicates that improved classification results could be obtained if the width and orientation could be extracted more reliably.

In summary, the algorithms presented in this paper provide an automatic technique for locating and successfully classifying anatomically important linear structures of which spicules were used as an example. Such classification can be employed to verify automatically detected potential abnormalities such as micro-calcification clusters, spiculated lesions and architectural distortions. In addition, the technique can be used to provide strength images relating to specific classes of abnormality; spicule strength images can for example be used to improve the accuracy of spiculated lesion detection algorithms [1, 4, 5]. The technique can also be used to reduce the required computation time by examining only those pixels that are classified into a given class.

References

1. R. Zwiggelaar, T.C. Parr, J.E. Schumm, I.W. Hutt, S.M. Astley, C.J. Taylor, and C.R.M. Boggis. Model-based detection of spiculated lesions in mammograms. *Medical Image Analysis*, 3(1):39–62, 1999.
2. S.M. Astley, R. Zwiggelaar, C. Wolstenholme, and C.J. Taylor. Prompting in mammography: how accurate must prompt generators be? 4th *International Workshop on Digital Mammography*, Nijmegen, The Netherlands:347–354, 1998.
3. H.-P. Chan, K. Doi, C.J. Vyborny, R.A. Schmidt, C.E. Metz, K.L. Lam, T. Ogura, Y. Wu, and H. MacMahon. Improvement in radiologists' detection of clustered microcalcifications on mammograms. *Investigative Radiology*, 25(10):1102–1110, 1990.
4. W.P. Kegelmeyer, J. Pruneda, P. Bourland, A. Hills, M. Riggs, and M. Nipper. Computer-aided mammographic screening for spiculated lesions. *Radiology*, 191:331–337, 1994.
5. N. Karssemeijer and G.M. te Brake. Detection of stellate distortions in mammograms. *IEEE Transactions on Medical Imaging*, 15(5):611–619, 1996.
6. L. Tabar and P.B. Dean. *The Mammographic Teaching Atlas*. Georg Thieme Verlag, Stuttgart, 1985.
7. T. Ema, K. Doi, R.M. Nishikawa, Y. Jiang, and J. Papaioannou. Image feature analysis and computer-aided diagnosis in mammography: reduction of false-positive clustered microcalcifications using local edge-gradient analysis. *Medical Physics*, 22(2):161–169, 1995.
8. R. Zwiggelaar, T.C. Parr, and C.J. Taylor. Finding orientated line patterns in digital mammographic images. In *Proceedings of the 7th British Machine Vision Conference*, pages 715–724, Edinburgh, UK, 1996.
9. J. Suckling, J. Parker, D. Dance, S. Astley, I. Hutt, C. Boggis, I. Ricketts, E. Stamatakis, N. Cerneaz, S. Kok, P. Taylor, D. Betal, and J. Savage. The mammographic images analysis society digital mammogram database. In Dance Gale, Astley and Cairns, editors, *Digital Mammography*, pages 375–378. Elsevier, 1994.

Conformal Geometry and Brain Flattening

Sigurd Angenent[1], Steven Haker[2], Allen Tannenbaum[2], and Ron Kikinis[3]

[1] Department of Mathematics, University of Wisconsin, Madison, Wisconsin 53705
[2] Department of Electrical and Computer Engineering, University of Minnesota, Minneapolis, MN 55455 email: tannenba@ece.umr.edu
[3] Harvard Medical School, Brigham and Women's Hospital, Harvard University, Boston, MA 02115

Abstract. In this paper, using certain conformal mappings from complex function theory, we give an explicit method for flattening the brain surface in a way which is bijective and which preserves angles. The conformal equivalence arises as the solution of a certain elliptic equation on the surface. Then from a triangulated surface representation of the cortex, we indicate how the procedure may be implemented using finite elements. Further, we show how the geometry of the cortical surface and gray/white matter boundary may be studied using this approach. Hence the mapping can be used to obtain an atlas of the brain surface in a natural manner.

Keywords: Brain flattening, conformal maps, functional MRI, segmentation.

1 Introduction

The problem of flattening or unfolding a highly undulated surface is of major importance for a number of problems in 3D medical visualization. Recently a number of techniques have been proposed to obtain a flattened representation of the cortical surface; see, e.g., [5–7, 15, 20] and the references therein. Flattening the brain surface has uses in many areas including functional magnetic resonance imaging, in which it is important to visualize neural activity within the three dimensional folds of the brain, as well as the study of various types of brain pathology.

Our approach to flattening the brain surface is based on the use of a certain fact from the theory of Riemann surfaces, specifically, that a surface without any handles, holes or self-intersections can be mapped conformally onto the sphere, and any local portion thereof onto a disc. This mapping, known as a conformal equivalence, is conformal in the sense that angles are preserved. It is also bijective (onto and one-to-one) and thus there is no problem with triangles "flipping" or overlapping, and no cuts need be made on the surface.

We should note that our approach is quite different from the previous works cited above in brain flattening which typically consider locally area or length preserving deformations. For example, in the nice approaches of [6, 15], the authors fit a parameterized deformable surface whose topology is mappable to a sphere. Then, it is possible to represent the brain surface on a planar map by using spherical coordinates.

In our work, the key observation is that the flattening function may be obtained as the solution of a second order elliptic partial differential equation (PDE) on the surface to be flattened. For triangulated surfaces, there exist powerful, reliable finite element procedures which can be employed to numerically approximate the flattening function.

2   Flattening the Brain Surface

In this section, we sketch the mathematical justification of our brain flattening procedure. Full details appear in [1]. A basic assumption is that the brain surface is topologically a sphere. While this is is not exactly correct (there are some small holes where the ventricles connect to the outer surface), we can always fill these in by using, e.g., morphological dilation and erosion. This will not affect the structures in which we are interested in flattening, in particular the brain hemispheres. Let $\Sigma \subset \mathbf{R}^3$ represent this brain model which we assume is an embedded surface (no self-intersections) of genus zero. In this section, since we will be giving the analytical solution to the uniformization problem, we assume that Σ is a smooth manifold. For the finite element method described in the next section, it will be enough to take it as a triangulated surface. (We refer the reader to [10] for the basic theory of uniformization of Riemann surfaces, and to [16] for the solutions of elliptic PDE's and the Dirichlet problem.) Fix a point p on this surface. Let δ_p denote the Dirac delta (impulse) function at p, Δ the Laplace-Beltrami operator on $\Sigma \backslash \{p\}$, and i the square root of -1. The Laplace-Beltrami operator is the generalization of the usual Laplacian operator to a smooth surface. Let S^2 denote the unit sphere in $\mathbf{R}^3$ and let $\mathbf{C}$ be the complex plane.

The following result provides the analytical basis for our brain mapping procedure:

A conformal equivalence $z : \Sigma \backslash \{p\} \to S^2 \backslash \{\text{north pole}\}$ may be obtained by solving the equation

$$\Delta z = \left(\frac{\partial}{\partial u} - i \frac{\partial}{\partial v} \right) \delta_p. \tag{1}$$

Here, u and v are conformal coordinates defined in a neighborhood of p. Further, we are identifying $S^2 \backslash \{\text{north pole}\}$ with the complex plane in the standard way from complex analysis, say via stereographic projection. This result means that we can get the conformal equivalence by solving a second order partial differential equation on the surface. Fortunately, on a triangulated surface, this may be carried out using a finite element technique we will describe below.

3   Finite Element Approximation of Conformal Mapping

We now describe a numerical procedure for solving (1), assuming that Σ is a triangulated surface. Using the notation of the previous section, let $\sigma = ABC$ be the triangle in whose interior the point p lies.

3.1   Functional Interpretation

The first step in the solution of (1) is to interpret $\left(\frac{\partial}{\partial u} - i\frac{\partial}{\partial v}\right)\delta_p$ as a functional on an appropriate space of functions, in our case the finite-dimensional space $PL(\Sigma)$ of piecewise linear functions on Σ. For any function f smooth in a neighborhood of p, one has

$$\int\int_\Sigma f\left(\frac{\partial}{\partial u} - i\frac{\partial}{\partial v}\right)\delta_p dS = -\left(\frac{\partial f}{\partial u} - i\frac{\partial f}{\partial v}\right)|_p,$$

and for $f \in PL(\Sigma)$, this last quantity is completely determined by the value of f at $A, B,$ and C.

Choose the u and the v axes so that A and B are along the u axis, and the positive v axis points towards C. Let E be the orthogonal projection of C on AB. Then for $f \in PL(\Sigma)$, and $\theta = \frac{\langle C - A, B - A, \rangle}{\|B - A\|^2}$, we have

$$\int\int_\Sigma f\left(\frac{\partial}{\partial u} - i\frac{\partial}{\partial v}\right)\delta_p dS = \frac{f_A}{\|B - A\|} - \frac{f_B}{\|B - A\|} + i\frac{f_C - (f_A + \theta(f_B - f_A))}{|C - E\|}.$$

3.2   Finite Elements

We briefly outline the finite element method for finding our approximation to z. The heart of the method simply involves the solution of a system of linear equations [12].

One may show that z satisfies (1) if and only if for all smooth test functions f, we have

$$\int\int_\Sigma \nabla z \cdot \nabla f dS = \left(\frac{\partial f}{\partial u} - i\frac{\partial f}{\partial v}\right)|_p. \tag{2}$$

This formulation is the key to the finite element approximation of the solution to (1) on the triangulated surface Σ. We restrict our attention to $PL(\Sigma)$, and seek a $z \in PL(\Sigma)$ such that (2) holds for all $f \in PL(\Sigma)$.

For each vertex $P \in \Sigma$, let ϕ_P be the continuous function which is linear on each triangle, has the value 1 at P, and is zero at all other vertices. Then these ϕ_P form a basis for $PL(\Sigma)$, and we seek a z of the form $z = \sum z_P \phi_P$, for some vector of complex numbers $(z_P), P \in \Sigma$. Further, since (2) is linear in f, it is enough to show that (2) holds whenever $f = \phi_Q$ for some Q.

Thus we want to find a vector $z = (z_P)$ such that for all Q,

$$\sum_P z_P \int\int \nabla\phi_P \cdot \nabla\phi_Q dS = \frac{\partial\phi_Q}{\partial u}(p) - i\frac{\partial\phi_Q}{\partial v}(p). \tag{3}$$

3.3 Formulation in Matrix Terms

The formulation (3) is simply a system of linear equations in the complex unknowns z_P. Accordingly, we introduce the matrix (D_{PQ}), where

$$D_{PQ} = \int \int \nabla \phi_P \cdot \nabla \phi_Q dS,$$

for each pair of vertices P, Q. Note that $D_{PQ} \neq 0$ only if P and Q are connected
by some edge in the triangulation. Thus the matrix D is sparse.

Suppose PQ is an edge belonging to two triangles, PQR, and PQS. A formula
from finite-element theory [12], easily verified with basic calculus, says that

$$D_{PQ} = -\frac{1}{2} \{\cot \angle R + \cot \angle S\}, \quad P \neq Q, \tag{4}$$

where $\angle R$ is the angle at the vertex R in the triangle PQR, and $\angle S$ is the angle
at the vertex S in the triangle PQS. The formula for the diagonal elements of
D is (see [1])

$$D_{PP} = -\sum_{P \neq Q} D_{PQ}. \tag{5}$$

Introducing vectors $a = (a_Q) = (\frac{\partial \phi_Q}{\partial u}(p))$ and $b = (b_Q) = (\frac{\partial \phi_Q}{\partial v}(p))$, equation
(3), becomes, in matrix terms,

$$Dx = a, \quad Dy = -b, \tag{6}$$

where, using our formula for $(\frac{\partial}{\partial u} - i\frac{\partial}{\partial v}) \delta_p$ derived in Section 3.1, we have

$$a_Q - ib_Q := \begin{cases} 0 & Q \notin \{A, B, C\}, \\ \frac{-1}{\|B-A\|} + i\frac{1-\theta}{\|C-E\|} & Q = A, \\ \frac{1}{\|B-A\|} + i\frac{\theta}{\|C-E\|} & Q = B, \\ i\frac{-1}{\|C-E\|} & Q = C. \end{cases} \tag{7}$$

4 Experimental Results

We tested our algorithm by flattening the brain surface contained in a $256 \times 256 \times 124$ MR brain image provided by the Surgical Planning Laboratory of Brigham
and Women's Hospital in Boston. These consist of sagittal T1 weighted gradient
echo images of a patient with a brain tumor. We chose a brain with a tumor to
illustrate the effect of the flattening on both normal and pathological features
in an MR brain set.

First, using the segmentation algorithm of [4, 14, 18], we found the brain
cortical surface, i.e the gray matter/CSF interface. The VTK Toolkit [17] was
then used to obtain a triangularization of the surface, which we proceeded to
smooth slightly to reduce the effects of aliasing. This was done by using the
flow according to mean curvature. A morphological based method was used to
remove any minute handles on the surface formed by the segmentation process.

We then used the method described in the previous sections to find a flattening map to the plane and then composed this map with a map from the plane to the unit sphere using standard inverse stereographic projection. This composition gives us a bijective conformal map from the surface to the sphere.

Note that it is not practical to view the planar mapping directly in its entirety, because stereographic projection stretches areas near the north pole too much to be useful. In fact it is not possible to map a sphere, a nearly complete sphere, or any other similarly shaped surface to the plane in any way without major distortion. However, smaller surface patches may be mapped to the plane with a more reasonable amount of distortion, and in fact the "best" (in terms of length distortion) mapping to the plane from a sphere with a geodesic disk removed is known. In practice, we have not found the distortion of area near the north pole to be a problem in solving the linear equations for our flattening map. The method seems to be stable across a wide variety of surface shapes and varying fineness of triangulations.

After flattening the brain surface, we used mean curvature to color corresponding points on the two surfaces (the lighter the point the higher the mean curvature on the brain surface). This provided us with an effective way to see how the flattening process acted on the gyral lines of the brain surface. This is shown in Figure 2, which provides two views of the cortical surface and the corresponding areas on the sphere. Note the tumor on the right parietal lobe visible in the vertex view. It is interesting to see how the conformality of the mapping from the brain surface to the sphere results in a flattened image which is locally very similar in appearance to the original.

Next, we tested our process on the more highly convoluted surface which is defined by the boundary between the white and gray matter within the brain. To extract this boundary, we used a combination of the method based on smoothing posterior probabilities as described in [19], and the segmentation method described in [4, 14, 18]. (See also [13, 21, 22], and the references therein for other approaches to brain segmentation.) Once the surface was obtained, our flattening method was applied exactly as it was for the cortical surface. The result of this process is shown in Figure 3. Note that much of the white matter surface is hidden within its deep convolutions, but that such areas on the sphere are clearly visible.

We point out that inverting the flattening map allows us easily to establish orthogonal coordinates on the surface as is seen in Figure 4. Further, the method allows us to find north and south poles on a highly convoluted surface such as the brain, giving an alternative method to that discussed in [3].

5   Conclusions

In this paper, we described a general method based on a discretization of the Laplace-Beltrami operator for flattening a surface in a manner which preserves the local geometry. The approach can be carried out using a finite element method which takes into account the special boundary conditions. We also illustrated the technique on the brain surface and white matter of an MR brain data set.

In addition to flattening the cortical surface, we have several other applications in mind including 3D colon and bladder flattening, automatic texture mappings, and image registration. We are very hopeful that our techniques will be useful for such problems as well.

References

1. S. Angenent, S. Haker, A. Tannenbaum, and R. Kikinis, "Laplace-Beltrami operator and surface unfolding," submitted to *IEEE Trans. on Medical Imaging*.
2. S. Angenent, S. Haker, A. Tannenbaum, and R. Kikinis, "On area preserving mappings of surfaces with minimal distortion," in prepartion.
3. C. Brechbühler, G. Gerig, and O. Kübler, "Parametrization of closed surfaces for 3D shape description," Technical Report, Communication Technology Laboratory, ETH, Zürich, Switzerland, 1996.
4. V. Caselles, R. Kimmel, and G. Sapiro, , "Geodesic snakes," *Int. Journal of Computer Vision*, 1997.
5. A. Dale and M. Sereno, "Improved localization of cortical activity by combining EEG and MEG with MRI cortical surface reconstruction: a linear approach," *Journal of Cognitive Neuroscience* 5 (1993), pp. 162-176.
6. C. Davatzikos and R. N. Bryan, "Using a deformable surface model to obtain a shape representation of the cortex," *IEEE Transactions on Medical Imaging*, 15, (1996), pp. 785-795.
7. H. Drury, D. van Essen, C. Anderson, C. Lee, T. Coogan, and J. Lewis, "Computerized mappings of the cerebral cortex: a multiresolution flattening method and a surface-based coordinate system," *Journal of Cognitive Neuroscience* 8 (1996), pp. 1-28.
8. M. P. Do Carmo, *Differential Geometry of Curves and Surfaces*, Prentice-Hall, Inc., New Jersey, 1976.
9. S. Haker, S. Angenent, A. Tannenbaum, R. Kikinis, G. Sapiro, and M. Halle, "Conformal surface parametrization for texture mappings," Technical Report, Department of Electrical and Computer Engineering, University of Minnesota, January 1999.
10. H. Farkas and I. Kra, *Riemann Surfaces*, Springer-Verlag, New York 1991.
11. I. Hollander, "Cerebral cartography - A method for visualizing cortical structures," *Computerized Medical Imaging and Graphics*, 19, (1995), pp. 397-415.
12. T. Hughes, *The Finite Element Method*, Prentice-Hall, New Jersey, 1987.
13. T. Kapur, W. Grimson, W. Wells III, and R. Kikinis, "Segmentation of brain tissue from magnetic resonance images," *Medical Image Analysis* 1 (1996), pp. 109-127.
14. S. Kichenasamy, A. Kumar, P. Olver, A. Tannenbaum, A. Yezzi, "Conformal curvature flows: from phase transitions to active contours," *Archive Rational Mechanics and Analysis* 134 (1996), pp. 275-301.
15. D. MacDonald, D. D. Avis, A. C. and Evans, "Multiple surface identification and matching in magnetic resonance images," in *Visualization in Biomedical Computing,* edited by R. Robb, SPIE Publications, vol. 2359, 1994, pp. 160-169.
16. J. Rauch, *Partial Differential Equations*, Springer-Verlag, New York 1991.
17. W. Schroeder, H. Martin, B. Lorensen, *The Visualization Toolkit*, Prentice-Hall, New Jersey, 1996.

17. W. Schroeder, H. Martin, B. Lorensen, *The Visualization Toolkit*, Prentice-Hall, New Jersey, 1996.
18. K. Siddiqi, A. Tannenbaum, and S. Zucker, "Area and length minimizing flows for image segmentation," *IEEE Trans. Image Processing* **7** (1998), pp. 433-444.
19. P. Teo, G. Sapiro, and B. A. Wandell, "Creating connected representations of cortical gray matter for functional MRI visualization," *IEEE Transactions on Medical Imaging*, 1998.
20. B. Wandell, S. Engel, and H. Hel-Or, "Creating images of the flattened cortical sheet," *Invest. Opth. and Vis. Sci.* **36** (S612), 1996.
21. C. Xu, D. Pham, and J. Prince, "Reconstruction of the central layer of the human cerebral cortex from MR images," *Medical Image Computing and Computer-Assisted Intervention*, Springer-Verlag, pp. 481-488, 1998.
22. X. Zeng, L. Staib, R. Schultz, and J. Duncan, "Volumetric layer segmentation using coupled surfaces propagation," *Computer Vision and Pattern Recognition*, pp. 708-715, 1998.

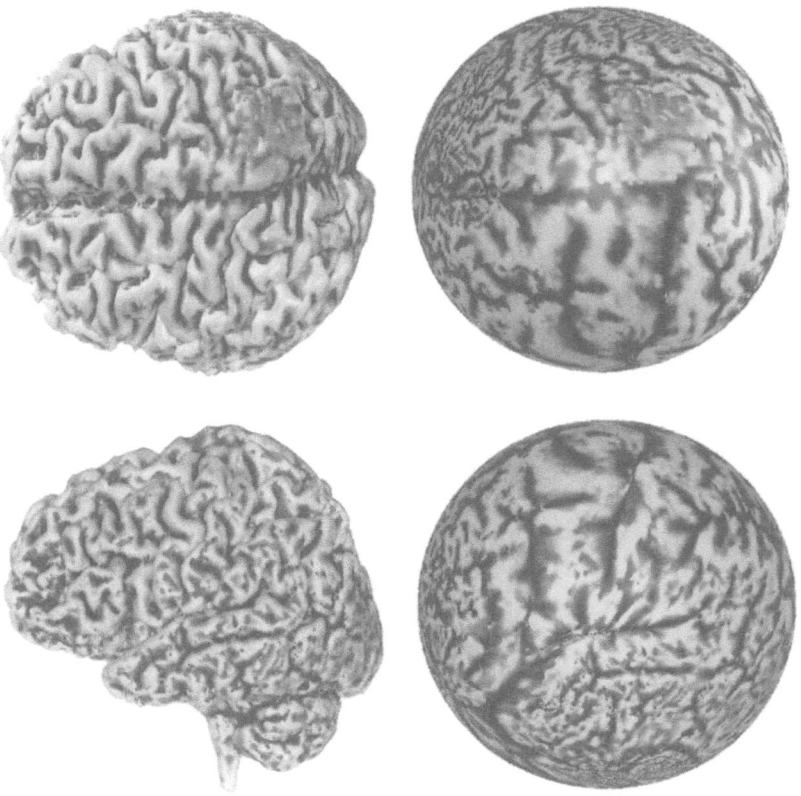

Fig. 1. Two Views of the Flattened Brain Surface

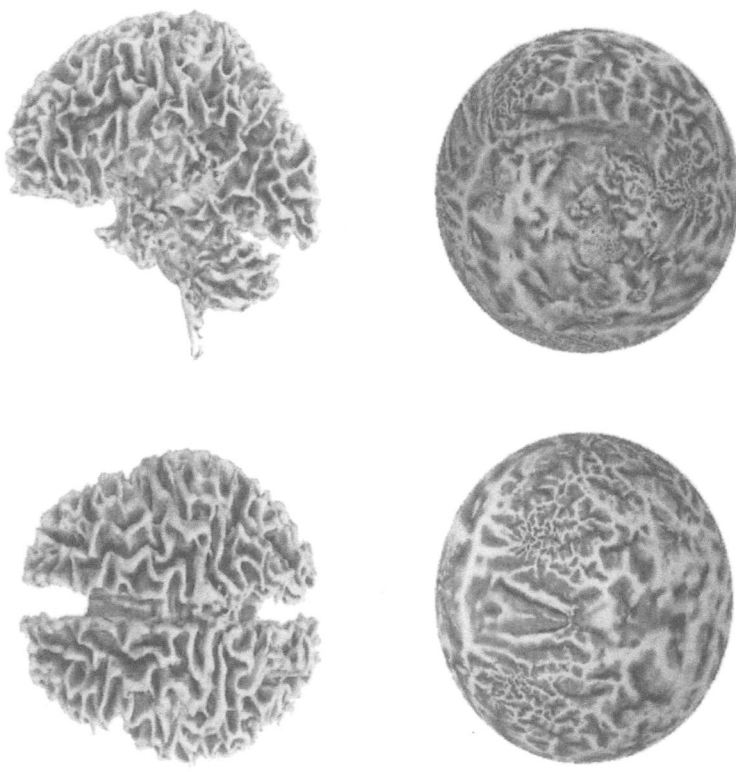

Fig. 2. Two Views of the Flattened White Matter

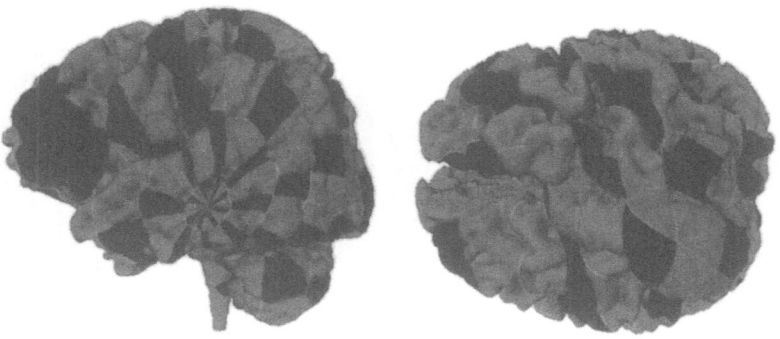

Fig. 3. Orthogonal Grid on Brain Surface

Quasi-Conformally Flat Mapping
the Human Cerebellum

Monica K. Hurdal[1], Philip L. Bowers[1], Ken Stephenson[2], De Witt L. Sumners[1], Kelly Rehm[3,4], Kirt Schaper[3], and David A. Rottenberg[3,4]

[1] Dept. of Mathematics, Florida State University, Tallahassee, FL 32306-4510, U.S.A.
mhurdal@math.fsu.edu   http://www.math.fsu.edu/~mhurdal
[2] Dept. of Mathematics, University of Tennessee, Knoxville, TN 37996-1300, U.S.A.
[3] PET Imaging Center, VA Medical Center, Minneapolis, MN, 55417, U.S.A.
[4] Dept. of Radiology, University of Minnesota, Minneapolis, MN, 55455, U.S.A.

Abstract. We present a novel approach to creating flat maps of the brain. It is impossible to flatten a curved surface in 3D space without metric and areal distortion; however, the Riemann Mapping Theorem implies that it is theoretically possible to preserve conformal (angular) information under flattening. Our approach attempts to preserve the conformal structure between the original cortical surface in 3-space and the flattened surface. We demonstrate this with data from the human cerebellum and we produce maps in the conventional Euclidean plane, as well as in the hyperbolic plane and on a sphere. Conformal mappings are uniquely determined once certain normalizations have been chosen, and this allows one to impose a coordinate system on the surface when flattening in the hyperbolic or spherical setting. Unlike existing methods, our approach does **not** require that cuts be introduced in the original surface. In addition, hyperbolic and spherical maps allow the map focus to be transformed interactively to correspond to any anatomical landmark.

1 Introduction

The human brain can be divided into regions based on function and anatomy [16]. These divisions are generally determined by the location of folds (gyri) and fissures (sulci) in the cortical surface. However, the surface of the brain is extremely convoluted, with considerable anatomical variability between individuals. The combination of fold complexity with anatomical variability makes it difficult to compare anatomical and functional information within and between subjects. Current visualization and comparison techniques do not satisfactorily overcome these difficulties. For example, functional (PET, fMRI, etc.) data can be projected onto a rendering of the cortical surface extracted from a coregistered magnetic resonance (MR) volume. Individual differences in cortical folding make it difficult to compare the location and extent of activated foci. Foci buried in deep sulci may appear on the cortical surface and widely separated foci on opposite walls of a sulcus may appear to be close together.

Interestingly, the surface representing the cortical grey matter is topologically equivalent to a two-dimensional sheet. Thus, it is possible to unfold or flatten this surface to create a 2D flat map of the cortex. This surface-based approach can assist in visualizing and comparing cortical folding patterns and help to resolve some of the problems which exist in traditional visualization techniques.

A number of computational tools have been developed to take advantage of this surface-based approach. Drury *et al.* [7] have developed an approach that attempts to reduce the areal and angular distortion between the original cortical surface in 3D space and the flattened surface in 2D space. This is accomplished by iteratively applying torsional and longitudinal forces to adjust the edge lengths in the mesh. Fischl *et al.* [8] create a flat map by reducing geodesic distance distortion while attempting to prevent folds in the flattened surface. Both techniques have been used successfully in several comparative and functional investigation studies [5, 6, 13–15].

In this paper we present a novel flat mapping approach that attempts to preserve the conformal structure between the original cortical surface and the flattened surface. There are two real advantages to using conformal flattening as opposed to others. First, it is completely canonical, meaning that such flattenings are uniquely determined once certain standard normalizations have been chosen. In particular, it requires no ad hoc cutting of the surface as do some of the previously described methods for surface flattening [7, 8]. Second, the flattening can be done in either the Euclidean plane or in the hyperbolic plane, and the surface can also be mapped conformally onto a sphere. Though the setting of the hyperbolic plane might seem merely incidental and of little practical value, its use allows the map origin to be transformed interactively so that different anatomical landmarks can be used as the map focus. This has the advantage of bringing into sharp relief areas of interest, but at the cost of relegating the region far removed from the origin to the periphery, where our Euclidean eyes cannot focus. The primary disadvantage of conformal flattening is that there is no attempt to control either the metric or areal distortion; indeed, there can be no such control as the conformal flattening is canonical and offers no such opportunity without the loss of conformality.

2   Quasi-Conformal Flattening

In constructing flat mappings of anatomical surfaces such as the cerebellum, one is faced with two major problems. The first is that one must take the raw 3D scan data and use it to produce a mesh of the 2D surface of interest. Computational triangulation methods usually result in a topologically complicated surface replete with local artifacts caused by several factors, including the peculiarities of certain standard algorithms and software packages (e.g. the marching cubes algorithm) and insufficient spatial resolution of the data. These local artifacts must be removed by slicing, patching and retriangulating the surface until a simply connected 2D mesh is obtained in 3D space that conforms to the surface of interest. In this section, we are concerned with the second major problem — that of flattening the highly convoluted mesh that conforms to the original surface once it has been converted into a topologically defect-free piecewise flat surface in 3D space. There is no way to flatten a curved 3D surface without metric and areal distortion [11]; however, there is one type of geometric information that, at least theoretically, can be preserved under flattening, namely conformal (angular) information encoded in the surface.

Our starting point is a piecewise flat triangulated surface in 3D space that is topologically a 2D disk. The 3D space coordinates of the vertices of each triangle of the mesh are given, and each edge of the mesh is either an interior edge contained in exactly two triangles, or a boundary edge contained in exactly one triangle. There is one boundary component — a single closed chain of boundary edges forming the boundary of the surface. Technically, this piecewise flat surface carries the structure of a Riemann surface (described below), and by the Riemann Mapping Theorem [1] it conformally maps onto any proper simply connected region in the complex plane. Our job is to describe a tool for producing (approximations to) these conformal mappings.

2.1   Riemann Surfaces

The technical description of a Riemann surface is in terms of a complex atlas: a collection of local mappings that provide local complex coordinates on the surface so that overlap mappings are analytic [2]. Rather than going into a detailed technical description for the uninitiated reader, it serves our purposes to understand that a Riemann surface provides a consistent way to measure angles that gives a full angle measure of 2π around each interior point, including interior vertices. For piecewise flat surfaces where all but the finitely many vertices have small neighborhoods isometric to disks in the Euclidean plane, the measure of an angle based at a point other than one of the triangle vertices is just the Euclidean measure of that angle. For an angle based at a vertex the measure determined by the complex atlas of the Riemann surface is the Euclidean measure linearly rescaled so that the total angle measure is 2π. Explicitly, denote by $\Theta(v)$ the **angle sum** about the vertex v, i.e. the sum of the Euclidean measures of the angles with vertex v from all of the triangles of the triangulation that contain v. The scale factor used at v for measuring angles is then $\frac{2\pi}{\Theta(v)}$. Hence, an angle with vertex v in our surface that has Euclidean measure θ will be found to have measure $\frac{2\pi\theta}{\Theta(v)}$ in the complex atlas of the Riemann surface. A **conformal mapping** of a Riemann surface to another one is a continuous locally one-to-one function that preserves all angle measures. Hence a conformal mapping from our piecewise flat surface to the complex plane is one that preserves the Euclidean angle measures at non-vertices, and maps neighborhoods of the vertices in such a way that the "market share" of angles is preserved, i.e. an angle based at vertex v of Euclidean measure θ has image an angle of Euclidean measure $\frac{2\pi\theta}{\Theta(v)}$ under any conformal mapping to the plane.

2.2   Approximating Conformal Mappings using Circle Packings

Our scheme for approximating conformal mappings of a piecewise flat surface to flat maps in the plane uses circle packings. Given a triangulation K of a disk, a

circle packing for K is a collection $\mathcal{C}_K = \{C(v): v \text{ is a vertex of } K\}$ of circles in the plane, one circle for each vertex v of K, with the property that circles $C(v)$ and $C(w)$ are tangent whenever the vertices v and w form an edge of K. The **Circle Packing Theorem** of [4] states that given any disk triangulation K and any assignment of positive numbers $r(v_1), \cdots, r(v_n)$ to the n **boundary** vertices $v_1, \cdots, v_n$ of K, there is a unique (up to Euclidean isometry) circle packing in the plane with boundary circle $C(v_i)$ having radius $r(v_i)$, for $i = 1, \cdots, n$.

Our first attempt to approximate conformal mappings uses these circle packings in the following way. Starting with a piecewise flat surface in 3D space, collect the combinatorial data from the surface in an abstract triangulation K. This is merely a list of the vertices of the surface (not their 3-space coordinates), the pairs of vertices in edges, and the (oriented) triples of vertices in triangular faces. Assign positive numbers to the boundary vertices (perhaps set all equal to one, or to the average of the lengths of the two edges containing a given vertex) and find the unique circle packing $\mathcal{C}_K$ guaranteed by the Circle Packing Theorem. The packing $\mathcal{C}_K$ serves the role of our flat mapping of the surface and the question is how well this **circle packing mapping** approximates a conformal mapping. We certainly do not expect the mapping to be conformal since none of the conformal data of the piecewise flat surface are used in constructing the circle packing — it is only the combinatorial data along with arbitrary boundary radii assignments that are used in constructing the circle packing. Nonetheless, the **Ring Lemma** of [12] applies to guarantee that this circle packing mapping is **quasi-conformal**, meaning that there is but a bounded amount of percentage angular distortion. To obtain closer approximations to the actual conformal mappings requires certain modifications of the circle packing routine that are designed to reduce the quasi-conformal distortion. Unfortunately, space considerations prevent a description of the necessary modifications and details will appear elsewhere.

2.3   Flat Maps in the Hyperbolic Plane

This approximation scheme works just as well in the hyperbolic plane as in the Euclidean plane (i.e. the complex plane $\mathbf{C}$). There is a version of the Circle Packing Theorem for the hyperbolic plane where hyperbolic radii are used as well as hyperbolic lines and triangles [4]. The **Poincaré disk** model of the hyperbolic plane [3] consists of the unit disk $\Delta = \{z \in \mathbf{C}: |z| < 1\}$ with metric determined by the line element $ds = \frac{2|dz|}{1-|z|^2}$, the Euclidean line element $|dz| = (dx^2 + dy^2)^{1/2}$ scaled by twice the reciprocal of $1 - |z|^2$. This means that the hyperbolic angle measures are the same as the Euclidean angle measures, but the hyperbolic distances are distorted when seen through our Euclidean eyes by constant hyperbolic lengths appearing smaller and smaller as the segment moves toward the unit circle boundary of Δ. We may apply the circle packing routine described previously, using hyperbolic measurements rather than Euclidean, and obtain quasi-conformal mappings of our piecewise flat surfaces to the hyperbolic plane. The portions of the flat mapping lying near the boundary unit circle are greatly distorted to our Euclidean eyes (though not so distorted to hyperbolic eyes), but the portions lying near the origin have small distortion in comparison. The nice feature of this is that one may arbitrarily choose what vertex of our surface should be mapped to the origin. This way, different portions of the original surface can be brought into focus with more distant portions relegated to the edges, and this can be automated easily to provide an interactive tool for viewing local features of interest on our surface. Extensions that allow interactive quasi-conformal spherical mappings are also available.

3   Flattening the Cerebellum

We obtained a high resolution MRI scan from the Montreal Neurological Institute, which was produced by registering and intensity averaging a series of 27 T1 weighted images from a single subject [9]. This volume is composed of isovoxels and has dimension 217^3. We chose to flatten the cerebellum in an effort to facilitate the description of activated cerebellar foci in functional neuroimaging.

The cerebellum was extracted from the MRI volume by defining a plane parallel to the posterior commissure-obex line and orthogonal to a plane passing through the vermal midline. Cortical regions defined by various lobes and fissures were color coded for identification purposes. We produced a triangulated surface representing the cerebellar surface using the marching cubes algorithm [10]. The output of this surface was checked for any topological errors and corrected as necessary. This triangulated mesh is topologically equivalent to a sphere as all edges in the surface occur exactly twice. This surface is composed of 41804 triangles with 20904 vertices and 62706 edges and is illustrated in Fig. 1. We introduced a single closed chain of boundary edges in the surface based around the brainstem and walls and apex of the fourth ventricle to act as the boundary of the flattened map. This mesh, representing the surface of the cerebellum, is a piecewise flat simply connected surface that is topologically equivalent to a disk.

Our quasi-conformal flattening procedure was applied to this surface to produce a number of flat maps. Firstly, in Fig. 2 we present the flat map that was created in the Euclidean plane. In this case, the circles for the boundary vertices were assigned a radius which was the average of the lengths of the two boundary edges containing that vertex. As with flat maps produced by other researchers [7,8], the shape of this map is largely determined by the length and number of edges in the chosen boundary and will vary in shape from map to map.

Fig. 2 also illustrates a spherical mapping, where two arbitrary points may be chosen as the north and south poles and no cuts need be introduced. This representation may be more natural for some anatomical shapes.

Flat maps that were created in the hyperbolic plane are illustrated in Fig. 3. There are a number of important features to note about these maps. Since we look at these maps with Euclidean eyes, portions of the map lying near the origin have small distortion and appear similar to those on a Euclidean map. However, regions of the map lying near the boundary of the unit circle (map border) are greatly distorted. Nevertheless, we are able to move the focus of the hyperbolic map to change the regions which are in focus and which are relegated to the map edges (with large distortion). This is the difference between the hyperbolic maps in Fig. 3. These transformations can be performed in real computation time by simply indicating the new map origin. Another feature of the hyperbolic maps is the boundary shape corresponds to the unit circle. This facilitates comparison of different maps. A coordinate system can easily be imposed by specifying two points, or a point and a direction. We do not need to introduce multiple cuts in the surface (other than the boundary); and perhaps most importantly, the maps are mathematically unique (up to certain transformations). The utility of quasi-conformal maps for studying functional imaging data is yet to be determined, but we believe these features will produce favorable results.

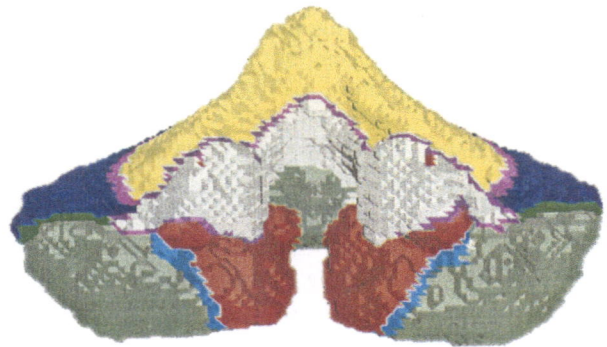

Fig. 1. Surface Representing the Cerebellum. Colors correspond to the following cortical regions: forest green = lobulus semilunaris, lobulus semilunaris inferior, lobulus biventer; red = tonsils, flocculus; yellow = lingula, lobus centralis, lobulus quadrangularis; blue = lobulus simplex, lobulus semilunaris superior; grey = white matter; bright green = fissura prima; cyan = fissura secunda; magenta = fissura horizontalis; purple = boundary used for flat maps.

4   Discussion

We have introduced a novel approach to unfolding and flattening the cortical surface which attempts to preserve the conformal structure of the original surface in 3-space. Our approach offers a number of advantages over existing approaches including:

- conformal mappings control and minimize angular distortion
- conformal mappings are canonical, and hence mathematically unique
- cutting of the original surface is not required to reduce distortion
- flattening can be done in the Euclidean and hyperbolic planes and mapping to a sphere is also possible

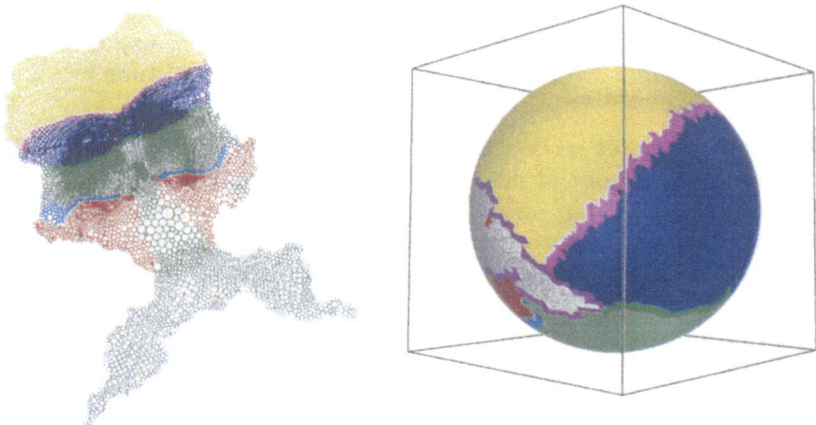

Fig. 2. Euclidean Flat Map and Spherical Map of the Cerebellar Surface. Colors correspond to regions shown in Fig. 1. A boundary is required to create a flap map of the cerebellum (left figure); however, the cerebellar surface is topologically equivalent to a sphere, so no boundary is required to quasi-conformally map it to the surface of sphere.

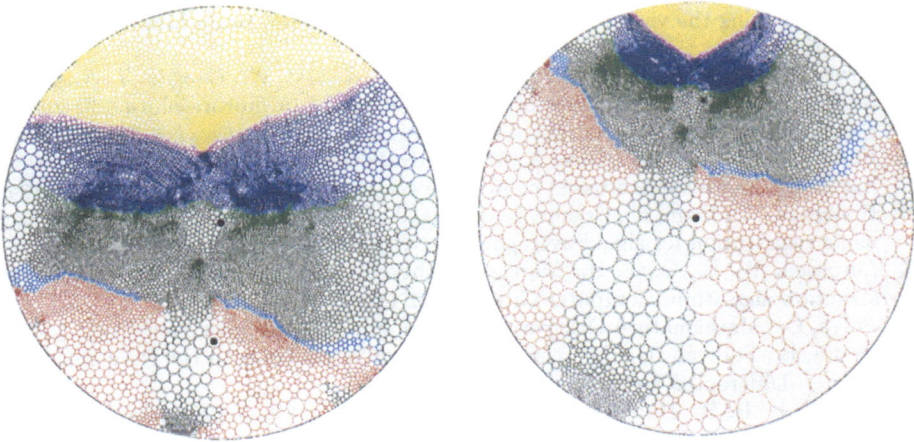

Fig. 3. Hyperbolic Flat Maps of the Cerebellar Surface. Colors correspond to regions shown in Fig. 1. The origin (map focus) is marked in black in the center of the maps. The map on the right has been transformed to a different map focus to display regions in the lower portion of the map. The black circle located near the bottom of the left map is used as the map origin in the right map. Similarly, the black circle located near the top of the right map corresponds to the map focus of the left map.

- a coordinate system can be easily imposed on the hyperbolic maps
- the map origin in the hyperbolic plane can be transformed interactively to change the map focus and alter the primary locations of map distortion
- computation times are on the order of minutes with real time user interaction.

Our approach produces quasi-conformal maps which may allow us to better localize functional regions of activation in normal subjects and patients with ataxia and other hereditary diseases. We are currently working on extensions that will produce closer approximations to the true conformal mapping.

This work is supported in part by NIH grants MH57180 and NS33718.

References

1. Ahlfors, L. V.: Complex Analysis. McGraw-Hill Book Company, New York, 1966
2. Beardon, A. F.: A Primer on Riemann Surfaces. Cambridge University Press, Cambridge, 1984, LMS Lecture Notes 78
3. Beardon, A. F.: An introduction to hyperbolic geometry, in Ergodic Theory, Symbolic Dynamics, and Hyperbolic Spaces, T. Bedford, M. Keane, and C. Series, eds., Oxford University Press, Oxford, 1991, ch. 11, pp. 1–34
4. Beardon, A. F., Stephenson K.: The uniformization theorem for circle packings. Indiana Univ. Math. J. **39** (1990) 1383–1425
5. Corbetta, M.: Frontoparietal cortical networks for directing attention and the eye to visual locations: Identical, independent, or overlapping neural systems? Proc. Natl. Acad. Sci. USA. **95** (1998) 831–838
6. Drury, H .A., Van Essen, D. C.: Functional specializations in human cerebral cortex analyzed using the visible man surface-based atlas. Hum. Brain Mapping 5 (1997) 233–237
7. Drury, H .A., Van Essen, D. C., Anderson, C. H., Lee, C. W., Coogan, T. A., Lewis, J. W.: Computerized mappings of the cerebral cortex: A multiresolution flattening method and a surface-based coordinate system. J. Cog. Neurosci. **8** (1996) 1–28
8. Fischl, B., Sereno, M. I., Dale, A. M.: Cortical surface-based analysis II: Inflation, flattening, and a surface-based coordinate system. Neuroimage **9** (1999) 179–194
9. Holmes, C. J., Hoge, R., Collins, L., Evans, A. C.: Enhancement of T1 MR images using registration for signal averaging. J. Neurosci. **3** (1996) S28, Part 2 of 2
10. Lorensen, W. E., Cline, H.: Marching cubes: A high resolution 3D surface construction algorithm. Computer Graphics **21** (1987) 163–169
11. Polya, G.: Mathematical Discovery, vol. 2. John Wiley & Sons, New York, 1968
12. Rodin, B., Sullivan, D.: The convergence of circle packings to the Riemann mapping. J. Differential Geometry **26** (1987) 349–360
13. Tootell, R. B. H., Hadjikhani, N. K., Vanduffel, W., Liu, A. K., Mendola, J. D., Sereno, M. I., Dale, A. M.: Functional analysis of primary visual cortex (V1) in humans. Proc. Natl. Acad. Sci. USA. **95** (1998) 811–817
14. Tootell, R. B. H., Mendola, J. D., Hadjikhani, N. K., Liu, A. K., Dale, A. M.: The representation of the ipsilateral visual field in human cerebral cortex. Proc. Natl. Acad. Sci. USA. **95** (1998) 818–824
15. Van Essen, D. C., Drury, H. A., Joshi, S., Miller, M. I.: Functional and structural mapping of human cerebral cortex: Solutions are in the surfaces. Proc. Natl. Acad. Sci. USA. **95** (1998) 788–795
16. Zeki, S.: A Vision of the Brain. Blackwell Scientific Publications, Oxford, 1993

Rendering the Unfolded Cerebral Cortex

Junfeng Guo[1], Alexandru Salomie[2], Rudi Deklerck[2], and Jan Cornelis[2]

[1] Shanghai Jiaotong University, Institute of IPPR, 200030 Shanghai, China
[2] Vrije Universiteit Brussel, Dept. ETRO-IRIS, Pleinlaan 2, 1050 Brussels, Belgium

Abstract. Classical volume rendering is computed by casting a bundle of parallel rays from a flat viewing plane onto the volume data set, and produces as such a spatially limited view of the objects in the data set. The method described in this paper is able to generate an overall planar view of an object that is topologically compatible with the sphere, by firing rays from a nearby surrounding surface and by unfolding this surface in a 2D plane, without introducing major distortions. It has been devised to facilitate the interpretation of the cerebral cortex. An initial surface consisting of two hemi-ellipsoids, one to cover the top and another one to surround the bottom of the brain, is interactively defined and deformed via a deformable model approach towards a dilated version of the cortical surface of the brain. During deformation, the nodes on the surface are continuously redistributed, to maintain a near homothetic mapping with the plane. Once the surface has converged to the dilated brain surface, rays are casted from the nodes, according to the normal of the surface at the node. The shading result, computed at the intersection of the rays with the original brain surface, is mapped via the near homothetic mapping to the plane. With this approach sulci can be followed in their entirety, so that it is much easier to derive their spatial relationship and to recognize them.

1 Introduction

The idea of producing two-dimensional cortical maps dates from the seventies [1][2]. At that time, a purely manual approach was used to attempt preserving measures of length, angle or area. Later on, computerised methods have been designed: Dale and Sereno [3] apply an iterated smoothing of the cortical surface, that only preserves neighbourhood relationships on the cortex. The most powerful methods are designed to keep geometric distortions as small as possible. Optimally, one should try to construct an isometric mapping, between the cortical surface and the plane, but as known from differential geometry this mapping only exists between surfaces which have the same Gaussian curvature K. As the plane has a constant Gaussian curvature K equal to zero and K is quite variable for the cortical surface, it is only possible to make an approximate isometric mapping.

Schwarz et al. [4][5] start from a triangular mesh and try to optimally preserve the metric structure of this mesh, represented as a distance matrix with elements

(i, j) equal to the shortest distance along the edges of the mesh between the vertices i and j. They use the Newton-Raphson method to maximise the goodness of fit between the distance matrix of the original surface and the distance matrix of the planar configuration. It is evident that this exhaustive calculation of all possible paths must lead to a good estimate of the global metrical characteristics of the surface, but this is achieved at the cost of an enormous computational load and combinatorial complexity. Therefore Schwartz et al. [4][5] divide the surface in overlapping patches of about 300 vertices.

Another solution to reduce the computational complexity, is to work only with first- or second-order nearest neighbour distances. However this approach is not always stable, as the normals of the patches may reverse in the planar configuration. In [6], this folding over of the facets in the plane is countered by introducing an additional error term in the residual energy functional. Since the distance matrix has now become a sparse matrix, a more efficient minimisation scheme based on the conjugate gradient approach can be devised.

Carman et al. [7] create two-dimensional maps of the cortex by modelling it as an elastic sheet whose internal forces act to preserve the topology and geometry of the sheet, while external forces act to unfold and flatten it. The unfolding force is designed to drive the overall surface into a planar configuration and to act against internal forces attempting to maintain intrinsic curvature or local folding. The internal forces are a longitudinal force and a torsional force which together model the elastic properties of the surface. The longitudinal force acts towards restoring the lengths between adjacent nodes of the triangular mesh to their reference values, while the torsional force attempts to preserve angles. All forces acting on a node N are based on a geometric relationship with the immediate neighbours of the node N.

In all the previously mentioned approaches the initial mesh on the cortical surface is constructed without taking into account any relationship with the plane, where it will be flattened. The flattening technique used in this paper, which is based on the concept of homothetic mapping described in [8], directly starts from a plane and keeps track how the points in the plane are distributing themselves on the cortical surface after several steps of deformation. This approach has the additional advantage that a very uniform triangular mesh can be obtained after convergence. Furthermore, the flat map has a rectangular boundary, whereas the procedure followed by [9] generates flat maps with an arbitrary shape.

2   Methods

2.1   Preprocessing, Segmentation

A T1-weighted MR image set of the brain of sufficient resolution (e.g. 100 slices with a size of 256×256) is segmented, i.e. all grey and white matter tissues are isolated via an approach based on the principles of seeded region growing, supervised clustering and morphological filtering[10]. The spinal cord is cut at the level of the bottom of the cerebellum. A dilated version of the binary volume is obtained by using an approximate spherical 7×7 mask.

2.2   Definition of the initial surface

Next, two hemi-ellipsoids are shaped interactively by adjusting their principle axes and common centre point, so that they fit as close as possible to the top and bottom parts of the brain. This interactive procedure is supported by a software, which provides three orthogonal views, arranged in a square four-window frame with the fourth window reserved for displaying the projection result. The axes of the ellipsoids are defined on the orthogonal sections of maximal brain extent.

Once the two hemi-ellipsoids are defined, the points (u, v) of a rectangular regular grid, defined in a planar space (i.e. our plane of projection), are attributed a corresponding point $\mathbf{x}(u, v)$ on the ellipsoidal surface, in a way that the centre of the original rectangle is mapped to the top of the hemi-ellipsoid and the points lying on the perimeter of the grid are moved towards the perimeter at the bottom of the hemi-ellipsoid.

This transform wraps the planar sheet around the hemi-ellipsoid. Yet this wrapping causes the distances between the points on the surface to be no longer uniform. In order to obtain good projection results, the distances are homogenised for the first time by the iterative method, described further on in section 2.4. For the sake of the speed of convergence, we only map a coarse regular subsample of the points defined in the (u, v) space to the hemi-ellipsoids. A fine-grain mapping is made, once the hemi-ellipsoid has deformed towards the dilated cortical surface. We find the hemi-ellipsoids leading to faster convergence and yielding better flattening results than the automatic approach based on hemispheres used in [8].

2.3   Deformation towards the surface

Once the points are homogenised, both the hemi-ellipsoidal surfaces are mapped towards the binary image of the brain (see Fig. 1) by means of a deformable surface model. The general formula of such a model is described in [11]:

$$
-\frac{\partial}{\partial u}\left(w_{10}\frac{\partial \mathbf{x}}{\partial u}\right) - \frac{\partial}{\partial v}\left(w_{01}\frac{\partial \mathbf{x}}{\partial v}\right) + 2\frac{\partial^2}{\partial u \partial v}\left(w_{11}\frac{\partial^2 \mathbf{x}}{\partial u \partial v}\right)
$$
$$
+ \frac{\partial^2}{\partial^2 u}\left(w_{20}\frac{\partial^2 \mathbf{x}}{\partial^2 u}\right) + \frac{\partial^2}{\partial^2 v}\left(w_{02}\frac{\partial^2 \mathbf{x}}{\partial^2 v}\right) = \mathbf{F}(\mathbf{x})
$$

The coefficients w_{ij} determine the mechanical properties of the surface. The elasticity (i.e. the stretching properties of the surface) is defined by (w_{10}, w_{01}), while the rigidity (i.e. the effort needed to bend the surface) depends on (w_{20}, w_{02}) and the resistance to twist is given by w_{11}. The term $\mathbf{F}(\mathbf{x})$ denotes the sum of external forces. When restricted to its first-order derivative terms, this model may be interpreted physically as a membrane, whereas the second order derivative terms model a thin plate. In order to simplify the computations, we prefer to omit the second order derivative terms and consider the surface acting as a

membrane. In this way we obtain the following equilibrium equation, including
the expanded external forces:

$$\beta(u,v)[\mathbf{x}_{uu}(u,v) + \mathbf{x}_{vv}(u,v)]$$
$$+ [1 - \gamma(u,v)] \cdot \{\mathbf{x}'(u,v) - \mathbf{x}(u,v)\} + \gamma(u,v)N(u,v) = 0 \tag{1}$$

where $\mathbf{x}'$ is defined in Fig. 1.

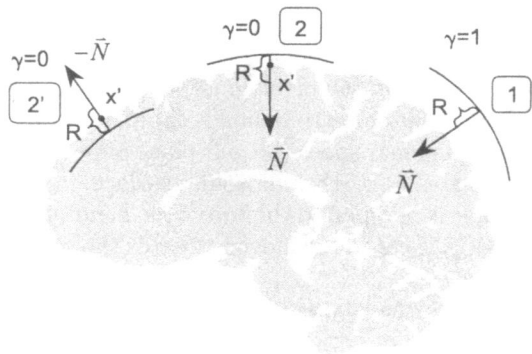

Fig. 1. External forces deforming the surface

In this model the elasticity is supposed to be isotropic and to be dependent
on the position in the membrane: i.e. $w_{10} = w_{01} = \beta(u,v)$. A similar formula is
used in [8], yet in their approach Davatzikos and Brian use a different restoring
force - based on a centre of mass function - that makes the surface converge
towards the centre of the cortical layer. In our approach, we are interested in
retrieving the exterior surface of the cortex and therefore repulse the surface,
once it enters the brain.

Instead of using a centre of mass function, that considers all the voxels within
a certain spherical neighbourhood around a node $\mathbf{x}(u,v)$ and which makes only
sense when there is a distinct grey-white matter border, we employ a modified
and simpler computational method, by only scanning voxels along the normal
direction within a certain distance R from $\mathbf{x}(u,v)$. When the node $\mathbf{x}(u,v)$ is lying
outside the brain and there is no intersection with the cortical surface found
within the distance R when scanning along the inner normal direction (case 1 in
Fig. 1), an attractive force $\mathbf{F}_{attr}(\mathbf{x})$, acting along $N(u,v)$ will be introduced: i.e.
$\mathbf{F}_{attr}(\mathbf{x}) = \gamma(u,v)N(u,v)$ by setting $\gamma(u,v) = 1$. As a consequence the restoring
force $\mathbf{F}_{rest}(\mathbf{x}) = (1 - \gamma(u,v))(\mathbf{x}'(u,v) - \mathbf{x}(u,v))$ will be inactive in this situation.
The force $\mathbf{F}_{rest}(\mathbf{x})$ can be either attractive or repulsive and will be made active
by imposing $\gamma(u,v) = 0$, when there is an intersection $\mathbf{x}'(u,v)$. In case 2, when
the node $\mathbf{x}(u,v)$ is lying outside the brain, the restoring force will further attract
the membrane towards the actual surface. In case 2', the scanning occurs in the
opposite direction and the derived restoring force will repel the node $\mathbf{x}(u,v)$.

Similar to $\gamma(u,v)$, $\beta(u,v)$ will take a different constant value when the node $\mathbf{x}(u,v)$ is close to the cortical surface (cases 2 and 2') or far way (case 1), as explained in [8].

In order to solve equation 1 numerically, we can consider its evolution equation:

$$
\begin{cases}
\beta(u,v,t)[\mathbf{x}_{uu}(u,v,t) + \mathbf{x}_{vv}(u,v,t)] + [1 - \gamma(u,v,t)] \cdot \{\mathbf{x}'(u,v,t) - \mathbf{x}(u,v,t)\} \\
+\gamma(u,v,t)N(u,v,t) = \alpha(u,v,t)\mathbf{x}_t(u,v,t) \\
\mathbf{x}(u,v,0) = \text{top or bottom hemi} - \text{ellipsoidal surface}
\end{cases}
$$

When the surface converges to its final position, $\alpha(u,v,t)\mathbf{x}_t(u,v,t)$ will tend towards zero, which also implies that the equilibrium equation 1 will be satisfied. By approximating the second order derivative with the finite difference formula $\mathbf{x}_{uu}^t(i,j) = \mathbf{x}_{i+1,j}^t - 2\mathbf{x}_{i,j}^t + \mathbf{x}_{i-1,j}^t$ and choosing $\alpha^t(i,j) = 4\beta_{ij}^t + 1 - \gamma_{ij}^t$, one can obtain the following iterative formula.

$$
\begin{aligned}
\mathbf{x}_{i,j}^{t+1} &= \frac{1}{4\beta_{ij}^t + 1 - \gamma_{ij}^t}[\beta_{ij}^t(\mathbf{x}_{i+1,j}^t + \mathbf{x}_{i-1,j}^t + \mathbf{x}_{i,j+1}^t + \mathbf{x}_{i,j-1}^t) \\
&+ (1 - \gamma_{ij}^t)\mathbf{x}_{ij}^{\prime t} + \gamma_{ij}^t N_{ij}^t]
\end{aligned} \tag{2}
$$

When the surface is far away from the cortex, γ_{ij}^t is equal to one, so that the iterative scheme is similar to the Point Jacobi Method [12]. Although it is possible to use a faster convergent scheme, such as the Successive Overrelaxation scheme used by [8], we found that for a large number of nodes, some of them might move among others, so that the distance homogenisation step, described in the next section, cannot be performed without making errors, due to local folding-over of the surface. Performing the distance homogenisation after each iteration, provides the additional advantage, that since the distances between the nodes remain more or less the same, the second order derivative, will be better approximated in the next step, than when the nodes are spread non-uniformly over the surface.

2.4   Homogenising distances

After each deformation step, the distances between the points are homogenised by an enhanced version of the Fixed-Point algorithm described in [8], to achieve a faithful visualisation of cortical anatomy later on. As stated before in the introduction, the optimal mapping is the isometric mapping, which preserves distances and angles everywhere. From differential geometry, we know that a mapping $\{u' = u'(u,v); \ v' = v'(u,v)\}$ is isometric when the first fundamental forms are identical at two corresponding points: $ds^2 = E(u,v)du^2 + 2F(u,v)dudv + G(u,v)dv^2 = E'(u',v')du'^2 + 2F'(u',v')du'dv' + G'(u',v')dv'^2 = ds'^2$

Two surfaces are locally isometric, if there is a local isometry at every point for each of the surfaces. However a local isometry may fail to be an isometry, when the surfaces have different topological properties (e.g. the cylinder and the plane, or the cortical surface and the plane). Even establishing a local isometry everywhere between the cortical surface and the plane is an impossible task, which is also true for the homothetic mapping, introduced in [8] to relax the condition on the distances, by requiring that they are preserved up to a global constant C : i.e. $E = C \cdot E'$, $F = C \cdot F'$, $G = G \cdot E'$. Note however, that once the homothetic mapping is known, the isometric mapping with the plane can be easily obtained by uniformly scaling the (u, v)-plane with C^{-1}. Since the fundamental form coefficients in the plane are $E = 1$, $F = 0$ and $G = 1$, the ideal homothetic mapping with the cortical surface is given by $E' = C$, $F' = 0$ and $G' = C$, in any point. As $E = \mathbf{x}_u \cdot \mathbf{x}_u$, $F = \mathbf{x}_u \cdot \mathbf{x}_v$ and $G = \mathbf{x}_v \cdot \mathbf{x}_v$, $\mathbf{x}(u, v_0)$ and $\mathbf{x}(u_0, v)$ will be constant speed curves, orthogonal to each other.

In [8], a regularisation of the positions of the nodes of the surface is obtained via alternatively adjusting all curves for constant $v = v_0$, i.e. $\mathbf{x}(u, v_0)$, and all curves for constant $u = u_0$, i.e. $\mathbf{x}(u_0, v)$ to make them equidistant between the nodes. An additional procedure is used to make the curves orthogonal to each other. We found that this heuristic approach, performs even better when the additional orthogonalisation step is replaced by two extra regularisation or homogenisation steps along both diagonal directions.

In our approach, the actual displacement $\Delta \mathbf{x}(u, v)$ of the nodes is only performed, when all the four regularisation steps have been accomplished and not after each step separately. It is the average of the four separate displacements: i.e. $\Delta \mathbf{x}(u, v) = \frac{1}{4} \sum_{k=1}^{4} \Delta \mathbf{x}_k(u, v)$. In order to ensure that the points move along the surface, the displacement is restricted to the tangent plane:

$$\Delta \mathbf{x}_{tp}(u, v) = \Delta \mathbf{x}(u, v) - \frac{< \Delta \mathbf{x}(u, v), N(u, v) >}{|N(u, v)|^2} \cdot N(u, v)$$

The above steps are repeated a number of times and we stop when all $\Delta \mathbf{x}_{tp}(u, v)$ are less than a certain tolerance factor, or the maximum number of iterations has been reached.

2.5   The coarse to fine approach

Once the surface has reached its final position, curves and nodes are added via interpolation to form a fine mesh. This fine mesh is deformed via the same strategy, as described in the sections 2.3 and 2.4, until it reaches its equilibrium state.

2.6   Shading the cortical surface

When the elastic deformation process has converged, a ray is fired for each point normal to the obtained dilated surface (defined in section 2.1). At the intersection of these rays with the original segmented brain, we compute the shading analogous to volume rendering and attribute the result to the corresponding (u, v) point in the plane. The planar images of both the upper and lower surface are laid next to one another and provide as such a continuous flat projection of the complete cortex. The formula we apply is a weighted sum of a contrast enhanced depth-shading term and a Phong-shading term[13].

$$I = \alpha(dc)^\gamma + (1 - \alpha) \cdot (I_a k_a + dc \cdot I_l(k_d(\boldsymbol{N}_{org} \cdot \boldsymbol{L}) + k_s(\boldsymbol{R} \cdot \boldsymbol{V})^n))$$
$$\text{with } dc = (1 - K\tfrac{depth}{depth_{MAX}}) \tag{3}$$

Since we compute a grey level intensity image only, we consider the ambient intensity I_a, the intensity I_l of the light source and the material constants k_a (ambient), k_d (diffuse), k_s (specular) to be the same for the three colour primaries (R,G,B). Further in this formula $\boldsymbol{N}_{org}$ stands for the normal at the intersection point with the original cortical surface, $\boldsymbol{L}$ is the direction of the light source, $\boldsymbol{R}$ is the reflection vector and $\boldsymbol{V}$ is the vector pointing towards the observer. The exponent n determines the spread of the specular reflections ($n \to \infty$ corresponds to the perfect mirror). Since, we have to compute the shading from every direction, it is better not to fix the position / direction of the observer and the light source in a global way, but to locally vary them for each element (u, v) that is shaded. A possible way of implementing this, is to assume that both $\boldsymbol{V}$ and $\boldsymbol{L}$, are oriented along the direction of the inner normal of the dilated surface $\boldsymbol{N}_{dil}(u, v)$. The inner product $\boldsymbol{R} \cdot \boldsymbol{V}$ then simplifies to $\boldsymbol{R} \cdot \boldsymbol{L} = 2(\boldsymbol{N}_{org} \cdot \boldsymbol{L})^2 - 1$. $\boldsymbol{N}_{org}(u, v)$ is computed via the grey-level gradient of the binary image [13].

In order to obtain useful results with the depth shading approach, we apply a non-linear contrast enhancement method based on γ-correction, since depth variations are usually very small, due to the fact that they are measured from the nearby dilated surface.

3   Results

Fig. 2 demonstrates the feasibility of the deformable surface and distance homogenisation approach. The results are produced for a $256 \times 256 \times 115$ T1 weighted MR set, that has been interpolated to obtain a $282 \times 388 \times 230$ volume. This operation is not really mandatory (other acceptable projections were obtained for a number of volume sets without interpolation). A grid of 361×401 points is defined in both (u, v) planes.

By connecting the (u, v) nodes in addition along one diagonal direction, one can directly obtain a triangular mesh for the mapped $\mathbf{x}(u, v)$ points at the surface. Fig. 2(a) shows a surface shaded view from the top, generated by means of a triangular mesh deformed towards the original cortical surface. A regular sample of constant speed curves has been overlaid on the surface. Note that distances and orthogonality are preserved rather well. The regularity of mapped nodes can also be directly inspected from the triangular mesh itself. Fig. 2(b) shows a very fine mesh of the dilated cortical surface. Even the very fine mesh is free from folded-over triangles, a problem that arises when the homogenisation pass is not performed after each deformation step.

Fig. 3 and Fig. 4 show renderings obtained for the entire unfolded cortex. Note that sulci can indeed be followed in their entirety. During our experiments we found that the Phong Shading component leads to very thick sulci, while pure depth shading might not visualise the smaller sulci well. By interactively adjusting the parameter α, the user can blend both results until he obtains a visually appealing and well interpretable image.

Currently with this number of points 722×401 and volume size $282 \times 388 \times 230$, such a rendering can be produced in about 5 minutes on a Pentium II 300 MHz, the interactive definition of the hemi-ellipsoids included. The deformation, including node regularisation, towards the dilated surface of a coarse grid consisting of 74×41 points, mapped initially on the hemi-ellipsoids, is performed in about 15 sec. Five extra steps of deformation and regularisation for the complete grid of 722×401 nodes takes about 3 minutes. After these steps, a well fitted surface is obtained for the dilated cortex. From this surface the rendering can be made in 4 sec.

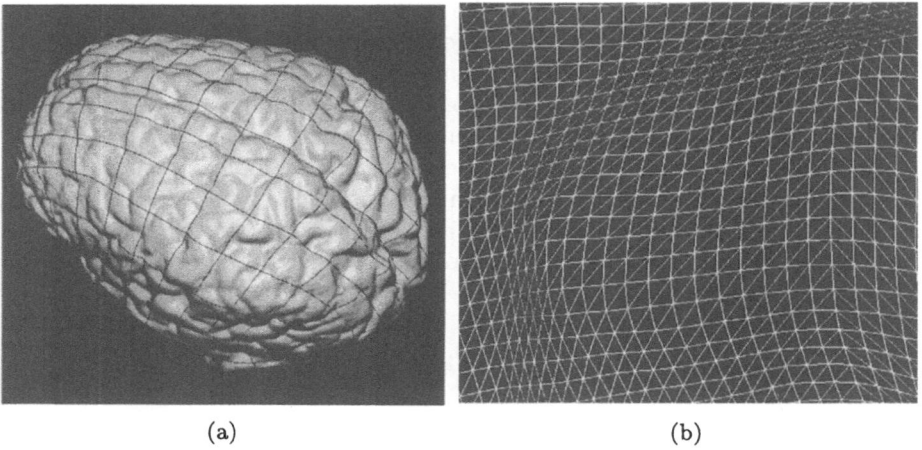

(a)   (b)

Fig. 2. Overlay of a sample of the constant speed curves on the original cortical surface (a) and The detailed mesh of a restricted area of the dilated cortical surface (b)

4   Discussion

The method proves to be quite robust. Its clinical value is currently evaluated. Since it takes only about 5 minutes to produce the rendering, it could even be envisaged to use such a kind of visualisation in clinical routine. Until now, we did not optimise the deformation and homogenisation algorithms in terms of computer instructions and register usage. Further, it is possible to consider a supplementary mesh, in between the coarse and fine mesh to further reduce the computation time. In addition one could try to derive the position and the size of the hemi-ellipsoids in an automatic way. While the approach could lead to a new practice to examine, analyse and visualise cortical anatomy, it also has the additional advantage to produce an extremely regular surface mesh of the

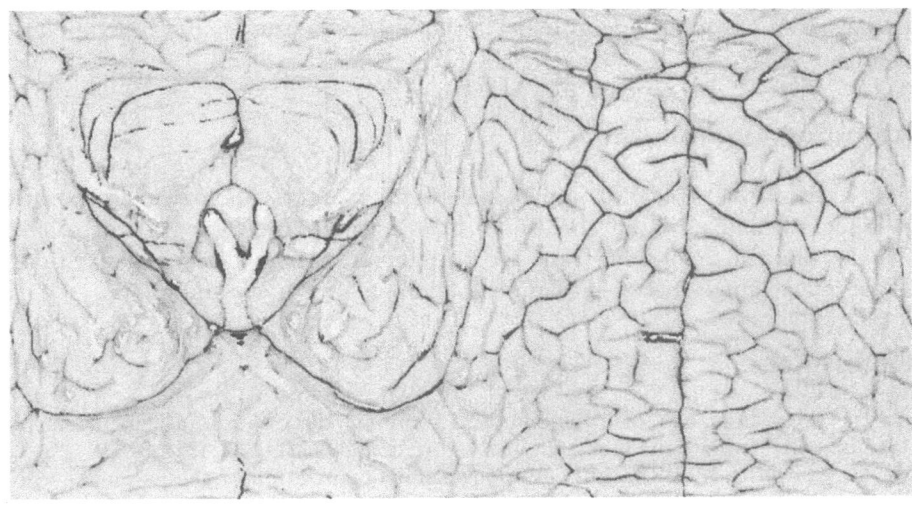

Fig. 3. Rendering of the unfolded cortical surface (emphasis on depth shading) $\alpha = 1.0, \gamma = 1, K_a = 0.1, K_d = 0.4, K_s = 0.5, K = 1, depth_{MAX} = 15$.

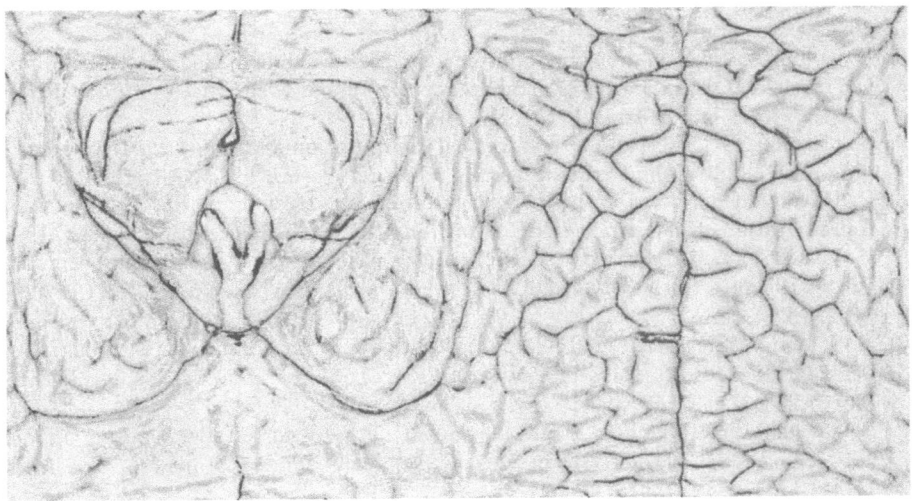

Fig. 4. Rendering of the unfolded cortical surface (depth and Phong shading) $\alpha = 0.7, \gamma = 1, K_a = 0.1, K_d = 0.4, K_s = 0.5, K = 1, depth_{MAX} = 15$.

cortical surface at any resolution (1.000 to 1.000.000 triangles) required by the user. Such a mesh could be used in finite-element studies or just for surface visualisation purposes (e.g. visualising the loci at the surface during stimulation studies).

Acknowledgements

This research was funded by a bilateral scientific and technological co-operation "Flanders-China" / Grant BIL97/72. The authors are very grateful to Prof. Pengfei Shi and Prof. Xin Yang for their co-operation in the organisation of scientific exchanges between Shanghai Jiaotong University and VUB.

References

1. D. Hubel and T. Wiesel. Laminar and columnar distribution of geniculo-cortical fibers in the macaque monkey. *J Comp Neurol*, 146:421–450, 1972.
2. D. Van Essen and S. Zeki. The topographic organization of rhesus monkey prestriate cortex. *J Physiol (Lond)*, 277:193–266, 1978.
3. A. Dale and M. Sereno. Improved localization of cortical activity by combining EEG and MEG with MRI cortical surface reconstruction: a linear approach. *J Cognit Neurosci*, 5:162–176, 1993.
4. E. Schwartz, A. Shaw, and E. Wolfson. A numerical solution to the generalized mapmaker's problem: flattening nonconvex polyhedral surfaces. *IEEE Trans Pattern Anal Machine Intell*, 11:1005–1008, 1989.
5. E. Wolfson and E. Schwartz. Computing minimal distances on arbitrary two-dimensional polyhedral surfaces. *IEEE Pattern Anal Machine Intell*, 11:1001-1005, 1989.
6. D. Tombeur. Investigations into Unitary and Non-Euclidean Geometry of Biomedical Images. Object Oriented Technology for Image Manipulation. *PhD Thesis, Vrije Universiteit Brussel*, 1994.
7. G. Carman, H. Drury, and D. Van Essen. Computational Methods for Reconstructing and Unfolding the Cerebral Cortex. *Cerebral Cortex*, 5:506–517, 1995.
8. C. Davatzikos and R. Bryan. Using a deformable surface model to obtain a shape representation of the cortex. *IEEE Trans. on Medical Imaging*, 15(6):785–795, 1996.
9. D. Van Essen and H. Drury. Structural and Functional Analyses of Human Cerebral Cortex Using a Surface-Based Atlas. *The Journal of Neuroscience*, 17(18):7079–7102, 1997.
10. A. Salomie, E. Nyssen, and J. Cornelis. Multivariate Techniques for Medical Image Segmentation. *Proceedings of the Signal Processing Symposium SPS 98*, Leuven, March 26-27, 155–158, 1998.
11. L. Cohen and I. Cohen. Finite element methods for active contour models and balloons for 2D and 3D images. *IEEE Trans Pattern Anal Machine Intell*, 15(11):1131–1147, 1993.
12. C. Hirsch. *Numerical Computation of Internal and External Flows. Volume 1: Fundamentals of Numerical Discretization*, Wiley, New-York, 1989.
13. U. Tiede, K. Höhne, M. Bomans, A. Pommert, M. Riemer, and G. Wiebecke. Investigation of Medical 3D-Rendering Algorithms. *IEEE Computer Graphics & Applications*, 41–52, 1990.

Tessellated Surface Reconstruction from 2D Contours

Chee Fatt Chan[†1], Chee Keong Kwoh[2], Ming Yeong Teo[1] and Wan Sing Ng[1]

[1]School of Mechanical and Production Engineering
[2]School of Applied Science
Computer Integrated Medical Intervention Laboratory
Nanyang Technological University, Nanyang Avenue, Singapore 639798
[†]p7105753d@ntu.edu.sg
http://mrcas.mpe.ntu.edu.sg/

Abstract. This paper presents a new triangulation method to define surfaces of 3D object from parallel 2D contours. These contours represent the boundary of a human organ segmented from 2D images acquired from radiological volumetric data using ultrasound (US), computer topography (CT) and magnetic resonance (MR) imaging. Many papers have identified and looked into the problems of generating surfaces from 2D contours. They are correspondence, tiling, branching and surface-fitting problems. Our new algorithm dealt with these problems in three steps. First, several adjacent contour mapping positions are used to reveal the correspondence of contours. Second, a tessellation algorithm approximates contours into line segments. Finally, surface meshes, in the form of strips and fans, use the gradient of line segments to optimise surface quality without affecting the rendering time.

1 Introduction

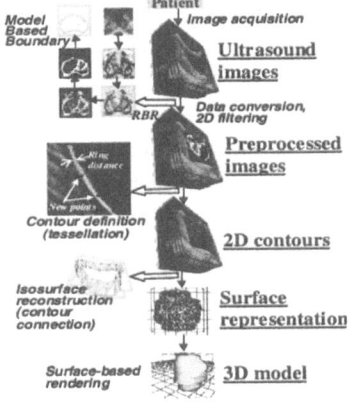

Fig. 1. URO-ART 3D-imaging pipeline.

3D models can provide more detailed and precise anatomical information than 2D image as they are important in determining the type of surgical indications, e.g. surgery planning, radiation therapy planning and volumetric measurements. Figure 1 shows a 3D-imaging pipeline approach in which a 3D prostate model is reconstructed from its contours from 2D-ultrasound images. Currently, this pipeline is implemented on a system called Augmented Reality for Therapy in Urology (URO-ART) where 3D prostate model is used for prostate cancer biopsy [1]. After the acquisition of a series of topographic images from a patient, the data usually undergo some pre-processing that

This work is supported by National Science and Technology Board (NSTB) in Singapore and the Ministry of Education (MOE) of Singapore for a joint funding under the strategic research grant JT ARC17/97.

include data conversion and image filtering. Then a set of object contours is defined on every topographic image. In our case, outlining the object boundary (e.g. prostate) of ultrasound images is done by employing a set of segmentation processes consisting of image pre-processing, edge enhancing using Radial Bas-Relief [2] followed by a model-based boundary extraction [3]. To form a 3D structure, the contours that use polygonal approximation [4] from adjacent cross sections are connected. One of the disadvantages of this approach is that ambiguities arise when attempts are made to connect equivalent points on contours. For medical visualisation, shapes are often complex and vary greatly from one cross section to the next. Furthermore, there is no guarantee that the edge segmentation will detect only one contour in each slice.

2   Reviewing 3D surface reconstruction techniques

It is common to extract from multiple parallel 2D slices of image into digitised 2D contours representing the object boundary. Ways to reduce the amount of points as to represent the 2D digitised contours are using polygonal approximation [4], contouring [5] and 2D marching squares [6]. 2D Marching squares algorithm (has been extended to 3D voxel known as 3D marching cubes) uses a divide-and-conquer technique that treat cells independently. After defining the 2D contours, the next step is to do edge linking. Running along the contours, surface triangles are constructed between adjacent planes. One of the different linking techniques available is proposed by Giraudon [7] based on an efficient data structure. Various conditions may be imposed: maximise the volume, minimise the surface, and minimise the edge length or angles, as proposed by Keppel et al. and Fuchs et al. [8,9]. However, their solutions are limited to one single contour on each cross section.

One of the difficulties in current techniques in surface modelling is that they are not efficient enough to handle complex topology of natural objects. For example, the surface reconstruction step throws away most of the valuable information on cross sectional images. Once the surface representation is created, there is no way of getting back to the original intensity values. Even simple volume cuts are meaningless because there is no information about the interior of an object. Furthermore, every change of surface definition criterion requires a recalculation of the whole data structure. However, as compared with volume reconstruction, surface reconstruction is fast in the creation of images for a wide variety of data and objects. A clear advantage of surface based methods is that a very high data reduction from volume to surface representations may be achieved. This affects both memory requirements and computing times. Computing times can be further reduced if the surface representations are based on common data structures such as triangle meshes, which are supported by computer graphics workstations. For a successful surface reconstruction, the following problems have to be resolved:

Tiling problem consists of finding the best set of triangulated facets to define the surface between a pair of connected contours in adjacent sections. Keppel et al. [8] proposes a graph search optimisation algorithm and Christiansen et al. [10] designs a heuristic approach to deal with this problem. The optimisation methods have computational overhead in comparison with the heuristic approach. On the contrary, the heuristic algorithms require pairs of contours that are to be aligned and similar in shape to work successfully. Base on Keppel's optimising algorithms to solve the problem of tiling two contours, Fuchs et al. [9] expresses the graph search using Euler tour of a toroidal graph. Ekoule et al. [11] develops an approach to tile two dissimilar contours on the assumption that their convex hulls are similar. Bajaj et al. [12] defines a set of criteria to constrain the undesired tiling and to allow detection of branching regions and dissimilar portions of a contour.

Correspondence problem involves finding the correct connections between the contours of adjacent slices. Meyers et al. [13] and Soroka [14] approximate the contours by fitting them with ellipses and then assembling them into cylinders to determine their correspondence. Bajaj et al. [12] addresses this problem assuming that reconstructed surface between adjacent slices can have at most one intersection with any line perpendicular to the slices. This limits some of the actual contours to correspond correctly in a topological manner.

Branching problem occurs when a contour in one slice can correspond to more than one contour in an adjacent slice. Boissonnat [15] uses Delaunay triangulation to compute vertices of contours in two adjacent slices. Lin et al. [16] combines surface interpolation to transform vertices of contours to create smooth surfaces that can handle the branching problem. This requires large number of triangles. Meyers et al. [13] and Ekoule et al. [11] use composite contours to connect the adjacent contours at the closed points. Their branch handling do not correspond well to the actual physical object. Bajaj et al. [12] dealt with branching problem by using a tiling algorithm that makes several passes. His initial few passes are able to tile as much of the surface as possible before tiling the "difficult" regions such as branching regions, holes and dissimilar areas of contours.

Surface fitting problem involves finding a smooth surface that either interpolates or approximates the vertices of the mesh and maintain the same topology. Miller et al. [17] approximates an isosurface of volume data by fitting a mesh homomorphic to a sphere that can be extended to finding of isosurfaces of topological type. Meyers et al. [13] uses a surface fitter on final constructed surface to regenerate surface. Bajaj et al. [12] uses 2D marching squares algorithm [6] to generate contour segments and links them to form simple polygons. The generated contour segments have coarsely spaced vertices for an accurate surface fitting of different types of curvature.

3   New reconstruction method

In this paper, we propose a new surface reconstruction algorithm based on the following general requirements:
1. Shorter computational time,
2. Maximise the use of triangular mesh and triangle strips,
3. Minimise the use of large sampling for a given set of points,
4. Surface quality can be maintain even data resolution is change or become spatial,
5. Restrain complexity of algorithm for easy implementation in an NT system.

   To obtain a topologically accurate surface model of an object using its stacks of parallel 2D contours, the model must approximate the physical boundary as well as possible. Ideally, this can happen if the distributing distance between surface vertices is small and the vertices are set on the 2D contour line. Therefore, for our implementation, we assume that our 3D-reconstruction method is built from accurate and complete (no opening and intersection of contours) 2D digitised contours that represented the boundary of the physical object. The digitised contours are extracted using segmentation methods such as the Model based RBR method [3] for ultrasound images, and global intensity threshold method (found in Materialise Mimics software[1]) for CT and MRI images. To ensure our tiling method is correct, our algorithm follows the guidelines stated in Bajaj et al. [12]:

1. For two dissimilar contours, tiling problem can occur when connecting every vertex of one contour to another contour,
2. Re-sampling of the reconstructed surface should yield the original contours.
3. Composite contours should not be formed; they do not correspond well to the actual physical object.

3.1   Contour Tessellation

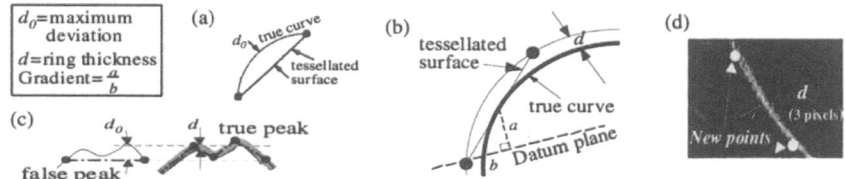

Fig. 2. (a) Principal of curve tessellation. (b) New contour tessellation. (c) Key advantage of new tessellation, showing the peak point, over the method of using only the deviated height. (d) New points created within 3 pixels error of ring thickness.

Figure 2(a) shows the basic principal of contour tessellation. Tessellated surface results because of the deviation (d_0) between the true curve and the tessellated straight line. Figure 2(b) shows the new approach of contour tessellation, this method can represent surfaces that deviation (d) from the straight line rather than representing the maximum deviation. The key step is by enlarging the true curve with a bounding ring thickness d. This new curve is set as a new boundary that can force the tessellation process to distribute a new set of point according to the curvature of the contour. One of the most important aspects of this new approach is that the topological consistency is checked by using gradient value ($\nabla = \frac{a}{b}$) of the true curve whenever a new point is set. Each vertex point is defined with reference to its neighbour linkage. Figure 2(c) shows the difference between curve tessellation and new approach of contour tessellation. The objective of this process is to use optimal number of line segment to represent a raster object data (e.g. point cloud data) without losing the shape and nature of the object. Advantages of this process to construct a surface are as follows:

1. It optimises the connecting of new vertices over a surface,
2. It uses an estimate of surface curvature to distribute more new vertices at regions of higher curvature.

---

[1] Mimics 6.0 is a trademark of Materialise Software

Let the true digitised curve to be approximated be detonated as P, $[p_1, p_2, ..., p_n]$. The tessellated curve is P', $[p'_1, p'_2,..., p'_m]$ such that m is significantly smaller than n, and the chain of line segments is defined as $[p'_1, p'_2], [p'_2, p'_3], ..., [p'_{m-1}, p'_m]$. The vertices of P' are ordered subsets of the vertices of P. The proposed tessellation algorithm starts at $[p_1, p'_1]$, which can be selected arbitrarily, until $[p_n, p'_m]$, or a new initial vertices causing the number of polygon sides to increase (This is explained in Section 3.3). In order to demonstrate the effectiveness of this new algorithm, the choice of method used to measure the error of approximation of curve P and P' are subject to the pixel density region error criterion. This criterion defines the goodness of fit in terms of pixel density deviations of the output curve P' from the input curve P. The error measure used is the pixel density (e = number of deviated pixels per line segment $[p'_{m-1}, p'_m]$) between a vertex of p and the line collinear with the corresponding approximating line segment. It is difficult to use mathematical functions to represent the digitised curve; the implementation is depended on the pixel resolution of the input data. Therefore, the idea of contour tessellation algorithm (illustrated in Figures 2(c) and (d)) can be divided into two-stages:
1. Sampling the true curve with a dynamic searching pixel mask (d × two pixels) within the bounding ring of thickness d.
2. Setting the new vertex point and joining line segments $[p'_{i-1}, p'_i]$ by sampling the optimal pixel gradient that satisfied any of the following situation:
   - Convex: p'_{i-1} on outer, p'_{i2} on inner and p'_i on outer ring positions.
   - Concave: p'_{i-1} on inner, p'_{i2} on outer and p'_i on inner ring positions.
   - Convex to concave: p'_{i-1} on outer, p'_{i2} on outer and p'_i on inner ring positions.
   - Concave to convex: p'_{i-1} on inner, p'_{i2} on inner and p'_i on outer ring positions.

3.2   Tiling using Triangle Strips and Fans

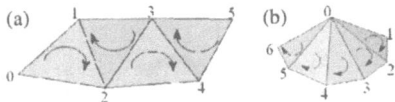

Fig. 3. (a) Triangle strip and (b) fan.

The speed of constructing triangulated surfaces for displaying is crucial to interactive visualisation; this is bounded by the rate at which triangulated data can be sent to the graphics subsystem for rendering. Each triangle can be specified using three vertices, but to maximise the use of the available data bandwidth, it is desirable to order the triangles so that the next triangle shares an edge. Using such an ordering, only the incremental change of one vertex per triangle need to be specified, potentially reducing the rendering time by factor of three by avoiding redundant clipping and transformation computations. Besides, such an approach also has benefits in compression for storing and transmitting models. Consider the triangulation in Figure 3(a). Without using triangle strips, this triangulation will be represented by specifying four triangles with three vertices each. By using triangle strips, as supported by the OpenGL[2] graphics library [18], the triangulation can use the strip (0,1,2,3,4,5). Such a sequential strip can reduce the cost to transmit n triangles from $3n$ to $n+2$ vertices. The problem of constructing quality triangle strips has received attention from both the graphics and the

---

[2] OpenGL 1.1 and SGI program are trademark of Silicon Graphics, Inc.

computational geometry communities. For example, Akeley et al. [19] has written a SGI² program that converts triangle meshes to triangle strips. According to Evans et al. [20], it is a "greedy" algorithm, which always chooses the triangle that is adjacent to the least number of neighbours (e.g. minimises the number of adjacencies) as the next triangle in a strip. Evans also describes other triangle strip generation algorithms as well as presenting some of the most effective techniques to date. He proposes an algorithm for constructing triangle strips from fully triangulated models. This has proved to be quite useful for generating efficient triangle strips for the OpenGL cost model. In the case of generating triangulated mesh from contours, the algorithm to determine sequential of strip can be simpler than Evans's algorithm. Figure 4 shows an example of linking a contour with concave arc and a straighten contour. This requires extension of tessellation gradient checking process that will close the connectivity surfaces between the low curve and the high curve. The connectivity surface can then be created through using one sequential triangle strip and one sequential triangle fan. Getting good sequences of triangle strips when multiple dissimilar contours are involved is discussed in the next Section.

3.3   Topological Consistency Checks

Fig. 4. Triangulating top contour to bottom contour by using one sequential triangle strip and one sequential triangle fan.

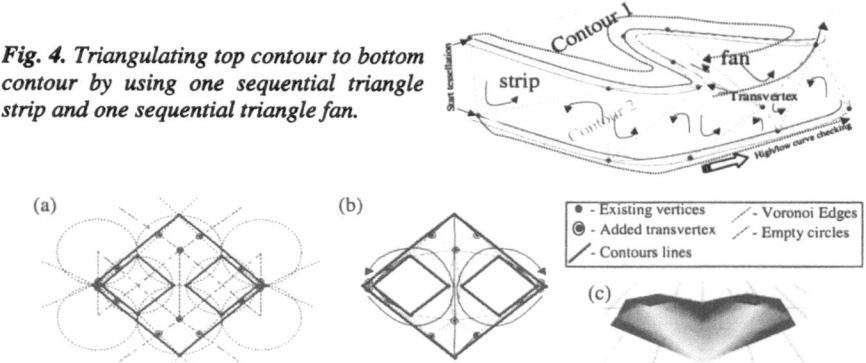

Fig. 5. Ttopological consistency checking. (a) Voronoi Diagram edges. (b) Triangulating top (2 diamond) to bottom contour (1 diamond) using two sequential strips. (c) Rendered model.

Gradient checking is used when tessellation shows that adjacent contour curvature has changed drastically. This change can be determined by the following conditions:
1. There is poor triangulation of any existing neighbour vertices that strayed away. This is checked using suspect line segments matching with Voronoi diagram [15] (Delaunay triangulation is not used) as a 2D template from the top, as shown in Figure 5(a). The Intersection of suspect line and Voronoi edge is used.
2. There is discontinuation of triangle strips along one contour.
3. When the triangulation meets the edge of a gap that is between two contours on the same slice or they are contours that overlapping one contour on an adjacent slice.
   If the above conditions are met during gradient checking, new vertices are needed to maintain the surface topological consistency. The additional vertex is named

Transvertex. In practice, Transvertex can be effective to handle branching and tiling problems as shown in Figure 4 and Figure 5. The automatic contour tessellation method, mentioned in Section 3.1, is able to create vertices for surface according the curvature of the contour. For instance, one contour may have a large number of vertices from an original description of an object while adjacent contour may have lesser vertices. By enforcing the use of triangle strips, one might face a problem of tempting to add new vertices on the adjacent tessellated contour line segment. This problem is also stated in Bajaj el al. [12] first guideline. Furthermore, if more vertices are added to an existing tessellated line segment, this will propagate more new vertices to other consecutive contours even though their existence do not represent the curvature of the surfaces. Figure 6 shows examples of connection paths with and without triangle strips (normal triangulation). Transvertices are used to fulfil the first guideline. Smooth shaded models demonstrate that using tessellated triangle strip has better topological surface appearance. For instance, Figure 6(d) shows concave cone stop at the middle without relying on the adjacent contour and 6(e) shows that the top straight line can be easily identified while the other seems bent in the shadow.

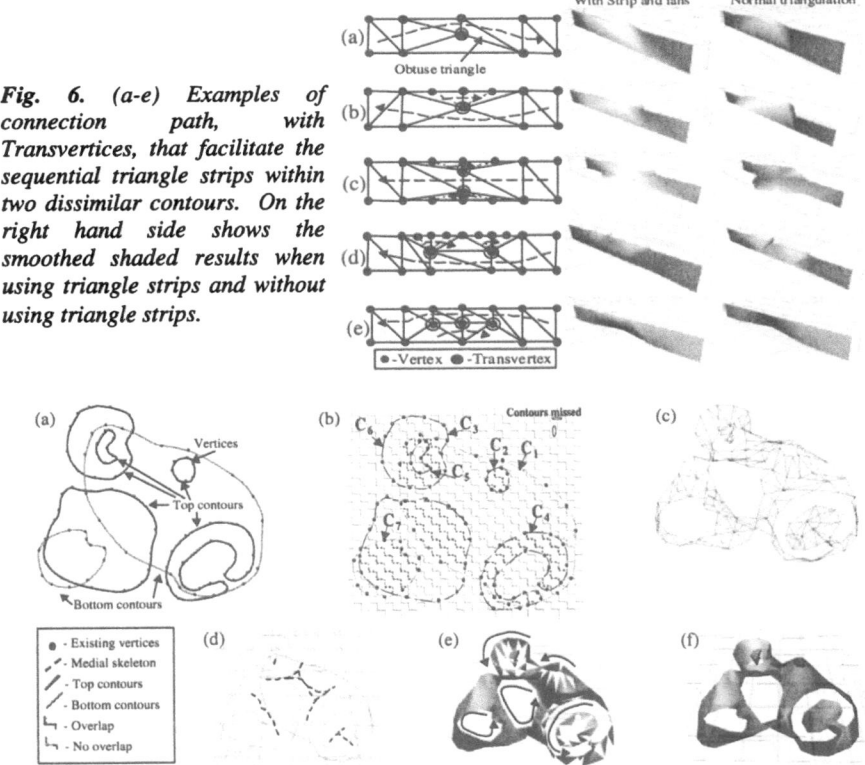

Fig. 6. (a-e) Examples of connection path, with Transvertices, that facilitate the sequential triangle strips within two dissimilar contours. On the right hand side shows the smoothed shaded results when using triangle strips and without using triangle strips.

Fig. 7. (a) Two slices, top and bottom, with complex contours (from [12]'s Figure 13(a)). (b) Top slice overlaps bottom slice into one slice for zigzag scan for contours intersection relationship. (c) Wireframe model. (d) Medial axis, the skeleton lines, are created for the canyon and concave terrain island. (e) 6 triangle strips (along C_2, C_3, C_4, C_5, C_7 and $C_1 \cup C_6$, represented by interval chain of blank triangles). (f) Smooth rendered results using algorithm.

The Voronoi diagram has the property that every vertex in the region around a site is closer to that site than to any of the other sites. This can also be used for approximation of the medial axis called Edge Voronoi Diagram (e.g. shown in Figure 7(d)). Medial axis of a polygon is the locus of points with equal distance to at least two contour points [15]. Calculating the real medial axis can assist the tiling of canyons, islands and any complex branching surfaces. It represents the metric and topological properties of shapes well. There is no composite contour form; therefore it fulfils Bajaj et al. [12] third guideline. Accurate medial axis is numerically difficult to achieve when existing contour vertices are far apart. Bajaj et al. [12] solves this problem using a rough medial axis. We use Bajaj's calculation of rough medial axis, but in our case, Transvertices need not be located on the medial axis, depending on where the running vertices of sequential triangle strips are. Figure 7 shows the result of our algorithm using two slices of contours of the shape used by Bajaj et al. [12]. Figure 7(e) shows an example of 3 strips meeting in-between canyons and additional transvertices are added by matching Voronoi diagram as mentioned earlier.

3.4   Correspondence of contours using contours cross-shadow mapping

Section 2 shows that many solutions for the correspondence problem use a global view of the data set and incorporate some assumptions about the objects to be reconstructed. This allows a reasonable solution to be generated where no uniquely correct solution is possible. These methods may become more difficult to implement if the distance between slices becomes large. Thus, automatic solution of the

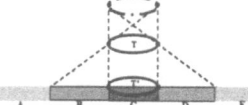

correspondence problem in its general form is difficult. Zigzag grid scan (Figure 7(b)) is used to define the location and the overlapping relationship of adjacent contours. Cross mapping (Figure 8) is used to solve the

Fig. 8. *Regions of cross mapping method.*

correspondence problem by satisfying the condition that: T is not connected to T' only if T' falls within the constraint,

$$S=AB+\overline{BCD}+DE \qquad (1)$$

For Example, (in Figure 9(h)), T is connected to right T' as $S=CDE$, but T is not connected to left T' as $S=AB$. Advantage of this method is that it takes the properties of similar triangles and the slope surface gradient from the last two adjacent contours are included to map the new correspondence region.

Fig. 9. The correspondence problem is solved by determining which of the contours from each section should be connected together. (a-p) Examples of different outcomes possible in using cross-shadow mapping method.

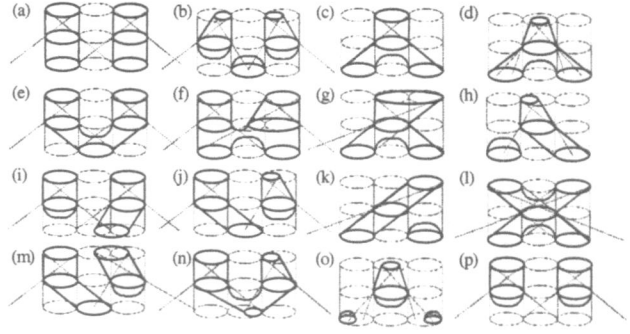

4   Preliminary Results of implementation

The algorithm has been implemented in Microsoft Visual C++ 5.0[3] using WindowNT 4.0[3] operating system. The graphics hardware of the system, Dual Intel Pentium II 333MHz TDZ2000 NT graphic workstation[4], is exploited by using the OpenGL library [18]. The new tessellation-meshing algorithm presented in this paper has been implemented to reconstruct a prostate gland (Figure 10). The model is generated from 19 slices of parallel-digitised 2D ultrasound images, each consisting of 256x256 elements of 8-bit depth, evenly spaced at 3 mm apart. 2D contours are segmented from these images without discontinuity using our new RBR model based method [3]. In order to illustrate and test the full practical detail features of the new algorithm, a human CT scanned pelvic bone is used. The pelvic images consisting of 83 slices (approximately 3mm for slice-to-slice thickness) from 512x512x512 with pixel size of 0.46mm, data are from Materialise's Mimics software (NV, Kapeldreef 60 B3001L). Only 38 slices with slice-to-slice thickness of 6mm are used. We used Mimic's intensity thresholding (range 1250 to 4095) to segment the pelvic bone. 2D Contours polylines (Figure 11(a)) and 3D models (Figure 11(b)) using 3D marching cube [6] are exported using Mimic's CTM to our software. The new tessellation algorithm is then tested to generate the smooth shaded pelvic model shown in 11(c).

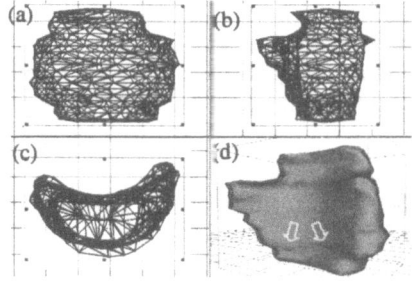

Fig. 10. A smooth rendered 3D prostate model using the new tessellation algorithm with 3 pixels error built from 19 slices of ultrasound images with a slice-to-slice thickness of about 3mm. 1118 facets are generated, with 78% of them in 20 triangle strips. The model takes 1-3 seconds to generate from the 2D contours. Arrows indicate the undesired artifacts. (Note: This model has only single branch for connection of contours.)

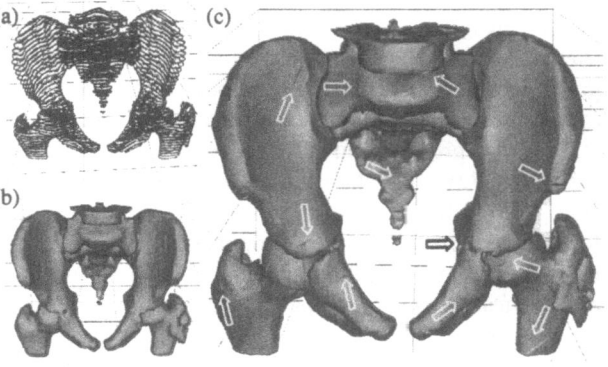

Fig. 11. (a) 38 cross-sections of a pelvis, slice-to-slice thickness 6mm. (b) model reconstructed using marching cube with 25572 facets. Approximately 16 seconds to generate in Mimics. (c) The model is generated using the new tessellation algorithm with 3-pixels error. 11329 facets with 67% of them in 194 triangle strips. Approximately 9 seconds to generate model from contours. Arrows indicate undesired artefacts.

---

[3] Microsoft Visual C++ 5.0 and WindowNT 4.0 are trademark of Microsoft Corporation.

[4] TDZ2000 is a trademark of Intergraph Corporation.

5   Limitations and Contributions

In the prostate model (Figure 10(d)) and pelvic model (Figure 11(d)), there are several deep "cut" artefacts that are denoted by a narrow and long shadow grove (indicated by block arrows). These are resulted by the triangulation strips used. We identified that the triangulation strips path used here are similar to the triangulation path as shown in the Figure 6(a). The middle Transvertex have located towards the left-hand side causing obtuse triangle to form. The "cuts" become longer if the upper contour line segment also has obtuse triangles. Obtuse triangles are caused during 2D contour tessellation. Different contours have different starting points that are dependent on the sequence of triangle strips. In some cases, this caused the last point to be located near the starting point.

The new tessellation algorithm generated the pelvic models with 28% less facets than marching cube model. The total running time for generating the pelvic model, using the new method without including segmentation time, has shown a significant improvement of only 9 seconds are needed to complete the whole task, while the marching cube model in Mimics uses 16 seconds. However, the running time may not indicate the performance of algorithm. E.g. the Mimic software may not be using OpenGL (graphical hardware supported). In terms of quality, our model shows much more topological surface details (visually examine) than the marching cube model. In terms of rendering speed, it is much faster than the marching cube model (all models are rendered on our software). This is because the graphics hardware handles 194 triangle strips instead of every facet. This results in the improvements in generating and rendering speed, and reduction in data handling.

6   Conclusion and Future directions

The new tessellation algorithm automatically determines the topological type of the surface, and the presence and location of the sharp features. In addition, the tessellated line segment defined between adjacent contour determines the choice of triangulation that can significantly impact the cost of the resulting strips. The gradient check also plays an important part when exercising a complete "walk" of triangle strips around a chosen contour. The algorithm is tested using ultrasound images of a prostate and CT images of a pelvic bone. The constructed pelvic model surface quality and data handling performance is compared with Lorensen's marching cube method [6]. It can be seen that the new algorithm is efficient for creating strips for polygon models that are supported by computer graphics workstations. This can be attributed largely to the first step of implementation of contour tessellation and the optimal use of triangle strips that can significantly reduce rendering time [20]. There are a number of areas for future research that include:

1. Eliminate obtuse triangulation; possible use of 3D delaunay triangulation or reversing of contour tessellation for the last few points.
2. Experiment with different sparse data. E.g. branching nerve or blood vessel.
3. Generate a graph consisting of running time (including rendering time) versus number of triangles used and the number of triangle strips used.
4. Determine the important of model's pixel error criterion with clinical application.

References

[1] C. F. Chan, C. G. Zhu, C. K. Kwoh, M. Y. Teo, W. S. Ng, Y. C. Weng, C. Cheng and K. T. Foo. Prostate Biopsy using Augmented Reality 3D-Visualisation. *18th Southern Biomedical Engineering Conference and 2nd International Conference on Ethical Issues in Biomedical Engineering, Clemson, U.S.A., May 21-23*, 1999. To appear.

[2] Y. J. Liu, W. S. Ng, M. Y. Teo and H. C. Lim. Computerised prostate boundary estimation of ultrasound images using radial bas relief method. *Medical Biology Engineering and Computing*, 35:445-454, 1997.

[3] R. Y. Wu, K. V. Ling, and W. S. Ng. Prostate Edge Strength Enhancement In Ultrasound Images Using New Radial Bas-Relief Method. *Technical report. Nanyang Technology University*, 1999.

[4] Y. Zhu and L. D. Seneviratne. Optimal polygonal approximation of digitised curves. *IEE Proceedings of Vision Image Signal Process*, 144(1):8-14, 1997.

[5] D. F. Watson. Contouring: A Guide to the Analysis and Display of Spatial Data. *Pergamon Press*, 1992.

[6] W. Lorensen and H. Cline. Marching cubes: a high-resolution 3D surface construction algorithm. *Computer Graphics*, 21:163-169, 1987.

[7] G. Giraudon. An efficient edge chaining algorithm. *Scandinavian Conference on Image Analysis, Stockholm*, 5(2):163-169, 1987.

[8] E. Keppel. Approximating complex surfaces by triangulation of contour lines. *IBM Journal Resolution Development*. 19(1):2-11, 1975.

[9] H. Fuchs, Z. M. Kedem and S. P. Uselton. Optimal surface reconstruction from planar contours. *Association for Computing Machinery*, 20(10):693-702, 1977.

[10] H. Christiansen and T. Sederberg. Conversion of complex contour line definitions into polygonal element mosaics. *Computer Graphics*, 12:187-192, 1978.

[11] A. B. Ekoule, F. C. Peyrin and C. L. Odet. A triangulation algorithm from arbitrary shaped multiple planar contours. *ACM Transition Graphics*, 10(2):182-199, 1991.

[12] C. L. Bajaj, E. J. Coyle and K. N. Lin. Arbitrary Topology Shape Reconstruction from Planar Cross Sections. *Graphical Models and Image Processing*, 58:310-319, 1996.

[13] D. Meyers, S. Skinner and K. Sloan. Surfaces from contours. *Association for Computing Machinery Transition Graphics*, 11(3):228-258, 1992.

[14] B. I.. Soroka. Generalised cones from serial sections. *Computer Vision Graphics and image Processing*, 15:154-166, 1981.

[15] J. D. Boisoonnat. Shape reconstruction from planar cross sections. *Computing Vision Graphics Image Proceeding*. 44(1):1-29, 1988.

[16] W. C. Lin and S. Y. Chen. A new surface interpolation technique for reconstructing 3D objects from serial cross-sections. *Computer Vision Graphics and image Processing*, 48:124-143, 1989.

[17] J. V. Miller, D. E. Breen, W. E. Lorensen, R. M. O'Bara and M. J. Wozn. Geomatrically deformed models: A method for extracting closed geometric models from volume data. *Computer Graphics, SIGGRAPH '91*, 24(4):217-226, 1991.

[18] OpenGL Architecture Review Board, OpenGL Reference Manual. *Addison-Wesley, Reading, MA*, 1993.

[19] K. Akeley, P. Haeberli and D. Burns. *C program on SGI developer's toolbox CD*, 1990.

[20] F. Evans, S. Skiena and A. Varshney. Optimizing Triangle Strips for Fast Rendering. *In Proceedings of Visualization '96*, 319-326, 1996.

Accurate Robust Symmetry Estimation

Stephen Smith and Mark Jenkinson

FMRIB (Oxford Centre for Functional Magnetic Resonance Imaging of the Brain)
Department of Clinical Neurology, University of Oxford
John Radcliffe Hospital, Headington, Oxford OX3 9DU, UK
Tel: +44 1865 222 726   Fax: +44 1865 222 717
{mark,steve}@fmrib.ox.ac.uk www.fmrib.ox.ac.uk

Abstract. There are various applications, both in medical and non-medical image analysis, which require the automatic detection of the line (2D images) or plane (3D) of reflective symmetry of objects. There exist relatively simple methods of finding reflective symmetry when object images are complete (i.e., completely symmetric and perfectly segmented from image "background"). A much harder problem is finding the line or plane of symmetry when the object of interest contains asymmetries, and may not have well defined edges.

A major area of interest is brain image analysis; there are various reasons why one would want to be able to automatically, robustly and accurately find the (sagittal) mid-plane from a 3D brain image. Example applications include pre-alignment (or sanity checking) for standard registration methods, mid-plane finding as part of symmetric probabilistic anatomical map generation, and, in particular, symmetry-based analyses (e.g., for schizophrenia research). This paper describes EROS - Extraction of Robust Orientation using Symmetry, which has been developed to solve this problem. It has been shown to work with MRI (T1, T2, EPI), PET, SPECT and CT, using robust measures to give accurate results even with images containing large asymmetries.

Keywords: Symmetry detection, robust registration, mid-plane.

Review

Much of the existing work concentrates on defining symmetry, and developing low-level symmetry operators. For example, in the symmetry work reported by Di Gesù et al. (e.g., [1]), applied to such problems as face detection and astronomical image analysis, the algorithm is specifically tuned to the characteristics of these problems. The emphasis is on finding small symmetric features, rather than finding symmetries in large complex objects. Similarly, in [4], Reisfeld et al. find points of symmetry - there is no attempt at robust (larger) object symmetry detection.

Other work has looked for larger-scale symmetry, but often using constraints on the symmetries looked for. For example, in [9], vertical symmetry axes only are looked for in the context of road scene understanding for autonomous vehicle control. Sun et al. (e.g., [5]) use the extended gaussian image (EGI) to find different types of symmetries in 2D and 3D images. The EGI, however, is derived by looking at image gradient directions or the orientation of sections of image edges, and is therefore intrinsically noisy compared with looking for symmetry by direct point matching. The method also relies on finding principal axes first, and may therefore not be very robust to asymmetries in objects.

Many methods depend on first finding image edges before proceeding to detect symmetries. Clearly there are applications which cannot provide such well-defined features - for example, see the PET and SPECT images below. The approach reported in this paper does not require edges to be found; even when processing images with high bias field (see discussion below), only edge enhancement is used, not edge detection.

There are few published methods for finding symmetry in brain images. Minoshima *et al.* [3] present a method which detects the symmetry plane in PET images, using zero-crossing counting (stochastic sign change). Whilst it is shown to be robust to large image asymmetries, it is hard to see how the method could be extended to overcome even small bias fields in MRI images. Thirion *et al.* [6] reflect the image about a pre-assumed symmetry plane, and then use registration to align the original and reflected images. From the estimated transformation the symmetry plane can be deduced. This is an impressive approach, but depends on the registration being able to cope perfectly with significant asymmetries in the brain image in order to function correctly - at the moment it appears that success is probably limited to cases of restricted asymmetry. The method is also dependent on having a very rough initial idea of where the symmetry plane is.

Method Detail

The method used to robustly find the plane of symmetry is now briefly outlined, followed by a more detailed explanation of the reasoning behind the system, and its implementation.

Preprocessing:

The image histogram is used to find robust estimates of the image "minimum" (5% into the cumulative histogram) and "maximum" (95%). Next a rough brain/background threshold is defined using these values; it is assumed to be $min + 0.1(max - min)$. Now a rough estimate of the position of the centre of gravity of the brain in the image is made, and an "average" brain radius is estimated by using the brain/background threshold and counting the number of voxels above this threshold. This radius is used to control subsampling when a multi-scale search for the optimal symmetry plane is carried out.

Symmetry search algorithm (3D case):

The main algorithm for the search for the symmetry plane is:

• For all possible mid-plane orientations (i.e., all angles α, β)
•   For all lines l perpendicular to mid-plane given by these angles (i.e., a 2D grid of lines through the mid-plane)
•   Find centre of symmetry ($s(x)$ is symmetry score at position x along line - find peak value, $s_l(x_p)$ for line l)
•   Add peak symmetry score into a total 1D array ($S(x_p) = S(x_p) + s_l(x_p)$)
•   Find peak in total array = score for these angles ($P_{\alpha,\beta} = MAX(S(x))$) - compare with peak found at other (α, β) so far.

See Figure 1 for example sets of lines perpendicular to a single choice of possible symmetry plane in each of three cases. (A single slice is shown, hence the symmetry plane is seen as a line.) The three cases are a "clean" image of a healthy brain, the "clean" brain with an incorrect choice of symmetry plane, and a brain with a large asymmetry superimposed. The position of the optimal centre of symmetry for each perpendicular line is shown. As a further clarification of how these positions are found, see Figure 2. In Figure 2 (left), the intensity profiles for three example lines in the "clean" and asymmetric cases are shown. Only one profile contains asymmetry - the final plot. In Figure 2 (right), the next processing stage for these plots is shown; the symmetry score at each possible centre of symmetry is given. Again, only the final plot shows asymmetry. Referring back to Figure 1, it is clear how the asymmetry has caused the marked centres of symmetry to shift.

Finally, all of the peak symmetry scores are combined across all perpendicular lines, into a single representative 1D array. Figure 3 (left) shows an example of this - the effect of the asymmetry is to give rise to non-aligned centres of symmetry in some of the perpendicular lines, causing the bulge on one side of the cumulative array. Figure 3 (right) shows these final arrays for the three cases shown earlier. When the mid-plane is incorrect, the peak symmetry scores will not all fall near the same x, so the total array will not contain as high a peak as when the plane is correct (the individual scores will be smaller as well, thus increasing the ability of the method to discriminate between correct and incorrect plane orientation).

Note that the lateral position of the symmetry plane, once the optimal angles have been selected, is immediately found from the position of the peak in the optimal cumulative 1D array. Clearly it would be easy to interpolate the values in this array if desired, to find a sub-voxel position.

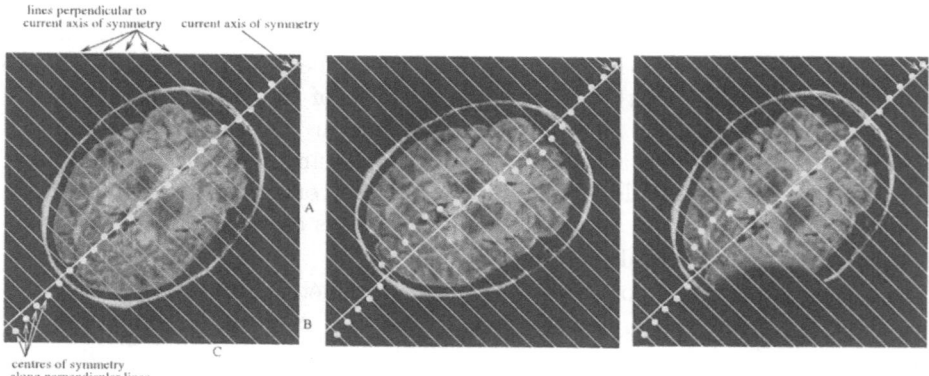

Fig. 1. Examples showing the set of lines perpendicular to proposed axes of symmetry in three cases with the position of centre of symmetry shown for each separate line.

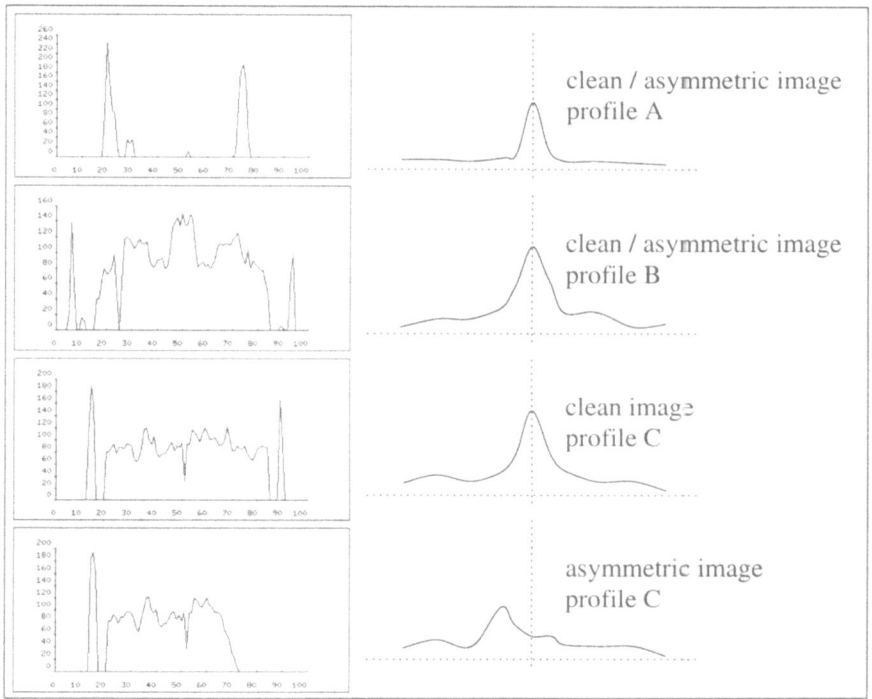

clean / asymmetric image
profile A

clean / asymmetric image
profile B

clean image
profile C

asymmetric image
profile C

Fig. 2. Left: Intensity profiles along perpendicular lines A, B and C for Figure 1.
Right: Symmetry score profiles along lines A, B and C; x is the position (along the
perpendicular line) of a proposed centre of symmetry, and y is the symmetry score for
that position.

Symmetry measure: The basic symmetry score used to find the centres of
symmetry along each perpendicular line is:

$$s(x) = \frac{\sum abs(I_{x+i} + I_{x-i}) - \sum abs(I_{x+i} - I_{x-i})}{\sum abs(I_{x+i} + I_{x-i}) + \sum abs(I_{x+i} - I_{x-i})} = \frac{even - odd}{even + odd}, \qquad (1)$$

where $even$ is a measure of the "evenness" (unnormalised symmetry) and odd is
a measure of the "oddness" (unnormalised asymmetry) of the intensity profile
about x. This formulation provides normalization for intrinsic variations in intensity contrast and noise across the image. However, it incorrectly assigns too
much weight to areas of the image which contain little signal. Thus a correction
is made:

$$s(x) = \frac{(even - odd) * l}{(even + odd) + g}. \qquad (2)$$

Correction l is derived from local contrast (i.e., within the current perpendicular
line), thus giving more weight to lines containing significant interest. Correction
g is a fraction of the global contrast, put here so that noise cannot have significant
influence when there is little signal - a problem in background regions.

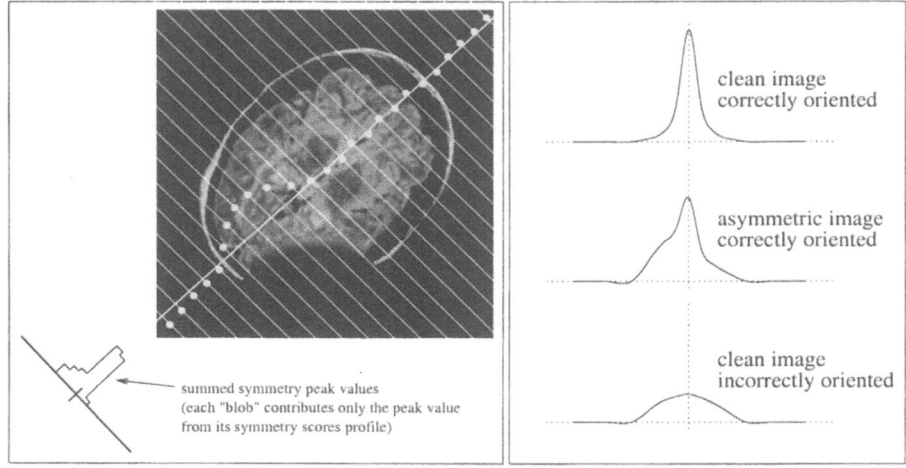

Fig. 3. Left: Example summed symmetry peak profile. **Right:** Example profiles for all images in Figure 1. As it is the position of the peak that matters, the asymmetry does not affect the estimate of the line of symmetry. The incorrectly oriented case gives a much lower peak than the correctly oriented case.

Robustness: EROS is robust to asymmetries (e.g., lesions or susceptibility artifacts) due to the method by which individual line symmetries are combined. The combination of all lines' symmetry positions into a single 1D array effectively produces a mode-like position statistic, although the robustness is increased even further than a true mode, where each peak would contribute an equal amount to the cumulative array. The contribution is the peak's value, not a constant, so that peaks derived from strong symmetries contribute more highly than those derived from weak symmetries.

A problem which has not been addressed thus far is that of a slowly varying additive or multiplicative field on top of the underlying image. This is common in MRI images, often termed bias field. EROS has been found to be robust to normal levels of bias field, i.e., still finds the correct plane of symmetry. However, with extreme bias field, simple symmetry does not exist - at optimal x, $I_{x+i} - I_{x-i}$ is not close to zero. In such cases, there is a very simple preprocessing stage which allows EROS to function correctly. By edge-enhancing the image (using a simple magnitude differential operator), the bias field is removed to first order. Successful mid-plane detection then results.

Computational efficiency measures: The calculations involved in robust symmetry detection are computationally expensive. A full search of all possible angles at full resolution is currently prohibitive. Therefore a multi-scale approach is taken - in practice, only two scales are used. Firstly, the image is smoothed and sub-sampled to give a smaller resulting image. Here the estimated brain size is used; it has been found empirically that a mean brain radius of 40 voxels in the subsampled image is the lowest resolution which still reliably gives a symmetry plane which is close to the "correct" solution. This solution is then used as the central point around which a restricted search is made at full (original) image resolution. The second measure to reduce computational cost is to only use a subset of all possible lines perpendicular to each tried symmetry plane. The spacing between these lines can be varied to speed up calculations. Currently, with these measures, EROS takes about 40 minutes to run on a typical MRI brain image, on a Silicon Graphics Origin 200.

Local detection: A particular application might either be more interested in the overall (global) optimal position for the plane of reflective symmetry (as has been assumed thus far), or, it may require more local detection, using only structures near the mid-plane to determine the exact position. The latter case is simple to accommodate - after the main algorithm, a final iteration can be applied, using only image points near the mid-plane in symmetry calculations, giving central detection instead of global.

Results, Conclusions and Future Work

Figure 4 shows example results from CT, SPECT and PET images respectively. These were 3D analyses - the central slice only is shown. The plane of symmetry thus shows as a line; the computed centre of gravity is also marked. Figure 5 (left) shows an MRI brain image with bad bias field artificially added. In order to allow EROS to succeed in finding the mid-plane, edge enhancement is carried out as a pre-processing step. Figure 6 (left) shows an MRI image with significant artificial asymmetries introduced. The simple non-robust solution is marked, as well as the robust one, which is correct. Figure 6 (right) shows symmetry detection on an image of the University of Ljubljani. The original image has been rotated and offset so that the symmetry line is not central in the image. The image was inverted so that the initial thresholding heuristics (easily alterable for different applications to brain analysis) would cause EROS to ignore the sky, and not the building!

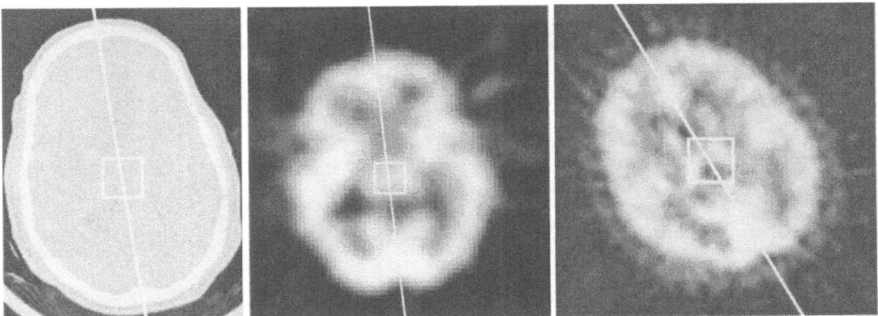

Fig. 4. Slice through 3D CT, SPECT and PET images after symmetry plane detection by EROS.

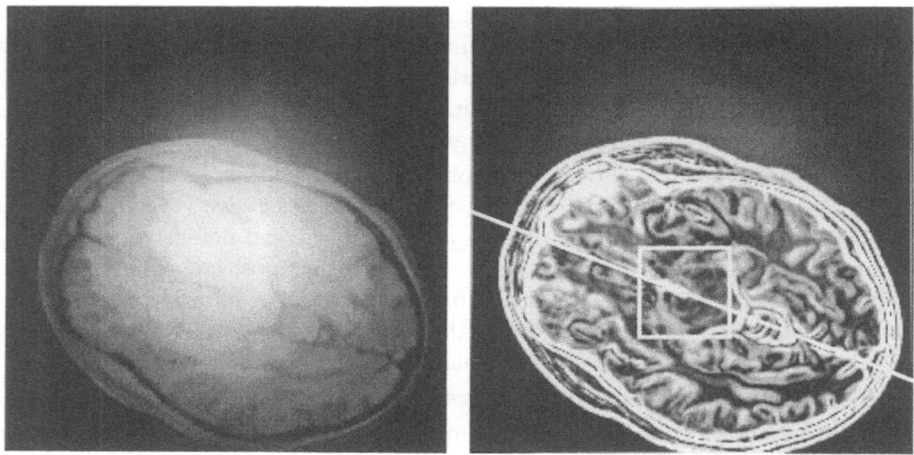

Fig. 5. An image badly corrupted by bias field after symmetry plane detection by EROS with edge enhancement pre-processing.

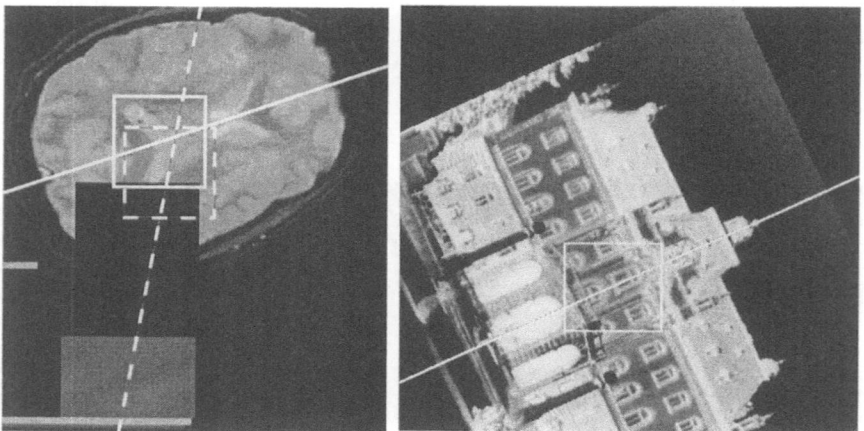

Fig. 6. Slice through 3D MRI (T2-weighted) image after symmetry plane detection by EROS. The image has been artificially corrupted to cause a large asymmetry. Non-robust symmetry detection fails completely (dashed line) whilst robust detection is successful.

EROS has not yet been found to fail to find the "correct" solution, except in investigations of how low, in resolution, the initial subsampled image can be. In terms of accuracy, the solution normally looks, by eye to be optimal at the voxel level. However, an area for future evaluation is a more quantitative investigation into the accuracy of results, compared with some kind of "gold standard", possibly defined manually by a group of investigators. In this way fine accuracy could be both optimised and quantified.

An example application of EROS is the pre-alignment of images before registration. Many existing registration methods carry out simple cost-function minimisation over a number of parameters without multiple starts - thus initial positioning often has a great effect on the success of the final registration. An example is the widely used AIR registration program [7, 8]. As part of a wider investigation into registration robustness [2], results from AIR were compared with the results given if EROS was used to pre-align the planes of symmetry from the two images. As Figure 7 shows, for almost all cases, using EROS improved the final registration quality greatly. In fact, EROS correctly aligned the symmetry plane in all cases; where the final registration was not correct after pre-alignment, the error was normally in rotation about the axis perpendicular to the mid-plane, which, obviously, is not at all constrained by finding the symmetry plane. Also, note that EROS is only used to provide a starting estimate to AIR - results could probably be improved if the plane alignment was actually used as a constraint during registration.

Figure 8 shows symmetry detection on two images of rotated shields. In the second case a large amount of noise was added but the result was still good.

An automatic, robust, accurate method has been developed. More work will be carried out to speed it up, and to address the question of rotation about the axis perpendicular to the mid-plane (this is a very different kind of problem). It will be straightforward to extend EROS to allow the estimation of a curved mid-"plane". There is scope for increasing the robustness of EROS by improving the lowest level measure of symmetry, based on means of absolute values. An alternative should be possible which is robust at even the lowest level to asymmetries, thus increasing even further the power to detect symmetry in objects with asymmetries. It is anticipated that the software will be made freely available from the FMRIB web site within a few months.

References

1. V. Di Gesù and C. Valenti. Symmetry operators in computer vision. *Vistas in Astronomy*, 40, 1996.
2. M. Jenkinson and S. Smith. Robustness issues in automatic brain image registration. *Proc. Int. Conf. on Medical Image Computing and Computer-Assisted Intervention*, 1999. submitted.
3. S. Minoshima, K.L. Berger, K.S. Lee, and M.A. Mintun. An automated method for rotation correction and centering of three-dimensional functional brain images. *Journal of Nuclear Medicine*, 33:1579–85, 1992.

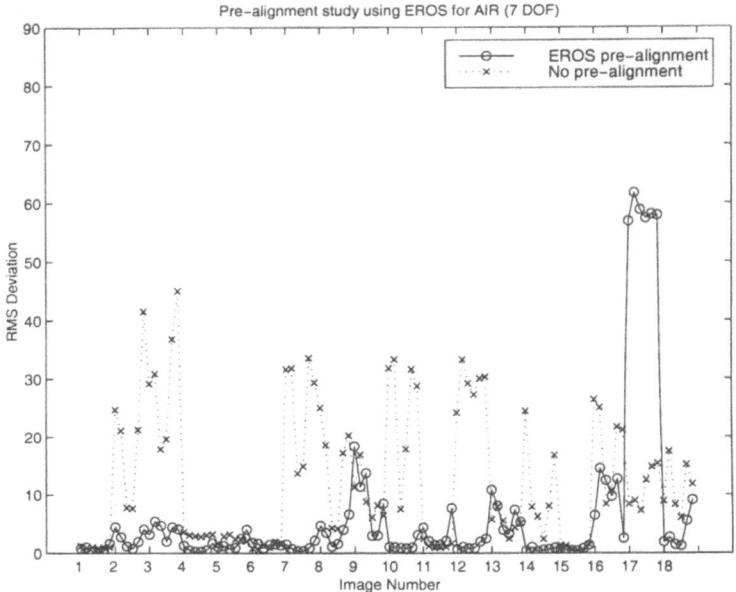

Fig. 7. Application of EROS to pre-alignment for registration - see text for details.

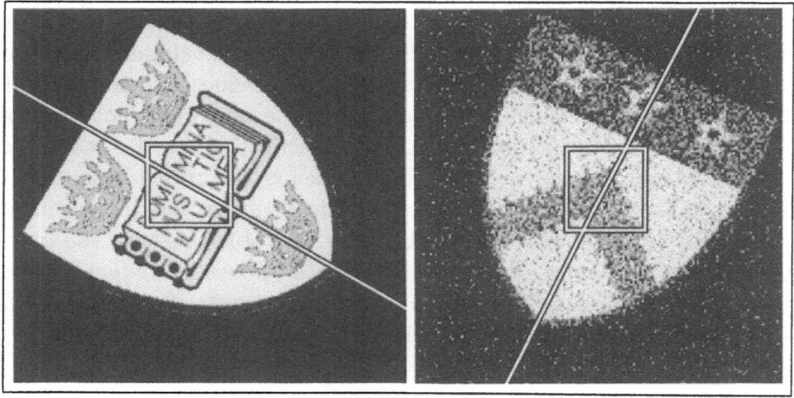

Fig. 8. Images of two shields after symmetry line detection by EROS. The second had Gaussian noise added (maximum image contrast = 255; noise standard deviation = 50).

4. D. Reisfeld, H. Wolfson, and Y. Yeshurun. Context free attentional operators: The generalized symmetry transform. *Int. Journal of Computer Vision*, 14:119–130, 1995.

5. C. Sun. Symmetry detection using gradient information. *Pattern Recognition Letters*, 16(9):987–996, 1995.

6. J.-P. Thirion, S. Prima, and G. Subsol. Statistical analysis of dissymmetry in volumetric medical images. Technical Report 3178, INRIA Sophia-Antipolis, 1997.
7. R.P. Woods, S.R. Cherry, and J.C. Mazziotta. Rapid automated algorithm for aligning and reslicing PET images. *Journal of Computer Assisted Tomography*, 16(4):620–633, 1992.
8. R.P. Woods, J.C. Mazziotta, and S.R. Cherry. MRI–PET registration with automated algorithm. *Journal of Computer Assisted Tomography*, 17(4):536–546, 1993.
9. T. Zielke, M. Brauckmann, and W. von Seelen. Intensity and edge-based symmetry detection applied to car-following. In *Proc. 2nd European Conf. on Computer Vision*, pages 865–873. Springer-Verlag, 1992.

Global Shape from Shading for an Endoscope Image

S.Y.Yeung[1], H.T.Tsui[1], and A.Yim[2]

[1] Department of Electronic Engineering
The Chinese University of Hong Kong
Shatin, Hong Kong
[2] Department of Surgery, Prince of Wales Hospital
ShaTin, Hong Kong

Keywords: Shape from Shading   Level set propagation   Endoscope image

Abstract. Okatani and Deguchi[13] proposed a local Shape from Shading (SFS) method for endoscope images by assuming the point light, which is close to the projection center, to be at the projection center. We extended and modified their method and devised a global SFS algorithm for the reconstruction of the complex shape of an internal organ. Since the surface of an organ is not Lambertian in general, we obtained the bi-directional reflection distribution function (BRDF) curve by calibration using a robot arm to achieve accurate endoscope orientation and positioning. Inspired by the idea of Kimmel and Bruckstein[8], global SFS method is based on the identification of singular points on the distance map, which each has the surface normal pointing towards the light source. Equal distance contours are propagated from each singular point using a level set method to get a local distance map of the surface. This is repeated for all singular points. After that, a set of local distance maps are selected to be merged together to construct a global distance map using a new scheme. The shape of the object can then be obtained from the global distance map. Simulated and real experiments were performed to verify the algorithm. Experimental result of global SFS from a single real endoscope image of a human lung is quite good.

1   Introduction

Shape from Shading (SFS) is a very useful technique for reconstructing 3D shape of an object from its single 2D grayscale image. When it was first introduced by Horn[4, 5], some assumptions were made to simplify the analysis. For example, the light source is supposed to be a single point light located at a great distance from the surface. The surface is of Lambertian, which means that the incident light is reflected evenly to all directions in a hemisphere by a Lambertian surface. The intensity of the surface in the image depends on the angle between local surface normal and the light source direction. Besides, this method suffers from the problem of topological ambiguities, which is known to be the problem of global shape from shading. We must solve this problem in order to get a correct global surface. These assumptions more or less limit the practical applications of Shape-from-Shading technique.

Many developments have been made to release these limitations. More accurate and complicated surface models are proposed to solve the problem of non-Lambertian surface. Torrance and Sparrow[18] proposed a theoretic reflectance model that takes specular reflection as well as diffuse reflection into consideration. Cook[3] extended the model by including ambient light and spectral dependencies. Bidirectional Reflection Distribution Function (or BRDF for short) is another model that can be used to describe conveniently the surface reflection by natural materials [7, 6, 11, 12].

It is very useful for morphological analysis of tumors on human inner organs if the global 3D shape can be reconstructed from endoscope image by SFS. However, the surface of human organ cannot be regarded as Lambertian. Okatani and Deguchi[13] used BRDF to describe the reflectance property to tackle this problem. They extended Kimmel and Bruckstein's SFS algorithm[10, 9] and introduced a notation of equal distance contour to recover the 3D shape by propagating the contour using a Level Set method[16]. Their algorithm also tackled the problem of a near light source quite well. But the algorithm can not reconstruct the shape if it has several hills and valleys. It is very important and significant to have a global SFS algorithm for endoscope image because the surface of human inner organ is often complicated in shape.

Bricault *et al.*[1] proposed a model-based SFS algorithm for transbronchial biopsy. Their algorithm can reconstruct global 3D surface. But pre-operative CT scan data is required as model for 3D reconstruction. Global SFS problem has also been studied by J.Oliensis and P.Dupuis[14, 15] and Kimmel [8]. Oliensis's algorithm is based on establishing the equivalence of shape from shading to a calculus of variations/optimal control problem. Kimmel's approach is based on classification of singular points according to topological properties of simple smooth surfaces. Both of the above algorithms assume a parallel light or a point light source distant from the surface. As far as we know, there is no method in the literature that can reconstruct global 3D shape from single grayscale image under a near light source. We extend Kimmel's algorithm and make it applicable to near light source.

The global SFS algorithm for endoscope image consists of three steps: First, starting from singular points, use a level set propagation algorithm to obtain distance maps from each surface point to the light source. This is the so-called local SFS problem for endoscope image. In this case, the singular points are those surface points that have local maximum intensity. Second, merge the distance maps together based on the classification of singular points. Third, project the distance map back to 3D coordinate to get the depth map of the object.

The rest of the paper is organized as follows. A brief review of local SFS algorithm for endoscope image by propagating equal distance contour proposed by Okatani etc.[13] is given in Section 2. In Section 3, the global SFS method for parallel light by Kimmel[8] is also reviewed, followed by the global SFS algorithm for endoscope image. The simulation and experiment results are shown in Section 4. Conclusion is given in Section 5.

2   Local SFS algorithm for endoscope image

A pinhole camera model is used for endoscope. In addition, since the surface of human inner organ is not Lambertian, a more general reflection model, BRDF is used to describe the reflection property of the surface, taking both the incident and reflection direction into consideration. The light of the endoscope can be approximated by a point light source located at the camera projection center[13]. This configuration simplifies the problem of near point light source and BRDF a lot.

2.1   Imaging system and brightness formulation

Here, we follow the derivation of Okatani and Deguchi[13]. The grayscale E in the image position (x, y) is given by,

$$E(x, \ y) = \delta \frac{F(\theta_i, \ \theta_r, \phi_r) \cos \theta_i}{r^2} \tag{1}$$

where $F(\theta_i, \ \theta_r, \phi_r)$ is the bidirectional reflectance distribution function[7] of the surface. ϕ_r is the azimuth angle between the incident light and the reflection light. r is the distance between the light source and the surface point, and δ is a constant depending on the intensity of light source and the camera parameters.

Since the light source and the view point is at the same position, the incident angle θ_i always equals to reflection angle θ_r, and ϕ_r is 0. Substitute the angles into Eq.1 yields,

$$E(x, \ y) = \delta \frac{F(\theta_i, \ \theta_i, 0) \cos \theta_i}{r^2} = \delta \frac{G(\cos \theta_i)}{r^2} \tag{2}$$

where $G(\cos \theta_i) = F(\theta_i, \ \theta_i, \ 0) \cos \theta_i$ is a monotonic increasing function with respect to $\cos \theta_i$. So given the image brightness $E(x, \ y)$ and the distance r, $\cos \theta_i$ can be uniquely determined by,

$$\cos \theta_i = G^{-1}(r^2 E(x, \ y)/\delta). \tag{3}$$

2.2   Equal distance contour propagation and shape reconstruction

Equal distance contour may be thought of as a curve on the object surface, where all points on that curve have the same distance to the light source. the contour can also be regarded as the intersection of the object with a sphere whose center is the light source. Given an initial equal distance contour, we can propagate it to construct a new equal distance contour $r + \delta r$, with δr small enough. Iteratively propagate the equal distance contour until each image point gets its distance to the projection center, the shape of the surface can then be represented by its distance map from the projection center of the endoscope. Starting from a small circle around a singular point as the initial equal distance contour $C(r_0)$, we define a function $\phi(x, y, r_0)$ on the image plane to be nagative inside the initial contour, and positive outside the contour. The equal distance contour at $r = t$ is given by

$$C(t) = (x, \ y)|\phi(x, \ y, \ t) = 0 \tag{4}$$

The contour can thus be propagated by updating the ϕ function with a velocity as

$$\phi_t = -\frac{G^{-1}(t^2 E(x, \ y)/\delta)}{f} \tag{5}$$

where f is the focal length of the endoscope.

Assume that the surface is smooth and simple and there is a point on the surface with the normal in the direction of the light source and has a minimum distance to the light. According to Eq.2, such a point can be selected by searching for the image point (x_0, y_0) with maximum brightness $E(x_0, y_0)$. The boundary of a small neighborhood of that singular point serves as the intial distance contour. The intial distance is given by,

$$r_0 = \sqrt{\delta G(1)/E(x_0, y_0)} \tag{6}$$

where the constant δ can be obtained by careful calibration.

3   Global SFS algorithm for endoscope image

Distance map is an alternative form to represent the shape of an object. If we can obtain the distance map of a global surface from its endoscope image, we can get the shape of the object easily. So the global SFS problem is now how to obtain a global distance map of the surface. Local SFS should be used to get locally correct distance map propagating from each singular point. The local distance maps are then merged together to obtain a global solution.

3.1   A global shape from shading algorithm for a parallel light

A simple global algorithm for SFS with a parallel light is proposed by Kimmel etc. see also [8]. Assuming that the surface is simple and smooth and can be described by a Morse function[2]. All singular points on that surface can be locally classified to be three types: Minima, Maxima and Saddle. The singular points are those that have surface normal in the direction of light source, and can be determined by considering the grid point of highest intensity within a connected area of pixels.

By propagating the equal height contour from a singular point m_i which is known to be a minima. we can obtain distance transform $D_i(x, y)$ of that singular point. The distance transform $D_i(x, y)$ is a relative depth map with respect to the singular point m_i. Given the absolute height $H(m_i)$ of each minima singular point on the depth map, the global surface $D_r(x, y)$ is given by [8],

$$D_r(x, y) = min(D_i(x, y) + H(m_i)) : i = 1 \ to \ N \qquad (7)$$

where N is the number of singular points which are minima. $D_i(x, y) + H(m_i)$ is the absolute height of the grid point (x, y) on the depth map.

It is difficult to use Eq.7 directly to get the global depth map of a surface because the absolute height $H(m_i)$ of the minima singular point m_i on the depth map is unknown. Besides, we cannot classify different types of singular points directly from the grayscale image, because all of the singular points are local brightest points. Kimmel proposed an iterative appoach to solve this problem. The inflection-type saddle point between two minima singular points should be identified. It serves as the merge point to merge two relative depth maps. The merging process goes on until a surface with no inflection-type saddle points is obtained. That surface is the global surface required. See [8] for detail.

3.2   The relationship between *depth map* and *distance map*

Let us first examine the relationship between depth map of a surface and distance map of that surface to the camera projection center. Take a simple surface of a hemisphere for example, as shown in the Fig.1. The radius of that hemosphere is R, and the light source and camera are located at the center of the hemisphere. All points on the surface have the same distance R to the light source. The corresponding distance map is shown in Fig.1(b). If on the depth map the surface normal at a point is in the direction of the light, its corresponding surface normal on the distance map is perpendicular to the $X - Y$ plane. It can be easily derived that propagating "equal distance contour" on the depth map is equivalent to the propagation of "equal height contour" on the distance map with a parallel light source coming from above and perpendicular to $X - Y$ plane. This equivalence helps to extend a global SFS algorithm for parallel light to a global SFS algorithm for a near light source.

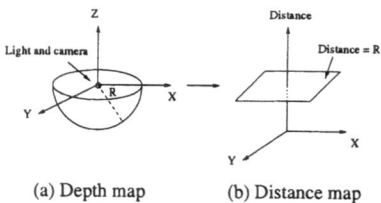

(a) Depth map   (b) Distance map

Fig. 1. Relationship of depth map and distance map

3.3   A global shape from shading algorithm for *endoscope* image

As mentioned before, the first step to reconstruct the global depth map of a surface from its endoscope image is to obtain its global distance map to the camera project center. We have discussed that propagating the equal distance contour on depth map is equivalent to propagating the "equal height contour" on the distance map. So the problem of obtaining global distance map for surface under endoscope is similar to the problem of obtaining global depth map for parallel light.

Assuming that the distance map is a simple and smooth surface. There are also three types of singular points: minima, maxima and saddle. (All singular points discussed below are on the distance map.) Starting from a minima singular point m_i, and using the Level set propagation, we can obtain a distance map $D_i(x, y)$. Since the absolute height of the point m_i on the distance map can be estimated by Eq.6, the distance map $D_i(x, y)$ is an absolute distance map. The global distance map $D_r(x, y)$ in this case is given by

$$D_r(x, y) = min(D_i(x, y)), i = 1 \ to \ N, \qquad (8)$$

The merging process is very simple. No iterative approach is needed. The resulting global distance map can be obtained from local distance maps in one step.

The key of this algorithm is to select all of the minima singular points on the distance map of the surface from the grayscale image. Let's have a look at the properties of three types of singular points on the distance map: Minima, Maxima and Saddle in the following.

Detecting maxima and saddle points According to mountaineers' theorem[17], the number of extrema located within a closed equal-height contour of a smooth surface exceeds by one the number of saddle points within that contour. Start propagating from a small circle around a minima singular point, the first singular point met by the equal-height contour must be a saddle point. Assuming there is a minima singular point m_i on the distance map, propagate equal-height contour from that point will yield a distance map $D_i(x, y)$. The first singular point met in the process of propagation must be a saddle point. Let us label the point as S. The height of that saddle point on the distance map can be correctly obtained from the distance map as $D_i(x_s, y_s)$, where (x_s, y_s) is the coordinate of point S in the image. As mentioned before, the surface normal at singular point will point in the direction of the light source. So $\cos\theta_i(S)$ equals 1. The distance from that singular point to the light source can be estimated by[13],

$$r_0(x_s, y_s) = \sqrt{\delta G(1)/E(x_s, y_s)} \qquad (9)$$

the value of $D_i(x_s, y_s)$ and $r_0(x_s, y_s)$ should match, i.e.

$$|D_i(x_s, y_s) - r_0(x_s, y_s)| < threshold \qquad (10)$$

The value of $|D_i(x_s, y_s) - r_0(x_s, y_s)|$ may not be zero because there may be some small error in estimating $r_0(x_s, y_s)$ and obtaining $D_i(x_s, y_s)$.

When the equal height contour on the distance map propagates through the saddle point S, there are two different cases. The contour will meet a maxima point(X) or a minima point(N). If the next singular point met is a maxima, the contour will be split into two parts: the inner part of the contour will end at the maxima singular point, and get the height of that maxima point on the distance map correctly. The height of that maxima point obtained from the distance map $D_i(X)$ should match the distance estimated by Eq.6, just like the case of the saddle. If the contour after passing the saddle point meets another minima point, there will be a topological error, the height of the next minima obtained from the distance map is not correct. The difference between $D_i(x_n, y_n)$ and $r_0(x_n, y_n)$ will be large. This helps to identify minima singular points from maxima and saddle points.

The proposed global SFS algorithm The procedure to get global distance map should be as follows:

step 1: Select singular points of distance map from the image by considering the local brightest point within a connected area of pixels in the image. These singular points, denoted as m_i, can fall into three types: minima, maxima and saddle.

step 2: Estimate the distance of each singular point m_i to the light by Eq.6. Use a small circle around the singular point to be an initial contour. Propagate the equal distance contour to get a local distance map D_i for each singular point.

step3: Use the obtained local distance maps to classify the singular points. Local distance maps propagated from maxima or saddle points must be deleted.

step 4: Merge the local distance maps starting from minima singular points together to get the global distance of the surface.

The procedure for the above step 2 is: For each singular point m_i, estimate its distance $r(m_i)$ to the light by Eq.6. Then search the distance map D_k starting from other singular point. If there is a distance map D_k such that $|D_k(m_i) - r(m_i)|$ is smaller than a threshold, then the singular point m_i is not a minima singular point. Then the corresponding distance map D_i should be deleted. The threshold we used in our experiments is $\frac{1}{2}(r(m_i) - r(m_k))$. The results are very good.

4   Simulations and experiments results

In the simulation, we use a software called Raytracing to simulate the endoscope lighting system and the camera. A complicated surface generated by matlab function $Z = PEAKS(X, Y)$ is used for testing. Its grayscale image taken by the simulated endoscope is shown in Fig.2(b). The global distance map was obtained first, as shown in Fig.2(c). The global depth map of the surface as shown in Fig.2(d) was then obtained by projecting the distance map back to 3D coordinate, . The result is very good.

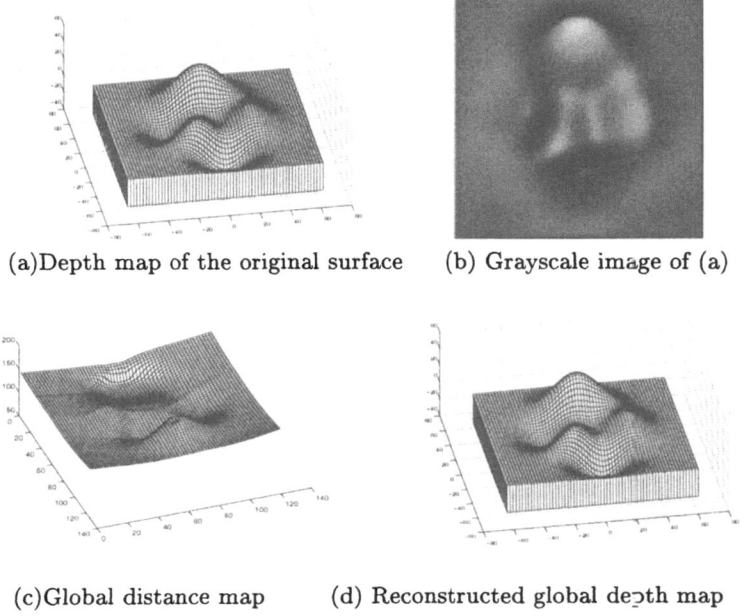

(a)Depth map of the original surface   (b) Grayscale image of (a)

(c)Global distance map   (d) Reconstructed global depth map

Fig. 2. Simulation result

Both Lambertian surface and nonLambertian surface are used in real experiments to verify the robustness of this algorithm. An image of a Lambertain model made of paper clay is taken by an real endoscope, as is shown in Fig.3(a). The reconstructed 3D surface of the model is shown in Fig.3(b). The BRDF for the Lambertian surface is degenerated to be $\cos \theta_i$. The result is satisfatory, except for little error due to interreflection between hills. Fig.4(a) shows the endoscope image of a patient's lung. Since the exact lung surface was not available for obtaining the BRDF, a similar surface was used to obtain the BRDF. A small piece of the surface was laid flat on the work table. The same endoscope was held by a robot arm to acquired images at viewing points forming a 90 degrees arc with the centre at the target object point. This allows us to compute a look up table for the function $G(\cos \theta_i)$. Shape of the lung was recovered using our global SFS method. Some liquid drops and blood drops are present on the image and had caused some unavoidable errors. In spite of this, the result is reasonably good.

5   Conclusion

In this paper, we have proposed a global SFS method for 3D reconstruction of an human internal organ from its endoscope image. Okatani and Deguchi[13] method is good only for local SFS. Unlike the method of Kimmel and Bruck-

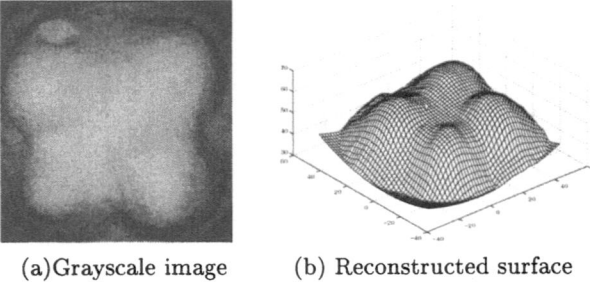

(a)Grayscale image   (b) Reconstructed surface

Fig. 3. Real experiment for Lambertian surface

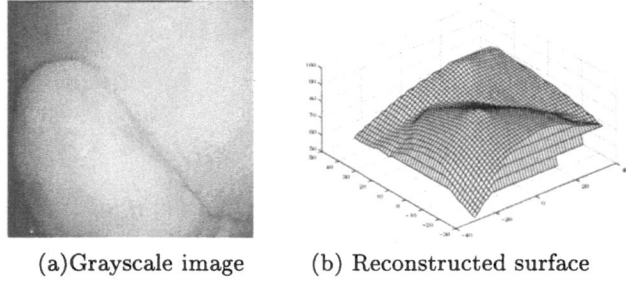

(a)Grayscale image   (b) Reconstructed surface

Fig. 4. Real experiment for non-Lambertian surface

stein[8] which used parallel light, our method used a near light model with the light assumed to be at the projection center. We obtained first a number of equal distance maps corresponding to the local minimum and merge them to form a global distance map. 3D shape is then derived from the global distance map. We did not assume the surface to be Lambertian. The BRDF of the surface is obtained by calibration with the help of a robot arm for accurate orientation and positioning of the endoscope. We have a different BRDF for different organ surface. Results from simulated experiments are very good. In the real images of organs, there are often bloods and liquid drops on the organ surface which have different surface reflectance properties. This heterogeneous surface is a major limitation of SFS in real applications. In spite of this, we managed to obtain quite good results. Better results may be expected if the blood and liquid can be removed from the image by image processing.

Acknowledgements

We thank Dr. T.W.Lee of the Prince of Wales Hospital for his help to get the real images for the experiment. This research was supported by the RGC research grants: CUHK 4162/97E and CUHK 4116/97E.

References

1. I. Bricault, G. Ferretti, and P. Cinquin. "Multi-level Strategy for Computer-Assisted Transbronchial Biopsy". In *Lecture Notes in Computer Science 1496, (MICCAI'98)*, pages 261–268, 1998.
2. J. W. Bruce and P. J. Giblin. *"Curves and Singularities"*. 2nd ed. Cambridge Univ. Press, Cambridge, UK, 1992.
3. R. L. Cook and K. E. Torrance. "A Reflectance Model for Computer Graphics". *Computer Graphics 15(3)*, pages 307–316, 1981.
4. B. K. P. Horn. *"Shape from Shading: A method for Obtaining the Shape of a Smooth Opaque Object from One View"*. MIT Project MAC Internal Report TR79 and MIT AI Laboratoru Technical Report 232, November.
5. B. K. P. Horn. *"Robot Vision"*. The MIT Press, 1986.
6. B. K. P. Horn and M. J. Brooks. *"Shape from Shading"*. The MIT Press, 1989.
7. B. K. P. Horn and R. W. Sjoberg. "Calculating the reflection map". *Applied Optics, 18*, pages 1770–1779, 1979.
8. R. Kimmel and A. Bruckstein. "Global Shape from Shading". *Computer Vision and Image Understanding, Vol. 62, No. 3*, pages 360–369, 1995.
9. R. Kimmel and A. Bruckstein. "Teacking Level Sets by Level Sets: A Method for Solving the Shape·from Shading Problem". *Computer Vision and Image Understanding, Vol. 62, No. 2*, pages 47–58, 1995.
10. R. Kimmel, K. Siddiqi, B. Kimia, and A. Bruckstein. "Shape from Shading: Level Set Propagation and Viscosity Solutions". *International Journal of Computer Vision, 16*, pages 107–133, 1995.
11. S. K. Nayar, K. Ikeuchi, and T. Kanade. "Surface Reflection: Physical and Geometrical Perspectives". *IEEE Transactions on Pattern Analysis and Machine Intelligence*, pages 611–634, 1991.
12. F. E. Nicodemus, J. C. Richmond, J. J. Hsia, I. W. Girsberg and T. Limperis. "Geometrical considerations and nomendature for reflectance". *NBS Monograph 160 (National Bureau of standards, Washington, D.C.)*, October 1997.
13. T. Okatani and K. Deguchi. "Shape Reconstruction from an Endoscope Image by Shape from Shading Technique for a Point Light Source at the Projection Center". *Computer Vision and Image Understanding, vol.66, No.2 May*, pages 119–131, 1997.
14. J. Oliensis. " Shape from Shading as a Partially Well-Constrained Problem". *CVGIP: Image Understanding, Vol. 54*, pages 163–183, 1993.
15. J. Oliensis and P. Dupuis. "A Global Algorithm for Shape from Shading". In *Proc. of the 4th ICCV*, pages 692–701, 1993.
16. S. Osher and S. A. Sethian. "Fronts propagating with curvature-dependent speed: Algorithms based on Hamilton-Jacobi formulations". *J. of Comput. Phys. 79*, pages 12–49, 1998.
17. E. Rouy and A. Tourin. "A viscosity solutions approach to shape-from shading". *SIAM J. Number. Anal. 29(3)*, pages 867–884, June 1992.
18. K. E. Torrance and E. Sparrow. "Theory for off-Specular Reflection from Roughened Surface". *J. Opt. Soc. Amer. 57*, pages 1105–1114, 1967.

The Measurement of Focal Diurnal Variation in the Femoral Articular Cartilage of the Knee

A. D. Brett, J. C. Waterton, S. Solloway, J. E. Foster, M. C. Keen, S. Gandy,
B. J. Middleton, R. A. Maciewicz, I. Watt, P. A. Dieppe and C. J. Taylor

[1] Division of Imaging Science, Manchester University, Manchester, UK
[2] Cardiovascular, Metabolism & Musculoskeletal Research Dept, AstraZeneca
Pharmaceuticals, Cheshire, UK
[3] Medical Physics & Bioengineering, United Bristol Healthcare Trust, Bristol, UK
[4] Safety of Medicines Dept., AstraZeneca Pharmaceuticals, Cheshire, UK
[5] Dept. Radiology, United Bristol Healthcare Trust, Bristol, UK
[6] Dept. Rheumatology, University of Bristol, Bristol, UK

Abstract. Our objective was to test the hypothesis that focal diurnal
changes occur in the femoral articular cartilage of the knee in asymptomatic young adults. Six volunteers each were scanned early in the
morning, and at the end of a working day spent mainly standing. This
protocol was repeated on three successive weeks. Femoral cartilage segmentations were obtained using a region-growing algorithm. These segmentations then were regridded onto a 500-pixel template, and differences in the resulting thickness maps were assessed. Analysis of variance
showed no significant diurnal variation in mean thickness. There were,
however, statistically-significant diurnal changes in the thickness maps.
Cartilage thickness decreased during the day in three specific locations
which suffer the greatest biomechanical force.

1 Introduction

Osteoarthritis (OA) is one of the principal causes of disability in elderly people.
The disease is characterised by focal structural changes, and eventual loss, of
articular cartilage. The knee joint is often most severely affected, and anatomical
locations suffering the highest biomechanical force are most likely to exhibit
cartilage damage.

Recently, it has become possible to measure accurately and precisely the
volume of the articular cartilage with MRI [13, 4]. Fat-suppressed 3D spoiled
gradient-echo MRI has been widely adopted, and provides good contrast with
reasonable scanning times. However, because of the shape of the cartilage, manual segmentation of the images is tedious, so that for large-scale studies, it is
desirable to develop semi-automatic techniques [6]. It now appears possible that
MRI assessment of cartilage volume will be accurate and precise enough to measure OA disease progression and therapeutic intervention in small-scale trials,
unlike the X-ray assessment of joint-space narrowing [3] which has poor statistical power. Before MRI can be employed in prospective controlled trials of

structure-modifying (cartilage-preserving) drugs, however, it will be essential to understand potential confounding factors, such as diurnal variation.

Recently, we have described [7] a study seeking evidence for diurnal variation in the volume of the femoral articular cartilage in young adults. In that work, there was no evidence for diurnal change in cartilage volume: the average volume change (PM MINUS AM) was -0.0010cm^3 (95% confidence interval -0.0945 to $+0.0745$), a decline of 0.1%. However, because OA is a disease of focal changes in the articular cartilage, we wished to determine whether regional diurnal changes could be detected in this data set. Further, we required a method of analysis which incorporated no preconceptions about the location or nature of the putative focal changes. It was therefore necessary to develop an objective method for significance testing of focal changes in a population of knees. The aims of this study were, therefore, to determine whether focal diurnal variations occur in the femoral articular cartilage of the knee.

2   Cartilage Data

Six volunteers (three male, three female), aged 21–25, without symptoms of any musculoskeletal disorder, were imaged in the morning (AM) at 07:45, and at 16:45 near the end of their working day (PM). Their days were spent predominantly in the laboratory, mostly standing at a bench. The imaging protocol, which is described below, was repeated on three consecutive weeks. One of the volunteers was not imaged at week two, giving a total of 34 scans.

2.1   Imaging Protocol

The MR parameters were [6]: field strength 1.0T (Siemens Impact); sagittal 3D spoiled gradient echo; fat saturation; TR 47 msec; TE 11 msec; flip angle 40°; 192 phase-encoding steps; 64 slice partitions; matrix zero-filled to 256×256; FOV 140 mm; no signal averaging, giving voxel dimensions $0.55 \times 0.55 \times 1.56$ mm.

2.2   Segmentation

There are various approaches to segmentation of the articular cartilage. This study employed a data-driven segmentation method ('Tosca' version 2.3) (IBM, Winchester, UK) [5] giving rapid and precise measurements of volume and thickness assessment at sub-voxel resolution. All segmentations were performed by the same operator (J.E.F) and all the femoral cartilage was included in the analysis. To segment the femoral articular cartilage, a seed-point was placed within the area to be analysed. A region grower algorithm [15] was then started using interactively-determined values for the cartilage. The procedure was repeated for each slice in the data set. To ensure anatomical accuracy, minor adjustments to the segmented regions were required occasionally. A proportion of the segmentations were checked by a musculoskeletal radiologist (I.W.). J.E.F.'s intra-observer coefficient of variation with this approach is 1.5% [6]. This semi-automatic technique was considerably faster than manual segmentation. The latter can be rather operator-dependent and, because of the time-consuming nature of the operation, prone to errors due to operator fatigue. Typically a complete semi-automatic cartilage volume measurement was produced in less than an hour.

3   Thickness Mapping

The 3D thickness distribution of the cartilage was obtained by a generalisation of a method previously used in 2D [16]. In 3D, the method consists of three stages:

1. Each of the contours of each of the cartilage segmentations was used as input data to an automatic landmark generation algorithm. This produced the same number of *corresponding* points on each of the contours across all cartilage examples.
2. Each of the cartilage examples was re-sampled by linear interpolation to contain the same number of corresponding slice contours, each with the same number of defining points.
3. Thickness measurements were made at a number of corresponding points defined by a medial axis for each slice of each cartilage example.

These stages will now be described in more detail below.

3.1   Generating Correspondence Between Contours

An automatic landmark generation algorithm [8] was used to create sets of corresponding landmarks on each of the slice contours of each of the segmented cartilage examples. This approach is possible because the topology of the slice contours does not change in a set of sagittal scans of the femoral cartilage. The algorithm is based upon a pair-wise corresponder which is used to match pairs of input shapes and measure the cost of these matches. The corresponder is used to produce a matrix of match costs between all pair combinations of the set of input shapes. The pairs with smallest matching costs are then merged to produce mean shapes. These mean shapes comprise the next level of a binary tree of merged pairs. Pairs of shapes are matched and merged at each level until a single mean shape exists at the root of the tree, the input shapes being the leaves of this tree, see Fig 1. A set of N_l landmarks may be placed upon the mean shape at the root using, for example, a critical point detection algorithm [17]. These landmarks may then be propagated through the branches of the tree to the leaves using the fact that correspondences exists between each pair and its mean. In this way, a set of N_l corresponding landmarks is produced on each of the input shapes.

The pair-wise corresponder takes a pair of densely sampled shape boundaries, **A** and **B**, and produces a sparse set of corresponding of point pairs on those boundaries in three stages:

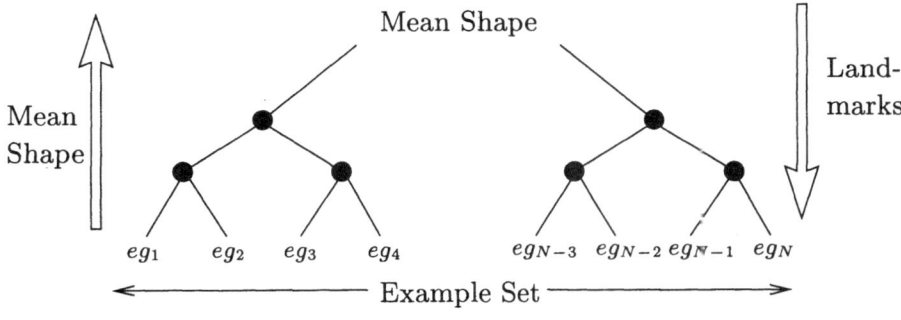

Fig. 1. A binary tree of merged shapes is produced using a pair-wise corresponder. Landmarks are propagated from a single mean shape at the root of the tree, to the example shapes at the leaves.

1. Sparse polygonal approximations to A and B, A'' and B'', are generated using the critical point detection algorithm of Zhu and Chirlian [17]. These are simply sparse representations of A and B - no correspondences are established at this stage and the two polygons will normally have differing numbers of vertices; $n_{A''} \neq n_{B''}$.
2. An initial estimate of corresponding sparse polygons, A' and B' are made. This stage uses a correspondence algorithm based on arc path length. The assumption is made that if a proportion of the boundary, say 5%, of the arc path length of A exists between two of the vertices of A'', then there should be 5% of the arc path length of B between the two points on B which correspond with those on A''. A least-squared Euclidean distance metric between sets of corresponding points is used to optimise this correspondence.
3. The initial set of correspondences generated in stage 2. is refined. This stage uses a greedy optimisation scheme to modify the correspondence pairs. This produces sparse polygons A' and B' which are similar in shape to one another and have similar representation errors with respect to their defining boundaries A and B.

3.2   Slice Interpolation

Correspondence between contours of each segmentation is not sufficient to produce a mapping between each segmentation example. We require correspondence between surfaces. This is achieved by linearly interpolating a new set of N_c slice contours between the first and last of the stack of contours representing each segmentation, see Fig 2. Each segmentation is now represented by a set of N_c contours, each having N_1 defining vertices.

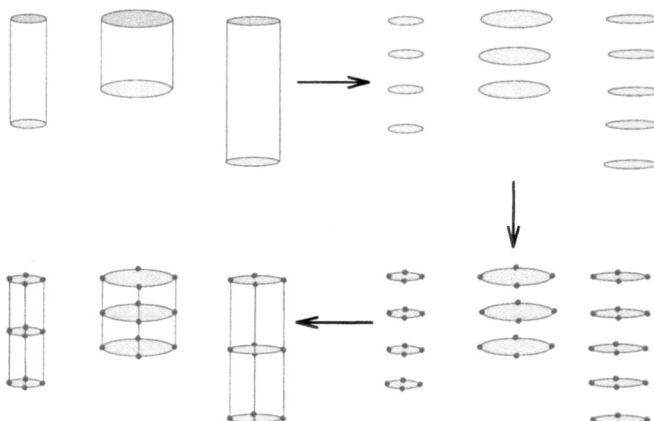

Fig. 2. Each example must have the same number of contours, each with the same number of defining vertices.

3.3   Thickness Computation

The medial axis of the points in each re-interpolated slice was found using the algorithm described by Shapiro [14]. A set of N_t equally-spaced points was generated along the medial axis. For each point, the thickness of the cartilage was given by the distance between the intercepts of the normal to the axis with the inner and outer surface, as shown in Fig 3.

The points, (x_j^i, y_j^i) and (y_j^o, x_j^o), of intersection of the normal to the jth point along the medial axis with the inner and outer surface respectively, are found by solving the equations,

$$
\begin{aligned}
(x_j^m - x_j^i)\cos\theta + (y_j^m - y_j^i)\sin\theta = 0 \\
(x_j^m - x_j^o)\cos\theta + (y_j^m - y_j^o)\sin\theta = 0
\end{aligned}
\tag{1}
$$

where $j = 1 \ldots N_t$. The thickness, t of the cartilage at each point is given by

$$
t_j = \sqrt{(x_j^i - x_j^o)^2 + (y_j^i - y_j^o)^2}.
\tag{2}
$$

This slice-by-slice method overestimates thickness where the slice plane is $< 90°$ to the surface, e.g. between the condyles: however since the thrust of our work is to measure differences in thickness, these small systematic errors should cancel. In any case most of the condylar surface, both load-bearing and non load-bearing is very close to 90% to the sagittal plane. By measuring the thickness with respect to the medial axis, the measurements are robust to small indentations on the cartilage surfaces.

3.4   Thickness Maps

The resulting thickness distribution maps are analogous to those obtained by other workers using different algorithms [12, 10]. Each 3D example was re-sampled

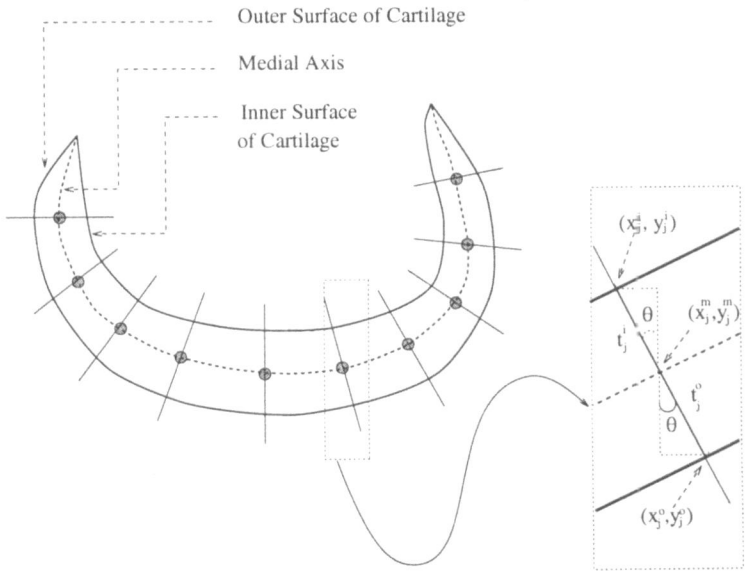

Fig. 3. Thickness measurements made in 2D along the medial axis of the contour defining the cartilage on one slice.

to produce a correspondence of $N_c = 25$ sagittal slices with $N_l = 38$ landmarks as defining vertices. The medial axis of each slice was sampled to give $N_t = 20$ thickness values so that a 25×20 point thickness map was generated. The diurnal change for each subject on each day was represented in the difference map, PM MINUS AM. The population mean diurnal difference was obtained from the mean of all seventeen PM MINUS AM maps. Additionally, a mean thickness value was calculated from each of the 34 thickness maps.

4   Statistical Analysis of Global Changes

Analysis of variance was used to test the hypothesis that there was a diurnal change in the mean thickness. The data were fitted using date, time of day and gender as fixed terms and subject-within-gender as random. To judge date, time of day, their interaction and how each interacts with gender, their interaction with subjects-within-gender were also fitted. The reproducibility of the method was assessed from the test-retest coefficient of variation (CoV). For each subject, i, the CoV is the standard deviation, σ_i, for a series of measurements on that subject, divided by the mean volume, μ_i, for the subject. The overall test-retest CoV for a group of N subjects is then $\sqrt{\sum_i (\sigma_i/\mu_i)^2/N}$. An assessment of the ability of the method to measure small weekly changes was obtained from the sum of the week-to-week term (i.e. variance for a volunteer of a given gender on a given date) $\sigma^2_{\text{subj(date}\times\text{sex)}}$ and the residual term $\sigma^2_{\text{residual}}$ in the analysis of variance: the CoV for a weekly difference is then

$$\frac{\sqrt{2(\sigma^2_{\mathrm{subj(date\times sex)}} + \sigma^2_{\mathrm{residual}})}}{\sum_i \mu_i/N}. \tag{3}$$

5 Statistical Analysis of Regional Changes

To test whether there was a statistically significant pattern of diurnal redistribution of the cartilage thickness, a principal component and linear discriminant analysis of the 34 thickness maps was performed. This analysis was undertaken without any prior assumptions about which locations might be most susceptible to diurnal change.

- With the assumption of identical covariance matrices for the two groups, a Principal Component Analysis (PCA) [9] on normalised thickness vectors, t, was performed, giving a set of eigenvectors, **P**.
- The original vectors were projected onto the eigenvector basis **P**, giving t**P**. This is a data reduction step which helps to reduce the complexity of the problem.
- A Linear Discriminant Analysis was performed on the projected vectors, using AM and PM thickness patterns as separate classes. This gave the vector, **d**, which provided the best discrimination between AM and PM.
- The eigenvectors, t**P**, were projected onto the discriminant vector **d**, giving t**Pd**.
- The scalar values derived from this projection for each thickness map were tested to see if there were significant differences between the AM and PM maps, using the two-tailed Student's t-test.

6 Results

6.1 Mean Thickness

Analysis of variance (Table 1) also showed no evidence of diurnal variation in mean thickness. There was a trend to thicker cartilage in males than females, consistent with previous observations from MRI in young people [2, 11].

6.2 Spatial Dependence of Thickness

We sought to test the hypothesis of focal diurnal changes in regional thickness, perhaps associated with regions of mechanical loading. Fig. 4 is a colour map showing the mean of all seventeen PM MINUS AM maps. Cartilage thickness decreased during the day in specific locations: in the patellofemoral compartment, in the lateral tibiofemoral compartment, and in the medial tibiofemoral compartment. Elsewhere cartilage volume was unchanged or became thicker. Projection of the original thickness vectors, t, onto the first two principal components of

Term	Cause of variation	Mean thickness / mm	
Fixed terms		Effect (95% confidence interval)	
sex	male minus female	0.52(1.07,-0.03)	P = 0.059
date	week 1 vs week 2 vs week 3	0.11(-0.24,0.36)	P > 0.05
time	AM minus PM	0.02(0.22,-0.17)	P > 0.05
Random terms		Contribution to total variance	
subj(sex)	given gender	53.8%	P = 0.036
subj(date×sex)	given gender on given date	25.5%	P = 0.006
subj(time×sex)	given gender at given time	12.4%	P = 0.02
residual		8.3%	

Table 1. Analysis of variance for mean thickness. For the fixed term date, data shown are for week 1 minus week 2; for week 1 vs week 3, and for week 2 vs week 3, (not shown) the effects were similar (all P > 0.05). Also included in the analysis of variance were the four cross terms (time×sex), (time×date), (date×sex) and (time×date×sex). These were fixed in the analyses, and none was significantly different from zero. P is the probability that a term contributed to the residual a significant additional source of variance. Although the terms 'subj(date×sex)' and 'subj (time×sex)' appear significant, the significance was lost when the outlying data from volunteer at week 3 were omitted.

the PCA analysis showed a clear separation between the different subjects, but did not separate the AM and PM images. However a significance test of the projection **tP** of the measurement vector onto the discriminant mode, giving **tPd**, showed that this diurnal change in the distribution of cartilage thickness was indeed statistically significant (p < 0.05). This discriminant vector is shown in Fig. 5.

7   Conclusions

Patients with OA lose cartilage not uniformly, but preferentially at certain locations, so that focal measurements of thickness will provide more information than volume alone, provided that good statistical power can be achieved. The method employed in this study allows multiple images from the same or different subjects to be regridded onto a standard template. Image analysis using this standard template allowed an objective evaluation of regional thickness changes common to our population, and allowed tiny physiological changes in articular cartilage thickness to be detected from data acquired using a standard clinical MRI protocol. A strength of the approach is that the evaluation is not influenced by prior expectations about which locations might be most likely to change. Nevertheless, diurnal cartilage thinning in this study was observed precisely at those sites known to be most susceptible to OA [1].

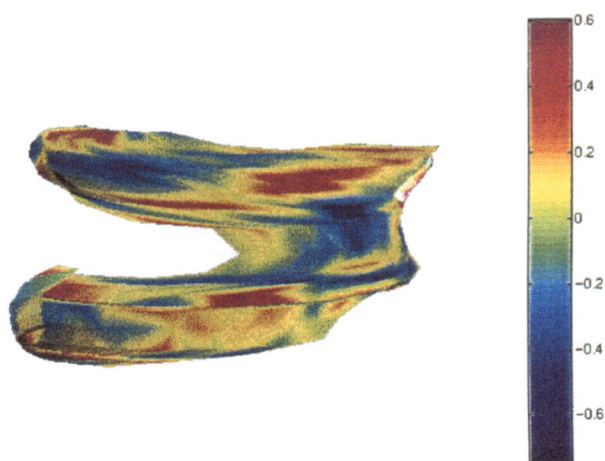

Fig. 4. Overall cartilage thickness difference map, i.e. the average of seventeen individual AM MINUS PM difference maps. The scale represents thickness change in mm. During the day, cartilage thickness decreased by ~ 0.5 mm in dark blue regions, while in red regions thickness increased by ~ 0.5 mm. Patellofemoral compartment is at right of figure, medial tibiofemoral compartment is bottom left in figure, lateral tibiofemoral compartment is top left.

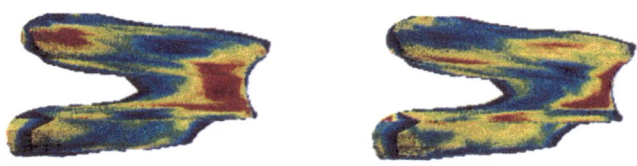

Fig. 5. Two instances of the principal components of the diurnal thickness variation. By moving along the vector which best discriminates between AM and PM measurements in the space of the principal components, we can examine the local changes to the cartilage thickness. These two figures show extremes in variation at +2 and -2 standard deviations from the mean of the cartilage thickness. The red areas are those which exhibit the greatest deviations from the mean, while the blue areas exhibit the least variation.

References

1. P. G. Bullough. Osteoarthritis and related disorders: pathology. In J. H. Klippe and P. A. Dieppe, editors, *Rheumatology*, volume 2, pages 8.3.1–8.8.8, London, 1998. Mosby Yearbook.
2. M. Cova, F. Frezza, I. Shariat-Razavi, M. Ukmar, R. S. P. Mucelli, and L. D. Palma. Valutazione con risonanza magnetica degli aspetti della cartilagini ialine articolari del ginocchio in funzione dell'età, del sesso e del peso corporeo. *Radiol. Med.*, 92:171–179, 1996.
3. P. A. Dieppe, J. Cushnaghan, and L. Shepstone. The Bristol 'OA500' study: Progression of osteoarthritis over three years and the relationship between clinical and radiographic changes at the knee joint. *Osteoarthr. Cartilage*, 6:87–97, 1997.
4. F. Eckstein, H. Sittek, S. Milz, and M. Reiser. The morphology of articular cartilage assessed by magnetic resonance imaging. *Surg. Radiol. Anat.*, 16:429–438, 1994.
5. P. J. Elliott, J. Diedrichsen, K. J. Goodson, R. Riste-Smith, and G. J. Sivewright. An object–oriented system for 3D medical image analysis. *IBM Systems Journal*, 35(1):5–24, 1996.
6. J. E. Foster, P. A. Dieppe, R. A. Maciewicz, J. Taberner, I. Watt, and J. C. Waterton. Quantification of cartilage volume and visualisation of osteoarthritis using a clinical MR system. *Arthr. Rheum.*, 39:s170, 1996.
7. J. E. Foster, M. C. Keen, I. Watt, P. A. Dieppe, R. A. Maciewicz, J. C. Waterton, and B. J. Middleton. Measurement of human articular cartilage volume: Diurnal effects on precision. In *Proc. ISMRM, 5th Meeting*, page 344, Vancouver, 1997.
8. A. Hill, A. D. Brett, and C. J. Taylor. Automatic landmark identification using a new method of non-rigid correspondence. In J. Duncan and G. Gindi, editors, 15th *Conference on Information Processing in Medical Imaging*, pages 483–488, Poulteney, VT, 1997. Springer-Verlag.
9. I. T. Jolliffe. *Principle Component Analysis*. Springer-Verlag, New York, 1986.
10. A. Lösch, F. Eckstein, M. Haubner, and K.-H. Englmeier. A non-invasive technique for three-dimensional assessment on articular cartilage thickness based on MRI part 1: development of a computational method. *Magn. Reson. Imaging*, 15:795–804, 1997.
11. S. Lukasz, R. Muhlbauer, S. Faber, K.-H. Englmeier, M. Reise, and F. Eckstein. Geschlechtsspezifische Analyse der Knorpelvolumina des Knieelenks - eine quantitative MRT-basierte Studie. *Anat. Anz.*, 180(6):487–93, 1998.
12. C. A. McGibbon, D. E. Dupuy, W. E. Palmer, and D. E. Krebs. Cartilage and subchondral bone thickness distribution with MRI. *Acad. Radiol.*, 5:20–25, 1998.
13. C. G. Peterfy, C. F. van Dijke, D. L. Janzen, C. C. Glüer, R. Namba, S. Majumdar, P. Lang, and H. K. Genant. Quantification of articular cartilage in the knee with pulsed saturation transfer subtraction and fat-suppressed MR imaging: Optimization and validation. *Radiology*, 192:485–491, 1994.
14. B. Shapiro and J. Sklansky. Skeleton generation from x,y boundary sequences. *Computer Vision, Graphics and Image Processing*, 15:136–153, 1981.
15. G. Sivewright and P. Elliot. Interactive Region and Volume Growing in MR and CT. *Medical Informatics*, 19(1):71–80, 1994.
16. S. Solloway, C. E. Hutchinson, J. C. Waterton, and C. J. Taylor. The use of active shape models for making thickness measurements of articular cartiage from MR images. *Magnetic Resonance in Medicine*, 37:943–952, 1997.
17. P. Zhu and P. M. Chirlian. On critical point detection of digital shapes. *IEEE Transactions on Pattern Analysis and Machine Intelligence*, 17(8):737–748, 1995.

Three-Dimensional Reconstruction and Quantification of Hip Joint Cartilages from Magnetic Resonance Images

Yoshinobu Sato[1], Tetsuya Kubota[1], Katsuyuki Nakanishi[2], Hisashi Tanaka[2], Nobuhiko Sugano[3], Takashi Nishii[3], Kenji Ohzono[3], Hironobu Nakamura[2], Takahiro Ochi[3], and Shinichi Tamura[1]

[1] Division of Functional Diagnostic Imaging, Biomedical Research Center
[2] Department of Radiology
[3] Department of Orthopaedic Surgery
Osaka University Medical School, Suita, Osaka, 565-0871, Japan
yoshi@image.med.osaka-u.ac.jp, http://www.med.osaka-u.ac.jp/image/yoshi

Abstract. A method for automated determination of the distribution of hip joint cartilage thickness from *in vivo* magnetic resonance (MR) images is described. Three-dimensional (3-D) filtering techniques are combined with the shape constraint of the ball and socket constitution of the hip joint to accurately detect and quantitate thin structures of cartilages. The method consists of three steps: 3-D cartilage enhancement filtering, detection, and quantification. First, the cartilage and articular space regions in MR images are effectively enhanced by 3-D radial directional second-derivative filtering based on the sphere approximation of the hip joint. Next, the initial regions of the cartilages and articular space are detected from the filtered images using thresholding and connectivity analysis. The boundaries of these regions provide the initial descriptions for the subsequent refinement processes. Finally, the boundaries of cartilage regions are accurately localized and quantitated three-dimensionally through subpixel edge searching. The effect of partial voluming on the accuracy of the estimated thickness is evaluated by means of software simulation studies, and the usefulness of the method is demonstrated through experiments using *in vivo* MR images of a normal volunteer and actual patients.

1   Introduction

Because determining the distribution of articular cartilage thickness is considered to be particularly important in the diagnosis of joint diseases, especially in their early stages, *in vivo* determination of cartilage thickness has received considerable attention. Magnetic resonance (MR) imaging is regarded as the most suitable modality for cartilage imaging because it provides inherently higher contrast with surrounding tissues than computed tomography (CT) [1]. Several successful results have been reported with respect to knee joint cartilage determination from *in vivo* [3],[4] as well as *in vitro* MR images [2]. In the case of hip joint cartilage, however, although *in vitro* thickness measurement have been studied [5],[6],[7],[8], no practical method applicable to *in vivo* MR images has yet been reported.

In the work reported in this paper, our aim was to develop a computerized method for the segmentation and thickness quantification of hip joint cartilage from *in vivo* MR images of the type that are obtained routinely. MR images are acquired during leg traction so as to clearly depict the articular space, which permits the discrimination of the femoral and acetabular cartilages [9]. Our intention is to use the method we have developed in clinical studies to investigate the relationship between the progress of joint diseases and cartilage thickness distribution, which will require its application to a large set of data obtained from patients and normal volunteers. This means that segmentation from surrounding tissues and thickness quantification need to be carried out without painstaking operator interaction yet with acceptable accuracy.

Our approach is to use three-dimensional (3-D) filtering techniques combined with the shape constraint of the ball and socket constitution of the hip joint to accurately detect and quantitate thin cartilage structures. The method consists of three steps: 3-D cartilage enhancement filtering, initial segmentation of cartilage regions, and accurate determination of cartilage edges for thickness measurement. Thin parts of cartilage are easily disposed to collapse due to noise, low resolution, and/or the partial volume effect. Filtering techniques designed to enhance small collapsed vessels in 3-D images, such as those obtained in MR and CT angiography, have been studied [10]. We use such a filter to enhance the cartilage regions and the articular space regions between femoral and acetabular cartilages, which enhances sheet-like structures but is modified based on the constraint of the spherical shape of hip joint. The subsequent cartilage segmentation is significantly improved using the filtered images. The boundaries of these segmented regions provide good initial points for final subpixel localization of cartilage edges.

2   Methods

The method fully utilizes the constraint of the hip joint shape. That is, it assumes that both the femoral and acetabular cartilages are distributed on a spherical surface. The thickness is measured radially from the center point of a sphere, which is an approximation of the femoral head. We define the locations of cartilage edges as the zero-crossing points of directional second derivatives of Gaussian-smoothed 3-D images. The directional second derivatives are taken in radial directions from the center point of the sphere that approximates the femoral head. The problem is how to search for and select the outer and inner edges of the femoral and acetabular cartilage regions from among all the zero-crossing points detected along each radial direction. Our approach is to extract the approximate cartilage and articular space regions so that their boundaries provide good initial points for the zero-crossing search. Multi-scale directional second-derivative filters are used to enhance the cartilages and the articular space between the femoral and acetabular cartilages, which facilitates segregation from surrounding tissues and the recovery of thin structures that have collapsed due to noise and/or the partial volume effect. Thresholding and connectivity analysis are then applied to extract the approximated cartilage and articular space regions. Even though the boundaries of these extracted regions do not exactly coincide with the zero-crossing positions, the search process successfully locates them by a simple ascending/descending method if the boundary is situated within the slope region that includes the zero-crossing we are seeking and does not include any local maxima and/or minima. In the following sections, each step of the method is described in detail.

2.1   Interpolation and Cartilage Enhancement Filtering

3-D MR images are interpolated using sinc interpolation [10] such that each voxel is isotropic in all three directions and, further, so the image size is doubled. Let $I(x)$ be the interpolated original 3-D MR image and $\nabla^2 I(x; \sigma)$ be the Hessian matrix of the 3-D MR image blurred by the isotropic Gaussian function with the standard deviation σ, which is given by

$$\nabla^2 I(x; \sigma) = \begin{bmatrix} I_{xx}(x;\sigma) & I_{xy}(x;\sigma) & I_{xz}(x;\sigma) \\ I_{yx}(x;\sigma) & I_{yy}(x;\sigma) & I_{yz}(x;\sigma) \\ I_{zx}(x;\sigma) & I_{zy}(x;\sigma) & I_{zz}(x;\sigma) \end{bmatrix}, \tag{1}$$

where partial second derivatives of the Gaussian blurred image $I(x; \sigma)$ are represented by expressions like $I_{xx}(x; \sigma) = \frac{\partial^2}{\partial x^2} I(x; \sigma)$, $I_{yz}(x; \sigma) = \frac{\partial^2}{\partial y \partial z} I(x; \sigma)$, and so on. Here, $I_{xx}(x; \sigma)$ is computed by $\{\frac{\partial^2}{\partial x^2} G(x; \sigma)\} * I(x)$, where $G(x; \sigma)$ is the 3-D isotropic Gaussian function and $*$ denotes the convolution.

Figure 1(a) shows a typical MR image of the hip joint cartilages. The bright regions of the femoral and acetabular cartilages are separated by the dark region of the articular space. Both the cartilage and articular space regions are typically sheet-like structures with spherical shapes in 3-D.

The cartilage and articular space enhancement filters are based on multi-scale directional second derivatives whose directions are the 3-D radial directions from the specified center point of a sphere that approximates the femoral head. Let c be the center of the spherical approximation of the femoral head. The cartilage enhancement filter to enhance bright structures is given by

$$I_{cartilage}(x) = \max_i \{-D(x; \sigma_i, c)\}, \tag{2}$$

where

$$D(x; \sigma_i, c) = r^\top \nabla^2 I(x; \sigma_i) r, \tag{3}$$

in which $r = \frac{x-c}{|x-c|}$.

Similarly, the articular space enhancement filter to enhance dark structures is given by

$$I_{space}(x) = \max_i D(x; \sigma_i, c), \tag{4}$$

Figure 1(b) shows a filter-enhanced image of the cartilages. During this stage of the process, operator interaction is necessary to specify the center point c of a sphere that approximates the femoral head, which is a simple task that does not involve trial and error.

2.2   Segmenting Cartilage and Articular Space Regions

The filtered images $I_{cartilage}(x)$ and $I_{space}(x)$ are thresholded, with the threshold values being determined through operator interaction. Using connectivity analysis, the approximated regions of the acetabular cartilage S_{acet}, the femoral cartilage S_{fem}, and the articular space S_{space} are extracted.

Figure. 1(c) shows the result of thresholding a cartilage-enhanced image. In Figs. 1(f) and (g), 3-D surface renderings of cartilage-enhanced and original MR images are respectively depicted. Comparison of these images clearly demonstrates the usefulness of cartilage enhancement filtering. Figure 1(d) shows the result of femur cartilage, acetabular cartilage, and articular space segmentation. Note that the boundaries of the cartilage regions provide good approximations of the inner edges (bone-attached) of the cartilages, while the articular space boundaries furnish outer edge approximations in the area where the acetabular and femoral cartilages overlap.

During this stage, operator interaction is needed to specify the threshold value and any one point included in the connected components. The operator often needs to manually remove unwanted connections to segments outside the regions.

2.3   Subpixel Edge Localization and Thickness Determination

The extracted 3-D cartilage regions are thinned to a width of one voxel by non-maximum suppression along the radial directions of filter-enhanced cartilage images. A cartilage thickness is assigned to each point of the thinned acetabular and femoral cartilage regions.

For each point of the thinned cartilage regions, the profile of the directional second derivative $D(x; \sigma_e, c)$ is reconstructed along the radial directional line that passes through this point and originates from center point, c, of the sphere approximating the femoral head. Here, σ_e is the standard deviation of the Gaussian blur combined with the second derivative computation. Similarly, binary profiles are reconstructed along the same radial directional line for the binary images of the segmented acetabular cartilage S_{acet}, femoral cartilage S_{fem}, and articular space S_{space}.

The profile reconstruction is performed at subpixel resolution by using a trilinear interpolation for the directional second derivative and a nearest-neighbor interpolation for the segmented cartilages and articular space images. Let $D(r)$ be the profile of the radial directional second derivative, and let $S_{acet}(r)$, $S_{fem}(r)$, and $S_{space}(r)$ be the profile of the segmented binary images. Here, r denotes the distance from the center of the sphere approximation, c.

Cartilage edges are localized in two steps: finding the initial point for the subsequent search using $S_{acet}(r)$, $S_{femur}(r)$, and $S_{space}(r)$, and then searching for the zero-crossing of $D(r)$. Figure 1(e) shows a zero-crossing map of $D(x; \sigma_e, c)$ as the binary image thresholded by zero.

In the edge localization of acetabular cartilage, the initial point of the inner edge, p_{in_0}, is given by the maximum value of r that satisfies $S_{acet}(r) = 1$ if it exists. Otherwise, the edge localization process terminates. The initial point of the outner edge, p_{out_0}, is given by the maximum value of r that satisfies $S_{space}(r) = 1$ if it exists. If $S_{space}(r) = 0$ and $S_{femur}(r) = 0$ for all r, p_{out_0} is given by the minimum value of r that satisfies $S_{acet}(r) = 1$. Otherwise, the edge localization process terminates.

Given the initial point of the search, if $D(p_{in_0}) < 0$, search outbound (the direction in which r increases) along the profile for the zero-crossing position p_{in}. Otherwise search inbound. Similarly, if $D(p_{out_0}) < 0$, search inbound toward the center along the profile for the zero-crossing position p_{out}. Otherwise search outbound. The thickness, t_{acet}, is given by $|p_{in} - p_{out}|$.

Localization of the femoral cartilage edges and thickness determination are done in a similar manner.

3   Experimental Results

3.1   Imaging Protocol and Implementation of the Method

3-D MR images of sagittal and coronal sections were obtained using 3-D-spoiled gradient-echo sequences (SPGR) with a surface coil [9]. Each 3-D MR image consists of 60 slices of a 256×256 matrix obtained with a 160-mm field of view (FOV) and a 1.5-mm slice thickness. Since $\frac{160}{256} = 0.625$ (mm), the original voxel size was $0.625 \times 0.625 \times 1.5$ (mm^3).

The original MR images were trimmed and then interpolated to make voxels isotropic and to double the resolution as described in Section 2.1. In the cartilage enhancement filtering, the three standard deviations of Gaussian blurring were used; their values were $\sigma_i = 2^{(i-1)/2}$ (pixels), where $i = 1, 2, 3$. Here, one pixel corresponded to $\frac{160}{2 \times 256} \simeq 0.31$ (mm) since the resolution was doubled. Details of the implementation of the second derivative computation combined with Gaussian blurring to obtain the Hessian matrix are described in [10]. In the cartilage edge localization, $\sigma_e = 1$ (pixel) was used for the zero-crossing search of the directional second derivative $D(x; \sigma_e, c)$.

3.2   Synthesized Images

To evaluate the accuracy limits of the method, we used 3-D synthesized images in which the partial volume effect was simulated. Each original synthesized image consisted of a $600 \times 600 \times 600$ matrix, which was reduced to $60 \times 60 \times 25$ by averaging a $10 \times 10 \times 24$ region to simulate partial voluming. We regarded the voxel size of an original image to be $0.0625 \times 0.0625 \times 0.0625$ (mm^3). Thus, the voxel size of the reduced image was $0.625 \times 0.625 \times 1.5$ (mm^3), which was the same voxel size as the real MR images. The images included a sheet structure with a bar profile of a constant thickness distributed on a sphere with a 40-mm diameter, which is a typical diameter of the femoral head. The reduced images were interpolated to obtain a $120 \times 120 \times 120$ matrix using sinc interpolation as described in Section 2.1. Other reduced images with $120 \times 120 \times 120$ matrices were also generated from the original synthesized images by averaging a $5 \times 5 \times 5$ region to simulate "high-resolution" MR imaging.

Figure 2(a) shows the mean of estimated thickness of sheet structures with a constant thicknesses in the slice passing through the sphere center, where the effect of partial voluming on accuracy should be minimal. Figure 2(b) shows the estimated thicknesses in the slice at a distance 12.5 mm from the center of the sphere (whose radius is 20 mm), where the effect of partial voluming should be considerable. Plots of thicknesses estimated from high-resolution synthesized images can be regarded as giving a good approximation of the inherent accuracy limitation of thickness estimation due to image resolution and σ_e value without partial voluming. Deviations from high-resolution image plots represent the effects of partial voluming on accuracy in Fig. 2(a) and (b). To observe the effect of partial voluming on accuracy, the variations in the estimated thicknesses were plotted against the distance between the slice plane and the sphere center (Fig. 2(c)). The plots for high-resolution image were almost ideal for every distance (not shown).

3.3 *In Vivo* MR Images

The method was applied to five sets of *in vivo* MR images, each containing two 3-D MR images of sagittal and coronal sections. One set was obtained from a normal volunteer; the others are patient data. Two of the sets are the left and right hip joints of the same subject. Figure 3 shows the thickness determinations using *in vivo* MR images for a patient with hip dysplasia. The results reconstructed from coronal and sagittal sections are well correlated, and from them, almost the entire cartilage distribution can be observed. Figure 4 shows thickness determinations for the normal volunteer, which reveal the acetabular cartilage distribution to be quite uniform (Fig. 4(b)). In contrast, abnormally thick areas of acetabular cartilage are clearly depicted in the distributions obtained for the patient with hip dysplasia (Fig. 3(a)).

Table 1 summarizes the segmentation results. Due to partial volume effects, the range of the reconstruction along the slice direction was typically around 30 mm while the diameter of the femoral head was around 42 mm. The amount of operator intervention was acceptable in all the cases.

4   Discussion and Conclusions

We have proposed a method for the segmentation and quantification of hip joint cartilages from *in vivo* MR images with a minimum amount of operator intervention. 3-D radial directional second-derivative filters with Gaussian blur enhance the cartilage and articular space regions to provide the initial descriptions for the subsequent refinement processes that accurately localize the cartilage edges. The accuracy limits of the method were evaluated using synthesized images, and it was successfully applied to five sets of *in vivo* MR images. Our goal is to apply the method we have developed to a large set of patient and normal volunteer data in a clinical study.

The only operator interventions required are the specification of the center point of the femoral head and the initial segmentation of cartilage and articular space regions. This initial segmentation potentially involves trial and error in order to determine an appropriate threshold value for obtaining the connected component without unwanted connections to other structures. The operator sometimes needs to manually remove unwanted connections. However, as shown in Table 1, such interventions are minimized by the effective enhancement of the cartilage and articular space regions.

The method assumes that the hip joint is spherical. As shown in Figs. 1(a) and 4(a), this assumption is appropriate for most subjects; an 18° error in the direction along which the thickness is measured results in an estimated thickness error of around 5 %, since $\cos(18°) \simeq 0.95$. Thus, small errors in direction will not seriously affect the thickness estimation. However, the assumption of sphericity is inappropriate in the cases of badly deformed hip joints. We are now planning to extend the method so as to incorporate automated estimation of the optimal direction.

In the previous reports, the estimated thicknesses were validated by comparison with the sections of specimen [2],[6],[8] or the manual traces by radiologists [3]. In contrast with previous work, we carried out software simulation studies to derive the basic characteristics relating to the effect of partial voluming on accuracy. The partial volume effect is more serious in the hip joint than the knee joint due to its spherical shape. We are now conducting *in vitro* studies using both normal and high-resolution real MR images of a resected femoral head to further corroborate the effect of partial voluming on accuracy.

Acknowledgements: The work described in this paper was partly conducted while the first author was a visiting researcher at the Surgical Planning Laboratory, Department of Radiology, Harvard Medical School and Brigham and Women's Hospital. He would like to thank Professor Ron Kikinis for providing a high-performance computing environment and Professor Ferenc Jolesz for continuous encouragement.

References

1. K. Jonsson, K. Buckwalter, M. Helvie, L. Niklason, and W. Martel, Precision of hyaline cartilage thickness measurements, *Acta Radiol,* **33**, 234–239 (1992).
2. F. Eckstein, A. Gavazzini, H. Sittek, M. Haubner, A. Losch, S. Milz, K-H Englmeier, E. Schulte, R. Putz, and M. Reiser, Determination of knee joint cartilage thickness using three-dimensional magnetic resonance chondro-crassometry (3D MR-CCM), *Magn Reson Med,* **36**, 256–265 (1996).

3. S. Solloway, C. E. Hutchinson, J. G. Waterton, and C. J. Taylor, The use of active shape models for making thickness measurements of articular cartilage from MR images, *Magn Reson Med*, **37**, 943–952 (1997).

4. S. Warfield, C. Winalski, F. Jolesz, and R. Kikinis, Automatic segmentation of MRI of the knee, *ISMRM Sixth Scientific Meeting and Exhibition*, Sydney, Australia, 563 (1998).

5. J. Hodler, D. Trundell, M. N. Pathria, and D. Resnick, Width of the articular cartilage of the hip: quantification by using fat-suppression spin-echo MR imaging in cadavers, *AJR Am J Roentgenol*, **159**, 351–355 (1992).

6. T. Kubota, T. Nishii, Y. Sato, K. Nakanishi, and S. Tamura, 3-D shape reconstruction of articular cartilage of femoral head from MR image on multiple plane, *IEICE Trans*, **J80-D-II**, 669–677 (1997).

7. T. Kubota, Y. Sato, K. Nakanishi, T. Ueguchi, T. Nishii, K. Ohzono, S. Tamura, T. Ochi, and H. Nakamura, 3D quantification and visualization of cartilage thickness of femoral head from MR Images of multiple slice axes, *Proc. Computer Assisted Radiology and Surgery (CAR '98)*, Tokyo, Japan, 861, (1998).

8. C. A. McGibbon, D. E. Dupuy, W. E. Palmer, and D. E. Krebs, Cartilage and subchondral bone thickness distribution with MR imaging, *Acad Radiol*, **5**, 20–25 (1998).

9. K. Nakanishi, H. Tanaka, T. Nishii, K. Masuhara, Y. Narumi, and H. Nakamura, MR evaluation of the articular cartilage of the femoral head during traction, *Acta Radiol*, **40**, 60–63 (1999).

10. Y. Sato, S. Nakajima, N. Shiraga, H. Atsumi, S. Yoshida, T. Koller, G. Guido, and R. Kikinis, Three-dimensional multi-scale line filter for segmentation and visualization of curvilinear structures in medical images, *Med Image Anal*, **2**, 143–168 (1998).

Table 1. Summary of segmentation results.

Subject (Left/Right) Age/Sex	Sagittal/ Coronal	Disease	Estimated femoral head diameter (mm)	Range of reconstruction along slice direction (mm)	# of manual operations: cartilage/space
A(L) 24/F	Sag Cor	Normal volunteer	42.0	30.625 37.5	1/0 0/0
B(R) 24/F	Sag Cor	Hip dysplasia bilateral	42.0	30.000 31.250	2/1 0/0
B(L) 24/F	Sag Cor	Hip dysplasia bilateral	42.0	28.125 31.250	3/1 0/0
C(R) 39/F	Sag Cor	After Chiari pelvic osteotomy	46.5	25.000 25.000	1/2 0/2
D(R) 43/F	Sag Cor	Osteoarthritis	42.0	31.250 31.250	0/2 0/0

The number of manual operations means the number of the operations that were necessary to remove unwanted connectivity by putting zero within a manually specified rectangular parallelepiped region during the interactive segmentation processes (Section 2.2), that is, the number of manual cutting operations needed to correctly segment out the cartilage and articular space regions.

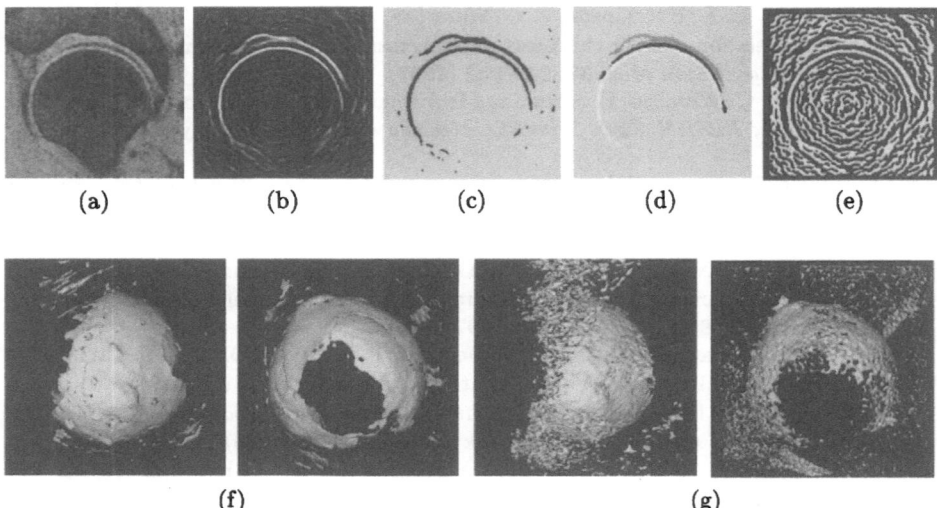

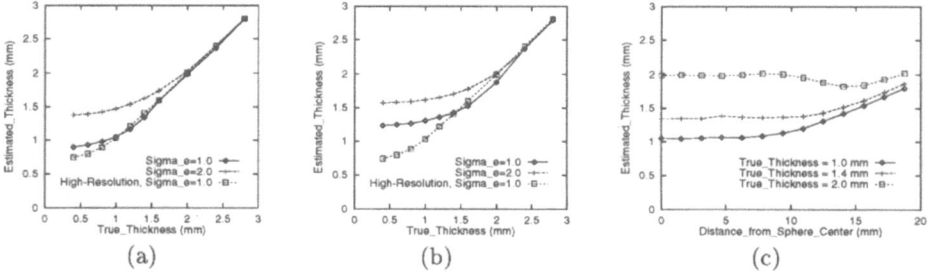

Fig. 1. Enhancement and segmentation of cartilage and articular space regions. (a) Original MR image. (b) Filter-enhanced cartilage image. (c) Binary image thresholded from filter-enhanced cartilage image. (d) Initial segmentation of cartilage and articular space regions (white: femoral cartilage, gray: acetabular cartilage, black: articular space). (e) Zero-crossing map of the directional second derivative $D(x; \sigma_e, c)$. (f) Surface rendering of filter-enhanced cartilage image (left: top view, right: side view). (g) Surface rendering of original MR image (left: top view, right: side view).

Fig. 2. Accuracy evaluation of estimated thickness. (a) Estimated thicknesses of sheet structures with constant thicknesses in the slice passing through the sphere center; $\sigma_e = 1$ pixel and $\sigma_e = 2$ pixels were used (1 pixel = 0.31 mm). The results for ten constant thicknesses were plotted (0.4, 0.6, 0.8, 1.0, 1.2, 1.4, 1.6, 2.0, 2.4, 2.8 (mm)). The estimated thickness for high-resolution synthesized images ($\sigma_e = 1$ pixel) is also shown. (b) Estimated thicknesses in the slice at a distance of 12.5 mm from the center of the sphere whose radius is 20 mm. (c) Variations in the estimated thicknesses against the distance between the slice plane and the center of the sphere. $\sigma_e = 1$ pixel was used.

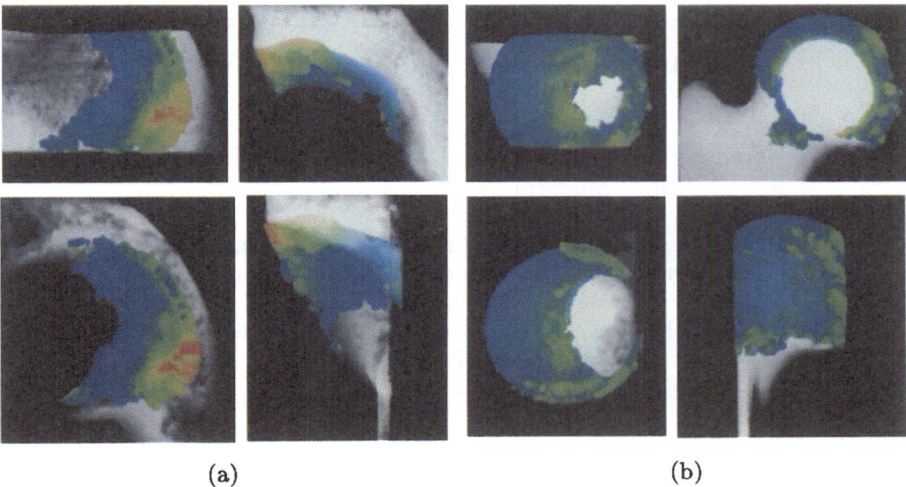

(a)   (b)

Fig. 3. Cartilage thickness distributions of a patient of with hip dysplasia (subject B(R) in Table 1). The original MR image and intermediate results are shown in Fig. 1. Thicker (thinner) cartilages are represented by red (blue) regions. Red: 16 pixels, green: 9 pixels, blue: 2 pixels (1 pixel = 0.31 mm). (a) Acetabular cartilage. Reconstruction results of coronal (upper) and sagittal (lower) sections are viewed from the inferior (left) and posterior (right) directions. (b) Femoral cartilage. Reconstruction results are viewed from the superior (left) and posterior (right) directions.

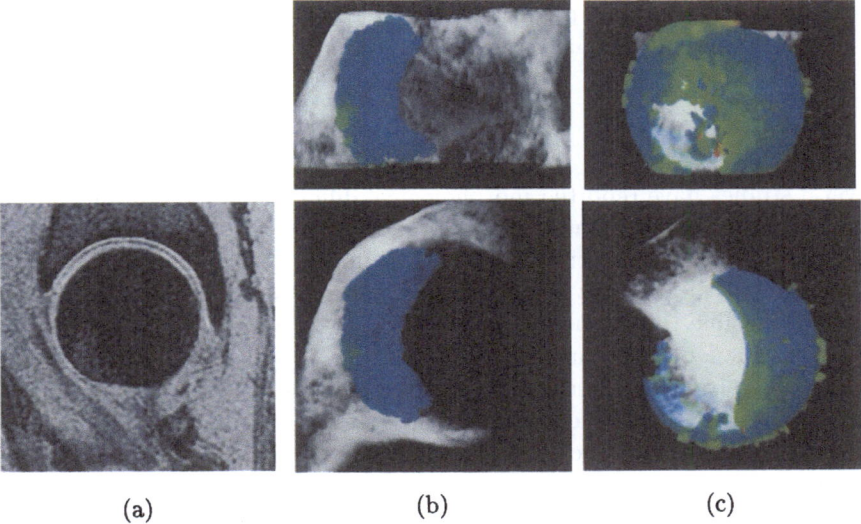

(a)   (b)   (c)

Fig. 4. Cartilage thickness distributions of a normal volunteer (subject A(L) in Table 1). (a) Original MR image. (b) Acetabular cartilage. Reconstruction results of coronal (upper) and sagittal (lower) sections are viewed from the inferior direction. (c) Femoral cartilage viewed from the superior direction.

Quantification of Cerebral Grey and White Matter Asymmetry from MRI

Frederik Maes[1], Koen Van Leemput[1], Lynn E. DeLisi[2],
Dirk Vandermeulen[1], and Paul Suetens[1]

[1] Katholieke Universiteit Leuven, Medical Image Computing (Radiology-ESAT),
UZ Gasthuisberg, Herestraat 49, B-3000 Leuven, Belgium
Frederik.Maes@uz.kuleuven.ac.be
[2] SUNY Stony Brook, Department of Psychiatry, Health Sciences Center,
Stony Brook, N.Y. 11794, USA
ldelisi@ccmail.sunysb.edu

Abstract. We present a completely automated procedure for measuring left and right hemispheric asymmetry in cerebral grey and white matter volumes from MR images using a chain of state-of-the-art image analysis algorithms. After bias correction and tissue classification, left and right hemispheres are separated by non-rigid registration to a template image in which both hemispheres have been carefully segmented. Volume renderings of each hemisphere separately demonstrate the high quality of the resulting segmentations. Because all steps in the procedure are completely automated and do not require user specified parameters, the results are highly reproducible and consistent. We present quantitative results obtained from a database of MR images of 40 schizophrenic patients and 31 normal controls.

1 Introduction

Several studies have reported morphological differences in the brains of schizophrenic patients when compared to normal controls [1], including decreased or reversed cerebral asymmetries. Current MR imaging techniques allow to acquire 3D images of the brain with high resolution and signal to noise ratio, which makes it feasible to measure brain morphology *in vivo*. But slice by slice manual delineation of structures of interest in 3D images by a human expert is tedious and usually subject to large inter- and intra-observer variability and poor reproducibility. This deteriorates the statistical significance of the reported morphological findings and may also explain some inconsistencies across studies. Moreover, in longitudinal studies aiming at detecting morphological changes over time, the quality of historical images is generally inferior to what is possible today. Hence the need for automated computer methods for image based morphometry which yield accurate, consistent and reproducible results and which are robust against imaging imperfections in historical data.

In this paper, we present a method for quantifying cerebral grey and white matter asymmetry from MR images. The method consists of bias field correction, tissue segmentation and atlas-based separation of left and right hemispheres and relies on state-of-the-art algorithms for rigid and non-rigid image registration and intensity-based voxel classification. Because all steps in the procedure are completely automated and do not require interactive intervention or user specified parameters, the results are highly reproducible and consistent. We present quantitative results obtained from a database of MR images of schizophrenic patients and normal controls within the scope of the European BIOMORPH Project [2].

2   Method

Bias correction and tissue classification   White and grey matter are segmented after bias correction by the intensity-based tissue classification algorithm of Van Leemput [3]. The method models the single or multi-channel MR signal as the realization of a random process, the intensities of each channel within each tissue class being drawn from a Gaussian distribution, but which is corrupted by a polynomial intensity inhomogeneity or bias field. The algorithm maximizes the a posteriori likelihood of the model parameters given the data by an Expectation-Maximization procedure, iteratively alternating between tissue classification, class intensity distribution estimation and bias field estimation. The method, which is fully automated, is initialized with a priori spatial distribution maps for grey matter, white matter and csf obtained from a digital brain atlas that is distributed with the SPM software package [4]. The atlas image is normalised to the space of the study image by an affine transformation which is computed automatically by maximizing mutual information between both images [5]. Only voxels to which the atlas assigns a non-zero a priori brain tissue probability are considered during segmentation.

Left/right hemispheric separation   Separation of the computed white and grey matter probability maps into left and right halves is achieved by non-rigid registration of the study image to a template MR image in which left and right hemispheres have been carefully segmented. This image and the segmentations were retrieved from the IBSR [6]. The delineations of left and right hemispheres were transformed into binary label images, which were subsequently edited by morphological operations to match the brain envelope rather than the individual gyri and sulci to be more robust against differences in local cortical topology (figure 1). The template image is matched to the study image by a combination of affine and locally non-rigid transformations, using the non-rigid intensity-based matching algorithm of Thirion [7]. The same transformation is then applied to the label images, which yields matched outlines of both hemispheres that allow to separate left and right halves in the tissue segmentations and, at the same time, to remove non-relevant structures such as the cerebellum and brain stem.

White and grey matter volumetry   Finally, volumes for grey and white matter for each brain half separately are computed by integrating the corresponding probability maps within the brain regions of interest defined by the matched template image.

350   F. Maes et al.

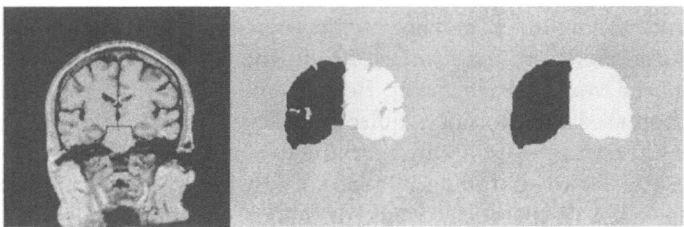

Fig. 1. Template of left and right hemispheres. Left: original MR image slice in which left and right hemispheres have been carefully segmented manually by a trained expert. Middle: conversion of the original contours into a binary template image. Right: the template image is edited to match the brain envelope rather than the individual gyri and sulci to be more robust against differences in local cortical topology.

3   Results

3.1   3D MPRAGE

Figure 2 illustrates the performance of the method on high quality high resolution data, consisting of a single sagittal T1-weighted image (Siemens Vision 1.5 T, 3D MPRAGE, 256 × 256 matrix, 1.25 mm slice thickness, 128 slices, FOV = 256 mm, TR = 11.4 ms, TE = 4.4 ms) with good contrast between grey matter, white matter and the tissues surrounding the brain. The grey and white matter segmentation maps obtained from the original images are correctly split in separate maps for left and right hemispheres by non-rigid registration with the labeled template image. The high quality of the segmentations and of the left/right separation is clearly illustrated by volume renderings of the grey and white matter maps of each brain half.

3.2   BIOMORPH schizophrenia data

The method was applied to a database of MR images, available within the BIOMORPH project [2], that was collected at SUNY, Stony Brook, N.Y, USA, as part of a prospective follow-up study of brain morphology in schizophrenic patients. Left and right white and grey matter volumes were segmented from a single coronal T1-weighted MR scan (GE Signa 1.5 T, 3D GRASS, 256 × 256 matrix, 1.5 mm slice thickness, 124 slices, FOV = 240 mm, TR = 24 ms, TE = 5 ms) for a group of 40 patients (26 males, 14 females, mean age was 27.7 ± 6.0) and 31 controls (18 males, 13 females, mean age was 30.6 ± 7.9).

A typical segmentation result in shown in figure 3. Normalising the multiplicative bias field to a mean value of 1, bias correction factors within the brain region typically range from 0.7 to 1.4 with a standard deviation of 0.06, which is clearly not negligible. The apparant symmetry of the resulting segmentations illustrates that the segmentation procedure is indeed capable of correcting for significant bias. Note that some voxels outside of the brain are erroneously classified as grey or, to a lesser extent, white matter. These voxels were assigned a

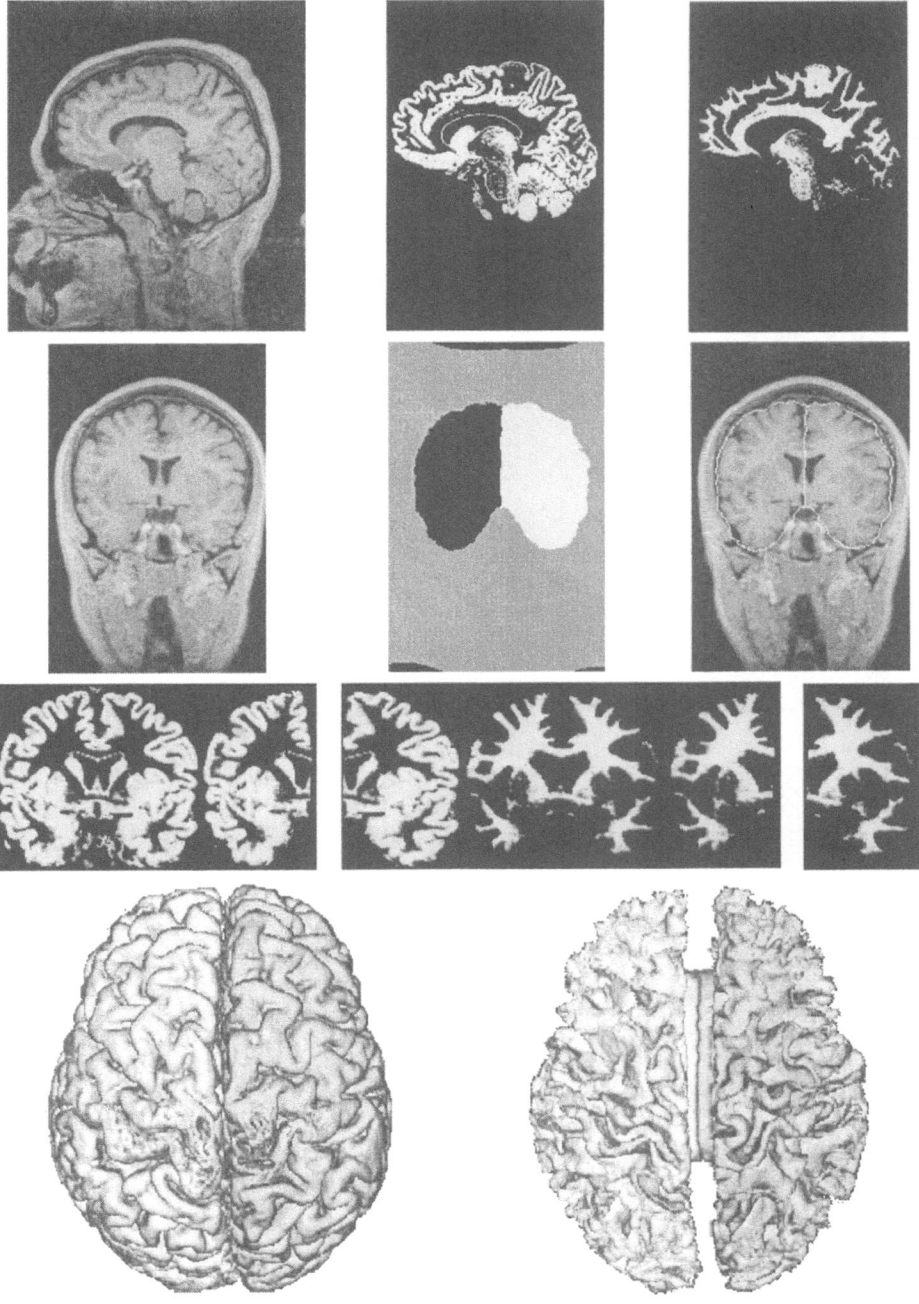

Fig. 2. Top: original sagittal MPRAGE image and grey and white matter segmentations. Middle: coronal cross section with matched labeled template and grey and white matter segmentations before and after hemispheric separation. Bottom: volume renderings of grey and white matter segmentation maps for each hemisphere separately.

non-zero a priori probability for these classes by the atlas used to initialize the segmentation process and because their intensity in these images is similar to those of the true grey or white matter voxels, the classification algorithm, which treats each pixel independently, is not able to discriminate between them.

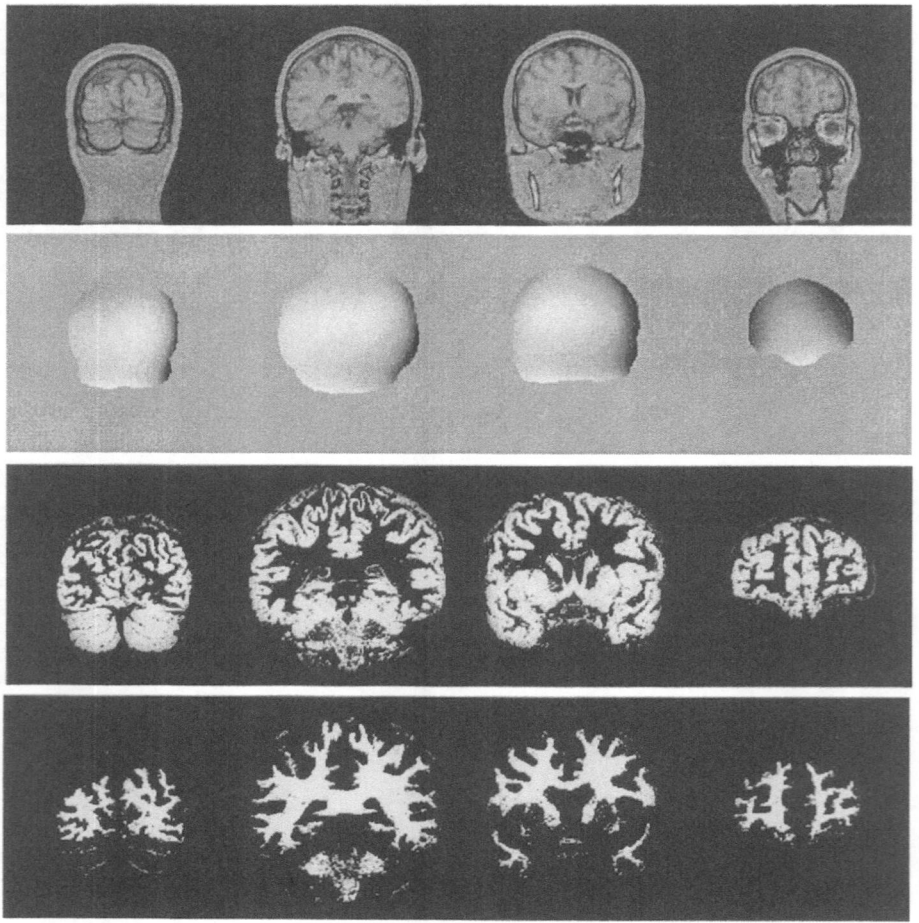

Fig. 3. Original T1-weighted image, estimated bias field and resulting grey and white matter segmentation for a typical BIOMORPH schizophrenia data set.

Grey and white matter segmentations for each hemisphere separately obtained after non-rigid registration of the labeled template image are shown in figure 4. Inspection of the results shows that separation of both brain halves, aswell as of cerebellum and brain stem, is generally excellent. This is also illustrated by volume renderings of the grey and white matter probability maps. The non-rigidly matched template image provides a more precise brain mask than the one used for segmentation, such that most of the wrongly classified non-brain voxels are removed when separating both brain halves.

3.3   Volume measurements

Grey and white matter volume measurements obtained from the BIOMORPH database of patients and controls are summarised in figure 5 and table 1. Volumes are obviously larger in males than in females and both grey matter and white matter show the tendency to be decreased in patients versus controls. We also found a slight difference between grey matter volumes left and right (about 2.5 cm^3 or 0.8% on average), both in schizophrenics and controls. Statistical analysis of these results and correlation with diagnosis, age, sex and dexterity is currently in progress.

		Patients		Controls	
		Males	Females	Males	Females
Number of subjects		26	14	18	13
Grey matter:	left:	331.3	285.6	339.2	299.2
	right:	329.5	282.2	337.2	296.6
White matter:	left:	198.2	169.6	203.1	174.1
	right:	199.5	169.5	203.1	173.1

Table 1. Mean left and right cerebral grey and white matter volumes (in cm^3) for the BIOMORPH database of patients and controls for males and females separately.

4   Discussion

Our grey and white matter segmentation method has been validated on simulated MR images with known ground truth and on real MR images by comparison with expert delineations [12]. We found that the automated and the manual segmentations consistently show excellent overlap (average overlap metric [13] values of 95%, 83% and 82% for total brain, grey matter and white matter respectively) and that differences mainly occur at the white matter/grey matter and grey matter/csf interfaces, which can be attributed to partial volume effects on the one hand and to the tendency of the automated method to more meticulously follow tissue borders than the manual tracer on the other hand. For 2 patients and 3 controls in the BIOMORPH database, two scans were available at two time points about one year apart. The mean difference between corresponding measurements at different time points was 1% for controls and 4% for patients. While real changes over time may be neglected in controls but can not be excluded in patients, we estimate the reproducibility of the method to be about 1%.

Various authors have presented various techniques to separate the brain hemispheres by the so-called mid-sagittal plane, defined as the plane that best fits the

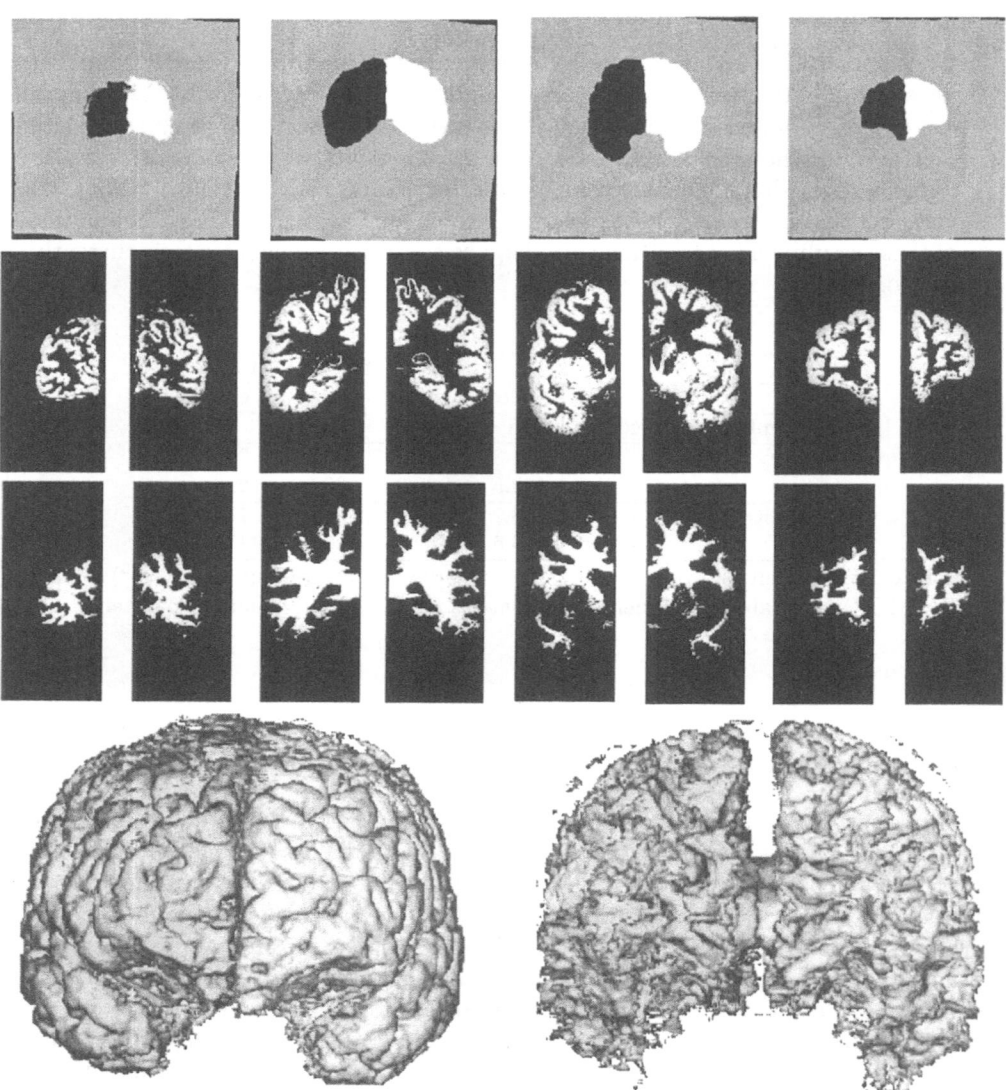

Fig. 4. After non-rigid registration with the labeled template image (top), the original grey and white matter segmentations can be separated into left and right alves and non-relevant structures, such as the cerebellum and the brain stem, can be removed.

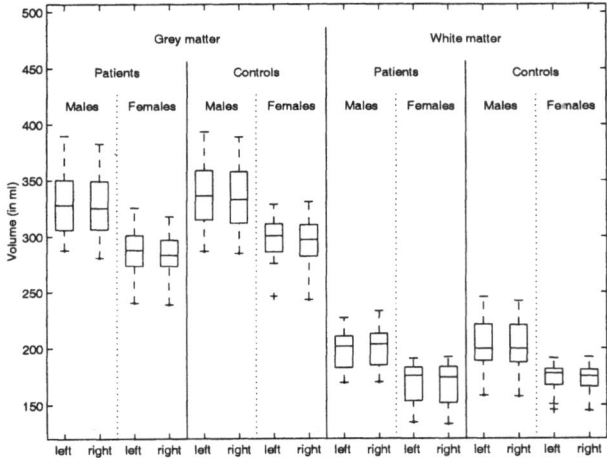

Fig. 5. Left and right cerebral grey and white matter volumes (in cm^3) for the BIOMORPH database of patients and controls for males and females separately.

inter-hemispheric fissure of the brain [8] or as the plane that maximizes similarity between the image and its reflection relative to this plane [9, 10]. The advantage of our approach of intensity-driven non-rigid registration to a labeled template image is that it doesn't assume the boundary between both hemispheres to be planar. Dawant [11] used exactly the same algorithm for automated atlas-based segmentation of internal brain structures and found that, for large scale structures such as the brain or the cerebellum, the resulting contours are virtually indistinguishable from outlines drawn by an experienced radiologist. The same technique can be applied to analyse asymmetry in subregions such as the frontal or temporal lobe.

Our approach assumes that differences in (dis)symmetry between the template image and the study images are completely resolved by the non-rigid registration. If this is not the case, bias may be introduced in the measurements due to the (dis)symmetry of the template image itself, which we derived from a single subject's scan. Such bias could be detected by doing the measurements again with the left/right axis in the template image reversed. Alternatively, an unbiased virtual brain template could be created by averaging images of several individuals and their reflected versions and delineating the average image.

Disturbing in the analysis of the BIOMORPH data is the influence of non-brain pixels that are falsely classified as grey matter, due to a lack of contrast between true grey matter and some non-brain tissues in these images. If additional MR channels were available that would allow to differentiate between these tissues, the problem would be solved by multi-channel segmentation. Incorporating spatial constraints in the classification, such as prohibiting grey matter pixels to be surrounded by non-brain pixels [12], improved the single-channel classification of the BIOMORPH data slightly, but still showed important misclassifications.

While non-rigid registration to the template image allows to exclude many of the misclassified non-brain pixels, the same non-rigid registration approach could be used to generate much sharper a priori tissue probability maps than the ones we are using now to initialize the segmentation process. We expect that non-rigid registration of such an atlas to the study images will yield a better brain mask and improved segmentations. Alternatively, the problem may be solved by straightforward morphological processing of the segmentation maps, including erosion/dilation and largest component selection.

5   Summary and conclusions

We presented a completely automated procedure for consistent and reproducible quantification of left and right cerebral white and grey matter volumes from MR images, which combines state-of-the-art algorithms for tissue classification and atlas-based segmentation. The method has been applied on a database of high resolution images of schizophrenic patients and normal controls. Further work will focus on reducing the influence of falsely classified non-brain pixels and on extending the approach to smaller subregions in the brain.

6   Acknowledgments

This work was supported by the EC-funded BIOMORPH project 95-0845 (Development and Validation of Techniques for Brain Morphometry), a collaboration between the Universities of Kent and Oxford (UK), ETH Zürich (Switzerland), INRIA Sophia Antipolis (France) and KU Leuven (Belgium), and by the Research Fund KU Leuven GOA/99/05 (Variability in Human Shape and Speech). The template image and its manual segmentation was provided by the Center for Morphometric Analysis at Massachusetts General Hospital, Charlestown, MA, USA, and is available at *http://neuro-www.mgh.harvard.edu/cma/ibsr*. The non-rigid registration software was provided by Jean-Philippe Thirion.

References

1. L.E. DeLisi, W. Tew, S. Xie, A.L. Hoff, M. Sakuma, M. Kushner, G. Lee, K. Shedlack, A.M. Smith, and R. Grimson. A prospective follow-up study of brain morphology and cognition in first-epsiode schizophrenic patients: preliminary findings. *Biol Psychiatry*, 38:349–360, 1995.
2. Development and validation of techniques for brain morphometry (BIOMORPH). Biomed Project No. 95-0845. Partners in the BIOMORPH project are: University of Kent at Canterbury, Kent, UK; ETH, Zürich, Switzerland; University of Oxford, Oxford, UK; INRIA, Nice, France; K.U. Leuven, Leuven, Belgium.
3. K. Van Leemput, F. Maes, D. Vandermeulen, and P. Suetens. Automatic segmentation of brain tissues and MR bias field correction using a digital brain atlas. In W.M. Wells, A. Colchester, and S. Delp, editors, *Medical Image Computing and Computer-Assisted Intervention (MICCAI'98)*, volume 1496 of *Lecture Notes*

in Computer Science, pages 1222–1229, Cambridge, MA, USA, October 1998. Springer.

4. J. Ashburner, K. Friston, A. Holmes, and J. Poline. *Statistical Parametric Mapping*. The Wellcome Department of Cognitive Neurology, University College London.

5. F. Maes, A. Collignon, D. Vandermeulen, G. Marchal, and P. Suetens. Multi-modality image registration by maximization of mutual information. *IEEE Transactions on Medical Imaging*, 16(2):187–198, April 1997.

6. Internet Brain Segmentation Repository (IBSR). Maintained by Andrew Worth at the Center for Morphometric Analysis, Massachusetts General Hospital, Charlestown, MA, USA. http://neuro-www.mgh.harvard.edu/cma/ibsr.

7. J.-P. Thirion. Fast non-rigid matching of 3D medical images. In *Medical Robotics and Computer Aided Surgery (MRCAS'95)*, pages 47–54, Baltimore, MD, USA, November 1995.

8. P. Marais, R. Guillemaud, M. Sakuma, A. Zisserman, and M. Brady. Visualising cerebral asymmetry. In K.H. Höhne and R. Kikinis, editors, *Visualization in Biomedical Computing*, volume 1131 of *Lecture Notes in Computer Science*, pages 411–416, Hamburg, Germany, September 1996. Springer.

9. Y. Liu, R.T. Collins, and W.E. Rothfus. Automatic bilateral symmetry (midsagittal) plane extraction from pathological 3D neuroradiological images. In K.M. Hanson, editor, *Medical Imaging 1998: Image Processing*, volume 3338 of *Proc. SPIE*, pages 1528–1539, San Diego, CA, USA, February 1998.

10. S. Prima, J.-P. Thirion, G. Subsol, and N. Roberts. Automatic analysis of normal brain dissymmetry of males and females in MR images. In W.M. Wells, A. Colchester, and S. Delp, editors, *Medical Image Computing and Computer-Assisted Intervention (MICCAI'98)*, volume 1496 of *Lecture Notes in Computer Science*, pages 770–779, Cambridge, MA, USA, October 1998. Springer.

11. B.M. Dawant, J.-P. Thirion, F. Maes, D. Vandermeulen, and P. Demaerel. Automatic 3D segmentation of internal structures of the head in MR images using a combination of similarity and free-form transformations. In K.M. Hanson, editor, *Medical Imaging 1998: Image Processing*, volume 3338 of *Proc. SPIE*, pages 1528–1539, San Diego, CA, USA, February 1998.

12. K. Van Leemput, F. Maes, D. Vandermeulen, and P. Suetens. Automated model-based tissue classification of MR images of the brain. Submitted to IEEE Trans. Medical Imaging, January 1999.

13. A. Zijdenbos, B. M. Dawant, R. A. Margolin, and A. C. Palmer. Morphometric analysis of white matter lesions in MR images: Method and validation. *IEEE Transactions on Medical Imaging*, 13(4):716–724, December 1994.

Quantitation of Vessel Morphology from 3D MRA

A. F. Frangi, W. J. Niessen, R. M. Hoogeveen,
Th. van Walsum, M. A. Viergever*

Image Sciences Institute, Utrecht Medical Center (UMC)
Room E.01.334, Heidelberglaan 100, 3584 CX Utrecht, The Netherlands

Abstract. Three dimensional magnetic resonance angiographic images (3D MRA) are routinely inspected using maximum intensity projections (MIP). However, accuracy of stenosis estimates based on projections is limited. Therefore, a method for quantitative 3D MRA is introduced. Linear vessel segments are modeled with a central vessel axis curve coupled to a vessel wall surface. First, the central vessel axis is determined. Subsequently, the vessel wall is segmented using knowledge of the acquisition process. The user interaction to initialize the model is performed in a 3D setting. The method is validated on a carotid bifurcation phantom and also illustrated on patient data.

1   Introduction

Accurate determination of vessel width is necessary for grading vascular stenoses, which is important in diagnosis and treatment planning in, for instance, stroke patients. Studies have revealed that patients with a severe ($> 70\%$) symptomatic stenosis in the carotids should be operated while patients with stenoses smaller than 30% should not undergo surgical treatment [1, 2].

MRA is increasingly used for vascular diagnosis. Although evaluation by radiologists is mainly performed on 2D maximum intensity projections (MIP) [3], it is known that these lead to vessel width underestimation and decreased contrast-to-noise ratio (CNR) [3–5].

In order to improve grading of stenoses we suggest a novel scheme for quantitative vessel analysis from 3D MRA. Hereto we use a 3D B-spline deformable model of a vessel segment which consists of a central vessel axis coupled to a vessel wall surface. The use of a B-spline representation for the curve and surface models enables the use of already existing, powerful interaction mechanisms inherited from Computer Assisted Design (CAD). For initialization, which is an important step in segmentation schemes based on deformable models, we suggest a technique based on an iso-surface rendering of the vasculature which allows for intuitive and efficient interaction in a 3D setting. In the fitting procedure, information of the image acquisition process is used to accurately define the vessel boundaries. The method is validated on MR phantom data and compared to operator performance. Results on patient data of the carotids are also shown.

---

* This research was sponsored by the Dutch Ministry of Economic Affairs (Program IOP Beeldverwerking, Project IBV97009) and EasyVision Advanced Development at Philips Medical Systems Nederland B.V.

2   Model-based vessel segmentation

A two-step vessel segmentation procedure is proposed. First, a representation of the central vessel axis is obtained, which is subsequently used as a reference for extracting the boundaries of the vessel.

The central vessel axis, $\mathbf{C}(t)$, is modeled using a B-spline curve of degree n with $s + 1$ control points. This representation enforces the lumen line to be connected

$$\mathbf{C}(t) = \sum_{i=0}^{s} N_{in}(t)\mathbf{P}_i \tag{1}$$

Here $\mathbf{P}_i$ are the control points, $N_{in}(t)$ is the i-th B-spline basis function of order n [6] and $t \in [0, 1]$. The model (sometimes referred to as *snake*) deforms towards the center of the vessel by minimizing an energy functional, $\mathcal{E}^C$, containing terms associated with the smoothness of the spline and the image content [7,8]

$$\mathcal{E}^C = \mathcal{E}_{ext}^C + \gamma^C \mathcal{E}_{int}^C \tag{2}$$

where $\mathcal{E}_{int}^C$ provides a regularization term depending on the first and second order parametric derivatives of the curve [9] and is weighted by a factor γ^C. The external energy, $\mathcal{E}_{ext}^C$, is used to attract the curve towards points which have a high likelihood of lying at the central vessel axis. For this purpose, a new filter was previously developed [10] which is based on the eigenvalues ($|\lambda_1| \le |\lambda_2| \le |\lambda_3|$) of the Hessian matrix computed at each voxel of the image.

$$\mathcal{V}(\mathbf{x}, \sigma) \triangleq \begin{cases} 0 & \text{if } \lambda_2 > 0 \text{ or } \lambda_3 > 0, \\ \left[1 - \exp\left(-\frac{\mathcal{R}_\mathcal{A}^2}{2\alpha^2}\right)\right] \exp\left(-\frac{\mathcal{R}_\mathcal{B}^2}{2\beta^2}\right) \left[1 - \exp\left(-\frac{\mathcal{S}^2}{2c^2}\right)\right] & \text{otherwise} \end{cases} \tag{3}$$

$$\mathcal{R}_\mathcal{A} \triangleq \frac{|\lambda_2|}{|\lambda_3|} \qquad \mathcal{R}_\mathcal{B} \triangleq \frac{|\lambda_1|}{\sqrt{|\lambda_2 \lambda_3|}} \qquad \mathcal{S} \triangleq \sqrt{\sum_j \lambda_j^2} \tag{4}$$

The filter can be interpreted as follows. For a bright, tubular structure we expect two eigenvalues which are large, negative, and of similar magnitude, and one eigenvalue which is small. Thus $\mathcal{R}_\mathcal{B}$, which is the smallest eigenvalue over the geometric average of the two larger eigenvalues, should be small. Moreover $\mathcal{R}_\mathcal{A}$, which measures the anisotropy in the cross-sectional plane should be close to one. Finally, in order to only measure tubular structures above the noise level, $\mathcal{S}$ measures the degree of "image content". The parameters α, β and c tune the sensitivity of the filter to deviations in $\mathcal{R}_\mathcal{A}$, $\mathcal{R}_\mathcal{B}$ and $\mathcal{S}$, relative to the ideal behavior for a line structure[1].

The Hessian matrix is computed using Gaussian derivative operators at multiple scales, in order to span the range of expected vessel widths of the imaged

---

[1] For further details of the filter and typical parameter settings we refer to [10].

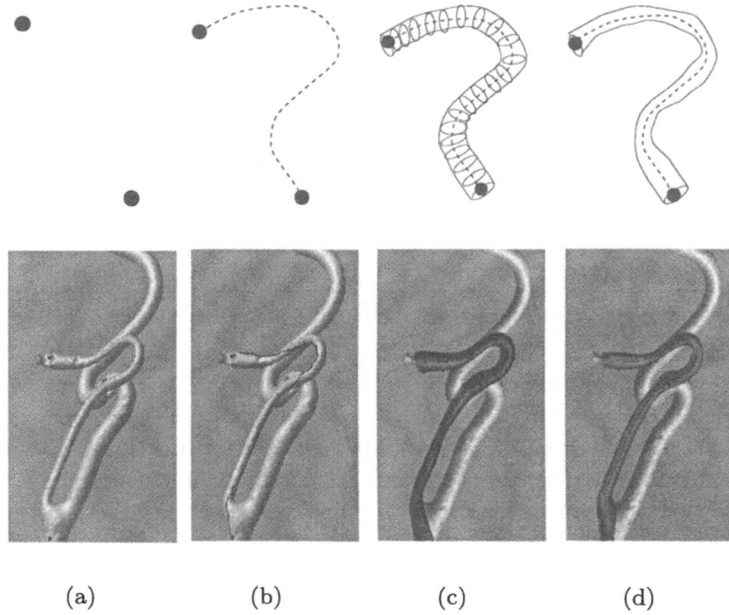

Fig. 1. Interaction scenario. *a)* A user initializes two (or more) points on the surface. *b)* From these seeds, a geodesic path is computed. *c)* The geodesic path is deformed until the central vessel axis is determined. Using the distance between the newly obtained vessel axis and the original geodesic path, a circular cross-section is swept along the axis to generate an initialization of the vessel wall model. *d)* Vessel wall (after deformation) and central vessel axis.

anatomy ($\sigma \in [\sigma_{min}, \sigma_{max}]$). In order to provide a unique filter response, the outputs of the filters at different scales undergo a *scale selection* procedure [11] –Equation (5). Different vessel sizes can be detected at their corresponding scales; therefore, both small and large vessels will be captured with the same scheme.

$$\mathcal{V}(\mathbf{x}) = \max_{\sigma_{min} \leq \sigma \leq \sigma_{max}} \mathcal{V}(\mathbf{x}, \sigma) \tag{5}$$

The designed filter has the properties that *i.* it filters out non tubular structures, *ii.* it is maximum at the center of the vessel while the output of the filter decreases slowly towards the boundaries, and *iii.* it is sensitive to vessels of different sizes [10]. The filter is therefore suited as an image force to attract the curve towards the central vessel axis. The external energy we propose is given by

$$\mathcal{E}_{ext}^C = -\frac{1}{\ell} \int_0^1 \mathcal{V}(\mathbf{C}(t)) \, \|\partial_t \mathbf{C}(t)\| \, dt \tag{6}$$

where ℓ denotes the length of the central vessel axis.

Once the central vessel axis is computed, we proceed to determine the vessel wall. Hereto, the vessel wall is modeled using a tensor product B-spline surface [12]

$$\mathbf{W}(t, u) = \sum_{j=0}^{q} \sum_{k=0}^{r} N_{jl}(u) N_{km}(t) \mathbf{P}_{jk} \qquad (7)$$

where $\mathbf{P}_{jk}$ are $((q + 1) \times (r + 1))$ control points, $N_{jl}(u)$ is the j-th B-spline periodic basis function of order l, and $u \in [0, 2\pi)$; $N_{km}(t)$ is the k-th B-spline non-periodic basis function of order m, and $t \in [0, 1]$. The parameters u and t traverse the surface in the circumferential and longitudinal directions respectively. We have deliberately coupled the longitudinal parameter (t) of the vessel wall and the central vessel axis since both span the vessel in the longitudinal direction. This coupling makes it possible to relate central vessel axis points with the corresponding boundary points.

To fit the vessel wall model in a smooth fashion we use an approach similar to the one applied for the central vessel axis, extending the concept from curves to surfaces. The wall model is deformed in a way that minimizes the following energy criterion

$$\mathcal{E}^{W} = \mathcal{E}_{ext}^{W} + \gamma^{W} \mathcal{E}_{int}^{W} \qquad (8)$$

where the internal energy term, $\mathcal{E}_{int}^{W}$, takes into account the stretching and bending energies of the vessel wall model. The stretching energy term can be physically interpreted as an approximation to the energy of a thin plate under tension while the bending energy is related to the rigidity of the deformable surface [9]. Both energies can be expressed as a combination of first and second order parametric derivatives of the surface, respectively.

For the external image force we use knowledge of the MR acquisition protocol. In previous work we showed that the optimal criterion for vessel width estimation depends on the MRA acquisition [13]. If $i.$ the resolution is sufficiently high (at least 3 pixels/dim.), $ii.$ saturation due to slow inflow at the borders is limited (for TOF), and $iii.$ flow artifacts are suppressed, the boundaries in Time-Of-Flight (TOF) and Contrast Enhanced (CE) acquisitions can be determined using the full-width-half-maximum (FWHM) criterion, while for Phase Contrast (PC) acquisitions the full-width-10%-maximum (FWTM) should be used (all with respect to the maximum luminal signal) [13]. These criteria can be casted into an energy function in the following way

$$\mathcal{E}_{ext}^{W} = \frac{1}{S} \int_{0}^{1} \int_{0}^{2\pi} \left| \tau_{acq} - \frac{L(\mathbf{W}(t, u))}{L(\mathbf{C}(t))} \right| \| \partial_t \mathbf{W} \times \partial_u \mathbf{W} \| \, dt du \qquad (9)$$

where $L(\mathbf{x})$ is the image grey-level at position $\mathbf{x}$, S is the vessel wall area, and τ_{acq} is a threshold that introduces the knowledge about the type of MRA imaging technique. This constant equals 0.5 for TOF and CE, and 0.1 for PC MR angiography. Notice that the weight $\| \partial_t \mathbf{W} \times \partial_u \mathbf{W} \|$ takes into account possible departures from chord-length parameterization in the surface.

To start the fitting procedure, first an initialization of the central vessel axis is required. Initialization and interaction of 3D deformable models is still an open problem. However, proper initialization is a requirement to find the correct local minimum for most deformable model approaches. We suggest the use of an iso-surface rendering for interactively inspecting the vascular anatomy and for selecting the target segment. In Figure 1, the steps of the procedure are highlighted. First, an iso-surface rendering of the angiogram is generated (Figure 1(a)) using *marching cubes* [14]. Secondly, the operator defines a vessel segment by clicking two points on the iso-surface which define the end-points of a geodesic path (minimum length path *on* the surface; this is the *only* step in the algorithm where user interaction is required). This path is used for initializing the central vessel axis after it has been converted into B-spline form using a least squares approximation –Figure 1(b). Thirdly, once the central vessel axis has been determined, the vessel wall is initialized with *no extra* user interaction by computing a radius function as the distance between the central vessel axis and the geodesic path. This distance provides a rough approximation of the vessel radius at every point along the center line. Using a standard CAD technique known as *swept surfaces* [12] the vessel model is initialized by sweeping a circle of the estimated radius orthogonally along the central vessel axis–Figure 1(c). Figure 1(d) shows the final result of the fitting procedure.

3   Results

In order to assess the performance of the algorithm we addressed the problem of diameter measurements for stenosis grading in an MR compatible, carotid bifurcation phantom with an asymmetric stenosis (R.G. Shelley Lt., North York, Ontario). A photograph of this phantom is shown in the left frame of Figure 2. The phantom is embedded in a rigid, transparent acrylic and manufactured to reproduce normal dimensions in the human vasculature [15].

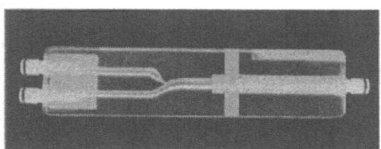 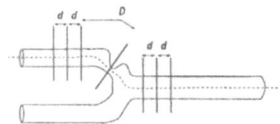

Fig. 2. Left: Carotid bifurcation phantom with an asymmetric stenosis (Courtesy of R.G. Shelley Lt., North York, Ontario, Canada). **Right:** Manual measurement protocol. In this study we used $D = 15$ mm and $d = 5$ mm.

Images were acquired on a 1.5 Tesla MR imaging system (Philips Gyroscan ACS-NT, Philips Medical Systems, Best, The Netherlands) with a quadrature head-neck receiver coil. Imaging parameters were as follows. Three-dimensional TOF acquisition: echo time (TE) 1.9 ms, repetition time (TR) 25.0 ms and flip angle (α) 15°, slice thickness 1.0 mm. CE acquisition: TE 2.0 ms, TR 6.6 ms, α 40°, slice thickness 1.0 mm. Both acquisitions: FOV 256 mm, scan matrix

256×256. Flow was regulated by a computer-controlled pump (Quest Image Inc., London, Ontario). Water was guided through the phantom with constant velocity (5 ml/s). For CE acquisitions a 5 mM solution of gadopentetate dimeglumine (Magnevist, Schering, Berlin, Germany) was used under the same flow conditions as the 3D TOF acquisition.

We assessed the performance of the algorithm in comparison with human operators and the ground truth as gold standard. The degree of stenosis was graded by two experts following a manual procedure. This is based on visual inspection of vessel dimensions on a multi planar reformatted (MPR) image generated by manually drawing a central vessel axis and computing the plane perpendicular to it. This procedure was performed on a clinical workstation (EasyVision, Philips Medical Systems, Best, The Netherlands).

In order to compare the measurements provided by the experts and the results obtained with our algorithm, a measurement protocol was defined as indicated in the right frame of Figure 2. The degree of stenosis was computed using the NASCET index (stenosis=1-(minimal residual lumen/distal ICA lumen diameter)x100%)[1]), and the CC index (with reference taken at the *common carotid artery*). To incorporate operator variability, the protocol required that the distal diameter was measured at $D = 15$ mm from the center of the stenosis and for two other successive planes separated by $d = 5$ mm. For each plane, the minimum and maximum observed diameters were recorded. All measurements were done twice by the same expert with enough delay to disregard any possible bias in the second measurement. The average stenosis grade and the 99% confidence interval (CI) were computed for each observer, for both observers and for the proposed algorithm. The statistics of stenosis grading with the model based approach were computed based on all possible values of the degree of stenosis for a region of 2 mm around the stenosis and a region of $2d = 10$ mm centered at a distance $D + d = 20$ mm from the stenosis. This yields a measure of stability of the model-based measurements in the region where the operators performed the manual analysis. In Figure 3, the average diameter measurements are shown (the average diameter in the orthogonal plane, at a given location along the central vessel axis). For comparison purposes, it also includes, at three points, diameter values from the specifications of the phantom [15].

In Table 3, the statistics of the stenosis grading are summarized. The phantom has a stenosis index of 69.2% according to NASCET and 78.5% according

Criterion	Code	WO_1 %D ± $CI_{99\%}$	WO_2 %D ± $CI_{99\%}$	BO_{12} %D ± $CI_{99\%}$	MB %D ± $CI_{99\%}$
CC (78.5% ±0.65%)	3D-TOF-1.0	69.8 ±3.47	62.8 ±5.30	66.3 =3.20	76.7 ±0.20
	3D-CEA-1.0	68.4 ±1.40	62.8 ±4.10	65.6 =2.30	76.0 ±0.22
NASCET (69.2% ±0.95%)	3D-TOF-1.0	55.2 ±4.10	39.1 ±7.52	47.2 =5.21	67.6 ±0.14
	3D-CEA-1.0	55.8 ±3.30	48.3 ±5.25	52.1 =3.38	65.9 ±0.19

Table 1. Stenosis Grading Summary: carotid bifurcation phantom with asymmetric stenosis. Within (WO_1, WO_2) and between observer (BO_{12}) variability of two experts compared to the model-based approach (MB). The stenosis is given according to two stenosis indexes: the *common carotid artery* (CC) and NASCET indexes. The true values are indicated in the first column.

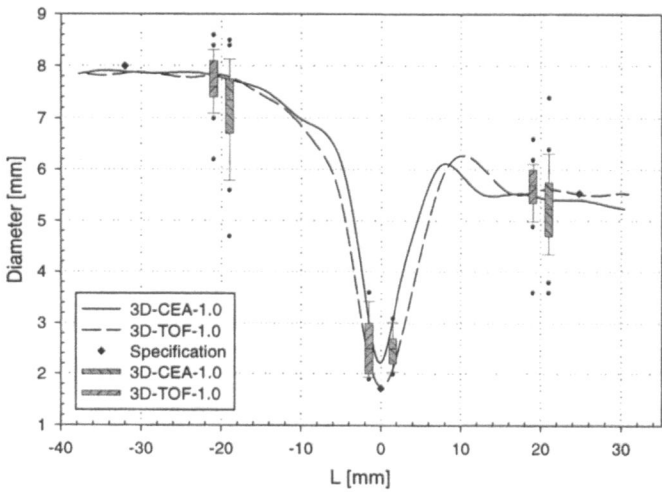

Fig. 3. Average diameter plots for the carotid bifurcation phantom starting at the common carotid artery and upstream to the stenoted branch. The diameter of the phantom (estimated from phantom specifications [15]) and the box-and-whisker plots corresponding to the measurements performed by two experts are also included. Two acquisitions were considered in this experiment, 3D TOF and CE MRA.

to CC (estimated from the manufacturer's specifications [15]). The table shows that the method significantly improves stenosis grading with an absolute error smaller than 3.3% for both criteria. Moreover reproducibility is better in the model based approach.

We also tested the method on patient data. Figure 4(a) and 4(b) show MIPs of 3D TOF angiograms of the left (mild stenosis) and right (severe stenosis) carotids of the same patient, respectively. Figure 4(c) shows the left carotids of a second patient with a mild stenosis. The in-plane resolution of the 3D TOF sequence was 0.5 mm, with a slice thickness of 1.0 mm and a slice gap of 0.5 mm.

A summary of quantitative results for stenosis grading of these data is given in Table 3. In the same table, stenosis grades assessed by a radiologist from 3D TOF MIPs and 2D DSA projections are also included for comparison. Our model based method correlates better with DSA, which is the gold standard in many radiological studies, than the manual assessment from 3D TOF. Note that since we have not assumed a circular vessel shape, other shape characteristics such as the minimum/maximum diameters and cross-sectional area of the vessel can be computed, yielding additional quantitative information. Although the performance has to be evaluated on a larger set, the algorithm performs well for non-severe stenoses or in absence of large flow artifacts. In Figure 4(b) we included an example of a severe stenosis. In this case, post-stenotic flow artifacts and poor luminal signal showed that the almost fully automated method does not yield accurate results if the original data are of poor quality (note that in

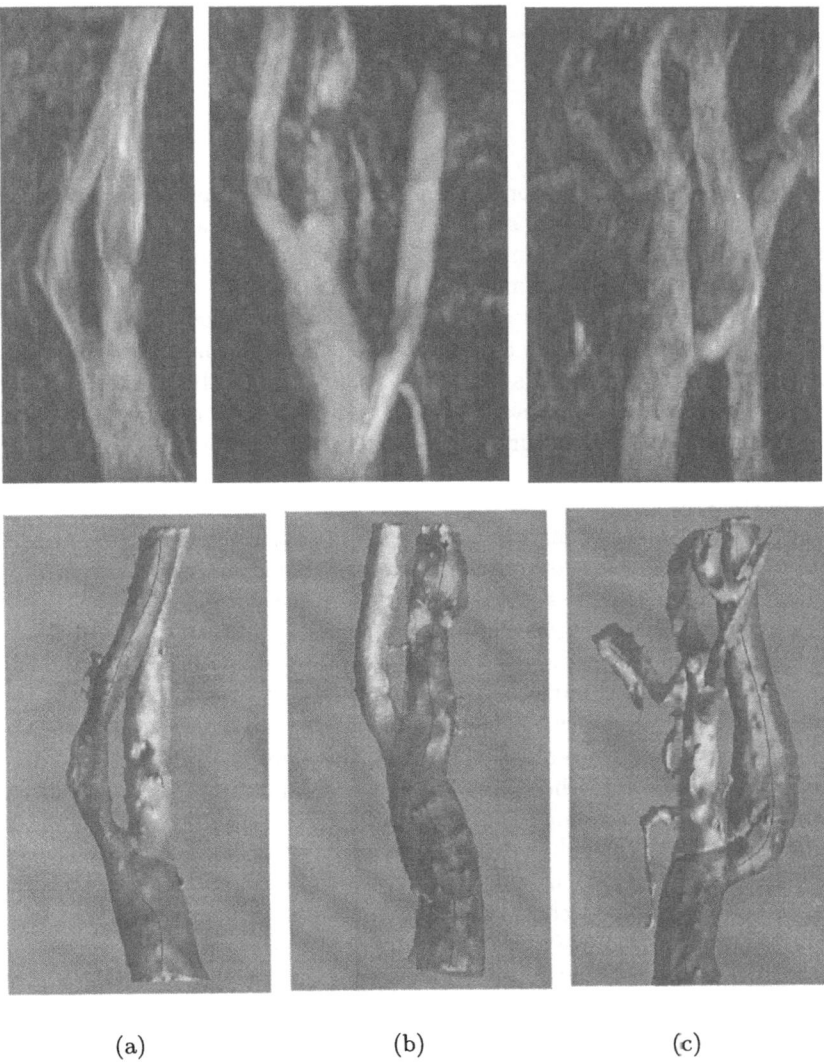

(a)   (b)   (c)

Fig. 4. Illustration on clinical data. The top row shows maximum intensity projections of 3D TOF datasets of the *internal carotid artery* (ICA). *a)* and *b)* correspond to the right and left ICA of the same patient and *c)* corresponds to the left ICA of a second patient. In the lower row we show the corresponding vessel models. The models are quite accurate for the two left ICA cases shown. For the right ICA, however, the presence of flow artifacts at the place of the severe stenosis (90% graded on MRA and 53% on DSA according to NASCET) precluded following the vessel axis in the stenosis.

this case the measurements of the operators in the 3D TOF and 2D DSA also show a large difference).

4 Discussion

We devised a method to perform quantitative diameter assessment at sub-voxel precision. The method shares some features with multiscale vessel enhancement algorithms based on eigenvalue analysis of the Hessian originally proposed by Koller et al. [16] and further modified by Sato et al. [17] and Lorenz et al. [18]. However, in these approaches a segmentation of the vasculature is obtained by estimating the vessel width as a function of the scale of maximum response. The accuracy of these algorithms is therefore a priori limited by the discretization of the scale parameter. This limits the applicability of these methods to give a general overview of the vasculature; for stenosis grading a more accurate approach is required. Aylward et al. [19] have suggested a method for vessel segmentation based on tracking the intensity ridges. The local vessel width is estimated using a line search technique to compute the scale of maximum response of a medialness function. Although this method can overcome the scale discretization problem, it still assumes that the vessel has a circular cross-section.

We have applied an algorithm which estimates the boundaries of the vessels using a flexible B-spline model which can be initialized using a small number of mouse clicks in a 3D surface display, and incorporates knowledge of the MR image acquisition. Whereas the algorithm contains a scale selection procedure in the determination of the central vessel axis, this does not influence the diameter assessment. Also, the method can model a wide class of cross-sectional shapes. Although often it is assumed that vessels have a circular cross-section, ex vivo measurements [20] have shown that this assumption is rather simplistic and, especially at the stenosis, a wide variety of geometric shapes can be observed. Three dimensional approaches, as the one presented in this work, provide a basis for both the description of the actual cross-sectional shape and its quantification. They also allow definition of stenosis indexes based on cross-sectional area reduction which are more robust than those based on diameter reduction.

The method has been illustrated on phantom and patient data. In the phantom data the method obtained diameter and stenosis measurements with an accuracy which was significantly better than the experts. Results on the TOF MRA data of patients are promising. However, this imaging technique is prone to flow artifacts. A larger evaluation study, including state-of-the-art acquisition

Patient	3D TOF	2D DSA	3D TOF (MB)
	%D	%D	%D
Fig. 4(a)	28%	36%	38%
Fig. 4(b)	90%	53%	NA
Fig. 4(c)	53%	34%	28%

Table 2. Stenosis grading of the carotids. Comparison of manual (3D TOF and DSA) and model-based (3D TOF). The stenosis index follows the NASCET criterion.

techniques like CE or blood pool agent (BPA) MRA which are less susceptible to flow artifacts, is planned to assess in which cases the proposed procedure can be used for reliable stenosis grading. The results presented in this study indicate that the proposed method has higher reproducibility and is more accurate than the laborious manual procedure of stenosis grading.

References

1. North American Symptomatic Carotid Endarterectomy Trial (NASCET) Steering Committe, "North American symptomatic carotid endarterectomy trial," *Stroke*, vol. 22, pp. 711–720, 1991.
2. European Carotid Surgery Trialists' Collaborative Group, "Randomised trial of endarterectomy for recently symptomatic carotid stenosis: final results of the MRC European Carotid Surgery (ECST)," *The Lancet*, vol. 351, pp. 1379–87, 1998.
3. H. Cline, C. Dumoulin, W. Lorensen, S. Souza, and W. Adams, "Volume rendering and connectivity algorithms for MR angiography," *MRM*, vol. 18, pp. 384–394, 1991.
4. C. M. Anderson, J. S. Saloner, D. Tsuruda, L. G. Shapeero, and R. E. Lee, "Artifacts in maximum-intensity-projection display of MR angiograms," *Am. J. Roent.*, vol. 154, pp. 623–629, 1990.
5. S. Schreiner, C. B. Paschal, and R. L. Galloway, "Comparison of projection algorithms used for the construction of maximum intensity projection images," *JCAT*, vol. 20, no. 1, pp. 56–67, Jan–Feb 1996.
6. G. Farin, *Curves and Surfaces for Computer Aided Geometric Design: A Practical Guide*, Academic Press, 1990.
7. M. Kass, A. Witkin, and D. Terzopoulos, "Snakes: Active contour models," *IJCV*, vol. 1, no. 4, pp. 321–331, 1987.
8. T. McInerney and D. Terzopoulos, "Deformable models in medical image analysis: a survey," *Med. Im. Anal.*, vol. 1, no. 2, pp. 91–108, 1996.
9. W. Wesselink, *Variational Modeling of Curves and Surfaces*, Ph.D. thesis, Utrecht University, Computer Science Department, 1996.
10. A. F. Frangi, W. J. Niessen, K. L. Vincken, and M. A. Viergever, "Multiscale vessel enhancement filtering," in *MICCAI98*, A. Colchester W. M. Wells and S. Delp, Eds., 1998, vol. 1496 of *LNCS*, pp. 130–137.
11. T. Lindeberg, "Feature detection with automatic scale selection," *IJCV*, vol. 30, no. 2, pp. 79–116, Nov. 1998.
12. L. Piegl and W. Tiller, *The NURBS Book*, Monographs in Visual Communication. Springer, 1996.
13. R. M. Hoogeveen, C. J. G. Bakker, and M. A. Viergever, "Limits to the accuracy of vessel diameter measurement in MR angiography," *J. Magn. Reson. Imag.*, vol. 8, pp. 1228–35, 1998.
14. W. E. Lorensen and H. E. Cline, "Marching cubes: a high resolution 3D surface reconstruction algorith," *Proc. SIGGRAPH'87*, vol. 21, pp. 163–169, 1987.
15. R. F. Smith, B. K. Rutt, A. J. Fox, R. N. Rankin, and D. W. Holdsworth, "Geometric characterization of stenoted human carotid arteries," *Acad. Radiol.*, vol. 3, pp. 898–911, 1996.
16. Th. Koller, G. Gerig, G. Székely, and D. Dettwiler, "Multiscale detection of Curvilinear Structures in 2-D and 3-D Image Data," in *Proc. ICCV95*, 1995, pp. 864–869, IEEE Computer Society Press.
17. Y. Sato, S. Nakajima, N. Shiraga, H. Atsumi, S. Yoshida, T. Koller, G. Gerig, and R. Kikinis, "Three-dimensional multi-scale line filter for segmentation and visualization of curvilinear structures in medical images," *Med. Im. Anal.*, vol. 2, no. 2, pp. 143–163, June 1998.
18. C. Lorenz, I.-C. Carlsen, Buzug T.M., C. Fassnacht, and J. Weese, "Multi-scale line segmentation with automatic estimation of width, contrast and tangential direction in 2D and 3D medical images," in *Proc. CVRMed-MRCAS'97*, J. Troccaz, E. Grimson, and R. Mösges, Eds., 1997, LNCS, pp. 233–242, Springer-Verlag.
19. S. Aylward, E. Bullit, S. Pizer, and D. Eberly, "Intensity ridge and widths for tubular object segmentation and description," in *Proc. IEEE/SIAM Workshop on Math. Meth. in Biomed. Im. Anal.*, 1996, pp. 131–8.
20. X. M. Pan, D. Saloner, L. M. Reilly, J. C. Bowersox, S. P. Murray, C. M Anderson, G. A. Gooding, and J. H. Rapp, "Assessment of carotid artery stenosis by ultrasonography, conventional angiography, and magnetic resonance angiography: correlation with *ex vivo* measurements of plaque stenosis," *J. Vasc. Surg.*, vol. 21, pp. 82–89, 1995.
21. O. E. H. Elgersma, P. C. Buijs, A.F.J. Wüst, Y. van der Graaf, B. C. Eikelboom, and W. P. Th. M. Mali, "Assessment of maximum internal carotid artery stenosis: Rotational vs. conventional intra arterial digital substraction angiography," *Radiol.*, accepted, 1999.

A Patient-Specific Computer Model for Prediction of Clinical Outcomes in the Cerebral Circulation Using MR Flow Measurements

M.E. Clark[1], Meide Zhao[1], Francis Loth[1,2], Noam Alperin[1,3], Lewis Sadler[1], Kern Guppy[1], and Fady T. Charbel[1]

[1]Division of Neurovascular Research (CANVAS Program), Department of Neurosurgery, University of Illinois at Chicago, Chicago, IL.
[2]Department of Mechanical Engineering, University of Illinois at Chicago, Chicago, IL.
[3]Department of Radiology, University of Illinois at Chicago, Chicago, IL.
m-clark4@uiuc.edu, mzhao@uic.edu, fcharbel@uic.edu,
floth@uic.edu, alperin@uic.edu

Abstract. A patient-specific, computer model of the cerebral circulation to predict cerebral blood flow and pressure is presented. The model is based on a previously reported numeric model consisting of a network of distensible vessels with pulsatile flow. The enhanced model uses a sector scheme to determine the efferent resistance distribution for a specific patient. An iterative algorithm was developed to determine the patient-specific efferent resistance distribution from *in vivo* cerebral blood flow measurements obtained using phase contrast magnetic resonance angiography (PCMRA). In comparison with PCMRA flow measurements and clinical outcomes, the enhanced model shows its ability to predict cerebral flow well in three patients who underwent a balloon occlusion of the carotid artery. A model that accurately predicts cerebral blood flow for different treatment scenarios can provide the surgeon with an invaluable tool in the management of complex cerebral vascular disorders.

1. Introduction

Computer simulation of the cerebral circulation, based on fluid-dynamic relations, has been carried out for more than three decades [1-2]. It offers the convenience of predicting flows and pressures at any desired section in the vessel network. Moreover, it not only can be used to estimate the flow and pressure in both normal and disease situations, but it also can be used to predict the result of treatment procedures [3-5]. However, simulating the patient-specific cerebral circulation presents a range of challenging problems. In the fluid-dynamic area, these problems include the proper modeling of the pulsatile flow, the vessel wall distensibility, and the efferent resistance distribution. In medical imaging, there are problems associated with the automatic extraction of the patient's vasculature, accurate measurement of vessel diameters, and quantification of blood flow and pressure. The interaction of these factors makes the simulation task complex. Although much effort has been expended in the last three decades towards solving these problems, patient-specific fluid-dynamic simulations have not yet reached the clinical utilization stage.

Cerebral circulation computer modeling can be done with various assumptions. The basic model applies the linear governing equations of steady flow and rigid vessels [1-2]. Models that incorporate the effects of pulsatile flow and distensible vessels [3-5] more accurately describe the physical behavior of blood flow in arteries. Several other cerebral circulation studies using pulsatile flow in distensible vessels have been reported [6-11]. To simulate the rupture condition of an aneurysm, Duros, et al. [5], used a 108-vessel model that not only contained the cerebral arteries but also the main systemic arteries, reasoning that they played an important role in wave propagation and overall flow distribution (Fig. 1).

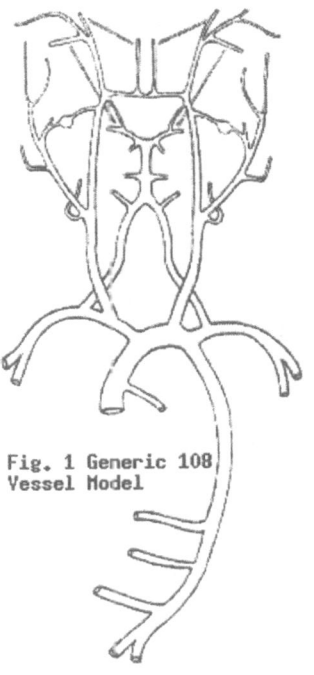

In previous work [12], a computer model of cerebral blood flow was developed using angiographic determination of vessel sizes and a generic pattern for the efferent terminal resistance. This simulation was used to analyze patients with different disease states that affect the cerebral circulation. The results have correlated qualitatively with the clinical outcomes, indicating the predictive value of these simulations. In addition, the predicted blood flow patterns correlate with various test results in these patients, such as single photon emission computerized tomography (SPECT), electroencephagraphy (EEG), cerebral oxygen saturation (rSO2), and transcranial Doppler (TCD).

The generic model results, obtained using the individual patient's vessel sizes (obtained from digital subtraction angiography (DSA)) and a generic pattern of peripheral resistance, indicate satisfactory accuracy for some, but not all, vessel flows. In order to improve the simulation, patient-specific information is needed regarding the peripheral resistance distribution. To achieve this patient-specificity, the flows in certain crucial cerebral arteries must be obtained from phase contrast magnetic resonance angiography (PCMRA). A patient-specific pattern of resistance can then be calculated. To this end, the original computer program has been modified so that all the efferents to a cerebral sector are melded into one terminal efferent vessel and a measured input flow to that sector is then used to determine its resistance. Seven such sectors have been identified in the cerebral macrovasculature. By combining the sector concept with PCMRA and DSA angiography, enhanced simulations of normal, diseased, and surgeon-modified cerebral configurations are being produced.

Fig. 1 Generic 108 Vessel Model

2. The Generic Model

The behavior of the cerebral arterial network with its pulsatile flow occurring in compliant arteries is mimicked using a computer algorithm for unsteady flow in a network of elastic vessels. The primary vessels of the cerebral macrovasculature are included in the network along with a skeleton of vessels, including the heart efferent, to represent the systemic vasculature. The circle acts as an invaluable distribution center for cerebral blood but the distribution decisions are initiated in the aortic arch and subclavians.

The numeric algorithm that is used to generate the pressures and flows at all locations within the vessel network and at all times during the heart pulse period is a one-dimensional, staggered, explicit finite-difference scheme [3], based on a conservation of mass relation to calculate the pressures, and a Navier-Stokes momentum equation to calculate the flows.

Not all or even most of the arteries in the cerebral circulation can be included in the model. Some judicious choice must be made as to where to terminate the model. The terminal boundary condition imposed on all efferents of the chosen network is, therefore, most crucial to the flow distributions predicted by the model and is the main thrust of this paper. A lumped parameter resistance-capacitance-resistance (RCR) combination was used in which the upstream resistance (R_1) was set equal to the characteristic impedance of the efferent [3].

The forcing function for the model is imposed at the root of the ascending aorta and is in the form of a normal pressure-time diagram there. A set of initial conditions, required to get the numeric process started, is given by setting all nodal pressures equal to the venous pressure and all nodal flows equal

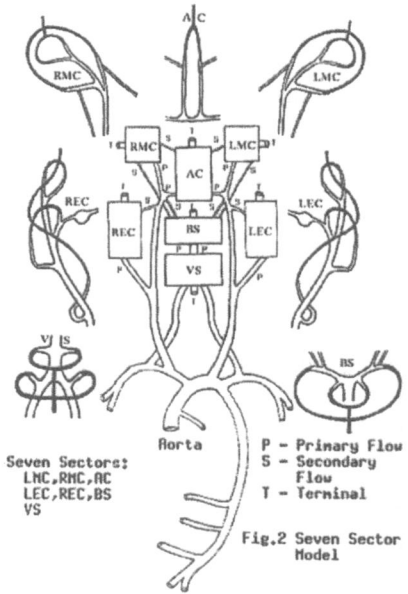

Fig.2 Seven Sector Model

to zero. Ten to fifteen pulse periods of calculations are required to bring the pressures and flows into steady-state pulsatility. Computation time for a typical run on a 400 MHz personal computer is approximately three minutes.

3. Sector Model

With the advent of PCMRA, the non-invasive measurement of cerebral artery flow has become a reality. This advance provided a means by which cerebral circulation simulations could be made more patient-specific. The crucial unknowns in such simulations are the terminal resistances of the modeled vessels. If time in the MRI machine were not a factor, the flow in each individual efferent of the model could be measured and a corresponding resistance could be calculated. To limit machine time and the number of flows to be determined for the patient, a sector model of the cerebral circulation was devised in which all of the terminal vessels in any sector were melded into one terminal vessel. Seven such sectors are shown in Fig.2 along with the primary and secondary flow inlets and/or outlets and with the terminal efferent for each sector. To determine this one terminal resistance, it is necessary to be able to define the flow into and/or out of the sector.

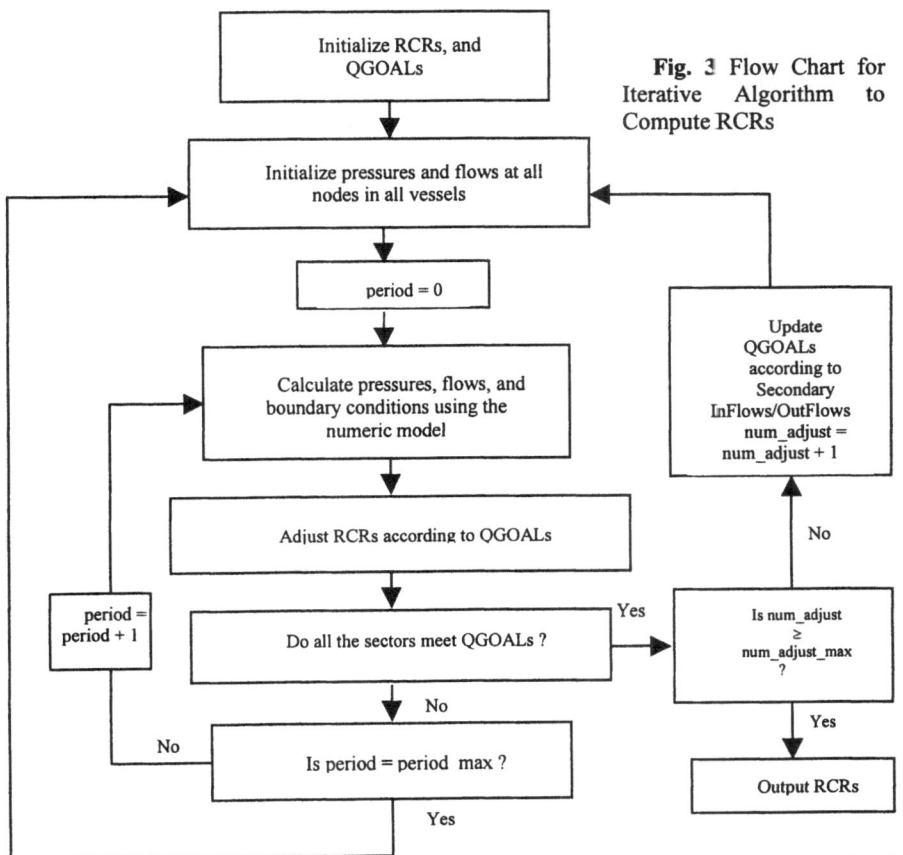

Fig. 3 Flow Chart for Iterative Algorithm to Compute RCRs

This requirement takes different forms for different sectors. For the left middle cerebral sector (LMC), there are three possible flow inlets (M1, the main middle cerebral vessel, and two small secondary collaterals or anastomoses) and one terminal resistance efferent. This single efferent takes the place of four efferents used in the original generic model (Fig.1) and has been formed by melding together these original efferents. The secondary anastomoses are not present in all cases and, when present, it is difficult to measure their flows. Therefore, the M1 flow represents the primary input to this sector and its mean flow value over a pulse period is required via PCMRA. The secondary flows are accounted for in the simulation by means of their current calculated values as described later.

To start the computations for the sector model (Fig.3), the assumption is made that the flow (QGOAL in Fig.3) in the terminal efferent for the sector is the same as the PCMRA measured flow in the primary input flow vessel, ignoring, for this first set of calculations, the other secondary inflows or outflows. A plausible set of terminal resistances are needed to start the calculations and can be concocted from either from a steady flow model of the vessel system or from a previous similar simulation. After each (pulse) period of calculation, the program adjusts the resistance for each sector terminal efferent by multiplying its current resistance by the ratio of the current calculated terminal flow to the goal (PCMRA) flow for that terminal. This procedure would correctly adjust any one terminal flow but, since all the other terminal resistances are adjusted concurrently, errors are introduced and many adjustments are needed in subsequent periods. This process continues for up to a user-specified number of pulse periods of calculations (period_max in Fig.3). A check is made at the end of each period to see if the measured sector flow goal has been achieved by the adjustment of the resistance of the terminal efferent. If all seven sector flow goals are achieved within the period limit, the program proceeds to the next step. If the goals are not met after the maximum number of periods, the program starts over with the current efferent resistances and the original initial conditions of zero flow and venous pressure at all nodes in all vessels.

The next step in the procedure is the adjustment of the flow goals (QGOALs in Fig.3) so as to account for the secondary inflows and/or outflows. Since all vessels in the model are involved in the calculations discussed above, the secondary flows have been continually updated in this process. In this set of calculations, the flow in the terminal efferent is set equal to the primary PCMRA flow adjusted for the flows in the secondary inlets and/or outlets. For the left middle cerebral sector, this amounts to adjusting the M1 flow for the inflow or outflow contributions of the two secondary anastomoses. For the basilar sector, the contributions of the posterior communicating arteries and the two secondary anastomoses must be considered with proper signs. For the left external carotid sector, the ophthalmic flow must be combined with the left external carotid PCMRA flow in subsequent calculations. These adjustments are made only at the beginning of a period_max run, which can be cut short if all sector flow goals are met. When a user-specified number of adjustments have been made, the program ends.

At this stage of the simulation, a patient-specific set of resistances has been generated from patient DSA angiograms and measured PCMRA sector flows. This resistance pattern can now be assumed to be invariant in additional simulations of this patient. Modifications in system configuration can be made, say, by inserting a bypass vessel between the external and internal carotid arteries or by vessel occlusion in the treatment of an aneurysm. The neurosurgeon can now play "what if?" games with the computer program to plan the best strategies for his/her treatment of the patient.

4. Cerebral Blood Flow Quantification

Flow quantification with PCMRA provides a powerful tool to non-invasively analyze blood flow [15]. It has been shown to do well in assessing both *in vitro* and *in vivo* flow velocities and volumetric flow rates (VFR) [16]. Accuracy of blood flow measurements is influenced by many MR parameters : among these are the partial volume [17] and the curved flow effect [18].

A three-dimensional (3D) vessel localization algorithm has been developed by Zhao, et al. [18] for the determination of slice selections and slice orientation to improve the accuracy of flow measurement. The 3D localizer was developed based on a 1.5 Tesla MRI General Electric imager. A 3D time of flight MRA covering the circle of Willis is performed and the images are extracted and transferred to a SGI workstation. The 3D surface rendering of the vasculature is then reconstructed from these images using a marching-cube algorithm [18]. The coordinates obtained from the 3D localization based on the 3D surface rendering specify the position of an oblique cine PCMRA scan. A cine PCMRA is then performed based on those coordinates. The following parameters were used: TR, 33 ms; TE, minimum; flip angle, 30; number of excitations, 2; field of view, 16 cm; image matrix, 256 x 128; number of phases, 32; slice thickness and velocity encoding (VENC) are 5 mm and 100 cm/sec for carotids, VA, and BA, and 4 mm and 70 cm/sec for MCA and ACA. The vessel area is semi-automatically determined though a newly-developed interface on a SGI workstation [18]. The velocity and volumetric flow rate (VFR) can then be calculated over the time course of the pulse period.

5. Presentation of Results - Case Studies

To exhibit the efficacy and abilities of the sector model of the cerebral circulation, three cases relating to the balloon occlusion test (BOT) used in the treatment of non-operable cerebral aneurysms will be presented and discussed. When an aneurysm is to be treated by occluding the vessel to which it is attached, a temporary occlusion of the vessel is made with a balloon to test the clinical outcome of the patient to permanent occlusion. Since the BOT is not without risk, the patient would benefit if a BOT computer simulation could be substituted. The three cases presented for discussion are intended to show how well the model predicts the BOT outcome.

Case 1. A 51-year-old white male presented with a two-month's history of progressively worsening left pulsatile tinnitus. Angiogram and PCMRA studies showed that both the left and right posterior communicating arteries and the A1 segment of the left anterior cerebral artery were small. The left internal carotid artery contained a large aneurysm and a stenosis of 60 percent. These data were used as Baseline in the computer simulation. The patient subsequently passed a BOT. A permanent occlusion of the LICA was made with balloons trapping the diseased distal cervical segment of the LICA.

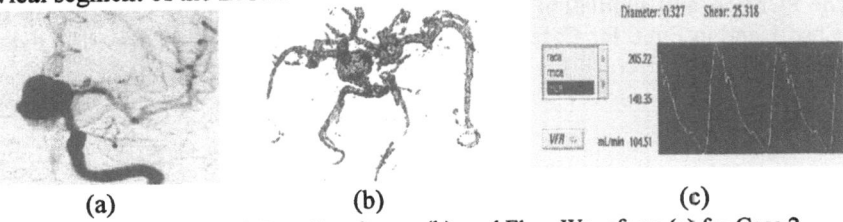

(a)   (b)   (c)

Fig. 4 Angiogram (a), 3D Localizer Image (b), and Flow Waveform (c) for Case 2.

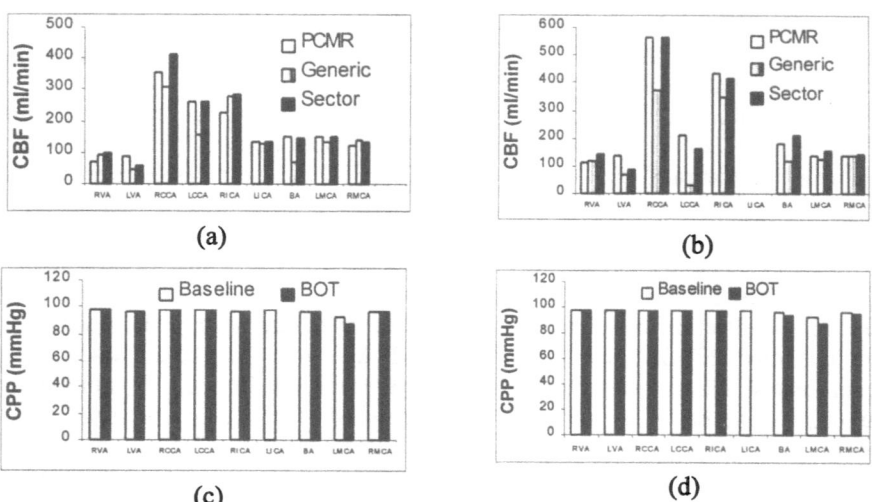

(a)   (b)

(c)   (d)

Fig.5 Results for Case 1: (a) Comparison of CBF (Cerebral Blood Flow) at Baseline and (b) post-BOT between PCMRA and simulations from Generic and Sector Models; Comparison of CPP (Cerebral Perfusion Pressure) between Generic (c) and Sector (d) simulations at Baseline and BOT

Case 2. A 56-year-old black female presented with a subarachnoid hemorrhage. Angiogram and PCMRA studies showed multiple aneurysms including a giant aneurysm at the left superior hypophyseal artery as well as a 40 percent stenosis in the left internal carotid artery. The patient failed the BOT under hypotensive challenge, becoming hemiparetic and aphasic during the test. SPECT also showed a massive difference between the two hemispheres with a significant decreased relative blood flow in the left hemisphere involving the frontoparietal, occipital and temporal lobes. A PCMRA CBF study was performed before the BOT. These data were used in the Baseline simulation.

Case 3. A 71-year-old white female presented with persistent headache. Angiogram and PCMRA studies showed a large right carotid-ophthalmic aneurysm as well as occlusions of both left and right posterior communicating arteries, occlusion of the anterior communicating artery, and a 40 percent stenosis in the left anterior cerebral artery. These data were considered as the Baseline in the computer simulation. A PCMRA CBF study was performed before the BOT. During the BOT in the right internal carotid artery, an immediate failure ensued when left side hemiparesis developed.

A typical angiogram, 3D localizer image, and flow waveform are presented in Fig. 4. The PCMRA and simulation results are shown in the form of bar graphs in Fig.5 for Case 1 and in Fig.6 for Cases 2 and 3. These results will be discussed in detail in the next section.

6. Discussion and Conclusions

The purpose of this paper is to demonstrate the efficacy of a novel simulation technique, the sector model, in the patient-specific prediction of clinical outcomes accompanying surgical intervention. The specific intervention considered here is the treatment of inoperable aneurysms by permanent occlusion of a carotid artery. The patient's tolerance of such an occlusion is determined by temporarily occluding the artery, the balloon occlusion test (BOT). Since this test is not without risk, it would be beneficial for the patient to substitute a valid computer simulation for it.

The PCMRA flow measurements along with the sector and generic model results are displayed in Fig. 5 and 6. For case 1, the Baseline results in Fig. 5a show excellent agreement between the PCMRA flow and the sector model results for most vessels. This result was expected since the PCMRA flow measurements were used in the RCR adjustments to satisfy the iterative process of Fig. 3. Once the RCR pattern had been determined for this patient, it was used independently to predict the post-BOT results shown in Fig.5b. Here again, the agreement between the PCMRA and the sector model results is excellent (with the possible exception of the LVA). The generic model compared well with the PCMRA measurements for some vessels, but not as

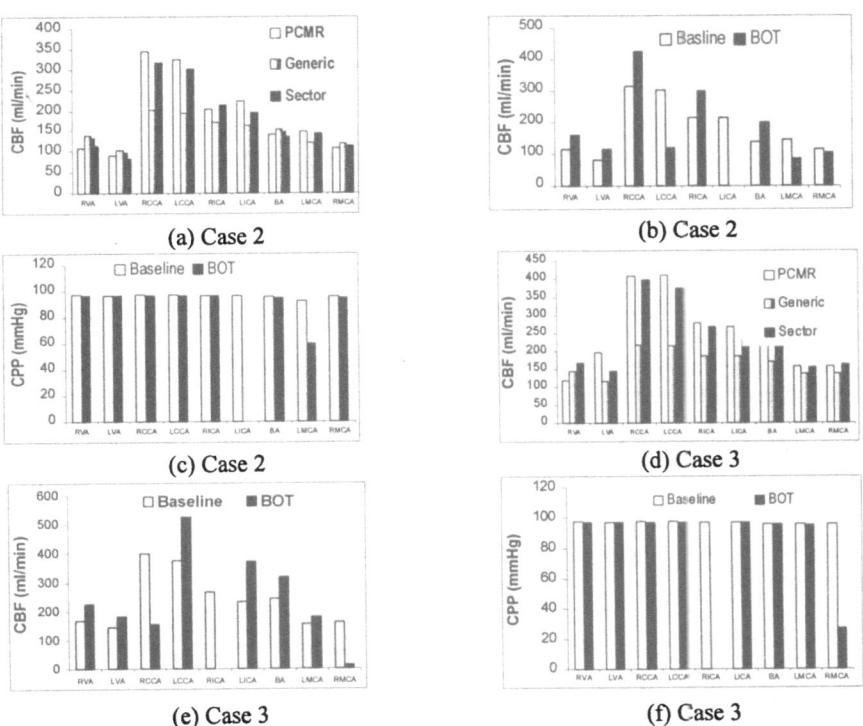

(a) Case 2

(b) Case 2

(c) Case 2

(d) Case 3

(e) Case 3

(f) Case 3

Fig. 6. Results for Case 2 (a)-(c) and Case 3 (d)-(f): Comparison of CBF at Baseline in Case 2 (a) and Case 3 (d) between PCMRA and simulations from Generic and Sector Models; Comparison of CBF in Case 2 (b) and Case 3 (e) and CPP in Case 2 (d) and Case 3 (f) between simulations at Baseline and BOT

consistently as the sector model. For cerebral perfusion pressure (CPP) results in Fig. 5c and 5d, both sector and generic models give comparable predictions for Baseline and BOT with no dramatic pressure drops during the test. Since the patient passed the test, these results are also compatible with the clinical outcome.

Similar results were obtained for Cases 2 and 3 for Baseline CBF as shown in Fig. 6a and 6d. Since both patients failed the BOT test, there are no post-BOT PCMRA data to compare with the simulation results. Therefore, only calculated Baseline and BOT CBF values are shown in Fig.6b and 6e for Cases 2 and 3, respectively. These cases have drastically different flow patterns in the carotid vessels (RCCA, LCCA, RICA, LICA) because of the balloon closure of the LICA and RICA in Cases 2 and 3, respectively. For the BOT simulation, the reduction in flow values for the LMCA in Case 2 and the RMCA for Case 3 in comparison with the Baseline values is compatible with the clinical outcome of BOT failure. A similar result for CPP values for these arteries is shown in Fig. 6c and 6f. The reduction in flow and pressure for Case 2 was not as pronounced as that for Case 3 because Case 2 failed the BOT only under hypotensive challenge. In Case 3, the reduction in flow is nearly 100 percent and the pressure is reduced to venous pressure levels in the RMCA.

For Case 3, when the seven-sector model was used to simulate the BOT, an anomaly was discovered in the AC sector. All possible inflow paths to the RMC and AC sectors were seemingly blocked by the occlusions indicated in Section 5. However, the sector model found the one unblocked path. That path started by following the LAC up to the junction of the terminal efferent. Since only part of the available LAC flow was needed to satisfy that efferent, the rest passed down the RAC and went on to satisfy the RMC sector. To correct this implausible solution and to prevent the anomaly, an eight-sector model was used with two separate AC sectors. However, the resulting RAC and RMC sectors had no connection to the forcing function in the ascending aorta except for minor contributions from the small ophthalmic and two secondary anastomoses. The results of the new simulation showed essentially zero flow and venous pressure levels in these sectors. The immediate left side hemiparesis in this patient is adequately explained by these simulation results.

In conclusion, patient-specificity has been achieved in the simulation and analysis of the three BOT patients. These results demonstrate a significant advance in computer modeling of the cerebral circulation through the introduction of the sector model. While the present study only examined three cases, the results clearly demonstrate the working hypothesis of this sector model. Further work using the model in a variety of surgical interventions and with a large population of patients is necessary before it is ready for clinical use. Current work is underway to obtain these validation data. Many improvements are envisioned for future models: the forcing function can be made more patient-specific; the systemic portions of the model can be made into sectors and governed by PCMRA measurements; and the autoregulatory aspects of the cerebral arterioles can be added to the simulation. In addition, the model can be generalized to other regions of the cardiovascular system like the coronary circulation or the circulation in the extremities. A model that can accurately predict cerebral blood flow will provide an invaluable tool for the surgeon in managing complex cerebral problems.

References

1. Himwich, W.A, Knapp, F.M., Wenglarz, R.A., Martin, J.D., and Clark, M.E.: The circle of Willis as simulated by an engineering model, Arch. of Neurology, (1965) 13: 164-172
2. Clark, M.E., Himwich, W.A., and Martin, J.D.: Simulation studies of factors influencing the cerebral circulation, Acta Neurol. Scandinav., (1967) 43: 189-204
3. Kufahl, R.H., and Clark, M.E.: A circle of Willis simulation using distensible vessels and pulsatile flow, J. of Biomechanical Engineering, (1985) 107: 112-122
4. Clark, M.E., Kufahl, R.H., and Zimmerman, F.J.: Natural and surgically-imposed anastomoses of the circle of Willis, Neurological Research, (1989) 11: 217-230
5. Duros, J., Clark, M.E., Kufahl, R.H., and Nadvornik, P.: On the rupture of an aneurysm, Neurological Research, (1991) 13: 217-223
6. Ling, S.C., and Atabek, H.B.: A nonlinear analysis of pulsatile flow in arteries, J. of Fluid Mechanics, (1972) 55: 493-511
7. Cooper, L.: Pulsating flow in a network with application to the circle of Willis, (1970) Ph.D. thesis, Washington University, St.Louis, MO
8. Chao, J.C., and Hwang, N.H.: Function dynamics of the circle of Willis, J. of Life Science, (1972) 2: 3-81
9. Himwich, W.A., and Clark, M.E.: Simulation of flow and pressure distributions in the circle of Willis. In: J. Cervos-Navarro, eds., Pathology of Cerebral Microcirculation, NY, Walter de Gruyter, (1974) 140-152
10. Clark, M.E., and Kufahl, R.H.: Simulation of cerebral macrocirculation. In: Proc of 1st Int. Conf. Cardiovascular System Dynamics, MIT Press, Boston (1978) 380-390
11. Hillen, B., Gaasbeek, T., and Hoogstraten, H.W.: A mathematical model of the flow in the posterior communicating arteries, J. of Biomechanics, (1982) 15: 441-448
12. Charbel, F.T., Misra, M., Clark, M.E., and Ausman, J.I: Computer simulation of cerebral blood flow in Moyamoya and the results of surgical therapies, Clinical Neurology and Neurosurgery, (1997), Suppl.2.
13. Charbel, F.T., Clark, M.E., Misra, M., Hannigan, K., Hoffman, W.E., and Ausman, J.I.: The application of a computerized model of the cerebral circulation in skull base surgery. 2nd Intern. Skull Base Congress, San Diego, (1996) 210
14. Raines, J.K., Jaffrin, M.Y., and Shapiro, A.H.: A computer simulation of the human artery system, Proc. of the 1971 Summer Computer Conference, (1971), 2, 171-178
15. Moran, P.R.: A flow velocity zeugmatographic interlace for NMR imaging in humans, Magnetic Resonance Imaging, (1982) 1, 197-203
16. Hofman, M.B.M., Visser, F.C., Vanrossum, A.C., Vink, G.Q.M., Sprenger, M., and Westerhof, N.: *In Vivo* validation of magnetic resonance blood volume flow measurements with limited spatial resolution in small vessels, Magnetic Resonance in Medicine, (1995), 33, 778-784
17. Tang, C., Blatter, D., and Parker, D.: Accuracy of phase-contrast flow measurements in the presence of partial-volume effects, JMRI, (1993) 3, 377-385
18. Frank, L., and Buxton, R.: Distortions from Curved Flow in magnetic Resonance Imaing, JMRI, (1992) 2, 82-93
19. Zhao, M., Charbel, F.T., Loth, F., and Alperin, N.: Improved Phase Contrast Quantification by 3D Vessel localization, (1998) Xth Annual International Workshop on Magnetic Resonance Angiography, Park City, Utah; Submitted to JMRI.

Exploratory Factor Analysis in Morphometry

A. M. C. Machado[1,3], J. C. Gee[2], and M. F. M. Campos[1]

[1] DCC, Federal University of Minas Gerais, Belo Horizonte, Brazil
{alexei,mario}@dcc.ufmg.br
[2] Department of Radiology, University of Pennsylvania, Philadelphia, USA
gee@rad.upenn.edu
[3] DCC, Pontifical Catholic University of Minas Gerais, Belo Horizonte, Brazil

Abstract. In this paper, we present an exploratory factor analytic approach to morphometry in which a high-dimensional set of shape-related variables is examined with the purpose of finding clusters with strong correlation. This clustering can potentially identify regions that have anatomic significance and thus lend insight to the morphometric investigation. The analysis is based on information about size difference between the differential volume about points in a template image and their corresponding volumes in a subject image, where the correspondence is established by non-rigid registration. The Jacobian determinant field of the registration transformation is modeled by a reduced set of factors, whose cardinality is determined by an algorithm that iteratively eliminates factors that are not informative. The results show the method's ability to identify gender-related morphological differences without supervision.

1 Introduction

This work presents a novel method for exploring the relationship among morphometric variables and the possible anatomic significance of these relationships. Our approach is based on the analysis of high-dimensional sets of vector variables obtained from non-rigidly deforming a template image so as to align its anatomy with the subject anatomy of a group, depicted in MRI studies. The resultant individualized templates provide an anatomic labeling of the subject data. In addition, information about regional shape can be extracted from the alignment transformations. This information—in the form of differential size differences among subject anatomies—is statistically analyzed to yield a reduced set of common *factors* that correspond to new variables with possible anatomic significance. In this way, the methodology more naturally facilitates hypothesis-driven explorations of regional differences in the data and lends deeper insight to the morphometric investigation.

An important and commonly used method for shape representation is the principal component analysis (PCA) of variance [10]. In this approach, a new set of variables is determined as linear combinations of the original variables, in such a way that they account for most part of the variance presented in the sample.

Marcus [9] and Cootes *et al.*[2] showed how PCA could be used to construct models based on manually chosen landmarks. The analysis was focused on the variable domain, since the number of subjects in the sample was usually larger than the number of variables being measured. Generalizing the use of PCA to high-dimensional variables, Le Briquer and Gee[7] applied the method directly to the mappings, registering an atlas to the subject anatomies.

Although PCA is efficient in summarizing variability in a dataset, the principal components are generally difficult to interpret. Factor analysis differs from PCA in that it provides a basis transformation from the variables into a factor domain that preserves the correlation among original variables. Factor analysis accounts for the covariance among these variables instead of representing principal modes of variance. In this sense, the information about the dependency among variables is preserved.

The use of factor analysis in morphometry has been examined by Marcus [9] and Reyment and Jöreskog [11] in the context of analyzing general scalar variables, presenting a wide discussion on the factor analysis of landmark data. Scalar features such as landmark distances and curvatures were considered in the analysis of ostracod species, where the displacements between landmarks were modeled as deformations of a thin-plate spline.

In this paper, we extend the exploratory factor analytic approach to high-resolution MRI morphometry, where the set of measurement variables are of very high dimension. The method is applied to the study of the corpus callosum and compared to previous published results [3, 8].

2   Methods

The displacement fields representing the spatial warps between the reference and the subjects' images are obtained from a Bayesian generalization of the Bajcsy and Kovačič elastic matching technique [1] and its finite element implementation [5]. The process comprises a global and local registration which account, respectively, for rigid transformations and continuous one-to-one mapping according to the elasticity theory principles.

2.1   Atlas-based MRI morphometry

The amount of scaling applied to an infinitesimal area around a point x in the template, when it is deformed to match a subject, can be evaluated by computing the Jacobian determinant of the mapping function between corresponding points. The pointwise Jacobian determinants for two populations can be compared by computing an *effect size*:

$$e(x) = [\mu_1(J(x)) - \mu_2(J(x))]/\sqrt{\sigma^2(J(x))}, \qquad (1)$$

where $\mu_p(J(x))$ is the mean pointwise Jacobian determinant of a population p and $\sigma^2(J(x))$ is the unbiased variance for populations 1 and 2 combined. These comparisons show shape differences between populations, reflected in the amount of compression or dilatation of a region-of-interest in the reference image.

2.2   Factor analysis

The purpose of factor analysis is to reduce the dimensionality of a problem by exploring the correlation among its variables. A set of p original variables, $\mathbf{y}$, is represented as linear combinations of m new variables called factors:

$$\mathbf{y} = \boldsymbol{\mu} + \boldsymbol{\Lambda}\mathbf{f} + \boldsymbol{\epsilon}, \tag{2}$$

where $\mathbf{y} = (y_1, \ldots, y_p)^T$ are the variables observed from a sample of a population with mean vector $\boldsymbol{\mu} = (\mu_1, \ldots, \mu_p)^T$ and covariance matrix $\boldsymbol{\Sigma}$; $\mathbf{f} = (f_1, \ldots, f_m)^T$ are the factors; $\boldsymbol{\epsilon} = (\epsilon_1, \ldots, \epsilon_p)^T$ are the error terms which account for the portion of $\mathbf{y}$ that is not common to the other variables; and $\boldsymbol{\Lambda} = ((\lambda_{11}, \ldots, \lambda_{1m}), \ldots, (\lambda_{p1}, \ldots, \lambda_{pm}))^T$ is the loading matrix. The coefficients λ_{ij}, called *loadings*, express the covariance between variable y_i and factor f_j.

The model and purpose of factor analysis lead to some assumptions regarding the behavior of $\mathbf{f}$ and $\boldsymbol{\epsilon}$. Since the expected value $\mathcal{E}(\mathbf{y} - \boldsymbol{\mu})$ is the null vector, $\mathcal{E}(\mathbf{f})$ and $\mathcal{E}(\boldsymbol{\epsilon})$ must also be $\mathbf{0}$. In order for the factors to account for all the correlation among the variables $\mathbf{y}$, the covariance among error terms and factors must be 0 and the covariances among error terms are represented by the diagonal matrix $\boldsymbol{\Psi} = diag(\psi_1, \ldots, \psi_p)$. The diagonal entries of $\boldsymbol{\Psi}$, ψ_i, are called *specific variances*. It is also assumed that the covariance matrix for factors is the identity matrix, so that the variance of y_i can be expressed as

$$var(y_i) = \sum_{j=1}^{m} \lambda_{ij}^2 + \psi_i. \tag{3}$$

The summation in (3) is called the *communality* or *common variance*. Based on the independence between $\boldsymbol{\Lambda}\mathbf{f}$ and $\boldsymbol{\epsilon}$, and considering $cov(\mathbf{f}) = \mathrm{I}i$, the relationship between $\boldsymbol{\Sigma}$, $\boldsymbol{\Lambda}$ and $\boldsymbol{\Psi}$ can be written as

$$\boldsymbol{\Sigma} = cov(\boldsymbol{\mu} + \boldsymbol{\Lambda}\mathbf{f} + \boldsymbol{\epsilon}) = cov(\boldsymbol{\Lambda}\mathbf{f}) + cov(\boldsymbol{\epsilon}) = \boldsymbol{\Lambda}cov(\mathbf{f})\boldsymbol{\Lambda}^T + \boldsymbol{\Psi} = \boldsymbol{\Lambda}\boldsymbol{\Lambda}^T + \boldsymbol{\Psi}. \tag{4}$$

An interesting characteristic of the loading matrix $\boldsymbol{\Lambda}$ is that it can be multiplied by an orthogonal matrix and still be able to represent the covariance among factors and original variables. Since any orthogonal matrix $\mathbf{Q}$ multiplied by its transpose leads to the identity matrix, the basic model for factor analysis in (2) can be written as

$$\mathbf{y} = \boldsymbol{\mu} + \boldsymbol{\Lambda}\mathbf{Q}\mathbf{Q}^T\mathbf{f} + \boldsymbol{\epsilon} = \boldsymbol{\mu} + \boldsymbol{\Lambda}^*\mathbf{f}^* + \boldsymbol{\epsilon},$$

where $\boldsymbol{\Lambda}^* = \boldsymbol{\Lambda}\mathbf{Q}$ and $\mathbf{f}^* = \mathbf{Q}^T\mathbf{f}$. If $\boldsymbol{\Sigma}$ in (4) is expressed in terms of $\boldsymbol{\Lambda}^*$, we have

$$\boldsymbol{\Sigma} = \boldsymbol{\Lambda}^*\boldsymbol{\Lambda}^{*T} + \boldsymbol{\Psi} = \boldsymbol{\Lambda}\mathbf{Q}(\boldsymbol{\Lambda}\mathbf{Q})^T + \boldsymbol{\Psi} = \boldsymbol{\Lambda}\mathbf{Q}\mathbf{Q}^T\boldsymbol{\Lambda}^T + \boldsymbol{\Psi} = \boldsymbol{\Lambda}\boldsymbol{\Lambda}^T + \boldsymbol{\Psi}, \tag{5}$$

showing that the original loading matrix $\boldsymbol{\Lambda}$ and the rotated matrix $\boldsymbol{\Lambda}^*$ yield the same representation of $\boldsymbol{\Sigma}$. The rotation of loadings plays an important role in factor interpretation, as it is possible to obtain a rotated matrix that assigns a few high loadings for each variable, keeping the other loadings small. If such matrix is obtained, each variable will be related to a single factor (or at least to a few ones), which can potentially be given a morphological interpretation.

2.3   Analysis of effect size

The effect size expression shown in (1) can be formulated in the factor domain, where for each point x_i, $y_i = J(x_i)$. In this way, the comparison between two populations can be performed based exclusively on the reduced set of factor values (*scores*) which completely represent each subject in the new basis. From the factor analysis model in (2) and the definition of variance in (3), we have that

$$e(x_i) = [\mu_1(y_i) - \mu_2(y_i)]/\sqrt{\sigma^2(y_i)}$$

$$= [\frac{1}{n1}\sum_{k=1}^{n1}(\sum_{j=1}^{m}\lambda_{ij}f_{jk} + \epsilon_{ik} + \mu(y_i)) - \frac{1}{n2}\sum_{k=1}^{n2}(\sum_{j=1}^{m}\lambda_{ij}f_{jk} + \epsilon_{ik} + \mu(y_i))]/\sqrt{\sigma^2(y_i)}$$

$$= [\sum_{j=1}^{m}\lambda_{ij}(\mu_1(f_j) - \mu_2(f_j)) + \mu_1(\epsilon_i) - \mu_2(\epsilon_i)]/(\sum_{j=1}^{m}\lambda_{ij}^2 + \psi_i)^{1/2},$$

where $\mu_1(y_i)$ and $\mu_2(y_i)$ are the mean Jacobian determinant values for the two populations; $\mu(y_i)$ and $\sigma^2(y_i)$ are the mean and variance for populations 1 and 2 combined; $n1$ and $n2$ are the respective number of subjects in each sample; m is the number of factors; λ_{ij} is the loading for variable i and factor j; f_{jk} is the j-th factor score of subject k; $\mu_p(f_j)$ is the mean value of factor j in the population p; $\mu_p(\epsilon_i)$ is the mean value of the error term i; and ψ_i the associated variance.

2.4   Implementation

In factor analysis, it is necessary to first define the number of factors to be considered. We present next an iterative algorithm that determines the number of factors based exclusively on the characteristics of the data set, instead of subjective considerations. The first step in the process is the computation of the covariance matrix Σ. Since the purpose of factor analysis is to represent the covariance among variables, the expression for Σ presented in (5) is simplified to $\Sigma = \Lambda\Lambda^T$, as Ψ is diagonal and does not affect the covariance values. Σ is then decomposed into

$$\Sigma = L\Theta L^T = (L\Theta^{1/2})(L\Theta^{1/2})^T,$$

where $\Theta^{1/2} = diag(\sqrt{\theta_1}, \ldots, \sqrt{\theta_p})$ is the diagonal matrix with the square root of the eigenvalues of Σ and L is the matrix of the corresponding eigenvectors. The loading matrix can thus be estimated based on the sample covariance matrix as $\Lambda = L\Theta^{1/2}$. The number of factors (number of columns in Λ) can be initialized to the number of eigenvalues greater then 1, since they account for the variance in at least one variable.

The computed loading matrix is then rotated so that each variable will exhibit high loading for only a few factors. This can be achieved by finding a sequence of rotations that maximizes the variance of the squared loadings in each column of Λ (*varimax* algorithm) [6]. The resultant loading values represent the correlation between variables and factors. The following algorithm reduces the initial number of factors by discarding factors which do not have high correlation with at least two variables. Since the absolute value for correlation ranges from 0 to 1, we consider factors to be informative when they have loadings with absolute value greater or equal to 0.5. Convergence is achieved when the number of factor m_t at iteration t equals the number of factors m_{t-1} computed in the previous iteration. The algorithm is summarized below:

Begin
    Compute sample covariance matrix Σ;
    Decompose Σ into its eigenvectors $\mathbf{L}$ and eigenvalues Θ;
    Set initial number of factors m_t to the number of eigenvalues
        with value greater then 1;
    Repeat until $m_t = m_{t-1}$
        $m_{t-1} \leftarrow m_t$;
        Estimate loadings as $\Lambda = \mathbf{L}\Theta^{1/2}$;
        Rotate loadings based on varimax *algorithm;*
        $m_t \leftarrow 0$;
        For $j \leftarrow 1$ to m_{t-1} do
            nvar $\leftarrow 0$;
            For $i \leftarrow 1$ to p do if $\lambda_{ij} \geq 0.5$ then nvar $\leftarrow$ nvar $+ 1$;
            If nvar > 1 then $m_t \leftarrow m_t + 1$;
End

3   Experimental Results

The set of MRI images used in the study is composed of 12 male and 16 female normal controls recruited as part of an ongoing study on schizofrenia being conducted at the Mental Health Clinical Research Center of the University of Pennsylvania. The subjects are right-handed with average age of 27 years (σ=5.8) for the male group and 28 years (σ=9.4) for the female. The images were acquired on a GE 1.5 Tesla instrument, using a spoiled GRASS pulse sequence optimized for high resolution, near isotropic volumes (flip angle = 35°, TR = 35 ms, TE = 6 ms, field of view = 24 cm, 0.9375×0.9375 mm^2 in-plane resolution, 1.0 mm slice thickness, no gap). The images were obtained in the axial plane and the midsagittal slice extracted and reformatted into 256×256 8-bit images (Fig. 1).

The subject images were rigidly registered to a female template by identifying 3 pairs of corresponding points and applying least-square optimization. The callosa were segmented using the K-means clustering algorithm and extracted by manual delineation. Local registration was performed by elastically matching the template to each globally aligned subject callosum. The resulting displacement fields were used to compute the determinant Jacobian values to which factor analysis was applied.

Fig. 2 shows the identified factors. The algorithm took 5 iterations to converge from 27 to 18 factors which were highly correlated with at least 2 variables. The

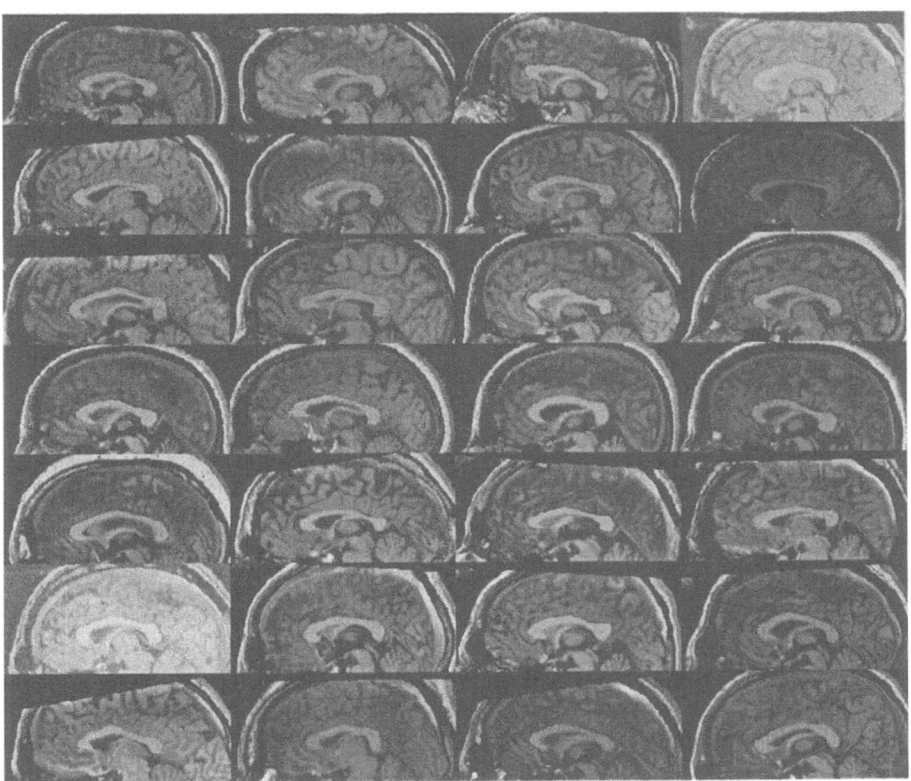

Fig. 1. Female (top) and male (bottom) subjects.

images show the absolute loading values that are greater than 0.5, for each informative factor. The gray levels are proportional to the absolute correlation, where pure white corresponds to complete correlation and the gray intensity shown in the background corresponds to a value of 0.5. These results can be compared with the findings of Gee *et al.* [4], who examined the same data set by computing the effect size between female and male populations. The comparison of Fig. 2 with Fig. 3 reveals an interesting relationship between the factors and the areas in which female and male morphology differ. The second factor shown in Fig. 2 coincides with the splenium and is is related to the major gender-related difference in the callosal anatomy, that has been observed in previous work [3, 8]. The inferior portion of the splenium can be divided into 2 parts: the right half does not seem to discriminate the two populations, as can be seen in Fig. 3b, whereas the left region is actually larger in the female group. These two regions are clearly separated into two factors (factors 14 and 11, respectively) as can be seen in Fig. 2. Other callosal parts that contribute to shape difference between females and males are indicated by factors 5, 9 and 15. Factor 15 is of particular interest, since it appears isolated in the right-most portion of the splenium (Fig. 3a), representing a region where the effect size is greater than 0.75.

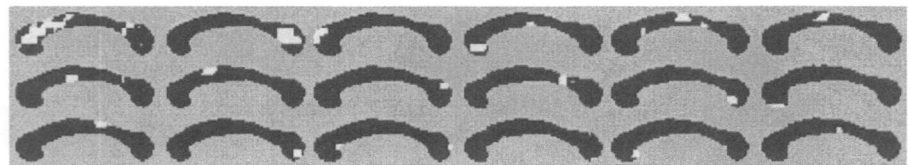

Fig. 2. Factor analysis of callosal morphology. For each factor, voxels that are highly correlated are highlighted in white. Factors are numbered from 1 to 18, left to right and top to bottom.

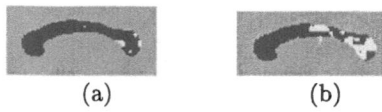

(a)   (b)

Fig. 3. Effect size analysis of callosal morphology. Voxels are highlighted where the effect size for area differences (female − male) are greater than 0.75 (a) and 0.5 (b).

4   Conclusion

A novel approach to morphometry was presented, in which the relationship among anatomic substructures are explored. The method is based on the factorial analytic model, where the covariance among variables is represented in a new basis of lower dimension. This enables more parsimonious descriptions and allows exploratory analysis of correlations which may reveal relationships between regions of interest that have not yet been observed. Factors can be visually identified as regions that embed strong correlation. The issue of determining the number of factors can be related to the desired degree of detailing in the analysis — fewer factors are expected to encompass greater regions with coarse correlation, whereas larger factor sets may represent smaller regions with stronger correlation. An algorithm was presented, which iteratively reduces the number of factors based on their contribution to the covariance representation of variable clusters. The ability of factor analysis to explore the relationship between parts of structures is a powerful tool for morphometry and a vast field for future work.

References

1. R. Bajcsy and S. Kovačič. Multiresolution elastic matching. *Computer Vision, Graphics and Image Processing*, 46:1–21, 1989.
2. T. Cootes, C. Taylor, D. Cooper, and J. Graham. Active shape models: Their training and applications. In *Computer Vision and Image Understanding*, pp. 38–59, 1995.
3. C. Davatzikos, M. Vaillant, S. Resnick, J. Prince, S. Letovsky, and R. Bryan. A computerized approach for morphological analysis of the corpus callosum. *Journal of Computer Assisted Tomography*, 20(1):88–97, 1996.

4. J. C. Gee, B. Fabella, S. Fernandes, B. Turetsky, R. C. Gur, and R. E. Gur. New experimental results in atlas-based brain morphometry. In *Proceedings of the SPIE Medical Imaging 1999: Image Processing*, San Diego, 1999. Bellingham.

5. J. C. Gee and D. R. Haynor. Numerical methods for high-dimensional warps. In A. Toga, editor, *Brain Warping*. Academic Press, San Diego, 1999.

6. H. Harman. *Modern Factor Analysis*. University of Chicago Press, 1976.

7. L. Le Briquer and J. C. Gee. Design of a statistical model of brain shape. In *XV International Conference on Information Processing in Medical Imaging*, pp. 477–482, 1997.

8. A. Machado and J. C. Gee. Atlas warping for brain morphometry. In *Proceedings of the SPIE Medical Imaging 1998: Image Processing*, Bellingham, pp. 642-651, 1998.

9. L. Marcus. Traditional morphometrics. In *Proceedings of the Michigan Morphometrics Workshop*, pp. 77–122. The University of Michigan Museum of Zoology, 1990.

10. A. Rencher. *Methods of Multivariate Analysis*. John Wiley & Sons, 1995.

11. R. Reyment and K. Jöreskog. *Applied Factor Analysis in the Natural Sciences*. Cambridge University Press, 1996.

Potential Usefulness of Curvature Based Description for Differential Diagnosis of Pulmonary Nodules

Y. Kawata[1], N. Niki[1] H. Ohmatsu[2], M.Kusumoto[3], R.Kakinuma[2], K.Mori[4],
K.Eguchi[5], M. Kaneko[3], N. Moriyama[3]

[1] Department of Optical Science, Tokushima University, Japan
[2] National Cancer Center Hospital East, Japan
[3] National Cancer Center Hospital,Japan
[4] Tochigi Cancer Center,Japan
[5] National Shikoku Cancer Center Hospital, Japan

Abstract. This paper examines the problem of obtaining a representation of the three-dimensional(3-D) pulmonary nodule images, which is a key problem in discriminating benign and malignant nodules for differential diagnosis of the lung cancer using thin-section CT images. A curvature based approach is developed with the aim of characterizing internal intensity structures of benign and malignant nodules. This approach makes use of curvature indexes to represent locally each voxel in a three-dimensional (3-D) pulmonary nodule image. From the distribution of curvature indexes and CT value over the 3-D pulmonary nodule image a set of histogram features is computed for global characterization of benign and malignant nodules. Linear discriminant analysis is used for classification and leave-one-out method is used to evaluate the classification accuracy. Compared with the performance of experienced physicians the potential usefulness of the curvature based features in the computer-aided differential diagnosis is demonstrated by using receiver operating characteristic (ROC) curves as the performance measure.

1 Introduction

Recently the detection rate of small peripheral pulmonary nodules has increased due to advances in imaging technology such as helical CT scanner [1]. For small nodules, the differential diagnosis by means of transbronchial or percutaneous biopsies can be difficult. There has been a considerable amount of interest in the use of thin-section CT images to observe small pulmonary nodules for differential diagnosis without invasive operation [1, 2]. In assessing the malignant potential of small pulmonary nodules in thin-section CT images, it is important to examine the condition of nodule interface, the nodule internal intensity, and the relationships between nodules and surrounding structures such as vessels, bronchi, and spiculation [1, 2]. Several techniques have been developed to quantify the pulmonary nodules. Nodule density analysis from CT value was employed in early investigations[3, 4]. The pattern classification approach incorporating multiple features, including measures of density, density distribution, and texture, was proposed to classify suspicious areas into malignant and benign lesions using slice images[5]. To quantify the relationships between nodules and surrounding structures the 3-D concentration index was derived [7] and classification approach between pulmonary artery and vein was proposed [6]. To analyze nodule surfaces, curvatures were introduced [8, 9] and fractal features were utilized [10].

In medical image analysis, several approaches have been investigated to represent local intensity structure directly computing the geometrical characteristics from gray-level 3-D medical images[16–18]. We have been investigating to analyze internal intensity structure of pulmonary by using curvature indexes and CT values [11]. The curvature indexes consist of the shape index and the curvedness [14]. In this paper we present histogram features of curvature indexes and CT values to characterize the internal intensity structure for he sake of classifying benign and malignant pulmonary nodules. Compared with the performance of experienced physicians the potential usefulness of the curvature based features in the computer-aided differential diagnosis is demonstrated by using a receiver operating characteristic (ROC) curves [22] as the performance measure.

2   Nodule Segmentation

The 3-D chest images used in this paper are reconstructed from thin section CT images obtained by the helical CT scanner (Toshiba TCT900S Superhelix). The thin-section CT images are measured under the following conditions; beam width: 2mm, table speed: 2mm/sec, tube voltage: 120kV, tube current :200mA and 250mA. For the scan duration, patients held their breath at full inspiration. Per patient, about 60 slices through the pulmonary nodule center at 1mm intervals are obtained. The range of pixel size in each square slice of 512 pixels is between 0.3x0.3 mm^2 and 0.4x0.4 mm^2, and the slice contains an extended region of the lung area. The 3-D chest image is reconstructed from the thin section CT images by a linear interpolation technique to make each voxel isotropic. Our segmentation algorithm is described in previous publication[8]. Briefly, the segmentation of the 3-D nodule image consists of three steps; 1) extraction of lung area, 2) region of interest(ROI) selection including the nodule region, 3) nodule segmentation based on the geometric approach. This lung area extraction step plays an essential role when part of a nodule in the peripheral lung area touches the chest wall [12]. The ROI including the nodule is selected interactively. The 3-D deformable surface model proposed by Casselles [13] is utilized.

3   Curvature based representation

Each voxel in the region of interest(ROI) including the pulmonary nodule is locally represented by a vector description which relies on the CT value and two curvature indexes that decouples the shape attribute and the curvature magnitude. By assuming that each voxel in the ROI lies on the surface which has the normal corresponding to the 3-D gradient at the voxel, we compute directly the curvatures on each voxel from the first and second derivatives of the gray level image of the ROI. To compute the partial derivatives of the ROI images, the ROI images are blurred by convolving with a 3-D Gaussian function of width σ. Herein, the width σ is represented as a scale. At each voxel the principal curvatures $\kappa_1(x;\sigma)$ $(\kappa_1(x;\sigma) \geq \kappa_2(x;\sigma))$ are computed by using the approach poposed by Thirion and Gourdon [16].

The voxel x in the ROI image is locally described by curvature indexes and CT value. The curvature indexes consists of the shape index and the curvedness[14, 15]. The original shape index defined by Koenderink and van Doorn [14] gives a continuous distribution of surface types between -1 and 1. To introduce the shape spectral function of the object's surface patch, Dorai and Jain [15] have modified the original definition of the shape index so that the shape index maps the surface types on the interval between 0 and 1. The definition of shape index used here is based on the modified definition [15] and the shape index with scale σ at the voxel x is given by

$$S_I(x;\sigma) = \frac{1}{2} + \frac{1}{\pi} arctan \frac{\kappa_1(x;\sigma) + \kappa_2(x;\sigma)}{\kappa_1(x;\sigma) - \kappa_2(x;\sigma)}. \tag{1}$$

The curvedness $R(x;\sigma)$ [14] is given by

$$R(x;\sigma) = \sqrt{\frac{\kappa_1(x;\sigma)^2 + \kappa_2(x;\sigma)^2}{2}}. \tag{2}$$

The curvedness quantifies how highly curved a surface is, and is inversely proportional to the size of the object.

4   Feature extraction and classification

In order to characterize globally the pulmonary nodule images through the local description, we use the shape spectrum which is originally proposed for object recognition in a range image by Dorai and Jain[15]. The shape spectrum measures the amount of the voxel which has a particular shape index value to characterize the 3-D pulmonary nodule image. The shape spectrum with scale σ is given by

$$H(h;\sigma) = \frac{1}{V} \int\int\int_O \delta\left(S_I(x;\sigma) - h\right) dO \tag{3}$$

where V is the total volume of the specified region O, dO is a small region around x, and δ is the Dirac delta function. In practice, a discrete definition of the shape spectrum is given by dividing the shape index range into B bins and counting the number of point falling in each bin k:

$$H\left(h = \frac{k}{B}; \sigma\right) = \frac{1}{N} \sum_{i=1}^{N} \chi_k \left(S_I(x_i; \sigma) - h\right) \qquad (4)$$

where x_i is a point on the object's surface, N is the total number of points on object's surface, and χ_k is the characteristic function of the kth bin:

$$\chi_k(x) = \begin{cases} 1 \ \frac{k-1}{B} \leq x < \frac{k}{B} \\ 0 \ otherwise. \end{cases} \qquad (5)$$

The objective in defining the shape spectrum is to measure the amount of the point which has a particular shape index value h. Thus, the shape spectrum is called the shape histogram [15]. For computational purposes, such as comparing spectra of different nodules, the shape histogram is normalized with respect to the volume of nodule. The normalized number of voxel falling in each bin represents the value of the shape histogram feature. The similar equations for the curvedness and CT value are obtained in the same manner. The domains of curvedness and CT value are specified $[0, C_{max}]$, $[I_{min}, I_{max}]$. A voxel in which the curvedness value is larger than C_{max} is considered as a voxel with curvedness value C_{max}. For the CT value the similar process is performed.

The linear discriminant analysis [19] is used to classify benign and malignant nodules based on the extracted features. A forward stepwise feature selection procedure [21] with the minimization of Wilks'lambda is used as an optimization criterion to select effective predictor variables. A leave-one-out method [20] is adapted to evaluate classification accuracy. In this method, one nodule image is left out from the classifier design group and a linear discriminant function is formed using the design group. The discriminant score is computed for the left-out case by using the resulting liner discriminant function. This process cycles through the data set until every nodule image is used. The discriminant scores are analyzed using receiver operating characteristic (ROC) method [22]. The discriminant scores of the malignant and benign nodules are used as the decision variable in the LABROC1 program which fit the ROC curve based on maximum likelihood estimation.

5   Results and Discussion

In this section, we present classification results with a set of histogram features derived from the curvature based representation of pulmonary nodules. The thin-section CT images of peripheral pulmonary nodules used in this study were provided by the National Cancer Center Hospital East. The data set included 128 nodule images from 128 patients. Of the 128 cases, 95 contained malignant nodules and 33 contained benign nodules. Lesions that showed no change or decreased in size over a 2-year period were considered benign. Other lesions were cytologically or histologically diagnosed. The performance of a set of

Table I. Classification results of histogram features based on CT values.

Feature space	HCT1	HCT2	HCT3
Num. of bins	25	50	100
Num. of features	2	3	3
Error rate (%)	36.7	35.2	28.9

Table II. Classification results of histogram features based on curvedness.

Feature space	HCV1	HCV2	HCV3
Num. of bins	25	50	100
Num. of features	1	1	3
Error rate (%)	38.3	36.7	26.2

Table III. Classification results of histogram features based on shape index.

Feature space	HSH1	HSH2	HSH3
Num. of bins	25	50	100
Num. of features	1	1	2
Error rate (%)	22.7	22.7	20.3

Table IV. Classification results for selected combination of feature spaces

Combined feature spaces	Num. of features	Error rate (%)
HCT3 HCV3 HSH3	12	12.5
HCT3 HSH3	7	13.3
HCV3 HSH3	4	15.6
HCT3 HCV3	6	26.6

histogram features was evaluated using our dataset. Table I, II, and III present the classification results for the histogram features based on CT value, curvedness, and shape index, respectively. In each table the histogram feature space name, the number of bins, error rate, and the number of features selected are presented. It is necessary to select appropriate scale for the effective description of nodules internal structure [23]. We selected a scale which provided the high classification rate over the specified discrete scales and assigned the value 2 to the scale in this study.

The benign/malignant classification results for the selected combinations of feature spaces are given in Tables IV. The results for only some of the interesting combinations tried were reported. The classification result of shape histogram features HSH3 achieved better accuracy than that of CT value and curvedness histogram features. For the selected combinations of feature spaces the combined feature spaces HCT3, HCV3, and HSH3 gave the best performance. The selected features provide an information which bins contribute to discriminate malignant cases from benign cases.

In order to comparison between physicians and computerized classification, the probability of malignancy of each pulmonary nodule in thin-section CT images which were printed on films was ranked by 11 physicians on a scale of

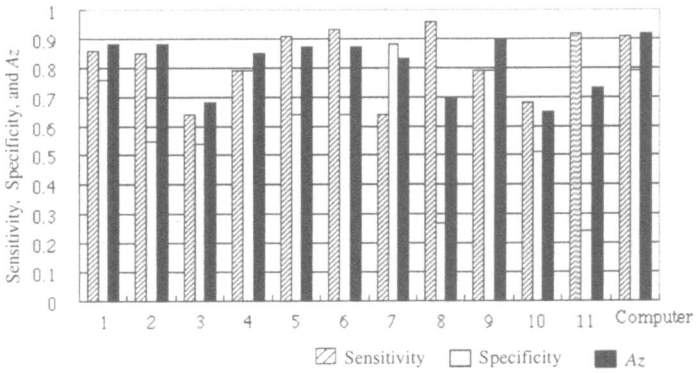

Fig. 1. Sensitivity, specificity, and Az value of each physician and the computerized classification with the combined feature space HCT3, HCV3, and HSH3.

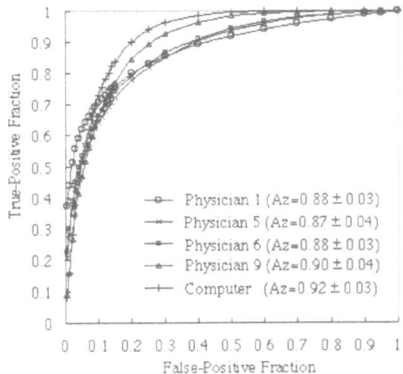

Fig. 2. ROC curves of four experienced physician and the computerized classification with the combined feature space of HCT3, HCV3, and HSH3.

1 to 10, where a ranking of 1 corresponded to the nodules with the most benign cases. Based on these ranking, sensitivity, specificity, and A_z value, which denotes area under the ROC curve, were computed. Fig.1 compares the performance of the attending 11 physicians and computerized classification with the combined features space of HCT3, HCV3, and HSH3. Physicians 1, 5, 6, and 9 have 15, 17, 13, 12 years of experience in Chest radiology. The computerized classification performance is close to that of the experienced physicians. Fig.2 shows the ROC curves obtained by four experienced physicians and the computerized classification with the combined features space of HCT3, HCV3, and HSH3. The ROC curves and A_z values do not necessarily reflect the accuracy expected to be obtained under clinical conditions. Additionally, since there are several types of benign and malignant nodules a few feature parameters to characterize pulmonary nodule images are not enough to discriminate overall benign and malignant cases automatically. Still, these results are promising that the features

derived from the curvature based representation quantify one of the important clues for the differential diagnosis of the small pulmonary nodule images.

6 Conclusions

An important problem in the analysis of medical image data is the representation and characterization of normal and pathology variation in anatomical shape. In this paper, focusing on the small pulmonary nodule images, we have developed a curvature based representation of internal intensity structure of pulmonary nodules in thin-section CT images. The results of our classification study indicate that a set of histogram features derived from the curvature based representation are useful in differencing the benign and malignant pulmonary nodules. Although these results were obtained with a relatively small data set, they demonstrate the potential of using CAD techniques to analyze pulmonary nodules and to assist physicians in making diagnostic decisions. A simple prototype has been developed with good results, and ongoing work deals with characterizing the relationship with the surrounding structure of pulmonary nodules. Further studies need to be performed with a lager database to investigate the generalizability of our approach.

Acknowledgments

Authors are grateful to physicians cooperating to the reading test. The authors would like to thank Prof. Charles E. Mets for the LABROC1 program.

References

1. M. Kaneko, K. Eguchi, H. Ohmatsu, R. Kakinuma,T. Naruke, K. Suemasu, N. Moriyama, "Peripheral lung cancer: Screening and detection with low-dose spiral CT versus radiography," *Radiology*, vol.201, pp.798-802, 1996.
2. K. Mori, Y. Saitou, K. Tominaga, K. Yokoi, N. Miyazawa, A. Okuyama, M. Sasagawa, "Small nodular lesions in the lung periphery: New approach to diagnosis with CT," *Radiology*, vol.177, pp.843-849, 1990.
3. S. S. Siegelman, E. A. Zerhouni, F. P. Leo, N. F. Khouri, F. P. Stitik, "CT of the solitary pulmonary nodule," *AJR*, vol.135, pp.1-13, 1980.
4. A. V. Proto and S. R. Thomas, "Pulmonary nodules studied by computed tomography," *Radiology*, vol.156, pp.149-153, 1985.
5. M. F. McNitt-Gray, E. M. Hart, J. Goldin, C. W. Yao, and D. R. Aberle, "A pattern classification approach to characterizing solitary pulmonary nodules imaged on high resolution computed tomography," *Proc. SPIE*, vol.2710, pp.1024-1034, 1996.
6. T. Tozaki, Y. Kawata, N. Niki, H. Ohmatsu, K. Eguchi, N. Moriyama, "Pulmonary organs analysis for differential diagnosis based on thoracic thin-section CT images," *IEEE Trans. Nuclear Science*, vol.45, pp.3075-3082, 1998.
7. Y. Hirano, Y. Mekada, J. Hasegawa, J. Toriwaki, H. Ohmatsu, and K. Eguchi, "Quantification of vessels convergence in three-dimensional chest X-ray CT images with three-dimensional concentration index," *Medical Imaging Tchnology*, vol.15, pp.228-235, 1997.

8. Y.Kawata, N.Niki, H.Ohmatsu, R.Kakinuma, K.Eguchi,¡¡M.Kaneko,¡¡N.Moriyama, "Quantitative surface characterization pulmonary nodules based on thin-section CT images" *IEEE Trans. Nuclear Science*, vol. 45, pp.2132-2138, 1998.

9. H. Kitaoka, R. Takaki, K. Itho, H. Kobatake, H. Ohmatsu, N. Moriyama, and K. Eguchi, "Shape analysis of pulmonary nodules in 3D-CT images with a new method of curvature estimation," *Proc. Computer Assisted Radiology and Surgery (CAR'98)*, H.U.Lemke, M.W.Vannier, and K.Inamura, Eds., pp.51-56, 1998.

10. J. Bejer, T. Liebig, R. C. Bittner, P. Wust, E. Fleck, R. Felix, "Surface analysis of pulmonary lesions using fractal features," *Proc. Computer Assisted Radiology and Surgery (CAR'97)*, H.U.Lemke, M.W.Vannier, and K.Inamura, Eds., pp.228-233, 1997.

11. Y. Kawata, N. Niki, H. Ohmatsu, R. Kakinuma, K. Mori, K. Eguchi, M. Kaneko, N.Moriyama, "Curvature base analysis of internal structure of pulmonary nodules using thin-section CT images" *Proc. IEEE Int. Conf. Image Processing*, vol.III, pp.851-855, 1998.

12. J. Hasegawa, K. Mori, J. Toriwaki, H. Anno, K. Katada, "Automated extraction of lung cancer lesions from multi-slice chest CT images by using tree-dimensional image processing," *IEICE Trans.*, vol.J76-D-II, pp.1587-1594, 1993.

13. V. Caselles, R. Kimmel, G. Sapiro, and C. Sbert, "Minimal surfaces: A three-dimensional segmentation approach," Technion Technical Report, 973, Israel, 1995.

14. J. J. Koenderink and A. J. Van Doorn, "Surface shape and curvature scales," *Image and Vision Computing*, vol.10, pp.557-565,1992.

15. C. Dorai and A. K. Jain, "COSMOS-A Representation scheme for 3D free-form objects," *IEEE Trans. Pattern Anal. Machine Intell.*, vol.19, pp.1115-1130,1997.

16. J. -P. Thirion and A. Gourdon, "Computing the differential characteristics of isointensity surfaces," *Comput. Vision and Image Understanding*, vol.61, pp.190-202, 1995.

17. S. Aylward, S. Pizer, E. Bullitt, D. Eberly, "Intensity ridge and widths for tubular object segmentation and description," *Proc. Mathematical Methods in Biomedical Image Analysis*, pp.131-138, 1996.

18. Y. Sato, S. Nakajima, H. Atsumi, T. Koller, G. Gerig, S. Yoshida, and R. Kikinis "Three-dimensional multi-scale line filter for segmentation and visualization of curvilinear structures in medical images," *Medical Image Analysis,*, vol.2, pp.143-163, 1998.

19. R.O. Duda and P.E. Hart "Pattern classification and scene analysis" *John Wiley & Sons*, 1973.

20. K. Fukunaga, "Introduction to statistical pattern recognition," *Academic Press, Inc., Second Edition*, 1990.

21. M.C. Costanza and A.A. Afifi, "Comparison of stopping rules in forward step wise discriminant analysis," J. of the American Statistical Association,vol.74, pp.777-785,1979.

22. C.E. Metz "ROC methodology in radiologic imaging," *Investigative Radiology*, vol.21, pp.720-733, 1986.

23. T.Lindeberg, "Detecting salient blob-like image structures and their scales with a scale-space primal sketch: A method for focus-of-attention," *Int. J. Computer Vision*, vol.11, pp.283-318, 1993.

Pulmonary Organs Analysis Method and Its Evaluation Based on Thoracic Thin-Section CT Images

Tetsuya Tozaki[1], Akira Tanaka[2], Yoshiki Kawata[2], Noboru Niki[2],
Hironobu Ohmatsu[3], Ryutaro Kakinuma[3], Kenji Eguchi[4],
Masahiro Kaneko[5], and Noriyuki Moriyama[5]

[1] Dept. of Electronic Eng., Kobe City College of Tech.,
8-3 Gakuen-higashi-machi, Nishiku, Kobe 651-2194, JAPAN
tozaki@kobe-kosen.ac.jp
[2] Dept. of Optical Science, Univ. of Tokushima,
2-1 Minami-josanjima-cho, Tokushima 770-8560, JAPAN
{atanaka,niki,kawata}@opt.tokushima-u.ac.jp
[3] National Cancer Center Hospital East,
[4] National Shikoku Cancer Center Hospital,
[5] National Cancer Center Hospital,

Abstract. To diagnose the lung cancer as to determine if it has malignant or benign nature, it is important to understand the spatial relationship among the abnormal nodule and other pulmonary organs. But the lung field has very complicated structure, so it is difficult to understand the connectivity of the pulmonary organs using thin-section CT images. This method consists of two parts. The first is the classification of the pulmonary structure based on the anatomical information. The second is the quantitative analysis that is then applicable to differential diagnosis, such as differentiation of malignant or benign abnormal tissue.

1 Introduction

The lung area has very complicated structure, so it is difficult to understand the spatial relationships among the pulmonary organs and the abnormal nodules. Because of this, a new Computer Assisted Diagnosis system for lung cancer becomes necessary [1].

In this paper, we describe a 3D analysis method of the lung based on thin-section CT images, and we aim to support the differential diagnosis of lung cancer. Our pulmonary organs analysis method consists of four parts. The first is the extraction of the regions of interest (ROI) based on the segmentation of the lung field. The second is the division of ROI into the bronchus and the blood vessels, and the third is the identification of the pulmonary artery and the pulmonary vein using anatomical information and 3D image processing technology [2, 3]. The last is a quantitative analysis of the spatial relationships among the abnormal nodules and other pulmonary organs to support the differential diagnosis of lung cancer, such as differentiation of malignant or benign nodules.

2 Extraction of the Bronchus, the Pulmonary Artery, and the Pulmonary Vein

2.1 Bias Correction

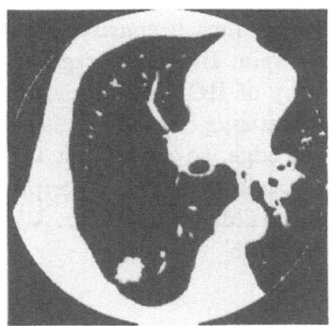
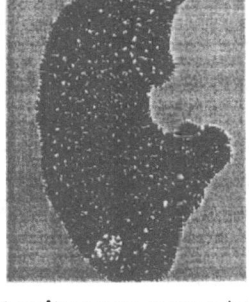

(a) thin-section CT image   (b) Intensity curve segmentation

Fig. 1. Thin-section CT image and the result of intensity curve segmentation. (a) shows a thin-section CT image, (b) shows a result of intensity curve segmentation against (a).

Fig.1 (a) shows a thin-section CT image at measurement condition, tube voltage, 150kV, tube current 200mA, beam width 2mm, table speed 2mm/s. Thin-section CT images have a large smooth bias component caused by various artifacts or diseases. To get high quality ROI images, we must remove this bias component. The correction method of the bias component is based on the segmentation of the lung field using Gaussian curvature and mean curvature. Calculation of Gaussian curvature K and mean curvature H are expressed in Eqs.(1) and (2) [4, 5].

$$K = \frac{1}{2h^2}(f_{xx}f_{yy} + f_{xy}f_{yx}) \tag{1}$$

$$H = \frac{1}{2h^{\frac{3}{2}}}(f_{xx} - 2f_x f_{xy} f_y + f_{xx}f_y{}^2 + f_{yy} + f_x{}^2 f_{yy}) \tag{2}$$

where f is the smoothed image by Gaussian filter, $h = 1.0 + f_x{}^2 + f_y{}^2$ and subscripts denote partial differentiation at the (x, y).

We segment the lung field into four regions based on the combination of the sign of two curvature. Each region express features such as pit surface ($K > 0$ and $H > 0$), peak surface ($K > 0$ and $H < 0$), saddle ridge ($K < 0$ and $H < 0$), saddle valley ($K < 0$ and $H > 0$) [6]. Fig.1 (b) shows a result of the intensity curve segmentation. In this figure, white regions are peak surface, green regions are pit surface, blue regions are saddle ridge, and red regions are saddle valley. We separate the segmented image into background regions and the ROI. Background regions are expressed by pit surfaces because of beam hardening effect, and ROI are expressed by peak surface, saddle ridge, and saddle valley. We approximate the bias component with a bicubic spline function, and the control points are on pit surface region. Then we subtract these estimated bias field from the original thin-section CT images.

2.2   Extraction of ROI

Peak surface, saddle ridge, and saddle valley are mostly consisted of the bronchus, the pulmonary artery, and the pulmonary vein. But these regions also include background of lung field near the boundary of ROI. To extract only ROI, we apply thresholding technique and edge emphasizing to bias corrected image. Core of ROI have relatively high CT value than edge, so we extract these region by thresholding technique. We use edge emphasizing to extract peripheral ROI. As the edge emphasizing filter, we apply Marr-Hildreth operator. We extract the edge of these regions by zero-crossing method [7].

2.3   Bronchus and Blood Vessels

The bronchus is described as a tree-like tube filled with air. CT values inside the tube are almost equal to the low CT values of air and CT values of the bronchus wall are as high as the blood vessels. The difference of CT values among the bronchus wall, the pulmonary artery, and the pulmonary vein is not distinctable. We present an algorithm to differentiate the bronchus based on the extraction of the air region inside the bronchus.

To get a high quality image of the bronchus and the blood vessels, we must extract the air regions inside the peripheral bronchus. We cannot, however, extract these air regions inside the peripheral bronchus by a simple thresholding algorithm because these parts have higher CT values than in the trunk bronchus. This is due to artifacts such as the partial volume effect. We extract the air region inside peripheral bronchus using the following procedures [8].

Step 1) Extraction of the initial air region based on threshold technique.

Step 2) Growth initial air region.

Step 3) Extraction of the air region inside the peripheral bronchus using intensity curve segmentation information.

In step 1), we use the extraction method described by K.Mori et al.. [9]. In Step 2), we emphasize the edge of air region using Laplacian Operator, and grow the initial air region obtained by Step 1) until it correspond to edge using region growing method morphologically. In Step 3), we use the intensity curve segmentation information to get the air region inside peripheral bronchus. On Thin-section CT images, the peripheral bronchus is expressed as a ring shape. In this case, inside the ring shape becomes an isolated small Pit Surface region through the intensity curve segmentation method that has smoothing process by small filter size. It is based on the fact that the inside of the peripheral bronchus has a pit feature in small region on the intensity curve field. We extract these pit Surface regions which connect to the air region obtained by Step 2) as the air regions inside peripheral bronchus.

2.4 Extraction of the Pulmonary Artery and the Pulmonary Vein

The pulmonary artery runs along the bronchus. The identification procedure of the pulmonary artery and the pulmonary vein is as follows [8].

Step 1) We obtain the initial blood vessels image at relatively high CT values from pulmonary blood vessels.

Step 2) We obtain centerline structures of the initial blood vessels using a 3D thinning algorithm [10].

Step 3) We represent the centerline structures as the set of branches.

Step 4) We classify the branches of the initial blood vessels into two classes based on the running direction of the branches against the bronchus.

Step 5) We identify blood vessel to the pulmonary artery and the pulmonary vein based on classified centerline structure using spatial connectivity of the blood vessels.

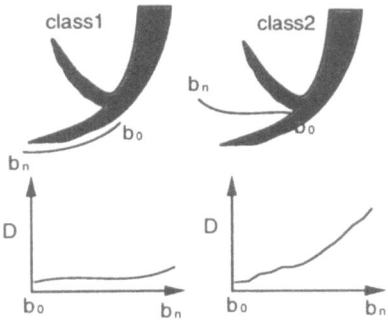

Fig. 2. Classification criterion

In Step 1), we extract the 3D main structure of blood vessels to keep the skeleton information of pulmonary blood vessels, and remove contact parts among the peripheral pulmonary artery and the peripheral pulmonary vein.

In Step3), we remove small branches caused by the irregular shape of the blood vessels, and we represent the centerline structure as the set of branches after removing the branching points of centerline structures.

In Step 4), we calculate the relationship among blood vessels branches and bronchus, and we classify the blood vessel branches into two classes. To represent the relationship among blood vessels and bronchus, we use the graph pattern as shown in Fig.2. In this figure, horizontal axis shows the sequential voxel number from the edge of the interesting branches, and vertical axis shows the minimum spatial distance D_i from the interesting voxel to the bronchus. If this graph has little change of spatial distance D_i and the value of D_i is lower than T, this branch is classified as pulmonary artery, otherwise if the value of D_i increases or decreases with the change of the interesting point, this branch is classified as pulmonary vein. Based on these graph pattern, we classify blood vessels branches into pulmonary artery or pulmonary vein.

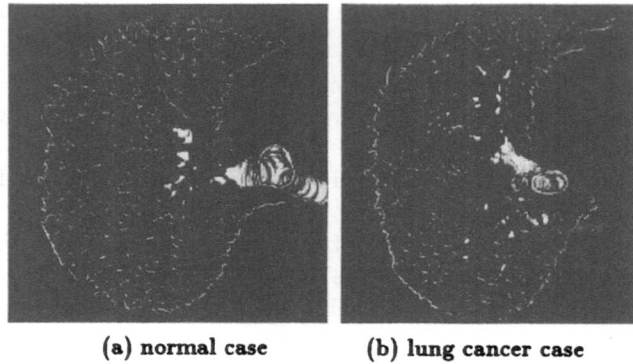

(a) normal case   (b) lung cancer case

Fig. 3. Classified lung organs

Fig.3(a) and (b) shows the whole pulmonary organs image consisted of the bronchus, the pulmonary artery, the pulmonary vein and the tumor. (a) shows the analysis result of normal lung, and (b) shows the lung cancer case. Red organ are the pulmonary artery, blue are the pulmonary vein, yellow are the bronchus, and green are the abnormal nodule extracted by interactive operation.

3   Quantitative Analysis

From the classified pulmonary organs images, we make quantitative analysis for differential diagnosis of lung cancer against follows items to support determination such as malignant or benign nature.

1) The number of connections among the pulmonary blood vessels and the abnormal nodule. 2) The direction of the blood vessels which connect to the abnormal nodule.

As the typical feature of malignant lung cancer, we can observe that the pulmonary blood vessels around the tumor are drawn in irregularly by the lung cancer tissue. We represent these malignant features using centerline of blood vessels obtained by 3D thinning algorithm. Understanding of the connection number is operated as follows. Firstly, we extract the abnormal nodule and the pulmonary blood vessels that connect to this abnormal nodule. Next, we apply a 3D thinning algorithm only to pulmonary vessels. Then we count the connection of the abnormal nodule and the centerline of the blood vessels each pulmonary artery and pulmonary vein.

The direction of the blood vessels that connect to the abnormal nodule is calculated as follows. Now the unit direction vector of the interesting blood vessels branch is $\hat{d}_P$ which is represented by the tangent direction at the connection point, and the unit direction vector from the connection point P to the center point of the abnormal nodule Q is $\hat{d}_Q$. Then we define the direction of the blood vessels that connect to the abnormal nodule as $V = \hat{d}_P \cdot \hat{d}_Q$ If V is larger than 0.9, we guess this branch are drawn in by the abnormal nodule irregularly.

Table1 (a) shows the result of the quantitative analysis against four malignant lung cancer cases, and (b) shows the result against four benign cases. Columns of each case show the connection number of the final pulmonary blood vessels. These columns show the complexity of state among these organs. A numerator shows the number of the blood vessels which head to the center of the abnormal nodule, a denominator shows the number of the blood vessels that connect to the abnormal nodule. "P.V." means the pulmonary vein connection. "P.A." means the pulmonary artery connection. We can understand there are obvious difference among malignant and benign cases. In malignant cases, the numbers of the blood vessels that head to center of the abnormal nodule are very large. And further, graph 1,2,3 understand there are more obvious difference among malignant and benign cases. Graph 1,2,3 show blood vessels connection in malignant cases is larger than that in benign cases, and show the ratio of the blood vessels which head to center of the abnormal nodule are very large.

Table 1. Application of the quantitative analysis.

(a) malignant cases

(b) benign cases

Cases	P.V.	P.A.	Total	ratio	Cases	P.V.	P.A.	Total	ratio
Case1	4/4	2/5	6/9	0.667	Case1	2/7	0/2	2/9	0.222
Case2	8/12	3/5	11/17	0.647	Case2	2/3	0/1	2/4	0.5
Case3	3/8	3/13	6/21	0.286	Case3	1/3	1/2	2/5	0.4
Case4	9/13	10/17	19/30	0.633	Case4	1/10	3/13	4/23	0.174

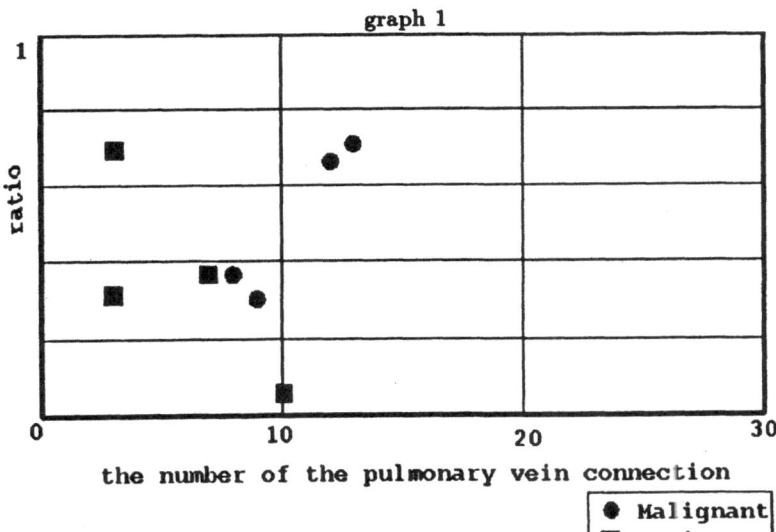

graph 1

the number of the pulmonary vein connection

● Malignant
■ Benign

graph 2

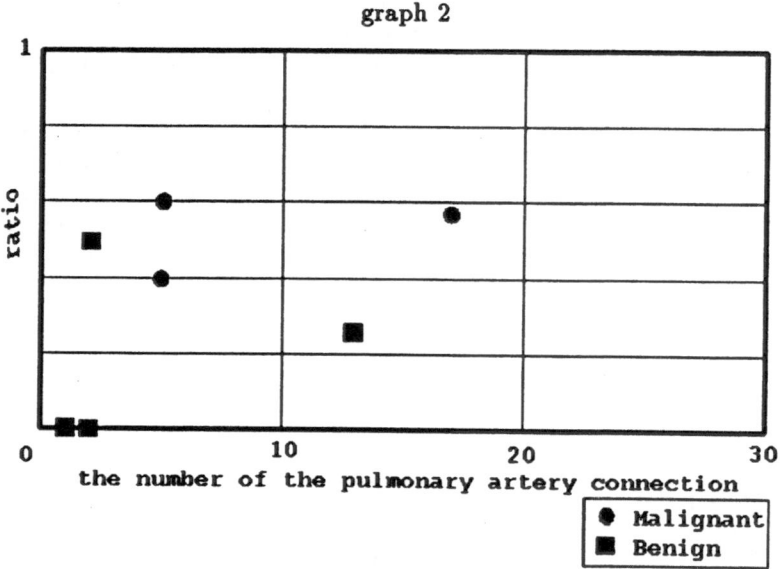

the number of the pulmonary artery connection

● Malignant
■ Benign

graph 3

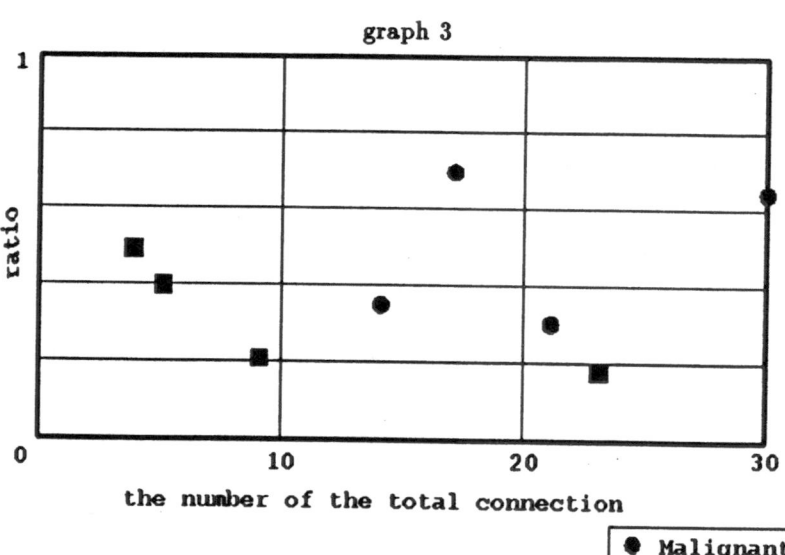

the number of the total connection

● Malignant
■ Benign

4 Conclusion

In this paper, we described a 3D image analysis method of the pulmonary organs structure based on thin-section CT images, and we applied this method to some normal lung and patient cases. By the segmentation of the lung filed using Gaussian curvature and mean curvature, we can extract peripheral ROI. Using anatomical informations of lung, we can classify the pulmonary organs to the bronchus, the pulmonary artery, and the pulmonary vein. We also applied these analysis results to a differential diagnosis of lung cancer. We could understand the spatial connectivity among the pulmonary organs and the abnormal nodules easily. A quantitative analysis of the relationship between the pulmonary organs and the abnormal nodules, can be expected to support differential diagnosis for a malignant or benign decision on the abnormal nodule. In future work, we will extract the bronchus, the pulmonary artery, and the pulmonary vein using more detailed anatomical information, and we will develop this image analysis method to support the differential diagnosis of lung cancer in the clinical medicine.

References

1. K. Kanazawa, M. Kubo, N. Niki, H.Satoh, H.Ohmatsu, K.Eguchi, N. Moriyama, "Computer Aided Screening System for Lung Cancer Based on Helical CT Images", proc. 4th VBC, Hamburg, vol.1131, pp.223-228, 1996.
2. T.Tozaki, Y.Kawata, N.Niki, H.Ohmatsu, K.Eguchi, N.Moriyama, "Three dimensional analysis of lung areas using thin slice CT images", SPIE Medical Imaging, Vol.2709, pp.2-11, 1996.
3. T. Tozaki, Y. Kawata, N. Niki, H.Ohmatsu, R.Kakinuma, K. Eguchi, N. Moriyama, "Pulmonary Organs Analysis for Differential Diagnosis Based on Thoracic Thin-section CT Images", IEEE Trans. on NUCLEAR SCIENCE, vol.45, pp.3075-3082, NO.6, 1998.
4. R.Deriche, "Recursively Implementing the Gaussian and Its Derivatives", In Proc. Second Int. Conf. On Image Processing, pp.263-267, 1992.
5. O. Monga, R. Lengagne, R. Deriche, "Crest lines extraction in volume 3D medical images: a multi-scale approach", INRIA RR2338, 1994.
6. Y.Kawata, N.Niki, T.Kumazaki, "Feature Extraction of Convex Surface on Blood Vessels Using Cone-Beam Images", IEEE International Conference on Image Processing, Vol.3, pp.315-318, 1996.
7. D. Marr, E. Hildreth, "Theory of edge detection", In Processing of the Royal Society of London, pp.187-217, 1980.
8. T.Tozaki, Y.Kawata, N.Niki, H.Ohmatsu, R.Kakinuma, K.Eguchi, M.Kaneko, N.Moriyama, "Pulmonary organs analysis method and its application to differential diagnosis based on thoracic Thin-section CT images", SPIE Medical Imaging, Vol.3338, pp.1459-1469. San Diego, 1998.
9. K.Mori, J.Hasegawa, J.Toriwaki, H.Anno, K.Katada, "Recognition of Bronchus in Three-Dimensional X-ray CT Images with Application to Virtualized Bronchoscopy System", proc. 13th ICPR, vol. III, Track C, pp528-532, Vienna, 1996.
10. N.Niki, Y.Kawata, T.Kumazaki, "3D Diagnostic Imaging of Blood Vessels Using an X-Ray Rotational Angiographic System", AAAI 1994 spring symposium, Stanford University, pp.169-172, 1994.

An Automatic Approach for 3-D Facial Shape Change Analysis by Combination of ASM and Morphometric Tools

Z. Mao and A. J. Naftel

Department of Physics, Astronomy and Mathematics
University of Central Lancashire, Preston PR1 2HE, UK

Abstract. This paper presents a new approach for automatic facial shape change analysis by combining a stereo-assisted active shape model (ASM) with morphometric tools. We firstly describe how to extend the 2-D ASM to 3-D space by stereo correspondence search and disparity map interpolation for automatic facial landmark extraction. Morphometric techniques such as generalized Procrustes analysis, principal component analysis and thin plate spline decomposition are then reviewed and applied to the quantitative analysis of shape changes in 2-D facial midline profiles and 3-D facial landmarks. The proposed method is validated both statistically and visually by characterizing bite-block induced shape changes in a heterogeneous sample of young orthodontic patients.

1 Introduction

Morphological changes in facial surface shape may occur as a result of growth processes, pathology or from soft tissue movements following corrective treatment. Techniques for three-dimensional analysis of morphological changes resulting from surgical correction have recently been proposed [1,2]. Among the existing non-landmark based shape analysis methods, the most successful approach applied to facial imaging is the use of surface curvature methods [3]. However, the calculation of surface curvature is unavoidably noise-sensitive and pre-processing techniques such as smoothing and local surface fitting must be carried out beforehand, which may remove surface detail. Recent advances in the rapidly maturing field of geometric morphometrics [4,5] offer an effective means for landmark-based shape analysis. Yet to date, morphometric tools have largely relied on expert knowledge for the manual detection of landmarks or curving outlines to segment anatomical regions of interest. In this paper, we present a new approach for automatic 3-D facial shape change analysis by combining 2-D active shape models (ASM) [6] with stereo disparity analysis for the automatic extraction of 3-D facial landmarks. These landmarks can then be subjected to morphometric analysis. The proposed method is applied to the shape analysis of group differences in a heterogeneous sample of young patients attending an orthodontic clinic. Anterior and lateral facial landmark shapes are analyzed using morphometric techniques with a view to characterising the differences in a geometrically and statistically meaningful way.

2   Materials

We collected frontal view facial stereo image pairs of 61 patients (aged 10 to 26 years; mean 16 years) attending a weekly orthodontic clinic at the Royal Preston Hospital. To test the efficacy of the proposed method, a deliberate gross change in the shape of the jaw of the patient was produced by means of a bite block. This induces 3-D morphological changes in the soft tissue having a similar order of magnitude to that which could be achieved clinically by functional orthodontic appliances or by surgical correction. Twenty-five facial images of patients were used to train a 2-D ASM for feature extraction. Metric 3-D facial surface reconstructions were obtained using an area-based stereo matching technique [7]. The 3-D data sets were then divided into two groups; group I to denote shape data prior to insertion of the bite block and group II after insertion. A morphometric analysis of facial shape change was then carried out using randomly selected patients to evaluate differences between groups I and II.

3   Method

3.1   Automatic 3-D facial landmark detection by ASM and stereo correspondence

ASM [6] is a statistical-based technique for building compact models of the shape and appearance of a flexible object to automatically locate new instances of the object in 2-D images.

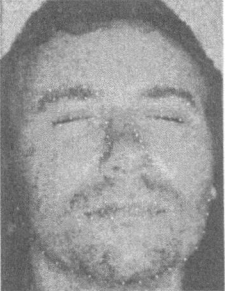

Fig. 1. Shape model points for 2-D feature detection

Initially, 107 facial landmark points were defined to represent the 2-D facial features as shown in Fig. 1. They were manually located on 25 grey-level training images from our facial database and Procrustes aligned to compute a mean shape and build the point distribution model (PDM). Principal component analysis on the covariance matrix of deviations from the mean shape was carried out to yield a set of basis vectors describing the main modes of shape variation in the training data. At the same time, the grey-level appearance models about each shape point were constructed in the same way as for the PDM. After the training procedure was completed, the average grey level profiles were used to drive and deform the shape model iteratively to locate 2-D facial features for stereo intensity images outside the training set.

To ensure correct convergence, an initial position of the PDM, defined by the scale and translation parameters, was calculated by locating the horizontal and vertical edges of the facial borders (Fig. 2) using the integral projection of the intensity image. The vertical integral projection $V(x)$ and horizontal projection $H(y)$ of an image $I(x,y)$ in a rectangular region $[x_1, x_2] \times [y_1, y_2]$ are defined by:

$$V(x) = \sum_{y=y_1}^{y_2} I(x,y), \qquad H(x) = \sum_{x=x_1}^{x_2} I(x,y) \tag{1}$$

A Sobel horizontal edge filter was applied to the intensity image followed by the vertical projection of the filtered image. Fig. 3 depicts the vertical projection of the horizontal edge, where L and R indicate the left and right facial borders. By finding the minimum and maximum values along the horizontal axis, the left and right facial borders were located. A similar operation was carried out to locate the upper facial border and the vertical position of the eyes and eyebrows (Fig. 2) and this information was then used to determine the initial scale and pose. Based on this initialization, 2-D facial landmark detection in the left stereo image was carried out. A maximum limit of 50 iterations was imposed when searching for the optimum position.

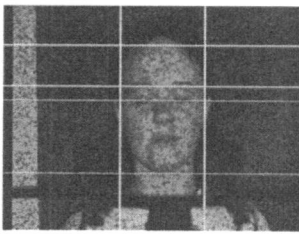

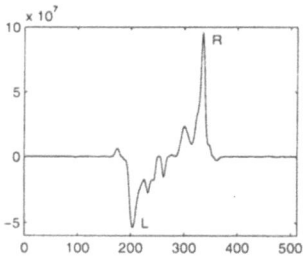

Fig. 2. Intensity image used for feature detection and stereo matching with detected borders

Fig. 3. The vertical integral projection of the filtered intensity image

After accurately locating the 2-D features in a left stereo image, area-based stereo matching [7] was performed to obtain the correspondence between stereo image pairs. If the corresponding point for a left feature point could not be found in the right image by the matching algorithm, the missing match was interpolated from the known neighbouring disparity values using an adjustable matching window and a thin-plate spline (TPS) mapping function. A smaller window size can be used in regions where the disparity map is dense, whilst a larger window is needed for regions containing sparse data. In our experiments, if the number of known disparity values was less than 40% of the total in a selected window, then the window size was automatically increased until the number of the known value reached a preset minimum of 20 values. Once all the disparity values had been obtained, these point correspondences were converted into 3-D space using a set of camera parameters obtained from a metric calibration rig [8]. Here, only 90 3-D facial feature landmarks (Fig. 4) are used for further morphometric analysis, whilst the detected landmarks on the facial border are used purely for the purpose of segmenting the face from the background.

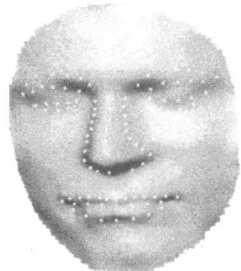

Fig. 4. Automatically detected facial landmarks on a 3-D facial model

3.2   Morphometric techniques for the shape analysis

Three main approaches for analysing facial shape change were employed; 1) Generalized Procrustes analysis (GPA), 2) principal components analysis (PCA) in the tangent space and 3) thin plate spline (TPS) interpolation for visualizing shape deformation.

Generalized Procrustes analysis is primarily used for estimating an average shape [5]. It registers sets of landmark configurations by removing translational and rotational differences and scaling them until they most closely match. The registered landmark configurations constitute Kendall's shape manifold [5] with Procrustes distance as metric. The dimension of Kendall's shape space is lower than that of the original figure space because the translation, rotation and scale differences have been removed. For k landmarks in 2-D, the shape space has dimension of $2k - 4$ and in 3-D, $3k - 7$. After Procrustes registration, standard multivariate analyses such as tests of group differences and PCA can be carried out directly on the tangent coordinates.

Principal components analysis in the tangent plane provides an effective means of investigating the structure of shape variability [5] and reducing the dimensionality of the shape data prior to multivariate analysis. Since the PCs are orthogonal, they each represent statistically independent modes of variation in the sample. When these PCs are sorted in descending order of eigenvalues for the covariance matrix, main modes of shape variation can be described by the first few significant PCs.

Shape deformation can be further interpreted using the TPS together with a Cartesian transformation grid to exactly map the biological shape change between two homologous 2-D data sets with minimum bending energy. The associated principal warps [4] decompose shape change into local and global components of successively increasing scale analogous to a Fourier analysis.

4   Result

ASM-assisted landmark detection was tested on 25 facial images outside the training set and a success rate of more than 80 percent was obtained. These landmarks were then converted into 3-D coordinate space by stereo correspondence information and disparity map interpolation. Metric reconstruction accuracy have previously been established using a calibration object with precisely determined ground truth. The average root mean square (RMS) error for stereo matching is 0.26 pixel yielding a RMS error of 0.28mm in 3-D spatial coordinates for target check points. Ninety three-dimensional landmarks were automatically located for both group I and group II shapes. Midline profiles were then obtained by a facial symmetry plane registration method [9] and resampled to produce 39 pseudo-landmark positions for each 3-D image model.

The morphometric analysis of facial shape change was first carried out on the 2-D midline profiles of 16 randomly selected patients. Fig. 5 illustrates the scatter plots of these profiles which were partially Procrustes aligned using the unchanged (upper 25) landmarks. The solid lines indicate the Procustes averaged profiles for groups I and II. As expected, the mouth and lower jaw region for the group II sample has been displaced forward and slightly downward by the bite block. This shape change can be depicted more clearly in Fig. 6 by a Cartesian transformation grid calculated using TPS deformation. The left and right pictures are the average profiles for group I and group II respectively.

GPA was then used to align the set of midline profiles followed by PCA on the Procrustes tangent coordinates to reveal the main modes of shape variation. The shape variation represented by the first three PCs is illustrated in Fig. 7. The largest shape differences were found in the mouth region captured in PC 1. This is largely due to the effect of bite block insertion and hence the simulated surgical correction. PCs 2 and 3 reveal combined effects of variation in nose shape which is expected given the age range in our sample (10-26 years). The first two PCs resulting from this analysis are plotted in Fig. 8. It can be seen that the two groups have been partially separated by the plot with group I ('o') largely occupying the bottom right half and group II ('*') the top left half of the figure. The percentages of variability accounted for by the first 3 PCs are 35.1%, 16.9% and 16.1%. Performing a two-sample Hotelling's T^2 test on Procrustes tangent coordinates on the first two PCs (sample size 20) yields a test statistic of 8.673 ($p = 0.025$). Hence, there is good evidence that the mean shapes are different and that this has not been masked by the heterogeneous nature of the patient sample. This indicates that the apparatus is sufficiently sensitive to detect relatively small changes in facial shape.

However, the midline profiles only utilise 2-D shape information. For a more revealing picture, the full 3-D landmark data set derived from the stereo correspondence search are chosen. Assigning landmark data to groups I and II as

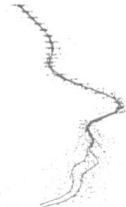 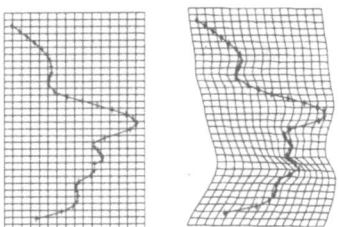

Fig. 5. Scattered plot of midline files. Solid lines indicate the aver profiles.

Fig. 6. The deformation of midline profiles viewed using a thin-plate spline deformation.

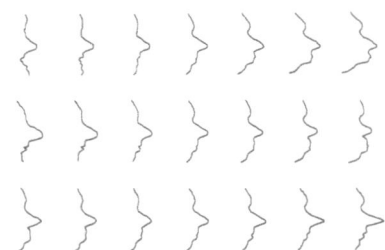

Fig. 7. Shape variation explained by first 3 PCs. Each row denotes the ith PC ($i = 1,2,3$) and each column displays a multiple c of the standardised PC scores ($c = -3, -2, -1, 0, 1, 2, 3$). $c = 0$ corresponds to the Procrustes averaged form. Row i corresponds to ith PC.

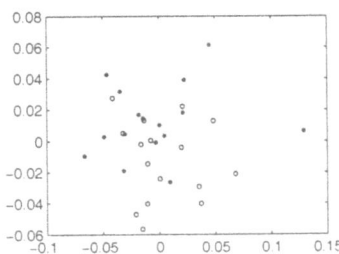 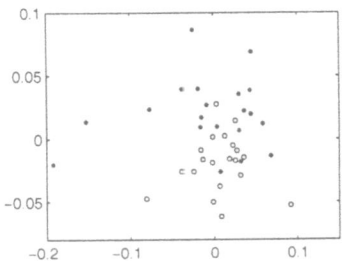

Fig. 8. Plot of PC 1(horizontal axis) vs PC 2 for group differences in midline profile, 'o' denotes group I (before bite block insertion) and '*' denotes group II (after insertion).

Fig. 9. Plot of PC 1(horizontal axis) vs PC 2 for group differences in 3-D landmarks, 'o' denotes group I (before bite block insertion) and '*' denotes group II (after insertion).

before, the extracted data were submitted to three-dimensional GPA and PCA. In this case the first 3 PCs account for 33.92%, 12.19% and 9.28% of the total variation in the combined sample. As shown in Fig. 9, the groups I and II are well separated signifying a clear difference in shape. Hotelling's T^2 test on the first 3 PCs (sample size 20) gave a statistically significant group difference at $p \sim 0.00029$. The evidence of difference in mean shape for 3-D landmark data is not in doubt and is clearly stronger than for 2-D data.

Investigating 3-D landmarks in the mouth region alone and projecting into the frontal facial plane, we can attempt to visualise the shape differences as a deformation from group I to group II, using TPS and principal warps decomposition. The results are illustrated in Fig. 10 and 11. Fig. 11 depicts the decomposition of deformation (i.e. shape difference) at successively larger scales. It provides an alternative picture of the basis space to PCA in tangent space coordinates. It was found that principal warp 3 acounts for 63.1% of the total bending energy. The weights for each principal warp (partial warp scores) and the affine contribution was calculated. Hotelling's T^2 test on these partial warp scores gave a statistically significant group difference at $p < 0.00001$.

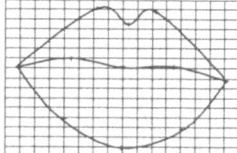 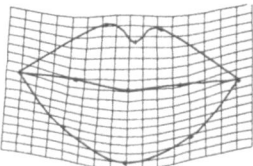

Fig. 10. Deformation from group I to group II as a thin plate spline. Averaged landmark configuration of group I(left), averaged landmark configuration of group II(right).

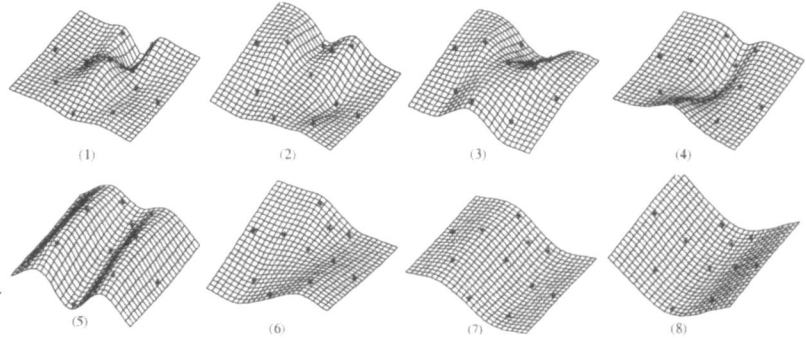

Fig. 11. Principal warps for the landmark configuration shown in Fig.10 (left).

5   Conclusion

We have developed an effective means for automatic landmark-based 3-D facial shape change analysis which combines stereo-assisted ASM with morphometric tools. The experiment results signify a relative displacement of the average shape of the mouth and lower jaw forwards and slightly downwards after insertion of the bite block. This is the desired effect of surgical treatment on patients presenting class II and class III abnormalities. We have shown that such changes can be validated statistically. It suggests that the proposed method may be useful for auditing clinical treatment of class II and class III abnormalities with respect to its effects on facial soft tissue morphology.

Acknowledgements

We would like to thank Dr Michael Trenouth of Royal Preston Hospital for providing access to orthodontic patients and the University of Central Lancashire for funding this work through an overseas research studentship award.

References

1. A. M. McCance, J. P. Moss, W. R. Fright, A. D. Linney and D. R. James. Three-dimensional analysis techniques. II Laser scanning: A quantitative 3-D soft-tissue analysis using a colour-coding system. *Cleft Palate-Craniofacial Journal*, 34(1):46–51, 1997.
2. J. P. Moss, A. M. McCance, W. Fright, A. D. Linney and D. R. James et al. A 3-Dimensional soft-tissue analysis of 15 patients with class-II, division-1 malocclusions after bimaxillary surgery. *American Journal of Orthodontics and Dentofacial Orthopedics*, 105(5):430–437, 1994.
3. A. M. Coombes, R. Richards, A. D. Linney, V. Bruce and R. Fright. Description and recognition of faces from 3D data. *Proceedings of SPIE - The International Society for Optical Engineering*, 1766:307–319, 1992.
4. F. L. Bookstein. Shape and the information in medical images: A decade of the morphometric synthesis. *Computer Vision and Image Understanding*, 66(2):99-118, 1997.
5. I. L. Dryden and K. V. Mardia. *Statistical Shape Analysis*, John Wiley & Sons, 1998.
6. T. F. Cootes, A. Hill, C. J. Taylar and J. Haslam. The use of active shape models for locating structures in medical images. *Image and Vision Computing*, 12(6):355–366, 1994.
7. Z. Mao and A. J. Naftel. Improved area-based stereo matching using an image segmentation approach for 3-D analysis of facial soft tissue changes. *Medical Image Understanding and Analysis '97*, University of Oxford, pp.209-212, 1997.
8. R. Y. Tsai. A versatile camera calibration technique for high-accuracy 3D machine vision metrology using off-the-shelf TV cameras and lenses. *IEEE Journal of Robotics and Automation*, 3(4):323-44, 1987.
9. Z. Mao and A. J. Naftel. 3D image analysis of facial shape changes using depth from stereo. *Nobless Workshop on Non-linear Model Based Image Analysis*, Glasgow, pp.283-288, 1998.

Segmentation of Echocardiographic Image Sequences Using Spatio-temporal Information

Einar Brandt, Lars Wigström and Bengt Wranne
einbr@imv.liu.se

Department of Medicine and Care, Clinical Physiology, Linköping University, Sweden

Abstract. This paper describes a new method for improving border detection in image sequences by including both spatial and temporal information. The method is based on three dimensional quadrature filters for estimating local orientation. A simplification that gives a significant reduction in computational demand is also presented. The border detection framework is combined with a segmentation algorithm based on active contours or 'snakes', implemented using a new optimization relaxation that can be solved to optimality using dynamical programming. The aim of the study was to compare segmentation performance using gradient based border detection and the proposed border detection algorithm using spatio-temporal information. Evaluation is performed both on a phantom and *in-vivo* data from five echocardiographic short axis image sequences. It could be concluded that when temporal information was included weak and incomplete boundaries could be found where gradient based border detection failed. Otherwise there was no significant difference in performance between the new proposed method and gradient based border detection.

1 Introduction

Endocardial delineation in echocardiographic images could be a strong clinical tool for quantification of wall motion abnormalities and global ventricular function. Manual delineation is however very time consuming and operator dependent [1]. Automatic processing of echocardiographic data is difficult due to the poor image quality of echocardiographic images. The most important degradation mechanisms include sidelobes and grating lobes, blur, acquisition on polar coordinates, poor contrast, artifacts and speckle noise [2].

Several methods and approaches for segmenting echocardiographic image sequences have been suggested, such as active contours [3], probabilistic frameworks [2], mathematical morphology [4], simulated annealing [5], combining edge-based deformable models and region-based segmentation [6], and using M-mode echocardiograms [7]. Despite all these efforts automatic segmentation remains as a difficult problem.

This paper describes a new method using local orientation estimated with quadrature filters for improving border detection by incorporating temporal information in the border detection. The idea of using temporal information in segmentation of echocardiographic image sequences is not new; it is proposed and discussed among others in [3, 5, 8].

2   Method

The overall strategy for segmentation used in this paper is to first compute a border probability image and then use an optimization algorithm to find the most probable segmentation. The objective is to find a border probability image sequence using both spatial and temporal information. In other words, we are looking for border-like structures that are continuous in time. The images in the image sequence are stacked to form a 3D (2D+T) image volume, see Figure 1 a). Consider a slowly moving plane in an image sequence. This is illustrated in Figure 1 b). The angle between the local orientation of a planar structure and the time axis depends on the velocity and continuity in time of the structure. We are searching for borders that are continuous in time, having an orientation approximately orthogonal to the time axis.

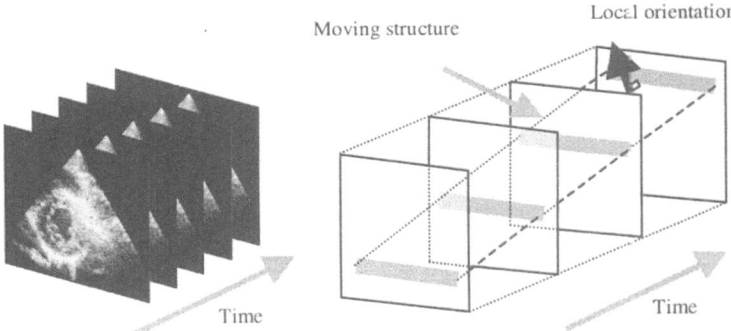

Fig. 1. a) Images are stacked to form an image volume. b) A slowly moving plane in an image sequence. The black arrow indicates the local orientation of the moving structure in the image volume. Note that the orientation of the structure is almost orthogonal to the time axis.

2.1   A 3D local orientation estimate

Mulet-Parada et al. proposed a filter bank consisting of 21 Log-Gabor filters to find a local orientation estimate [8] in an echocardiographic image sequence. An alternative way of estimating local orientation is using quadrature filters and a local orientation tensor concept described by Hans Knutsson [10]. A quadrature filter is a filter with a zero transfer function in one half plane of the frequency domain. The normal vector of that plane is said to be the orientation of the quadrature filter. The quadrature filter is a complex valued filter where the real part detects boundaries and the imaginary part detects borders. For calculating a local orientation estimate in 3D a set of minimally six quadrature filters is required [9]. The directions of the quadrature filters should be evenly distributed in space. In 3D this is accomplished when each quadrature filter is pointing at nodes of a hemi-icosahedron, as illustrated in Figure 2.

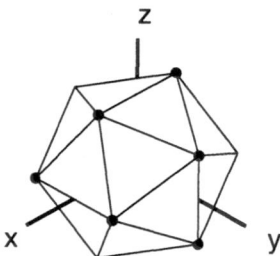

Fig. 2. An Icosahedron, the points on the icosahedron indicates the direction of the quadrature filters.

A tensor describing the local orientation can be constructed as [9]:

$$\mathbf{T_e} = \sum_k q_k \left(\frac{5}{4} \hat{n}_k \hat{n}_k^T - \frac{1}{4} \mathbf{I} \right) \tag{1}$$

Where q_k is the output from quadrature filter k, $\hat{n}_k$ is the direction vector of quadrature filter k, and $\mathbf{I}$ is the identity tensor.

In the 3D case, the tensor is a 3x3 matrix. The eigenvectors and eigenvalues of the tensor describes the nature of the orientation in a local neighborhood. The eigenvector with the largest eigenvalue gives an estimate of the dominant local orientation in the neighborhood. The idea is now that we can suppress structures that are not continuous in time by projecting the estimated orientation vector on a plane normal to the time axis. Remember that a non-moving plane has a normal vector (orientation) orthogonal to the time axis, see Figure 1b. A border probability estimate is therefore:

$$g = \|\lambda_1\| \left\| \begin{bmatrix} 1 & 0 & 0 \\ 0 & 1 & 0 \\ 0 & 0 & 0 \end{bmatrix} \begin{bmatrix} e_{1x} \\ e_{1y} \\ e_{1t} \end{bmatrix} \right\| \tag{2}$$

where g is the border probability. The matrix is a projection matrix (projection on a plane normal to the time axis), λ_1, the vector is the eigenvector corresponding to the largest eigenvalue λ_1 of the tensor $\mathbf{T_e}$.

It is also possible to weight the different border orientations by changing the projection matrix. More important is, however, the ability to distinguish between lines and edges. In our case we are looking for edges that goes from dark to bright (transition between blood pool and myocardium). This is done by only looking at the imaginary part of the eigenvalue.

2.2 Computational simplification

Instead of calculating a local orientation estimate and projecting the resulting orientation we can directly project the set of quadrature filters. The problem is then reduced to find the local orientation in a 2D plane. Finding local orientation in 2D can be accomplished with only three quadrature filters [9]. In addition, the eigenvalue calculation will be much faster. Note, however, that the quadrature filters are still three dimensional, but fewer filters are required. When four quadrature filters are used in 2D it is possible to directly calculate the local orientation without calculating the eigenvalues and eigenvectors [9].

3 Optimization

The border detection algorithm results in a "border probability" image. From this image we need to find the most probable border using an optimization algorithm. As a foundation for the optimization, the concept of active contours where chosen. Active contours are a common choice for segmenting medical images, since they capture anatomical irregularities well [11]. The border is modeled as a physical string with rigidity and elasticity. The contour is positioned so that its energy is minimized. This approach is usually referred as 'snakes' in the literature [11]. Modeling the border as a string results in the following optimization problem [12]:

$$\min_{f} \int \left(g(f(s)) + \alpha f'(s)^2 + \beta f''(s)^2 \right) ds \qquad (3)$$

Where f is the active contour, g is the energy from the border probability image, α and β are elasticity and rigidity, respectively. This optimization problem can not be solved to a guaranteed optimum. Therefore, a reformulation of the optimization problem is required. The problem can be solved by an iterative process such as simulated annealing similar to what Friedland et al. suggested [5]. Iterative algorithms do not give any guarantees about optimality of the result in finite time. Instead, we propose a reformulation of the problem to a combinatorial optimization problem. This reformulation is possible if we can restrict the active contour to a proper discrete function $y(x)$. This restriction can be accomplished by resampling the original image (see section 3.1). The optimization problem in Equation 3 can now be approximated by [12]:

$$\min_{y_i \in 1...M} \begin{cases} \sum_{i=1}^{L} \sum_{j=y_{i-1}}^{y_i} \left(\frac{\|y_i - j\|}{\|y_{i-1} - y_i\| + 1} g(i-1, j) + \frac{\|j - y_{i-1}\|}{\|y_{i-1} - y_i\| + 1} g(i, j) \right) + \\ \\ \sum_{i=1}^{L-1} \alpha(y_i - y_{i+1})^2 + \sum_{i=2}^{L-1} \beta(-y_i + 2y_{i+1} - y_i)^2 \end{cases}$$

$$(4)$$

Where g is the border probability image, α is the elasticity term, β is the rigidity term, L is the number of layers (columns) in the discrete grid, M is the number of rows in the discrete grid, and the active contour f is represented by the discrete function $f : \{y_i\}$.

The first term of Equation 4 simply describes a sum of linear interpolations in the border probability and the two last terms describes the rigidity and elasticity terms. The main advantage with this new reformulation is that the physical interpretation of treating the contour as a physical string is kept, including rigidity The other advantage is that it can be solved to optimality by a fast dynamic programming algorithm. The problem is solved with an algorithm very similar to Dijkstra's shortest path algorithm. This is possible since y_{i-1} is implicitly known when calculating forward vertices in Dijkstra's algorithm. Details on solving the optimization problem can be found in [12]. Dynamical programming has earlier been used for segmentation of echocardiographic images by among others [3] and [7].

3.1   Resampling

The reformulation of the optimization problem restricts the segmented contour to a proper one-dimensional function $y(x)$. The resampling of the original image was performed before border detection. In the consecutive frames the resampling is performed along the delineated contour in the previous frame (resampling line, indicated in black in Figure 3 below). In this manner the function $y(x)$ can be used to represent the delineated contour for the next frame, assuming a similarity.

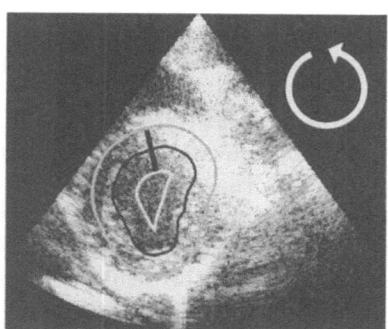

Resampled image

Fig. 3. Left: Original image with resampling direction is indicated by a white arrow. Right: The resampled image.

A delicate question is how to weight temporal and spatial scale. The following idea was used to establish an approximate scale. During one heart beat in a normal heart a point on the endocardium moves approximately 10 mm before it returns to its original position. There are approximately 50 frames in one heartbeat. Therefore 50 frames should correspond to 10 mm.

4   Validation

The segmentation performance using gradient based border detection and local orientation border detection was compared. The optimization parameters where kept constant ($\alpha = 0.001$ and $\beta = 0.005$). The border probability image was normalized prior to the optimization process. For gradient based border detection a 5x10 median filter, followed by two orthogonal gradient filters (1 0 -1) were applied. The orientation filter size was 9x9x9 pixels with a bandwidth of one octave and a center-frequency of $\pi/5$.

First, an artificial image sequence consisting of a moving border in a fair amount of noise was used to evaluate the two border detection methods. The image sequence was 100x100x9 pixels, and the amplitude of the border was 1/5 in a fully developed Gaussian multiplicative speckle noise. The phantom image sequence is shown in Figure 5.

To quantitatively assess the accuracy of the segmentation process, image sequences from three normals and two patients were used. The images were acquired from parasternal short axis view. The number of frames per heartbeat were not resampled, and varied between 39 to 70. The original image was resampled to 50x300 pixels (orthogonal to resampling line and along resampling line respectively). User interaction was limited to setting region of interest on the first image. The same region of interest was used for both border detection methods. The segmentation result was compared with a manual delineation performed by two different observers on 10 images per image sequence. Papillary muscles where included in the delineation, if they where connected to the wall in the imaged plane.

Quantitative analysis of segmentation performance on *in-vivo* data is a difficult task since there is no gold standards available [1]. Two measures were used for comparison, delineated cavity area and symmetrical difference. Symmetric difference is an error metric defined as the area of a pixelwise XOR comparison on those pixels enclosed by the different segmentations, see Figure 4. The difference was calculated in 10 images per heart beat evenly distributed in time and in six segments in each image.

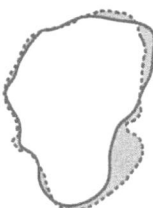

Fig. 4. The symmetric difference between two delineations — dashed and solid lines respectively, is marked in gray color.

5   Results

In the case of the phantom, no consistent border could be found at all with the gradient border detection algorithm. When temporal information was included, the border could be detected with good accuracy, see Figure 5.

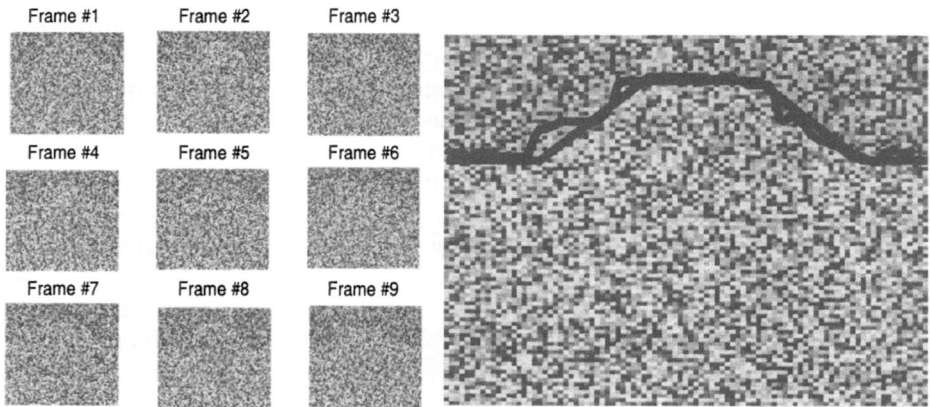

Fig. 5. Left: Test image sequence with a slowly moving border with a fair amount of noise. Right: Border detected in frame #5 of the image sequence. The 'straight' line is the true border and the 'wigged' line is the border detected by the algorithm.

For the *in-vivo* image sequences, cavity area was used for determination of systematic errors and symmetric difference was used to determine in which segment the differences were most pronounced. In one of the image sequences with poor image quality it was not possible to perform fully automatic segmentation using the gradient border detection algorithm, while the local orientation succeeded well. This sequence was removed from further statistical analysis. The differences in mean cavity area and mean symmetric difference in different segments for the two border detection methods compared to the two observers are illustrated in Figure 6. A Bland Altman analysis [13] was performed to find out if manual segmentation could be replaced with automatic segmentation, see Figure 7.

6   Discussion

The border detection method proposed in this paper is easily expanded to higher dimensions such as 3D+T. Images from different modalities can easily be used such as MRI or 3D ultrasound. In 3D+T, the computational simplification presented is extra valuable since it reduces the number of quadrature filters required from 24 to 6. One improvement applicable to the segmentation process proposed in this paper would be to optimize the contour for all frames in parallel (i.e. a 2D+T deformable model for the entire image volume) [14]. Unfortunately the

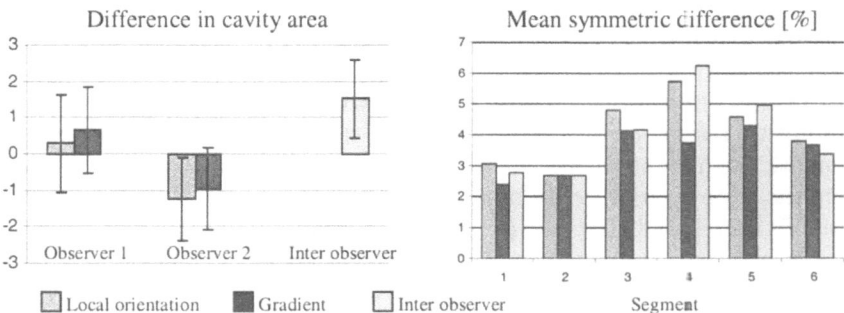

Fig. 6. Left: The difference in cavity area measured with the two border detection methods compared to the two observers. Note the systematic difference between the two observers. Right: Symmetric difference in different segments for the two border detection methods compared to manual delineation. The segments are anterior wall (1), anterior septal (2), posterior septal (3), posterior (4), posterior lateral (5), and anterior lateral (6). As a reference inter-observer symmetric difference is also plotted.

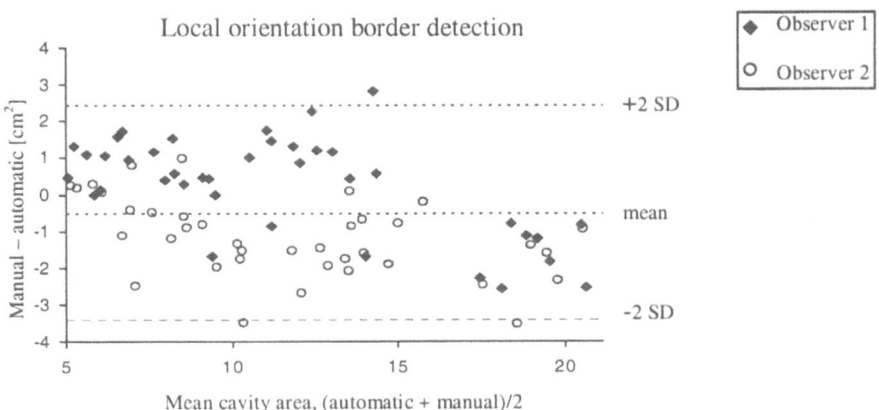

Fig. 7. Bland Altman plot where segmentation using local orientation border detection is compared with the manual delineation by the two observers.

reformulation of the optimization algorithm proposed here can then no longer be used and an iterative algorithm has to be used for the optimization.

7 Conclusion

The fact that endocardial border detection of echocardiograhic image sequences is a difficult task is clearly illustrated with the large inter-observer difference. Automatic segmentation has the advantage of good reproducibility. Therefore automatic segmentation could be a method to reduce variability. Further investigation is necessary before it is possible to say that automatic segmentation statistically can replace manual segmentation. The mean symmetric difference for the six segments corresponds well to the symmetric difference for inter-observer delineations. This suggests that the differences in measured cavity area between computer and manual delineations arose in the same segments as where the human observers had difficulties. It can be concluded that when temporal information is included weak and incomplete boundaries (such as in the phantom and one of the image sequences) can be found where gradient based border detection fails.

References

1. V. Chalana and Y. Kim: A methodology for evaluation of boundary detection algorithms on medical images. IEEE Trans Med Imaging, vol. 16, pp. 642–52, 1997.
2. J. M. B. Dias and J. M. N. Leitão: Wall Position and Thickness Estimation from Sequences of Echocardiographic Images, IEEE Transactions on Medical Imaging, vol. 15, pp. 25-38, 1996.
3. B. B. Luc Maes, Paul Suetens, Frans Van de Werf: Automated contour detection of the left ventricle in short axis view in 2D echocardiograms, Machine Vision and Applications, vol. 6, pp. 1-9, 1993.
4. J. W. Klingler, Jr., C. L. Vaughan, T. D. Fraker, Jr., and L. T. Andrews: Segmentation of echocardiographic images using mathematical morphology, IEEE Trans Biomed Eng, vol. 35, pp. 925-34, 1988.
5. N. Friedland and D. Adam: Automated ventricular boundary detection from sequential ultrasound images using simulated annealing, IEEE Transactions on Medical Imag, vol. 4, pp. 344-353, 1989.
6. A. Chakraborty, L. H. Staib, and J. S. Duncan: Deformable Boundary Finding in Medical Images by Integrating Gradient and Regional Information, IEEE Transactions on Medical Imaging, vol. 15, pp. 859-870, 1996.
7. M. Unser, G. Pelle, P. Brun, and M. Eden: Automated Extraction of Serial Myocardial Borders from M-Mode Echocardiograms, IEEE Transactions on Medical Imaging, vol. 8, pp. 96-103, 1989.
8. M. Mulet-Parada and J. A. Noble: 2D+T Acoustic Boundary Detection in Echocardiography presented at MICCAI-98, Cambridge, 1998.
9. G. Granlund and H. Knutsson: Signal Processing for Computer Vision, Linköping: Kluwer Academic Publishers, 1995.

10. H. Knutsson: Representing local structure using tensors, presented at the 6th Scandinavian Conferance on Image Analysis, pp 244-251, Oulo, Firland, June 1989.

11. T. McInery and D. Terzopoulos: Deformable models in medical image analysis: a survey, Medical Image Analysis, vol. 1(2), 1996.

12. E. Brandt: Segmentation Techniques for Echocardiographic Image Sequences, LiTH-ISY-EX-1934, 1998, Department of Electrical Engineering, Linköpings Universitet, Sweden.

13. J. M. Bland and G. D. Altman: Statistical methods for assessing agreement between two methods of clinical measurent, The Lancet, February 8, pp. 307-310, 1986.

14. D. Kucera and R. W. Martin: Segmentation of sequences of echocardiographic images using a simplified 3D active contour model with region-based external forces, Comput Med Imaging Graph, vol. 21, pp. 1-21, 1997.

3D Cardiac Deformation from Ultrasound Images

Xenophon Papademetris[1], Albert J. Sinusas[23], Donald P. Dione[3]
and James S. Duncan[12]

[1] Departments of Electrical Engineering, [2] Diagnostic Radiology, and [3] Medicine,
Yale University New Haven, CT 06520-8042
papad@noodle.med.yale.edu

Abstract. The quantitative estimation of regional cardiac deformation from 3D image sequences has important clinical implications for the assessment of viability in the heart wall. Such estimates have so far been obtained almost exclusively from Magnetic Resonance (MR) images, specifically MR tagging. In this paper we describe a methodology for estimating cardiac deformations from 3D ultrasound images. The images are segmented interactively and then initial correspondence is established using a shape-tracking approach. A dense motion field is then estimated using an anisotropic linear elastic model, which accounts for the fiber directions in the left-ventricle. The dense motion field is in turn used to calculate the deformation of the heart wall in terms of strain in cardiac specific directions. The strains obtained using this approach in open-chest dogs before and after coronary occlusion related to changes in blood flow, show good agreement with previously published results in the literature. This proposed method provides quantitative regional 3D estimates of heart deformation from ultrasound images.

1 Introduction

The fundamental goal of many efforts in the cardiac imaging and image analysis community is to assess the regional function of the left ventricle (LV) of the heart. The general consensus is that the analysis of heart wall deformation provides quantitative estimates of the location and extent of ischemic myocardial injury. There have been considerable efforts within the medical image analysis community aimed at estimating this deformation, almost exclusively using magnetic resonance (MR) images, primarily MR tagging [13, 7, 11], and to a lesser extent, MR phase contrast [9, 14] velocity images.

In this paper we describe and test an approach to estimate the regional deformation of the left-ventricle from ultrasound left ventricular images. We use a biomechanical model to describe the myocardium and shape-based tracking displacement estimates on the epi and endo-cardial walls to generate the initial displacement estimates. These are integrated in a Bayesian estimation framework and the overall problem is solved using the finite element method. This method produces *quantitative regional* 3D cardiac deformation estimates from ultrasound images which up-to now was thought to be only possible using magnetic resonance and especially MR tagging. The fast improving quality of ultrasound images with the introduction of harmonic imaging [6] and contrast agents [15] should make it possible to obtain even more accurate estimates of 3D left ventricular deformation in the future.

2 Our Approach

We estimate a dense displacement field within a Bayesian estimation framework which consists of a data term and a model term. These are described in sections 2.1 and 2.2 respectively.

2.1 Obtaining Initial Displacement Data

Image Acquisition The images were acquired using an HP Sonos 5500 Ultrasound System with a 3D transducer (Transthoracic OmniPlane 21349A (R5012)). The 3d-probe was placed at the apex of the left-ventricle of an open-chest dog using a small ultrasound gelpad (Aquaflex) as a standoff as shown in figure 1. Each acquisition consisted of 13-17 frames per cardiac cycle depending on the heart rate. The angular slice spacing was 5 degrees resulting in 36 image slices for each frame.

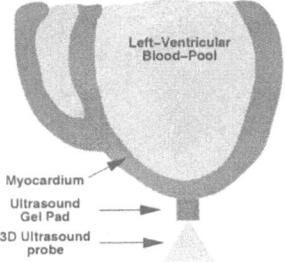

Fig. 1. Image acquisition geometry.

Image Segmentation The endo- and epi- cardial surfaces were extracted interactively using a software platform [16] originally developed for MR image data and subsequently modified to allow for the different geometry and image characteristics of ultrasound. For the automated part of the segmentation, for each image slice, we used an integrated deformable boundary method whose external energy function consisted of the standard intensity term and a texture-based term similar to the integrated method proposed in [3], although in our case the contours were parameterized as b-splines to allow for easy interaction. This produced reasonable results as shown in figures 2 and 3. We are currently looking into more sophisticated techniques for generating the external energy maps, including those suggested by Mulet-Parada et al [10].

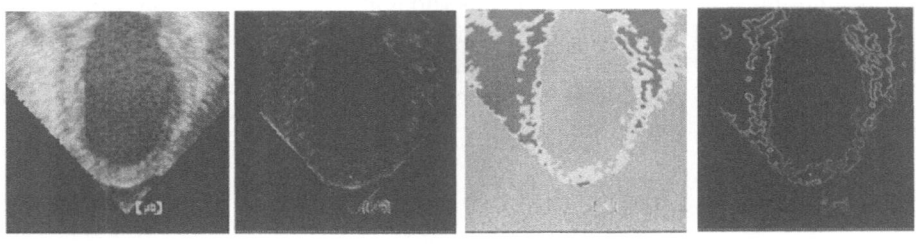

Original Image   **Texture Based**   **Texture+Intensity**   **Intensity Energy Map**
                  MRF Segmentation   **Energy Map**

Fig. 2. External Energy Functions for intensity and intensity+texture snakes. Note that the intensity only energy function is very noisy inside the left-ventricular blood-pool which creates many local minima for the deformable contour. The use of the texture eliminates most of these minima.

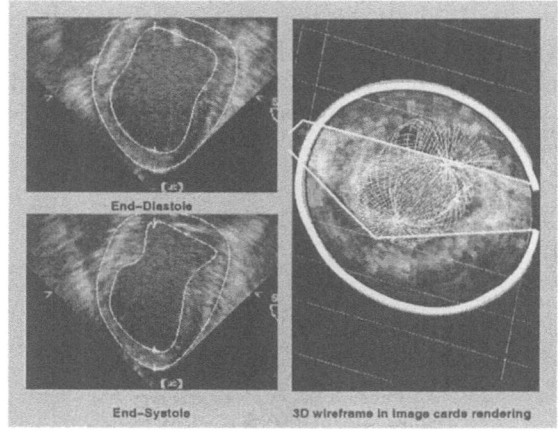

Fig. 3. Images and superimposed extracted contours. Only two of the eight frames are shown. The 3D rendering on the right shows all the wire-frame contours superimposed on a long axis (original) and a short-axis (interpolated) image slices.

Shape-Tracking Displacement Estimates In this work, the original displacements on the outer surfaces of the myocardium were obtained by using the shape-tracking algorithm whose details were presented in [12]. The method tries to track points on successive surfaces using a shape similarity metric which tries to minimize the difference in principal curvatures and was validated using implanted markers [12].

For example, consider point p_1 on a surface at time t_1 which is to be mapped to a point p_2 on the deformed surface at time t_2. First, a search is performed a physically plausible region W_2 on the deformed surface and the point $\hat{p}_2$ which has the local shape properties closest to those p_1 is selected. The shape properties here are captured in terms of the principal curvatures κ_1 and κ_2. The distance measure used is the bending energy required to bend a curved plate or surface patch to a newly deformed state. This is labeled as d_{be} and is defined as:

$$d_{be}(p1, p2) = A \left(\frac{(\kappa_1(p_1) - \kappa_1(p_2))^2 + (\kappa_2(p_1) - \kappa_2(p_2))^2}{2} \right) \tag{1}$$

The displacement estimate vector for each point p_1, u_1^m is given by

$$u_1^m = \hat{p}_2 - p_1 \quad , \quad \hat{p}_2 = \frac{\arg\min}{p_2 \in W_2} \left[d_{be}(p1, p2) \right]$$

Confidence Measures in the match: The bending energy measures for all the points inside the search region W_2 are recorded as the basis to measure the *goodness* and *uniqueness* of the matching choices. The value of the minimum bending energy in the search region between the matched points indicates the goodness of the match. Denote this value as m_g, we have the following measure for matching goodness:

$$m_g(p_1) = d_{be}(p_1, \hat{p}_2) \tag{2}$$

On the other hand, it is desirable that the chosen matching point is a unique choice among the candidate points within the search window. Ideally, the bending energy value of the chosen point should be an outlier (much smaller value) compared to the values of the rest of the points. If we denote the mean values of the bending energy measures of all the points inside window W_2 except the chosen point as $\bar{d}_{be}$ and the standard deviation as σ_{be}^d, we define the uniqueness measure as:

$$m_u(p_1) = \frac{d_{be}(p_1, \hat{p}_2)}{\bar{d}_{be} - \sigma_{be}^d} \tag{3}$$

This uniqueness measure has a high value if the bending energy of the chosen point is small compared to some smaller value (mean minus standard deviation) of the remaining bending energy measures. Combining these two measures together, we arrive at one *confidence measure* $c^m(p_1)$ for the matched point $\hat{p}_2$ of point p_1:

$$c^m(p_1) = \frac{1}{k_{1,g} + k_{2,g} m_g(p_1)} \times \frac{1}{k_{1,u} + k_{2,u} m_u(p_1)} \tag{4}$$

where $k_{1,g}, k_{2,g}, k_{1,u}$, and $k_{2,u}$ are scaling constants for normalization purposes. We normalize the confidences to lie in the range 0 to 1.

Modeling the initial displacement estimates: Given a set of displacement vector measurements u^m and confidence measures c^m we model theses estimates probabilistically by assuming that the noise in the individual measurements us normally distributed with zero mean and a variance equal to $\frac{1}{c^m}$. In addition we assume that the measurements are uncorrelated, although this is an assumption that is not strictly correct and we are presently working on this. Given these assumptions we can write the measurement probability for each point as:

$$p(u^m|u) = \frac{1}{\sqrt{2\pi\sigma^2}} e^{\frac{(u-u^m)^2}{2\sigma^2}} \qquad (5)$$

2.2 Modeling the myocardium

The passive properties of the left-ventricular myocardium are captured using a biomechanical model. We use an anisotropic linear elastic model which allows us to incorporate information about the preferential stiffness of the tissue along fiber directions from [5]. These fiber directions are shown in figure 4. The model described in terms of an internal or strain energy function of the form:

$$W = \epsilon' C \epsilon \qquad (6)$$

where ϵ is the strain and C is the 6×6 matrix containing the elastic constants which define the material properties. This is described in more detailed in continuum mechanics textbooks such as Malvern [8].

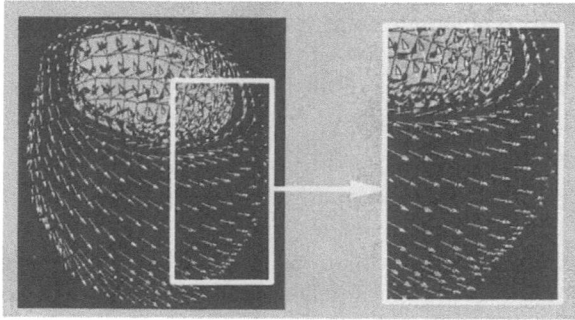

Fig. 4. Fiber direction in the left ventricle as defined in Guccione et al [5].

Deformation and Strain: Consider a body $B(0)$ which after time t moves and deforms to body $B(t)$. A point X on $B(0)$ goes to a point x on $B(t)$ and the transformation gradient F is defined as $dx = FdX$. The deformation is expressed in terms of the strain tensor ϵ. Because the deformations to be estimated in this work are larger than 5%, we use a finite strain formulation implemented using a logarithmic strain ϵ^L, which is defined as: $\epsilon = ln\sqrt{F.F'}$. Since the strain tensor is a 3×3 symmetric 2nd-rank tensor (matrix), we can re-write it in vector form as, $e = [\epsilon_{11}\ \epsilon_{22}\ \epsilon_{33}\ \epsilon_{12}\ \epsilon_{13}\ \epsilon_{23}]'$. This will enable us to express the tensor equations in a more familiar matrix notation.

Strain Energy Function: The mechanical model can be defined in terms of a strain energy function. The simplest useful continuum model in solid mechanics is the linear elastic one which is of the form: $W = e'Ce$ where C is a 6×6 matrix and defines the material properties of the deforming body. The left ventricle of the heart is specifically modeled as a transversely elastic material to account for the preferential stiffness in the fiber direction, using the matrix C:

$$C^{-1} = \begin{bmatrix} \frac{1}{E_p} & \frac{-\nu_p}{E_p} & \frac{-\nu_{fp}}{E_f} & 0 & 0 & 0 \\ \frac{-\nu_p}{E_p} & \frac{1}{E_p} & \frac{-\nu_{fp}}{E_f} & 0 & 0 & 0 \\ \frac{-\nu_{fp}E_f}{E_p} & \frac{-\nu_{fp}E_f}{E_p} & \frac{1}{E_f} & 0 & 0 & 0 \\ 0 & 0 & 0 & \frac{2(1+\nu_p)}{E_p} & 0 & 0 \\ 0 & 0 & 0 & 0 & \frac{1}{G_f} & 0 \\ 0 & 0 & 0 & 0 & 0 & \frac{1}{G_f} \end{bmatrix} \tag{7}$$

where E_f is the fiber stiffness, E_p is cross-fiber stiffness and ν_{fp}, ν_p are the corresponding Poisson's ratios and G_f is the shear modulus across fibers. ($G_f \approx E_f/(2(1 + \nu_{fp}))$. If $E_f = E_p$ and $\nu_p = \nu_{fp}$ this model reduces to the more common isotropic linear elastic model. The fiber stiffness was set to be 3.5 times greater than the cross-fiber stiffness [5]. The Poisson's ratios were both set to 0.4 to model approximate incompressibility. This model was previously used in [17].

A probabilistic description of the model: As previously demonstrated by Christiansen et al [4] there is a correspondence between an internal energy function and a Gibbs-Prior. If the mechanical model is described in terms of an internal energy function $W(C, u)$, where C represents the material properties and u the displacement field, then we can write an equivalent prior probability density function $p(u)$ (see equation 9) of the Gibbs form:

$$p(u) = k_1 \exp(-W(C, u)) \tag{8}$$

2.3   Integrating the Data and Model Terms

Having defined both the data term model (equation 5) and the model term (equation 8) in terms of probability density functions we naturally proceed to write the overall problem in a Bayesian estimation framework as follows: Given a set of noisy input displacement vectors u^m and the associated noise model $p(u^m|u)$ (data term) and a prior probability density function $p(u)$ (model term), find the best output displacements $\hat{u}$ which maximize the posterior probability $p(u|u^m)$. Using Bayes' rule we can write.

$$\hat{u} = \frac{\arg\max}{u} p(u|u^m) = \frac{\arg\max}{u} \left(\frac{p(u^m|u)p(u)}{p(u^m)} \right) \tag{9}$$

The prior probability of the measurements $p(u^m)$ is a constant once these measurements have been made and therefore drops out of the minimization process.

Taking logarithms in equation (9) and differentiating with respect to the displacement field u results in a system of partial differential equations, which we solve using the Finite Element Method [2]. The first step in the finite element method is the division or tessellation of the body of interest into elements; these are commonly tetrahedral or hexahedral in shape. Once this is done, the partial differential equations are written down in integral form for each element, and then the integral of these equations over all the elements is taken to produce the final set of equations. For more information one is referred to standard textbooks such as Bathe [2]. The final set of equations is then solved to produce the output set of displacements. In our case the myocardium is divided into approximately 2,500 hexahedral elements.

For each frame between end-systole (ES) and end-diastole (ED), a two step problem is posed: (i) solving equation (9) normally and (ii) adjusting the position of all points on the endo-and epi-cardial surfaces so they lie on the endo- and epi-cardial surfaces at the next frame using a modified nearest-neighbor technique and solving equation (9) once more using this added constraint. This ensures that there is no bias in the estimation of the radial strain.

3   Results

To evaluate the efficacy of using image-derived *in vivo* deformation estimates to measure regional LV function we conducted experiments on fasting, anesthetized, open chest, adult mongrel dogs with approval of the Yale University Animal Care and Use Committee. In this preliminary work, we report results from three animals. The 3D ultrasound images were obtained either before (dog1) or after occlusion of the left anterior descending coronary artery (dog2 and dog3). Coronary occlusion created an area of dysfunction which we call the risk area. Also regional blood flow in the heart wall was determined using a radio-labeled microsphere technique. Here, radioactively labeled microspheres were injected into the left atrium and reference blood samples were drawn from the femoral arteries. Regional myocardial blood flow was calculated using a method previously described in Sinusas et al [1]. The blood flow measurements are used to identify the risk area and play no further role in this work.

The images were segmented interactively and the surfaces sampled to 0.5 voxel resolution, at which point curvatures were calculated and the shape-tracking algorithm was used to generate initial displacement estimates. The heart wall was divided into 2500 hexahedral elements and the anisotropic linear elastic model was used to regularize the displacements. The computational time after the segmentation was of the order of 3-4 hrs/dog (depending on the heart rate and hence the number of image frames) on a Silicon Graphics Octane with an R10000 195 Mhz processor and 128 MB RAM,

For the purpose of analyzing the results, the left-ventricle of the heart was divided into 4 cross-sectional slices, slice 1 being at the bottom or apex of the ventricle and number 4 being at the top or base of the ventricle. Each slice was further subdivided into 8 sectors, as shown in figure 5. A sector was labeled as being in the risk area if the endocardial mircrosphere flow was less than $0.25ml/min/g$. The normal region was defined by 5 transmural sectors located in the posterior lateral wall at the base of the heart (sectors 5,6,7 of the basal slice and sectors 6,7 of the mid-basal slice). We report the average of radial and circumferential strains for the risk areas and the normal regions.

Study	Norm RR %	Risk RR %	Norm CC %	Risk CC %	Norm LL %	Risk LL %
dog1	17.7	n/a	-13.4	n/a	-4.3	n/a
dog2	22.4	- 4.3	- 8.4	1.9	-3.4	-0.7
dog3	17.2	-13.7	-12.4	-7.3	-3.1	-2.0

Table 1. Summary of results for three animal studies (Norm=Normal Region, Risk= Risk Area, RR=Average Radial Strain, CC=Average Circumferential Strain, LL=Average Longitudinal Strain).

The results are summarized in Table 1. Function in the risk area, which was independently defined by microsphere flow, was markedly reduced compared to non-affected regions and the control normal animal. The radial strain is notably smaller in the risk area after coronary occlusion. The circumferential strain becomes less negative also indicating a loss of function. There was a small decrease in the longitudinal strain as well. The progressive development of regional radial and circumferential strains for 'dog2' is shown in figure 6.

Croisille et al [11] reported similar values (Radial=23.2%, Circum. = −10.5% and Long.=−7.5%) for strains in the normal regions of dog hearts using three-dimensional tagged MRI. However, they observed smaller reductions in strains post-occlusion, which can be attributed to coronary re-perfusion in their model and significantly delayed imaging after the occlusion (2 days later as opposed to 15-20 minutes in our case). This probably allowed for partial recovery of function in the risk region.

4   Conclusions

In this work we have demonstrated that estimates of 3D cardiac deformation can be obtained from ultrasound images, which are consistent with regional blood flow measurements. The estimated strains are also consistent with values reported in the literature using MR tagging [11]. In the future we hope to validate these estimates of regional deformation directly by comparing them to strains concurrently measured from implanted sonomicrometers.

Acknowledgments

The first author would like to thank Farah Janzad for her help with segmenting the images. Additional thanks to Jason Soares and Jennifer Hu for tissue processing and surgical preparation respectively. We also would like to acknowledge support from the National Institutes of Health and the American Heart Association.

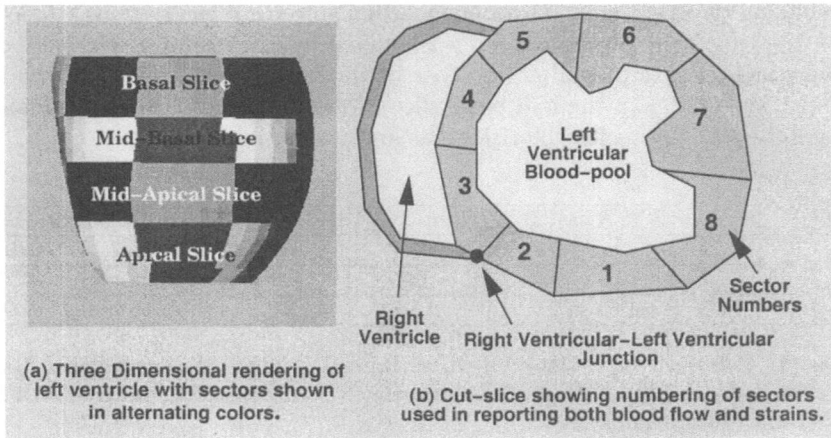

Fig. 5. Division of a slice of the heart for the purpose of reporting results. Each sector consists of approximately 75 elements in the finite element mesh.

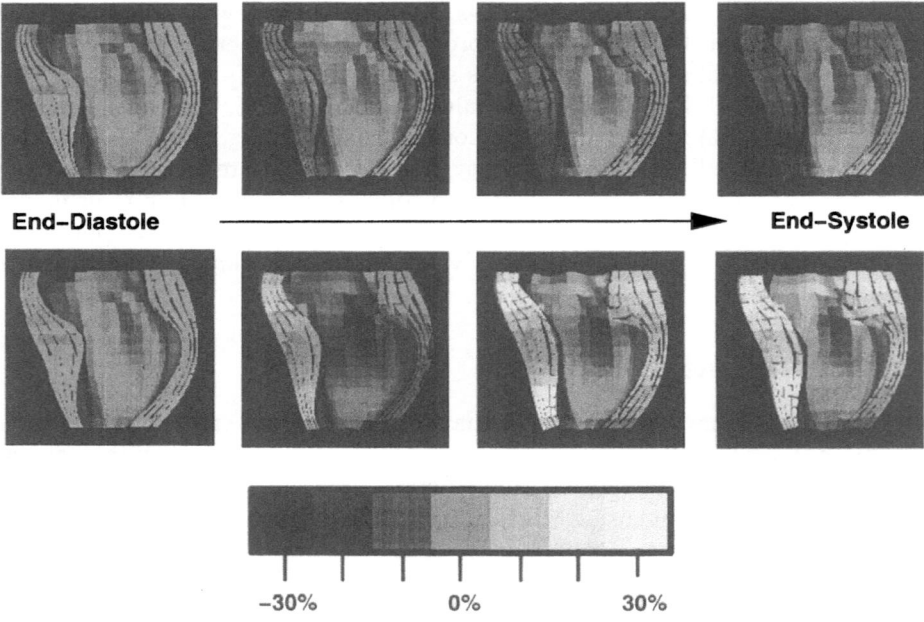

Fig. 6. A long-axis cut-away sectional view of the left ventricle showing circumferential(top) and radial(bottom) strain development in a dog following left anterior descending coronary artery occlusion (on the lower right half of the heart). Note the normal behavior in the left half of the heart. There was positive radial strain (thickening) and negative circumferential strain (shortening) as we move from End Diastole to End Systole. The lower right half of the heart where the affected region was located showed almost the opposite behavior, as expected.

References

1. Sinusas A.J., Trautman K.A., Bergin J.D., Watson D.D., Ruiz M., Smith W.H., and Beller G.A. Quantification of area of risk during coronary occlusion and degree of myocardial salvage after reperfusion with technetium-99m methoxyisobutyl isonitrile. *Circulation*, 82:1424-37, 1990.
2. K. Bathe. *Finite Element Procedures in Engineering Analysis*. Prentice-Hall, New Jersey, 1982.
3. A. Chakraborty, M. Worring, and J.S. Duncan. On multi-feature integration for deformable boundary finding. *Proceedings of the International Conference on Computer Vision*, pages 846–851, 1995.
4. Christiansen G. E., Rabbitt R. D., and Miller M. I. 3D brain mapping using deformable neuroanatomy. *Physics in Medicine and Biology*, 39:609–618, 1994.
5. J. M. Guccione and A. D. McCulloch. Finite element modeling of ventricular mechanics. In P. J. Hunter, A. McCulloch, and P. Nielsen, editors, *Theory of Heart*, pages 122–144. Springer-Verlag, Berlin, 1991.
6. Caidahl K., Kazzam E., Lingberg J., Andersen G. N., Nordanstig J., Dahlqvist S.R., Waldenstro A, and Wikh R. New concept in echocardiography: harmonic imaging of tissue withoug use of contrast agent. *The Lancet*, 352:1264-1270, 1999.
7. Prince J. L. and McVeigh E. R. Motion estimation from tagged mr image sequences. *IEEE Transactions on Medical Imaging*, 11:238–249, June 1992
8. Lawrence E. Malvern. *Introduction to the Mechanics of a Continuous Medium*. Prentice-Hall, Englewood Cliffs, New Jersey, 1969.
9. F. G. Meyer, R. T. Constable, A. G. Sinusas, and J. S. Duncan. Tracking myocardial deformation using spatially constrained velocities. In *Information Processing in Medical Imaging*. Kluwer, 1995.
10. Mulet-Parada Miguel and Noble J. Alison. 2d+t acoustic boundary detection in echocardiography. In *MICCAI*, Boston, Massachusetts, October 1998.
11. Croissile P., Moore C.C., Judd R.M., Lima J.A.C, Arai M., McVeigh E.R., Becker L.C., and Zerhouni E.A. Differentiation of viable and nonviable myocardium by the use of three-dimensional tagged mri in 2-day-old reperfused infarcts. *Circulation*, 99:284-291, 1999.
12. Shi P., Sinusas A.J., Constable R.T., Ritman E., and Duncan J.S. Point-tracked quantitative analysis of left ventricular motion from 3D image sequences. *IEEE Transactions on Medical Imaging*, in-press.
13. J. Park, D. Metaxas, and L. Axel. Volumetric deformable models with parameter functions: a new approach to the 3D motion analysis of the LV from MRI-SPAMM. In *Fifth International Conference on Computer Vision*, pages 700–705, 1995.
14. P. Shi, G. Robinson, A. Chakraborty, L. Staib, R. T. Constable, A. Sinusas, and J. Duncan. A unified framework to assess myocardial function from 4D images. In *Lecture Notes in Computer Science: First International Conference on Computer Vision, Virtual Reality, and Robotics in Medicine*, pages 327–337, 1995.
15. Porter T.R., Xie F., , Kricsfeld A., Chiou A., and Dabestani A. Improved endocardial border resolution using dobutamin stress endocardiography with intravenous sonicated dextrose albumin. *J. Am College of Cardiology*, 23:1440-43, 1994.
16. Papademetris X., Rambo J., Dione D.P., Sinusas A.J., and Duncan J.S. Visually interactive cine-3D segmentation of cardiac mr images. *Suppl. to the J. Am. Coll. of Cardiology Vol. 31, Number 2 (Suppl. A)*, February 1998.
17. Papademetris X., Shi P., Dione D.P., Sinusas A.J., and Duncan J.S. Recovery of soft tissue object deformation using biomechanical models. In *Information Processing in Medical Imaging*, Visegrad, Hungary, June 1999.

Directional Representations of 4D Echocardiography for Temporal Quantification of LV Volume

Elsa ANGELINI[1], Andrew LAINE[1], Shin TAKUMA[2], Shunichi HOMMA[2]

[1] Department of Biomedical Engineering,
Fu Foundation School of Engineering and Applied Science
Columbia University, New York, NY
laine@bme.columbia.edu
[2] Department of Medicine, Echocardiography Laboratories,
College of Physicians and surgeons, Columbia-Presbyterian Medical Center
Columbia University, New York, NY

Abstract. Real-time acquisition via four-dimensional (3D plus time) ultrasound obviates the need for slice registration and reconstruction, leaving segmentation as the only barrier to an automated, rapid, and clinically applicable calculation of accurate left ventricular cavity volumes and ejection fraction. Speckle noise corrupts ultrasound data by introducing sharp changes in an image intensity profile, while attenuation alters the intensity of equally significant cardiac structures, depending on orientation with respect to the position of the ultrasound beam. These properties suggest that measures based on phase information rather than intensity are appropriate for denoising and boundary (surface) detection. Our method relies on the expansion of temporal volume data on a family of basis functions called Brushlets. These basis functions decompose a signal into distinct patterns of oriented textures. Projected coefficients are associated with distinct "brush strokes" of a particular size (width) and orientation (direction). Brushlet decompositions are invariant to intensity (contrast range) but depend on the spatial frequency content of a signal. Preliminary results of this directional space-frequency analysis applied to both phantoms and clinical data are presented. The method will be used to clinically evaluate 4D data and to extract and quantify heart LV volumes.

1 Introduction

Cardiologists are excited about the opportunity for improved clinical and diagnostic performance via new 3D and 4D cardiac acquisition techniques, as they can view a heart at any angle with only one acquisition sequence. This represents a great potential cost savings for health care management as a patient would not need to be recalled in case a traditional echoplanar view did not reveal some crucial aspect of heart function. Also, cardiologists believe that a new visualization tool for displaying volumes in time would improve their diagnostic accuracy regarding tissue characterization and performance measures, such as cardiac output (CO) and ejection fraction (EF), by reducing the (inter-physician) variability of these measures.

Motivation: A diversity of modalities allows for the acquisition of dynamic sequences of cardiac volumes such as CT, Tagged MRI, SPECT and ultrasound. Echocardiography is the fastest, least expensive, and least invasive method for imaging the heart. The simplest and most useful clinical parameter used to assess cardiac function is ejection fraction (EF), calculated as the difference between end diastolic and end systolic left ventricular volumes. However, accurate calculations of ventricular volume from standard echocardiographic data are tedious and costly to employ clinically. This is because existing methods require time to digitize endocardial borders on a series of two-dimensional images, then register the image set and reconstruct each cavity volume.

Real-time acquisition via three-dimensional ultrasound obviates the need for slice registration and reconstruction, leaving segmentation as the remaining barrier to an automated, rapid, and therefore *clinically applicable calculation of accurate left ventricular cavity volumes and ejection fraction.*

Because it provides such a rich description of the temporal and spatial environment of any area of interest, three-dimensional ultrasound also offers the potential for *increased sensitivity* in detecting subtle wall motion abnormality indicative of ischemia (for example during an exercise stress test), compared to fast MRI techniques.

Existing Methods: State of the Art. Extraction of cardiac volume and quantitative analysis of wall deformation is of great interest to researchers in the field of medical imaging. Multigated radionuclide angiography (MUGA) and 2D echocardiography (2DE) are traditional screening techniques used in echocardiography. The main drawback of MUGA is that it requires the injection of a radiopharmaceutical agent. The 2D echocardiography technique is limited by its geometric resolution and by low signal-to-noise ratios (SNR) intrinsic to ultrasound images. Advanced invasive techniques such as Xray-CT and high cost nuclear modalities such as Tagged MRI and SPECT offer excellent resolution in space and time.

The majority of the volume extraction methods are based on prior models of the entire heart or of the left ventricle only. The parametrization of the model generally uses Finite Element models where the volume is constructed after deformation of the model following physics based constraints for equilibrium. Movement of the cardiac wall extracted from temporal data requires some parametrization of the model. Duncan et al. used contour shape descriptors in [1], Ayache; Cohen et al. [2] have used superquadratics. The nature of the constraints varies between models and can take a wide range of properties, including differential constraints [3], displacement and velocity constraints [4] as well as other constraints allowing for non-rigid movements.

Temporal Quantification: A dynamic Measure of CO. As a precursor for volume extraction, our data required some preprocessing to increase available SNR. Indeed it seems that any effort to build a 3D model and apply some deformation to isolate the LV volume from the raw data would be pointless because of the poor signal available for feature analysis. Following this statement, we employed multiscale denoising as a preprocessing step to volume extraction. The design principle of our denoising method relies on the expansion of temporal volume data on a family of basis functions called Brushlets, introduced in 1997 by Meyer and Coifman [5].

These basis functions offer a decomposition of a signal into distinct patterns of oriented textures. In 2D, depending on the tilling of the L^2 domain chosen prior to analysis, the projected coefficients are associated with distinct "brush strokes" of a particular size (width) and orientation (direction). Final denoising is achieved with the construction of gradient maps, thresholding of selected coefficients and reconstruction of an "enhanced/denoised" volume. The reconstructed data serves as an initial guess for volume extraction. The potential of the proposed methodology resides in the mathematical assertion that the problem of 3D surface denoising and detection is more constrained, more accurate in localization (time and space) and more robust when compared to traditional methods of 2D denoising and segmentation.

2 Motivation and Methodology

Raw data acquired from 4D ultrasound has specific characteristics relevant to problems in segmentation. Feature detection should be robust to speckle noise and attenuation artifacts. Speckle noise corrupts the data by introducing sharp changes in an image intensity profile, while attenuation alters the intensity of equally significant cardiac structures, depending on their orientation with respect to the position of the ultrasound beam. *These acquisition properties suggest that measures based on phase information rather than intensity might be more appropriate for denoising and edge detection.* This idea was first expressed and developed on ecocardiography images in a paper by Noble et al. [6, 7]. Their work showed promising results and improvement in the quality of edges detected in the spatio-temporal domain in comparison to the Deriche intensity-based method [8]. Moreover, it is interesting to note that the brushlet decomposition is invariant to intensity and contrast range of an image but depends on the spatial frequency content of a signal. This makes it a very attractive and powerful basis for the analysis of 4D cardiac ultrasound where choosing a single global intensity-based edge threshold is not possible due to position dependent attenuation.

Powerful denoising and segmentation methods have been developed in the context of wavelet analysis [9, 10]. The intuitive principle used in this framework is to consider a domain where features of interest in a signal can be decorrelated from noise allowing for a selective reconstruction of the signal features alone. Wavelet basis functions are characterized by finite time support and localized spectrum in the Fourier domain. Wavelet orthogonal bases are constructed by scaling and translating a single "mother wavelet function". This framework introduces the notion of shift in time and scale, providing a time-scale representation of a signal via wavelet coefficients. Brushlet functions have similar mathematical properties to wavelet functions. A wavelet scale is analogous to a brushlet "brushstroke" characterized by a specific size and an orientation. A brushlet decomposition is carried out on subquadrants of the Fourier domain, where tiling of the domain is analogous to the shifting of wavelet functions, and strong gradient in the transform domain means a discontinuity of pattern orientation. The coefficients do not rely on pixel intensity but on spatial frequency alone.

An overcomplete scheme is essential for accurate preservation of spatial information (features) in the original data set [11].

Brushlet Basis

Brushlet functions are complex valued and well localized in the frequency domain. Their construction is based on a windowed Fourier transform of the Fourier transform of an image. A windowed Fourier basis of the Fourier plane provides a more flexible angular resolution than wavelet packets [12]. The projection on this orthonormal basis of $L^2(\Re)$ provides a decomposition of an image along distinct texture orientations. The initial idea motivating the construction of the brushlet is the desire to build an orthonormal basis of transient functions with good time-frequency localization. For this purpose, windowed complex exponential functions have been used for many years in the context of the sine and cosine transforms. Similarly, Meyer and Coifman introduced a division of the real axis into the subintervals $[a_n, a_{n+1}]$, and a new set of basis functions:

$$u_{j,n}(x) = b_n(x - c_n)e_{j,n}(x) + v(x - a_n)e_{j,n}(2a_n - x) - v(x - a_{n+1})e_{j,n}(2a_{n+1} - x) \quad \text{With}$$

c_n equal to the middle value of $[a_n, a_{n+1}]$, b_n and v are two window funtions, and

$e_{j,n}$ the complex value exponential defined as:. $e_{j,n}(x) = \dfrac{1}{\sqrt{l_n}}e^{-2i\pi\frac{(x-a_n)}{l_n}}$

The windowing functions b_n and v and the basis function $u_{j,n}$ are displayed in Figure 1.

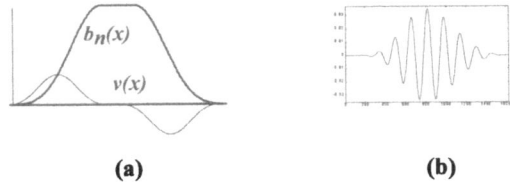

(a)   **(b)**

Figure 1: (a), Windowing function b_n, and bump function v defined on the interval $[a_n-\varepsilon, a_{n+1}+\varepsilon]$. (b), real part of brushlet basis funtion $u_{j,n}$ defined for $j=5$, $l_n=8$, and $\varepsilon=4$.

Suppose we call f a given signal and $\hat{f}$ its Fourier transform. We can project $\hat{f}$ on a brushlet basis, $\hat{f} = \sum_n \sum_j \hat{f}_{n,j} u_{n,j}$ with $u_{n,j}$ the brushlet basis function and $\hat{f}_{n,j}$ the brushlet coefficients. By applying an inverse Fourier transform, we can compute a decomposition of f, $f = \sum_n \sum_j \hat{f}_{n,j} w_{n,j}$ on the orthonormal basis $w_{n,j}$, the inverse Fourier transform of $u_{n,j}$.

The projection of $\hat{f}$ on $u_{n,j}$ is efficiently implemented by a folding technique described by Wickerhauser in [13] and fast Fourier transform (FFT). The reconstruction is simply computed in the same manner by an inverse Fourier transform and unfolding operation.

The 2D and 3D implementations are a direct extrapolation of the 1D projection computation using a tensor product structure. For the 2D brushlet function basis, the x and y axis are divided into subintervals and on each interval, we define a set of orthonormal 2D basis functions $u_{j,n} \otimes u_{m,k}$ and their inverse Fourier transform pair $w_{j,n} \otimes w_{m,k}$.

An illustration of sample 1D and 2D brushlet basis functions computed in this fashion is shown in Figure 2, below. We can observe the difference in spatial and frequency resolution obtained with two different window sizes of b. A good spatial resolution corresponds to a window with small support and is associated with less frequency resolution as shown in Figure 2(a.2-b.2-c.2). Good frequency resolution corresponds to a window with small support and is thus associated with less spatial resolution as shown in Figure 2(a.1-b.1-c.1).

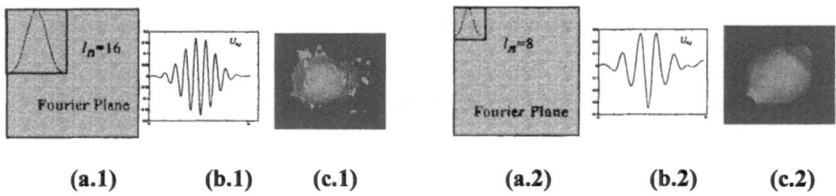

| (a.1) | (b.1) | (c.1) | (a.2) | (b.2) | (c.2) |

Figure 2: Two-dimensional *brushlet* basis functions $u_{n,j} \otimes u_{m,k}$ for $j=5$, $\varepsilon=4$, (a) $l_n=16$, (b) $l_n=8$. (a.1-a.2), Selection of size of the quadrants in the Fourier plane for windowing with b. (b.1-b.2), Real part of 1D brushlet basis function . (a.3-b.3), Real part of 2D brushlet basis .

As the number of quadrants increases, the frequency resolution and the number of distinct brushlet orientations represented increases, while the size of the brush stroke and its spatial resolution decrease at the same time. This tradeoff between spatial and frequency resolution is analogous to the Nyquist uncertainty principle for spectral analysis. We illustrate these theoretical properties in Figure 3 with the use of two mathematical phantoms. To best demonstrate the directional selectivity of a brushlet quadrant we chose as a first example, in Figure 3(a.1 -b.1), a non-specific oriented circular pattern with variable spatial frequency in every direction (concentric circular bands of variable size and gray values). The second phantom, in Figure 3(a.2-b.2), is a 2D representation of a chirp signal.

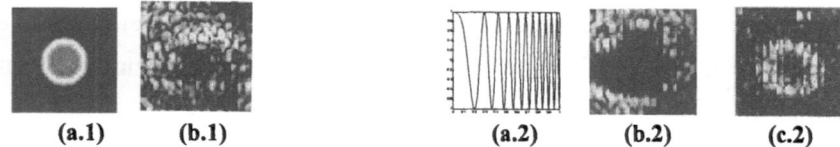

| (a.1) | (b.1) | (a.2) | (b.2) | (c.2) |

Figure 3: (a.1), A mathematical phantom with concentric bands of variable size and gray value. (a.2), Chirp signal in 1D. (b.2), Cross-product of the 1D signal displayed as an image. (b.1 - c.2), Modulus of the brushlet coefficients for a tiling of the Fourier domain into 4 quadrants (b.1) and 16 quadrants (c.2). Note the different pattern orientations in distinct quadrants.

The implementation of this analysis in three dimensions is straightforward. The tensor product structure of the basis allows a direct extrapolation of the 1D case to both 2D and 3D. In terms of implementation, for a given volume data, its 3D Fourier transform is first computed, then each sub-block is folded along the three directions and finally expanded into a 3D exponential basis by a 3D Fourier Transform.

Multiscale Analysis

As described above, the brushlet serves as a basis for analysis of the Fourier transform of the original signal and not the signal itself. The number of subintervals along each dimension of the signal (3 for a volumetric data set) and their position in transform space determine the size and the orientation of the brushstroke. The notion of tiling of the Fourier domain of the signal prior to analysis is illustrated in Figure 4.

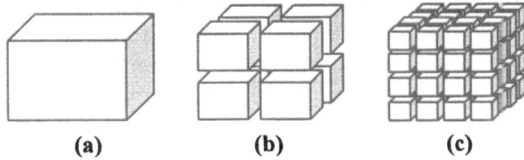

(a)   (b)   (c)

Figure 4: Tiling of the Fourier domain prior to projection on the brushlet basis. (a), Original Fourier Transform of the volume data. (b), Tiling of the Fourier domain into 4 quadrants by dividing each direction in two. Each cube is half the dimension of the original data in each direction. (c), Tiling of the Fourier domain into 64 cubes by dividing each direction by four. Each cube is thus four times smaller than the original volume.

The tiling of the Fourier sub-spaces determines the number distinct directional brushlet basis used for the analysis and their size (i.e., the more quadrants defined, the more *angular directions* for a particular brush stroke are available). The coefficient domain is the same size as the sub-cubes for each brushstroke. Therefore, the smaller the quadrants, the more precise is the frequency resolution of the analysis and the better the resolution at each spatial frequency, or scale. It is important to note that the improvement in frequency resolution implies a loss in spatial resolution as the number of coefficients influencing the reconstruction of the whole signal diminishes with the size of the cube.

The notion of multiscale decomposition can be extended with the brushlet basis by analogy to the wavelet structure. In this context, we analyze our signal with different tiling and manipulate independently different scales for different orientations. Coifman and Meyer exploited this property for optimal compression. In this study, we have used it for denoising and enhancement by eliminating the most outer quadrants as high-frequency noisy components and reconstructing with selected low frequency (inner-quadrants) coefficients. More precisely, in the example displayed in Figure 4, the eight cubes of the tiling in (b) correspond in terms of direction and frequency to the eight inner cubes of the finer tiling shown in (c). The frequency resolution in (b) is less than in (c) but the spatial resolution is inversely finer. Multiscale analysis in this context consists of tracking directional patterns within the eight cubes of (b) corresponding to the eight inner cubes of (c), at a lower scale of analysis.

Overcomplete Framework

Recall that the size of the cubes created with the tiling of the Fourier domain determines the size of the coefficient domain associated with each characteristic brushstroke of a cube. The diminution of dimension between the spatial domain and the transform domain is analogous to a two-fold downsampling in dyadic wavelet analysis. This downsampling is problematic when manipulating transform coefficients, because there is not a homomorphism between the original signal and coefficient domains.

The theory of overcomplete multiscale analysis has been developed to overcome this mathematical limitation. Overcomplete multiscale representations are well suited for image analysis and denoising/enhancement, because they avoid aliasing effects introduced by critically sampled representations [14] and yield a shift invariant representation. In our case, the aliasing effect arises from the selection of overlapping subintervals on the Fourier plane that are expanded into a local Fourier basis. To avoid this and increase the number of coefficients within the same subinterval size, we project onto an extended Fourier basis. This increases the matrix size of the projection domain without changing the original signal. The overcomplete projection is efficiently implemented by padding the original signal with zeros and computing its FFT. Since padding a signal will increase the resolution of the FFT, overcomplete projections increase the number of coefficients for the same interval and therefore the resolution in the transform (coefficient) plane as illustrated in Figure 5.

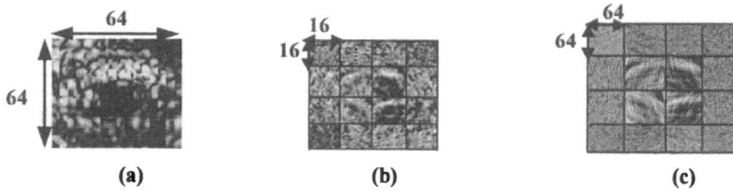

(a)   (b)   (c)

Figure 5: (a) Original cardiac ultrasound slice (64 × 64 pixels) from 4D data. (b-c), Real part of coefficients for a 16-quadrant tiling of the Fourier plane in the non-overcomplete case (b), and overcomplete case (c). In (b), the dimension of each quadrant is four times smaller than the original image matrix size . In (c), each coefficient quadrant has the same dimension as the original image matrix.

Thresholding for Denoising

Images formed with coherent energy such as ultrasound suffer from speckle noise. This type of noise consists of a granular pattern and is correlated with the surface characteristics of an organ and orientation of the beam. The resulting image degradation has a significant impact on image quality, interpretation and post processing.

More recently several spatial and frequency based denoising techniques have been investigated for echoplanar ultrasound images [15], [16], [17]. However, these traditional methods often reduce noise at the cost of blurring edge features. For this reason multiscale analysis has been intensively tested as a denoising tool [9, 18]. The general scheme for denoising is achieved by lowering or eliminating noise energy via coefficient thresholding or 'shrinkage". Of particular interest to us is the recent work of Zong, Laine and Geiser [19], using non-linear thresholding on dyadic wavelet coefficients for speckle reduction. It showed a significant advantage by reducing interphysician variability in quantification of cardiac areas, leading to an improved accuracy in the diagnosis of coronary disease. Thresholding is based on the assumption that the noise component can be isolated in certain projection coefficients while energy of a signal is largely concentrated in separate coefficient sets (sub-spaces). This approach has been successfully applied for many years within wavelet decompositions via frames [20], [9].

In our study, we used the threshold selection method for coefficient shrinkage in an orthonormal basis developed by Donoho and Jonhstone [21] and investigated by Mallat in [20]. After projecting original data on a selected basis, we applied a hard thresholding on the projected coefficients in the transform domain as defined below.

The value of the threshold level was empirically deduced from distinct image properties and the projection coefficients' distribution. After the thresholding operation, the denoised signal was simply reconstructed with the new set of coefficients.

Results

Volume analysis with brushlet basis and gradient volume visualization was tested on three different volumes of increasing complexity: (1) a mathematical phantom with three intensity levels of gray, (2) a contrast echocardiogram and, (3) a clinical volume data set.

The 3D-ultrasound acquisition machine used in this study was the Model 1 RT3D (Volumetric Medical Imaging Inc, Durham, NC), originally developed at Duke University [22]. A single volumetric data acquisition cycle requires around 70ms at a depth setting between 10 and 15 cm. A transthoracic 2.5 MHz matrix array transducer scans the 3D volume electronically. The resolution of the acquisition is 64×64 pixels in the short axis plane and an average of 300 pixels in the long axis plane. The clinical volume processed in this study was of size $64 \times 64 \times 64$, and the phantom volumes were made to match these same dimensions.

The three volumes were analyzed with the brushlet basis for a tiling of the Fourier domain in eight cubes with overcomplete representations. This analysis provided a decomposition of four brushstrokes represented by paired diagonal cubes. The brushstroke orientation in each of the three directions was +/-45° for each cube.

Visualization in 3D used isosurfaces and isovolumes at selected levels. The level was set as the maximum value of each gradient volume, in the transform domain. The "marching cube" algorithm was used for the isovolume computation [23].

1.   A **mathematical phantom** created with three gray levels is illustrated in Figure 6(a.1-b.1-c.1-d.1). It consists of two ovoid shapes, one inside the other one. The initial geometry of the phantom is known *a priori*. The edges were blurred with a median filter, prior to processing. This example is provided to clearly visualize the concept of a gradient volume in the transform domain. The maximum gradient values were located in the inter-space between the two ovoid objects. Reconstruction after hard tresholding returned the original volume with negligible numerical error.

2.   An *in-vitro* **contrast echocardiogram phantom** that consists in a balloon, filled with human albumin and sonicator bubbles as a contrast agent, immerged in a water tank is shown in Figure 6. A volume was recorded with the same 3D-ultrasound machine used in clinical screenings. A typical slice (64×64 pixels) of the volume data is

displayed in Figure 6(a.2) below. The inner black cavity corresponds to the albumin tissue inside the balloon. The surrounding white layer is an artifact created by the bubble accumulation on the inner surface of the balloon wall. The corresponding gradient volume in the transform space is displayed in Figure 6(b.2-d.2). We observed a very efficient outline of the inner cavity of albumin from the outside of the balloon.

3.   A **clinical volume data** set was acquired with the same clinical 3D-ultrasound transducer. The patient lied on a gantry during the screening examination and an apical view of the left ventricle and atrium is acquired by placing the beam on his/her lateral costal margin. The data are presented in Figure 6(a.3-c.3).

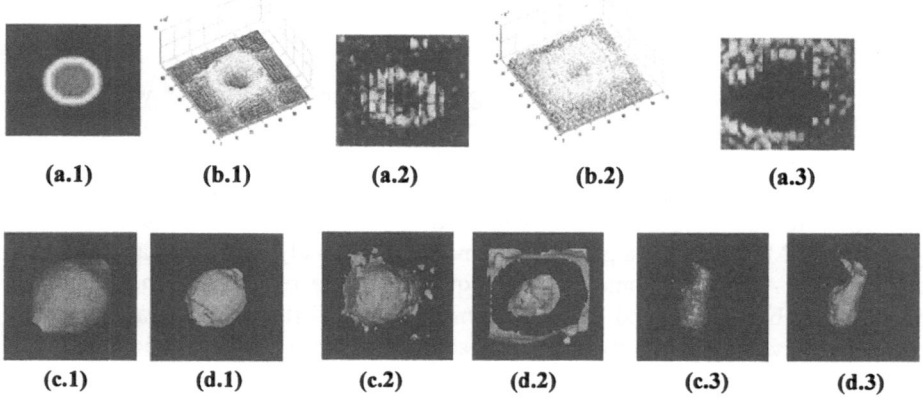

| (a.1) | (b.1) | (a.2) | (b.2) | (a.3) |

| (c.1) | (d.1) | (c.2) | (d.2) | (c.3) | (d.3) |

Figure 6: (a.1-b.1-c.1-d.1), Mathematical phantom. (a.2-b.2-c.2-d.2), Contrast echocardiogram phantom. (a.3-c.3-d.3), Clinical volume data. (a.1-a.2-a.3), 2D slice in cross section of the volume data. (c.1-c.2), Volume visualization of the phantoms. (c.1). (b.1-b.2), Plot of the gradient in the transform plane for one slice of the domain. (d.1-d.2), Isosurface of the maximum gradient in the transform domain. (c.3-d.3), Volume visualization of the gradient in the transform plane for an 8-cubes (c.3) and 64-cubes (d.3) tiling of the Fourier domain.

Validation of Gradient volumes in Transform Domain In order to validate our gradient volumes as a "valid" representation of the data in terms of feature shapes and locations we asked an expert in echocardiography to manually digitize the volume data of the contrast phantom and the clinical echocardiograms. The manual segmentation was performed on sixty four 2D slices of the volumes (64×64×64 pixels). The result of the superposition of the gradient volumes and the manually segmented volumes is displayed in Figure 7. Regarding the phantom data in Figure 7(a), the match between the gradient data (isosurface of maximum value) in the transform domain and the manually segmented volume of the albumin cavity is excellent. Please note that the isosurface describes the inner albumin cavity and the outer balloon wall separated by the bubble layer. Indeed the gradient in directional information between the two layers is high. The match for the clinical data, as displayed in Figure 7(b), is also very impressive. The most striking result in the transform domain is our *ability to isolate information from the ventricular papillary muscles and the wall muscular* *pattern*. The sample manual segmentation did not trace the papillary muscles. This difference in contour is distinguishable in Figure 7(b) at the "neck" of the gradient volume, where the papillary muscles insert (see arrow). This is a remarkable result since systematic errors usually prohibit visualization of papillary muscles in 3D from traditional 2D gated data.

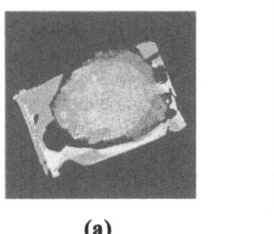   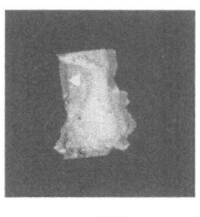

(a)   (b)

Figure 7: Comparison between manually segmented contours and gradient isosurfaces at maximal values for echocardiographic phantom (a) and clinical data (b). (a), Volume visualization of the gradient inner isosurface surrounded by the manually extracted volume of the balloon. (b), Volume visualization of the gradient isosurface at maximum value surrounded by manually extracted volume of the left ventricle. The papillary muscles were not segmented manually but are correctly isolated by the gradient surface.

Denoising Performance. Denoising performance via hard tresholding was evaluated for an empirical threshold value of 20% of the maximum coefficient values of each cube. The clinical data set was decomposed into an eight-cube ($2 \times 2 \times 2$) tiling of the Fourier domain. Quantitative measurements of image quality improvement are difficult. We plan to follow the validation approach of Laine et al. [19] by using cardiologist performance for denoising quality assessment. A first observation of the denoised volume data showed improvement in the smoothness of the LV edges. However a loss in contrast was observed in the reconstructed voxels.

Conclusion

Our method for feature extraction used a hybrid technique to combine model based and directional denoising and segmentation in three dimensions by identifying efficient projection coefficients within sets of redundant articulated (orientation rich) bases. The results of our method will be used to clinically evaluate new 4D ultrasound (3D plus time) acquisition techniques and provide an accurate method to quantify heart volumes from this type of data. This is a very exciting challenge since this type of data is totally new. A future study will aim at modeling the heart volume at systole and diastole and then study of myocardium deformation patterns to characterize and isolate areas of ischemic tissue. The development of non- invasive measurement techniques of cardiac tissue stress and strain is of major clinical importance. The result of our proposed analysis would provide a valuable imaging tool for modeling cardiac volumes.

References

[1]   J. Duncan, R. Owen, L. Staib, and P. Anandan, "Measurement of non-rigid motion using contour shape descriptors," presented at Computer Vision and Pattern Recognition, 1991.

[2]   Eric Bardinet, Laurent D. Cohen, and N. Ayache, "Tracking and motion analysis of the left ventricle with deformable superquadratics," *Medical Image Analysis*, vol. 1, pp. 129-149, 1996.

[3]   S. Benayoum, C. Nastar, and N. Ayache, "Dense non-rigid motion estimation in sequence of 3D images using differential constraints," presented at Conference on ComputerVision , Virtual Reality and Robotics in Medicine, Nice, France, 1995.

[4]   P. Shi, G. Robinson, C. Constable, A. Sinusas, and J. Duncan, "A model-based integrated approach to track myocardial deformation using displacement and velocity constraints.," presented at IEEE International Conference on Computer Vision, Cambridge, MA, 1995.

[5]   F. Meyer and R. R. Coifman, "Brushlets: A tool for directional image analysis and image compression," *Applied and computational harmonic analysis*, vol. 4, pp. 147-187, 1997.

[6]   Miguel Mulet-Parada and J. A. Noble, "2D+T acoustic boundary detection in ecocardiography," presented at Medical Image Computing and Computer-Assisted Intervention-MICCAI'98, Boston, MA, 1998.

[7]   G. Jacob, J. A. Noble, M. Mulet-Parada, and A. Blake, "Evaluating a robust contour tracker on echocardiographic sequences," *Medical Image Analysis*, vol. 3, pp. 63-75, 1999.

[8]   R. Deriche, "Fast algorithms for low-level vision.," *Patter Analysis and Machine Intelligence*, vol. 12, pp. 78-87, 1990.

[9]   D. L. Donoho and I. Jonhstone, "Ideal denoising in an orthonormal basis chosen from a library of bases," *Comptes Rendus de l'Academie des Sciences, Paris, Serie I*, vol. 319, pp. 1317-1322, 1994.

[10]   J. Fan and A. F. Laine, "Multiscale contrast enhancement and denoising in digital radiographs," in *Wavelets in Medicine and Biology*, A. Aldroubi and M. Unser, Eds. Boca Raton, FL: CRC Press, 1996, pp. 163-189.

[11]   A. F. Laine, J. Fan, and W. Yang, "Wavelets for contrast enhancement of digital mammography," *IEEE Engineering in Medicine and Biology Society Magazine*, vol. 14, pp. 536-550, 1995.

[12]   M. V. Wickerhauser, "Smooth localized orthonormal bases," *Comptes Rendus de l'Academie des Sciences, Paris I*, pp. 423-427, 1993.

[13]   P. Ausher, G. Weiss, and M. V. Wickerhauser, "Local sine and cosine bases of Coifman and Meyer and the construction of smooth wavelets," in *Wavelets- A tutorial in Theory and Applications*, vol. 2, *Wavelet Analysis and its Applications*, C. K. Chui, Ed. San Diego: Academic Press, 1992, pp. 237-256.

[14]   S. Mallat, "A theory for multiresolution signal decomposition: The wavelet representation," *IEEE Transactions on Pattern Analysis and Machine Intelligence*, vol. 11, pp. 674-693, 1989.

[15]   E. A. Geiser, D. C. Wilson, G. L. Gibby, J. Billet, and D. A. Conetta, "A method for evaluation of enhancement operations in two-dimensional echocardiographic images," *Journal of the American Society of Echocardiography*, vol. 4, pp. 235-246, 1991.

[16]   S. M. Collins, D. J. Skorton, E. A. Geiser, J. A. Nichols, D. A. Conetta, N. G. Pandian, and R. E. Kerber, "Computer-assisted edge detection in two-dimensional echocardiography: comparison with anatomic data," *Journal of the American Society of Echocardiography*, vol. 53, pp. 1380-1387, 1984.

[17]   M. J. Lester, J. F. Brenner, and W. D. Selles, "Local transforms for biomedical image analysis," *Computer Graphics, Image Processing*, vol. 13, pp. 17-30, 1980.

[18]   D. L. Donoho and I. M. Johnstone, "Threshold selection for wavelet shrinkage of noisy data," presented at 16th Annual Int. Conference of the IEEE Engineering in Medicine and Biology Society, 1994.

[19]   Xuli Zong, Andrew F. Laine, and E. A. Geiser, "Speckle reduction and contrast enhancement of echocardiograms via multiscale nonlinear processing," *IEEE Transactions on Medical Imaging*, vol. 17, pp. 532-540, 1998.

[20]   S. Mallat, *A Wavelet Tour of Signal Processing*, 1998.

[21]   D. L. Donoho and I. M. Johnstone, "Ideal spatial adaptation via wavelet shrinkage,"*Biometrika*, vol. 81, pp. 425-455, 1994.

[22]   S. W. S. Olaf T. Von Ramm, "Real time volumetric ultrasound imaging system," *Journal of Digital Imaging*, vol. 3, pp. 261-266, 1990.

[23]   A. V. S. Inc., "AVS/Express, Developer Edition," , 4.1 ed. Waltham, MA, 1998.

Image Processing for Diffusion Tensor Magnetic Resonance Imaging

C.-F. Westin, S.E. Maier, B. Khidhir, P. Everett, F.A. Jolesz, and R. Kikinis

Surgical Planning Lab, Radiology, Brigham and Women's Hospital,
westin@bwh.harvard.edu, Harvard Medical School, Boston

Abstract. This paper describes image processing techniques for Diffusion Tensor Magnetic Resonance. In Diffusion Tensor MRI, a tensor describing local water diffusion is acquired for each voxel. The geometric nature of the diffusion tensors can quantitatively characterize the local structure in tissues such as bone, muscles, and white matter of the brain. The close relationship between local image structure and apparent diffusion makes this image modality very interesting for medical image analysis.

We present a decomposition of the diffusion tensor based on its symmetry properties resulting in useful measures describing the geometry of the diffusion ellipsoid. A simple anisotropy measure follows naturally from this analysis. We describe how the geometry, or shape, of the tensor can be visualized using a coloring scheme based on the derived shape measures. We show how filtering of the tensor data of a human brain can provide a description of macrostructural diffusion which can be used for measures of fiber-tract organization. We also describe how tracking of white matter tracts can be implemented using the introduced methods. These methods offers unique tools for the *in vivo* demonstration of neural connectivity in healthy and diseased brain tissue.

1 Introduction

Diffusion Tensor Magnetic Resonance Imaging (DT-MRI) is a recent MR imaging modality. In Diffusion Tensor MRI, a tensor describing local water diffusion is acquired for each voxel. Diffusion in tissue can be anisotropic depending on the characteristics of the tissue. For example in the white matter fiber tracts the diffusion is mainly in the direction of the fibers. In areas with fluid, such in the CSF filled ventricles, the diffusion is spherical, i.e. isotropic. The advent of robust diffusion tensor imaging techniques has prompted the development of quantitative measures for describing the diffusion anisotropy. A good review by Basser and Pierpaoli can be found in [1].

Since MRI methods in general always obtain a macroscopic measure of a microscopic quantity which necessarily entails intravoxel averaging, the voxel dimensions influence the measured diffusion tensor at any particular location in the brain.

Factors which would affect the shape of the apparent diffusion tensor (shape of the diffusion ellipsoid) in the white matter include the density of fibers, the degree of myelination, the average fiber diameter and the directional similarity of the fibers in the voxel. The geometric nature of the measured diffusion tensor within a voxel is thus a meaningful measure of fiber tract organization.

With current conventional proton magnetic resonance imaging (MRI) techniques, the white matter of the brain appears to be a remarkably homogeneous tissue without any suggestion of the complex arrangement of fiber tracts. Although the individual axons and the surrounding myelin sheaths cannot be revealed with the limited spatial resolution of *in vivo* imaging, distinct bands of white matter fibers with parallel orientation may be distinguished from others running in different directions if MRI techniques are sensitized to water diffusion and the preferred direction of diffusion is determined.

Water diffusion in tissue due to Brownian motion is random but some structural characteristics of tissues may limit diffusion. In the white matter, the mobility of the water is restricted in the directions perpendicular to the axons which are oriented along the fiber tracts. This anisotropic diffusion is due to the presence of tightly packed multiple myelin membranes encompassing the axon. Myelination is not essential for diffusion anisotropy of nerves as shown in studies of nonmyelinated garfish olfactory nerves [3] and anisotropy exists in brains of neonates before the histological appearance of myelin [16] but myelin is widely assumed to be the major barrier to diffusion in myelinated fiber tracts. Therefore the demonstration of anisotropic diffusion in brain by magnetic resonance has opened the way to explore noninvasively the structural anatomy of the white matter *in vivo* [8, 4, 1, 10].

2   Materials and Methods

In this work we applied a modified version of the recently proposed Line Scan Diffusion Imaging (LSDI) technique [7]. This method, like the commonly used diffusion-sensitized, ultrafast, echo-planar imaging (EPI) technique [12] is relatively insensitive to bulk motion and physiologic pulsations of vascular origin. But unlike EPI, LSDI exhibits minimal image distortion, does not require cardiac gating, head restraints or post-processing image correction, and can be implemented without specialized hardware on all standard MRI scanners.

Here, we present a quantitative characterization of the geometric nature of the diffusion tensors, a method for characterization of marcostructural diffusion properties, and a display method for showing clear and detailed *in vivo* images of human white matter tracts. The orientation and distribution of most of the known major fiber tracts can be identified using these methods.

2.1   Imaging Parameters

Our data were acquired at the Brigham and Women's Hospital on a GE Signa 1.5 Tesla Horizon Echospeed 5.6 system with standard 2.2 Gauss/cm field gradients. The time required for acquisition of the diffusion tensor data for one slice was 1 min; no averaging was performed. Imaging parameters were: effective TR=2.4 s,

TE=65 ms, b_{high}=750 s/mm^2, b_{low}=5 s/mm^2, field of view 22 cm, effective voxel size 4.8×1.6×1.5 mm^3, 6 kHz readout bandwidth, acquisition matrix 128×128.

The gradient cycle in the LSDI interleaving scheme was modified to provide acquisition of more gradient directions and to allow elimination of the crusher gradients. Instead of alternating merely between high and low gradient strengths, the modified sequence cycled through eight configurations of the diffusion gradients. In all other respects it was identical to the sequence described in [7].

2.2   Calculation of Tensors

For each slice, eight images are collected with different diffusion weightings and noncollinear gradient directions. If S_0 represents the signal intensity in the absence of a diffusion-sensitizing field gradient and S the signal intensity in the presence of gradient $\mathbf{g} = (g_x, g_y, g_z)^T$, the equation for the loss in signal intensity due to diffusion is given by the Stejskal-Tanner formula:

$$\ln(S) = \ln(S_0) - \gamma^2\delta^2(\Delta - \delta/3)\mathbf{g}^T\mathbf{D}\mathbf{g}, \tag{1}$$

where γ is the gyromagnetic ratio of hydrogen ^{1}H (protons), δ is the duration of the diffusion sensitizing gradient pulses and Δ is the time between the centers of the two gradient pulses. The eight images provide eight equations for S in each voxel which are solved in a least-squares sense for the 6−1 unknowns: the six independent components of the symmetric diffusion tensor, $\mathbf{D}$, and S_0. In the LSDI sequence, it is easy to show that cross terms between the slice select gradient for the 180° pulse and the diffusion sensitizing gradients account for less than 0.1% of the diffusion weighting, and have therefore been neglected here. Diffusion attenuation due to imaging gradients is already factored into S_0, as is T$_2$ weighting.

2.3   Geometrical Measures of Diffusion

In order to relate the measure of diffusion anisotropy to the structural geometry of the tissue a mathematical description of diffusion tensors and their quantification is necessary [1]. First, a complete diffusion tensor, $\mathbf{D}$, is calculated (Equation 1) for each voxel. Using the symmetry properties of the diffusion ellipsoid we decomposed the diffusion tensor, and from the tensor basis assigned scalar measures, describing the linearity and the anisotropy, to each voxel [15].

The diffusion tensor can be visualized using an ellipsoid where the principal axes correspond to the directions of the eigenvector system. Let $\lambda_1 \geq \lambda_2 \geq \lambda_3 \geq 0$ be the eigenvalues of the symmetric tensor $\mathbf{D}$, and let $\hat{\mathbf{e}}_i$ be the normalized eigenvector corresponding to λ_i.

$$\mathbf{D} = \lambda_1\hat{\mathbf{e}}_1\hat{\mathbf{e}}_1^T + \lambda_2\hat{\mathbf{e}}_2\hat{\mathbf{e}}_2^T + \lambda_3\hat{\mathbf{e}}_3\hat{\mathbf{e}}_3^T \tag{2}$$

Diffusion can be divided into three basic cases depending on the rank, of the representation tensor:

1) Linear case ($\lambda_1 \gg \lambda_2 \simeq \lambda_3$): diffusion is mainly in the direction corresponding to the largest eigenvalue,

$$\mathbf{D} \simeq \lambda_1 \mathbf{D}_l = \lambda_1 \hat{\mathbf{e}}_1 \hat{\mathbf{e}}_1^T. \tag{3}$$

2) Planar case ($\lambda_1 \simeq \lambda_2 \gg \lambda_3$): diffusion is restricted to a plane spanned by the two eigenvectors corresponding to the two largest eigenvalues,

$$\mathbf{D} \simeq 2\lambda_1 \mathbf{D}_p = \lambda_1 (\hat{\mathbf{e}}_1 \hat{\mathbf{e}}_1^T + \hat{\mathbf{e}}_2 \hat{\mathbf{e}}_2^T). \tag{4}$$

3) Spherical case ($\lambda_1 \simeq \lambda_2 \simeq \lambda_3$): isotropic diffusion,

$$\mathbf{D} \simeq 3\lambda_1 \mathbf{D}_s = \lambda_1 (\hat{\mathbf{e}}_1 \hat{\mathbf{e}}_1^T + \hat{\mathbf{e}}_2 \hat{\mathbf{e}}_2^T + \hat{\mathbf{e}}_3 \hat{\mathbf{e}}_3^T). \tag{5}$$

In general, the diffusion tensor $\mathbf{D}$ will be a combination of these cases. Expanding the diffusion tensor using these cases as a basis gives:

$$\begin{aligned}
\mathbf{D} &= \lambda_1 \hat{\mathbf{e}}_1 \hat{\mathbf{e}}_1^T + \lambda_2 \hat{\mathbf{e}}_2 \hat{\mathbf{e}}_2^T + \lambda_3 \hat{\mathbf{e}}_3 \hat{\mathbf{e}}_3^T \\
&= (\lambda_1 - \lambda_2) \hat{\mathbf{e}}_1 \hat{\mathbf{e}}_1^T + (\lambda_2 - \lambda_3)(\hat{\mathbf{e}}_1 \hat{\mathbf{e}}_1^T + \hat{\mathbf{e}}_2 \hat{\mathbf{e}}_2^T) \\
&\quad + \lambda_3 (\hat{\mathbf{e}}_1 \hat{\mathbf{e}}_1^T + \hat{\mathbf{e}}_2 \hat{\mathbf{e}}_2^T + \hat{\mathbf{e}}_3 \hat{\mathbf{e}}_3^T) \\
&= (\lambda_1 - \lambda_2) \mathbf{D}_l + (\lambda_2 - \lambda_3) \mathbf{D}_p + \lambda_3 \mathbf{D}_s
\end{aligned}$$

where $(\lambda_1 - \lambda_2)$, $(\lambda_2 - \lambda_3)$ and λ_3 are the coordinates of $\mathbf{D}$ in the tensor basis $\{\mathbf{D}_l, \mathbf{D}_p, \mathbf{D}_s\}$. A similar tensor shape analysis has proven to be useful in a number of computer vision applications [13, 14, 6].

As described, the relationships between the eigenvalues of the diffusion tensor can be used for classification of the diffusion tensor according to geometrically meaningful criteria. By using the coordinates of the tensor in our new basis measures are obtained of how close the diffusion tensor is to the generic cases of line, plane and sphere. The generic shape of a tensor is obtained by normalizing with a magnitude measure of the diffusion. Here we define this magnitude as the largest eigenvalues of the tensor. This gives for the linear, planar and spherical measures:

$$c_l = \frac{\lambda_1 - \lambda_2}{\lambda_1} \tag{6}$$

$$c_p = \frac{\lambda_2 - \lambda_3}{\lambda_1} \tag{7}$$

$$c_s = \frac{\lambda_3}{\lambda_1} \tag{8}$$

$$c_l + c_p + c_s = 1 \tag{9}$$

An anisotropy measure describing the deviation from the spherical case is achieved as follows:

$$c_a = c_l + c_p = 1 - c_s = 1 - \frac{\lambda_3}{\lambda_1} \tag{10}$$

2.4   Relaxation of Data

For many medical image analysis procedures preprocessing of the data in order to reduce the image noise level is important [5]. For diffusion data, regularization based on a Markov model was used to achieve more stable directionality information for tracking white matter fiber tracts [11].

In this paper we argue for staying in the tensor domain when processing simplifies cleaning up of the data. Simple averaging of the tensor components has proven to be a robust relaxation method. One reason for the usefulness of this approach is that tensors have more degrees of freedom compared to scalars and vectors. This is illustrated in Figure 1. Adding two vectors (a) and (b) results in a new vector (c). The data (a) and (b) and the result (c) are of the same order. However, adding two rank 1 tensors (d) and (e), e.g. diffusion tensors from two differently oriented white matter tracts, results in a rank 2 tensor (f), i.e. the output has more degrees of freedom than the input tensors and describes the plane in which diffusion is present. Averaging of tensors are different from averaging a vector field:

- The average of a set of vectors gives the "mean event"
- The average of a set of tensors gives the "mean event" and the "range of the present events"

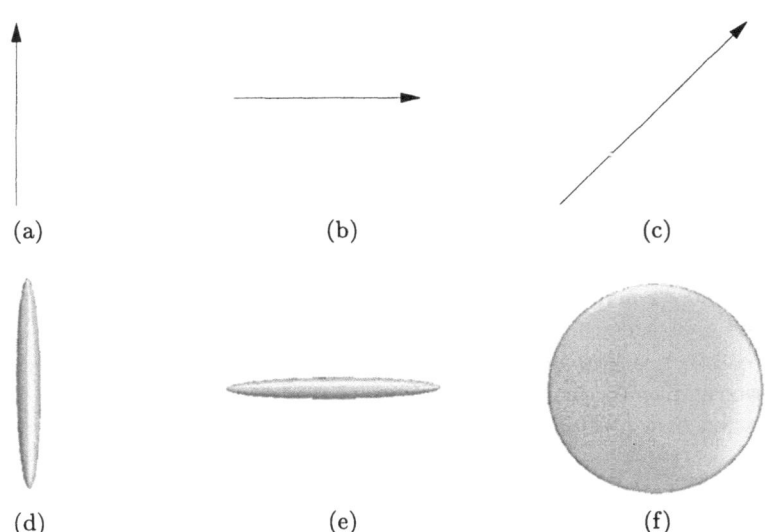

Fig. 1. Vector and tensor summation. Two vectors, (a) and (b), and their sum (c). Two diffusion tensors, (d) and (e), of rank close to 1 visualized as ellipsoids with eigenvectors forming principal axes. The summation of the two tensors gives a rank 2 tensor (f).

Figure 2 shows two stylized 2D examples illustrating the effect of relaxation of a diffusion tensor field. (a) Relaxation of a field that contains inconsistent data (left) gives a result of almost round ellipses (right). In (b) relaxation of a field containing data with a clear bias in one direction resulting in a more stable estimate of the directionality of the field.

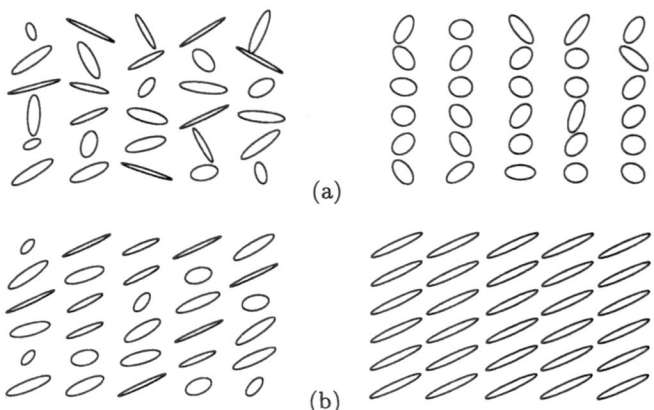

(a)

(b)

Fig. 2. Stylized 2D examples illustrating the effect of relaxation of a diffusion tensor field. (a) Relaxation of a field that contains inconsistent data (left) gives a result of almost round ellipses (right). (b) Relaxation of a field containing data with a clear bias in one direction.

2.5   Macrostructural Diffusive Similarities

In the previous section we characterized diffusion isotropy and anisotropy within a voxel. Here, we will introduce a new method for examining the pattern or distribution of diffusion within an image volume.

Basser and Pierpaoli proposed a scalar measure for macrostructural diffusive similarity based on summing tensor inner products between the center voxel tensor and its neighbors [2]. As in a vector case, the inner product between two tensors measures their degree of similarity.

We will use this idea, and show that averaging the diffusion tensor field has a close relation to this approach. A weighted linear sum of tensor inner products operation over an image volume can be expressed as

$$\sum_k \langle \mathbf{D}(\mathbf{x}), a(\mathbf{x}_k)\mathbf{D}(\mathbf{x}_k)\rangle = \langle \mathbf{D}(\mathbf{x}), \sum_k a(\mathbf{x}_k)\mathbf{D}(\mathbf{x}_k)\rangle = \langle \mathbf{D}(\mathbf{x}), \mathbf{D}_a(\mathbf{x})\rangle \quad (11)$$

where the brackets denote inner product, $a(\mathbf{x}_k)$ is a spatial mask defining the local image volume of interest around $\mathbf{x}$, k is an index ordering the voxel in this volume. $\mathbf{D}_a$ is a weighted average of the tensors in the neighborhood under the mask a, $\sum_k a(\mathbf{x}_k)\mathbf{D}(\mathbf{x}_k)$. Or, in other words, the filtered output from applying

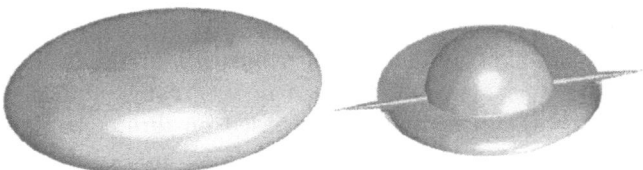

Fig. 3. Comparison of an ellipsoid and a composite shape depicting the same tensor with eigenvalues $\lambda_1 = 1$, $\lambda_2 = 0.7$, and $\lambda_3 = 0.4$.

the filter $a(\mathbf{x}_k)$ to the data $\mathbf{D}(\mathbf{x}_k)$. Note that averaging of a diffusion tensor field and then deriving a scalar measure from the averaged field is *not the same* as averaging a scalar field derived from the original field.

Equation 11 shows that the scalar macrostructural measure is an inner product between a diffusion tensor with a blurred version of itself. This can be seen as inner products between tensors in a scale pyramid where the tensors with highest spatial resolution, and tensors at a level in the scale pyramid corresponding to the size of interest (scale obtained by blurring with mask a). Figure 4 (rightmost column) shows three level of such a pyramid.

The rank of the average tensor $\mathbf{D}_a$ describes the complexity of the macroscopic diffusion structure. If the rank is close to one, the structure is highly linear which will be the case in regions of bundles of fibers having the same direction. If the rank is two, fibers are crossing in a plane, or the underlying diffusitivity is planar. Instead of carrying out the inner product in Equation 11, to get a scalar value for similarity, we use the tensor $\mathbf{D}_a$ as a description of macrostructural diffusion.

2.6 Visualization of Diffusion Tensors

A 3D diffusion tensor can be visualized using an ellipsoid where the principal axes correspond to the tensor's eigenvector system. However, it is difficult to distinguish between an edge-on, flat ellipsoid and an oblong one using the surface shading information. Similar ambiguity exists between a face-on, flat ellipsoid and a sphere. We propose two techniques for the visualization of tensor fields that overcome the problems with ellipsoids. Figure 3 compares the ellipsoidal representation of a tensor with a composite shape whose linear, planar, and spherical components are scaled according to c_l, c_p, and c_s.

Additionally, coloring based on the shape measures c_l, c_p, and c_s can be used for visualization of shape. Figure 6 shows a coloring scheme where the color is interpolated between the blue linear case, the yellow planar case, and the red spherical case.

2.7   Eigenvalue Transformations

Smoothing a diffusion tensor field removes high frequency noise and as discussed above stabilizes the field. In this section we discuss methods that changes the eigenvalues of the tensors in a way that further can stabilize the data. Let $\mathbf{D} = \sum_{k=1}^{3} \lambda_k \hat{\mathbf{e}}_k \hat{\mathbf{e}}_k^T$. The first method is based on direct manipulation of the eigenvalues λ_k.

$$\mathbf{T} = \sum_{k=1}^{3} f_k(\lambda_k) \hat{\mathbf{e}}_k \hat{\mathbf{e}}_k^T \tag{12}$$

where f_k are scalar functions. The function f can for example be a thresholding operator which results in decreased rank of the tensors when the eigenvalues are smaller than the specified threshold. Another method is a "max shape" operator,

$$\mathbf{T} = \begin{cases} c_l \mathbf{D}_l & \text{if} \quad c_l > c_p, c_s \\ c_p \mathbf{D}_p & c_p > c_l, c_s \\ c_s \mathbf{D}_s & c_s > c_l, c_p \end{cases} \tag{13}$$

This operation forces the tensor into the closest of the three generic shapes line, plane, and sphere.

2.8   Tracking White Matter Tracts

This section gives a sketch of a tracking algorithm that uses the diffusion tensors as operators. Let $\mathbf{x}_0$ be the initial seed point, and $\mathbf{v}_0$ be the seed direction, e.g. the eigenvector corresponding to the largest eigenvalue. A tracking sequence $\{\mathbf{x}_0, \mathbf{x}_1, ...\}$ can then be obtained by the following iteration formula:

$$\mathbf{x}_{k+1} = \mathbf{x}_k + \alpha \hat{\mathbf{v}}_k \tag{14}$$

$$\mathbf{v}_{k+1} = \mathbf{T}(\mathbf{x}_{k+1}) \mathbf{v}_k \tag{15}$$

where $\mathbf{T}(\mathbf{x}_{k+1})$ is the tensor in spatial position $\mathbf{x}_{k+1}$. The idea here is based on that $\mathbf{v}_k$ will turn towards the largest eigenvector of the tensor $\mathbf{T}(\mathbf{x}_{k+1})$. When the tensor has lower than full rank, it will act as a projection operator. When rank one, the vector $\mathbf{v}_k$ will be projected onto $(\mathbf{e}_1)_{k+1}$. Further, when the tensor is spherical, $\mathbf{v}_k$ will not turn since all vectors are eigenvectors.

3   Results

When applied to white matter, the linear measure, c_l, reflects the uniformity of tract direction within a voxel because it will be high only if the diffusion is restricted in two orthogonal directions. The anisotropy measure, c_a, indicates the relative restriction of the diffusion in the most restricted direction and will emphasize white matter tracts which within a voxel exhibit at least one direction of relatively restricted diffusion. Figure 4 shows the three geometrical measures and the anisotropy index. Major white matter tracts such as the corpus callosum show high linearity. In Figure 5 a diffusion tensor field from an axial slice of the brain is shown (left) and the averaged tensor field (right). The window, a, used was a $5 \times 5 \times 3$ Gaussian window with standard deviation equal to 1, defined in the in-plane resolution of the image. Since the out-of-plane resolution is slightly less than half the in-plane resolution, there is almost no smoothing performed between the slices. The original field (left) and the averaged field (right) have been weighted with their linear diffusion measure, c_l (Equation 8), respectively. This procedure can be used to measure fiber tract organization quantitatively. The size of the filter should be chosen in relation to the size of the fiber tracts of interest.

Figure 7 shows the effect of the two eigenvalue operations described in section 2.7. The left image shows the input data, a simulated tensor field of crossing white matter tracts. Due to partial voluming effects, the tensors in the area where the fibers are crossing have planar shape. The middle image shows the effect of smoothing the field with a 5×5 Gaussian kernel followed by a remapping the eigenvalues when f is a thresholding operator (Equation 12). The threshold was set to 20% of the largest eigenvalue, $0.2\lambda_1$. The right image shows the effect of the max shape operator on the same input data.

Figure 8 shows the result of tracking three crossing fiber tracts. A $5 \times 5 \times 5$ Gaussian operator followed by the max shape operator was used to stabilize the data. Each trace line is a composition of the results from both seed directions e_1 and $-e_1$ joined together.

4   Conclusions

We have proposed measures classifying diffusion tensors into three generic cases based on a tensor basis expansion. When applied to white matter the linear index shows uniformity of tract direction within a voxel while the anisotropic index quantifies the deviation from spatial homogeneity. The non-orthogonal tensor basis chosen is intuitively appealing since it is based on three simple, yet descriptive, geometrically meaningful cases.

We have described how tensor diffusion data can be processed without reverting to the use of only scalar measures of the tensor data. By staying in the tensor domain, cleaning up of the data can be done meaningfully with simple methods such as smoothing. We discuss addition of tensors geometrically and argue that adding tensors and vectors are different in that tensor summation gives more than the "mean" event due to more degrees of freedom. By using the geometric diffusion measures on locally averaged tensors local directionality consistency can be determined (e.g. existence of larger fiber tracts). We have proposed that this averaging approach can be used to derive a tensor field that can be used to describe macrostructural features in the tensor diffusion data. The linear measure c_l derived from the averaged tensor field can for example be used for quantitative evaluation of fiber tract organization. We also have described how non-linear operations can be used to remap the eigenvalues of the diffusion tensors and given a sketch of how this can be used for tracking white matter tracts.

linear   planar   spherical   tensor map

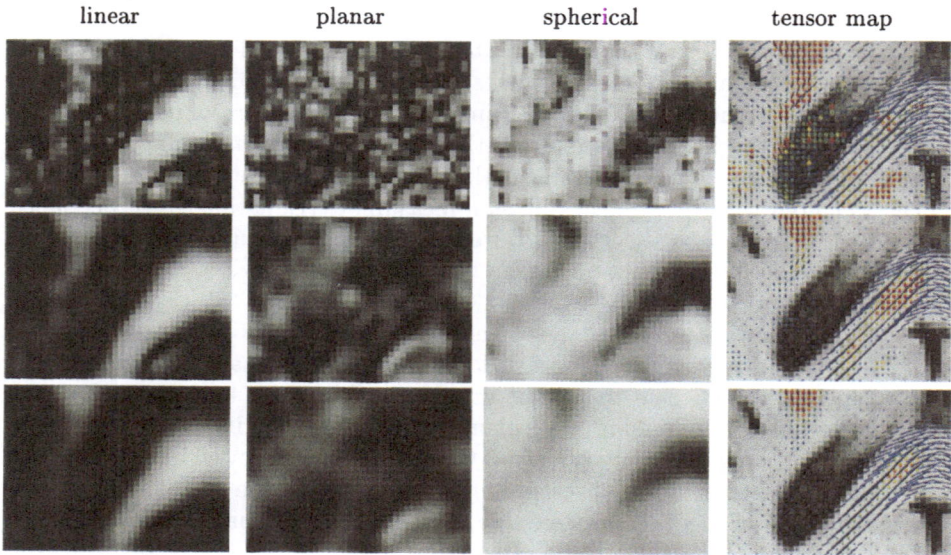

Fig. 4. Axial brain images showing the three geometrical measures and diffusion tensor maps with three different smoothing parameters. **Top:** shows the geometrical measures and the tensor map derived from the original data. **Middle:** shows the same measures derived from data that has been averaged with 9x9x3 Gaussian kernel. **Bottom:** from data averaged with a 15x15x5 Gaussian kernel. The rightmost column shows the tensors. The blue headless arrows represent the in-plane components of $c_l \hat{e}_1$. The out-of-plane components of $c_l \hat{e}_1$ are shown in colors ranging from green through yellow to red, with red indicating the highest value for this component. Display technique from [9]

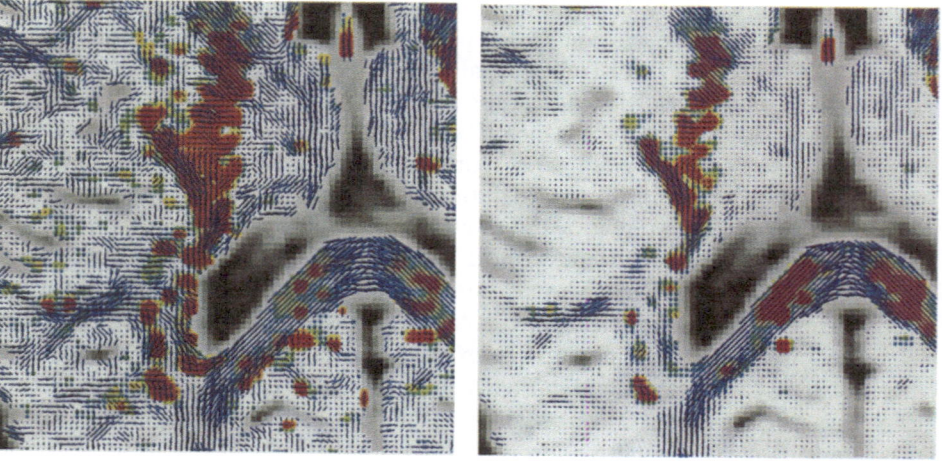

Fig. 5. Left: Diffusion tensors, weighted with their linear measure c_l, from an axial slice of a human brain. **Right:** Averaged diffusion tensors using a 5x5x3 Gaussian kernel weighted with their linear measure c_l.

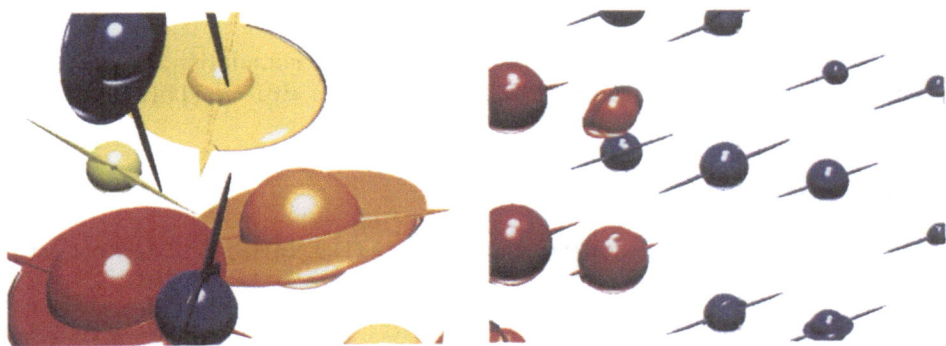

Fig. 6. Visualization of diffusion tensors. The tensors are color coded according to the shape: linear case is blue, planar case is yellow, and spherical case is red. The radius of the sphere is the smallest eigenvalue of the diffusion tensor, the radius of the disk is second largest and the length of the rod is twice the largest eigenvalue.

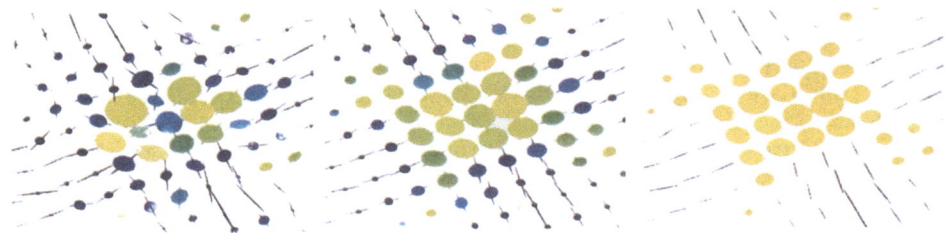

Fig. 7. Left: Simulated diffusion tensor data of two crossing white matter tracts. **Middle** The effect of thresholding the eigenvalues at 20 % of λ_1. **Right**: The effect of the max shape operator.

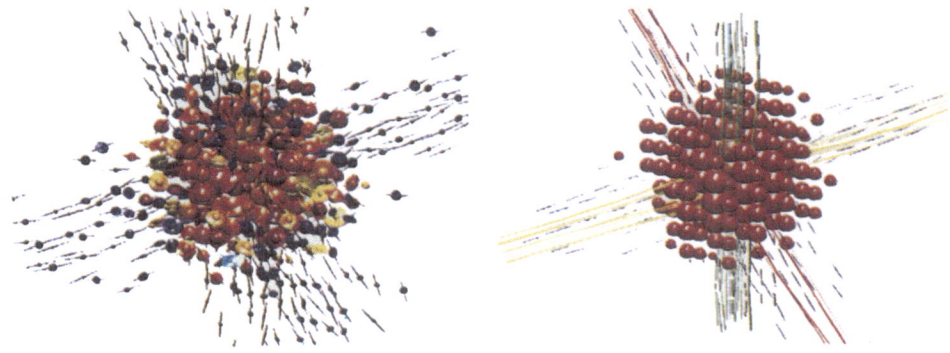

Fig. 8. Left: Original tensor data. **Right:** Tracking fibers after applying the max shape operator. 10 points were randomly seeded at one end of each of the three branches. Note how the stream lines "tunnel" trough the area in the center where the information of directionality is uncertain.

Acknowledgements

This work was funded in part by the Wenner-Gren Foundation, Sweden, the Whitaker Foundation, NIH grants P41-RR13218-01, R01-RR11747-01A, P01-CA67165-03.

References

1. P.J. Basser. Inferring microstructural features and the physiological state of tissues from diffusion-weighted images. *NMR in Biomedicine*, 8:333–344, 1995.
2. P.J. Basser and C. Pierpaoli. Microstructural and physiological features of tissues elucidated by quantitative-diffusion-tensor MRI. *J. Magn. Reson. Ser. B*, 111:209–219, 1996.
3. C. Beaulieu and P.S. Allen. Determinants of anisotropic water diffusion in nerves. *Magn. Reson. Med.*, 31:394–400, 1994.
4. T. L. Chenevert, J. A Brunberg, and J. G. Pipe. Anisotropic diffusion in human white matter: Demonstration with MR techniques in vivo. *Radiology*, 177:401–405, 1990.
5. G. Gerig, O. Kübler, R. Kikinis, and F.A. Jolesz. Non-linear anisotropic filtering of MRI data. *IEEE Transaction on Medical Imaging*, 11(2):221–232, June 1992.
6. G. H. Granlund and H. Knutsson. *Signal Processing for Computer Vision*. Kluwer Academic Publishers, 1995. ISBN 0-7923-9530-1.
7. H. Gudbjartsson, S. E. Maier, R. V. Mulkern, I. Á. Mórocz, S. Patz, and F. A. Jolesz. Line scan diffusion imaging. *Magn. Reson. Med.*, 36:509–519, 1996.
8. M. E. Moseley, Y. Cohen, J. Kucharczyk, J. Mintorovitch, H. S. Asgari, M. F. Wendland, J. Tsuruda, and D. Norman. Diffusion-weighted MR imaging of anisotropic water diffusion in the central nervous system. *Radiology*, 176:439–445, 1990.
9. S. Peled, H. Gudbjartsson, C-F. Westin, R. Kikinis, and F.A. Jolesz. Magnetic Resonance Imaging shows Orientation and Asymmetry of White Matter Tracts. *Brain Research*, 780(1):27–33, January 1998.
10. C. Pierpaoli, P. Jezzard, P. J. Basser, A. Barnett, and G. Di Chiro. Diffusion tensor MR imaging of the human brain. *Radiology*, 201:637, 1996.
11. C. Poupon, J.-F. Mangin, F. Frouin, J. Régis, F. Poupon, M. Pachot-Clouard, D. Le Bihan, and I. Bloch. Regularization of mr diffusion tensor maps for tracking brain white matter bundles. In *Proceedings of MICCAI'98*, number ISSN 0302-9743 in Lecture Notes in Computer Science 1496. Springer Verlag, 1998.
12. R. Turner, D. le Bihan, J. Maier, R. Vavrek, L. K. Hedges, and J. Pekar. Echo planar imaging of intravoxel incoherent motions. *Radiology*, 177:407–414, 1990.
13. C-F. Westin and H. Knutsson. Extraction of local symmetries using tensor field filtering. In *Proceedings of 2nd Singapore International Conference on Image Processing*. IEEE Singapore Section, September 1992.
14. C-F. Westin and H. Knutsson. Estimation of Motion Vector Fields using Tensor Field Filtering. In *Proceedings of IEEE International Conference on Image Processing*, Austin, Texas, November 1994. IEEE.
15. C-F. Westin, S. Peled, H. Gudbjartsson, R.Kikinis, and F.A Jolesz. Geometrical diffusion measures for MRI from tensor basis analysis. In *ISMRM '97*, Vancouver, Canada, April 1997.
16. D. M. Wimberger, T. P. Roberts, A. J. Barkovich, L. M. Prayer, M. E. Moseley, and J. Kucharczyk. Identification of "premyelination" by diffusion-weighted MRI. *J. Comp. Assist. Tomogr.*, 19(1):28–33, 1995.

Inferring the Brain Connectivity
from MR Diffusion Tensor Data

C. Poupon[12], C.A. Clark[1], V. Frouin[1], D. LeBihan[1], I. Bloch[2], and J.-F. Mangin[1]

[1] SHFJ, CEA, 91401 Orsay, France
cpoupon@shfj.cea.fr
WWW home page: http://www-dsv.cea.fr/
[2] ENST, 75013 Paris, France

Abstract. Magnetic resonance diffusion tensor imaging (DTI) has become an established research tool for the investigation of tissue structure and orientation. In this paper, we are interested in the connectivity induced by white matter fibers in the living human brain. Considering the data resolution, this question has to be addressed at the level of fascicles made up by a bunch of parallel fibers. We propose first an algorithm dedicated to the fascicle tracking in a direction map inferred from diffusion data. This algorithm takes into account the usual fan shaped merge of several fascicles in one larger bundle. Then, we propose a way of inferring a regularized direction map from diffusion data in order to get a robust tracking. The regularization stems from a priori knowledge on the white matter geometry embedded in a model of the bending energy of an equivalent spaghetti plate. Finally, we propose a study of the tracking behaviour according to the weight given to the regularization and some examples of the tracking results with real data.

1 Introduction

Up to now, information on brain anatomical connectivity has only been obtained from post mortem studies. Many anatomical methods have been designed for this purpose. Among all possible approaches, chemical tracers which are transported by the axons from a point of injection either anterogradely or retrogradely, have become the method of choice [1]. These methods have yielded detailed brain connectivity maps in different species like the cat and the monkey. However, major disadvantages of these techniques are the required animal sacrifice and the cumbersome 3D reconstruction of the serial sections. Therefore, there has been increasing interest in the development of MRI-based in vivo tract tracing tools. One direction of research relies on magnetic resonance diffusion imaging for the *in vivo* study of the human brain.

Calculation and subsequent diagonalization of the water apparent diffusion tensor yields its eigenvalues and eigenvectors. The eigenvector corresponding to the largest eigenvalue may be considered to represent the main direction of diffusion in a voxel. Given that one may ascribe diffusion anisotropy in white matter to a greater hinderance or restriction to diffusion across the fiber axes than along them, the principal eigenvector may be considered to point along the direction of a putative fiber bundle crossing this voxel. Considering the orientation of the principal eigenvector in neighbouring voxels, it may be deduced whether the fibers in those voxels are connected or not. While this has been used to segment large white matter structures of the brain such as the corpus callosum and pyramidal tract [2], it is necessary to refine this methodology in order to assert which cortical areas or grey nuclei are connected by fascicles embeded in white matter bundles. The first part of this paper describes a fascicle tracking algorithm dealing with fascicle junctions. This algorithm input is a direction map made up for instance by the tensor first eigenvector. Then we propose a model to compute a regularized direction map from the tensor data in order to improve the robustness of the tracking algorithm. Results with real tensor data show that this model improves the consistency of the tracking.

2   Methods

DTI was performed on a 1.5T Signa Echospeed MRI system (General Electric, Milwaukee). Image parameters were: image matrix=128 × 128 pixels, 56 slices, in plane resolution=1.875mm, slice thickness=2.8mm. A standard T1-weighted image was also acquired.

A first step of the tracking approach consists in defining a volume of interest (VOI) on which will be restricted all the methods described in the following. This VOI, which is made up by the voxels belonging to white matter, is automatically extracted from the T1-weighted image using an algorithm developed in our institution [3]. A morphological dilation is then applied to this segmentation in order to be robust to potential distortions between the echo-planar diffusion images and the high resolution T1-weighted image.

2.1   A simple fascicle tracking algorithm

The diffusion tensor and subsequently the eigen system are calculated for each voxel of the VOI [4]. Then, different approaches can be chosen to try to infer the brain connectivity from the DT data. The simplest idea consists in defining a connectivity rule between adjacent white matter voxels in order to define the major bundles as different connected components [2]. This approach can not really deal with brain connectivity because a bunch of bundles bound to cross the same white matter bottleneck (corpus callosum, internal capsule) belong to the same connected component. In this paper, we develop a different idea which consists in partitioning the white matter domain in a set of putative fascicles represented by chains of linked voxels. Using this approach, the largest bundles are split into a set of fascicles which allows for instance the study of the connectivity induced by the fibers of the corpus callosum. This idea could be related to the notion of tractography introduced by Basser [5].

The partitioning of white matter in a set of fascicles relies on a simple rule to link voxels. This rule is defined from a direction map, namely an image of unitary vectors. In a first approach, this direction map is simply the image of the eigen vector of the diffusion tensor associated with the largest eigenvalue. Let $d(M)$ denotes the direction of voxel M. Each voxel M is endowed with a forward

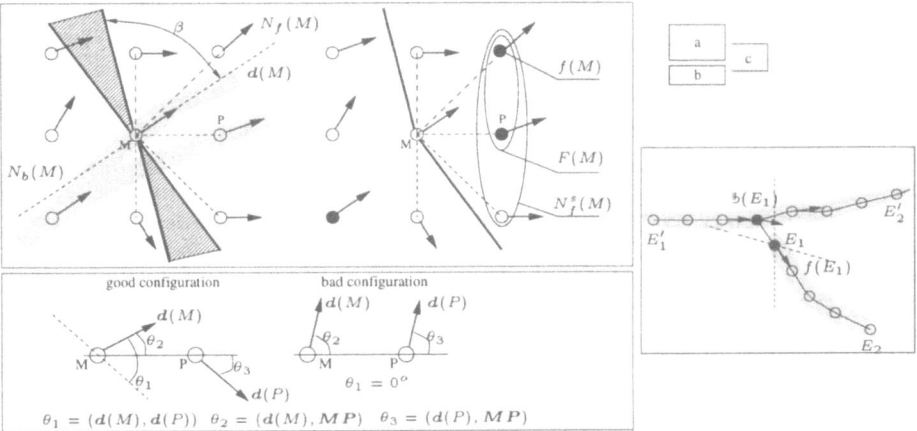

Fig. 1. (a) : construction of the extended neighborhoods of a site M (see text); some underlying fascicles are represented in gray; (b) : the 3 angles used to compute the low curvature criterion $s(M, P)$ (cf. Eq. 1); (c) : fan shaped fascicle split leading to the definition of junctions.

and a backward conic neighborhood $\mathcal{N}_f(M)$ and $\mathcal{N}_b(M)$ defined from $\boldsymbol{d}(M)$ (see Fig. 1a). The conic neighborhood $\mathcal{N}_f(M)$ (respectively $\mathcal{N}_b(M)$) is defined as the subset of M 26-neighbors belonging to the half-cone whose apex is M, whose direction is $\boldsymbol{d}(M)$ (resp. $-\boldsymbol{d}(M)$) and whose aperture angle is β (typically set to $45°$). A voxel M can be linked to at most one voxel $f(M)$ (resp. $b(M)$) of $\mathcal{N}_f(M)$ (resp. $\mathcal{N}_b(M)$). The linked forward neighbor $f(M)$ is defined if the set $\mathcal{N}_f^s(M) = \{P \in \mathcal{N}_f(M), M \in \mathcal{N}_f(P) \cup \mathcal{N}_b(P)\}$ is non empty. Simply speaking, this constraint is related to the fact that a consistent connectivity relationship has to be symmetrical. If we define the function (see Fig. 1b):

$$s(M, P) = \frac{\mathbf{max}^2 \left((\boldsymbol{d}(M), \boldsymbol{u}_{MP}), (\boldsymbol{d}(P).\boldsymbol{u}_{MP}), (\boldsymbol{d}(M).\boldsymbol{d}(P))\right)}{\|MP\|}, \qquad (1)$$

where $\boldsymbol{u}_{MP} = \frac{MP}{\|MP\|}$ and $(\boldsymbol{u}, \boldsymbol{v})$ denotes the angle between directions $\boldsymbol{u}$ and $\boldsymbol{v}$, then the definition of $f(M)$ is (see Fig. 1a):

$$f(M) = \mathbf{Arg\ min}_{P \in \mathcal{N}_f^s(M)} s(M, P) \qquad (2)$$

Hence, $f(M)$ is the best forward neighbor according to a criterion taking into account the three angles between $\boldsymbol{d}(M)$, $\boldsymbol{d}(P)$ and the direction MP (see Fig. 1). This criterion endows the locally tracked fascicle with the lowest possible curvature. The best backward neighbor $b(M)$ is defined in the same way:

$$b(M) = \mathbf{Arg\ min}_{P \in \mathcal{N}_b^s(M)} s(M, P), \qquad (3)$$

where $\mathcal{N}_b^s(M) = \{P \in \mathcal{N}_b(M), M \in \mathcal{N}_f(P) \cup \mathcal{N}_b(P)\}$ has to be non empty.

The partition of white matter in fascicles stems from the definition of a connectivity rule $\mathcal{C}$ between adjacent voxels. Two voxels M_1 and M_2 are connected

$(M_1 \; \mathcal{C} \; M_2)$ if and only if they are symetrically best neighbors to each other: $(M_1 = f(M_2)$ or $M_1 = b(M_2))$ and $(M_2 = f(M_1)$ or $M_2 = b(M_1))$. The fascicles are the connected components defined by this connectivity rule. Since a voxel can not be endowed with more than two neighbors with this rule, simple topological considerations lead to the fact that each fascicle can be represented by a chain of voxels $(M_1, M_2, ..., M_n)$, where $M_i \; \mathcal{C} \; M_{i+1}$ for $i \in \{1, 2, ..., n-1\}$. In fact two different kinds of chains can exist. The simple chains whose extremities M_1 and M_n are respectively endowed with only one neighbor for the rule $\mathcal{C}$ correspond to the natural anatomical notion of fascicle. In the following such chains will be denoted unambigously by their extremity pair $\{M_1, M_n\}$. The second kind of potential chains corresponds to the closed loops without real extremities for which $M_n \; \mathcal{C} \; M_1$. Such pathological chains should not exist from an anatomical point of view.

2.2   Towards brain connectivity

The partition of white matter in such mathematically defined fascicles is not sufficient to get access to the brain connectivity level. Indeed, we have to deal with the configurations where a fascicle extremity E_1 is not located on the boundary but inside white matter, which is a nonsense from an anatomical point of view. Let us assume without loss of generality that the extremity voxel E_1 is linked to its fascicle $\{E_1, E_2\}$ by $f(E_1)$ $(f(E_1) \in \{E_1, E_2\})$ (see Fig. 1c). Two different cases can occur.

1. If $b(E_1)$ exists, $b(E_1)$ belongs to another fascicle $\{E'_1, E'_2\}$. This configuration can be interpreted anatomically as a "fascicle merge". In the case of two parallel fascicles, such a merge can be related to a decrease of the diameter of the underlying bundle implying a higher fiber density. When the two fascicles follow relatively different directions, the merge occurs at a location where the underlying bundle is split in a fan shaped fashion. In order to deal with this fascicle merge notion, we have to extend the initial linking rule $\mathcal{C}$ to allow the existence of junction voxels. This extension consists in the introduction of two sets of linked forward and backward neighbors, respectively $\mathcal{F}(M)$ and $\mathcal{B}(M)$, for each voxel M. For the simple voxels, $\mathcal{F}(M) = \{f(M)\}$ and $\mathcal{B}(M) = \{b(M)\}$. For the junctions, these sets can include more voxels. Let us go back to the configuration introduced above. Since $b(E_1) \in \mathcal{N}_b^s(E_1)$, either $E_1 \in \mathcal{N}_f(b(E_1))$ or $E_1 \in \mathcal{N}_b(b(E_1))$. The first case naturally leads to the addition of E_1 in $\mathcal{F}(E_1)$, the second case leads to the addition of E_1 in $\mathcal{B}(E_1)$.
2. If $b(E_1)$ does not exist, we face a very unplausible anatomical situation which should be rare but manageable in the future. This situation does not lead to linked neighbor sets extension.

The above considerations have led to the design of an extended set of linked neighbors $\mathcal{F}(M)$ and $\mathcal{B}(M)$. It should be noted that the construction of these neighbor sets does not require the computation of the fascicles which have been mainly introduced for the sake of clarity:

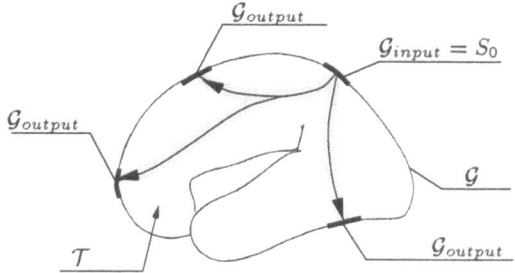

Fig. 2. tracking process; the tracking starts at a subset $\mathcal{G}_{input}$ of the boundary $\mathcal{G}$ between white and gray matter; it uses $\mathcal{F}(M)$ and $\mathcal{B}(M)$ sets to propagate through white matter $\mathcal{T}$ until a cortical or basal $\mathcal{G}_{output}$ region is reached.

- if $\mathcal{N}_f^s(M) \neq \emptyset$:

$$\mathcal{F}(M) = \{f(M)\} \cup \{P \in \mathcal{N}_f^s(M) \mid f(P) = M \text{ or } b(P) = M\},$$

  otherwise $\mathcal{F}(M) = \emptyset$;
- if $\mathcal{N}_b^s(M) \neq \emptyset$:

$$\mathcal{B}(M) = \{b(M)\} \cup \{P \in \mathcal{N}_b^s(M) \mid f(P) = M \text{ or } b(P) = M\},$$

  otherwise $\mathcal{B}(M) = \emptyset$.

With these definitions we are now able to define clearly the way of inferring the brain connectivity through tracking.

The VOI related to white matter is made up by three kinds of voxels. Let $\mathcal{G}$ denote the set of voxels located at the boundary of the VOI (see Fig. 2). A simple point of view leads us to consider this set as the gate to gray matter. Let $\mathcal{T}$ denote a second set of voxels which verify $\mathcal{F}(M) \neq \emptyset$ and $\mathcal{B}(M) \neq \emptyset$. These voxels located inside white matter are endowed with a way of tracking forward and backward using $\mathcal{F}(M)$ and $\mathcal{B}(M)$. Finally, let $\mathcal{P}$ denote the set of the remaining voxels for which at least one of the two neighbor sets is empty. These voxels are pathological because if one of them is reached during a tracking process, this process is stopped before reaching the set $\mathcal{G}$.

Asking a question about brain connectivity amounts to selecting a subset $\mathcal{G}_{input}$ of $\mathcal{G}$ and performing a tracking process from this subset. The tracking process simply consists in the construction of a sequence of subsets $\{\mathcal{S}_0, \mathcal{S}_1, ..., \mathcal{S}_n\}$ of the VOI using the following rules (see Fig. 2):

- $\mathcal{S}_0 = \mathcal{G}_{input}$;
- $\mathcal{S}_1 = \{M \mid \exists M_{-1} \in \mathcal{S}_0 \text{ with } M \in \mathcal{F}(M_{-1}) \text{ or } M \in \mathcal{B}(M_{-1})\}$;
- for each $i \in \{2, 3, ..., n\}$, $\mathcal{S}_i = \{M \mid \exists M_{-1} \in \mathcal{S}_{i-1} \text{ and } \exists M_{-2} \in \mathcal{S}_{i-2} \text{ with } (M \in \mathcal{F}(M_{-1}) \text{ and } M_{-2} \in \mathcal{B}(M_{-1})) \text{ or } (M \in \mathcal{B}(M_{-1}) \text{ and } M_{-2} \in \mathcal{F}(M_{-1}))\}$.

The third rule assures that the tracking is always performed in the same direction along the underlying fascicles. Once this sequence has been computed, the answer to the brain connectivity question is the new subset $\mathcal{G}_{output}$ of $\mathcal{G}$ defined by:

$$\mathcal{G}_{output} = \mathcal{G} \cap \bigcup_{i \in \{1, 2, ..., n\}} \mathcal{S}_i$$

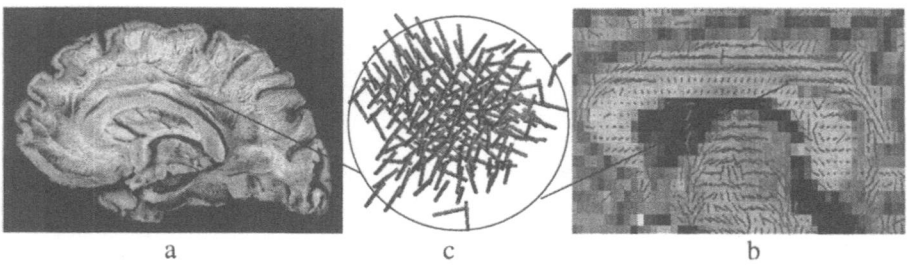

Fig. 3. geometry of white matter fascicles; (a) dissection of a human brain (The Virtual Hospital); (b) sagittal slice of anatomical MRI with projection of directions $d(M)$; (c) example of noisy DTI region; each cylinder represents the direction $d(M)$.

More sophisticated questions can be answered using the same kind of ideas.

2.3   Direction map regularization

During the design of the previous tracking method, potential pathological configurations which could perturb the inference of the brain connectivity have been highlighted. In fact, with a noisy direction map, such configurations are bound to be very usual. Indeed, the simple tracking approach introduced above can not tolerate even a one voxel gap in the middle of a fascicle. Unfortunately, DTI contains noise. Moreover, the low resolution of DT images relatively to the usual fiber bundle diameters leads to an important partial volume effect. When a voxel includes several fiber directions, the tensor is very difficult to interpret. In such situations, the main eigen vector can follow a "mean direction" largely different from the directions of the underlying fascicles.

In order to overcome the difficulties induced by noise and partial volume effect, a first idea consists in developing a tracking algorithm dealing with potential gaps using longer links. In fact such a solution seems rather difficult to design in a consistent way. Indeed, the general tracking problem turns out to be relatively "ill-posed", which means that two different diffusion tensor acquisitions of the same brain could lead to two highly different fascicle sets because of noise.

In fact, the tracking difficulties are not induced by the tracking algorithm proposed in the first part of this paper, but by the noisy nature of the direction map made up by the tensor first eigenvectors. Therefore, this direction map has to be restored before applying the tracking. We have recently introduced a class of Markovian models dedicated to such a restoration [6]. In this paper, we focus on one specific model of this class which appears especially adapted to the tracking problem.

The geometry of white matter illustrated by Fig 3. is highly similar to the geometry of spaghetti plates. This analogy between fascicles and spaghetti will help us to introduce the mathematical model underlying the construction of the regularized direction map. Let us consider a single spaghetti. Before any cooking, this spaghetti can be considered as a straight line. Put in hot water, the spaghetti becomes a bended curve. The highest the water temperature is, the highest is the spaghetti curvature. A simple way to assess the cooking effect on the spaghetti geometry would consist in integrating the curvature to get some kind of spaghetti bending energy E:

$$E(spaghetti) = \int_0^{length} \frac{\mathcal{K}}{2} c^2(s) ds \; ; \tag{4}$$

where s is simply a curvilinear abcisse along the spaghetti, $c(s)$ is the spaghetti curvature at abcisse s and $\mathcal{K}$ is the stress rigidity. This energy, well known in chemistry as Kratky-Porod model of semi-flexible polymeres [7], can be extended in a straighforward way to a whole spaghetti plate. The fascicle tracking algorithm introduced previously is searching locally for the fascicle with the lowest curvature. This local point of view is not robust to noise in the direction map. This weakness can be overcome if a global point of view is chosen: searching for the fascicle set with the lowest energy of the equivalent spaghetti plate.

The computation of the regularized direction map can be classically interpreted in a Bayesian framework. The optimal direction map D_{opt} has to maximize the a posteriori probability $p(D/T)$, where T denotes the diffusion tensor data and D denotes a random field which realization scope covers all possible direction maps.

2.4 Markovian model

The realizations of the random variables $d(M)$ of the field D are unitary vectors with any 3D direction. Let us consider a voxel M of the VOI. This voxel has to belong to one fascicle. $d(M)$ is the putative local direction of this fascicle for a realization of the field. Since fascicles can not end up inside white matter, we have to find neighboring voxels, forwards and backwards, with similar fascicle directions (or perhaps the boundary of white matter). Moreover, this property is sufficient to define the whole geometry of a plausible fascicle set. In the next section, we will propose a Markovian model whose deep local minima correspond to fascicle sets with low curvatures, or spaghetti plates with low energy. Because of this analogy, we will refer to this model as the spaghetti plate model.

The optimal direction map D_{opt} is a trade-off between the measured tensor data and the *a priori* knowledge on the low curvature of fascicles. The Bayesian framework leads to the definition of D_{opt} as the global minimum of the energy $U(D)$:

$$U(D) = U_S(D) + \alpha U_T(D) = \sum_M V_S(M, D) + \alpha \sum_M V_T(M, D) \tag{5}$$

where $U_S(D)$ is the regularizing energy related to the analogous spaghetti plate and $U_T(D)$ is a quadratic distance to the maximal potential diffusion along spaghetti of the direction map. The constant α allows us to weight the influence of the *a priori* knowledge. The potentials $V_S(M, D)$, which are defined on interaction cliques made up by the 26-neighborhood, are inspired by the spaghetti bending energy introduced above (see Eq. 1 and 4):

$$V_S(M, D) = s(M, f_{90}(M)) + s(M, b_{90}(M)) \tag{6}$$

where $f_{90}(M)$ and $b_{90}(M)$ are best linked neighbors related to half-cones with $\beta = 90°$ aperture angle, covering the whole 26-neighborhood. The potentials $V_T(M, D)$, which are constructed from the tensor dot product, measure the discrepancy between diffusion in the direction $d(M)$ and the diffusion in the direction of the tensor first eigenvector $e_1(M)$:

$$V_T(M, D) = \left(\frac{d(M)^t T(M) d(M) - e_1(M)^t T(M) e_1(M)}{\|T(M)\|} \right)^2 \qquad (7)$$

The discrepancy is normalized by the tensor norm [8] in order to get rid of all diffusion-based information apart from anisotropy.

3   Results

The state space of the random variables $d(M)$ has been descretized in 162 uniformly distributed directions. A deterministic ICM like algorithm is used to get the $U(D)$ local minimum nearest to the $e_1(M)$ direction map. Regularization has been performed with eleven different values of the weighting parameter α. Then, in order to study the influence of regularization on the fascicle set geometry, several subsets of points have been defined from the construction of $\mathcal{F}_{45}(M)$ and $\mathcal{B}_{45}(M)$ extended neighborhoods. It should be noted that the 90° cone aperture is only used during regularization in order to penalize the worst configurations. In return, during a tracking operation, the aperture angle is largely reduced in order to forbid anatomically meaningless links. The evolution relatively to α of the cardinals of four specific sets of points has been studied (see Fig. 4):

Fascicle nodes: sites endowed with exactly one forward neighbor and one backward neighbor ($\mathcal{B}(M) = \{b(M)\}$ and $\mathcal{F}(M) = \{f(M)\}$);

Junctions: sites related to the merge (or split) of several fascicles made up of points of the previous type ($cardinal(\mathcal{B}(M)) \times cardinal(\mathcal{F}(M)) > 1$);

Gate to gray matter: sites leading to gray matter ($N_f(M) = \emptyset$ or $N_b(M) = \emptyset$);

Pathological sites: sites endowed with forward (or backward) basic neighbors, but no forward (or backward) symmetrical neighbors, *i.e.* pathological sites (($N_f^s(M) = \emptyset$ and $N_f(M) \neq \emptyset$) or ($N_b^s(M) = \emptyset$ and $N_b(M) \neq \emptyset$)).

Fig. 4 presents the evolution from no regularization (right asymptotes) to high regularization (left). First, the number of pathological sites (see Fig. 4.3) decreases dramatically with the regularization which demonstrates the efficiency of the model. Second, the regularization leads to a decrease of the number of junctions and to a dramatic increase of the number of simple fascicle nodes. This effect is mainly due to a reorganization of the fascicles inside larger bundles (see Fig. 4.1) which corresponds to the usual underlying anatomical reality. Indeed, the chronotopic establishment of the connections leads to topographically ordered bundles [9]. Hence, the large bundles are endowed with somatotopic organizations, which means that different parts of the bundle section include axons connecting different brain areas. Finally, the number of sites leading to gray matter decreases slightly which is related to the fact that with a 90° cone

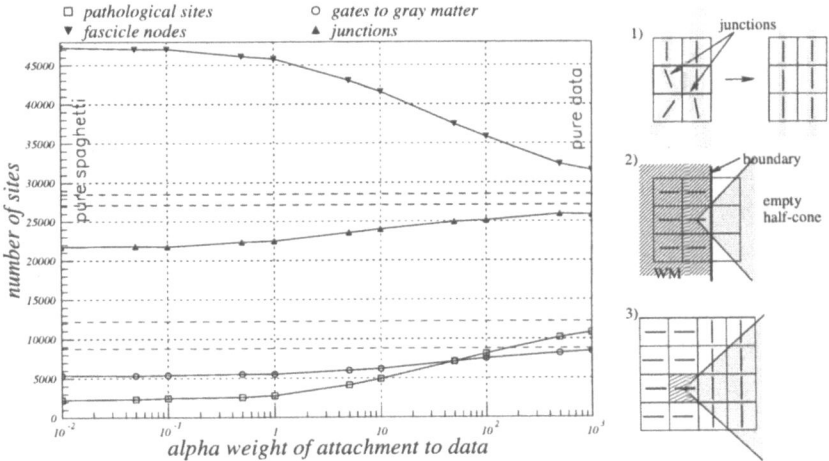

Fig. 4. (left) evolution of the numbers of four different types of configurations; (right) 1) fascicle mixing inside a bundle before regularization versus a bunch of aligned fascicles after regularization; 2) sites of white matter leading to gray matter; 3) pathological site without tracking possibility.

aperture during the regularization, only convex areas of the boundary (see Fig. 4.2), namely cortical gyri, are not penalized. While, these areas are the main cortical connexion locations, this effect call for refinements of the regularizing model. All the curve evolutions reach limits beyond which no more topological effect is observed on the fascicle set. This observation suggests that the weight $\alpha = 1$ is a reasonable trade-off between regularization and attachment to the data which has been used for further experiments.

In order to illustrate the impact of the regularization on the fiber tracking procedure in a more visual way, we have applied the idea exposed in Fig. 2 with two different inputs (see Fig. 5), one in the motor area (yellow), the other one in the frontal lobe (green). One additional threshold parameter has been added to the tracking process in order to give the user the possibility to focus on fascicles endowed with lower maximal curvature than the one allowed by the tracking cone aperture ($\beta = 45°$): all best neighbors which do not verify $s(M, f(M)) < \gamma^2$ are suppressed. In the following γ has been fixed to 20°. Fig. 5 presents the tracking results before and after regularization. Two kinds of problems occur before regularization. For the yellow input, in spite of the low threshold, the tracking invades the whole bundles and follows very unplausible trajectories. For the green input, the tracking stops immediately in the middle of white matter while with a higher threshold, the same problem as with the yellow input occurs. In return, after regularization, the tracking yields much more plausible results, even if a real anatomical validation is currently not available.

4   Conclusion

This paper outlines the opening of a new research domain for the image analysis community. Indeed, dealing with tensor images calls for the development of com-

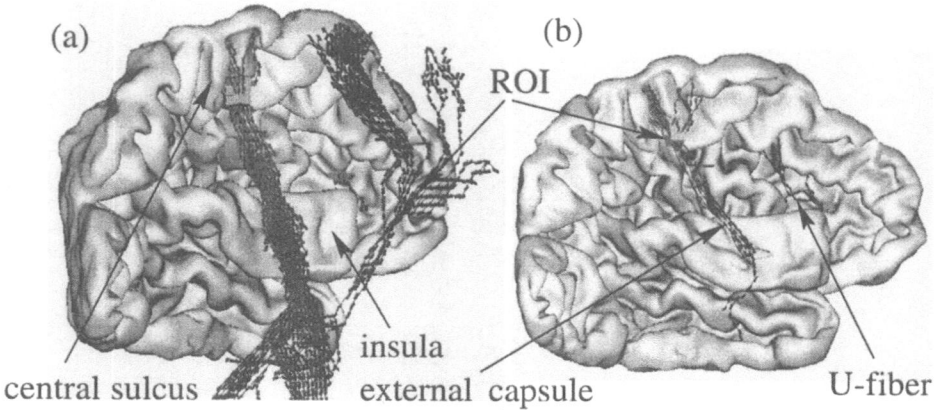

Fig. 5. tracking of fascicles from 2 different inputs [motor area and frontal area]; (a) before regularization; (b) after regularization.

pletely new algorithms. This direction of research could lead to the first method giving access *in vivo* to the human brain connectivity, Such a method would have a great impact both on brain mapping and on pathological studies. Indeed, it should be noted that the connectivity of the human brain and especially of the human cortex is still relatively ill-defined. One of the challenge to take up rapidly is the design of reliable validation approaches using for instance animals and standard anatomical methods.

References

1. M.P. Young, J.W. Scannell, and G. Burns. *The Analysis of Cortical Connectivity*. Neuroscience Intelligence Unit. Springer Verlag, 1995.
2. D.K. Jones, A.Simmons, S.C.R. Williams, and M.A. Horsfield. Non-Invasive Assessment of Structural Connectivity in White Matter by Diffusion Tensor MRI. In *Proceedings of the 6th ISMRM, Sydney*, vol. 1, 1998, pp. 531.
3. J.-F. Mangin, V. Frouin, I. Bloch, J. Régis, and J. Lopez-Krahe. From 3D Magnetic Resonance Images to Structural Representations of the Cortex Topography using Topology Preserving Deformations. *Journal of Mathematical Imaging and Vision*, vol. 5, 1995, pp. 297–318.
4. P.J. Basser, J. Mattiello, and D. LeBihan. Estimation of the Effective Self-Diffusion Tensor from the NMR Spin Echo. *Journal of Magnetic Resonance*, no. 103, 1994, pp. 247–254.
5. P.J. Basser. Fiber-Tractography via Diffusion Tensor MRI (DT-MRI). In *Proceedings of the 6th ISMRM, Sydney*, vol. 2, 1998, pp. 1226.
6. C. Poupon et al. Regularization of MR Diffusion Tensor Maps for Tracking Brain White Matter Bundles. *LNCS 1496, MICCAI'98*, Springer-Verlag, MIT Boston, October 1998, pp. 489–498.
7. P.M. Chaikin and T.C. Lubensky. *Principles of Condensed Matter Physics*. Cambridge University Press, 1995.
8. P.J. Basser and C. Pierpaoli. Microstructural and Physiological Features of Tissues Elucidated by Quantitative-Diffusion-Tensor MRI. *Journal of Magnetic Resonance*, no. 111, 1996, pp. 209–219.
9. Z. Molnár *Development of thalamocortical connections*. Springer Verlag, 1998.

Strategies for Data Reorientation during Non-rigid Warps of Diffusion Tensor Images

D.C. Alexander, J.C. Gee, and R. Bajcsy.

GRASP Lab. and Dept. Radiology, University of Pennsylvania, 3401, Walnut St., Philadelphia. PA 19104, USA.

Abstract. This paper describes work on the registration of diffusion tensor images of the human brain. An existing registration algorithm, the multi-resolution, elastic matching algorithm, [1-3], has been adapted for this purpose. One problem with the application of such a method to this new data type is that transformations of the image affect the DT values at each voxel, as the orientation can change with respect to the surrounding anatomical structures. Three methods for the estimation of an appropriate reorientation of the data from the local displacement field, which describes the image transformation, are presented and tested. Results indicate that the best matches are obtained from a reorientation strategy that takes into account the effects of local shearing on the data as well as the rigid rotational component of the displacement. The methods presented here may be useful for the computation of region based similarity measures of single valued intensity images, which also vary with local image orientation.

1 Introduction

Diffusion tensor (DT) imaging is a recent innovation in MRI (magnetic resonance imaging), [4]. In DT imaging, the measurement acquired at each voxel in an image volume is a symmetric second order tensor, which describes the local water diffusion properties of the material being imaged. The DT may be thought of as a Gaussian density describing the probability of the final position of a molecule, initially at the centre of a voxel, after some fixed time. DT imaging of the human brain has provoked particular interest because of the added insight it provides into the structure of white matter regions. Neuronal axons are fibres that form the connections between different cells of the brain. In these axons water is free to diffuse along the fibre, but diffusion in perpendicular directions is greatly restricted by the cell wall. DT measurements taken from areas in the brain where large numbers of parallel axons are bundled together, for example the white matter tracts, thus tend to exhibit a high degree of anisotropy and the principal direction (PD) of the DT points along the axes of the bundled fibres. By associating neighbouring voxels according to the PD of their DTs, connection pathways within the brain can be traced and mapped, see for example [5], although the resolution at which these images can currently be obtained is such that only major pathways can be extracted reliably. There are an increasing number of clinical applications of DT imaging, for example, the analysis of stroke and multiple sclerosis, [6].

Three images derived from a slice of a DT image of the human brain are shown in Figure 1. The larger image on the left shows a line at each pixel, which indicates the PD of the DT projected into the xy plane. For pixels at which the PD is close to the z-direction, these lines are less meaningful and are drawn in correspondingly lighter colours. The two images on the right show two common indices that are derived from the DT. The lattice anisotropy, [7], image (top) is hyperintense in white matter regions where the diffusion is strongly weighted in one direction. In the PD image, the crescent shaped regions of high anisotropy at the top and bottom of the image have configuration that suggests they are bundles of fibres running from one side of the brain to the other. The DT trace (bottom) is a measure of the total diffusion at a point and thus tends to be largest in areas where the diffusion is unrestricted in all directions such as regions of CSF (cerebro-spinal fluid).

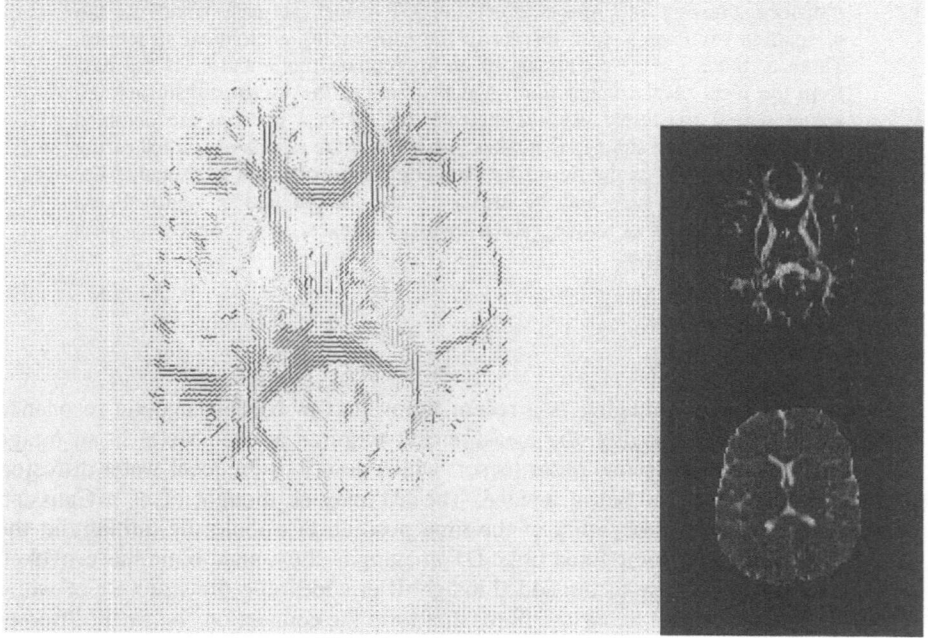

Figure 1 Images derived from a slice of a DT image. Left: principal DT eigenvector projected into the xy-plane. Lighter lines indicate greater z-component in the PD. No line is drawn at points where the anisotropy falls below a certain threshold. Top right: lattice anisotropy image. Bottom right: DT trace image.

Here we consider spatial normalisation of DT images and, in particular, the adaptation of the elastic matching algorithm, [1-3], to work with this new data type. Adaptation of the algorithm is complicated by the fact that each DT has an associated orientation. Image transformations tend to change the orientation of DTs with respect to the surrounding anatomical structure of the image. For a simple image transformation, such as rigid rotation, DT orientation can be preserved by applying a similar transformation to each DT. However, more complex transformations are generally required for accurate spatial normalisation of brain images. The elastic matching algorithm, [1-3], provides spatial normalisation via high dimensional warps described by a displacement field. The required reorientation of the DTs is dependent on the local properties of the displacement field. In this paper, we discuss strategies for estimation of this reorientation.

Motivation for this work is twofold. Firstly, spatial normalisation of MR images from large groups of patients is of great benefit in clinical studies of anatomical variation over population groups. Spatial normalisation of DT images is required to assist clinical studies of the variation of diffusion properties. It may also be of use in the analysis of the variation of pathways within the brain once the technology to extract these pathways reliably is available. Secondly, the added structure in DT images may allow better anatomical matches to be made between images acquired from different patients, than can be obtained by matching on single valued intensity images. Statistical models of accurate matches based on detailed information, such as combinations of the DT with complementary structural information, could be used to constrain spatial normalisations computed using less expressive data. We also note that the reorientation strategies outlined here may be useful for the computation of region based similarity measures for single valued intensity images undergoing non-rigid transformations. Such measures have already proved effective for image matching, but further improvements might be obtained if the effects of local image reorientation on their values are taken into account.

In the next section, the elastic matching algorithm is described briefly and some issues of its application to DT imagery are discussed. In section 3, we present three strategies for estimating the required reorientation of the DTs during an image transformation. Some experiments to compare these strategies are detailed in section 4 and quantitative results are provided. Finally, conclusions are drawn in section 5.

2 Elastic Matching of DT Images

In this section, we give a brief description of the elastic matching algorithm. Details of the algorithm can be found in, [1-3]. Issues concerning is application to DT imagery, in particular the requirement for reorientation of the data as image transformations are applied, are then discussed.

2.1 Elastic Matching Algorithm

The elastic matching algorithm computes a displacement field describing a warp of one image, which aligns it with another similar image. The warp is computed by iteratively minimising an energy function. The basic energy function contains two terms: a term derived from the similarity of the image data at corresponding points in the fixed target and warped source images, and a term that expresses the amount of deformation caused by the warp.

To provide a starting point for the algorithm that is close to the final solution, a global affine transformation is first applied to the source image. We use Wood's AIR (Automated Image Registration) algorithm, [8,9], to compute the global transformation. Elastic matching is then applied at consecutive levels of a multi-resolution pyramid, from low resolution to high resolution, to find a warp that optimises the balance between pointwise similarity of the image data and deformation of the source image.

2.2   Application to DT Images

Two issues arise with the application of the elastic matching algorithm to this new type of data. Firstly, how to define the similarity between data at corresponding positions in the two images and secondly, consistency of DT orientations.

For intensity images, for example proton density, T1- or T2-weighted images, it is common to use the squared intensity difference or the cross-correlation of the two images as the measure of local similarity. A detailed discussion of the similarity measures that can be used for comparing DTs is beyond the scope of this paper. We have found that a similarity measure, S_T, based on the magnitude of tensor difference produces good results. Experimental justification of this choice, as opposed to other tensor comparison measures, matching on PD alone or cross correlation of indices derived from the DT, is presented in [10]. For two DTs, $\mathbf{D_1}$ and $\mathbf{D_2}$, S_T is given by

$$S_T = -\frac{1}{\sigma}\sqrt{trace\left[(\mathbf{D_1} - \mathbf{D_2})^2\right]}. \tag{1}$$

The expression in the square root is equivalent to the sum of squared differences of the elements of the DT matrix, and σ is a weighting parameter. S_T is used as the similarity measure in all the experiments presented in this paper.

Here we are concerned with the issue of DT orientation. In the next section we present various strategies for extracting the appropriate reorientation of the DT from the local displacement gradient. In doing so, the image transformation is modelled as locally affine and so we will first consider how we expect basic affine transformations of an image region to affect the DTs at voxels within the region. An affine transformation is comprised of the following components:

- **Rigid translation** of an image region should have no effect on the DTs in the region, since the measured diffusion is not dependent on absolute position.
- **Rigid rotation** of a piece of tissue with respect to a laboratory frame would cause the diffusion characteristics of that tissue to be rotated by the same amount with respect to the laboratory frame of reference. Thus rigid rotation of an image region should be accompanied by a similar transformation of the DTs.
- **Scaling** part (or all) of an image is analogous to changing the size of a particular tissue region. Such a change in size of a region of tissue would generally correspond to an increased number of cells comprising the region. We would not expect the microscopic structure of the tissue to be affected and thus we do not expect the point-wise diffusion properties of the material to change.
- **Shear** of an image region, in general, has the both stretching and rotational effects. Stretching can be viewed in a similar way to scaling and we assume that it does not affect the DT values. The rotational effect of a shear is more complex than the effects of rigid rotation, since its effect on a DT depends on the DTs original orientation with respect to the shear. The orientation of a fibre whose axis is in the same direction as a shearing force would be unaffected by the deformation, but if the axis is in a perpendicular direction the fibre would undergo some reorientation. We thus expect to observe similar effects in the orientation of DTs in image regions undergoing these transformations. This is illustrated in 2D in Figure 2.

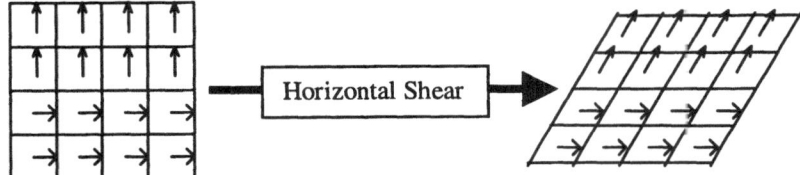

Figure 2 Illustration on the effects of image shear on the orientation of DTs. The arrow in each square of the grid represents the PD of a DT before and after a shear is applied.

We assume throughout that the fundamental diffusion characteristics at any point in the image are unaffected by an image transformation, i.e., the shape of the DT is unaffected so its eigenvalues are preserved. The only change that occurs as a result of the transformation is a reorientation of the axes of the tensor. If T_1 is the DT matrix at a point in an undeformed image, then the matrix, T_2, of the DT in the transformed version of the image is the same matrix after a similarity transform has been applied to rotate the frame of reference of the measurement:

$$T_2 = R^T T_1 R , \tag{2}$$

where R is an appropriate rotation matrix, estimations for which are discussed in the next section.

3 DT Reorientation Strategies

In this section, three strategies are detailed for the extraction of the appropriate reorientation of the DT at each point, i.e., estimation of the rotation matrix, R, in (2). The first two strategies use methods from classical continuum mechanics, which extract the rigid rotation component from the local displacement gradient. The third method accounts for the additional effects of local shearing forces, which is ignored in the first two strategies, by applying the local displacement directly to the principal axes of the DT.

3.1 Small Strain Strategy

Suppose we have two image volumes, I_1 and I_2, and a displacement field, $\underline{u}(\underline{X}) = (u_x(X,Y,Z), u_y(X,Y,Z), u_z(X,Y,Z))$, that describes the warp between the two images, so that if $\underline{x} = \underline{X} + \underline{u}$, then $I_2(\underline{x}) = I_2(\underline{X} + \underline{u}) = I_1(\underline{X})$. The *displacement gradient*,

$$J_u = \frac{d\underline{u}}{d\underline{X}} = \begin{bmatrix} \dfrac{\partial u_x}{\partial X} & \dfrac{\partial u_x}{\partial Y} & \dfrac{\partial u_x}{\partial Z} \\ \dfrac{\partial u_y}{\partial X} & \dfrac{\partial u_y}{\partial Y} & \dfrac{\partial u_y}{\partial Z} \\ \dfrac{\partial u_z}{\partial X} & \dfrac{\partial u_z}{\partial Y} & \dfrac{\partial u_z}{\partial Z} \end{bmatrix}, \tag{3}$$

at a point, describes the relative displacements of local points and can be decomposed into a rigid rotation component and pure deformation component. If we adopt elastic body models for the two image volumes, as in the elastic matching algorithm, and further assume that the strain on the elastic volume is everywhere small, then a simple additive approximation to this decomposition can be used: $\mathbf{J_u} = \mathbf{E} + \mathbf{\Omega}$. In this decomposition, $\mathbf{E}$, is a symmetric matrix that represents the pure deformation component and $\mathbf{\Omega}$ is the skew-symmetric matrix, given by,

$$\Omega = \begin{bmatrix} 0 & \dfrac{1}{2}\left(\dfrac{\partial u_x}{\partial Y} - \dfrac{\partial u_y}{\partial X}\right) & \dfrac{1}{2}\left(\dfrac{\partial u_x}{\partial Z} - \dfrac{\partial u_z}{\partial X}\right) \\ -\dfrac{1}{2}\left(\dfrac{\partial u_x}{\partial Y} - \dfrac{\partial u_y}{\partial X}\right) & 0 & \dfrac{1}{2}\left(\dfrac{\partial u_y}{\partial Z} - \dfrac{\partial u_z}{\partial Y}\right) \\ -\dfrac{1}{2}\left(\dfrac{\partial u_x}{\partial Z} - \dfrac{\partial u_z}{\partial X}\right) & -\dfrac{1}{2}\left(\dfrac{\partial u_y}{\partial Z} - \dfrac{\partial u_z}{\partial Y}\right) & 0 \end{bmatrix}. \tag{4}$$

Ω represents the relative displacements due to the rigid rotation component at point $\underline{X}$=(X,Y,Z) in the undeformed image I_1. It can be shown, [11], that Ω is the relative displacement matrix equivalent to a rotation about axis $\underline{\omega}$, through angle $|\underline{\omega}|$, where

$$\underline{\omega} = -\Omega_{yz}\,\underline{i} - \Omega_{zx}\,\underline{j} - \Omega_{xy}\,\underline{k}. \tag{5}$$

Ω_{nm} in equation (5) is the entry in the n-th row and m-th column of the matrix Ω and $\underline{i}$, $\underline{j}$, and $\underline{k}$ are unit vectors in the directions of the axes of the original co-ordinate frame, $\underline{X}$.

The transformation matrix, $\mathbf{R}$, corresponding to this rotation can be obtained from the general formula for rotation through angle θ about an axis given by the unit vector (r_x, r_y, r_z), [12]:

$$\mathbf{R} = \begin{bmatrix} r_x^2(1-\cos\theta)+\cos\theta & r_x r_y(1-\cos\theta)-r_z\sin\theta & r_x r_z(1-\cos\theta)+r_y\sin\theta \\ r_x r_y(1-\cos\theta)+r_z\sin\theta & r_y^2(1-\cos\theta)+\cos\theta & r_y r_z(1-\cos\theta)-r_x\sin\theta \\ r_x r_z(1-\cos\theta)-r_y\sin\theta & r_y r_z(1-\cos\theta)+r_x\sin\theta & r_z^2(1-\cos\theta)+\cos\theta \end{bmatrix} \tag{6}$$

When the transformation is described locally by a displacement vector field, $\mathbf{J_u}$ is obtained by numerical differentiation of $\underline{u}$. For a global affine transformation, described by a matrix $\mathbf{G}$, $\mathbf{J_u}$, and consequently $\mathbf{R}$, is constant over the entire image volume and $\mathbf{J_u}$ can be obtained directly from $\mathbf{G}$.

3.2   Finite Strain Strategy

Malvern, [11], states that the small strain assumption is justified if the angle of rotation is small compared to one radian. The displacement gradient can always be decomposed into deformation and rigid rotation components, but the additive approximation to this decomposition is inaccurate for larger angles of rotation. In such cases, called "finite strain" cases, [11], a more complex decomposition must be used. Here we just give the expression for the rigid rotation matrix, a derivation of this expression can be found in [11]. For the finite strain case, $\mathbf{R}$ is given by:

$$\mathbf{R} = \mathbf{F}.\left(\mathbf{F}^T.\mathbf{F}\right)^{-\frac{1}{2}}. \tag{7}$$

Where **F** is the *deformation gradient* given by,

$$\mathbf{F} = \frac{d\underline{x}}{d\underline{X}} = \mathbf{I} + \mathbf{J}_U. \tag{8}$$

Computation of **R** in the finite strain case is more computationally complex, since an eigen-decomposition is required to compute the matrix power in (7), [11].

3.3   Eigenvector Deformation Strategy

The deformation component of the displacement gradient includes transformations such as shearing and non-uniform scaling. As illustrated in Figure 2, these transformations can also affect the orientation, but both the previous strategies discard the deformation component. An alternative approach is to consider the action of the displacement directly on unit vectors in the principal diffusion directions.

There are a number of possible strategies that could be adopted to estimate the appropriate reorientation of the DT in this way. In general, the action of the displacement on a particular elliptical contour of the DT will yield a contour that is no longer elliptical. We wish to preserve the fundamental shape of the DT and, furthermore, the property we are most concerned with preserving is the PD. Thus, in the method we have chosen to use here, we ensure that the PD is mapped perfectly to its image under the local displacement. Orientation of the DT in the orthogonal directions is computed in such a way as to ensure that the other eigenvectors of the DT are as close as possible to their images. The method proceeds as follows:

- Compute unit eigenvectors, $\underline{e}_1$, $\underline{e}_2$, $\underline{e}_3$, of the DT.
- Apply the local deformation gradient, **F**, to the principal eigenvector, $\underline{e}_1$, to find its image in the deformed configuration, $\mathbf{F}(\underline{e}_1)$.
- Compute the rotation matrix, $\mathbf{R}_1$, that maps $\underline{e}_1$ onto a unit vector in the direction of $\mathbf{F}(\underline{e}_1)$. The axis and angle of this rotation are obtained from the vector and scalar products of $\underline{e}_1$ and $\mathbf{F}(\underline{e}_1)$, and $\mathbf{R}_1$ can then be calculated using equation (6).

A secondary rotation is required to map the second principal eigenvector, $\underline{e}_2$, from its position *after* the first rotation to a direction as close as possible to its image under **F**.

- Find the images of $\underline{e}_2$ under transformations **F** and $\mathbf{R}_1$.
- Find the projection, $P(\underline{e}_2)$, of $\mathbf{F}(\underline{e}_2)$ onto a plane perpendicular to $\mathbf{R}_1(\underline{e}_1)$. Note that the 2nd principal eigenvector of the rotated DT, $\mathbf{R}_1(\underline{e}_2)$, already lies in this plane.
- Compute a second rotation, $\mathbf{R}_2$, that rotates $\mathbf{R}_1(\underline{e}_2)$ onto a unit vector in the direction of $P(\underline{e}_2)$. The axis of this rotation is $\mathbf{R}_1(\underline{e}_1)$ and the angle is found from the dot product of $\mathbf{R}_1(\underline{e}_2)$ with $P(\underline{e}_2)$.

Note that in this scheme, the DT reorientation is not constant for global affine transformations, unlike the previous two methods. Although the deformation gradient, **F**, is constant, its effect on the eigenvectors of the DT depends on the orientation of $\underline{e}_1$ and $\underline{e}_2$, so a separate reorientation must be computed at every voxel.

4   Experiments and Results

In this section, a set of experiments is described, which test the performance of the different DT reorientation strategies proposed in the previous section. Experiments are performed over a single pair of DT images of the human brain. Details of data acquisition are given first, followed by a description of the experiments and, finally, results from these experiments and some discussion.

4.1   Data

Both images are taken from young female subjects. The general image acquisition methodology is identical to that reported in [4]. Images were acquired using a 1.5T GE Signa Horizon EchoSpeed spectrometer. Each DT image consists of 33 contiguous axial slices, with slice thickness 3.5mm, 220mm field of view and 128x128 in-plane resolution. Six gradient directions were sampled and 4 images were acquired for each direction. Four images with no diffusion weighting were also acquired and so a total of 28 T2-weighted acquisitions were made per slice of the DT image volume.

Brain regions were extracted from the background by hand in both images and background voxels are set to a value outside the measurement range.

4.2   Experiments

In all the experiments, the elastic matching algorithm is run at four resolutions from one sixteenth to one half of the full, isotropic, 1mm^3, volume, which is interpolated from the original image. The weighting of the deformation term in the elastic matching energy function is varied from 1.0 to 0.125, through successive negative powers of two for successive levels of the pyramid.

In order to select an optimal value for σ, which controls the weighting of the similarity term of (1), a number of landmark correspondences were defined in each image. For each reorientation strategy, the value of σ was chosen to be that for which the summed distance between landmarks after matching is minimal. For the match obtained with σ set at this optimum value, a second measure is computed, which indicates the similarity of PDs at corresponding points. Care must be taken with measures of this type, as the PD is poorly defined in regions where the diffusion is isotropic, and the difference cannot be relied upon as a measure of match quality. For this reason, the final measure of match quality, E_{PD}, is an average of the dot product of the two PDs weighted by the geometric mean of their lattice anisotropies.

$$E_{PD} = \frac{\sum \sqrt{v(\mathbf{D}_1).v(\mathbf{D}_2)}.(pd(\mathbf{D}_1).pd(\mathbf{D}_2))}{\sum \sqrt{v(\mathbf{D}_1).v(\mathbf{D}_2)}}. \tag{9}$$

The sums are taken over the region within both hand extracted brain regions. $\mathbf{D}_1$ and $\mathbf{D}_2$ are the DTs in corresponding positions of the two images, $v(\mathbf{D})$ represents the lattice anisotropy of $\mathbf{D}$ and $pd(\mathbf{D})$ is a unit vector in the PD of $\mathbf{D}$.

4.3   Results

Separate matches are computed using each of the DT reorientation strategies and once more with no DT reorientation. The quality of each match is assessed using E_{PD} and results are given in Table 1. We also give the magnitude of the tensor difference (-σS_T

of (1)) averaged over the overlap region to give a measure, E_T, in each case. Note that *higher* values of E_{PD} indicate better match quality, whereas *lower* values of E_T are more desirable.

Table 1 Quality measures for the matches between the pair of brain volumes computed using each of the DT reorientation strategies.

Reorientation strategy	Small Strain	Finite Strain	Eigenvector deformation.	No reorientation.
E_T	627.8	625.3	622.2	623.4
E_{PD}	0.768	0.768	0.772	0.771

The optimal value of the similarity weighting parameter, σ, was found to be around 200 for each strategy. The value of the landmark distance measure is noisy in the vicinity of this minimum point and no significant differences in this measure can be observed between the difference reorientation strategies. The values of E_{PD} and E_T, however are more stable and the differences in these values observed in Table 1 are consistent in the vicinity of $\sigma=200$. With σ set this value, we find that both the small strain and finite strain reorientation strategies produce poor performance and the matches obtained with them are worse than with no reorientation at all. The eigenvector deformation strategy is the only strategy that improves the quality of match over the control case in which no reorientation is applied.

5   Conclusions

We have presented three methods for estimation of the appropriate reorientation of DTs in image volumes undergoing non-rigid transformations, which we model as locally affine. Of the three methods the best results were obtained from the eigenvector deformation strategy, which explicitly computes the effects of the local displacement field on vectors along the principal axes of the diffusion ellipsoid. This is the only method of the three presented that takes into account the reorientation effects of the deformation component of the image transformation.

The numerical differences in the results above are small. This fact may reflect that the structure of these particular brains is such that little reorientation is required during matching, or it may be that the reorientation is not correct throughout the matched image volume. Experiments on an extended data set are planned. Simple experiments with synthetic data can verify that for a known displacement field, the expected reorientation of the data is extracted correctly by the methods described above. However, we cannot verify that a good voxel-voxel anatomical match is made for the real data.

Although the orientation of the DTs is updated throughout the matching process, there is currently no explicit term in the energy function for their orientation. The inclusion of such a term should allow the elastic matching algorithm to exploit the correspondence of orientational information in the DTs while computing the match and so should further improve the quality of the matches obtained. As mentioned in the introduction, this issue also arises when matching intensity images using region based similarity measures and the improvement of these matches is added motivation for continued investigation in this area.

References

1. R. Bajcsy and S. Kovacic, "Multi-Resolution Elastic Matching", Computer Vision, Graphics and Image Processing, Vol., 46, pp. 1-21, 1989.

2. J.C. Gee and D.R. Haynor, "Numerical Methods for High Dimensional Warps". Chapter in "Brain Warping", ed. A.W. Toga, Academic Press, 1998

3. J.C. Gee and R.K. Bajcsy, "Elastic Matching: Continuum Mechanical and Probabilistic Analysis". Chapter in "Brain Warping", ed. A.W. Toga, Academic Press, 1998

4. C. Pierpaoli, P. Jezzard, P.J. Basser, A. Barnett, G. Di Chiro, "Diffusion Tensor MR Imaging of the Human Brain", Radiology, Vol. 201, No. 3, pp. 637-648, 1996.

5. C. Poupon, J.-F. Mangin, V. Frouin, J. Regis, F. Poupon, M. Pachot-Clouard, D. LeBihan, and I. Bloch, "Regularisation of MR Diffusion Tensor Maps for Tracking White Matter Bundles", Proc. MICCAI'98, MIT, Boston, 1998.

6. M.A. Horsfield, H.B.W. Larsson, D.K. Jones, A. Gass, "Diffusion magnetic resonance imaging in multiple sclerosis", Journal of Neurology, Neurosurgery and Psychiatry, Vol. 64 (Supplement), pp S80-S84, 1998.

7. C. Pierpaoli and P.J. Basser, "Toward a Quantitative Assessment of Diffusion Anisotropy", Magnetic Resonance Medicine, Vol. 36, pp. 893-906, 1996.

8. R.P. Woods, S.T. Grafton, C.J. Holmes, S.R. Cherry and J.C. Mazziotta, "Automated Image Registration: I General Methods and intra-subject intra-modality validation", Journal of Computer Assisted Tomography, Vol. 22 pp. 141-154, 1998.

9. R.P. Woods, S.T. Grafton, J.D.G. Watson, N.L. Sicotte and J.C. Mazziotta, "Automated Image Registration: II Inter-subject validation of linear and non-linear models", Journal of Computer Assisted Tomography, Vol. 22 pp. 155-165, 1998.

10. D.C. Alexander, R. Bajcsy and J.C. Gee, "Elastic Matching of Diffusion Tensor MRIs", accepted for publication in Computer Vision and Image Understanding, 1999.

11. L.E. Malvern, "Introduction to the Mechanics of a Continuous Medium", Prentice-Hall, Inc. Englewood Cliffs, N.J., 1969.

12. K.S. Fu, R.C. Gonzalez and C.S.G. Lee, "Robotics: Control, Sensing, Vision and Intelligence", New York: McGraw-Hill, 1987.

Analysis of Functional MRI Data
Using Mutual Information [*]

Andy Tsai[1], John W. Fisher III[1,2], Cindy Wible[3,4],
William M. Wells III[2,3], Junmo Kim[1], and Alan S. Willsky[1]

[1] Laboratory for Information and Decision Systems,
Massachusetts Institute of Technology,
Cambridge, MA, USA
{atsai, junmo, willsky}@mit.edu
http://ssg.mit.edu/
[2] Artificial Intelligence Laboratory,
Massachusetts Institute of Technology,
Cambridge, MA, USA
{fisher, sw}@ai.mit.edu
http://ai.mit.edu/
[3] Department of Radiology,
Brigham and Women's Hospital,
Harvard Medical School,
Boston, MA, USA
cindy@bwh.harvard.edu
http://splweb.bwh.harvard.edu:8000/
[4] Department of Psychiatry,
Brockton/West Roxbury VAMC,
Harvard Medical School,
Brockton, MA, USA

Abstract. A new information-theoretic approach is presented for analyzing *f*MRI data to calculate the brain activation map. The method is
based on a formulation of the mutual information between two waveforms—
the *f*MRI temporal response of a voxel and the experimental protocol
timeline. Scores based on mutual information are generated for all voxels
and then used to compute the activation map of an experiment. Mutual
information for *f*MRI analysis is employed because it has been shown to
be robust in quantifying the relationship between any two waveforms.
More importantly, our technique takes a principled approach toward calculating the brain activation map by making few assumptions about the
relationship between the protocol timeline and the temporal response of
a voxel. This is important especially in *f*MRI experiments where little is
known about the relationship between these two waveforms. Experiments
are presented to demonstrate this approach of computing the brain activation map. Comparisons to other more traditional analysis techniques
are made and the results are presented.

[*] This work was supported by ONR grant N00014-91-J-1004 and by subcontract
GC123919NGD from Boston University under the AFOSR Multidisciplinary Research Program on Reduced Signature Target Recognition.

1   Introduction

We present a novel method based on an information-theoretic approach to find
the brain activation maps for fMRI experiments. In this method, mutual information is calculated between the temporal response of a voxel and the protocol
timeline of the experiment. This value can then be used as a score to quantify
the relationship between the two waveforms. Mutual information is appropriate
for fMRI analysis because it has been shown to be more robust than other methods in identifying complex relationships (i.e. those which are nonlinear and/or
stochastic). More importantly, our nonparametric estimator of mutual information requires little *a priori* knowledge of the relationship between the temporal
response of a voxel and the protocol timeline. Over the past few years, mutual
information has been used to solve a variety of problems [2, 8, 9].

2   Background

2.1   Functional Magnetic Resonance Imaging

Functional magnetic resonance imaging is a powerful new imaging modality with
the ability to noninvasively generate images of the brain that reflect brain tissue
hemodynamics. Brain tissue hemodynamics are spatially related to the metabolic
demands of the brain tissue caused by neuronal activity. Therefore, indirectly,
this imaging modality can capture brain neuronal dynamics at different sites
while being activated by sensory input, motor performance, or cognitive activity.

The specific area of fMRI analysis we address in this paper is the identification of those voxels in the fMRI scan which are functionally related to the
experimental stimuli. This entails determining whether the acquired temporal
response of a voxel during the scan is related to the experimental protocol timeline that is used during the scan. This relationship is difficult to establish for the
following reason: it is known from single unit recording studies that the response
characteristics of neurons differ between brain regions *and* in relationship to different stimuli. Some neurons may respond to stimuli with brief transient activity,
whereas others might show more sustained activity to the same stimulation. As
cognitive and psychological variables such as habituation and attention are added
to the equation, the relationship between brain activity and stimuli becomes even
more complex [7]. This, coupled with the fact that fMRI measurements–which
do not directly measure brain activities–are many steps removed from single unit
recordings, makes the relationship between the two waveforms even harder to
establish. Because of the complex, most certainly nonlinear and perhaps stochastic, nature of the relationship between the two waveforms, it has been difficult
to find a suitable metric to quantify the dependencies. The technique we present
in this paper can be used to overcome such obstacles.

2.2   Popular Strategies for Analysis of fMRI data

Currently, the popular analysis methods used to obtain the activation map includes direct subtraction [5], correlation coefficient [1, 10], and the general linear

model [4]. Quantitative comparisons of these methods are difficult given the absence of ground truth, little knowledge about human brain activation patterns, and the indirect role fMRI plays in capturing brain activation. The following is a short description of the popular fMRI analysis techniques.

Direct Subtraction (DS) This method involves calculating two mean intensities for each voxel–one mean value calculated based on averaging together all the temporal responses acquired during the "task" period, and the other mean value calculated based on averaging together all the temporal responses acquired during the "rest" period of an experiment. To determine whether a voxel is activated or not, one mean intensity is subtracted from the other. Voxels with significant difference in the mean intensities of the two data groups are identified as being activated. To yield a statistic to identify significant difference in the intensities, a Student's t-test is employed. This test determines whether the means of the two data groups are statistically different from one another by utilizing the difference between the means relative to the variabilities of the two data groups. The t-value this method generates, for a temporal response y, is calculated as

$$t = \frac{\bar{y}_{on} - \bar{y}_{off}}{\sqrt{\frac{\sigma_{y_{on}}^2}{N_{on}-1} + \frac{\sigma_{y_{off}}^2}{N_{off}-1}}}$$

where y_{on} and y_{off} denote the set of data points in the temporal measurements that correspond to the "task" and the "rest" periods, respectively, and N_{on} and N_{off} denote the number of time points that corresponds to the "task" and the "rest" periods, respectively. The mean and variance of the data group y_{on} are denoted as $\bar{y}_{on}$ and $\sigma_{y_{on}}^2$, respectively. Likewise, the mean and variance of the data group y_{off} are denoted as $\bar{y}_{off}$ and $\sigma_{y_{off}}^2$, respectively. The major shortcoming associated with this method is that it relies heavily on the assumption that temporal measurements of a given voxel can be partitioned into two data groups, each normally distributed according to a different mean and variance.

Correlation Coefficient (CC) The correlation coefficient ρ_{xy} is a normalized measure of the correlation between the reference waveform x and the measurement waveform y, and is defined by

$$\rho_{xy} = \frac{\sum(x - \bar{x})(y - \bar{y})}{\sqrt{\sum(x - \bar{x})^2 \sum(y - \bar{y})^2}}$$

where $\bar{x}$ and $\bar{y}$ denote the means of x and y, respectively. The summation is taken over all the time points in the waveform. It is easy to establish that $-1 \leq \rho_{xy} \leq 1$. Voxels with large $|\rho_{xy}|$s are considered to be activated. For this method, $|\rho_{xy}|$ is used as the test statistic for statistical inference. This method critically depends on the choice of the reference waveform. Various waveforms have been used [1, 10]; however, in light of the many unknown factors affecting measurement of brain activation, reference waveform design poses a serious obstacle, especially for more complicated protocols.

General Linear Model (GLM) The statistical models used for parameter modeling in the two previously described analysis methods are both special cases of the general linear model. This model is a framework designed to find the correct linear combination of explanatory variables (such as hemodynamic response, respiratory and cardiac dynamics) that can account for the temporal response observed at each voxel during an experiment. Assume that there exists T number of time point measurements per voxel in the fMRI data set. Let y_t denote the measurement at some voxel at time t, and let ϵ_t denote the error term associated with the linear model fit at that same voxel at time t, with $1 \leq t \leq T$. Here, $\epsilon_t \sim \mathcal{N}(0, \sigma^2)$. Suppose there are J number of explanatory variables in the linear model. Let x_{jt} denote the value of the jth explanatory variable at time t with $1 \leq j \leq J$. Also let β_j denote the scaling parameter for the jth explanatory variable. With these definitions, the general linear model can be written as

$$\begin{bmatrix} y_1 \\ y_2 \\ \vdots \\ y_T \end{bmatrix} = \begin{bmatrix} x_{11} & x_{12} & \dots & x_{1J} \\ x_{21} & x_{22} & \dots & x_{2J} \\ \vdots & & \ddots & \vdots \\ x_{T1} & x_{T2} & \dots & x_{TJ} \end{bmatrix} \begin{bmatrix} \beta_1 \\ \beta_2 \\ \vdots \\ \beta_J \end{bmatrix} + \begin{bmatrix} \epsilon_1 \\ \epsilon_2 \\ \vdots \\ \epsilon_J \end{bmatrix}.$$

The above equation can be written succinctly in matrix notation as $Y = X\beta + \epsilon$. In general, X is full rank and the number of explanatory variables J is less than the number of observations T indicating that the method of least squares can be employed to find the scaling parameters β. Since $X^T X$ is invertible, the least squares estimate for β, which we denote by $\hat{\beta}$, is $(X^T X)^{-1} X^T Y$. Then $\hat{\beta}$ is used to test whether it corresponds to the model of an activation response (as specified in X) or the null hypothesis. One of the major problems associated with this method is in the design of X. As mentioned earlier, little is known about the relationship between fMRI temporal response and brain stimulation. Hence, it is difficult to identify the necessary explanatory variables that can account for the temporal responses seen in fMRI measurements.

3   Description of Method

3.1   Mutual Information and Entropy

Mutual information (MI) and entropy are concepts which underly much of information theory [3]. They cannot be adequately described within the scope of this paper. Suffice it to say that MI is a measure of the information that one random variable (RV) conveys about another, and entropy is a measure of the average uncertainty in a RV. Both quantities are expressed in terms of bits of information. Here, we demonstrate the appropriateness of MI for fMRI analysis.

The mutual information, $I(u, v)$, between the RVs u and v, is defined as [3]

$$I(u, v) = h(v) - h(v|u) = h(u) - h(u|v), \quad (1)$$

where the entropy, $h(v)$, quantifies the randomness of v and the conditional entropy, $h(v|u)$, quantifies the randomness of v conditioned on observations of

u. These terms are described by the following expectations:

$$h(v) = -E_v \left[\log_2(P(v))\right]$$
$$h(v|u) = -E_u \left[E_v \left[\log_2(P(v|u))\right]\right].$$

where P denotes probability density. It is clear from (1) that MI is symmetric. That is, the information that u conveys about v is equal to the information that v conveys about u. Furthermore, since u is a discrete RV in our case and conditioning always reduces uncertainty $(h(u|v) \leq h(u))$, v can convey at most $h(u)$ bits of information about u (and vice versa). We can therefore lower and upper bound the MI between u and v by 0 and $h(u)$, respectively.

3.2 Calculation of Brain Activation Map by MI

We present nonparametric MI as a formalism for uncovering dependencies in calculating the fMRI activation map. Recall that in our specific application, we seek at most one *bit* of information (whether or not a voxel is activated). This impacts our choice of the reference waveform. The reference waveform need be no more complicated than our hypothesis space (1 bit). The protocol timeline shown in Fig. 1 is the simplest model of our hypothesis space and is sufficient as the reference waveform when using MI as the basis for comparison. More elaborate waveforms can be employed, but they imply more information than is necessary. The consequence of this is that complicated waveform design in unnecessary; the reference waveform need only adequately *encode* the hypothesis space.

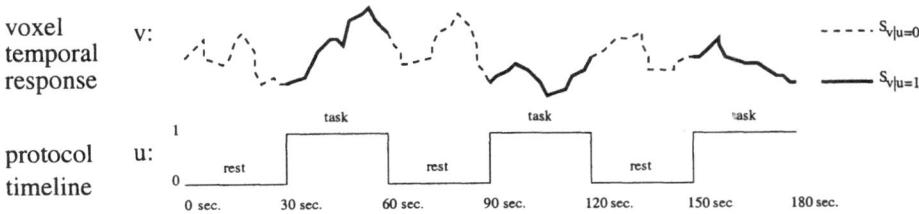

Fig. 1. Illustration of the Protocol Timeline, $S_{v|u=0}$, and $S_{v|u=1}$.

In the following derivation, we will refer to the temporal response of a voxel as v, and the reference waveform as u. We have already established the appropriateness of using the protocol timeline as the reference waveform u. As such, u only takes on two possible values, 0 and 1, so we can rewrite equation (1) as

$$I(u,v) = h(v) - P(u = 0)h(v|u = 0) - P(u = 1)h(v|u = 1) \qquad (2)$$

where $P(u = 0)$ and $P(u = 1)$ are the *a priori* probabilities of u taking on the values of 0 and 1, respectively. This reference waveform is chosen because it is the simplest encoding of the actual hypothesis (task vs. rest) with equal probabilities reflecting the relative frequencies of samples during each state.

478   Andy Tsai et al.

As an illustrative example, suppose v is a scaled and biased version of u (i.e. $v = cu + d$ where $c, d \in \Re$ and $c \neq 0$). Then

$$h(v|u = 0) = -E_v\left[\log_2(P(v|u = 0))\right] = -E_v\left[\log_2(1)\right] = 0 \text{ bits},$$

$$h(v|u = 1) = -E_v\left[\log_2(P(v|u = 1))\right] = -E_v\left[\log_2(1)\right] = 0 \text{ bits},$$

$$h(v) = -E_v\left[\log_2(P(v))\right] = -E_v\left[\log_2(0.5)\right] = -\log_2(0.5) = 1 \text{ bit},$$

so that $I(u, v) = 1$ bit. This is the maximum MI that can be achieve between the square wave u and *any* other waveform v. Since only 1 bit of information is encoded in u, only 1 bit of MI can exist between u and *any* v.

3.3   Estimating Entropies

Evaluating equation (2) requires computing $h(v)$, $h(v|u = 0)$, and $h(v|u = 1)$ which are integral functions of the densities $P(v)$, $P(v|u = 0)$, and $P(v|u = 1)$. In general, these must be estimated. We choose the nonparametric Parzen window method [6] to estimate the densities and the sample means to estimate the entropy terms. The Parzen density estimate (with leave-one-out) is defined as

$$\hat{P}(v) = \frac{1}{(N_{S_v} - 1)}\left[\sum_{v_j \in S_v} G_\sigma(v - v_j) - G_\sigma(0)\right]$$

where N_{S_v} is the number of data points in the sample set S_v, G_σ is an admissible kernel function (we use the Gaussian kernel, other kernels are possible), and σ is the standard deviation of the density function. The set S_v is composed of *all* the data points from v. Our estimate for the conditional $P(v|u = 0)$ is

$$\hat{P}(v|u = 0) = \frac{1}{(N_{S_{v|u=0}} - 1)}\left[\sum_{v_j \in S_{v|u=0}} G_\sigma(v - v_j) - G_\sigma(0)\right]$$

where $N_{S_{v|u=0}}$ is the number of data points in the sample set $S_{v|u=0}$. The set $S_{v|u=0}$ is composed of the subset of data points from v with time points corresponding to when $u = 0$. Similarly, the estimate for $P(v|u = 1)$ is identical to $\hat{P}(v|u = 0)$ only taken over the subset of samples from v with time points corresponding to when $u = 1$.

Kernel size (in our case the standard deviation, σ of the Gaussian kernel) is an issue for the Parzen window density estimator. Consistent with our information-theoretic approach, we choose the kernel size which maximizes the likelihood of the data [3]. For example, the kernel size $\hat{\sigma}_{ML}$ used to estimate $h(v)$ is

$$\hat{\sigma}_{ML} = \arg\max_\sigma\left\{\frac{1}{N_{S_v}}\sum_{v_j \in S_v} \log \hat{P}(v_j)\right\}.$$

As direct evaluation of the entropy terms is computationally prohibitive we approximate them with their sample means [8,9]. For example, $h(v)$ is approximated by

$$h(v) \approx -\frac{1}{N_{S_v}} \sum_{v_j \in S_v} \log_2 \left(\frac{1}{N_{S_v} - 1} \sum_{v_i \in S_v} G_\sigma(v_j - v_i) - G_\sigma(0) \right)$$

The conditional terms, $h(v|u = 0)$ and $h(v|u = 1)$, are defined similarly using the previously defined subsets $S_{v|u=0}$ and $S_{v|u=1}$, respectively.

4   Experimental Results

We applied the above described fMRI analysis method to a single fMRI data set that examines right-hand movements. The data set contains 60 whole brain acquisitions with each whole brain acquisition containing 21 slice images.

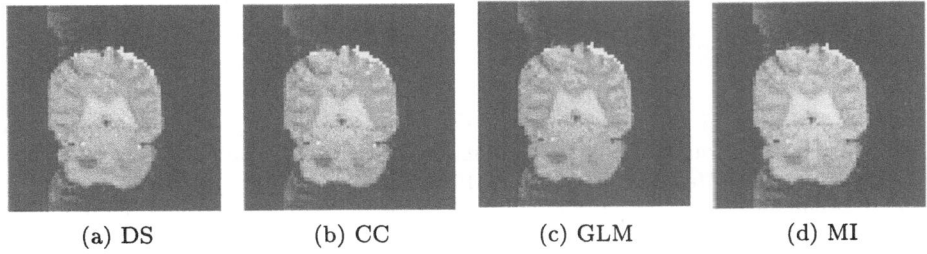

(a) DS   (b) CC   (c) GLM   (d) MI

Fig. 2. Comparison of fMRI Analysis Techniques.

Only the analysis results from the 10th coronal slice of the whole brain acquisition are shown in Fig. 2. The figure provides a qualitative comparison of our analysis technique with other techniques previously mentioned in this paper. A quantitative comparison of these different methods is difficult since the ground truth is unknown. In keeping with the fairness of the comparison, the threshold (which determines whether a voxel is activated or not) that yields the "best" activation map for each analysis technique is used. For this particular fMRI data set, the "best" activation map is judged based on the prior expectation that brain activation is restricted to the left primary motor cortex and occurs in clusters. It is important to point out that MI is inherently a normalized measure so for our technique, the threshold can be specified meaningfully in terms of bits of information. Fig. 2(d) is obtained using a threshold of 0.7 bits. While the qualitative differences between the techniques as observed in Fig.2 is small the MI approach combines very few assumptions about the underlying data *and* an inherently normalized threshold (none of the other techniques have both of these properties). We believe that these results demonstrate the viability and efficacy of the MI approach for *f*MRI data analysis, although more extensive experimentation is warranted.

5   Summary

We have developed a theoretical framework for using MI to calculate the *f*MRI activation map. While there are many existing approaches to calculate the activation map, all of these techniques depend on some *a priori* assumptions about the relationship between the protocol timeline and the *f*MRI voxel temporal response. The strength of our approach is that it relies on sound theoretical principles, it is fairly easy to implement, and does not require strong assumptions about the nature of the relationships between the *f*MRI temporal measurements and the protocol timeline, while still retaining the ability to uncover complex relationships (beyond second-order statistics). In addition, experimental results confirmed that this information-theoretic approach can be as effective as other methods of calculating activation maps. Finally, from the clinical standpoint, nuisance variables are significantly reduced, that is, the protocol timeline need only encode the actual hypothesis test (e.g. waveform matching is unnecessary).

References

1. P.A. Bandettini, A. Jesmanowicz, E.C. Wong, and J.S. Hyde. Processing strategies for time-course data sets in functional MRI of the human brain. *Magnetic Resonance in Medicine*, 30:161–173, 1993.
2. F. Bello and A.C.F. Colchester. Measuring global and local spatial correspondence using information theory. In *Proceedings of the First International Conference on Medical Computing and Computer-Assisted Intervention*, 1998.
3. T.M. Cover and J.A. Thomas. *Elements of Information Theory*. John Wiley and Son Inc., 1st edition, 1991.
4. K.J. Friston, P. Jezzard, and R. Turner. Analysis of functional MRI time-series. *Human Brain Mapping*, 1:153–171, 1994.
5. O. Henriksen, H.B.W. Larsson, P. Ring, E. Rostrup, A. Stensgaard, M. Stubgaard, F Stahlberg, L. Sondergaard, C. Thomsen, and P. Toft. Functional MR imaging at 1.5T. *Acta Radiologica*, 34:101–103, 1993.
6. E. Parzen. On estimation of a probability density and mode. *Annals of Mathematical Statistics*, 33:1065–1076, 1962.
7. D.L. Schacter and R.L. Bucknew. On the relations among priming, conscious recollection,and intentional retrieval: evidence from neuroimaging research. *Neurobiology of Learning and Memory*, 70(1):284–303, 1998.
8. P. Viola and W.M. Wells III. Alignment by maximization of mutual information. *International Journal of Computer Vision*, 24(2):137–154, 1997.
9. W.M. Wells III, P. Viola, H. Atsumi, S. Nakajima, and R. Kikinis. Multi-modal volume registration by maximization of mutual information. *Medical Image Analysis*, 1(1):35–51, 1996.
10. G.K. Wood, B.A. Berkowitz, and C.A. Wilson. Visualization of subtle contrast-related intensity changes using temporal correlation. *Magnetic Resonance Imaging*, 12(7):1013–1020, 1994.

Statistical Segmentation of fMRI Activations Using Contextual Clustering

Eero Salli[1,2], Ari Visa[3], Hannu J. Aronen[1,2], Antti Korvenoja[2,4], and Toivo Katila[1,4]

[1] Laboratory of Biomedical Engineering, Helsinki University of Technology,
P.O.B. 2200, FIN-02015 HUT, Espoo, Finland
{Eero.Salli, Toivo.Katila}@hut.fi
[2] Department of Radiology, Helsinki University Central Hospital, P.O.B. 380,
FIN-00029 HYKS, Helsinki, Finland
Hannu.Aronen@huch.fi, Antti.Korvenoja@helsinki.fi
[3] Department of Information Technology, Lappeenranta University of Technology,
FIN-53851 Lappeenranta, Finland
Ari.Visa@lut.fi
[4] BioMag Laboratory, Helsinki University Central Hospital, P.O.B. 503, FIN-00029
HYKS, Helsinki, Finland

Abstract. A central problem in the analysis of functional magnetic resonance imaging (fMRI) data is the reliable detection and segmentation of activated areas. Often this goal is achieved by computing a statistical parametric map (SPM) and thresholding it. Cluster-size thresholds are also used. A new contextual segmentation method based on clustering is presented in this paper. If the SPM value of a voxel, adjusted with neighborhood information, differs from the expected non-activation value more than a specified decision value, the contextual clustering algorithm classifies the voxel to the activation class, otherwise to the non-activation class. The voxel-wise thresholding, cluster-size thresholding and contextual clustering are compared using fixed overall specificity. Generally, the contextual clustering detects activations with higher probability than the voxel-wise thresholding. Unlike cluster-size thresholding, contextual clustering is able to detect extremely small area activations, too Moreover, the results show that the contextual clustering has good segmentation accuracy, voxel-wise specificity and robustness against spatial autocorrelations in the noise term.

1 Introduction

The most common goal of the fMRI study is the recognition and segmentation of brain areas that respond to a given task or stimulus. Usually, it is required that the overall specificity of the recognition is high. On the other hand, the sensitivity of the process and good specificity in the neighborhood of activated areas are also important. The segmentation task is challenging due to low signal-to-noise ratio of activation related signal changes.

The analysis of an fMRI image series is most often based on the computation of the SPM and making statistical inferences from it. The SPM can be computed using general linear model [1]. Also non-parametric approaches like Kolmogorov-Smirnov [2] statistics are frequently used. Inferences from the SPMs are usually based on voxel-wise intensities above a threshold [3], on the spatial extent of contiguous voxels above a threshold (cluster-size thresholds) [4, 5] or on the combination of these two [6]. Usually the parameters of tests are chosen so that the probability of detecting a false activation in the whole volume (or in the search volume) is relatively small, e.g. 0.05.

In this paper, we present a new method for making statistical inferences and segmentation, called as contextual clustering, which uses both the original statistical value and current voxel classification in the neighborhood to determine the new voxel classification. Contextual clustering, voxel-wise and cluster-size thresholding methods are compared. Especially, sensitivity, segmentation accuracy and robustness against spatial correlations are studied.

2 Materials

The results of this study are based on simulated and measured fMRI data. First, noisy background data *(Data A)* was created by using Matlab's (The Mathworks, inc., Natick, MA, USA) pseudorandom generator. Voxel values were chosen from the Gaussian distribution with mean zero and variance one (Fig. 1(a)). For each simulation, 120 three-dimensional samples (images) were created. The matrix size of each sample was $32 \times 32 \times 16$. In total, 500 fMRI experiments were simulated, so that the total number of random values generated was $500 \times 120 \times 32 \times 32 \times 16$. The *Data A* was used to determine segmentation parameters and to estimate voxel-wise specificity of each segmentation method. Next, a simulation phantom of 12 spheres (Fig. 1(b)) was added into the samples $21 \ldots 40$, $61 \ldots 80$ and $101 \ldots 120$ of *Data A*. This operation formed *Data B* which was used to estimate the sensitivity and segmentation accuracy of the segmentation methods. The *Data* sets C and D were formed by spatially filtering *Data A* using a filter with $3 \times 3 \times 3$ Gaussian kernel of full width at half magnitude (FWHM) 0.6 voxels and 1.2 voxels, respectively. Data sets C and D were used to evaluate robustness of the various methods against spatial autocorrelations.

The measured data of a volunteer was acquired with a $1.5-T$ Siemens Magnetom Vision system (Siemens, Erlangen, Germany) using a gradient-echo echo-planar (EPI) sequence (TE 76 ms, TR 3.5 s, flip angle 90°), and a standard head coil. The right median nerve of a right-handed male volunteer was stimulated electrically with a 0.2 ms constant voltage pulse. The stimulus intensity was adjusted slightly above the motor threshold. The stimulation rate was 4 Hz. The subject kept eyes closed during the experiment. To minimize head movements, bite bar and supporting vacuum pillow were used.

A set of 240 images (matrix $128 \times 128 \times 16$, pixel size 2×2 mm, slice thickness 5 mm) was acquired with the baseline and stimulation condition alternating in blocks of ten images. The first three samples of each block were not taken into statistical analysis to account for the delay in the hemodynamic response.

3   Methods

3.1   Computation of a statistical parametric map

For the purposes of this segmentation study the simple t statistics is an adequate method to compute an SPM. In voxel i, the test statistics can be formulated [7]:

$$t_i = \frac{\overline{X}_{iB} - \overline{X}_{iA}}{\sqrt{\frac{(n_A-1)\sigma_{iA}^2+(n_B-1)\sigma_{iB}^2}{n_A+n_B-2}\left(\frac{1}{n_A}+\frac{1}{n_B}\right)}}, \tag{1}$$

where $\overline{X}_{iA}$ and $\overline{X}_{iB}$ are the means of the observed intensity values, σ_{iA}^2 and σ_{iB}^2 estimated variances and n_A, n_B the sizes of the task state (subindex A) and control state sets (subindex B). The t statistics can be formulated easily also using the general linear model [1]. Variable t_i has the Student's t distribution with $n_1 + n_2 - 2$ degrees of freedom under null hypothesis. The t-map is transformed to Gaussian distributed z-map using $z_i = q_{norm}(p_t(t_i. r))$, where q_{norm} is the normal inverse distribution function at x and $p_t(x, r)$ is the cumulative distribution function for t distribution with r degrees of freedom at x.

Often, prior to the computation of SPM, the image data are spatially filtered in order to increase the signal-to-noise ratio and sensitivity [3]. However, artifacts such as blurred edges result after low pass filtering. As our study concentrates on the segmentation of an already computed SPM, the filtering of image data is not studied here.

3.2   Segmentation methods

Voxel-wise thresholding (VWTH). The simplest segmentation method of an SPM is thresholding applied to each voxel separately. The voxel at location i is considered as active if and only if $z_i < T$, where T is a threshold. In our notation the activations have negative mean and T is chosen negative.

Cluster-size thresholding (CSTH). A cluster c is considered as active if and only if for all voxels within the cluster $z_i < T$ and the size of cluster c is at least T_{size} voxels [5]. In our study, the method is used in 3D with 26-connectivity.

Contextual clustering (CC). The algorithm of contextual clustering is: 1) Label the voxels with $z_i < T$ as *active* and other voxels as *non-active*. Voxels outside the image volume are considered as *non-active*. 2) Compute for all voxels i the number of *active* neighbor voxels, u_i. 3) Relabel the voxels for which

$$z_i + \frac{\beta}{T}(u_i - N/2) < T \tag{2}$$

as *active* and other voxels as *non-active*. The number of neighbor voxels equals to N. Using the 26-connectivity $N = 26$. The parameter β determines the weighting of the contextual information and is usually positive. If we set $\beta = 0$ we have the conventional context-free thresholding rule. 4) If the current labeling is same as the labeling in the previous cycle or in the cycle before that, then stop the iterations, otherwise return to the step 2).

It should be noted that from the mathematical point of view the algorithm is identical with iterated conditional modes (ICM) algorithm of two classes [8]. However, the 2-class ICM algorithm with on-line parameter updating is not applicable because each activation has its own density function. Therefore, actually the 4-class ICM should be used in our case of three different activation and one background distributions. In practice, the number of activation distributions is unknown and therefore the ICM algorithm cannot be used conventionally. Instead of trying to classify every voxel into most probable class, as is done with ICM, the algorithm is used in a completely new way: as a hypothesis testing technique. In other words, if the statistical parametric value of a voxel adjusted with contextual information differs from the null distribution more than a preset threshold, the null hypothesis is rejected. Using the parameter β the trade off between sensitivity and segmentation accuracy can be adjusted. One way to set the parameter β is to write $\beta = T^2/s$. Then s specifies the excess of activated voxels $(u_i - N/2)$ in the neighborhood required to classify a non-active voxel to the *active* class with the probability of 0.5.

3.3   Estimation of parameter values for common overall false activation probability and voxel-wise specificity

In order to compare the sensitivity of the methods the probability of observing false activation voxel(s) in a whole volume was fixed to value of 0.05. The parameter estimation was done by applying the algorithms to the *Data A* with different decision parameter values. A decision parameter value that gave a false activation in 25 images out of 500 (i.e. overall p-value 0.05) was chosen. Also the probability of false activation at voxel level was computed from the measured number of false activation voxels.

3.4   Sensitivity, segmentation accuracy and robustness

The 500 SPMs computed from the *Data B* were segmented with each segmentation method. The segmented images of each method were averaged separately. The resulting *mean image* shows the probability of detection at voxel-level.

In addition, in order to estimate the segmentation accuracy, the number of voxels falsely classified as active in the neighborhood of activation $R3C4$ (see Fig. 1(b)) was counted.

The robustness against spatial autocorrelations in the noise term was evaluated by segmenting *Data C* and *Data D*. If the overall probability of detecting false activation is significantly larger than the expected value of 0.05, the robustness of the method against spatial autocorrelations is low.

4   Results

The estimated decision parameter values and measured probabilities of false activations at voxel level for various segmentation methods are given in Table I. It is seen that although the overall specificity is fixed, there are differences in specificity at voxel level. Best voxel level specificity was achieved with voxel-wise thresholding and contextual clustering. An interesting observation was that all false activations detected with contextual clustering were only one voxel in size. We also studied the overall specificity with larger volume $64 \times 64 \times 16$ using the same decision parameters. In this case the achieved overall false activation rate was 0.23 ± 0.05.

Table 1. Estimated decision parameter values T for overall false activation rate 0.05 and measured probability of false activation at voxel level $P(f_v)$, probability of false activation voxels $P(f_{R3C4})$ in the neighborhood of activation $R3C4$ at voxel level and overall probability of false activation in the presence of spatial autocorrelations $P(f_{c1})$ (FWHM = 0.6 voxels) and $P(f_{c2})$ (FWHM = 1.2 voxels).

Method	Abbrev.	T	$P(f_v) \cdot 10^{-6}$	$P(f_{R3C4})$	$P(f_{c1})$	$P(f_{c2})$
Voxel-wise thresholding	VWTH	−4.490	3.05	0.000	0.05	0.04
Cluster-size thr., $T_{size} = 2$	CSTH:2	−3.269	6.35	0.001	0.08	0.19
Cluster-size thr., $T_{size} = 8$	CSTH:8	−2.066	27.5	0.019	0.18	0.51
Context. clust., $\beta = T^2/2$	CC:2	−0.597	3.05	0.006	0.05	0.05
Context. clust., $\beta = T^2/6$	CC:6	−1.415	3.05	0.001	0.05	0.05

The sensitivity of each segmentation method is shown in Fig. 1(c)-(g). The images are computed by averaging the segmentation results. It can be seen that the voxel-wise thresholding and contextual clustering can detect activations as small as only one voxel in size. On larger activations the cluster-size thresholding with $T_{size} = 8$ and contextual clustering are more sensitive than the voxel-wise thresholding. Cluster-size thresholding with $T_{size} = 2$ seems to be only slightly more powerful than voxel-wise thresholding but misses the smallest activations.

Activation $R3C4$ was used to evaluate segmentation accuracy, i.e. the specificity in the neighborhood of an activation. Also robustness against spatial autocorrelations was studied. The results are reported in Table I. Cluster-size thresholding with $T_{size} = 8$ had worst segmentation accuracy and robustness against autocorrelations.

As the last experiment, we analysed the measured fMRI data. Results on two subsequent slices are shown in Fig. 2. All methods found activations of primary sensorimotor cortex (SMI) and supplementary motor area (SMA). Large β or cluster-size threshold T_{size} decreases the ability to distinguish closely separated activations as multiple foci. This is most clearly seen in the area of SMI, where the clusters of activated voxels in the central sulcus and postcentral sulcus merge with $T_{size} = 8$ or $\beta = T^2/2$.

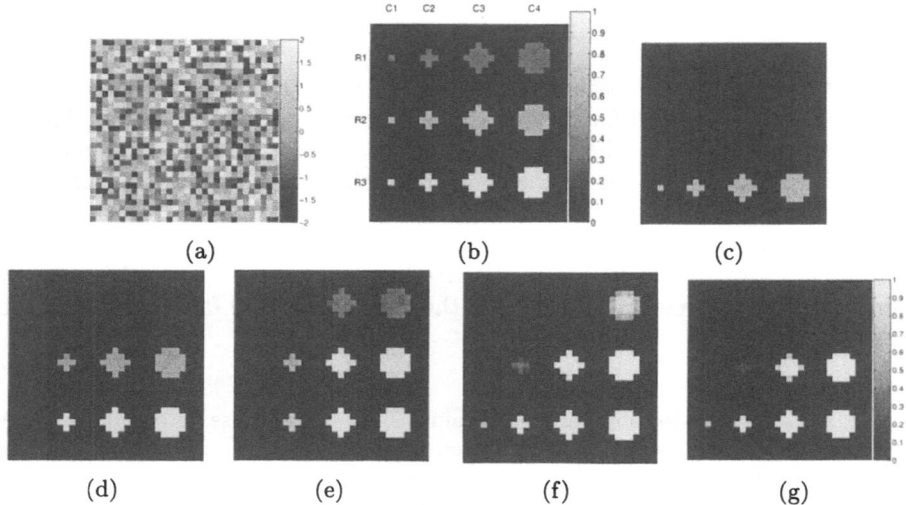

Fig. 1. (a) Gaussian noise image, (b) slice 8 of the phantom. (c)-(g) Probability of activation detection at voxel level. (c) VWTH, (d) CSTH:2, (e) CSTH:8, (f) CC:2, (g) CC:6. The scale for (c)-(g) is shown on the right side of (g).

5 Discussion

The methods for analysing fMRI data are often compared by power analysis only. Much less attention is paid to a segmentation accuracy and robustness. As we consider these properties equally important, they were included into this study.

Our parameter selection was based on a number of simulations. Although it is sometimes possible to approximately compute parameter values for chosen overall specificity [4], the simulation approach has some advantages. First, we are not forced to make any assumptions about the distribution of noise (e.g. smoothness or Gaussianity). The false activation rates can be estimated as precisely as needed, by simply increasing the number of simulations. The major drawback of the simulation approach, as compared to the theoretical one, is the large number of calculations required. However, with the relatively low matrix sizes of fMRI acquisitions, the parameter estimation can be done even with desktop computers in few hours.

One could criticize that in our simulations the time series of activation voxels follow simple box-car function corrupted with independent Gaussian noise. Some evidence exists that the assumptions about time series data being Gaussian distributed and time series samples being independent holds well in fMRI data [9], but the question is still debated. The hemodynamic response function is, of course, much more complicated than a simple box-car function. For the same reason, the SPMs are sometimes computed by using other methods than simple

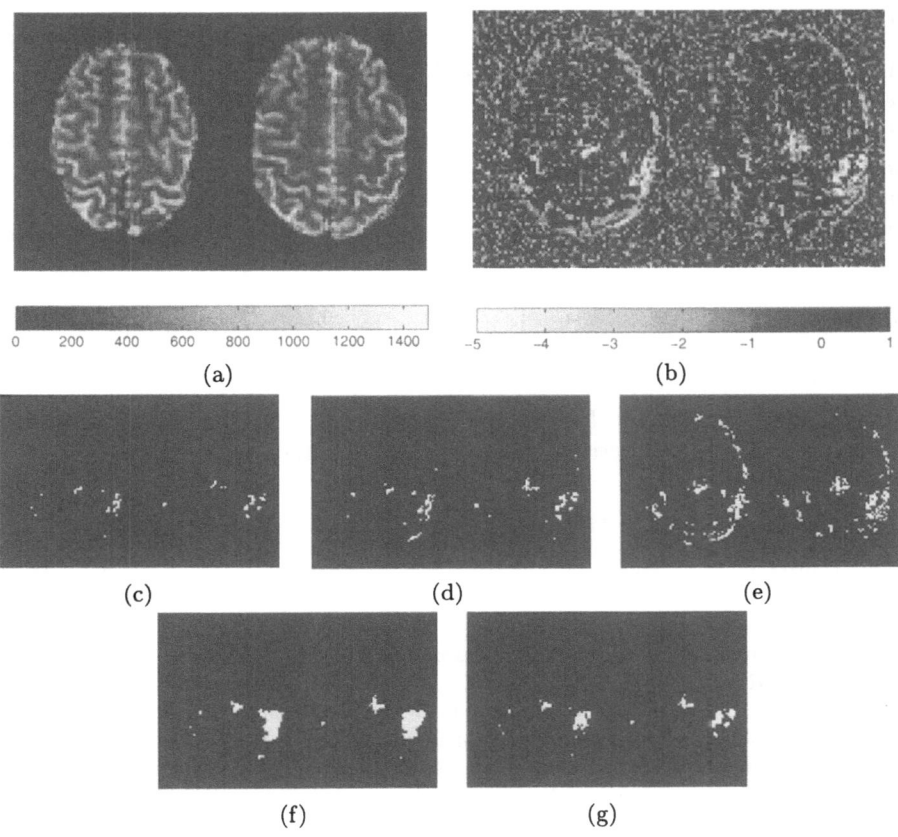

Fig. 2. Segmentation of fMRI data in two subsequent slices. (a) Two EPI slices at $t = 0$ s, (b)The corresponding SPM (z-map). Responses to stimulation of the right median nerve in the contra- and ipsilateral SMI and SMA can be seen as brighter areas in the SPM. In the SMI, activation is seen in two adjacent sulci (precentral and postcentral). Segmentation of the SPM by (c) VWTH, (d) CSTH:2 (e) CSTH:8, (f) CC:2 and (g) CC:6.

unpaired t test [10, 11]. We believe, however, that the limitations mentioned do not have any significant effects on the results of this segmentation study.

The spatial autocorrelations in the noise term may have effects on the performance of segmentation methods. If the structure of autocorrelations is known it can be taken into account in the estimation of decision parameters. In practice, the structure can not be estimated precisely. Therefore, a good robustness against spatial autocorrelations is a desirable feature of the segmentation method and this property was analysed in the present study.

6   Conclusions

Based on our results, the following conclusions can be made: 1) Generally, contextual clustering is more sensitive than voxel-wise thresholding. 2) Contextual clustering can detect, unlike cluster-size thresholding, activations that are only one voxel in size. 3) On detecting large activations, the precedence of contextual clustering and cluster-size threholding depends on the parameter values chosen of a method and the size and strength of an activation. 4) Contextual clustering has extremely good voxel-wise specificity, segmentation accuracy, and robustness against spatial autocorrelations. 5) The detection rate of large but weak activations with contextual clustering is increased by increasing β-parameter, but at the same time, the segmentation accuracy decreases.

In summary, a new contextual method to statistically segment fMRI activations, called as contextual clustering, has been developed. This clustering method appears to be very competitive with the other methods studied.

References

1. K. J. Friston, A. P. Holmes, K. J. Worsley, J. B. Poline, C. D. Frith, R. S. J. Frackowiak. Statistical parametric maps in functional imaging: a general linear approach. *Human Brain Mapping*, 2:189–210, 1995.
2. K. K. Kwong. Functional magnetic resonance imaging with echo planar imaging. em Magn. Reson. Q., 11:1–20, 1995.
3. J. Xiong, J.-H. Gao, J. L. Lancaster, P. T. Fox. Assessment and optimization of functional MRI analyses. *Human Brain Mapping*, 4:153–167, 1996.
4. K. J. Friston, K. J. Worsley, R. S. J. Frackowiak, J. C. Mazziotta, A. C. Evans. Assessing the significance of focal activations using their spatial extent. *Human Brain Mapping*, 1:213–220, 1994.
5. S. D. Forman, J. D. Cohen, M. Fitzgerald, W. F. Eddy, M. A. Mintun, D. C. Noll. Improved assessment of significant activation in functional magnetic resonance imaging (fMRI): Use of a cluster-size threshold. *Magn. Reson. Med.*, 33:636–647, 1995
6. J.-B. Poline, K. J. Worsley, A. C. Evans, K. J. Friston. Combining Spatial Extent and Peak Intensity to Test for Activations in Functional Imaging. *Neuroimage*, 5:83–96, 1997.
7. J. S. Milton, J. C. Arnold. Introduction to probability and statistics. Principles and applications for engineering and the computing sciences. 3rd edn. McGraw-Hill, Inc. New York, 1995.
8. J. Besag. On the statistical analysis of dirty pictures. *J. R. Statist. Soc. B.*, 48:259–279, 1986.
9. D. Ekatodramis, G. Székely, G. Gerig. Detecting and inferring brain activation from functional MRI by hypothesis-testing based on the Likelihood ratio. In: M. W. Wells, A. Colchester, S. Delp (eds.). Medical Image Computing and Computer-Assisted Intervention - MICCAI'98. *Lecture Notes in Computer Science*, Vol. 1496. Springer-Verlag. Berlin 578–589, 1998.
10. K. J. Friston, P. Jezzard, R. Turner. Analysis of functional MRI time-series. *Human Brain Mapping*, 1:153–171, 1994.
11. B. A. Ardekani, J. Kershaw, K. Kashikura, I. Kanno. Activation detection in functional MRI using subspace modeling and maximum likelihood estimation. *IEEE Trans. Medical Imaging*, 18:101–114, 1999.

Using Sulcal Basins for Analyzing Functional Activations Patterns in the Human Brain

G. Lohmann and D.Y. von Cramon

Max-Planck-Institute of Cognitive Neuroscience
Stephanstr. 1a, 04103 Leipzig, Germany
Ph: ++49-341-9940 217, Fax: ++49-341-9940 221
email: lohmann,cramon@cns.mpg.de

Abstract. In previous work, we have introduced the concept of sulcal basins. Sulcal basins are subdivisions of cortical folds that allow to establish a complete parcellation of the cortical surface into separate regions. In this paper, we present methods of using this concept to support the analysis of functional activation patterns in the human brain as measured by fMRI (functional magnetic resonance imaging) experiments. In particular, we present two methods of performing inter-subject averages. The first method uses a form of non-linear spatial normalization based on sulcal basin landmarks. The second method performs group averages using sulcal basins themselves as entities for averaging. This second approach has the advantage of ensuring that truly anatomically homologue entities enter the averaging process. In addition, it yields results that are immediately interpretable by a specialist.
The methods are presented in the context of an fMRI experiment in which 10 test subjects were asked to respond to various visual stimuli.

1 Introduction

In previous work, we have introduced the concept of sulcal basins [7],[5],[6]. Sulcal basins are subdivisions of cortical folds that allow to establish a complete parcellation of the cortical surface into separate regions. These regions are neuroanatomically meaningful and can be identified from MR data sets across many subjects.

In this paper, we present methods of using this concept to support the analysis of functional activation patterns in the human brain as measured by fMRI (functional magnetic resonance imaging) experiments. FMRI allows to create digital images that display local changes in blood flow with a spatial resolution of about 3 mm and a temporal resolution of up to 1 second. Since its invention a few years ago [1], it has become one of the most important technologies used in human brain mapping research.

The data produced by a typical fMRI experiment consist of a time sequence of digital images taken every n seconds. Each image contains several 2D slices where typically slices are about 5mm thick and gaps between slices are about 2mm wide. Usually, two or more experimental conditions are alternated within the same experiment. For instance, some baseline condition may be contrasted with a condition in which some visual or auditory stimulus is presented.

The aim of fMRI data analysis is threefold. The first aim is to detect image regions which display a significant difference in image intensity between various experimental conditions. We will refer to those regions as "activation areas". Secondly, the exact anatomical location of activation areas should be reported. And thirdly, some method of inter-subject averaging must be provided. At present, inter-subject averaging is usually performed by applying some form of spatial normalization to each individual data set using image warping techniques, and then computing pixel-wise averages in a stereotactic coordinate space [13].

In this paper, we will propose a method of inter-subject averaging that does not require spatial normalizations and warping. In fact, the sulcal basin model provides a means of performing inter-subject comparisons and group averages based on individual anatomy rather than on a stereotactic coordinate space.

However, if needed, the sulcal basin model can also used to perform a spatial normalization based on non-linear warping. In this paper, we will present both methods of inter-subject averaging. We present the warping method primarily for the purpose of validating the basin concept.

2 fMRI data analysis

2.1 Experimental data

We will describe our methods in the context of an fMRI experiment described by Pollmann et al. [14]. In this experiment, 10 healthy test subjects were asked to respond to various visual stimuli while fMRI data were being recorded.

Sixteen fMRI slices with a thickness of 5mm, interslice distance 2mm, 19,2cm FOV and an image matrix of 64x64 were collected at a 3T Bruker 30/100 Medspec (Bruker Medizintechnik GmbH, Ettlingen, Germany) using a gradient recalled EPI sequence (TR=2000ms, TE=40ms, flip angle=40). All 16 slices were recorded every 2 seconds. During the experiment, a baseline condition and an experimental condition alternated. At the same time, sixteen anatomical T1-weighted 2D slices were also recorded that were geometrically aligned with the functional data.

In addition to the fMRI data, we also obtained anatomical 3D MR data sets from all 10 subjects. The spatial resolution between planes was approx. $1.5mm$ and the within-plane resolution was set to approx. $0.95mm \times 0.95mm$. The images were resampled to obtain isotropic voxels of size $1mm \times 1mm \times 1mm$ so that each data set contained 160 slices with 200×160 pixels in each slice. All 3D data sets were rotated into a stereotactic coordinate system such that the origin was halfway between CA and CP (see also [9]).

2.2 Statistical analysis

The analysis of the fMRI data proceeds in several steps [8]. After some pre-processing involving radiometric and geometric corrections, a statistical t-test is employed in order to identify image regions that show a significant difference in image intensities between the experimental conditions.

The result of this analysis is a map in which the fMRI image sequence is collapsed into one image where each pixel encodes the degree of significance with which the image intensity differs between the experimental conditions. The degree of significance is represented by p-values that are given as normalized z-scores. Therefore, these maps are often called a "zmap". We obtained such a zmap for each test subject.

2.3 Spatial normalization

In order to facilitate group studies, the zmaps from various test subjects must be geometrically aligned in 3D space. This is achieved in two steps: co-registration and spatial normalization.

During co-registration the zmaps are rotated and shifted into correspondence with the 3D anatomical MR data set acquired from each subject. Remember that the 3D anatomical data sets are already rotated and translated into a common stereotactic coordinate system. Thus, co-registration also aligns the zmaps.

The co-registration was achieved as follows. As noted before, during the experimental session we recorded not only functional MR slices but also 2D anatomical MR slices that were geometrically aligned with the functional data. We used these antomical slices to compute rotational and translational parameters that maximized the correlation between the anatomical 2D data slices and the 3D reference data set. We then used these same parameters to register the zmaps as well. The co-registration algorithm is explained in more detail in [11].

After co-registration, all zmaps reside in a common stereotactic coordinate system. However, due to differences in individual anatomy, this does not guarantee that corresponding anatomical locations of different subjects occupy the same location within this coordinate system. Therefore, some form of spatial normalization is required.

Spatial normalization is frequently used in the context of human brain mapping in an effort to remove inter-subject or inter-modal variability. Generally, the aim is to geometrically align one data set with another such that corresponding brain locations are mapped onto each other and spatial variability is diminished([3],[13]).

The simplest form of spatial normalization is a linear scaling that brings all data sets into a common standard size. More sophisticated methods involve non-linear warping techniques that seek to warp individual data sets onto some reference atlas. Spatial normalization approaches can be loosely classified into two major groups: intensity-driven and landmark-driven approaches. Intensity driven approaches try to match locally corresponding image regions of similar grey value intensity (e.g. [2],[4],[10],[18]). Landmark-driven approaches use anatomical landmarks such as curves[17] or surfaces [16][19] to guide the warping. For a complete reference on spatial normalization and registration see [20],[12].

In the following, we will propose a new method of spatial normalization based on the concept of sulcal basins.

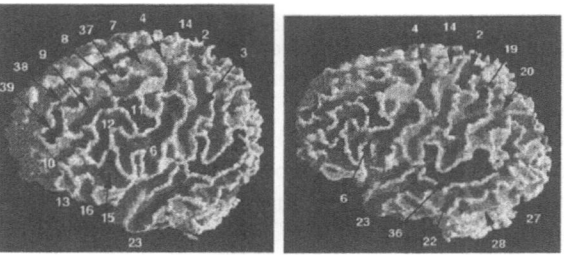

Fig. 1. The result of a segmentation and labelling of sulcal basins. The numbers indicate neuroanatomical labels, e.g. '3' is the label for the inferior part of the central sulcus. The anatomical model contains 38 left-hemispheric basins.

3 Sulcal basins

Sulcal basins are concavities on top of the white matter surface (after removal of the cortical compartment) that are bounded by convex ridges that separate one basin from the next so that adjacent sulcal basins meet at the top of the ridge. The entire white matter surface is covered by such concavities so that a decomposition into sulcal basins yields a complete parcellation of the surface.

A method for segmenting and labelling sulcal basins was introduced in [7]. Figure 1 shows the resulting labelled basins. The numbers indicate neuroanatomical labels. Our present model contains 38 left-hemispheric basins.

The sulcal basin model facilitates a new approach to non-linear spatial normalization. The basic idea is to guide a surface based warping mechanism by sulcal basin landmarks.

The surface to be warped is the morphological closure of the white matter which is obtained by applying a 3D morphological closing filter to the white matter image. The surface to be warped is the surface of the morphological closure (figure 2c).

To normalize brain shapes, we first selected a "model" brain from our 10 data sets to which all other brains were subsequently deformed. All data sets were initially subjected to a linear scaling in the x, y and z-directions so that they all had the same bounding box. We then use a quadratic polynomial F to perform an additional non-linear deformation that uses sulcal basin information. Note that all voxels belonging to the surface of the morphological closure are also elements of some sulcal basin so that every surface voxel inherits a basin label from the basin to which it belongs. The quadratic polynomial F has the form:

$$F(x,y,z) = \begin{pmatrix} a_{00} + a_{01}x + a_{02}y + a_{03}z + a_{04}xy + a_{05}xz + a_{06}yz + a_{07}x^2 + a_{08}y^2 + a_{09}z^2 \\ a_{10} + a_{11}x + a_{12}y + a_{13}z + a_{14}xy + a_{15}xz + a_{16}yz + a_{17}x^2 + a_{18}y^2 + a_{19}z^2 \\ a_{20} + a_{21}x + a_{22}y + a_{23}z + a_{24}xy + a_{25}xz + a_{26}yz + a_{27}x^2 + a_{28}y^2 + a_{29}z^2 \end{pmatrix}.$$

The deformation parameters a_{lk} pertaining to the quadratic polynomial F are estimated using the following definition of pairwise discrepancy. For each

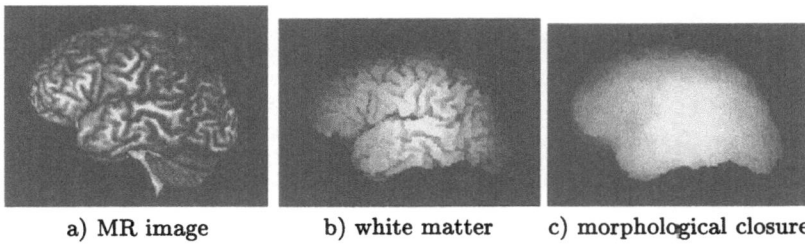

a) MR image   b) white matter   c) morphological closure

Fig. 2. Extracting a surface for subsequent warping

node $p_i \in \mathbb{R}^3, i = 1, ..., n$ in one data set, we select the corresponding node q_i in the model data set. The corresponding node must have the same basin label and it must be the node whose Euclidean distance $\|q_i - p_i\|$ from p_i is minimal. The deformation parameters a_{lk} are then chosen such that the following term is minimized:

$$\sum_{i=1}^{n} (q_i - F(p_i; a_{lk}))^2.$$

The minimization was performed using Powell's optimization method ([15]). We selected the model brain by computing pairwise discrepancies between all data sets, and choosing the one whose average discrepancy to all other brains was the least in this group.

4   Experiments

4.1   Results of spatial normalization and averaging

We applied the spatial normalization to the co-registered zmaps of our 10 test subjects. Comparing the effects of the sulcal basin normalization with the simple linear normalization, we found that the sulcal basin normalization does indeed decrease the inter-subject variance of the zmaps.

Let z_j^i denote the jth voxel in the zmap of the ith subject, and let

$$\mu_j = \frac{1}{10} \sum_{i=1}^{10} z_j^i, \quad \sigma_j^2 = \frac{1}{10-1} \sum_{i=1}^{10} (\mu_j - z_j^i)^2$$

denote the inter-subject average and standard deviation at each voxel. When using a simple linear normalization, we found that the variance σ_j across subjects at each voxel is larger on average than when using the sulcal basin normalization. The mean standard deviation $\sum_{j=0}^{n} \sigma_j$ using linear normalization was 1.233 (σ =0.776) compared to 1.187 (σ=0.776) ($p < 0.0001, t = 51.28$).

When performing a voxel-by-voxel comparison of inter-subject variance we found that 54.8 percent of the voxels had a larger inter-subject variance when using linear instead of sulcal basin normalization. Figure 3 shows the zmap

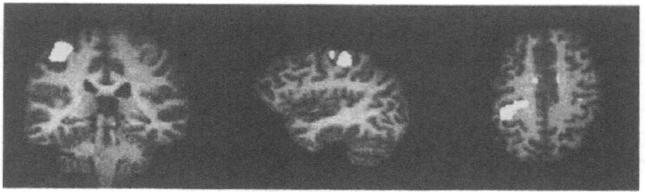

Fig. 3. Activation areas thresholded at z=2.25 and superimposed on an anatomical MR data set.

averaged across subjects after non-linear normalization and superimposed onto one anatomical data set. It was thresholded at $z = 2.25$.

Since the inter-subject variance is decreased by spatial normalization, the functional activation areas become more pronounced and more easily identifiable. In our context, activation areas are defined as connected components of the thresholded zmap. Table 1 shows two listings of activation areas obtained after linear and non-linear normalization.

	size	sum	location
a	942	3102.40	(-9, -12, 53)
b	857	2559.49	(-39, -34, 49)
	2	5.51	(-45, -37, 44)
d	23	65.02	(-21, -24, 42)
c	877	2670.00	(0, -78, -15)
	40	112.83	(-12, -85, -17)
	3	8.29	(-14, -90, -15)
	2744	8523.54	

a) linear normalization

	size	sum	location
a	874	2877.10	(-10, -10, 53)
b	1221	3772.57	(-41, -33, 49)
	12	33.58	(-42, -22, 52)
a	23	64.74	(-11, 0, 46)
d	32	90.38	(-22, -24, 42)
	3	8.32	(-28, -26, 42)
c	767	2389.69	(0, -78, -14)
	1	2.75	(7, -89, -14)
	2933	9239.14	

b) sulcal basin normalization

Table 1. Listing of activation areas with z-values thresholded at z=2.75. Activation sizes are given in mm^3. The location is given as Talairach-Fox coordinates of the voxel with the highest z value. The sum represents the sum over all z-values within the area. Note that by using non-linear normalization the total sum increases by about 9 percent (from 8523.54 to 9239.14). Corresponding areas are labelled by a letters a,b,c,d in both tables. For some smaller areas correspondences could not be identified.

4.2   Results of group averages not using stereotactic coordinates

In the previous section, we have described a method of obtaining group averages using spatial normalization. However, the main advantage of the sulcal basin model is that is allows to perform group averages using anatomical locations rather than stereotactic coordinates.

Table 2 lists the 38 basin locations and the average funczional activations found in each basin. This time however, the average is obtained by summing across corresponding basins of all subjects, not across corresponding locations in the stereotactic coordinate space. The activation level of a basin (within one subject) is defined as the mean z-score within this basin. To determine whether a significant level of activation is present in a basin, we average activation levels across subjects and perform a t-test against the null hypothesis that no activation is present in the basin. In this experiment, we found a significant level of activation ($p < 0.05$) in 10 basins.

The important point here is that activations are now averaged in an anatomically meaningful manner, and the result is listed in a way that is immediately interpretable by a specialist. The results listed in table 1 correspond to the results listed in the table 2 (with the exception of right hemispheric and median activations). For instance, area "a" corresponds to basins 4,14. Note that due to the thresholding of z-values inherent in table 1, one major activation area (basin 24) is missing altogether in table 1 as the z-scores were just below the threshold.

basin	activation level	p		basin	activation level	p
2	0.732	0.064		21	0.154	0.288
3	1.096	0.002 *		22	0.507	0.062
4	1.103	0.005 *		23	0.472	0.046 *
5	1.291	0.027 *		24	0.332	0.103
6	0.495	0.018 *		25	0.123	0.295
7	0.193	0.160		26	0.489	0.008 *
8	0.253	0.233		27	-0.111	0.353
9	-0.410	0.023 *		28	-0.161	0.191
10	-0.065	0.416		29	0.143	0.107
11	0.065	0.450		30	0.027	0.402
12	0.098	0.451		31	0.605	0.045 *
13	-0.857	0.117		32	0.380	0.160
14	0.533	0.042 *		33	0.085	0.362
15	-0.097	0.390		34	0.089	0.387
16	0.058	0.396		35	-0.049	0.429
17	-0.125	0.380		36	-0.131	0.227
18	0.855	0.016 *		37	0.421	0.082
19	0.586	0.078		38	0.044	0.460
20	0.213	0.108		39	-0.348	0.237

Table 2. Listing of average functional activations levels across 10 subjects. Basins with significant levels of activations ($p < 0.05$) are marked by a star. The p-values resulted from a t-test against the null hypothesis that the activation level is zero. Only basins of the left lateral hemisphere are listed. The basin labels correspond to the labels displayed in figure 1.

5   Discussion

We have introduced a new approach to spatial normalization and inter-subject averaging using the sulcal basin model. The prime advantage is that this model allows inter-subject comparisons on the basis of the individual anatomy rather than on a somewhat arbitrary stereotactic coordinate space. Thus, image warping might not even be necessary for inter-subject averaging as averaging can be performed using the sulcal basins instead of voxels in some coordinate space.

This new approach offers three advantages over the standard spatial normalization and pixel-wise average approach. Firstly, in averaging across sulcal basin locations instead of voxels in stereotactic coordinate space, it is guaranteed that truly corresponding entities are matched and averaged. Secondly, the results are displayed in a way that is much more useful to the specialist as it is based on an established neuro-anatomical vocabulary. A third advantage is that this method does not depend on any form of thresholding of z-values as is required by standard averaging methods. Thresholding of significance values is often quite arbitrary and might lead to misinterpretations. Using sulcal basins, we can directly report the presence or absence of an activation in a basin together with a significance level.

The fact that a spatial normalization based upon sulcal basins reduces the variance in the zmap-average is evidence that this model is indeed anatomically and functionally valid although further proof is warranted. The fact that the improvement in zmap-variance is only moderate is not surprising. Had we obtained drastically different results, then we would have to disbelieve either our previous results obtained by the standard linear normalization method, or be would have to doubt our new results.

The spatial normalization using second-order polynomials is a somewhat crude approach and was introduced primarily for the purpose of demonstrating the validity of the sulcal basin concept. Other methods of using sulcal basins as landmarks for warping are conceivable and will be tested in the future.

Acknowledgments

We would like to thank Dr. Volker Bosch for valuable discussions about the statistical aspects of this paper, and Dr. Stefan Pollman for providing the fMRI data.

References

1. J.W. Belliveau, D.N. Kennedy, R.C. McKinstry, B.R. Buchbinder, R.M. Weisskopf, M.S. Cohen, J.M. Vevea, T.J. Brady, B.R. Rosen. Functional mapping of the human visual cortex by magnetic resonance imaging. *Science*, 254:716–719, 1991.
2. G.E. Christensen, R.D. Rabbitt, M.L. Miller. Deformable templates using large deformation kinematics. *IEEE Transactions on Image Processing*, 5(10):1435–1447, 1996.

3. P.T. Fox. Spatial normalization origins: objectives, applications, and alternatives. *Human Brain Mapping*, 3:161–164, 1995.
4. K.J. Friston, J. Ashburner, C.D. Frith, J.B. Poline, J.D. Heather, and R.S.J. Frackowiak. Spatial registration and normalization of images. *Human Brain Mapping*, 2:165–189, 1995.
5. G.Lohmann, D.Y.v.Cramon. Automatic detection and labelling of the human cortical folds in magnetic resonance data sets. In *ECCV (European Conference on Computer Vision)*, Freiburg,Germany, June 2-6 1998.
6. G.Lohmann, D.Y.v.Cramon. Automatic labelling of the human cortical surface using sulcal basins. *Medical Image Analysis*, (submitted), 1998.
7. G.Lohmann, D.Y.v.Cramon. Sulcal basins and sulcal strings as new concepts for describing the human cortical topography. In *IEEE workshop on biomedical image analysis*, Santa Barbara, CA, June 1998.
8. F. Kruggel, G.Lohmann. BRIAN (Brain Image Analysis) - a toolkit. In *CAR 96*, Paris, June 1996.
9. F. Kruggel, G.Lohmann. Automatical adaptation of the stereotactical coordinate system in brain MRI data sets. In J. Duncan, editor, *Int. Conf. on Information Processing in Medical Imaging (IPMI 97)*, Poultney, Vermont, USA, June 9–13 1997.
10. J.L. Lancaster , T.G. Glass, B.R. Lankipalli, H. Downs, H. Mayberg, P.T. Fox. A modality-independent approach to spatial normalization of tomographic images of the human brain. *Human Brain Mapping*, 3(3):209–223, 1995.
11. G. Lohmann. Registration of functional mri data to 3d structural mr reference images. Technical report, Max-Planck-Institute of Cognitive Neuroscience, Leipzig, Germany, 1998.
12. J.B.A. Maintz, M.A. Viergever. A survey of medical image registration. *Medical Image Analysis*, 2(1), March 1998.
13. J.C. Maziotta, A.W. Toga, A. Evans, P. Fox, J. Lancaster. A probabilistic atlas of the human brain: theory and rationale for its development. *Neuroimage*, 2:89–101, 1995.
14. S. Pollmann R. Weidner, H.J. Müller, D.Y. von Cramon. Brain areas involved in visual dimension weighting. In *5th International Conference on Functional Mapping of the Human Brain (submitted)*, 1999.
15. W.H. Press, S.A. Teukolsky, W.T. Vetterling, B.P. Flannery. Numerical Recipies in C. Cambridge University Press, 2nd Edition, 1992.
16. S. Sandor, R. Leahy. Surface-based labeling of cortical anatomy using a deformable atlas. *IEEE Transactions on Medical Imaging*, 16(1):41–54, Feb. 1997.
17. G. Subsol, J-P Thirion, and N. Ayache. A General Scheme for Automatically Building 3D Morphometric Anatomical Atlases: application to a Skull Atlas. *Medical Image Analysis*, 2(1), March 1998.
18. J.-P. Thirion. Image matching as a diffusion process: an analogy with Maxwell's demons. *Medical Image Analysis*, 2(3), 1998.
19. P. Thompson, A.W. Toga. A surface-based technique for warping three-dimensional images of the brain. *IEEE Transactions on Medical Imaging*, 15(4):402–417, 1996.
20. A.W. Toga. *Brain Warping*. Academic Press, San Diego, CA, 1999.

Comparison of Land-Mark-Based and Curve-Based Thin-Plate Warps for Analysis of Left-Ventricular Motion from Tagged MRI

A. A. Amini, Y. Chen, and D. Abendschein

CVIA Laboratory, Campus Box 8086, 660 S. Euclid Ave.
Washington University Medical Center
St. Louis, MO 63110, USA
Email: amini@cauchy.wustl.edu
WWW: http://www-cv.wustl.edu/

Abstract. MRI is unique in its ability to non-invasively and selectively alter tissue magnetization, and create tagged patterns within a deforming body such as the heart muscle. The resulting grid patterns define non-invasive tissue markers, providing a mechanism for *in-vivo* measurement of tissue motion and strain. In this paper, we report on objective comparison of thin-plate spline warps in reconstructing true deformations when using homologous land-mark points and when using homologous curves from tagged MR-image sequences of a cardiac motion simulator. In addition, the number of corresponding land-mark points as well as the number of corresponding curves are varied in order to determine the effect on accuracy of reconstructions. Finally, application of the developed techniques to computing LV tissue motion and strain in systole from short-axis tagged images of a porcine model with anterior myocardial infarction (MI) are given.

1 Introduction

Non-invasive techniques for assessing the dynamic behavior of the human heart are invaluable in the diagnosis of heart disease, as abnormalities in the myocardial motion sensitively reflect deficits in blood perfusion [9, 17]. MRI is a non-invasive imaging technique that provides superb anatomic information with excellent spatial resolution and soft tissue contrast. In MR tagging, the magnetization property of selective material points in the myocardium are altered in order to create tag grid patterns within a deforming body such as the heart muscle [17, 7]. During tissue contractions, the grid patterns move, allowing for visual tracking of the land-mark grid intersections over time. The intrinsic high spatial and temporal resolutions of such myocardial analysis schemes provide unsurpassed information about local contraction and deformation in the heart wall which can be used to derive local strain and deformation indices from different myocardial regions.

A number of researchers have developed different approaches to analysis of tagged MRI data [16, 11, 10]. An unanswered question is whether more accuracy is gained in utilizing complete curve-grid information in reconstructing LV deformations, or whether use of tag intersections (i.e., landmarks) alone is sufficient. In this paper, we report on comparisons of land-mark-based and curve-based warps, and describe conditions under which thin-plate reconstructions using complete tag grid information would be preferred. We also apply the reconstruction algorithm to obtain dense strain maps from tagged MRI in a porcine model with anterior MI.

2   Constrained Thin-Plate Spline Warps

Tracking tissue deformations with SPAMM using snake grids provides 2D displacement information at tag intersections and 1D displacement information along other 1D snake points [1–4]. The displacement measurement from tag lines however are sparse; interpolation is required to reconstruct a dense displacement field from which strain, torsion, and other mechanical indices of function can be computed at all myocardial points.

To proceed more formally, the vector field which warps the *deformed image* into the *undeformed image* is assumed to be C^1 continuous. This smoothness requirement is achieved by minimizing an objective function which combines spatial derivatives of both components of the reconstructed displacements

$$\Phi_1 = \int \int u_{xx}^2 + 2u_{xy}^2 + u_{yy}^2 \, dx dy + \int \int v_{xx}^2 + 2v_{xy}^2 + v_{yy}^2 \, dx dy \qquad (1)$$

characterizing approximating thin-plate splines. It should be noted that although thin-plate warps have been used in the past for other medical imaging applications ([8]), they have only been utilized to interpolate a warp given homologous landmark points. Assuming 2D tissue motion (as is roughly the case towards the apical end of the heart [13]), two possible physical constraints (in addition to (1)) can be considered:

1. Corresponding homologous land-marks obtained from intersecting horizontal and vertical tag grid lines should come into correspondence after application of the thin-plate warp. The intersection of two tag grid lines are "pulled" towards one another by minimizing

$$\Phi_2 = \sum (u - u_{int})^2 + (v - v_{int})^2 \qquad (2)$$

   where u_{int} and v_{int} are the x and y components of displacement at tag intersections.

2. Corresponding homologous curves should come into correspondence, that is, any point on a deformed tag in frame n must be warped to lie on its corresponding undeformed tag in frame 0 of the sequence. For a vector field to perform such a warp, $h(u,v)$ of figure 1 must be minimized. Let $P_1 = P_1(u,v) = (x,y) + (u,v)$ as in figure 1, and let P_2 be any point on the

undeformed tag line. The following term is then summed over all deformed horizontal and vertical grid points:

$$\Phi_3 = \sum (h(u,v))^2 = \sum \{(\boldsymbol{P}_1(u,v) - \boldsymbol{P}_2) \cdot \boldsymbol{n}\}^2 \tag{3}$$

where the summation is performed on all points (x,y) on the deformed grids.

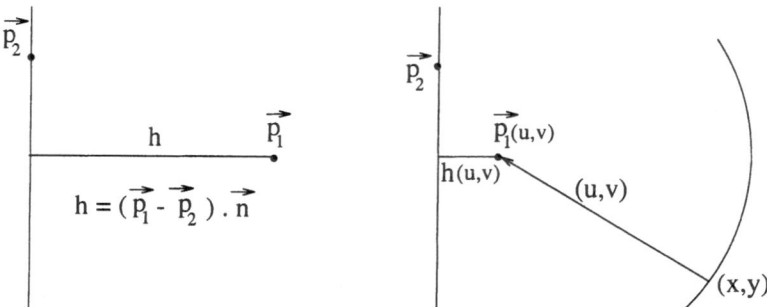

Fig. 1. Distance of a point P_1 to a straight line can easily be calculated with knowledge of *any* point, P_2, on the line and the normal vector (left). The residual distance from a *warped point* of a deformed tag line to its corresponding undeformed tag line in frame 0 of the sequence, $h(u,v)$, can similarly be calculated (right).

In order to compare curve-warps with land-mark warps, an objective function maybe formed by a linear combination of the terms in (1), (2), and (3),

$$\Phi = \lambda_1 \Phi_1 + \lambda_2 \Phi_2 + \lambda_3 \Phi_3 \tag{4}$$

where $\lambda_1, \lambda_2, \lambda_3$ are non-negative weights. The following test cases can then considered: **I.** $\{\lambda_1 > 0, \lambda_2 > 0, \lambda_3 = 0\}$, and **II.** $\{\lambda_1 > 0, \lambda_2 = 0, \lambda_3 > 0\}$. Additionally, within each of case **I** (land-mark-based warps) and **II** (curve-based warps), the number of homologous land-mark points/curves may be varied to determine the effect on accuracy of reconstructions. In order to optimize Φ with Conjugate-Gradient Descent, partial derivatives of Φ_1 can be calculated using the computational molecule approach discussed in [14] and also used in [4]. Partial derivatives of (2) can easily be obtained. Finding partial derivatives of Φ_3 is also straightforward:

$$\nabla \Phi_3 = 2 \sum \{(\boldsymbol{P}_1(u,v) - \boldsymbol{P}_2) \cdot \boldsymbol{n}\} \cdot \boldsymbol{n} \tag{5}$$

As maybe concluded from the last paragraph, minimization of (4) leads to a system of linear equations with full rank under non-trivial deformations. Therefore, (4) is a convex objective function, with a global minimum. It should be noted that in comparison to [4], in the present article we describe thin-plate techniques which require knowledge of homologous landmark points and/or curves;

though with an additional constraint, namely that one set of the homologous curves should be straight. This is a modification of the framework in [4], making the objective function convex, bypassing local minima, and resulting in reduced computational costs.

3   Land-Mark-Based vs. Curve-Based Warps

An environment based on a 13 parameter kinematic model of Arts et al. [6] has been implemented as was described in [15] for simulating a time sequence of tagged MR images at arbitrary orientation. Based on user-selected discretization of the space between 2 concentric shells and by varying the canonical parameters of the model, both a sequence of tagged MR images as well as a "ground truth" vector field of actual material point deformations are available [4]. The parameters of the motion model, referred to as k-parameters, and the transformations to which they correspond are: k_1: Radially dependent compression, k_2: Left ventricular torsion, k_3: Ellipticalization in long-axis (LA) planes, k_4: Ellipticalization in short-axis (SA) planes, k_5: Shear in x direction, k_6: Shear in y direction, k_7: Shear in z direction, k_8: Rotation about x-axis, k_9: Rotation about y-axis, k_{10}: Rotation about z-axis, k_{11}: Translation in x direction, k_{12}: Translation in y direction, and k_{13}: Translation in z direction. For the purposes of comparing 2D displacement field reconstructions, we have used the parameters k_2, k_4, k_5, and k_{10} for generating 2D deformations of the geometric model, based on which simulated tagged images and 2D displacement vector fields of *actual* material points are produced. The error norms used in comparing the ground truth vector field (V_g) with the vector field measured by the warp algorithms (V_m) are: $\varepsilon_{rms} = \sqrt{\frac{1}{N} \sum |V_m - V_g|^2}$ and $\varepsilon_{dist} = \sqrt{\frac{1}{N} \sum (h(u,v))^2}$ where N is the total number of deformed grid points on the myocardial region, the summation in ε_{rms} is performed on entire myocardial regions, and the summation in ε_{dist} is performed on all points (x, y) on the deformed grid (figure 1).

In order to test the accuracy of reconstructions as a function of the number of homologous landmarks and homologous curves, a number of experiments were carried out. The experiments were designed to determine the effect of number of homologous land-mark points vs. number of homologous curves on the accuracy of thin-plate spline reconstruction of deformations. The cardiac simulator was used to generate a sequence of SA tagged images in addition to ground-truth displacement vector fields. The imaging parameters chosen resulted in 7 × 7 image tag grids. The intersections of the tag lines in the myocardial area yielded all of the available land-mark points, and the tag segments which were in the myocardial region yielded all of the available curves for warping. In order to vary the number of homologous land-marks and curves, the 7 × 7 grid was subsampled to a 1 × 1, 2 × 2, 3 × 3, 4 × 4, and the original 7 × 7 grid. To compare land-mark based and curve-based warps, for each subsampled grid considered, the intersections of the corresponding grids were used as the land-mark points. The findings for parameter k_4 (short-axis ellipticalization) are displayed in figures 2 and 3 (plots for k_2, k_5, and k_{10} generally follow the same patterns). Please note

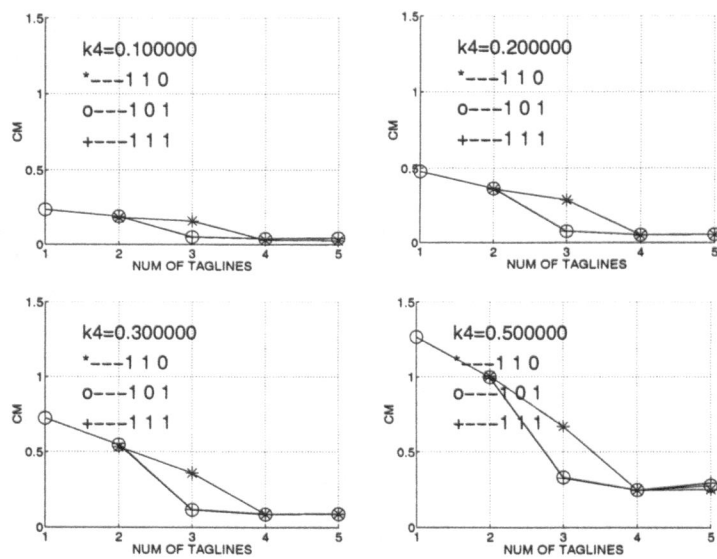

Fig. 2. Plots of ε_{rms} as a function of number of tag lines used in thin-plate spline reconstruction of deformations. Different plots correspond to different values of k_4, ellipticalization in short-axis plane.

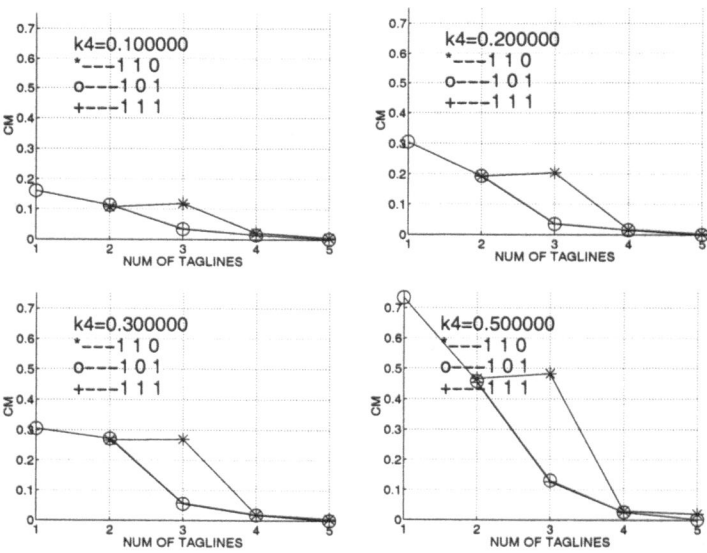

Fig. 3. Plots of ε_{dist} as a function of number of tag lines used in thin-plate spline reconstruction of deformations. Different plots correspond to different values of k_4, ellipticalization in short-axis plane.

that for these figures, there are no land-marks for the 1×1 grid, and additionally the results of the 7×7 grid are labeled as case "5" on the x-axis of the plots. For the plots, "1 1 0" corresponds to $\lambda_1 = 1$, $\lambda_2 = 1$, $\lambda_3 = 0$. Similarly, "1 0 1" corresponds to $\lambda_1 = 1$, $\lambda_2 = 0$, $\lambda_3 = 1$, and "1 1 1" corresponds to $\lambda_1 = 1$, $\lambda_2 = 1$, $\lambda_3 = 1$.

The plots indicate that for small deformations, there is no significant difference between using curve-based, and land-mark based warps, but that for larger deformations, there is more graceful degradation of curve-based warps in reconstruction of true deformations in comparison to land-mark based warps. There are also no significant differences between curve-based and land-mark based warps when the number of land-marks/curves increase. In the rest of the article, $\{\lambda_1 = 1, \lambda_2 = 0, \lambda_3 = 1\}$ was used for analysis of the *in-vivo* data.

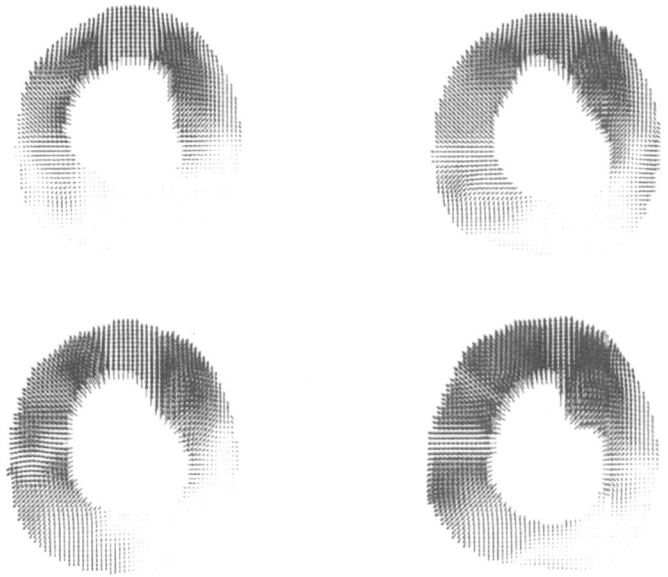

Fig. 4. Four displacement vector fields for the post-MI study corresponding to 202, 225, 247, and 270 *msec* after the ECG trigger. Segmental motion of all myocardial points can easily be quantitated and visualized from the location, direction, and length of the displayed vectors. An akinetic area in the lower-right area is indicated.

4   Myocardial Strains

Starting at any time point during the cardiac cycle, the heart's motion is viewed here as a mapping which warps the *deformed* tag configuration into the *unde-*

formed configuration: $\mathbf{X} = \Gamma(\mathbf{x})$. Equivalently, with $\mathbf{X} = V(\mathbf{x}) + \mathbf{x}$, the deformation gradient tensor can be written as $\mathbf{F} = \nabla\Gamma(\mathbf{x}) = \nabla V(\mathbf{x}) + \nabla\mathbf{x}$ where V is the computed displacement vector field. Therefore, assuming little or no through-plane motion, the strain tensor can be computed from spatial derivatives of displacements:

$$\mathbf{E} = \frac{1}{2}(\mathbf{F}^T\mathbf{F} - \mathbf{I})$$
$$= \begin{pmatrix} u_x + \frac{1}{2}(u_x^2 + v_x^2) & \frac{1}{2}(u_y + v_x + u_x u_y + v_x v_y) \\ \frac{1}{2}(u_y + v_x + u_x u_y + v_x v_y) & v_y + \frac{1}{2}(u_y^2 + v_y^2) \end{pmatrix} \tag{6}$$

Once a displacement vector field is available, the strain of deformation can be computed at all myocardial points within a short-axis slice. Furthermore, the quantity $\mathbf{M}^T\mathbf{E}\mathbf{M}$ will give the value of strain for the direction $\mathbf{M}$.

5   *In-Vivo* Imaging

A SPAMM pulse sequence was used to collect images from a porcine model of myocardial infarction. The repetition time (TR) of the imaging sequence was approximately 7.1 msec, the echo time (TE) was 2.9 msec, and the rf pulse flip angle was 15 degrees. Other imaging parameters were: field of view = $300mm$, data acquisition matrix size = 250×256 (phase encoding by readout), in-plane resolution = $1.2 \times 1.17mm^2$, slice thickness = $7mm$, and tag spacing = $7mm$.

5.1   Results

Figure 4 shows 4 displacement vector fields ($\mathbf{V}$) computed from grids in tagged short-axis images at 202, 225, 247, and 270 *msec* after the ECG trigger in a pig after inducing an anterior MI. The magnitude of the motion fields for each of these figures can easily be computed. Although the infarct zone can readily be recognized from the vector fields, these zones more clearly stand out in the vector field magnitude maps [5]. The next pair of figures: figure 5 and figure 6 show the radial and circumferential strains for the post-MI study after application of a median filter for reducing noise. Finally, figure 7 shows the picture of a stained histological slice of the LV roughly corresponding to the position of image slices for the porcine model.

   In summary, the areas of the myocardium which lack motion can be recognized from either the magnitude of the displacement vectors or from the patterns of radial and circumferential strain maps. These areas appear to correlate well with the stained tissue.

6   Conclusions

We have compared land-mark based and curve-based thin-plate warps for reconstruction of dense displacement vector fields from SPAMM grids. Using the

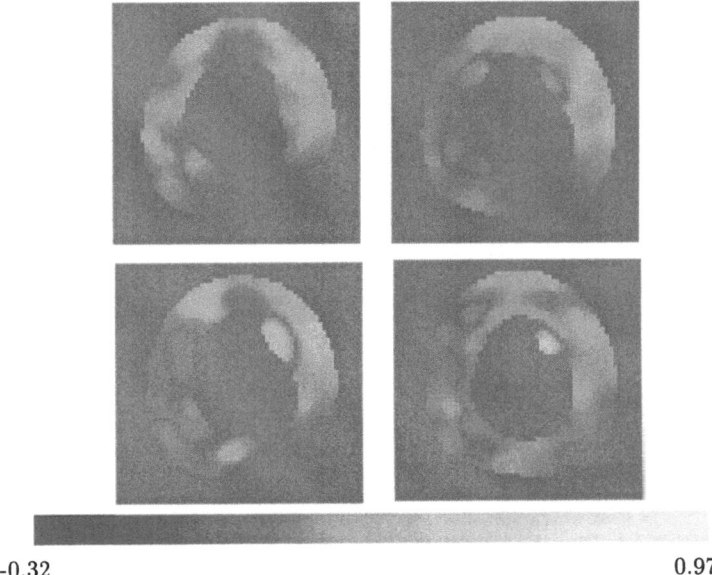

-0.32   0.97

Fig. 5. This figure shows radial strains for the post MI study (corresponding to the same time points as in figure 4). Notice that the lower-right area consistently has small strain values.

Cardiac Motion Simulator, it was found that for larger deformations, land-mark based warps fail when few homologous land-mark points are available, but that performance gracefully diminishes for curve-based warps when the number of homologous curves are decreased. In addition, preliminary results from application of methods to *in-vivo* data of a porcine model of myocardial infarction were given. Although we have not taken into account motion in the out-of-plane direction, we are encouraged by the in-plane results obtained thusfar.

Acknowledgements

This work was supported in part by a grant from the Whitaker Biomedical Engineering Foundation, grant IRI-9796207 from the NSF, and grant HL-57628 from the NIH.

References

1. A. A. Amini. Automated techniques for measurement of cardiac motion from MR tagging. Proposal funded by The Whitaker Foundation, 1992.
2. A. A. Amini and et al. MR physics-based snake tracking and dense deformations from tagged MR cardiac images. In *AAAI Symposium on Applications of*

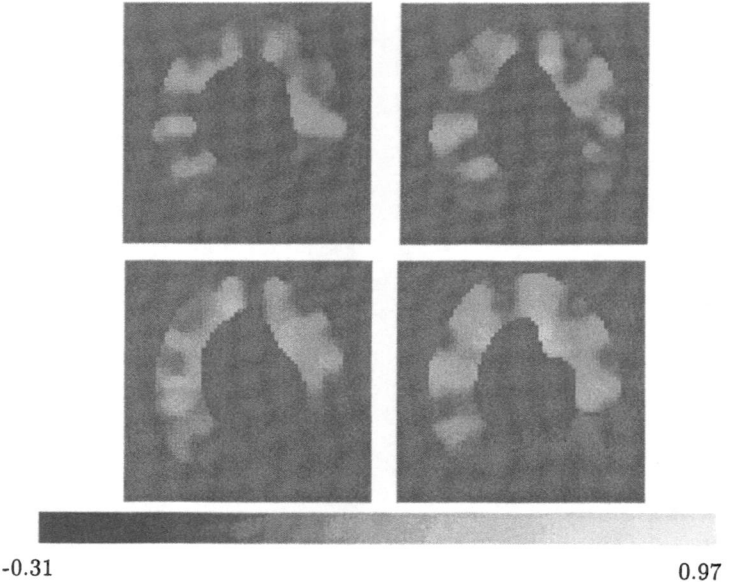

-0.31   0.97

Fig. 6. This figure shows circumferential strains for the post MI study (same time points as in figure 4). Once again, the lower-right area consistently has small strain values.

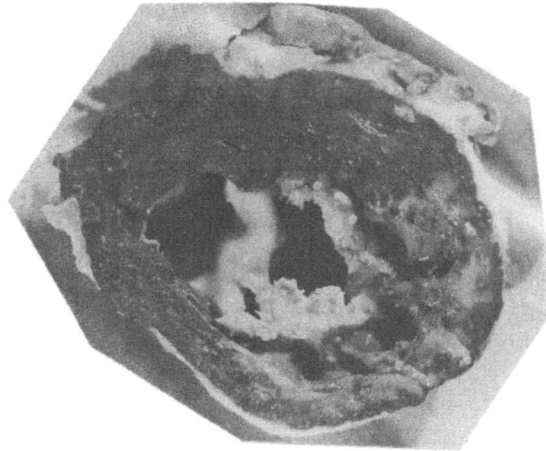

Fig. 7. Stained histological slice of the pig's LV; roughly corresponding to collected short-axis image slice positions. The area in the lower right (between 2 and 7 o'clock locations) of the picture with no dye uptake (bright region) is the infarct zone. Note also the distinct narrowing of the myocardial regions in these areas.

Computer Vision to Medical Image Processing, Stanford University, Stanford, California, March 1994.

3. A. A. Amini, R. W. Curwen, and J. C. Gore. Snakes and splines for tracking non-rigid heart motion. In *European Conference on Computer Vision*, pages 251–261, University of Cambridge, UK, April 1996.

4. A. A. Amini, Y. Chen, R. Curwen, V. Mani, and J. Sun. Coupled B-Snake Grids and Constrained Thin-Plate Splines for Analysis of 2D Tissue Deformations from Tagged MRI. *IEEE Trans. on Medical Imaging*, 17(3):344-356.

5. A. A. Amini, Y. Chen, D. Abendschein. Comparison of Land-Mark-Based and Curve-Based Thin-Plate Warps for Analysis of Left-Ventricular Motion from Tagged MRI. CVIA Lab Internal Report. March 1999.

6. T. Arts, W. Hunter, A. Douglas, A. Muijtjens, and R. Reneman. Description of the deformation of the left ventricle by a kinematic model. *J. Biomechanics*, 25(10):1119–1127, 1992.

7. L. Axel and L. Dougherty. MR imaging of motion with spatial modulation of magnetization. *Radiology*, 171(3):841–845, 1989.

8. F. Bookstein. Principal warps: Thin-plate splines and the decomposition of deformations. *IEEE Transactions on Pattern Analysis and Machine Intelligence*, PAMI-11:567–585, 1989.

9. W. Grossman. Assessment of regional myocardial function. *J. of Amer. Coll. of Cardiology*, 7(2):327 – 328, 1986.

10. S. Gupta and J. Prince. On variable brightness optical flow for tagged MRI. In *Information Processing in Medical Imaging (IPMI)*, pages 323–334, 1995.

11. J. Park, D. Metaxas, and L. Axel. Volumetric deformable models with parameter functions: A new approach to the 3d motion analysis of the LV from MRI-SPAMM. In *International Conference on Computer Vision*, pages 700–705, 1995.

12. P. Radeva, A. Amini, and J. Huang. Deformable B-Solids and implicit snakes for 3d localization and tracking of SPAMM MRI data. *Computer Vision and Image Understanding*, 66(2):163–178, May 1997.

13. N. Reichek. Magnetic resonance imaging for assessment of myocardial function. *Magnetic Resonance Quarterly*, 7(4):255–274, 1991.

14. D. Terzopoulos. *Multiresolution Computation of Visible Representation*. PhD thesis, MIT, 1984.

15. E. Waks, J. Prince, and A. Douglas. Cardiac motion simulator for tagged MRI. In *Proc. of Mathematical Methods in Biomedical Image Analysis*, pages 182–191, 1996.

16. A. Young, D. Kraitchman, L. Dougherty, and L. Axel. Tracking and finite element analysis of stripe deformation in magnetic resonance tagging. *IEEE Transactions on Medical Imaging*, 14(3):413–421, September 1995.

17. E. Zerhouni, D. Parish, W. Rogers, A. Yang, and E. Shapiro. Human heart: Tagging with MR imaging – a method for noninvasive assessment of myocardial motion. *Radiology*, 169:59–63, 1988.

Contour Tracking in Echocardiographic Sequences without Learning Stage: Application to the 3D Reconstruction of the Beating Left Ventricule

Marie-Odile Berger[1], Goetz Winterfeldt[1], and Jean-Paul Lethor[2]

[1] Loria/Inria-Lorraine, BP 101,
F-54600 Villers-les-Nancy, France
email:{berger@loria.fr}
[2] CHU Brabois, Nancy, France

Abstract. In this paper we present a contour tracker on echographic image sequences. To do this, we use a hierarchical approach: we first compute a global estimation of the ventricular motion. Then we use a fine tuning algorithm to adjust the detection of the ventricular wall. The global estimation is based on a parametric motion model with a small number of parameters. This allows us to compute the motion in a robust way from the velocity computed at each point of the contour.
Results are presented demonstrating tracking on various echographic sequences. We conclude by discussing some of our current research efforts.

1 Introduction

Parameters of cardiac functions can be drawn from the analysis of echocardiographic image sequences, especially the motion of the ventricular wall, heart wall thickness and shape parameters. These analyses are based on the detection of the left ventricular internal wall edge. Usually, the ventricular edges are manually traced by the physician but this operation is time consuming if an entire cardiac cycle must be analyzed. Hence, there is considerable interest in developing methods to perform automatic extraction of the ventricular contours in a sequence.

Several authors have recently proposed contour trackers which rely on a preliminary learning stage [3]. This allows them to restrict the class of allowable motion (shape deformations) to an admissible set that has been learned on a training data set of the patient to be examined. As the variability of the ventricular deformation between patients can be large, the allowable deformations for a given patient is likely to be not suited for another one.

That is the reason why we attempt to measure cardiac motion directly on grey level images. Within the computer vision community, considerable attention has been given to tracking and understanding object motion. Methods for computing motion can roughly be categorized as either differential or matching methods. However, the performance of these techniques are not the same:

the accuracy, reliability and density of the computed velocity field can differ significantly according to the technique used.

- **differential techniques**: the common assumption is that the observed intensity is constant over time. The constant brightness assumption can be formally stated as $I(x, y, t) = I(x + \delta x, y + \delta y, t + \delta t)$. Expanding the image brightness function in a Taylor'e series around the points (x, y) we obtain the *gradient constraint equation*:

$$\nabla I(x, y, t).v + I_t(x, y, t) = 0 \qquad (1)$$

It is a single equation which allows us to compute the normal optical flow $v^\perp$. Due to the finite differences used to approximate derivatives in the consistancy equation (1), differential techniques are thus inacurrate for large displacements. This may cause problems to track the mitral valve because this structure is thin and can undergo large motions.

- **matching techniques** [5]: such approaches define velocity v as the shift that yields the best fit between image regions at different times. Finding the best match amounts to minimize a similarity measure over v such as the sum of squared differences:

$$v = argmin_{\{v=(v_x, v_y)\}} \sum_{i=-w}^{i=w} \sum_{j=-w}^{j=w} [I(x+i, y+j, t) - I(x+i+v_x, y+j+v_y, t+1)]^2$$

However, as there are no specific points on the ventricular wall, the peak of the correlation is not always clearly discernible. It is therefore difficult to estimate point wise motion. Consider for instance Fig.1: The left image shows the ventricular wall traced by an expert. The right image shows the correspondences given by the correlation (original points are drawn in black and the detected points are drawn in white). In regions where gradient information is missing (right part of the ventricle), results are of course very poor. On the left side, the computed motion is more reliable. In contrast to differential techniques, large displacements can be handled with correlation based methods provided that the size w of the window correlation is large enough. However, the reliability of the computed motion is not very good.

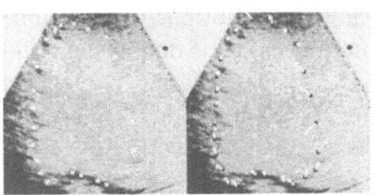

Fig. 1. Correspondences given by correlation: (a) the ventricular wall in a given frame (b) the motion computed with correlation in the next frame.

To conclude, due to the weak signal to noise ratio in echocardiographic images, the computed velocity is not relevant at several places of the contour. These measurements can not therefore be used as is for the ventricular wall detection. Following previous works on deformable structures [2] we therefore use a hierarchical algorithm; we first compute a global estimation of the ventricular deformation. Then we use a fine tuning deformation to adjust the details. The global estimation is based on a parametric motion model with a small number of parameters (4, 5 or 6). These parameters are estimated in a robust way from the velocity field computed at each point of the contour. From this estimation, active contours models are used to detect the ventricular wall.

The motion models we use are described in section 2. The overview of our tracker is given in section 3. Section 4 describes our method for computing motion. Finally, we show in section 5 experimental results that demonstrate the validity of our approach.

2   Which motion model?

In order to describe the ventricular wall motion properly, we tested three motion models: similarity, affinity and affine model. The similarity model

$$X = s\ cos\theta x - s\ sin\theta y + t_x$$
$$Y = s\ sin\theta x + s\ cos\theta y + t_y$$

describes a contraction ($s < 1$) or an expansion ($s > 1$) of the ventricle with respect to a central point.

The affinity model:

$$X = s_1 cos\theta x - s_2 sin\theta y + t_x$$
$$Y = s_1 sin\theta x + s_2 cos\theta y + t_y$$

uses two different scale factors s_1 and s_2 in two orthogonal directions. At first sight, this is well suited for describing the ventricle motion: indeed, the main motion of the ventricle is perpendicular to the long axis of the ventricle. In addition, there is a small motion along the long axis.

The affine model:

$$X = ax + by + t_x$$
$$Y = cx + dy + t_y$$

is more general and allows various motions to be handled.

In the following, the motion model is denoted f_p where p is the set of parameters models. $p = [s, \theta, t_x, t_y]$ for a similarity, $p = [s_1, s_2, \theta, t_x, t_y]$ for an affinity and $p = [a, b, c, d, t_x, t_y]$ for an affine model. The advantages and drawbacks of these three models are discussed in the section devoted to the results.

3   Overview of tracker

The tracker is initialized with the contour traced by the expert in the first frame of the sequence. Once initialized, the tracker operates in a loop following three major steps: prediction, motion computation and adjustment (Fig. 2).

```
1. Computation of an initial guess using correlation based
   methods.
2. Iterative computation of the velocity field using motion
   model.
3. Adjustment of the ventricular wall with snakes.
```

Fig. 2. Block diagram of the tracker

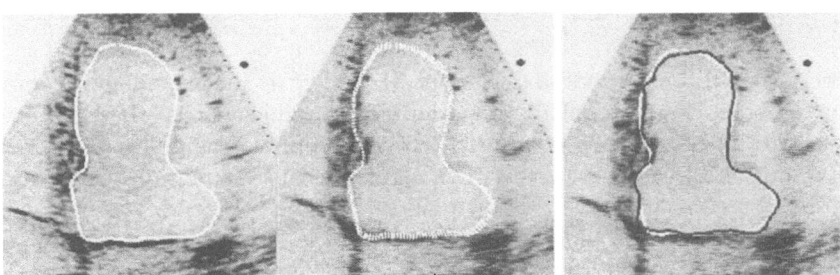

Fig. 3. The main steps of the tracker: (a) the contour detected in a given frame (b) the computed motion (c) prediction (in white) and result of the detection (in black).

The first step aims at computing an initial guess in order to overcome problems stemming from small structures undergoing large motion as the mitral valve. Let $\{M_i\}_{1<i\leq N}$ be the points of the contour detected in a given frame. Using cross correlation, these points can be matched with points P_i in the next frame. If f_p is the motion model used, a first estimation of the ventricle in the next frame is obtained by minimizing the distance between the two curves $C = \{f_p(M_1), ...f_p(M_N)\}$ and $C' = \{P_1, ..., P_N\}$. As the correspondence given by the correlation process is not always relevant, we use the *closest point* distance and we compute the optimal parameters p minimizing

$$min_p \sum distance(f_p(M_i), C')$$

where $distance(f_p(M), C') = min_i||f_p(M), P_i||$. Hence, $\{f_p(M_-), ...f_p(M_n)\}$ is a first rough estimation of the ventricular wall.

From this initial guess, the ventricle motion is computed iteratively using only normal optical flow. This computation is described in section 4.

Finally, snakes [4] are used from the predicted position of the ventricle. In most cases, this position is sufficiently close to the ventricular boundary so that the snake converges successfully.

The main steps of our algorithm are illustrated in figure 3. Fig. 3.a shows the ventricle border detected in a given frame. Fig. 3.b exhibits the motion (Step 1+2) computed between the two frames using the affinity model. Fig. 3.c shows the results of the adjustment after the snake process.

4 Motion computation

Let C be the ventricular contour detected in a given frame I_1 . Our aim is to compute the motion of C between two consecutive frames I_1 and I_2.

We implemented a weighted least squares fit of local first-order constraint (1) to a global model of v on the ventricular contour by computing $\hat{p}_0$ which minimizes

$$\sum_{1 \leq i < N} |(\overrightarrow{M_i f_p(M_i)}.n_i)n_i - v^\perp(M_i)|^2 \tag{2}$$

where n_i is the unit normal to C at point M_i and $v^\perp$ is the normal flow computed from (1). This way, we calculate the motion $\hat{p}_0$ which yields the best fit with the motion measurements computed with differential techniques. The use of a global motion of the curve is very important because it permits us to override divergence trends at erroneous flow points.

As the optical flow does not match the true displacement, we refine the estimation iteratively in the following way: we compute the normal optical flow $v_1^\perp$ on the curve $f_{\hat{p}_0}(M_i)_{\{1 \leq i \leq N\}}$ between the registered image $I_1(f_{\hat{p}_0}^{-1})$ and I_2. Resolving (2) with $v = v_1$ then allows us to compute $f_{\hat{p}_1}$. Hence, $f_{\hat{p}_1} \circ f_{\hat{p}_0}$ is a better estimate of the motion and so on... Successive infinitesimal refinements $f_{\hat{p}_q} \circ ... \circ f_{\hat{p}_0}$ gives an accurate estimation of the motion field. The prediction obtained is generally close to the true ventricular wall and the snake process can be applied successfully.

5 Results

Our method has been tested within a project aiming at 3D reconstruction of the beating left ventricle [6]. The system consists of a probe rotating around its axis. For each rotation of the probe, an entire heart contraction is recorded at a 25 frames/sec rate. We then acquire a matrix of images. Its size is 8×9 because we only acquire images between end diastolic and end systolic (8 images) and the probe rotation is 20 degrees.

First, we compare the performance of the tracking algorithm using the three motion models we use: similarity, affinity and affine model. A frame by frame visual comparison of tracking using these three models showed that the affinity model generally gives superior results in term of how closely the tracker followed the ventricle. Indeed, it appears that the similarity model does not manage to encompass the variability of the shape deformation. On the other hand, the affine model is not sufficiently restrictive when the noise level is high and the prediction step may be erroneous. Hence, the use of affinity appears as a good compromise.

We tried to quantify the degree of improvement by comparing our results to the ventricle manually traced by an expert in some sequences. Note that these traces can only be considered as *indicative* and not as ground truth. Indeed, there is a large variability between the traces outlined by different experts [1].

Error Metric

We compare the areas enclosed by the expert detection and the computed detection. We think that this measure is more appropriate because the area of the ventricle is an important clinical parameter to evaluate the left ventricular function. More precisely, if $\mathcal{A}_{comp}$ (resp $\mathcal{A}_{expert}$) is the area enclosed by the computed (resp. expert) detection, the metric used is defined as

$$area\ error = \frac{\#\{x \in \mathcal{A}_{comp}\ and\ x \notin \mathcal{A}_{expert}\} \cup \{x \notin \mathcal{A}_{comp}\ and\ x \in \mathcal{A}_{expert}\}}{\#\mathcal{A}_{expert}}$$

where $\#E$ denotes the cardinal number of E.

Tracking experiments

Four matrix database have been outlined by the expert. This amounts to outline the ventricle in 8×9 images for each patient. In order to test our algorithm, we considered the contour $c_{i \times j}$ traced by the expert in frame i of the sequence which corresponds to the probe angle $j \times 20$ degrees. We computed the distance between the results given by the algorithm in the next frame to the contour $c_{i+1 \times j}$ traced by the expert. The results are averaged on all the images which have been outlined by the expert in the database.

This computation was performed for the three motion models and the results are shown in table 5. The area error in percentage is around 6%.

These results prove that the affinity model is slightly more appropriate than the two others. Not surprisingly, the affine model gives the worst results because of its excessive flexibility. The standard deviation is the highest for this model; when we look at the results (Fig.4, 6), we can see that results are sometimes very good with this models. Unfortunately they are sometimes poor for high noise level. We now give tracking results for different patients. Fig 4 shows snapshot views of tracking using the affinity models. The detected curve is shown in white whereas the expert trace is drawn with black points. The visual impression is good. Fig 5.a plots the evolution of the area errors with the three motions models. In this case, the area errors are rather similar and the results obtained in the last frame are close too (Fig. 5.b).

Fig. 6 shows tracking results for another patient. Tracking results are good except at the end of the sequence because the process is unable to handle the ventricular deformation in the right direction.

3D reconstruction Fig. 7 exhibits the 3D construction of the left ventricle with the patient used in Fig. 6.

Motion model	area errors (in %) Mean	area errors standard deviation	min error	max error
Similarity	6.0837	1.6884	3.6253	10.5606
Affinity	5.8903	1.5169	3.8013	10.0563
Affine	6.2169	1.9765	3.6323	14.1187

Table 1. Comparison of the tracking error for the three motion models.

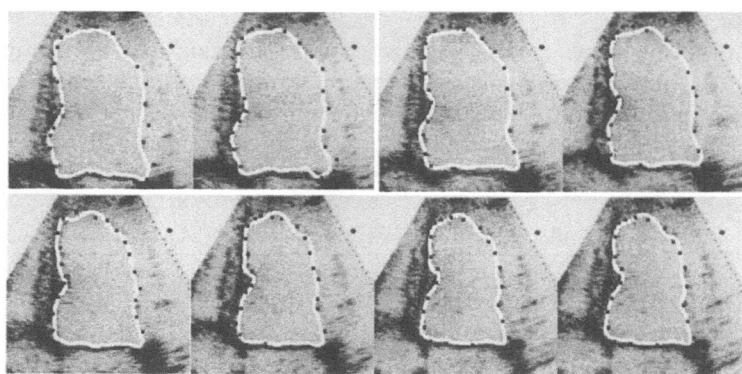

Fig. 4. Tracking results: the tracked ventricle is shown in white and the trace of the expert is shown with black points.

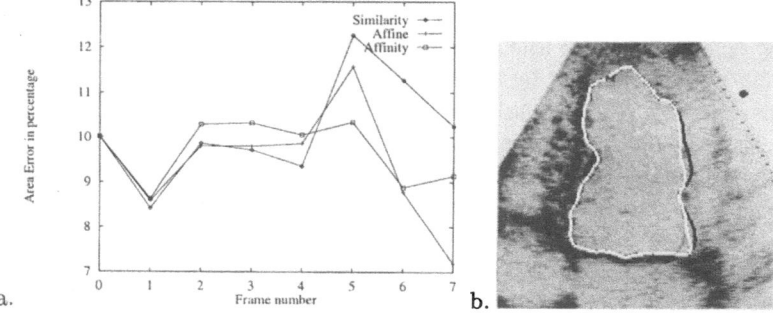

Fig. 5. (a) Plot of the area errors trough the sequence for the three motion models (b) results of the tracking in the last frame: similarity is in gray, affinity is in white and affine in black.

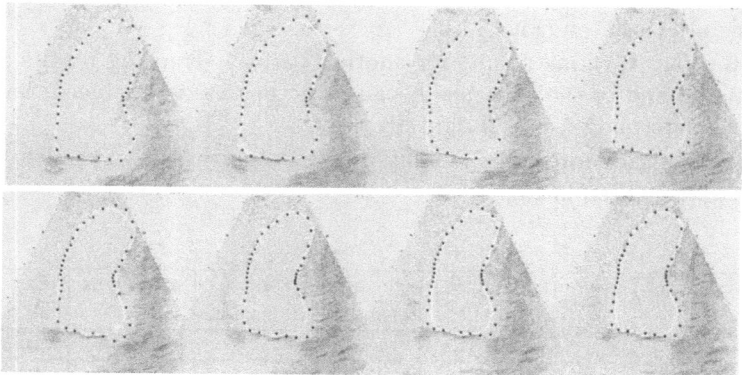

Fig. 6. Tracking results: the tracked ventricle is shown in white and the trace of the experts is shown with black points.

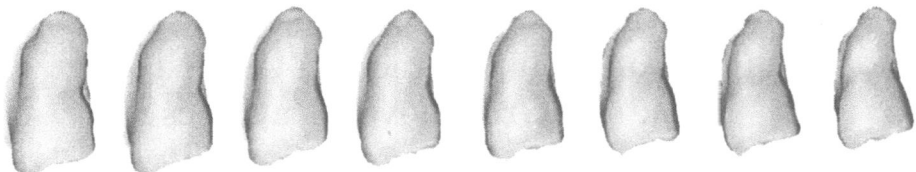

Fig. 7. 3D reconstruction of the beating left ventricle between end diastolic and end systolic.

6   Discussion and Conclusion

To conclude we have presented a new approach to tracking on echocardiographic images. Our approach, which combines both motion based approach and fine adjustment with snakes, give promising results. The use of this hierarchical approach allows us to compute a reliable estimation of the velocity which can be used successfully as initial guess for the adjustment stage.

It is clear that further investigation should be made into the problem of ventricular adjustment. In fact, the snakes can be attracted by structures which do not belong to the endocardium. Indeed, gradient information obtained from echographic images is always incomplete because of drop outs. This problem especially appears because of shadowing effect caused by the ribs. We currently investigate how the spatial coherency of our data can be used to overcome the above problems. Indeed, some structures of the endocardium which are missing in a scan plane are likely to be present in the neighbored scan planes. That is the reason why we want to achieve the adjustments stage in the 3D space instead of the 2D space.

References

1. V. Chalna and Y. Kim. A methodology for evaluation of boundary detection algorithms on medical images. *IEEE Transactions on Medical Imaging*, 16(5):642–652, December 1997.
2. M. Chen, T. Kanade, H. Rowley, and D.Pommerleau. Anomaly Detection through Registration. In *CVPR' 1998*, 1998.
3. G. Jacob, A. Noble, and A. Blake. Robust Contour Tracking in Echographic Sequences. In *ICCV 98, Bombay (India)*, pages 408–413, January 1998.
4. M. Kass, A. Witkin, and D. Terzopoulos. Snakes: Active Contour Models. *International Journal of Computer Vision*, 1:321–331, 1988.
5. C. Lamberti, P. Botazzi, and A. Sarti. Region Based Matching Field Computation in 2D Echocardiography. In *Computers in Cardiology, 1993*, pages 739–742, 1993.
6. J.-P. Lethor, G. Winterfeldt, M.-O. Berger, M. Handschuhmacker, and I. Marcon. A Fast automated System for Four Dimensional Reconstruction of the left Ventricle Using Transthoracic Echographic Images. In *Computers in Cardiology*, 1997.

Segmentation of Echocardiographic Data. Multiresolution 2D and 3D Algorithm Based on Grey Level Statistics

Djamal Boukerroui[1], Olivier Basset[1], and Atilla Baskurt[2] and Alison Noble[3]

[1] CREATIS, CNRS Research Unit (UMR 5515) and affiliated to INSERM,
INSA 502, 69621 Villeurbanne cedex, France
{djamal.boukerroui, olivier.basset}@creatis.insa-lyon.fr
[2] LIGIM (EA 1899), Claude Bernard University, Lyon, France
abaskurt@ligim.univ-lyon1.fr
[3] Departement of Engineering Science, University of Oxford,
Oxford OX1 3PJ, UK
noble@robots.ox.ac.uk

Abstract. We propose in this paper a robust adaptive region segmentation algorithm of dirty images in a Bayesian framework. A multiresolution implementation of the algorithm is performed using a wavelets basis. The algorithm can process both 2D and 3D data. In this work we focus on the adaptive character of the algorithm and we discuss how global and local statistics can be taken into account in the segmentation process. Results of segmentation performed on echocardiographic sequences (2D+T) and an evaluation of the performance of the proposed algorithm are presented.

1 Introduction

The first step toward automatic analysis or evaluation of a given image is generally considered to be successful segmentation. In recent years, many authors have applied Bayesian estimation techniques for image segmentation. These statistical approaches have improved the segmentation results of different image modalities (natural scenes [2], texture images [4], ultrasonic images [1], [10], ...). The segmentation results depend largely on the estimation of the model region parameters that can be based on local/global statistics and can be adaptive. In previous work [1], we have presented an adaptive segmentation algorithm based on texture characterisation. This paper proposes an improvement on the adaptivity by introducing an enhancement to control the adaptive properties of the segmentation process.

The paper is organised as follows. Section 2 describes, briefly, t he mathematical framework of our approach and the proposed improvement to take into account both global and local statistics of the data in the optimisation process. A brief description of the algorithm and its implementation is given in Sect. 3. Section 4 presents the segmentation results on echocardiographic sequence images and a comparison of the computer-generated boundaries to the hand-outlined by a medical expert. The paper's conclusions are summarised in Sect. 5.

2   Modelling

We assume that the observed data Y is a random field defined on a 2D (3D) rectangular grid S. Y_s denotes the value of Y at the site $s \in S$. A segmentation of the image (volume) into regions will be noted by X, where $X_s = i$ means that the pixel (voxel) at s belongs to region i. The probability $P(X = x)$ is written as $P(x)$. The number of different regions in X is k. The conditional density function of Y given X is assumed to exist and to be strictly positive and is denoted by $P(y \mid x)$. The image may be segmented by estimating the pixel classification X given the observed image Y using the maximum *a posteriori* (MAP) estimation of X. Hence, once the distributions of $P(y \mid x)$ and $P(x)$ are defined, the problem of segmenting an image is reduced to that of minimising an energy function.

We use a Markov Random Field to model the region process X, due to its restriction to local interaction. With this assumption, according to Hammersley-Clifford theorem [9], and for a given neighbourhood system, the prior density $P(x)$ can be written as a Gibbs density where:

$$\ln P(x) \cong \sum_{c \in C} V_c(x) \ , \tag{1}$$

$$\text{and} \ \ V_c(x) = V_{<s,t>} = \beta_{<s,t>} \left(1 - 2\delta \left(x_s, x_t \right) \right) \ . \tag{2}$$

Here, $V_c(x)$ are the clique potentials and δ is the Kronecker delta function.

We use a 8-connected (6-connected) spatial neighbourhood for 2D (3D) lattice. $\beta_{<s,t>} = \beta$ if the clique $< s, t >$ is horizontal or vertical and $\beta_{<s,t>} = \beta / \sqrt{2}$ if the clique $< s, t >$ is right or left diagonal. The Gibbsian parameter β is positive, so that two neighbouring pixels are more likely to belong to the same class than to different classes. Increasing β value increases region size and leads to excessive smoothing of boundaries.

The conditional density distribution $P_s(y_s \mid x_s = i)$ of the observed grey level intensity at a site s is assumed to be Gaussian, with mean μ_s^i and variance $(\sigma_s^i)^2$. The local class mean μ_s^i is a slowly varying function of s. These assumptions lead to the following energy function:

$$U(x \mid y) = \sum_s \left(\ln(\sigma_s^{x_s}) + \frac{1}{2(\sigma_s^{x_s})^2} \left(y_s - \mu_s^{x_s} \right)^2 \right) + \sum_{<s,t>} V_{<s,t>}(x) \ . \tag{3}$$

This function has two components. The first term constrains the region intensity to be close to the data and the second is a regularisation term, which imposes a smoothness constraint. Computation of the exact minimum of the energy function is time consuming. As an alternative to Simulated Annealing

[11], the *Iterated Conditional Mode* algorithm [8] has been used, which does not guarantee a global minimum of the energy function but is a fast deterministic algorithm. Starting from an initial segmentation x_0 the algorithm updates the label of sites in x in order to maximise the conditional density function at each site knowing the labels values at its neighbourhood and the observation y.

2.1   Parameter estimation

A rectangular window is used for the estimation of the local class means and variances for all region types i and at each site s. Given the region labels x, μ_s^i and σ_s^i are the average and the standard deviation of pixels (voxels) of the region i inside a window of width W centred at s. This is achieved using the Maximum Likelihood Estimation. Initially, for robust estimation, the window size W is equal to the whole image (volume) and then, as the algorithm progresses, the segmentation becomes better and smaller windows give more reliable and accurate estimations. Thus, the algorithm fits progressively to local characteristics of each region. In our implementation, as in [2], the window size is reduced by a factor of two until a final value $W_{\min}$. This gives the adaptive character to the algorithm. A major difficulty of this algorithm, as it stands, is that it takes into account the global statistics of the regions only in the first few iterations. Indeed, when the algorithm starts from a bad initial solution or when the statistics of image regions are not Gaussian (due to the presence of multiplicative noise, gradient of intensity, outliers,...) the adaptive properties decrease the robustness of the algorithm and detain it to converge to the optimal solution.

2.2   The proposed energy function

We propose, in this paper, to weight the energy function to take into account the global statistics of the image. Then the energy function becomes:

$$U(x|y) = \sum_s \frac{\varphi(W_s^{x_s})}{N_s^\varphi} \left(\ln(\sigma_s^{x_s}) + \frac{1}{2(\sigma_s^{x_s})^2} (y_s - \mu_s^{x_s})^2 \right) + \sum_{<s,t>} V_{<s,t>}(x) \ , \quad (4)$$

where $W_s^{x_s}$ is a weighting coefficient which measures the similarity between the local statistics of the region x_s and the global ones. φ is a transformation function and N_s^φ is a normalised constant of the function φ at the site s defined by the following condition:

$$\sum_{x_s} \varphi(W_s^{x_s}) = k \ . \quad (5)$$

Here, as already noted, k is the number of regions.

In the case of a segmentation problem, the similarity measure that is largely used to compare two distributions is the Kolmogorov-Smirnov distance [3], [4], [5]. So we take $W_s^{x_s} = D\left(y(x_s), y(s, x_s)\right)$; where D is the Kolmogorov-Smirnov distance between the cumulative distribution functions of the whole sites of the class x_s and the sites of the same class in the analysed window W centred at s. The introduction of the transformation function φ aims to control the adaptive term and the weighted one. We define φ as:

$$\varphi(W_s^{x_s}) = A_s + (W_s^{x_s})^b \tag{6}$$

$$\text{and} \quad \frac{A_s}{\displaystyle\max_{all\ class}\left[(W_s^{x_s})^b\right] - \min_{all\ class}\left[(W_s^{x_s})^b\right]} = a \quad \forall s\ , \tag{7}$$

where a is a positive constant.

Thus, at each site s, the constant a controls the contribution of the adaptive term A_s (local statistics) and the weight $(W_s^{x_s})^b$ which, takes into account the global statistics. The influence of the control parameters a and b on the φ function is illustrated Fig. 1 (For example for $a \gg 1$, (4) is equivalent to (3)). We use $b = 1$ in the following.

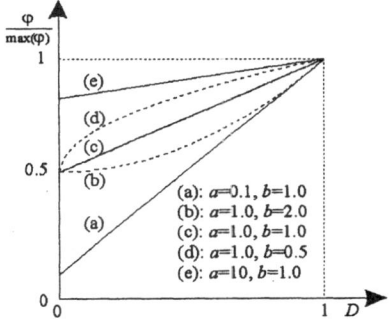

Fig. 1. The influence of the control parameters a and b.

3   Algorithm

In Sect. 2, the conditional density distribution of the observed grey intensity at a site s is assumed to be Gaussian. Clearly this assumption is not true in many cases, especially for displayed ultrasound data. We make use of the Central Limit Theorem as in [10], which states that the distribution of the mean of a large number of independent random observations tends toward a Gaussian distribution centred to their collective mean. This assumption is reasonably acceptable for low-pass filtered and decimated images that are originally governed by non-Gaussian statistics and leads us to a multiresolution implementation of our algorithm.

Hence, a hierarchical structure has been used to implement our algorithm [1], [6]. Starting from the highest resolution image, a multiresolution pyramid is built using the Discrete Wavelet Transform (DWT) approach. The coarsest resolution is initially segmented and the result of the segmentation is passed on to the next finer level of resolution and so on, until the finest resolution image is segmented. So a lattice point at one resolution will correspond to four (eight) points at the next finer resolution in the case of 2D (3D) data. An initial solution of the minimisation problem, at the coarsest resolution, is obtained with the K-means clustering algorithm. Starting from this segmentation, the algorithm alternates between the estimation of region labels and model parameters and is stopped when no further changes in the labels occur. The Gibbsian parameter at each scale is derived from the full resolution one according to the multiscale approach proposed in [7]. In this work, the number of regions k and the Gibbsian parameter β at the full resolution are not estimated. For more detailed description of the hierarchical implementation see [1], [7].

4   Results

In this section we present the results of applying our new algorithm on a long-axis echocardiographic sequence of 106 images (2D+T). In the segmentation process the sequence is considered as a 3D volume to enable temporal continuity to be use in the segmentation process. All the results presented in the following are obtained for 3 classes, $\beta = 1$ at the full resolution and for 3 levels of decomposition of the Discrete Wavelet Transform.

Figure 2 shows the segmentation results (superimposed on the original data) for 4 frames (1–4) and for 3 different values of the control parameter a (A, B, C). Images A were obtained for $a = +\infty$ i.e using the energy function in (3). B and C are obtained with $a = 10$ and $a = 1$ respectively. A deviation with respect to the actual boundaries is observed in the left part of the images (right ventricle) when the adaptive character is emphased (Fig. 2 A), whereas a good detection was obtained when global statistics are included in the segmentation process (Fig. 2 C). As expected, the segmentation is better when both global and local statistics are included in the segmentation process. Our formulation of the problem allows us to control the effective contribution of each statistics by varying the parameter a. There is little difference between results A and B, probably

Table 1. Perimeter and area error measures of the computer-generated segmentation of the left ventricle relative to measurement made by hand by a medical expert. The minus sign indicates that our estimation is larger than the medical expert's.

	$a = +\infty$	$a = 10$	$a = 1$
Perimeter (pixel size)	$\mu = -28.83\,\%$ $\sigma = 8.22\,\%$	$\mu = -25.38\,\%$ $\sigma = 7.17\,\%$	$\mu = -19.52\,\%$ $\sigma = 4.99\,\%$
Area (pixel size)^2	$\mu = -6.29\,\%$ $\sigma = 6.91\,\%$	$\mu = -6.03\,\%$ $\sigma = 6.92\,\%$	$\mu = -7.59\,\%$ $\sigma = 6.71\,\%$

because in experiment B the global statistic is taken with only 10 percent in comparison with the local one. This allows us to have grown some insight into the importance of the parameter a.

An evaluation of the computer detection of the boundary of the left ventricle has been made. The validation of a segmentation algorithm is an important and difficult task. First we computed 2 classical measures (Perimeter and Area) on the 106 frames of the computer-generated and the hand-outlined boundaries. The results are summarised in Table 1. We can see that the perimeter shows us that a little improvement is made when global statistics are involved. However it is quite difficult to make a conclusion using only these two measures.

Recently, a more applicable methodology for evaluation of boundary detection algorithm has been proposed [12]. This methodology uses essentially two distance measures: The Hausdorff Distance (HD) and the Average Distance (AD). The HD between two curves is defined as the maximum of the Distance to the Closest Point's (DCP) between the two curves. The DCP associates each point on both curves to a point on the other curve, and the HD finds the largest distance between the associated points. The AD is the average of all distances between the correspondence points between the curves. This allow us to analyse the regional differencies between the curves.

Table 2 shows the minimum, the maximum, the mean and the standard deviation of the two distances over the whole range of the data. Here also we can see that the HD does not show any significant difference between the performance of the three algorithms. However the AD shows clearly that the third algorithm is better than the two others ($p < 0.0001$ for the Friedman's rank test [12]).

5   Conclusion

In this paper, we have proposed an adaptive region segmentation algorithm based on global and local statistics in a Bayesian framework. The enhancement we developed can be regarded as a generalisation of previous work [1], [10]. The formulation of the segmentation problem allows us to control the effective contribution of each statistic. Segmentation results performed on a long-axis echocardiographic sequence (2D+T) has been presented. A comparison of the computer-generated boundaries of the left ventricle to the hand-outlined by a

Table 2. Direct comparison of the computer-generated boundaries of the left ventricle to the hand-outlined by a medical expert.

		$a = +\infty$	$a = 10$	$a = 1$
Hausdorff Distance	(min , max)	(8.06 , 23.53)	(8.06 , 23.53)	(8.48 , 22.56)
	(μ , σ)	(14.21 , 3.91)	(13.63 , 3.74)	(13.64 , 3.48)
Average Distance	(min , max)	(2.49 , 17.13)	(2.45 , 15.80)	(1.82 , 11.75)
	(μ , σ)	(8.78 , 3.09)	(8.19 , 2.94)	(5.96 , 2.20)

medical expert has been made. Our experiments indicate that taking into account the global statistic, in an adaptive algorithm, improves the segmentation results.

The first results obtained with our algorithm on echocardiographic data gives satisfying segmentation. However, a comparison of the segmentation results with boundaries outlined by multiple observers will be an important future step to confirm this conclusion. It would be also interesting to compare or to associate our approach with high-level model-guided segmentation, using "deformable-templates" for instance, which includes *a prior* knowledge about the object structure is in the segmentation process.

The proposed method is general and can be applied to other adaptive image segmentation problems that can be posed in a Bayesian framework. Other similarity measures and φ functions could be used.

References

1. D. Boukerroui, O. Basset, N Guérin, and A. Baskurt. Multiresolution texture based adaptive clustering algorithm for breast lesion segmentation. *European Journal of Ultrasound*, 8(2):135–144, 1998.
2. T. N. Pappas. An adaptive clustering algorithm for image segmentation. *IEEE Transactions on Signal Processing*, SP-40(4):901–914, 1992.
3. R. Muzzolini, Y.-H. Yang, and R. Pierson. Multiresolution texture segmentation with application to diagnostic ultrasound images. *IEEE Transactions on Medical Imaging*, 12(1):108–123, 1993.
4. C. Kervrann and F. Heitz. Segmentation non supervisée des images naturelles texturées: approche statistique. *Traitement du signal*, 11(1):31–41, 1994.
5. D. Geman. Random fields and inverse problems in imaging. *Ecole d'été de probabilités de Saint-Flour XVIII, Hennequin, P.L., (eds.) (1988), Vol. 1427. Springer-Verlag, Lecture Notes in Mathematics, Berlin*, 161–172, 1990.
6. B. C. Vemuri, S. Rahman, and J. Li. Multiresolution adaptive K-means algorithm for segmentation of brain MRI. *Intl. Compu. Sci, Conf. On Image Analysis and Comp. Graphics, Hong Kong*, 347–354, 1995.
7. F. Heitz, P. Perez, and P. Bouthemy. Multiscale minimization of global energy functions in some visual recovery problems. *CVGIP: Image Understanding*, 59(1):125–134, 1994.
8. B. J. Besag. On the statistical analysis of dirty pictures. *Journal of the Royal Statistical Society B*, 48(3):259–302, 1986.
9. B. J. Besag. Spatial interaction qnd the statistical analysis of lattice systems. *Journal of the Royal Statistical Society B*, 26(2):192–236, 1974.
10. E. A. Ashton and K. J. Parker. Multiple resolution Bayesian segmentation of ultrasound images. *Ultrasonic Imaging*, 17(2):291–304, 1995.
11. S. Kirkpatrick, C. Gelatt, and M. Vecchi. Optimization by simulated annealing. *Science*, 220:671–680, 1983.
12. V. Chalana and Y. Kim. A methodology for evaluation of boundary detection algorithm on medical images. *IEEE Transactions on Medical Imaging*, 16(1):642–652, 1997.

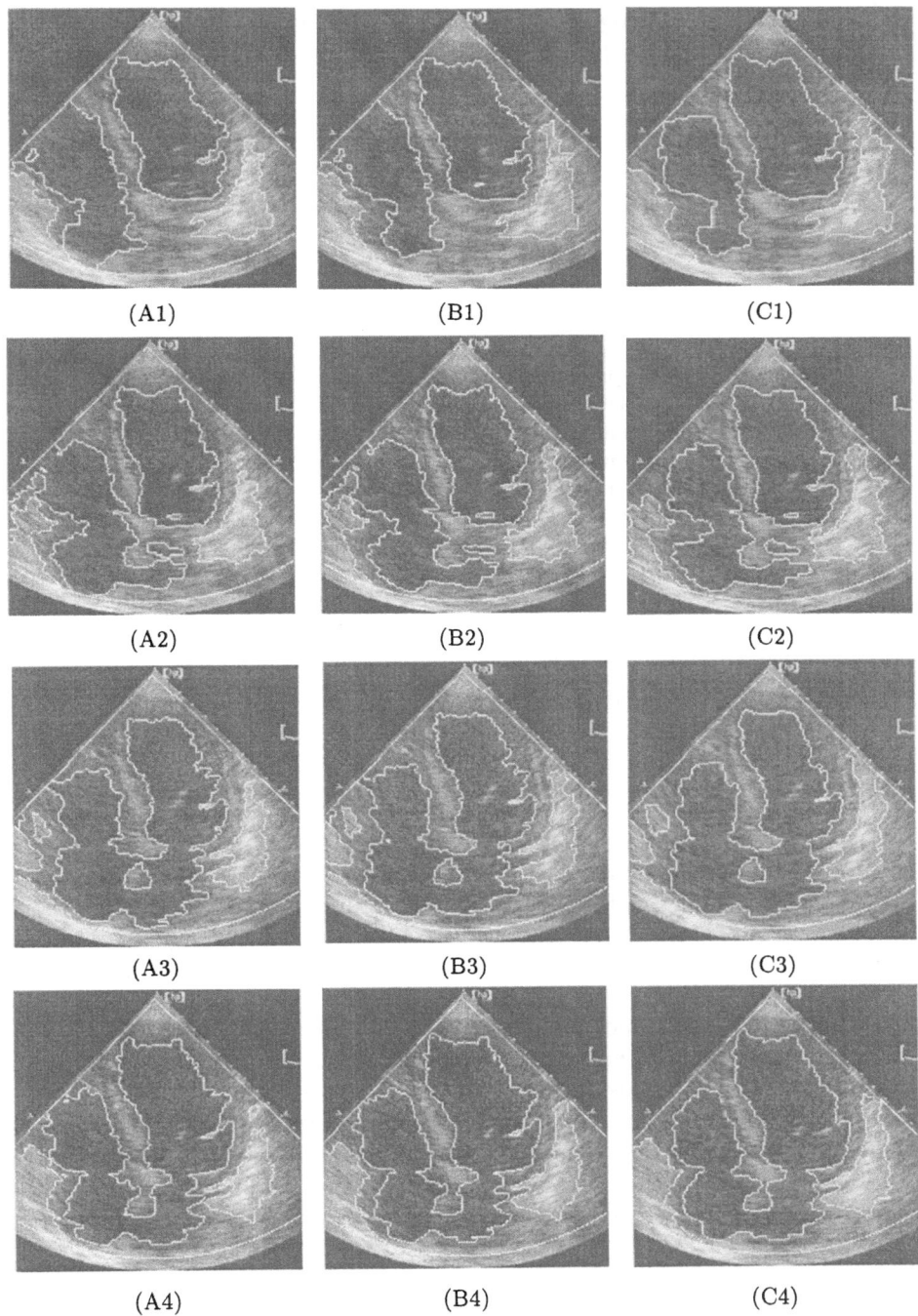

(A1)   (B1)   (C1)

(A2)   (B2)   (C2)

(A3)   (B3)   (C3)

(A4)   (B4)   (C4)

Fig. 2. Segmentation results for 3 different values of the control parameter a : from left to right $a = +\infty$, $a = 10$ and $a = 1$; frames 1 and 2 : systole, frames 3 and 4 : diastole.

Locating Motion Artifacts in Parametric fMRI Analysis

A.J.Lacey, N.A.Thacker, E. Burton, and A.Jackson

Division of Imaging Science and Bio-medical Engineering, University of Manchester,
Manchester, M13 9PT
a.lacey@man.ac.uk
http://www.niac.man.ac.uk

Abstract. In this paper we assess rigid body co-registration in terms of residual motion artifacts for the different correlation approaches used in fMRI. We summarise, from a statistical perspective, the three main approaches to parametric fMRI analysis and then present a new way of visualising motion effects in correlation analysis. This technique can be used both to select regions of relatively unambiguous activation and to verify the results of analysis. We demonstrate the usefulness of this visualisation technique on fMRI data sets suffering from motion correlated artifacts. We use it in our assesment of rigid body co-registration concluding that it is an acceptable basis for re-alignment, provided that correlation is done using a measure which estimates variance from the data at each voxel.

1 Introduction

Subject motion during the time course of functional activation studies has been shown to cause spurious signals which can mimic "true" activation [1, 2]. Motion correction using image registration software is therefore common practice in functional imaging and many groups now routinely make use of rigid body co-registration using software packages such as Automatic Image Registration (AIR) [3–5]. However, depending on the details of the data capture, the assumption of a rigid body may be inappropriate. In some cases slices of image data may undergo different amounts of motion and in other cases the data may suffer from motion blurring. These processes could leave residual motion artifacts in the data which bias subsequent interpretation.

Previous workers have demonstrated the potential problems of motion in fMRI analysis [1, 2] using data sets with simulated movement. The estimation of this effect shows the likely scale of this contribution to an fMRI signal. We have found no paper which attempts to quantify directly the affect on the computed correlation measures.

The objective of this work was to develop a technique to test whether rigid body co-registration successfully removes motion effects to a statistically acceptable level. We first review the statistical characteristics of published analysis techniques in order to design a test for the effectiveness of rigid-body co-registration which is applicable to the range of current approaches. We then go on to demonstrate the effects of motion and co-registration on the common statistical correlation forms used for analysis.

2   fMRI Analysis Techniques

There have been many approaches to the analysis of functional NMR images proposed in the literature. Considered from a statistical point of view these techniques can be grouped as either non-parametric or parametric. It is generally accepted that whilst non-parametric techniques are initially more robust, parametric techniques will ultimately have better discriminability once the analytical models have been refined. Generally, parametric analysis can be decomposed into two stages; the application of a voxel by voxel time dependent analysis, followed by a regional analysis of clusters [6, 7]. The first of these is designed as a significance test, the hypothesis being that the data seen in the image can be accounted for entirely by random noise fluctuations. The second is a significance test based on the probability of observing particular sized regions failing the first test. This process is well suited to removing isolated "fake" activations but doesn't perform well on larger connected regions such as those often presented by motion. Thus it is the performance of the first test with which we are concerned.

The voxel based null hypothesis test is generally implemented as a correlation measure between the image signal and a normalised wave-function which models the activation paradigm. The details of this correlation measure vary in the literature, but all successful measures have the same fundamental statistical origins; some measure of correlation C is normalised by it's expected variance $var(C)$ in order to produce a measure which can be treated like a 't test' or 'Z score' [7]. As regards the selection of a wave-function, although the ability to extract signal will be strongly dependent on having the correct functional form and phase, the technique of error propagation can be used to show that any normalised wave-function will produce a set of correlation measures with an identical distribution for the null hypothesis. Thus we choose to work with a square wave for simplicity.

Three measures, chosen to cover a set of statistically distinct possible approaches, were used for this investigation;

$$C_j^1 = \sum_{t=1}^{T} I_{tj}.W_t$$

A simple correlation measure with no explicit (fixed) normalisation, where W is a normalised correlation waveform ($|W|^2 = 1$) and I_j is a mean subtracted temporal data set at voxel j . This correlation measure can be converted into a simple null hypothesis statistic by dividing by a pooled estimate of the standard deviation on the measure $\sqrt{var(C)}$ and will behave in the same way as any measure which makes the basic assumption of constant uniform image noise, including Fourier approaches. While we accept that such a simple measure is unlikely to be used unmodified in serious fMRI analysis we have included it here for completeness.

$$C_j^2 = \frac{\sum_{t=1}^{T} I_{tj}.W_t}{1/(T-1)\sqrt{\sum_t^T (I_{tj} - W_t.C_j^1)^2}}$$

A measure with individual voxel variance estimation which we believe to be statistically equivalent to that used in SPM [8], where the numerator is the estimate of variation about the assumed model. This technique will behave in the same way as any measure which estimates variance from the data, such as 't-tests' and 'z-scores'.

$$C_j^3 = \frac{\sum_{t=1}^{T} I_{tj}.W_t}{\sqrt{\sum_t^T I_{tj}^2}}$$

A normalised correlation measure as used in STIMULATE [9]. This measure is normalised between -1 and 1 but cannot be interpreted as a standard null hypothesis statistic unless the numerator approaches that of C_j^2, which will only happen when the noise dominates the observed signal distribution (i.e. C_j^1 is small).

3   Experiments

Experiments were performed on 6 healthy volunteers. Volunteers A,B and C were scanned at rest and volunteers D, E and F performed a motor activation paradigm (finger tapping) during scanning. Head movements were minimised using foam padding and a velcro strap and a bite bar with a groove was used to provide a reference to minimise out of plane movements. For each subject 18 dynamic acquisitions of $50 \times 3mm$ contiguous transverse slices covering the whole head using a T2*-weighted gradient echo sequence were acquired.

Our investigation involves the following steps:

- **Calculate rigid body motion for genuine null hypothesis data (no activation) for two groups of three subjects.** One group performing the motion stimulus paradigm and the others at rest. All data were registered to a base volume for each volunteer using the Woods algorithm [3, 4]. The main automated image registration (AIR) parameters were set as follows: intensity threshold = 275, initial sampling interval = 81, final sampling interval = 1 pixel, sample increment decrement ratio = 3, convergence criteria = 0.0005, maximum number of iterations for each sampling density = 300, no spatial smoothing was used, interpolation to standard voxel size was active.
- **Compute simulated data from the motion vectors.**
  The motion parameters were used to interpolate a set of data from the first volume with equivalent motion vectors to those estimated by the AIR package.

- **Demonstrate the effects of motion on the correlation measures used in real data.**
  As the effects of motion are expected to be proportional to local image gradient, we plot correlation scores against this quantity. Here we define image gradient G_j as follows;

$$dI_{x,y}/dx = (I'_{x+1} - I'_{x-1})/2$$

$$dI_{x,y}/dy = (I'_{y+1} - I'_{y-1})/2$$

$$G_j = \sqrt{((dI_j/dx)^2 + (dI_j/dy)^2)}$$

where x and y are image indices and I' is the first input image of the temporal sequence smoothed with a unit Gaussian kernel. The smoothing process sets the scale for the range of applicability of the linear assumption and allows the gradient information to be estimated from a single temporal slice. Averaging of the temporal data set to produce a mean gradient would also be possible and perhaps even preferable for very large motions, but was not found necessary for this work.
  For data without motion artifact, this plot is expected to show the correlation score, distributed normally around zero correlation with variable density along the image gradient axis. For this case a fixed threshold value will have the same affect in terms of rejecting the null hypothesis for all values of image gradient. Any variation from this distribution shows itself as increased broadening or non-ideal structure perpendicular to the image gradient axis.
- **Demonstrate that these effects are also visible in the simulated data.**
  The simulated data, being effectively noise free, does not yield sensible variance estimates in the denominator terms of the standard correlation measures, C^2 & C^3. However, the individual estimates of the denominators are expected to be quite constant across the dataset. As a consequence C^1 is used to analyse the simulated data as it is expected to behave in a very similar fashion to the other two measures.
- **Demonstrate that these effects are removed by rigid body co-registration in the real data by repeating the analysis for motion corrected data.**
- **Simulate the effect of isolated failures of co-registration by shifting an image in each co-registered sequence.**

4   Results and Discussion

The standard deviations on the estimated motions are shown in figure 1 for the two groups of three subjects (A,B,C and D,E,F). For the group with no stimulus these results are close to the expected accuracy of the AIR software and the *motion scatter plots*, figure 2(a), show no unexpected structure or observable correlation between edge contrast and the correlation score for any of the three

	Pitch	Roll	Yaw	X	Y	Z
A	0.20 °	0.22 °	0.30 °	0.49 pixels	0.31 pixels	0.06 pixels
B	0.22 °	0.49 °	0.16 °	0.25 pixels	0.50 pixels	0.11 pixels
C	0.22 °	0.33 °	0.18 °	0.28 pixels	0.30 pixels	0.09 pixels
D	0.90 °	0.60 °	0.38 °	0.96 pixels	0.84 pixels	0.31 pixels
E	0.85 °	0.06 °	0.41 °	0.45 pixels	0.57 pixels	0.16 pixels
F	0.39 °	0.12 °	0.37 °	0.37 pixels	0.41 pixels	0.17 pixels

Fig. 1. Standard deviations on estimated movement for each subject calculated using AIR

measures. In contrast subjects D, E & F show significant movement, figure 1, and generate plots with distinct structure, figure 2(b). Notice the broadening of the data in the y-dimension (correlation score) towards the end of the x-axis where the image gradient is largest (at edges).

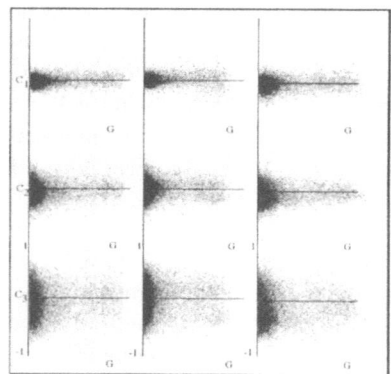

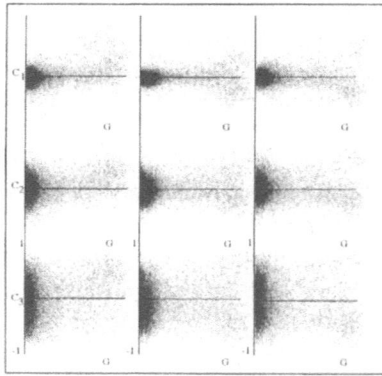

(a) No stimulus subjects A, B and C (columns)

(b) Motion stimulus subjects D, E and F (columns)

Fig. 2. Correlation scores v edge contrast (G) plots. Correlation scores are rows C^1, C^2, C^3 from top to bottom

Applying motion vectors estimated using the AIR software to the genuine null hypothesis data (no activation) gives the plots of figure 3(a). The distributions we see in these plots are entirely consistent with rigid body motion plus random noise. In contrast the plots of co-registered data, figure 3(b), show that this correlation has been significantly reduced by the process of co-registration. C^1 shows a gradual increasing instability (broadening) of the correlation score with edge contrast when compared to C^2 and C^3. C^3 is marginally less affected by motion than the conventional null hypothesis statistic because the denominator term is increased by the variation in the image data induced by motion. While C^3 may be adequate for visually identifying relative large measures, the lack of a meaningful scaling makes this correlation score more difficult to interpret.

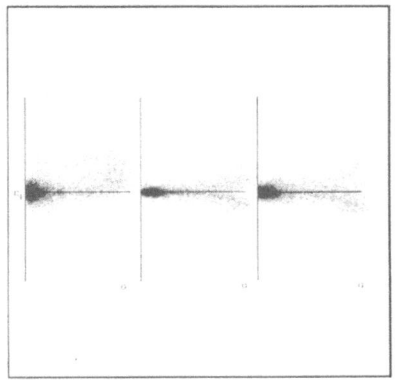

(a) Simulated stimulus

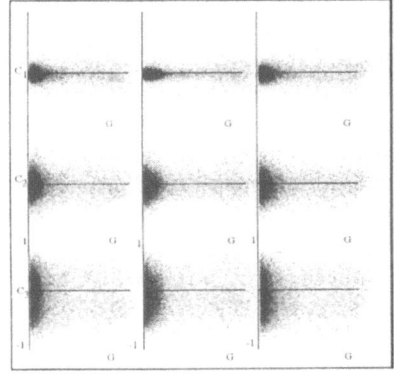

(b) Motion corrected stimulus

Fig. 3. Correlation scores v edge contrast (G) plots for subjects D, E and F (columns). Correlation scores are rows C^1, C^2, C^3 from top to bottom (only C^1 is shown in the left plot)

Subject	D	E	F
C^1	1.27	1.21	1.13
C^2	1.00	0.98	1.05
C^3	1.01	1.03	1.04

(a) Intermediate and low gradient correlations

Subject	D	E	F
C^1	1.31	1.58	1.21
C^2	0.96	0.99	0.93
C^3	0.96	0.98	0.95

(b) Intermediate gradient correlations for offset data

Fig. 4. Dimensionless measures of relative standard deviation $(\sqrt{var(C_{1/8})}/var(C_{0/8}))$

The majority of problems occur when motion artifacts mimic the effects of signal by correlating with the stimulus response function (see figure 2(b)). No motion correction procedure can be perfectly accurate and some residual errors are to be expected. This can be observed after motion correction by calculating the ratio of variances for the correlation measures for two ranges of image gradient, figure 4(a). The ratio of the variance is calculated between the first eighth (corresponding to brain tissue) and second eighth (corresponding to the boundary between brain tissues) of the dynamic range of image gradients (x-axis). The accuracies of these ratios are of the order of 1%. Figure 4(a) shows that C^1 in particular is badly affected by the increased instability around edges.

When performing rigid body alignment with an iterative automated system there is always a chance that the alignment algorithm will fail. When this happens (if it is not picked up by a validation process) it will generate isolated temporal data points at each voxel which will reduce the overall correlation scores for measures such as C^2. We can illustrate this by offsetting the first image in each sequence of data by two pixels and recomputing the variances for gradients corresponding to tissue boundaries, figure 4(b). In general, any motion correction technique, even a poor one, removing the majority of the motion from the data set and leaving only residual behaviour which is uncorrelated with the stimulus response curve, will not invalidate (statistically) the conclusions of any study using such a measure. Thus our results suggest that rigid body co-registration does effectively remove false correlations caused by motion correlated to the stimulus response.

5   Use of Motion Correlation Plots in fMRI Quality Control

Figure 5(a) shows a motion correlation plot for data generated during analysis (C^2). Activations are present in this data at both high and low level image gradient. In itself this would not be unduly worrying, but there is also a general broadening of the underlying distribution for positive correlation values at high gradient. On closer inspection this data set was found to have systematic shift artifacts at the level of 0.5 pixels in almost half of the re-sliced data set due to failure of the automatic co-registration software. The manually selected region of relatively unambiguous activation is shown as a rectangle. The new analysis technique allowed us not only to identify genuine activation, figure 5(b) but also perform quality control on our software analysis chain.

6   Conclusions

We have analysed the affect of motion on fMRI analysis. Given the broad range of approaches in the literature we have concentrated this analysis on the common statistical foundations of the parametric methods, which are the use of correlation measures. Our results are expected to be independent of the details of the shape of the correlation stimulus and should generalise to all fMRI studies based on assessing levels of significance from correlation scores.

We have constructed a method for visualising the effects of motion on fMRI analysis. As the effects of motion are expected to be proportional to the local image gradient, a scatter plot of correlation function versus image gradient

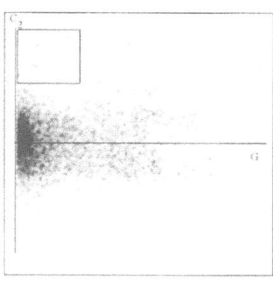
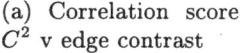

(a) Correlation score
C^2 v edge contrast

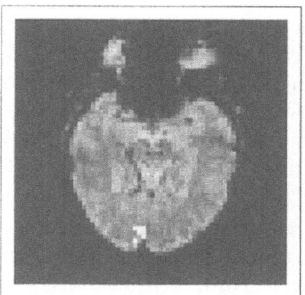

(b) fMRI image with superimposed activation

Fig. 5. Quality control of fMRI analysis showing the activation corresponding to unambiguous correlations (data within manually selected box)

separates the effects of motion across the plot. This distribution is self scaling, easily visually interpreted and can be used as a general tool to check the relative accuracy of different motion correction procedures. Such a method could also be used with non-normalised correlation measures (i.e. C^1) in order to assess the adequacy of particular co-registration procedures in the absence of ground truth.

In this study we have used the new technique to visualise the effects of motion in a typical fMRI study for three correlation approaches. The results indicate that motion artifacts are manifest in motion based experiments. These effects are significantly reduced after motion correction but still observable in simple correlation analyses which assumed pooled variance. Finally, null hypothesis based correlation methods which estimate the variance from the data at each voxel are unaffected by motion provided that any resulting residual motion, is uncorrelated with the stimulus. As we see no residual correlation with the stimulus response curve following rigid body re-alignment, we consider the rigid body assumption an acceptable basis for motion correction for these measures. In general, it will never be possible to remove all stimulus correlated motion completely, but techniques, such as those described here, could be used to monitor the success or failure of attempts to do so.

Our **TINA** software system is available as open source, including the algorithms discussed in this paper, from http://www.niac.man.ac.uk/Tina

References

1. J V Hajnal, I R Young, and G M Bydder. Contrast mechanisms in functional mri of the brain. In W G Bradley and G M Bydder, editors, *Advanced MR Imaging Techniques*, pages 195–207. Martin Dunitz Ltd London, 1997.

2. K J Friston, J Ashbuner, C D Frith, J B Poline, J D Heather, and R S J Frackowiak. Spatial registration and renormalisation of images. *M.R.M.*, 2:165–188, 1995.

3. R P Woods, S R Cherry, and J C Mazziotta. Rapid automated algorithm for aligning and reslicing pet images. *JCAT*, 16:620–633, 1992.

4. R P Woods, J C Mazziotta, and S R Cherry. Mri-pet registration with an automated algorithm. *JCAT*, 17:536–546, 1993.

5. A Jiang. Motion detection and correction in functional mr imaging. *H.B.M.*, 3:224–235, 1995.

6. K J Friston, A Holmes, J B Poline, C J Price, and C D Frith. Detecting activations in pet and fmri: Levels of inference and power. *Neuroimage*, 40:223–235, 1996.

7. N Lange. Tutorial in biostatistics, statistical approaches to human brain mapping by functional magnetic resonance imaging. *Statistics in Medicine*, 15:389–428, 1996.

8. K J Friston, R J Dolan, and R S J Fackowiak. Statistical parametric mapping, 1991. MRC Cyclotron Unit, Hammersmith Hospital, London, England.

9. J P Strupp. Stimulate: A gui based fmri analysis software package. *Neuroimage*, 3, 1996.

Non-rigid Registration by Geometry-Constrained Diffusion

Per Rønsholt Andresen[1,2] and Mads Nielsen[2,3]

[1] Department of Mathematical Modelling, Technical University of Denmark
pra@imm.dtu.dk   http://www.imm.dtu.dk/~pra
[2] 3D-Lab, School of Dentistry, University of Copenhagen, Denmark
http://www.lab3d.odont.ku.dk
[3] IT-University of Copenhagen, Denmark
http://www.it.edu

Abstract. Assume that only partial knowledge about a non-rigid registration is given so that certain points, curves, or surfaces in one 3D image map to certain certain points, curves, or surfaces in another 3D image. We are facing the aperture problem because along the curves and surfaces, point correspondences are not given. We will advocate the viewpoint that the aperture and the 3D interpolation problem may be solved *simultaneously* by finding the *simplest* displacement field. This is obtained by a geometry-constrained diffusion which yields the simplest displacement field in a precise sense. The point registration obtained may be used for growth modelling, shape statistics, or kinematic interpolation. The algorithm applies to geometrical objects of any dimensionality. We may thus keep any number of fiducial points, curves, and/or surfaces fixed while finding the simplest registration. Examples of inferred point correspondences in a longitudinal growth study of the mandible are given.

Keywords: Aperture-problem, automatic landmark detection, diffusion, kD-tree, non-rigid registration, simplest displacement field, homology.

1 Introduction

In a registration, we wish to establish the spatial correspondence of points in two images. Correspondence is defined through the concept of homology except in pathological cases. In general, homologous points will, dependent on the medical task, reflect similar anatomy, functionality, or geometry, etc. In this paper, we assume that homologous *objects* have been defined *a priori*. Therefore, we seek an automatic method for establishing *point* correspondences based on *object* correspondences. Pursuing this, we presume that: 1) The optimal registration is a mapping between homologous points, 2) The underlying biological process is smooth and homologous points do not "change place" i.e., the ordering of the anatomical structures is preserved. Formally: the registration field must not fold or be torn apart. It is then a homeomorphism.

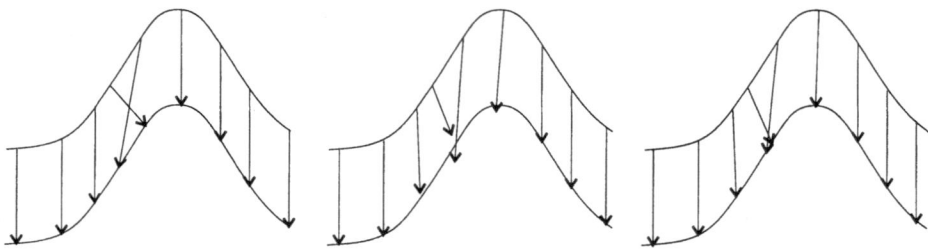

Fig. 1. *The images show schematically how the diffusion algorithm works on the deformation field. The Cartesian components of the initial deformation field (arrows in the left image) are Gaussian smoothed. Some of the links have now diverged from the surface (middle image) and must be projected back on to the surface (right image). The fold (the two crossing arrows) is removed by repeating the steps until the field does not change.*

In other words, within the objects, a solution to the generalized *aperture problem* must be chosen. In this paper, we introduce the concept of *geometry-constrained diffusion* for solving the interpolation and aperture problems simultaneously.

When performing shape statistics or analyzing (longitudinal) shape development, the tools from shape statistics (see e.g., [4]) require point matches. That is, to perform a statistical analysis of the variation of shapes we must identify homologous *points* on the shape samples. When having only a few landmarks the registration may be performed manually, but for thousands of points it becomes tedious and practically impossible. In many cases punctual landmarks are hard to establish in images, and the process requires considerable prior anatomical knowledge.

Automated methods using geometrical features such as crest-lines [9] are powerful, but do not provide a *dense* field, and may give problems in regions where shape features change topology so that correct matching is not possible. We propose using *geometry-constrained diffusion* for inferring the locally simplest non-rigid object registration.

The result of *geometry-constrained diffusion* is a dense, continuous, invertible displacement field (a homeomorphism). Many fields may fulfill the geometrical constraints given by the objects. The diffusion process gradually simplifies an initial registration field. In general, diffusion is a gradient ascent in entropy. That is, locally it changes the registration field so as to remove its structure as fast as possible. An unconstrained diffusion in this way leads to an affine registration. The geometry-constrained diffusion also simplifies the registration field as fast as possible, but is limited locally so as to preserve the object mappings (see Fig. 1).

In section 3, the theory of geometry-constrained diffusion is summarized. Section 4 describes the implementation. Examples of the simplification of an initial crest-line-based non-rigid registration are shown in section 5.

2   Related Work

In the literature, many algorithms for non-rigid registration exist. In this paper, we address the equally important problem of measuring the complexity of the geometrical deformation in a non-rigid registration. This measure may be introduced either by having only a finite number of semi-local low parameter registrations, or a viscous fluid or elasticity constraint, or a deformation energy of which the thin-plate spline energy is the canonical example (see [6] for a survey). Feldmar and Ayache's approach[5] resembles ours the most.

Feldmar and Ayache[5] perform a surface registration based on a distance measure including local geometrical properties of the surfaces The surface registration is a collection of local affine registrations. The parameters of these registrations are spatially blurred so as to construct a smoothly varying registration. A difference to our approach is that we do not make a collection of local affine frames, but a global registration field. Secondly, and most importantly, we do not exploit any metric properties of the surfaces, but look for a globally simple registration field. This also creates a tendency to match points of similar geometry since the field otherwise must be more complex.

In principle, the geometry-constrained diffusion could also have been formulated as a geometry-constrained gradient descent in displacement energy [3]. Hence, we here present a general technique for handling under-determined geometrical constraints in conjunction with variational approaches for non-rigid registration.

3   Geometry-constrained Diffusion

A registration field may be diffused simply by diffusing the Cartesian components independently. The geometry-constrained diffusion is constructed such that it preserves certain fiducial mappings during the diffusion. Assume that the identification of some fiducial points, curves and/or surfaces is given *a priori*. In order to handle this partial geometrical knowledge in the general non-rigid registration problem, we propose geometry-constrained diffusion which in a precise sense simplifies the displacement field while preserving fiducial points, curves, and/or surfaces.

Given two images $I_1 : \mathbb{R}^3 \mapsto \mathbb{R}$ and $I_2 : \mathbb{R}^3 \mapsto \mathbb{R}$, we define the registration field $R : \mathbb{R}^3 \mapsto \mathbb{R}^3$. Along the same line we define the displacement field $D : \mathbb{R}^3 \mapsto \mathbb{R}^3$ such that $R(x) = x + D(x)$. We may then define:

Definition 1 (Displacement diffusion). *The diffusion of a displacement field* $D : \mathbb{R}^3 \mapsto \mathbb{R}^3$ *is an independent diffusion in each of its Cartesian components:*

$$\partial_t D = \triangle D$$

where the Laplacian, $\triangle = \frac{\partial^2}{\partial x^2} + \frac{\partial^2}{\partial y^2} + \frac{\partial^2}{\partial z^2}$, *is applied independently in the x-, y-, and z-component of D.*

The only difference between the registration and displacement field is the addition of a linear term. This term does not influence the diffusion so that registration diffusion is identical to the displacement diffusion.

This vector-valued diffusion has some obvious and important symmetries:

Proposition 1. *The displacement diffusion is invariant with respect to similarity transforms of any of the source or target images.*

Proof. The translational part of the similarity transform only adds a constant to the displacement field, and the diffusion is invariant to this. The displacement $y = D(x) + x$ is (up to a translation) similarly transformed such that $x' = s_1 R_1 x$ and $y' = s_2 R_2 y$ where R_1 and R_2 are 3×3 rotation matrices. Under $s_1 R_1$ the displacement is mapped to $D_1(x') = D(s_1^{-1} R_1^{-1} x') - x' + s_1^{-1} R_1^{-1} x'$. Applying $s_2 R_2$ also we find

$$D'(x') = s_2 R_2 [D(s_1^{-1} R_1^{-1} x') - x' + s_1^{-1} R_1^{-1} x']$$

The latter terms leave the diffusion unaltered since they only add terms of first order, and the diffusion depends only on terms of second order. Since the diffusion is linear, it is invariant to $s_2 R_2$. By re-mapping t the diffusion is known to be independent of similarity transforms of the base manifold.   •

Applying the displacement diffusion without further constraints, it reaches a steady state which is an affine registration. This is easily seen since only linear functions are in the null-space of the diffusion equation.

In the case where the same geometrical structures have been identified in both images we wish to make certain that the diffusion of the displacement field reflects these structures. Assume that a surface $S_1 : \mathbb{R}^2 \mapsto \mathbb{R}^3$ in the source image is known to map on to the surface $S_2 : \mathbb{R}^2 \mapsto \mathbb{R}^3$ in the target image. We thus define

Definition 2 (Surface-constrained diffusion). *The surface constrained diffusion of* $D : \mathbb{R}^3 \mapsto \mathbb{R}^3$ *mapping* $S_1 : \mathbb{R}^2 \mapsto \mathbb{R}^3$ *onto* $S_2 : \mathbb{R}^2 \mapsto \mathbb{R}^3$ *is given by*

$$\partial_t D = \begin{cases} \Delta D - n_{S_2} \frac{n_{S_2} \cdot \Delta D}{\|n_{S_2}\|^2} & \text{if } x \in S_1 \\ \Delta D & \text{if } x \notin S_1 \end{cases}$$

where n_{S_2} is the unit surface normal of $S_2(D(x) + x)$.

This corresponds to solving the heat flow equation with certain boundary conditions. In this case, however, we do not keep the solution fixed at the surface, but allow points to travel along the surface. This is a dual approach to the geometry-driven curve and surface diffusion by Olver, Sapiro, and Tannenbaum [8] and others. We keep only the tangential part of the diffusion along the surface whereas they diffuse the geometry of the surface maintaining only the normal flow. The surface normal n_{S_2} may simply be obtained as a length normalization of $n_{S_1} + J n_{S_1}$ where J is the Jacobean of D. In this way the formulation is no longer explicitly dependent on S_2. That is, given an initial (guess of the) displacement field and a surface in this source image to be preserved under diffusion, we may still apply the above equation without explicitly referencing to S_2.

Curve constraints and point constraints can be handled in a similar manner. For the curve problem, we project onto a curve by only taking the part of the diffusion which is along the curve tangent. Point constraints simply disregard the diffusion at these points. The three types of geometry-constrained diffusions may be combined in any fashion as long as the boundary conditions (the matches) do not contradict one another.

We make the following proposition:

Proposition 2 (Similarity Invariance (II)). *The geometry-constrained diffusion is invariant to similarity transforms of the source or target image.*

Proof. We have already shown that the unconstrained diffusion is similarity invariant. Both the surface normal and the curve tangent are also invariant under the similarity transform.   •

We will conjecture that the geometry-constrained diffusion removes any fold in the initial displacement. This means that, the steady state solution to the geometry-constrained displacement diffusion creates an invertible mapping.

Conjecture 1 (Invertibility). A geometry-constrained diffused displacement field induces a one-to-one mapping of $\mathbb{R}^3$.

The steady state displacement field will be a homeomorphism assuming the above invertibility-conjecture is valid since the constrained diffused displacements are continuous. It will also be smooth except on the constrained objects where it will generally not be differentiable across object boundaries, but will be differentiable along smooth objects.

It is evident that the scheme is not symmetric in the images. This is due to the change in local metric by the non-linear displacement field. This makes the ordering of the two images important. It is, however, not obvious (to us) that the steady states will differ.

The geometry-constrained diffusion can be implemented simply by applying an numerical scheme for solving a space and time discretized version of the diffusion. It is well known that the diffusion equation is solved by Gaussian convolution. That is, an unconstrained diffusion can be updated an arbitrarily long time-step, by applying a Gaussian of appropriate size. The geometry-constrained diffusion cannot be solved directly in this manner due to the constrains. In general, the finite time step diffusion (Gaussian convolution) makes the displaced source surface diverge from the target surface, so that it must be back-projected to the target surface. The back-projection may be performed to the closest point on the target surface (see Fig. 1). In this way, the algorithm resembles the iterative closest point algorithm [2, 10] for rigid registrations.

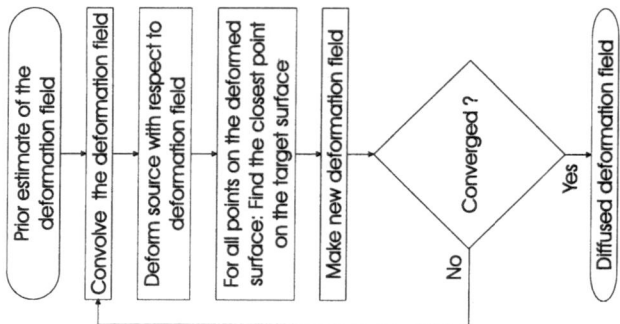

Fig. 2. *Flow diagram for the diffusion algorithm. See section 4 for details.*

4   Implementation

A time and space discretized solution the the geometry-constrained diffusion may be obtained by iterative Gaussian convolution and back-projecting the constrained surfaces.

The crux of the algorithm then becomes (see Fig. 2 for a flow chart):

1. **Initial displacement.** Construct an initial guess of the displacement field.
2. **Diffusion step.** Convolve the displacement field with a Gaussian kernel.
3. **Deform source.** Deform the source surface with respect to the displacement field.
4. **Matching (Projection onto the target surface).** For all points on the deformed surface: Find the closest point on the target surface.
5. **Update displacement field.** For all points on the deformed surface: Change the displacements according to the match.
6. **Convergence.** Is the displacement field stable? If not, go to 2.

Some of the steps are explained in greater detail below.

4.1   Diffusion step

We use the normalized Gaussian convolution [7]. For each of the Cartesian components of the displacement field, a Gaussian weighted average is constructed and divided with the sum of the weights. The standard deviation of the Gaussian σ is the only parameter in the numerical scheme (see section 4.4).

4.2   Matching

As in [10] we use a 3D-tree for finding the closest point on the target surface. As reference points on the triangulated target surface we use the center of mass (CM point) for each triangle. The three corners of the triangles are used for calculating a plane. Using also the surface normals, we construct the following

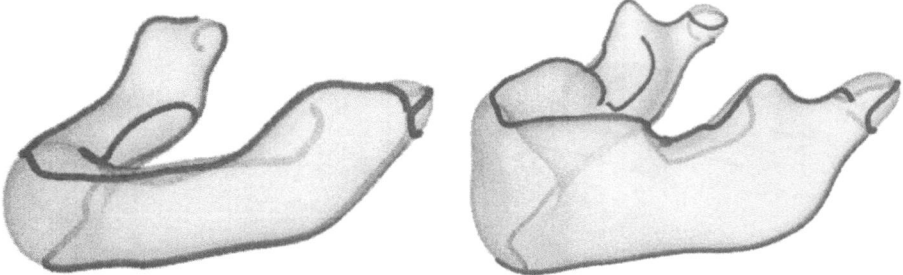

Fig. 3. *Iso-surface and crest-lines for a 3 (left) and 56 (right) month old mandible. The mandibles are Gaussian smoothed ($\sigma = 3mm$) in order to capture the higher scale features. The dimensions of the left and right mandibles are ($H \times W \times L$) $18 \times 57 \times 53mm$ and $31 \times 79 \times 79mm$, respectively. Surfaces are translucent.*

algorithm for finding the closest point: First, find the closest CM point using the Kd-tree. Secondly, calculate the closest point on the surface as the intersection of the corresponding triangle-plane and the line given by the deformed point and the normal at the CM point.

4.3   Convergence

The diffusion is stopped when

$$\sum_{p_i} \|D_n(p_i) - D_{n-1}(p_i)\|^2 < \epsilon, \tag{1}$$

where p_i is the points on the source surface, D_n is the displacement in the nth-iteration, and ϵ is a user-chosen parameter. Alternatively, a fixed number of iterations could be chosen. 5-10 iterations is normally enough.

4.4   Choice of Time Step σ

The Gaussian kernel size, σ, is the only parameter in the diffusion algorithm. It determines the time discretization step. A too large value of σ, may tear apart the surface since we diffuse too far before back-projecting. This problem occurs in regions of high surface curvature. A too small value of σ also gives problems since we have chosen a fast but imprecise back-projection algorithm. The error in the back-projection introduces some artificial "bumps" in the path along which we diffuse. This may be overcome by a more precise back-projection algorithm or in practice by choosing σ sufficiently large (see Fig. 4-6). Identical solution are obtained for an interval of σ's.

  In practice, we choose a small σ and increase it on the fly if folds persist.

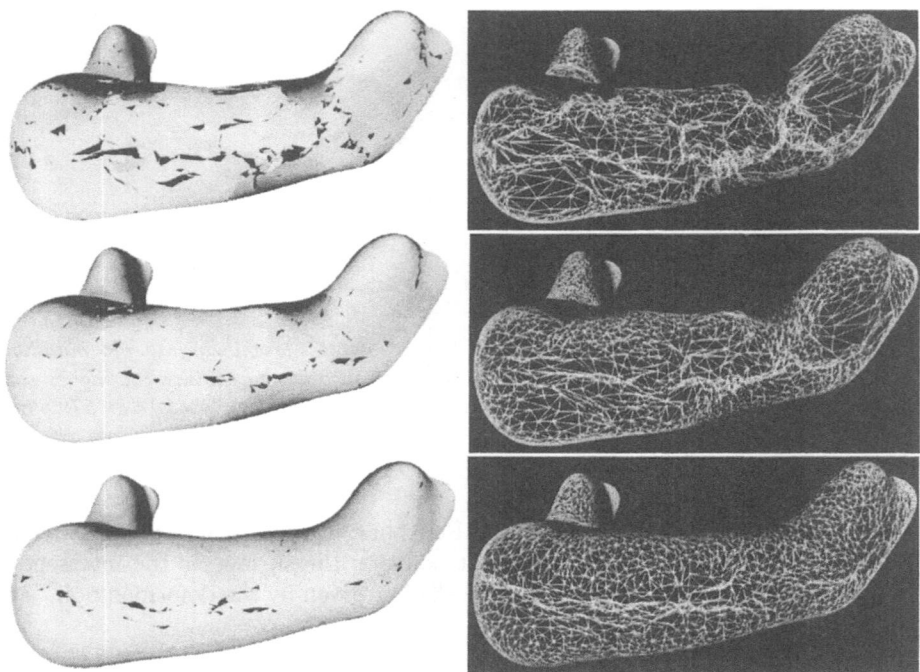

Fig. 4. *Result of running the diffusion algorithm ($\sigma = 2mm$) on the displacement field. Deformation of the 56 month old mandible to the 3 month old mandible (see Fig. 3). The surface and wire-frame of the deformed surface are shown to the left and right respectively. The initial displacement, one iteration with the diffusion algorithm, and the last iteration are shown from top to bottom, respectively. The foldings are a result of the imperfect initial registration (extremal-mesh registration extended to the whole surface by Gaussian regularization as in [1]). The final result is almost perfect, but some folds still exist, owing to the discretization of the surface and displacement field.*

5   Results

The method has been applied for registration of 31 mandibles from 6 different patient in a longitudinal growth study of the mandible. One mandible is chosen as the reference mandible. In order to propagate the landmarks, all mandibles are registered with the reference mandible and geometry-constrained diffusion is applied. The reference mandible is shown in Fig. 3-right. Fig. 3-left displays the target surface for all the subsequent figures, except for Fig. 6, which shows an example where the diffusion algorithm gives an erroneous result. The prior estimate of the displacement field is obtained by crest-line matching [1]. See Fig 7 for match between two sets of crest-lines.

As seen in Fig. 4 (top images) the initial deformation contains folds. Applying the diffusion algorithm removes almost all the folds, but some persist. By increasing σ (see section 4.4), these are removed (Fig. 5). As seen in Fig. 6, too large a value of σ will eventually tear apart the surface.

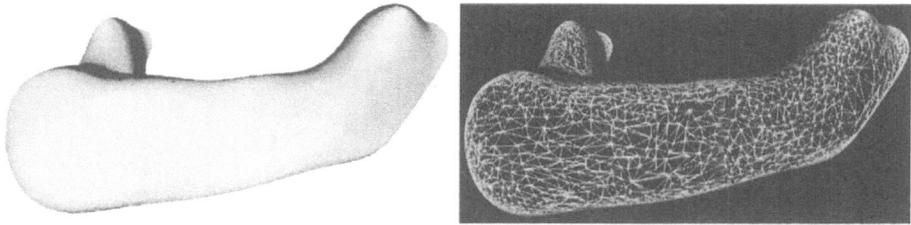

Fig. 5. *Converged diffusion algorithm with a high value of σ (σ = 10mm). The surface and wire-frame of the deformed surface are shown to the left and right respectively. We have forced the displacement field to be more smooth, by increasing σ.*

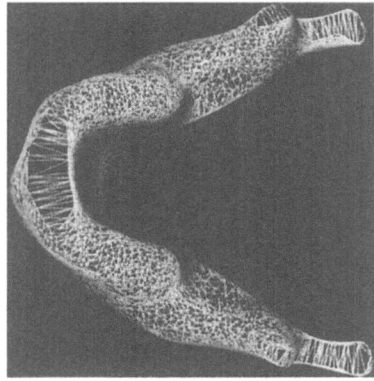

Fig. 6. *The deformation vectors are moved too far away from the surface (The value of σ is too high) resulting in a wrong projection back onto the surface.*

Very convincingly, Fig. 8 shows that the crest-lines are useful anatomical landmarks but only in areas where their topology stays fixed. Teeth eruption changes the crest-line topology of the mandible. We see two lines before teeth eruption on top of the mandible (Fig. 3 - left image) but only one after teeth eruption (Fig. 3 - right image). A pure (crest-) line matching algorithm is not able to handle such changes. Introducing the diffusion algorithm, the single crest-line (the green line on top of the mandible in Fig. 8) is able to perform correctly - i.e., be registered in between the two other lines (the two red lines on top of the mandible in the same figure) as seen in Fig. 8-right.

The same phenomenon is seen on the bottom of the mandible. A single line on the young mandible is split in two on the older mandible.

6   Conclusion

In the present paper we have proposed an algorithm for finding the simplest displacement field, which is conjectured to be a homeomorphism (1-1 continuous mapping).

The geometry-constrained diffusion in this paper serves to simplify the non-rigid registration of surface models. The result is a much smoother displacement

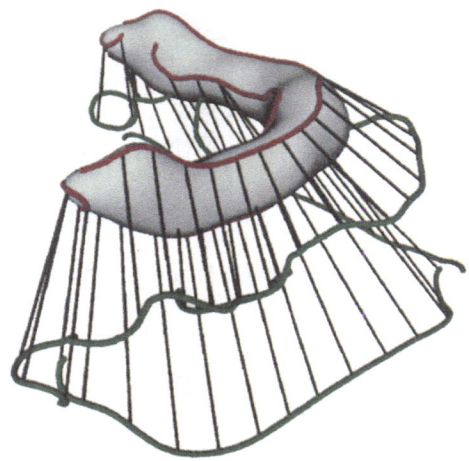

Fig. 7. *Match (lines in black) between the two sets of crest-lines (before applying the diffusion algorithm). The crest-lines in red and green are from the mandibles shown in Fig. 3. Only every 11th link is shown for visual clarity. We see that the matches to a very good extent connect homologous points.*

field. Volume registration is achieved by having more than one surface. It turns out that the algorithm itself is also very simple.

In theory, the method is parameter free, but implementations include parameters of space- and time-discretization and convergence threshold.

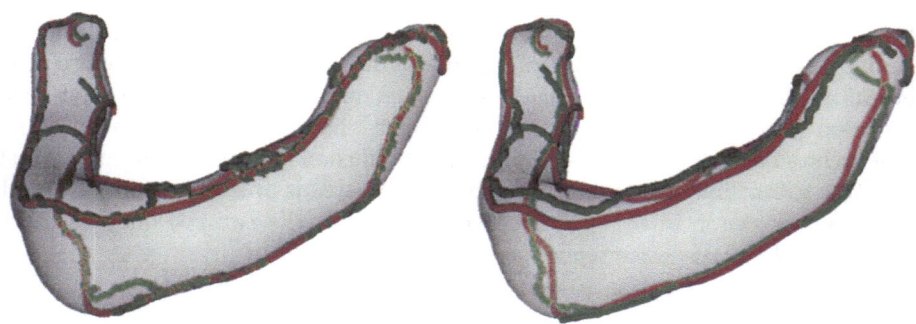

Fig. 8. *Left and right images show the deformed (in green) and the original (in red) crest-lines before and after applying the diffusion algorithm ($\sigma = 2mm$), respectively. In the initial registration crest-lines are registered with crest-lines. Where the topology does not change and away from umbilic points we see (almost) no movement of the green crest-lines. Teeth eruption changes the topology on "top of the surface" (see Fig. 3) therefore the green crest-lines move.*

We are currently using the method for registering a longitudinal growth study of the mandible in order to extract more than 14000 homologous points which again are used for inference of the growth. In that study, applying the geometry-constrained diffusion results in a very significant increase in the explained variance by the growth model.

7 Acknowledgments

The work was supported by the Danish Technical Research Council, grant number 9600452 to Per Rønsholt Andresen. The authors also thank Sven Kreiborg (School of Dentistry, University of Copenhagen, Denmark) and Jeffrey L. Marsh (Plastic and Reconstructive Department for Pediatric Plastic Surgery, Washington University School of Medicine at St. Louis Children's Hospital, St. Louis, Missouri, USA) for the CT data. Also thanks to Bjarne K. Ersbøll (Technical University of Denmark) and Andy Dobrzeniecki (3D-Lab, Denmark) for comments on the manuscript. The Visualization Toolkit (http://www.kitware.com) was used for the visualizations.

References

1. P. R. Andresen, M. Nielsen, and S. Kreiborg. 4D shape-preserving modelling of bone growth. In W. M. Wells, A. Colchester, and S. Delp, editors, *Medical Image Computing and Computer-Assisted Intervention (MICCAI'98)*, volume 1496 of *Lecture Notes in Computer Science*, pages 710–719, Cambridge, MA,USA, 1998. Springer. Electronic version: http://www.imm.dtu.dk/~pra.
2. P. J. Besl and N. D. McKay. A method for registration of 3-D shapes. *IEEE Transactions on Pattern Analysis and Machine Intelligence*, 14(2):239 – 255, 1992.
3. F. L. Bookstein. Landmark methods for forms without landmarks: localizing group differences in outline shape. In *Proceedings of the IEEE Workshop on Mathematical Methods in Biomedical Image Analysis*, pages 279–89, 1996.
4. F. L. Bookstein. Shape and the information in medical images: A decade of the morphometric synthesis. *Computer Vision and Image Understanding*, 66(2):97–118, 1997.
5. J. Feldmar and N. Ayache. Rigid, affine and locally affine registration of free-form surfaces. *International Journal of Computer Vision*, 18(2):99–119, 1996.
6. H. Lester and S. R. Arridge. A survey of hierarchical non-linear medical image registration. *Pattern Recognition*, 32:129–149, 1999.
7. M. Nielsen and P. R. Andresen. Feature displacement interpolation. In *IEEE 1998 International Conference on Image Processing (ICIP'98)*, pages 208–12, 1998. Electronic version: http://www.imm.dtu.dk/~pra.
8. P. J. Olver, G. Sapiro, and A. Tannenbaum. Invariant geometric evolutions of surfaces and volumetric smoothing. *SIAM Journal on Applied Mathematics*, 57(1):176–194, 1997.
9. J.-P. Thirion. The extremal mesh and the understanding of 3D surfaces. *International Journal of Computer Vision*, 19(2):115–128, 1996.
10. Z. Zhang. Iterative point matching for registration of free-form curves and surfaces. *International Journal of Computer Vision*, 13(2):147–176, 1994.

Wavelet Compression of Active Appearance Models

C. B. H. Wolstenholme and C. J. Taylor

Division of Imaging Science and Biomedical Engineering,
University of Manchester,
Manchester M13 9PT, U.K.
cbw@sv1.smb.man.ac.uk
http://www.isbe.man.ac.uk

Abstract. Active Appearance Models (AAMs) provide a method of modelling the appearance of anatomical structures in medical images and locating them automatically. Although the AAM approach is computationally efficient, the models used to search unseen images for the structures of interest are large - typically the size of 100 images. This is perfectly practical for most 2-D images, but is currently impractical for 3-D images. We present a method for compressing the model information using a wavelet transform. The transform is applied to a set of training images in a shape-normalised frame, and coefficients of low variance across the training set are removed to reduce the information stored. An AAM is built from the training set using the wavelet coefficients rather than the raw intensities. We show that reliable image interpretation results can be obtained at a compression ratio of 20:1, which is sufficient to make 3-D AAMs a practical proposition.

1 Introduction

Model-based interpretation of medical images provides an effective method of using prior knowledge of a class of images to achieve robust segmentation and anatomical labelling. We have recently described Active Appearance Models (AAMs) which provide a generic approach to modelling the shapes and grey-level appearance of the structures of interest in a class of images and for locating them automatically by matching the models to unseen images [1]. So far we have only described 2-D applications of AAMs [2, 3]. In principle AAMs could be straightforwardly extended to 3-D. However, although the approach is computationally efficient, the models are large - typically the size of 100 images. This is perfectly practical for most 2-D images, but is currently impractical for 3-D images.

Wavelet transforms provide a useful approach to image compression [4–6]. By transforming an image, they enable relatively high compressions with very little degradation to the original image. In medical images all information is potentially important, and the near lossless nature of wavelet compression lends itself well to medical image compression [7].

By combining the image search effectiveness of the AAM with the compression capabilities of wavelets, we hope to develop a 3D image search algorithm which is both efficient and robust.

2 Active Appearance Models

In this section we provide a brief outline of the standard AAM approach, and describe two models used to evaluate our new approach. For a more comprehensive description of the AAM algorithm, see [1].

2.1 Modelling Image Appearance

Active Appearance Models are generated using a statistical analysis of the shape and texture variation over a training set of images. Rather than model the complete image, a region of interest is first labelled using a set of landmark points that describe the shape of the labelled objects in each image. Each example in the training set is labelled with the same number of points marking out the same structures. After alignment with the mean shape, the coordinates of the landmark points are concatenated to form the shape vector $\mathbf{x}$ Figure 1 shows two examples of images labelled with landmark points.

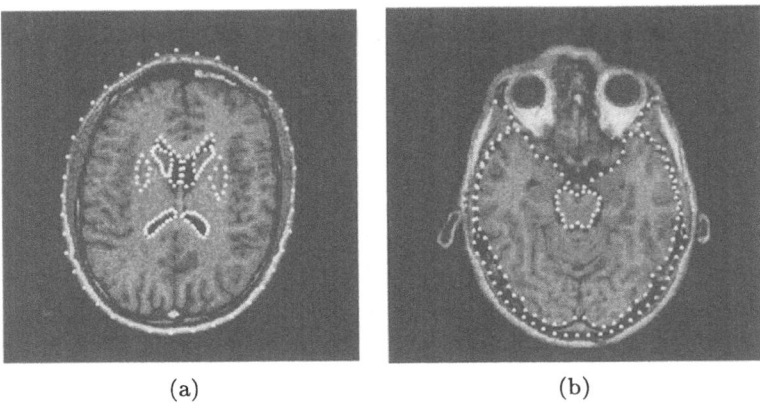

(a)   (b)

Fig. 1. Two examples of an MR brain slice labelled with landmark points. One around the ventricles, the caudate nucleus, the lentiform nucleus, and the outside of the skull (a), and the other around the brain stem, brain hull and inside of the skull (b)

The variation in shape across the set is described by applying Principle Component Analysis (PCA) to the landmark points, resulting in a Point Distribution Model (PDM). Full details of this method can be found in [8]. Any valid example of the shape modelled can then be approximated using:

$$\mathbf{x} = \bar{\mathbf{x}} + \mathbf{P_s b_s} \tag{1}$$

where $\bar{\mathbf{x}}$ is the mean shape vector, $\mathbf{P_s}$ is a set of orthogonal modes of variation, and $\mathbf{b_s}$ is a vector of shape parameters.

To build a statistical model of the grey-level appearance we sample points within the convex hull of the landmark points. This is a somewhat arbitrary choice which is appropriate for the examples show here. A more sophisticated sampling scheme could easily be devised. The samples are warped to the mean shape using a triangulation algorithm. Thus the warped images all match the mean shape. Grey level information $\mathbf{g_{im}}$ is then sampled from this shape normalised image. By applying PCA to the normalised data, we obtain a linear model that can approximate valid examples of grey-level appearance:

$$\mathbf{g} = \bar{\mathbf{g}} + \mathbf{P_g}\mathbf{b_g} \tag{2}$$

where $\bar{\mathbf{g}}$ is the mean normalised grey-level vector, $\mathbf{P_g}$ is a set of orthogonal modes of intensity variation, and $\mathbf{b_g}$ is a set of grey-level parameters.

By varying the vectors $\mathbf{b_s}$ and $\mathbf{b_g}$, the shape and grey-level of any example can be approximated. There may exist some correlation in the variances of shape and grey-level, so a further PCA can be applied to the data, concatenating the vectors, and obtaining a model of the form:

$$\begin{pmatrix} \mathbf{W_s}\mathbf{b_s} \\ \mathbf{b_g} \end{pmatrix} = \mathbf{b} = \begin{pmatrix} \mathbf{Q_s} \\ \mathbf{Q_g} \end{pmatrix} \mathbf{c} = \mathbf{Q}\mathbf{c} \tag{3}$$

where $\mathbf{W_s}$ is a diagonal matrix of weights for each shape parameter, correcting for the difference in units between the shape and grey-level models, $\mathbf{Q}$ is a set of orthogonal modes of appearance variation, and $\mathbf{c}$ is a vector of appearance parameters.

The linearity of the resulting model enables us to express shape and grey-levels as functions of $\mathbf{c}$

$$\mathbf{x} = \bar{\mathbf{x}} + \mathbf{P_s}\mathbf{W_s}\mathbf{Q_s}\mathbf{c} , \quad \mathbf{g} = \bar{\mathbf{g}} + \mathbf{P_g}\mathbf{Q_g}\mathbf{c} \tag{4}$$

where

$$\mathbf{Q} = \begin{pmatrix} \mathbf{Q_s} \\ \mathbf{Q_g} \end{pmatrix} \tag{5}$$

A synthetic image can be generated for a given $\mathbf{c}$ by first generating the shape-free grey-level image, $\mathbf{g}$, and warping it to match the known control points described by $\mathbf{x}$.

2.2   Appearance Models of the Brain

Two sets of images were labelled with landmarks to make up the training sets for two appearance models. Both used slices from T1 weighted MR images of the brain. The training set for the ventricle model ((a) in Figure 1) contained 36 labelled images each with 163 landmark points, and the brain stem model ((b) in Figure 1) contained 42 images in its training set, each with 145 landmark points.

The effect of varying parameters in the vector $\mathbf{c}$ in each model is shown in Figure 2, where the first two parameters, c_1 and c_2, are varied by ± 2 standard deviations.

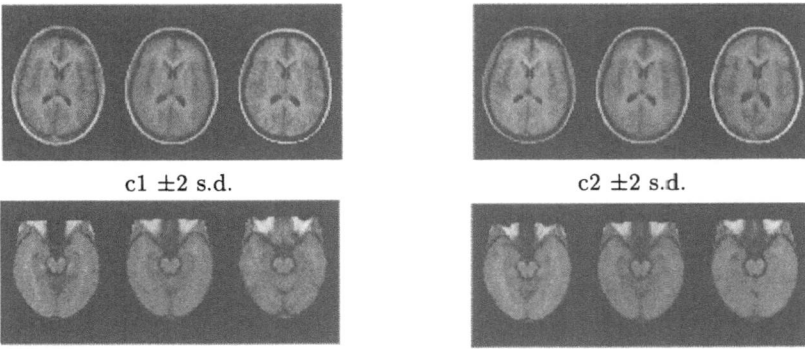

c1 ±2 s.d.   c2 ±2 s.d.

Fig. 2. The first two modes of appearance variation in the two models

2.3   Image Search

To complete the tests on the normal model, we built an AAM using both models, and tested them in a model search.

The AAM search algorithm tries to minimise the difference in the model frame between a sample, $\mathbf{g_s}$, from an image being searched, and a synthesised image, $\mathbf{g_m}$, by varying the appearance model parameters $\mathbf{c}$ which, for notational simplicity, is taken to include parameters for position, orientation and scale. This difference is given by:

$$\delta\mathbf{g} = \mathbf{g_s} - \mathbf{g_m} \qquad (6)$$

Remember the $\mathbf{c}$ parameter also vary the shape, which affects the way the sampled image $\mathbf{g_s}$ is acquired. A linear relationship between $\delta\mathbf{g}$ and $\delta\mathbf{c}$, the change in $\mathbf{c}$ required to minimise $|\delta\mathbf{g}|$, is learnt during a second training phase:

$$\delta\mathbf{c} = \mathbf{A}\delta\mathbf{g} \qquad (7)$$

The matrix $\mathbf{A}$ is obtained by applying linear regression using random displacements, $\delta\mathbf{c}$, from an image generated using the mean shape, pose and contrast. Equation (7) can then be used in an iterative matching algorithm by measuring the difference, δg, between an image generated by the current model parameters and predicting the change, $\delta\mathbf{c}$, required to minimise $|\delta g|$. Full details of this can be found in [1].

Figure 3 shows results of AAM image search in each of the models described above. Quantitative results are given in Section 3.4.

3   Compressing the Model's Least Variant Features

3.1   Wavelets

Wavelet analysis can be carried out using the Fast Wavelet Transform (FWT) algorithm developed by Stéphane Mallat [9]. This involves the decompositions

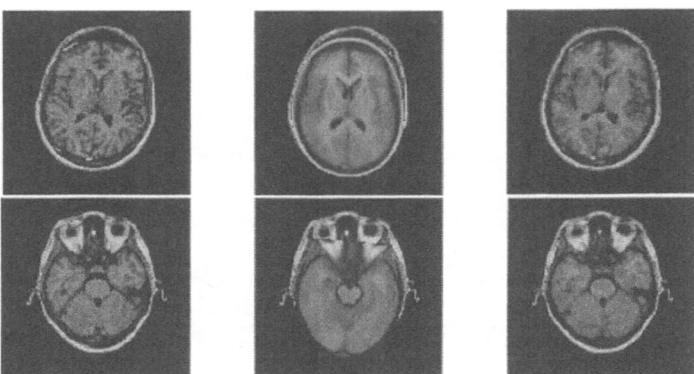

Fig. 3. Search results for the two brain models, showing the original image, the start position of the model, and the search result

of a signal by passing it through high-pass and low-pass filters. The wavelet coefficients are generated using a convolution of the high-pass and low-pass filters with the signal in turn. The low-pass filter gives rise to the *approximation* and the high pass filter gives rise to the *details*. The approximations, therefore, represent the low frequencies within the signal, which approximate the original signal, and the details represent the minor corrections to the approximation for the accurate reconstruction of the signal. As the signal is being passed through two filters, the result would be data of double the length of the original. Therefore, a further step is necessary. This step, *downsampling*, reduces the data by removing the coefficients at every second location.

In 2D signals, details are required in multiple directions - one horizontal, one vertical, and one diagonal. This is implemented using an extra bank of filters through the second dimension. Figure 4 shows this algorithm diagrammatically. To reconstruct the signal from the wavelet coefficients we need to reverse the process and replace the decomposition filters with reconstruction filters. Upsampling also replaces the downsampling in the diagram, so that zeros are inserted at every second position.

In the standard FWT, the filtering process can be applied to the approximation resulting from a previous pass, creating a multi-level tree. Further decomposition can be achieved using wavelet packet analysis. This is similar to the method described above, except that it not only decomposes the approximations at each level, but it also decomposes the details at each level, leading to a binary (one-dimesional decomposition) or quad- (two-dimensional decomposition) tree (Figure 5). As the details are the higher frequencies, which only add minor information to a signal or an image, then changing the values of small details has little effect on the reconstructed image. This is the basis of the wavelet compression. In standard wavelet compression, a threshold is set, and if a detail coefficient falls below that threshold, it is zeroed. The zeroed values can then be removed to reduce the data, provided a scheme for their replacement is devised.

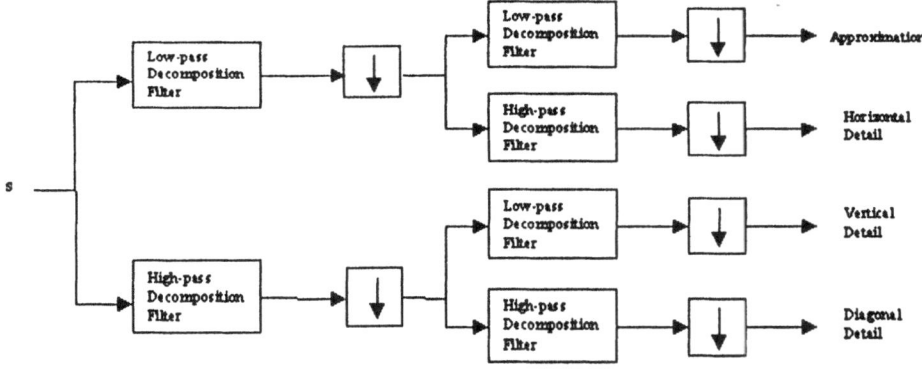

Fig. 4. 2D wavelet decomposition. The rows of the signal, s, are passed through high- and low-pass filters, then downsampled. The resulting columns of the signal are then passed through further filters to give the approximation and three sets of details.

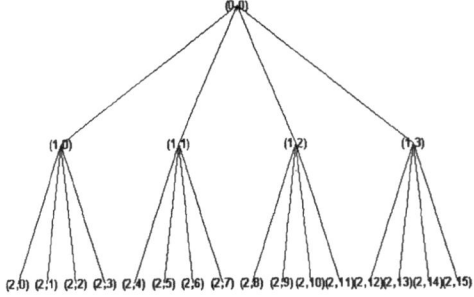

Fig. 5. A wavelet tree to two levels. Each node holds a set of coefficients giving a detail or approximation of the previous level

3.2 Compression Over an Image Set

When building an appearance model, a training set of images is used, each marked with the landmark points. After the shape model has been trained using the landmarks, the grey-level texture model is built. This is done by taking a convex hull around the landmarks, sampling from the training image, and warping the sampled data to the mean shape. This puts the grey-level samples in a shape free frame, as shown in Figure 6. In this shape free frame all the images are similar, so this is an ideal place to compress the images, since a standardised vector can be held for all the images detailing the decompression information. In the case of standard wavelet compression, zeroed coefficients that match throughout the image set, after the threshold is applied, can be zeroed. A vector containing the positions of the zero columns could be stored, and the zeros replaced at reconstruction time. The main problem with this method is

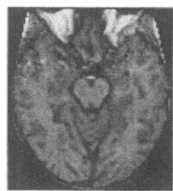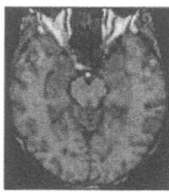

Fig. 6. The shape free samples taken from the first and second images in the brain stem model's image set

that the zeroed coefficients throughout the set rarely fall into line, giving only low rates of compression.

A better scheme, giving much higher rates of compression, is to remove the coefficients that show the least variance throughout the image set. Rather than zero these coefficients, they can be set to their mean to preserve any non-zero, but invariant values. A vector is then held which contains the means of all the positions that have been removed. This vector can be used during reconstruction to replace the mean values. The resulting vector can be passed through the wavelet reconstruction to recover the shape free image, with minimised loss of quality.

This method differs from the standard wavelet compression method in that compression can be applied to the approximation as well as the detail without much degradation of the images. This is possible as the coefficients are being set to the mean rather than being zeroed. The wavelet decomposition is still important to the method as most of the change is still in the detail coefficients. This is due to the fact that in the 2D analysis, the details outweigh the approximations by 3:1 at the first level of the analysis, and this increases at the lower levels. We use three levels of decomposition.

The Appearance Models can be trained on the sets of compressed wavelet coefficients instead of the original image information.

3.3 Improving the AAM Search with Wavelets

A multiresolution version of the AAM algorithm outlined in Section 2 has been described previously and shown to improve both speed and robustness [10]. The method requires extra training of the Appearance Model at each resolution at which the search is to be carried out. As the aim of the wavelet tranform is to compress the Appearance Model, the standard multiresolution algorithm could not be applied. One property of the wavelet decomposition, however, is the downsampling and repeated decomposition of the approximations. These approximations lie in the left hand nodes of the wavelet tree (Figure 5), such that node **n,0** is the approximation at level **n**. The images at these nodes can be reconstructed, and represent a multi-level decomposition of the approximations as shown in Figure 7

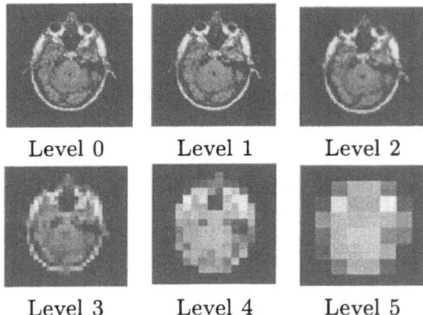

Level 0   Level 1   Level 2

Level 3   Level 4   Level 5

Fig. 7. Images recovered from the different levels of approximations in the wavelet tree, showing their multiresolution property

As the model is decomposed to three levels, then we can reconstruct at each level to represent that resolution of the model. Figure 8 shows the Appearance Model representation at four resolutions (level 0 being that of the normal Appearance Model). The AAM can also be trained using the multi-level model. The mean model is reconstructed at each level, and random model displacements are reconstructed at the same level to train a regression matrix at that level. This is repeated at each level in the tree. In image search, a wavelet transform identical to that of the model is applied to the image to be searched, and its approximations are reconstructed at each level in turn. The model then searches at each level from the lowest resolution to the highest, with the result of each level used as the starting displacement for the next.

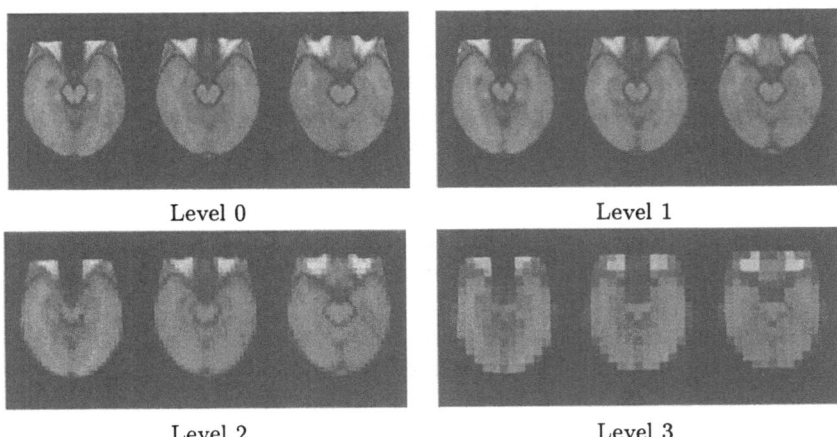

Level 0   Level 1

Level 2   Level 3

Fig. 8. The appearance model reconstructed at the different levels of approximations

3.4   Compressed Appearance Models of the Brain

Compressed appearance models were built using the sets of training images
labelled as shown in Figure 1 , and three levels of Haar wavelet decomposition,
The models were tested at 75%, 90% and 95% compression, giving compression
ratios of 4:1, 10:1 and 20:1 respectively. The first mode of appearance variation
resulting from the brain stem models is shown in Figure 9 together with the
uncompressed model.

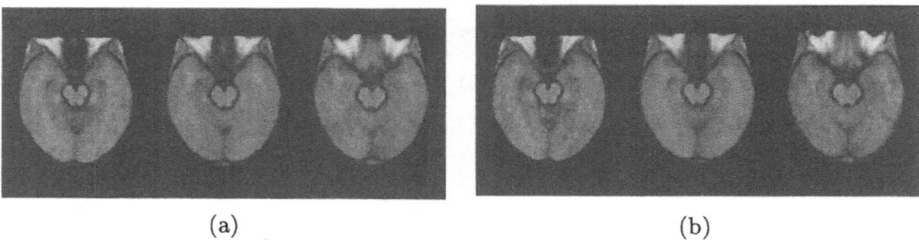

(a)   (b)

Fig. 9. The first mode of variation of the model of the brain stem compressed to 20:1
(a) compared to the normal model (b)

Since the models built using wavelet coefficients could still represent the appearance of the images, and could be reconstructed with reasonable accuracy,
AAMs of the models were built to test the compressed model's ability in image
search. Only the models at 10:1 and 20:1 compression were used for this experiment. 'Leave-all-in' and 'leave-one-out' tests were used to give estimated
upper and lower bands on search accuracy. Figure 10 shows an example result
from the tests using the 20:1 compressed model using the multilevel search, and
Table 1 shows the mean point to point errors between the search results and
the original training landmarks for the compressed and non-compressed models. All the models tested gave similar results in the leave-all-in tests, showing
that the compression had little effect on the AAMs search capabilities on previously seen image. In the leave-one-out tests, however, while the non-compressed
and compressed models using the standard search again gave similar results, the
multilevel search greatly improved the model's results. The non-compressed and
20:1 compressed models gave mean errors of 16.33 and 16.89 pixels respectively
at their worst (and these failed to locate the brain), while the multilevel model
at 20:1 compression resulted in a worst mean error of only 6.35 pixels, which
located the brain. The best mean error for the multilevel model in the leave-one-
out tests was also better at 1.72 pixels compared to the non-compressed (1.90
pixels) and 20:1 compressed (1.94 pixels) models.

4   Discussion and Conclusions

We have demonstrated a method for compressing the amount of data required
to describe an Appearance Model, while still retaining the necessary information

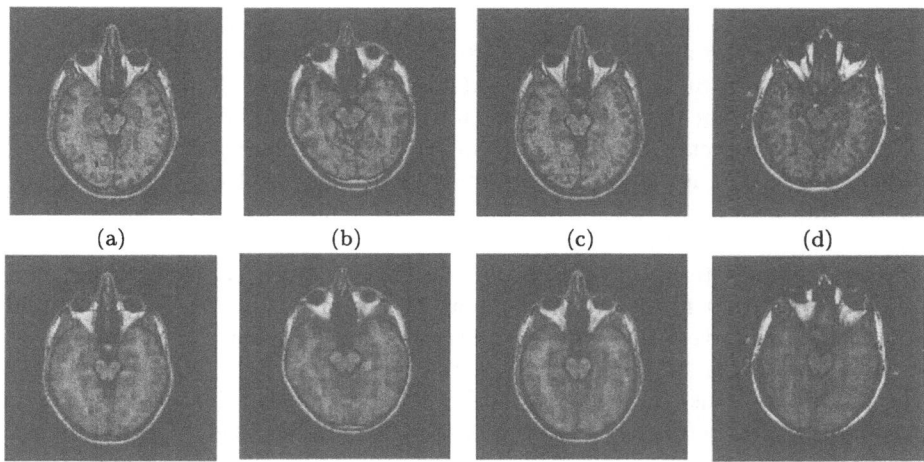

| | (a) | (b) | (c) | (d) |

Fig. 10. The search results of the 20:1 compressed brain stem model from 'leave-all-in' (best (a) and worst (b)) and the 'leave-one-out' (best (c) and worst (d)) tests using the multilevel search. The top row are the original images, and the bottom are the search results

Compression	Leave-all-in			Leave-one-out		
	% Successful	% Failure	P to P	% Successful	% Failure	P to P
None	100	0	3.03	92.86	7.14	4.47
20:1	100	0	3.11	90.48	9.52	4.78
Multi-res 20:1	100	0	3.25	100	0	3.89

Table 1. Search results from the leave-all-in and leave-one-out tests. The mean Point to Point error is measured between landmarks resulting from the reconstructed shape after search to the original landmarks in pixels.

for using the model successfully in the AAM search algorithm. The method uses wavelets to place the shape-free images used by the appearance model into a frame where compression can be carried out with minimal degradation to the images. The compression is achieved by removing the coefficients that vary least throughout the training set within the wavelet space. We have shown that the model is still effective when used as an Active Appearance Model in image search. The level of compression achieved (20:1) is sufficient to reduce a model, which uncompressed would be around 6 gigabytes, into a size manageable within the memory of a desktop computer.

The model loses detail as the compression increases, but it still searches accurately, and once the object is located in an image, the more detailed information can be retrieved directly from the image.

As the model building process is linear, a compression scheme using a linear transform has the advantage that the final model is equivalent to that which would have been built from the raw data. Wavelets provide one such scheme. Wavelets also have the advantage over more traditional compression methods such as the Discrete Cosine Transform (DCT) of avoiding blocking effects. A further advantage is the image-like property of the wavelet coefficients, which allows the use of the multi-level transform as a basis for the multi-resolution appearance model without the need for extra training.

It is a small step from our current results to accurately locating brains in 2D, a process that may be used to bootstrap some existing 3D brain stripping algorithms. However, the reason for studying compression is to enable us to extend the AAMs to 3D. If AAM search can be used for 3D MR images of the brain, then this could prove an effective, fully automatic method for brain stripping and structure segmentation, as well as proving useful in solving other medical imaging location and segmentation problems.

References

1. T F Cootes, G J Edwards, and C J Taylor. Active appearance models. In *Proceedings of the European Conference on Computer Vision*, volume 2, pages 484–498. Springer, 1998.
2. G J Edwards, C J Taylor, and T F Cootes. Learning to identify and track faces in image sequences. In *8th British Machine Vision Conference*, pages 130–139. BMVA Press, 1997.
3. T F Cootes, C Beeston, G J Edwards, and C J Taylor. A unified framework for atlas matching using active appearance models. In *Accepted for IPMI 1999*, 1999.
4. G Strang and T Nguyen. *Wavelets and Filter Banks*. Wellesley - Cambridge Press, Wellesley, 1997.
5. C K Chui. *Wavelet Analysis and Its Applications*. Academic Press, London, 1992.
6. I Daubechies. *Ten Lectures on Wavelets*. CBNS-NSF regional conference series in applied mathematics, Philadelphia, 1992.
7. A Zandi, J Allen, E Schwartz, and M Boliek. Crew: Compression with reversible embedded wavelets. In *IEEE Data Compression Conference*, pages 212–221, 1995.
8. T F Cootes, C J Taylor, D H Cooper, and J Graham. Image search using trained flexible shape models. *Advances in Applied Statistics*, pages 111–139, 1994.
9. S Mallat. A theory for multiresolution signal decomposition: the wavelet representation. *IEEE Pattern Analysis and Machine Intelligence*, 11:674–693, 1989.
10. T F Cootes, G J Edwards, and C J Taylor. A comparative evaluation of active appearance model algorithms. In *Proceedings of the British Machine Vision Conference*, volume 2, pages 680–689. BMVA Press, 1998.

Towards a Better Comprehension of Similarity Measures Used in Medical Image Registration

Alexis Roche, Grégoire Malandain, Nicholas Ayache, and Sylvain Prima

INRIA Sophia Antipolis - Epidaure Project
2004 Route des Lucioles BP 93
06902 Sophia Antipolis Cedex, France
{aroche,greg,na,sprima}@sophia.inria.fr

Abstract. While intensity-based similarity measures are increasingly used for medical image registration, they often rely on implicit assumptions regarding the physics of imaging. The motivation of this paper is to determine what are the assumptions corresponding to a number of popular similarity measures in order to better understand their use, and finally help choosing the one which is the most appropriate for a given class of problems. After formalizing registration based on general image acquisition models, we show that the search for an optimal measure can be cast into a maximum likelihood estimation problem. We then derive similarity measures corresponding to different modeling assumptions and retrieve some well-known measures (correlation coefficient, correlation ratio, mutual information). Finally, we present results of registration between 3D MR and 3D Ultrasound images to illustrate the importance of choosing an appropriate similarity measure.

1 Introduction

Over the last years, intensity-based (or iconic) techniques have been applied to a number of registration problems including monomodal as well as multimodal, and rigid as well as non-rigid registration [8]. Their basic principle is to maximize a criterion measuring the intensity similarity of corresponding voxels. Common to the many proposed similarity measures is the idea that, when matched, the images should verify a certain relationship; the similarity measure is intended to quantify how well this relationship is verified depending on the considered transformation between the images.

Choosing one measure adapted to a specific registration problem is not always straightforward for at least two reasons. First, it is often difficult to model the physical relationship that exists between two images. Second, most of the similarity measures rely on imaging assumptions that are not fully explicit. Existing similarity measures may be classified into four main kinds of hypotheses:

Identity relationship. The basic assumption is that when matched the images are identical. This includes a number of popular measures: the sum of squared intensity differences (SSD), the sum of absolute intensity differences, cross-correlation

[3], entropy of the difference image [4],... Although these measures are not equivalent in terms of robustness and accuracy, none of them is able to cope with relative intensity changes from one image to the other.

Affine relationship. The step beyond is to assume that the two images I and J to be registered are related by an affine mapping, i.e. $I \approx \alpha J + \beta$. The measures adapted to this situation are more or less variants from the correlation coefficient [3], defined as the ratio between the images' covariance and the product of individual standard deviations:

$$\rho(I, J) = \frac{\mathrm{Cov}(I, J)}{\sqrt{\mathrm{Var}(I)}\sqrt{\mathrm{Var}(J)}}. \tag{1}$$

The correlation coefficient is generally useful for matching images from the same modality. Nevertheless, the affine hypothesis is hardly valid for images from different modalities, and thus it has not provided convincing results in multimodal registration.

Functional relationship. For multimodal images, more complex relationships are involved. The approach we proposed in [15] was to assume that, at the registration position, one image could be approximated in terms of the other by applying some intensity function, $I \approx f(J)$. Making no assumption regarding the nature of the function, we derived a natural statistical measure, the correlation ratio:

$$\eta^2(I|J) = 1 - \frac{\mathrm{Var}(I - \hat{f}(J))}{\mathrm{Var}(I)}, \tag{2}$$

where $\hat{f}(J)$ is the least square optimal non-linear approximation of I in terms of J [11]. The correlation ratio is closely related to a very popular measure previously proposed by Woods et al.[23], and generalized using robust metrics in [10].

Statistical relationship. Finally, assuming a functional relationship is sometimes too restrictive. Then, it is more appropriate to use information theoretic measures, from which mutual information [7, 20] is today probably the most popular:

$$\mathcal{I}(I, J) = \sum_i \sum_j \log \frac{p(i, j)}{p(i)\, p(j)}, \tag{3}$$

where $p(i, j)$ is the intensity joint probability distribution of the images, and $p(i)$ and $p(j)$ the corresponding marginal distributions. This category is not fundamentally different from the previous one, as the ideal case is still perfect functional dependence; mutual information is however theoretically more robust to variations with respect to this ideal situation.

A number of comparison studies have shown that similarity measures yield different performances depending on the considered modality combinations [22, 2, 13, 10, 15]. There is probably no universal measure and, for a specific problem, the point is rather to choose the one that is best adapted to the nature of the images.

Up to now, the link between explicit modeling assumptions and similarity measures has not been made clear. After some authors [9, 5] proposed that image registration could be seen as a maximum likelihood estimation problem, Viola et al. [20, 21] suggested the analogy of this approach with registration using information theory. Remarkably, other teams had motivated information-theoretic measures by other arguments [7, 17].

In section 2, we propose to formulate image registration as a general maximum likelihood estimation problem. Then, deriving optimal similarity measures from specific modeling assumptions, we retrieve the correlation ratio and mutual information in section 3. Section 4 proposes to illustrate the practical differences between these two measures with results of registration between 3D MR and 3D Ultrasound images.

2 Formulation

2.1 Maximum likelihood registration

Two images I and J to be registered are related through the common anatomical reality that they measure. But the way anatomical structures are represented depends on the physics of imaging involved in each acquisition. Thus, modeling the relationship between the images requires the knowledge of both the underlying anatomy and the image formation processes. A convenient model of the anatomy will be an image called "segmentation" or "scene": by definition, a scene is any image for which the intensity of a given voxel represents directly the tissue class it belongs to.

Assuming that we know a scene, we can model indirectly the relationship between I and J based on image acquisition models. A standard approach is to interpret an image as being a realization of a random process that corrupts the scene. This means that the relationship between I and S (resp. J and S) is defined in terms of a conditional probability density function $P(I|S)$. The two following assumptions are usually stated:

- The voxels of the image are conditionally independent knowing the scene, that is:

$$P(I|S) = \prod_{x_k \in \Omega_I} P(i_k|S),$$

  where Ω_I denotes the voxel grid of I, and $i_k \equiv I(x_k)$ is the intensity of the voxel with coordinates x_k in a given frame attached to the grid Ω_I.
- The noise is context-free. In other words, the intensity of a voxel depends only on its homologous in the scene:

$$P(i_k|S) = P(i_k|s_k^\downarrow), \quad \text{with} \quad s_k^\downarrow \equiv S(T(x_k)) = (S \circ T)(x_k),$$

  where T is the spatial transformation that relates the coordinate frames of Ω_I and Ω_S, the grid of S. In the case where I and S are not supposed to be aligned, T has no reason to be the identity.

Under these assumptions, the conditional probability of I knowing the scene, S, and the transformation, T, is easily seen to be:

$$P(I|S,T) = \prod_{x_k \in \Omega_I} P(i_k|s_k^\downarrow). \tag{4}$$

We can model the relationship between J and S in the same manner. However, as we are interested only in the relative displacement between I and J, we will consider J as a "reference" image being already aligned with the scene, meaning that no transformation is involved in the conditional probability,

$$P(J|S) = \prod_{y_l \in \Omega_J} P(j_l|s_l), \quad \text{with} \quad j_l = J(y_l), \quad s_l = S(y_l), \tag{5}$$

$\Omega_J \equiv \Omega_S$ being the voxel grid of J, which coincides with that of S. Without knowledge of the scene, the probability of the image pair (I, J) is obtained by integrating over all possible realizations of S. Assuming that the two acquisitions are independent, we have $P(I, J|S, T) = P(I|S, T)\,P(J|S)$, and thus:

$$P(I, J|T) = \int P(I|S,T)\,P(J|S)\,P(S)\,dS = P(J) \underbrace{\int P(I|S,T)\,P(S|J)\,dS}_{P(I|J,T)}, \tag{6}$$

where the last step relies on Bayes rule. The transformation T appears as a parameter of this joint probability function, and it is natural to invoke the maximum likelihood principle to formulate registration, as already proposed for instance in [20, 6, 1, 9, 5]. It simply states that the most likely transformation between I and J is the one that maximizes the joint probability of (I, J),

$$\hat{T} = \arg\max_T P(I, J|T) = \arg\max_T P(I|J,T),$$

the last equivalence holding because J is independent of T.

Evaluating the integral of (6) may be somewhat cumbersome if the prior probability on S is a complex function. For mathematical convenience, we will assume that the voxels of the scene are independently distributed, yielding the factored form: $P(S) = \prod_{y_l} P(s_l)$. Thus, no auto-correlation is assumed for the scene: this is the minimal way to introduce prior anatomical information. Notice that this does not mean that the voxels are identically distributed, such that spatial dependences may be incorporated to the model. If this modeling is still insufficient, a maximum a posteriori (MAP) estimation strategy would be employed. This alternative, using for example a Gibbs-Markov random field prior, requires an explicit estimation of the scene that is computationally very expensive in the case of 3D images.

Under these assumptions, we show in [16] that $P(I|J, T)$ is of the same factored form as $P(I|S, T)$; letting $j_k^\downarrow \equiv J(T(x_k))$, we have:

$$P(I|J,T) = \prod_{x_k \in \Omega_I} P(i_k|j_k^\downarrow), \tag{7}$$

$$\text{with} \qquad P(i_k|j_k^\downarrow) = \int P(i_k|s_k^\downarrow = s)\,P(s_k^\downarrow = s|j_k^\downarrow)\,ds. \tag{8}$$

2.2   Estimating the conditional densities

In the framework where the transformation is found by maximum likelihood, the most natural way to estimate densities is also to use a maximum likelihood strategy. This means that we can search for the conditional densities $P(i_k|j_k^\downarrow)$ that maximize exactly the same criterion as in (7). Basically, this is a parametric approach: we assume that the $P(i_k|j_k^\downarrow)$' belong to a given class of distributions parameterized by a vector θ (regardless, for the moment, of what θ represents); then their maximum likelihood estimates, for a given estimate of the transformation T, are found by:

$$\hat{\theta}(T) = \arg\max_\theta \; P(I|J,T,\theta) = \arg\max_\theta \prod_{x_k \in \Omega_I} P_\theta(i_k|j_k^\downarrow).$$

The parametric form of $P(I|J,T,\theta)$ may be derived from the modeling assumptions presented in section 2.1 whenever all the components of the model, $P(I|S,T)$, $P(J|S)$, and $P(S)$ are themselves chosen as parametric densities. Then, from (8), the form of $P(I|J,T,\theta)$ can be known. In section 3, we will show that under some specific modeling assumptions, maximum likelihood density estimates can be computed explicitly.

For practical optimization, it is more convenient to consider the negative log-likelihood (to be minimized); thus, we will define the energy of a transformation T as:

$$U(T) = -\log \max_\theta P(I|J,T,\theta) = \min_\theta \left[-\sum_{x_k \in \Omega_I} \log P_\theta(i_k|j_k^\downarrow) \right]. \qquad (9)$$

2.3   Practical issues

In section 2.1, we have derived the likelihood registration criterion under the implicit assumption that the transformation T is searched among mappings from the floating image grid, Ω_I, to the reference image grid, Ω_J. This means that a given voxel of image I is always supposed to match a node of the reference grid. Therefore, the spatial resolution of the transformation is intrinsically limited by the resolution of the reference grid, and clearly this assumption cannot deal with sub-voxel accurate registration.

In order to manipulate continuous transformations, we can oversample the reference image using interpolation techniques [7]. But this is possible only if the transformed position of a voxel falls inside the reference domain. Since this domain has a finite extension in space, other voxels may fall outside, so that there is not enough information to extrapolate the intensity of their correspondent (see figure 1). The problem of how to treat these "outside" voxels plays an important role in voxel-based image registration. They are generally ignored by the registration criterion, which necessitates some heuristic normalization to avoid nasty effects such as disconnecting the images [18, 20, 15].

We discuss in [16] that ignoring these voxels would not be consistent with the maximum likelihood framework. Instead, a natural approach is simply to extend

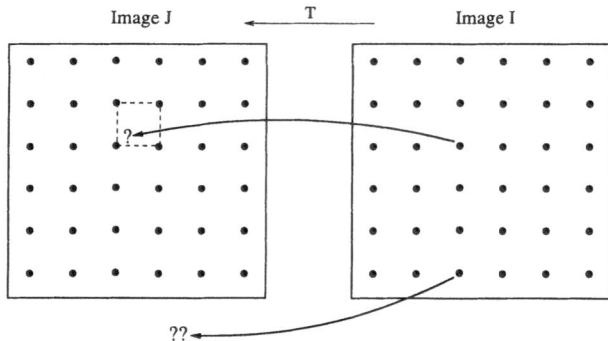

Fig. 1. Effects of applying a continuous spatial transformation. The point marked with ’?’ can be interpolated, unlike the point marked with ’??’. Instead, this latter point may be assigned an arbitrary intensity j^*.

the reference domain by assigning the external points to a constant and arbitrary intensity $J = j^*$. Although this is a computational artifice, this enables us to take into account every voxel of I at each iteration of the registration process.

3   From modeling assumptions to similarity measures

3.1   Gaussian channel

Perhaps the simplest model we can imagine is that the image J be a valid scene ($J = S$) and the image I be a measure of J corrupted with additive and stationary Gaussian white noise:

$$I(x_k) = f\left(J\left(T(x_k)\right)\right) + \epsilon_k,$$

where f is some unknown intensity function: each tissue class j is imaged in I with an average response value $f(j) = f_j$. Then, the conditional densities $P(i_k|j_k^\downarrow)$ are of the Gaussian form:

$$P(i_k = i|j_k^\downarrow = j) = \frac{1}{\sqrt{2\pi}\,\sigma}\, e^{-\frac{(i-f_j)^2}{2\sigma^2}},$$

and the parameter vector $\theta = (f_0, f_1, \ldots, \sigma)$ needs to be estimated. In order to minimize the negative log-likelihood (equation 9) with respect to θ, we group the voxels x_k that match the same class. Letting $N = \text{Card}\,\Omega_I$, $\Omega_I^j = \{x_k \in \Omega_I,\ j_k^\downarrow = j\}$, and $N_j = \text{Card}\,\Omega_I^j$, we have:

$$-\log P(I|J, T, \theta) = N \log \sqrt{2\pi}\,\sigma + \frac{1}{2} \sum_{x_k \in \Omega_I} \frac{(i_k - f(j_k^\downarrow))^2}{\sigma^2}$$

$$= N \log \sqrt{2\pi}\,\sigma + \frac{1}{2} \sum_{j} \sum_{x_k \in \Omega_I^j} \frac{(i_k - f_j)^2}{\sigma^2}. \qquad (10)$$

The optimal parameters are then easily found by differentiating the log-likelihood:

$$-\frac{\partial \log P}{\partial f_j} = -\frac{1}{\sigma^2} \sum_{\Omega_I^j} (i_k - f_j) \quad \Longrightarrow \quad \hat{f}_j = \frac{1}{N_j} \sum_{\Omega_I^j} i_k,$$

$$-\frac{\partial \log P}{\partial \sigma} = \frac{N}{\sigma} - \frac{1}{\sigma^3} \sum_j \sum_{\Omega_I^j} (i_k - f_j)^2 \quad \Longrightarrow \quad \hat{\sigma}^2 = \sum_j \frac{N_j}{N} \hat{\sigma}_j^2,$$

where $\hat{\sigma}_j^2 \equiv \frac{1}{N_j} \sum_{x_k \in \Omega_I^j} (i_k - \hat{f}_j)^2$ is the image variance corresponding to the iso-set Ω_I^j. The registration energy $U(T)$ is then obtained by substituting the optimal θ parameter:

$$U(T) = N \log \left[\sqrt{2\pi e} \sum_j \frac{N_j}{N} \hat{\sigma}_j^2 \right] = N \log \left[\sqrt{2\pi e} \operatorname{Var}(I - \hat{f}(J^\downarrow)) \right].$$

This result has a satisfying interpretation: $U(T)$ decreases with the variance of the difference image between I and the intensity corrected $\hat{f}(J)$. The intensity function $\hat{f}$ is nothing but a least-square fit of the image I in terms of the reference J: it is in fact the same fitting function as in the definition of the correlation ratio (equation 2) [15], and we see that the registration energy $U(T)$ is related to the correlation ratio $\eta^2(I|J^\downarrow)$ by:

$$\eta^2(I|J^\downarrow) = 1 - \frac{1}{k} e^{\frac{U(T)}{N}}, \qquad \text{with} \quad k = \sqrt{2\pi e} \operatorname{Var}(I).$$

In the original version of the correlation ratio [15], the quantities N and $\operatorname{Var}(I)$ were computed only in the overlap between the images, and thus they could vary according to the considered transformation. Their role was precisely to prevent the image overlap from being minimized. In the implementation proposed in section 2.3, N and $\operatorname{Var}(I)$ are independent of the considered transformation. Minimizing $U(T)$ is then strictly equivalent to maximizing the correlation ratio, although is not strictly equivalent to maximizing the original version of the correlation ratio. In our experiments, this distinction seemed to have very little impact on the results.

Another remark is that we can impose constraints to the intensity function f, e.g. to be polynomial [16]. Notably, if we constraint f to follow an affine variation with respect to j, i.e. $f(j) = \alpha j + \beta$, we get a similar equivalence with the correlation coefficient defined in (1):

$$\rho^2(I, J^\downarrow) = 1 - \frac{1}{k} e^{\frac{U(T)}{N}}, \qquad \text{with} \quad k = \sqrt{2\pi e} \operatorname{Var}(I).$$

3.2   Unspecified channel

A straightforward extension of the previous model would be to assume the reference image J to be also corrupted with Gaussian noise. Then, having defined the prior probabilities for the tissue classes, we could derive the analytical form of the conditional densities $P(i_k|j_k^\downarrow)$ from (8). This case has been investigated by Leventon and Grimson [6]: it turns out that there is probably nothing much faster than a EM algorithm to provide maximum likelihood estimates of the density parameters.

In order to get explicit density estimates, we can relax every formal constraint on the model. Then, the densities $P(i_k|j_k^\downarrow)$ are totally unspecified, and we will only assume that they are stationary, i.e. $P(i_k = i|j_k^\downarrow = j)$ is independent of the position x_k. For the sake of simplicity, we consider the case of discrete densities, but the study is similar for continuous densities. The problem is now to minimize

$$- \log P(I|J,T,\theta) = \sum_{x_k \in \Omega_I} - \log f(i_k|j_k^\downarrow),$$

with respect to $\theta = (f(0|0), f(1|0), \ldots, f(1|1), \ldots, f(2|0), \ldots)$ and under the constraints: $\forall j, \; C_j = \sum_i f(i|j) - 1 = 0$. We regroup the intensity pairs $(i_k, j_k^\downarrow)$ that have the same values:

$$\Omega_{i,j} = \{x_k \in \Omega_I, \; I(x_k) = i, \; J(T(x_k)) = j\}, \qquad N_{i,j} = \text{Card } \Omega_{i,j}.$$

Then, the negative log-likelihood becomes:

$$- \log P(I|J,T,\theta) = - \sum_{i,j} N_{i,j} \log f(i|j).$$

Introducing Lagrange multipliers, there exist constants $\lambda_0, \lambda_1, \ldots$, such that for any j:

$$0 = \frac{\partial \log P}{\partial f(i|j)} - \sum_{j'} \lambda_{j'} \frac{\partial C_{j'}}{\partial f(i|j)} = \frac{N_{i,j}}{f(i|j)} - \lambda_j.$$

Thus, taking into account the constraints $\sum_i f(i|j) = 1$, the optimal parameters verify:

$$\hat{f}(i|j) = \frac{N_{i,j}}{N_j} = \frac{p(i,j)}{p(j)},$$

where $p(i,j) \equiv N_{i,j}/N$ is the image normalized 2D histogram and $p(j) \equiv \sum_i p(i,j)$ the corresponding marginal distribution for $J^\downarrow$. From (3), we see that $U(T)$ is nothing but a decreasing function of mutual information:

$$U(T) = -N \sum_{i,j} p(i,j) \log \frac{p(i,j)}{p(j)} = N\left[H(I) - \mathcal{I}(I, J^\downarrow)\right],$$

where $H(I)$ is the entropy of image I and is constant in the implementation proposed in section 2.3. The same remark as in 3.1 holds for the distinction between the usual implementation of mutual information and the one considered here.

3.3   Comparison of measures

In the derivation of the correlation ratio (CR), it was assumed that the image to be registered is a measure of the reference corrupted with additive and stationary Gaussian white noise. In contrast, for deriving mutual information (MI), no assumption was made apart from stationarity and, of course, the general assumptions discussed in section 2. Does it make MI necessarily a better registration measure than CR ?

In principle, the answer is no whenever the assumptions of CR are verified by the images. Basically, these are reasonable if the reference image can be considered as a good anatomical model: in practice, this is seldom pefectly true. The problem then becomes to determine what is better between an over-constrained and an under-constrained measure, a question to which experiments can yield some insight, as will be illustrated in the next section.

4   Experiments

In order to illustrate the practical differences between CR and MI, we present results of 3D rigid registration between two brain images of the same patient: an MR, T1 weighted scan ($256 \times 256 \times 124$ voxels of $0.9 \times 0.9 \times 1.1$ mm), and an intra-operative 3D ultrasound (US) image ($180 \times 136 \times 188$ voxels of 0.95^3 mm). As the US image was acquired before opening the duramater, there is essentially a rigid displacement to find. In these experiments, we used a registration algorithm similar to MIRIT [7], using Powell's method as an optimization strategy and partial volume (PV) interpolation.

The correct registration position was found manually using an interactive matching tool, and then validated by a clinician. The estimated accuracy was 2 degrees in rotation and 2 mm in translation [12]. We took this result as a "ground truth" for subsequent experiments.

We then performed 200 automatic registrations by initializing the algorithm with random displacements from the "ground truth" position a rotation vector Δr with random direction and constant magnitude $\|\Delta r\| = 15$ degrees, and a translation Δt with random direction and constant magnitude $\|\Delta t\| = 20$ mm. These values correspond to the variation between the "ground truth" and the original position. For each random transformation, two registrations were performed using alternatively CR and MI.

Two kinds of results are observed: either the algorithm retrieves the "ground truth" transformation (yielding errors systematically lower than $\|\delta r\| = 2$ degrees and $\|\delta t\| = 2$ mm), or it converges to a local maximum (yielding errors systematically larger than $\|\delta r\| = 10$ degrees and $\|\delta t\| = 10$ mm). The main result is that CR fails in 14% cases while MI fails in 51% cases (see table 1). The RMS errors computed on successful registrations are lower than the expected accuracy of the "ground truth"; thus, they prove nothing but the fact that both CR and MI have a maximum in the neighborhood of the ideal registration transformation (this is probably also a global maximum). However, the percentages

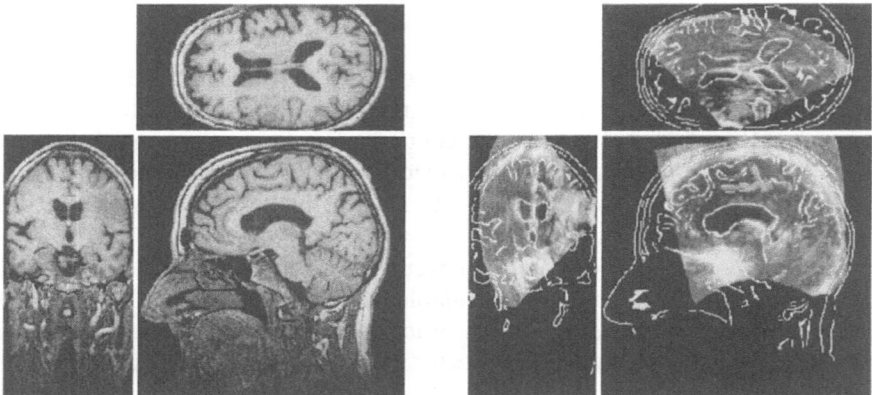

Fig. 2. Result of US/MR registration by maximization of CR. Left, three orthogonal views of a MR, T1 weighted image. Right, corresponding views of the registered US image with contours from the MR overlayed.

of success indicate that CR may have a wider attraction basin, an observation consistent with previous experiments with other modality combinations [15].

Table 1. RMS errors and percentages of failures in 3D US-MR rigid registration.

Reference Image	Similarity Measure	RMS		RMS (successes)		Failures (%)
		$\Delta\theta$ (deg)	Δt (mm)	$\Delta\theta$ (deg)	Δt (mm)	
Original MR	CR	11.49	23.33	1.11	0.42	14.0
	MI	19.07	47.14	1.27	0.64	51.0
Diffused MR	CR	12.64	26.29	0.92	0.52	12.5
	MI	17.35	27.41	1.35	0.82	28.0
Distorted MR	CR	28.51	18.08	3.21	2.04	36.0
($\sigma = 10\%$)	MI	44.23	45.06	1.84	1.36	90.0

To study the effect of noise in the reference image, we repeated the same experimental protocol twice, using as a reference image the MR pre-segmented by anisotropic diffusion [14], and the MR corrupted with Gaussian noise. The number of failures for both measures are clearly affected by the amount of noise, as can be seen on table 1. This comes as no surprise in the case of CR, since this measure has been derived under the assumption that there is no noise in the reference image (see section 3.1). This is more surprising for MI, as no such assumption was made.

We conclude that the attraction basin of the measures could be extended by denoising the reference image as a preprocessing step. Studying effects on accuracy would have been of great interest too, but this was not possible here because the "ground truth" was not accurate enough.

5   Conclusion

We have formalized image registration as a general maximum likelihood estimation problem and shown that several existing similarity measures may be reinterpreted in this framework. This enables us to better understand the implicit assumptions we make when using a particular measure, and hopefully help the selection of an appropriate strategy given a certain problem.

Experimental results of US/MR registration confirm (if needed) that similarity measures relating to different assumptions yield different performances. The CR measure was shown to be more robust than MI with respect to the initialization of registration. As CR relies on more restrictive hypotheses than MI, this suggests the importance of constraining the relationship between the images. On the other hand, the assumptions should also be founded, and we are aware that CR relies on a model that is simpler than realistic.

Because the presented work allows to systematically derive similarity measures from explicit modeling assumptions, this is a step towards taking into account more realistic models of image acquisition and anatomy. In the future, we plan to develop this approach for the challenging problem of US/MR registration.

Acknowledgments

The images were provided by ISM, Salzburg, Austria, for the US datasets, and the Max Planck Institute for Psychiatry, AG-NMR, Munich, Germany, for the MR datasets, as part of the EC-funded ROBOSCOPE project HC 4018, a collaboration between The Fraunhofer Institute (Germany), Fokker Control System (Netherlands), Imperial College (UK), INRIA Sophia Antipolis (France), ISM-Salzburg and Kretz Technik (Austria).

Part of this work was supported by la Région PACA (France).

Many thanks also to Sébastien Ourselin and Alexandre Guimond for constant interaction and countless suggestions.

References

1. R. Bansal, L. H. Staib, Z. Chen, A. Rangarajan, J. Knisely, R. Nath, and J. S. Duncan. A Novel Approach for the Registration of 2D Portal and 3D CT Images for Treatment Setup Verification in Radiotherapy. In *Proc. MICCAI'98*, pages 1075–1086, Cambridge, MA (USA), October 1998. LNCS.
2. M. Bro-Nielsen. Rigid Registration of CT, MR and Cryosection Images Using a GLCM Framework. *CVRMed-MRCAS'97*, pages 171–180, March 1997.
3. L. G. Brown. A survey of image registration techniques. *ACM Computing Surveys*, 24(4):325–376, 1992.
4. T. M. Buzug and J. Weese. Voxel-Based Similarity Measures for Medical Image Registration in Radiological Diagnosis and Image Guided Surgery. *Journal of Computing and Information Technology*, pages 165–179, 1998.

5. W. L. S. Costa, D. R Haynor, R. M. Haralick, T. K. Lwellen, and M. M. Graham. A Maximum-Likelihood Approach to PET Emission/Attenuation Image Registration. In *IEEE Nuclear Science Symposium and Med. Imag. Conference*, 1993.

6. M. E. Leventon and W. E. L. Grimson. Multi-modal Volume Registration Using Joint Intensity Distributions. In *Proc. MICCAI'98*, pages 1057–1066, Cambridge, MA (USA), October 1998. LNCS.

7. F. Maes, A. Collignon, D. Vandermeulen, G. Marchal, and P. Suetens. Multimodality Image Registration by Maximization of Mutual Information. *IEEE Transactions on Medical Imaging*, 16(2):187–198, 1997.

8. J. B. A. Maintz and M. A. Viergever. A survey of medical image registration. *MedIA*, 2(1):1–36, 1998.

9. M. S. Mort and M. D. Srinath. Maximum Likelihood Image Registration with Subpixel Accuracy. In *Proc. SPIE*, volume 974, pages 38–45, San Diego, 1988.

10. C. Nikou, F. Heitz, J.-P. Armspach, and I.-J. Namer. Single and multimodal subvoxel registration of dissimilar medical images using robust similarity measures. In *SPIE Conference on Medical Imaging*, volume 3338, pages 167–178, 1998.

11. A. Papoulis. *Probability, Random Variables, and Stochastic Processes*. McGraw-Hill, Inc., third edition, 1991.

12. X. Pennec and J.P. Thirion. A framework for uncertainty and validation of 3D registration methods based on points and frames. *IJCV*, 25(3):203–229, 1997.

13. G. P. Penney, J. Weese, J. A. Little, P. Desmedt, D. L. G. Hill, and D. J. Hawkes. A Comparison of Similarity Measures for Use in 2D-3D Medical Image Registration. In *Proc. MICCAI'98*, pages 1153–1161, Cambridge, MA (USA), 1998. LNCS.

14. P. Perona and J. Malik. Scale-Space and edge detection using anisotropic diffusion. *IEEE Trans. on Pattern Analysis and Machine Intelligence*, 12(7):629–639, 1990.

15. A. Roche, G. Malandain, X. Pennec, and N. Ayache. The Correlation Ratio as a New Similarity Measure for Multimodal Image Registration. In *Proc. MICCAI'98*, pages 1115–1124, Cambridge, MA (USA), October 1998. LNCS.

16. A. Roche, G. Malandain, and N. Ayache. Unifying Maximum Likelihood Approaches in Medical Image Registration. INRIA Research Report. *In press.*

17. C. Studholme, D. L. G. Hill, and D. J. Hawkes. Automated 3-D registration of MR and CT images of the head. *Medical Image Analysis*, 1(2):163–175, 1996.

18. C. Studholme, D. L. G. Hill, and D. J. Hawkes. An overlap invariant entropy measure of 3D medical image alignment. *Pattern Recognition*, 1(32):71–86, 1998.

19. P. Viola. *Alignment by Maximization of Mutual Information*. PhD thesis, M.I.T. Artificial Intelligence Laboratory, 1995.

20. P. Viola and W. M. Wells. Alignment by Maximization of Mutual Information. *Intern. J. of Comp. Vision*, 24(2):137–154, 1997.

21. W. M. Wells, P. Viola, H. Atsumi, and S. Nakajima. Multi-modal volume registration by maximization of mutual information. *MedIA*, 1(1):35–51, 1996.

22. J. West and al. Comparison and evaluation of retrospective intermodality brain image registration techniques. *J. of Comp. Assist. Tomography*, 21:554–566, 1997.

23. R. P. Woods, J. C. Mazziotta, and S. R. Cherry. MRI-PET Registration with Automated Algorithm. *J. of Comp. Assist. Tomography*, 17(4):536–546, 1993.

Entropy–Based, *Multiple–Portal–to–3DCT* Registration for Prostate Radiotherapy Using Iteratively Estimated Segmentation

Ravi Bansal[1], Lawrence H. Staib[1], Zhe Chen[2], Anand Rangarajan[1], Jonathan Knisely[2], Ravinder Nath[2], and James S. Duncan[1]

[1] Departments of Electrical Engineering and Diagnostic Radiology,
[2] Department of Therapeutic Radiology, Yale University, New Haven, CT 06520-8042

Abstract. In external beam radiotherapy (EBRT), patient setup verification over the entire course of fractionated treatment is necessary for accurate delivery of specified dose to the tumor. We develop an information theoretic minimax entropy registration framework for patient setup verification using *portal images* and the treatment planning 3D CT data set. Within this framework we propose to simultaneously and iteratively segment the portal images and register them to the 3D CT data set to achieve robust and accurate estimation of the pose parameters. Appropriate entropies are evaluated, in an iterative fashion, to segment the portal images and to find the registration parameters. Earlier, we reported our work using a single portal image to estimate the transformation parameters. In this work, we extend the algorithm to utilize dual portal images. In addition, we show the performance of the algorithm on real patient data, analyze the performance of the algorithm under different initializations and noise conditions, and note the wide range of parameters that can be estimated. We also present a coordinate descent interpretation of the proposed algorithm to further clarify the formulation.

1 Introduction

In external beam radiotherapy (EBRT) uncertainties due to patient setup errors can be reduced by registering the high contrast *simulator images*, obtained at diagnostic energies (40–100 KeV), to the low resolution, low contrast 2D *portal images*, which are obtained using the treatment energy X–rays (4–20 MeV). Two dimensional analysis of patient setup verification using single portal and simulator images is restricted to the verification of in–plane rotations and translations. Out–of–plane rotations and translations of the patient can degrade the accuracy of the image registration [13].

To account for out–of–plane rotations and translations, a *pair* of simulator and portal images of the same patient, obtained from different views, can be employed. However, such an analysis of the patient setup from 2D images can lead to inconsistencies in the determination of the transformation parameters [13]. Many treatment centers are moving towards offering full 3D conformal treatments that are initially planned from 3D CT datasets. Thus, for consistent and accurate three–dimensional analysis of the patient setup, it is necessary to register the 3D CT datasets to the 2D portal images. However, due to the poor quality of the portal images, automated registration of the portal images to the CT data set has remained a difficult task.

A number of methods have been proposed for both two dimensional and three dimensional analysis of the patient setup. Algorithms for two dimensional analysis include gray–level intensity based image alignment algorithms [3, 14], visual inspection by the physician [23] and the anatomical landmark–based approaches [5, 13, 20–22]. Studies which carry out three–dimensional registration of the treatment planning 3D CT data set to the 2D portal images include interactive determination of patient setup [12], silhouette based techniques [18], gray scale correlation–based methods [8, 19], a pattern–intensity based method [26], and a ridge–based method [11]. One of these approaches is interesting in that it also makes use of multi-scale medial information in the anatomical structure, using a strategy known as *cores* [10].

We have been developing an information theoretic registration framework, the initial form of which was reported in [1], where segmentation of a portal image and registration to the 3D CT data set is carried out iteratively and simultaneously. This framework is based on the intuition that if we have a rough estimate of the segmentation of the portal image, then it can help estimate the registration parameters. The estimated registration parameters can then in turn be used to better segment the portal image and so on. This framework is termed *minimax* entropy as it has two steps: the *max* step and the *min* step. In the entropy maximization step, the segmentation of the portal image is estimated, using the current estimates of the registration parameters. In the entropy minimization step, the registration parameters are estimated, based on the current estimates of the segmentation. The algorithm can start at any step, with some appropriate initialization on the other.

2   Mathematical Notations and Formulation

Let, $\mathbf{X} = \{\mathbf{x}(i)\}$, for $i = 1, \ldots, N^2$ denote the $N \times N$ random field from which the portal images are sampled. Let, $\mathbf{G} = \{\mathbf{g}(i)\}$, for $i = 1, \ldots, N^3$ denote the random field from which 3D CT images are sampled. Let $\mathbf{Y}(T) = \{\mathbf{y}(i, T)\}$ for $i = 1, \ldots, N^2$ denote the $N \times N$ random field from which the projections from the 3D CT data set are sampled, at a given set of transformation parameters $\mathbf{T} = T$. The projected 3D CT images are also called the *digitally reconstructed radiographs* (DRRs). We will assume that the pixels for all the random fields are independently distributed. Thus, the probability density function of the random field $\mathbf{X}$ can be written in the factored form as $p_{\mathbf{X}}(X) = \prod_i p_{\mathbf{x}_i}(x_i)$. Note that for notational simplicity, we shall now write $\mathbf{x}(i)$ as $\mathbf{x}_i$ and $\mathbf{y}(i, T)$ as $\mathbf{y}_i$.

Segmentation information is incorporated into the problem by considering the joint density function $p(x_i, y_i)$ as a mixture density. Let $A = \{bone, no-bone\} = \{1,2\}$, denote the set of classes into which the pixels are classified. The set of classes can also be denoted by a set of vectors, $\{(1,0),(0,1)\}$. Since X–rays pass through both bone and soft tissue, a pixel in portal image is classified as *bone* if the X–ray passes through at-least some bone tissue, rest of the pixels are classified *no–bone*. Let, $\mathbf{M} = \{\mathbf{m}(i)\}$, for $i = 1, \ldots, N^2$ denote the $N \times N$ random field on the segmentation of the portal images.

Let $\mathbf{Z}$ be the N^2 x 2 *classification matrix*, with each row $\mathbf{z}_i$ of the matrix defining a set of random variables $\mathbf{z}_i = (\mathbf{z}_{1i}, \mathbf{z}_{2i})$, defined to be:

$$\mathbf{z}_{1i} = \begin{cases} 1, & \text{if } \mathbf{m}_i = bone \\ 0, & \text{if } \mathbf{m}_i = no\text{--}bone \end{cases} , \mathbf{z}_{2i} = \begin{cases} 0, & \text{if } \mathbf{m}_i = bone \\ 1, & \text{if } \mathbf{m}_i = no\text{--}bone \end{cases}$$

The expected values of the random variables $\mathbf{z}_{ai}, \forall a$, denoted by $< z_{ai} > = P(\mathbf{m}_i = a)$, satisfy the constraint, $\sum_{a \in A} < z_{ai} > = 1$. Note that the random variables $\mathbf{z}_{1i}, \mathbf{z}_{2i}$ are negatively correlated random variables, with the random variable $\mathbf{z}_i$ taking only two possible values, $\{(1,0),(0,1)\}$.

For clarification, we first pose our problem in a *maximum a–posteriori* (MAP) framework where both the segmentation, $\mathbf{M}$, and the transformation parameters, $\mathbf{T}$, are being estimated explicitly. However, we note some restrictions with this approach for our problem and thus we propose a maximum likelihood (ML)/EM [7] framework to overcome these restrictions. For our problem, the EM approach has several restrictions, which lead us to propose our new minimax entropy strategy described (in section 3).

2.1 Maximum A–Posteriori (MAP) Formulation

An estimate of the segmentation of the portal image, $\mathbf{M}$, can be used to help estimate pose, $\mathbf{T}$, of the 3D CT data set based on a MAP formulation to simultaneously estimate the pose $\mathbf{T}$ and the portal image segmentation, $\mathbf{M}$, as follows:

$$(\hat{T}, \hat{M}) = \arg \max_{T,M} p(T, M | X, G) = \arg \max_{T,M} \sum_i \left(\sum_{a \in A} z_{ai} \ln p_a(x_i, y_i) - \ln p(y_i) \right) \quad (1)$$

where we assume each pixel is statistically independent, and the joint density function, $p(x_i, y_i)$, can be written as a mixture density, in terms of component density functions, $p_a(x_i, y_i)$, as, $p(x_i, y_i) = \sum_{a \in A} P(\mathbf{m}_i = a) \, p(x_i, y_i | \mathbf{m}_i = a) = \sum_{a \in A} P(\mathbf{m}_i = a) \, p_a(x_i, y_i) = \sum_{a \in A} P_i(a) \, p_a(x_i, y_i)$ where, $\mathbf{m}_i$ is the random variable denoting label at the ith pixel.

This formulation requires that the algorithm solve for a unique segmentation of the portal image, $\mathbf{M}$, for a unique estimate of the pose parameters, $\mathbf{T}$. An estimated segmentation will effect the estimate of the pose parameters. Since we feel that accurate segmentation of a portal image, in general, is quite difficult, we prefer instead not to commit the algorithm to a particular segmentation.

2.2 Maximum–Likelihood (ML) Formulation

Thus, instead of solving the MAP problem, we pose our problem in a ML framework, with segmentation labels appearing as hidden variables. Such an approach *could* be captured using an EM algorithm.

The ML/EM estimate [7] of the pose parameters can be formulated as:

$$\hat{T} = \arg\max_{T} \ln p(T|X,G) = \arg\max_{T} \sum_{i}\left(\sum_{a \in A} < z_{ai} >^k \ln p_a(x_i,y_i) - \ln p(y_i)\right) \quad (2)$$

where $< z_{ai} >^k = \left(\frac{<z_{ai}>^{k-1} p_a^{k-1}(x_i,y_i)}{\sum_{b \in A} <z_{bi}>^{k-1} p_b^{k-1}(x_i,y_i)}\right)$. We assume a uniform prior on the pose parameters, $\mathbf{T}$, and ignore the term $p(G|T)$, since the 3D CT data set, G, is statistically independent of the pose parameters, $\mathbf{T}$.

In the ML formulation of the problem, only the transformation parameters are being estimated, with a probability distribution on the segmentation labels being estimated. This allows the algorithm to not commit to a particular segmentation of the portal image.

There are two reasons why we need to move beyond the above listed idea to find an appropriate solution to our problem. First, the EM algorithm for the mixture model as formulated above, requires that the form of $p_a(x_i, y_i)$, $\forall a$ is known (i.e. one should know whether they are Gaussian, Rayleigh, exponential, etc.). For multi-modal image registration it is difficult, if not impossible, to know a priori the joint density function between the pixel intensities in the two images. Second, in the EM framework, the prior probabilities on each pixel, $P_i(a)$, are required to be known. If these probabilities are not known, then they can also be estimated within the EM framework, assuming that the segmentation labels on each pixel are independently and identically distributed (i.i.d.), i.e., $P_i(a) = \pi_a$, where π_a satisfy the constraint $\sum_{a \in A} \pi_a = 1$. For our problem, i.i.d. assumption does not hold.

3   Minimax Entropy Formulation

We overcome the restrictions of the ML formulation by borrowing the idea of averaging over the estimated density function from *mutual information* (MI). MI was first proposed and successfully applied for multi–modality image registration by two research groups [25, 6]. The proposed minimax algorithm [2] for solving the basic problem posed by equation (2), in a computational form similar to EM, has two steps, the *max step* and the *min step*, which are evaluated iteratively to determine the registration parameters and the probability distribution of the portal image segmentation. The *max* step is formulated as follows:
Max Step:

$$P^k(M) = \arg\max_{P(M)}\left[-\sum_{M} P(M) \ln P(M) + \sum_{M} P(M) \ln P(M|X, Y(T^{(k-1)}))\right] \quad (3)$$

under the constraint $\sum_{M} P(\mathbf{M} = M) = 1$, where $\mathbf{M}$ is the random variable whose domain is the set of possible segmentations of the portal image, where each pixel can be labeled from the set of labels A. We assume that pixel labels are statistically independent, i.e., $P(\mathbf{M} = M) = \prod_i P(\mathbf{m}_i = a) = \prod_i P_i(a)$. As formulated above, the max–step simply states that the maximum entropy estimate of the probability $P(\mathbf{M} = M)$ is the posterior probability on the segmentation of the portal image, i.e $P(M|X, Y(T^{(k-1)}))$, given the current estimate of the transformation parameters, $T^{(k-1)}$, the portal image, X, and the DRR, Y [4]. This simple formulation of the estimated probability of a segmentation of the portal image allows us to systematically put constraints on the segmentation probability function, as we show below. The analytical solution to equation (3) estimates the probability of a segmentation label at the ith pixel to be:

$$P_i^k(a) = \left(\frac{P_i^{k-1}(a) \ p_a^{k-1}(x_i, y_i)}{\sum_{b \in A} P_i^{k-1}(b) \ p_b^{k-1}(x_i, y_i)} \right)$$

where the component density functions, $p_a^{k-1}(x_i, y_i)$, are estimated from the previous step.

Note that the $P_i^k(a)$'s, in the kth iteration, form the weighing terms in the Parzen window estimates, in equation (6) below, of the component density functions, $p_a(x, y)$. The component density functions, in turn, are used to estimate the joint entropies, $H_a(x, y) = -\iint p_a(x, y) \ln p_a(x, y) \, dx \, dy$, which are minimized in the *min* step to estimate the registration parameters.

In order to better incorporate our initial uncertainty on the registration parameters into the problem, an annealing schedule [17] is imposed on the estimated probability of a segmentation of the portal image pixel. The modified *max step*, equation (3), can thus be written as:

$$P^k(M) = \arg \max_{P(M)} \left[-\frac{1}{\beta} \sum_M P(M) \ln P(M) + \sum_M P(M) \ln P(M|X, Y(T^{(k-1)})) \right] \quad (4)$$

under the constraint $\sum_M P(\mathbf{M} = M) = 1$, where $\beta = \frac{1}{t}$, and t is the *temperature*, which determines the annealing schedule. The annealing schedule is imposed to incorporate subjective information in estimating $P^k(M)$ [2].

To overcome the need of the EM algorithm for known component densities, we propose estimating $p_a(x_i, y_i)$ from the given data set at the current estimated transformation parameters. Note that we use *Parzen* window method [9] for non–parametric density function. However, these estimated joint density functions cannot be used in the EM algorithm. Instead, we evaluate the expected value of the objective function in the EM algorithm w.r.t. $p(x_i, y_i)$ which leads to the *min* step (see [2]):

Min Step : $$T^k = \arg \min_T \sum_{a \in A} \frac{1}{N^2} \left(\sum_{i=1}^{N^2} P_i^k(a) \right) H_a(x, y) - H(y) \quad (5)$$

which is joint conditional entropy $H(M, X|Y)$. The component density function for class a, $p_a(x, y)$, is estimated as the weighted sum of Gaussian kernels, $G_\psi(x) = (2\pi)^{\frac{-n}{2}} |\psi|^{\frac{-1}{2}} \exp(-\frac{1}{2} x^T \psi^{-1} x)$, using the Parzen window method as follows:

$$p_a^k(x, y) \approx \frac{1}{\sum_{(x_i, y_i) \in \mathbf{I}} P_i^k(a)} \sum_{(x_i, y_i) \in \mathbf{I}} P_i^k(a) \ G_{\Psi_a}(x - x_i, y - y_i) \quad (6)$$

where, $P_i^k(a) = P^k(\mathbf{m}_i = a)$ is the probability that the ith pixel in the portal image belongs to class a, estimated in the *max* step, equation (3), Ψ_a is 2–by–2 covariance matrix, which is assumed to be diagonal. Note that this assumption does not means that the random variables $\mathbf{x}$ and $\mathbf{y}$ are independent. $\mathbf{I}, \mathbf{J}$ denote sets of sizes N_I and N_J, respectively, of pixels sampled at random from the portal image, X, and the DRR, Y. The joint entropy functions, which are the expected value of the log of the joint probability density functions, are approximated as statistical expectations using the Parzen window density estimates as follows. $H_a(x, y)$

$$\approx \left(\frac{-1}{\sum_{w_j \in \mathbf{J}} P_j^k(a)} \right) \sum_{w_j \in \mathbf{J}} P_j^k(a) \ln \left(\frac{1}{\sum_{w_i \in \mathbf{I}} P_i^k(a)} \sum_{w_i \in \mathbf{I}} P_i^k(a) \, G_{\Psi_a}(w_j - w_i) \right)$$

where $w_i = (x_i, y_i)$. The entropy of the DRRs, $H(y)$, is estimated as in Viola and Wells [25]. While MI assumes that pixels are i.i.d., we avoid this assumption by using mixture densities. We note that Studholm et. al. [24], register images with mutual information as a match measure while incorporating segmentation information on one of the images. However, the image was pre–hand segmented. **Coordinate Descent Interpretation:** The minimax entropy algorithm above is developed within a probabilistic framework. However, within the optimization framework the algorithm can be viewed as a coordinate descent approach which seeks to optimize a cost function by iterative estimation of the parameters along different coordinates. Let

$$F(\tilde{P}, T) = -H(M, X|Y) + H(M)$$
$$= \iint dX \, dY \sum_M p(X, Y|M) \, \tilde{P}(M) \, \ln p(M, X|Y) - \sum_M \tilde{P}(M) \ln \tilde{P}(M)$$

Note that $F(\tilde{P}, T)$ is a functional (function of function) which is to be optimized to estimate density function $\tilde{P}(M)$ and the parameters, $\mathbf{T}$. Optimizing $F(\tilde{P}, T)$ using the coordinate descent approach leads to the following two steps:
Step 1: $\tilde{P}^k(M) = \arg\max_{\tilde{P}} F(\tilde{P}, T^{k-1})$,   under constraint $\sum_M \tilde{P}^k(M) = 1$
Step 2: $T^k = \arg\max_T F(\tilde{P}^k, T)$

Step 1, where the energy functional $F(\tilde{P}, T)$ is being optimized to estimate $\tilde{P}(M)$, utilizing the transformation parameters T^{k-1}, is equivalent to the *max* step. Thus, estimation of the density function $\tilde{P}(M)$, a variational calculus problem within the optimization framework, is interpreted as *maximum entropy* estimation of a density function within the probabilistic framework. Step 2, where we optimize $F(\tilde{P}, T)$ to estimate $\mathbf{T}$, utilizing current estimates of $\tilde{P}(M)$, is equivalent to the *min* step as the marginal entropy term, $H(M)$, is independent of the parameters $\mathbf{T}$.
Utilizing Dual Portal Images: It is expected that utilizing another portal image, typically the left–lateral (LL) portal image acquired in the orthogonal direction, will greatly enhance the accuracy of the estimated pose. Thus, we extend the algorithm to utilize two portal images, AP and LL, for the estimation of the pose. Both the min step and the max step are modified to incorporate this new information. While estimating the segmentations of the two

portal images, in the *max* step, we assume that the segmentations of the two portal images are statistically independent. Thus, in the max step for the 2–portal case, $P^k(M_{AP})$ and $P^k(M_{LL})$, are estimated by repeating equation (4) for the two portal images separately. Note that though there are two portal images, whose segmentation is being estimated separately, there is only one set of transformation parameters, $\mathbf{T}$, is to be estimated. In the initial formulation of the algorithm, the optimal pose parameters are thus estimated as $\hat{T}^k = \arg\min_T [H(M_{AP}, X_{AP}|Y_1) + H(M_{LL}, X_{LL}|Y_2)]$ where X_{AP}, X_{LL} denote the AP and the LL portal image respectively, and Y_1, Y_2 denote the DRRs obtained from the 3D CT data set in the AP and LL directions.

4   Results

In this section we evaluate the accuracy and robustness of the proposed minimax algorithm using both real and simulated data. A plexi–glass pelvic bone phantom is scanned to provide the 3D CT dataset. The phantom consists of real human pelvic bone encased in plexi–glass of density close to the density of soft–tissue. The phantom is then moved to the treatment room to obtain real portal images at the treatment energy X–rays (6 MV). The simulated portal images are obtained in the following fashion. First, the 3D CT voxel values are mapped from diagnostic energy values to the values at the treatment energy X–rays using attenuation coefficient tables [15]. Second, the 3D CT data set is transformed by known transformation parameters. Third, the digitally reconstructed radiographs (DRRs) are rendered, using perspective projection, from the CT data set, both in the anterior–posterior (AP) and the left–lateral (LL) directions. Two different testing sets of simulated portal images are then generated from the resulting DRRs. To obtain the first set of simulated portal images, varying amounts of i.i.d. Gaussian noise are added to the DRRs. To obtain the second set of simulated portal images, the DRRs are blurred using blurring kernels of increasing width, which simulates the finite size of the radiation source, and low contrast and low sharpness of the real portal images. Since the true registration parameters are known for the simulated portal images, these datasets are used to study the accuracy and robustness of the algorithm under increasing noise and blur in the images.

Our previous work [1] suggested that the proposed algorithm is not robust to the estimation of the out–of–plane transformation parameters when using only single AP portal images. The second portal image would be expected to improve this robustness. The in–plane translations for the AP portal image consists of translations along the X and Y axes and the in–plane rotation is the rotation about the Z–axis, θ_{XY}. For the lateral portal image, the in–plane translations are the translations of the 3D CT dataset along the Y and Z axis and the in–plane rotation is the rotation about the X–axis, θ_{YZ}. Note that by using two portal images, the rotation about the Y–axis, θ_{XZ}, is the only out–of–plane parameter to be estimated.

	t_x (vox)	t_y (vox)	t_z (vox)	θ_{YZ} (deg)	θ_{XZ} (deg)	θ_{XY} (deg)
True	15.0	5.0	0.0	0.0	0.0	10.0
Estd.	15.62	5.19	-0.06	0.43	0.21	10.85

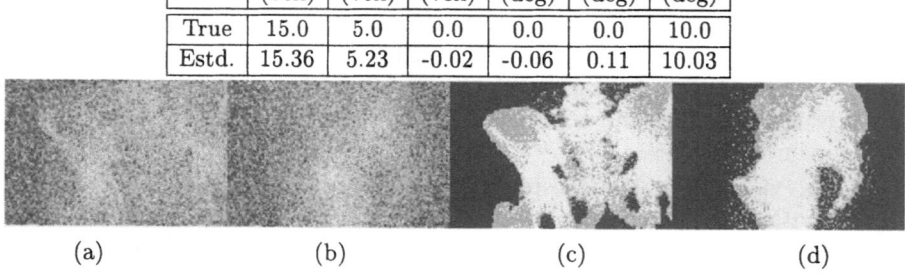

(a)   (b)   (c)   (d)

Fig. 1. (a) Simulated AP portal image. (b) Simulated left–lateral portal image. (c) Estimated segmentation of the AP portal image. (d) Segmentation of the LL portal image estimated by the algorithm. Estimated and the true parameters are shown in the table.

4.1 Dual Simulated Portal Data

The simulated portal images are obtained as explained above. The six transformation parameters to be estimated are denoted as t_x, t_y and t_z (along the x–axis, y–axis and z–axis respectively) and the three rotations are denoted as θ_{YZ}, θ_{XZ} and θ_{XY} (about the x–axis, y–axis and z–axis respectively).

The simulated dual portal images are blurred using a uniform blurring kernel of width 11 to obtain the portal images shown in figure 1 (a), (b). Figure 1 (c), (d) show the corresponding segmentation of the portal images estimated by the algorithm. The table in the figure shows the true and the estimated parameters. Note that the estimated translations are within 1 voxel of the true values, even in the presence of a blur of 11 pixels. The estimates of the rotation parameters are within 0.5^o, on average, of the true values.

	t_x (vox)	t_y (vox)	t_z (vox)	θ_{YZ} (deg)	θ_{XZ} (deg)	θ_{XY} (deg)
True	15.0	5.0	0.0	0.0	0.0	10.0
Estd.	15.36	5.23	-0.02	-0.06	0.11	10.03

(a)   (b)   (c)   (d)

Fig. 2. Simulated portal images with noise. (a) AP with std 30.0 (b) Left–lateral with std 30.0 Estimated segmentation of (c) AP portal image. (d) LL portal image. The table show the true and the parameters estimated by the algorithm.

Figure 2 (a), (b) shows the simulated portal images with Gaussian noise of standard deviation = 30.0. The dynamic range of the pixel intensities was 255. Note again the accuracy of the parameters estimated by the algorithm.

Figure 2 (c), (d) shows the segmentation of the portal images as estimated by the algorithm.

Performance under varying initializations: Figure 3 (a) and (b) shows the graphs of error in estimated parameters for varying amounts of rotational and translational setup variations, in the presence of Gaussian noise of standard deviation $(\sigma) = 20.0$ in the simulated portal images. To obtain these graphs, first, the 3D CT dataset is transformed by a known amount and, AP and LL DRRs are obtained. Then i.i.d. Gaussian noise of $\sigma = 20.0$ is added to the DRRs to obtain the simulated portal images. For the graph labeled θ_{YZ}, only the parameter θ_{YZ}, which denotes rotation about the X–axis, is varied to obtain the DRRs. All other parameters are kept fixed at the true values. The 3D CT is then reset to its untransformed position and the algorithm is run to estimate $\mathbf{T}$. The error in the estimated parameter is then plotted. The graphs show that, for this dataset, the algorithm could estimate the rotation angles up to 50° accurately. For the translations, the estimates for the three translations were accurate up to 25 or more voxels. These figures also show that either the algorithm is quite accurate in estimating the parameters or it breaks down completely, that is, the estimated parameters are totally different than the true parameters. This shows that the algorithm gets trapped into a local minimum if the global minimum is very far from the initial starting position.

Performance under varying noise: Figures 3 (c) and (d) show the performance of the algorithm under increasing noise. The AP and LL portal images, for example for the graph labeled θ_{XY}, are obtained by first rotating the 3D CT data by 15° about the Z–axis and then rendering the DRRs both in the AP and the LL directions. A varying amount of noise is then added to the DRRs to obtain the simulated portal images. The 3D CT data set is then initialized to its undeformed position and the algorithm is run to estimate $\mathbf{T}$. The graph shows the error in estimated BdT for various amounts of noise. Similarly, for the graphs labeled $\theta_{YZ}, \theta_{XZ}, t_x, t_y, t_z$, the 3D CT data set was transformed by 30°, 25°, 20 voxels, 20 voxels and 15 voxels respectively to obtain the DRRs.

4.2   Performance on Actual Patient Treatment Data

Figure 4 shows the results of running the proposed algorithm on real patient data. Figures 4 (a) and (b) show histogram equalized AP and LL portal images, respectively. The DRRs projected through the 3D CT data in its original pose are shown in the figures 4 (c) and (d). Running the algorithm estimates a new pose of the 3D CT dataset, which differs from the original pose by $\theta_{XY} = 3.2^o$, $\theta_{YZ} = 2.92^o$, $\theta_{XZ} = 1.93^o$, $t_x = 3.53$ voxels, $t_y = 12.5$ voxels and $t_x = 13.54$ voxels. The DRR projections in the new pose are shown in the figures 4 (e) and (f). Segmentations of the AP and LL portal images, estimated by the algorithm, are shown in the figures 4 (g) and (h), respectively. Due to poor quality of these *digitized portal film* images, the segmentation step was initialized manually in several regions to highlight the background. To assess the accuracy of the

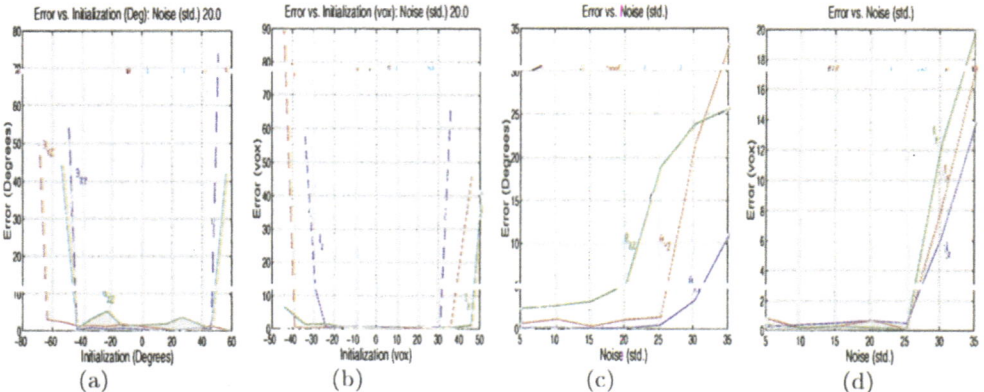

Fig. 3. (a) Error in estimated rotation angles. (b) Error in estimated translation. (c) Error in estimated angles with increasing noise. (d) Error in estimated translation with increasing noise.

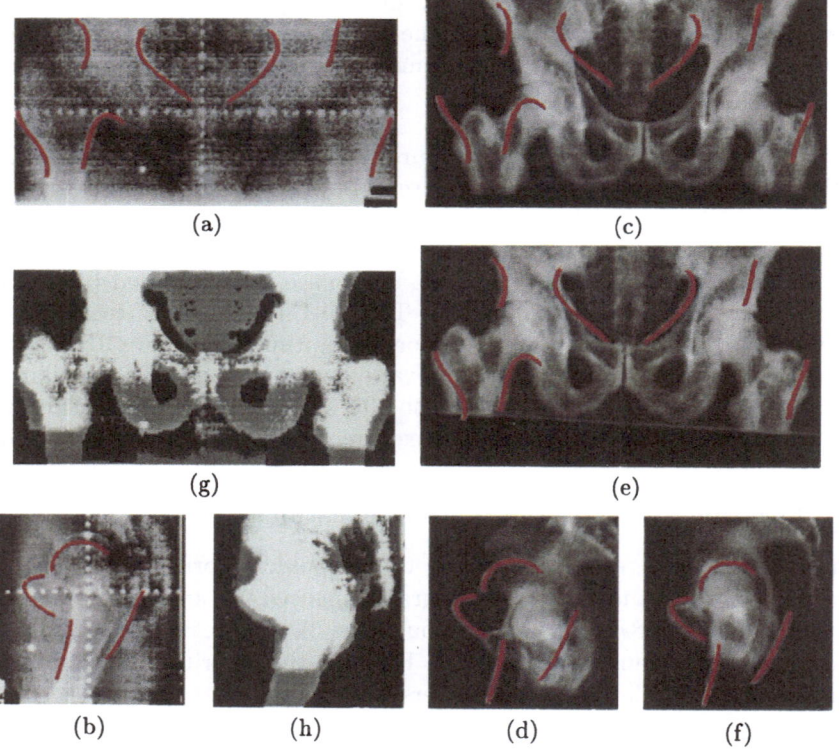

Fig. 4. Recovery of setup variation using *actual patient data*. (a,b) Portal images, (c,d) DRR's of 3D CT in original pose, (e,f) DRR's in corrected pose, (g,h) implicit segmentation of portals.

estimated pose of the 3D CT data set, contours are hand drawn on the portal images, matching visible features. These contours are then mapped onto the DRRs, in figures 4 (c), (d), (e), (f) undeformed. Note that the contours are used only to visually assess the goodness of the estimated pose. The contours match closely to the features in DRRs obtained at the pose estimated by the algorithm, although there is some remaining error, perhaps resulting from error in θ_{XZ} (out–of–plane rotation for both views).

5   Discussion and the Future Work

In this work we extended our algorithm [1] to utilize dual portal images to estimate the transformation parameters, note the performance of the algorithm utilizing real patient data, present experiments which demonstrate the extent of parameters algorithm can estimate, demonstrate the robustness of the algorithm under increasing noise, and present a coordinate descent interpretation of the algorithm.

Our future research includes algorithm speed–up, validation of the accuracy and robustness of the algorithm, especially in comparison to the mutual information based registration and the ridge based algorithm [11]. Effects of artifacts in the portal images, like air bubbles, unstable features, like movement of femurs w.r.t. pelvic bone and portal images with exposures only through the limited treatment field require further study. The inclusion of edges and whole boundary information will likely lead to more accurate results. Thus, we will extend our algorithm to incorporate such information into the same framework.

References

1. R. Bansal, L. Staib, Z. Chen, A. Rangarajan, J. Knisely, R. Nath, and J.S. Duncan. A novel approach for the registration of 2D portal and 3D CT images for treatment setup verification in radiotherapy. *Medical Image Computing and Computer–Assisted Intervention (MICCAI'98)*, LNCS–1496:1075–1086, 10–12 October 1998.
2. R. Bansal, L. Staib, et al. A minimax entropy registration framework for patient setup verification in radiotherapy: Evaluation and comparisons. Technical Report YALE–IPAG–TR–1999-01, Dept. of Electrical Engineering and Diagnostic Radiology, Yale University, Jan 1999.
3. Martin Berger and Guido Gerig. Motion Measurments in Low–Contrast X–ray Imagery. In W.M. Wells et al., editors, *Medical Image Computing and Computer–Assisted Intervention –MICCAI'98*, volume 1496 of *LNCS*, pages 832–841, 1998.
4. R. M. Bevensee. *Maximum Entropy Solutions to Scientific Problems*. P T R Prentice Hall, 1993.
5. J. Bijhold et al. Radiation field edge detection in portal images. *Phys. Med. Biol.*, 36(12):1705–1710, 1991.
6. A. Collignon, F. Maes, et al. Automated multimodality image registration using information theory. *Info. Proc. in Med. Imaging (IPMI)*, pages 263–274, 1995.
7. A. P. Dempster, N. M. Laird, and D. B. Rubin. Maximum likelihood from incomplete data via EM algorithm. *J. Royal Statistical Soc., Ser. B*, 39:1–38, 1977.

8. L. Dong and A. L. Boyer. An image correlation procedure for digitally reconstructed radiographs and electronic portal images. *Int. J. Radiation Oncol. Biol. Phys.*, 33(5):1053–1060, 1995.

9. R. O. Duda and P. E. Hart. *Pattern Classification and Scene Analysis*. John Wiley & Sons, 1973.

10. D. S. Fritsch et al. Core–based portal image registration for automatic radiotherapy treatment verification. *Int. J. Radiation Oncol. Biol. Phys.*, 33(5):1287–1300, 1995.

11. K. Gilhuijs. *Automated verification of radiation treatment geometry*. PhD thesis, Univ. of Amsterdam, Radiotherapy dept., the Netherlands, 1995.

12. K. Gilhuijs et al. Interactive three dimensional inspection of patient setup in radiation therapy using digital portal images and computed tomography data. *Int. J. Rad. Oncol. Biol. Phys.*, 34(4):873–885, 1996.

13. J. Hanley et al. The effects of out–of–plane rotations on two dimensional portal image registration in conformal radiotherapy of the prostate. *Int. J. Radiation Oncology Biol. Phys.*, 33(5):1331–1343, 1995.

14. D. H. Hiristov and B. G. Fallone. A gray–level image alignment algorithm for registration of portal images and digitally reconstructed radiographs. *Med. Phys.*, 23(1):75–84, Jan 1996.

15. J. H. Hubble. *Photon Cross Sections, Attenuation Coefficients, and Energy Absorption Coefficients From 10KeV to 100 GeV*. Nat. Stand. Ref. Data. Ser., Nat. Bur. Stand. (U.S.), August 1969.

16. E. T. Jaynes. Prior probabilities. In R. D. Rosenkrantz, editor, *E. T. Jaynes: Papers on probability, statistics and statistical physics*, volume 158, pages 114–130. D. Reidel Publishing Company, Boston. USA, 1983.

17. S. Kirkpatrick et al. Optimization by simulated annealing. *Science*, 220:671–680, 1983.

18. S. Lavallee, R. Szeliski, and L. Brunie. Anatomy–based registration of three–dimensional medical images, range images, X–ray projections, and three–dimensional models using octree–splines. In Russell H. Taylor et al., editors, *Computer–Integrated Surgery: Technology and Clinical Applications*, pages 115–143. The MIT Press, Cambridge, Massachusetts, 1996.

19. L. Lemieux et al. A patient–to–computed–tomography image registration method based on digitally reconstructed radiographs. *Med. Phys.*, 21(11):1749–1760, November 1994.

20. K. W. Leszczynski, S. Loose, and S. Boyko. An image registration scheme applied to verification of radiation therapy. *The British Journal of Radiology*, 71(844):413–426, 1998.

21. H. Meertens, J. Bijhold, and J. Strackee. A method for the measurement of field displacement errors in digital portal images. *Phy. Med. Biol.*, 35(3):299–323, 1990.

22. C. D. Mubata, A. M. Bidmead, et al. Portal imaging protocol for radical dose-escalated radiotherapy treatment of prostate cancer. *Int. J. Radiation Oncol. Biol. Phys.*, 40(1):221–231, 1998.

23. W. D. Neve, F. Heuvel, et al. Interactive use of on–line portal imaging in pelvic radiation. *Int. J. Radiation Oncology Biol. Phys.*, 25:517–524, 1993.

24. C. Studholme et al. Incorporating connected region labelling into automated image registration using mutual information. In *Proc. of MMBIA'96*, pages 23–31, 1996.

25. P. Viola and W. M. Wells. Alignment by maximization of mutual information. *Fifth Int. Conf. on Computer Vision*, pages 16–23, 1995.

26. J. Weese et al. 2D/3D registration of pre–operative ct images and intra–operative x–ray projections for image guided surgery. In H.Lemke et al., editors, *Comp. Assist. Rad. and Surg.*, pages 833–838. 1997.

Registration of Video Images to Tomographic Images by Optimising Mutual Information Using Texture Mapping

M. J. Clarkson, D. Rueckert, A. P. King, P. J. Edwards, D. L. G. Hill, and D. J. Hawkes

Division of Radiological Sciences and Medical Engineering
The Guy's, King's and St. Thomas' Schools of Medicine and Dentistry
Guy's Hospital, London SE1 9RT, UK

Abstract. In this paper we propose a novel tracking method to update the pose of stereo video cameras with respect to a surface model derived from a 3D tomographic image. This has a number of applications in image guided interventions and therapy. Registration of 2D video images to the pre-operative 3D image provides a mapping between image and physical space and enables a perspective projection of the pre-operative data to be overlaid onto the video image. Assuming an initial registration can be achieved, we propose a method for updating the registration, which is based on image intensity and texture mapping. We performed five experiments on simulated, phantom and volunteer data and validated the algorithm against an accurate gold standard in all three cases. We measured the mean 3D error of our tracking algorithm to be 1.05 mm for the simulation and 1.89 mm for the volunteer data. Visually this corresponds to a good registration.

1 Introduction

We consider the general problem of relating pre-operative MR/CT data to an intra-operative scene for image guided interventions. Registration of 2D video images to the 3D pre-operative data provides a link between what is currently visible in the intra-operative scene and the information present in the 3D pre-operative data. The potential applications of such a registration method will be in image guided surgery in which video, endoscopy or microscopy images are used. Clinical applications include neurosurgery, ENT surgery, spinal surgery, image guided laproscopy and high precision radiotherapy. We have previously considered registering video images taken from an operating microscope to CT data, using video image intensity directly [3]. We propose a novel method of updating the registration over a period of time using a tracking algorithm that incorporates texture mapping and describe work in progress in applying the algorithm to clinical data.

A video image is a projection of the 3D scene onto a 2D imaging plane. This can be characterised by the pinhole camera model [6]. Given a point in the 3D scene, denoted in homogeneous coordinates by $\mathbf{x} = (x, y, z, 1)$ the aim is to find the 3×4 transformation matrix $\mathbf{G}$ that relates $\mathbf{x}$ to a point on the 2D image denoted by $\mathbf{u} = (u, v, 1)$

$$k\mathbf{u}^T = \mathbf{G}\,\mathbf{x}^T . \tag{1}$$

The matrix $\mathbf{G}$ represents a rigid body transformation from 3D scene coordinates to 3D camera coordinates, followed by a projective transformation onto the 2D image plane and k represents a scale factor for homogeneous coordinates. The rigid body transformation describes the pose (position and orientation) of the camera relative to the scene, and has six degrees of freedom. The projective transformation is determined by the internal characteristics of the camera. Assuming fixed zoom and focus, the camera can be calibrated so that the projective transformation is known. This reduces the registration problem to finding the six rigid body parameters which determine the camera pose.

1.1   Previous Work

The problem of estimating the pose of a camera with respect to an object is an essential step in many machine vision applications. Pose estimation can be achieved through corresponding pairs of 2D and 3D features, such as points [8] or points and lines [11]. The accuracy of the pose estimation algorithm is determined by the number of features, the accuracy with which the 2D and 3D coordinates of the features are known and the accuracy of their correspondence. Often many features are required for an accurate estimate of the pose. Registration of 3D medical images to 2D video images of a patient using anatomical point based methods is likely to be inaccurate. The landmark points are often difficult to localise accurately in the 3D image due to limited resolution and contrast. In addition, localisation of landmarks can be difficult in the 2D image as some landmarks may be hidden or prone to movement. This leads to poor registration accuracy.

Colchester *et al.* [4] have described a system in which a light pattern is projected onto the skin surface. Video images from a pair of calibrated cameras are used to reconstruct the illuminated surface, which is then registered to a surface model derived from the 3D image. Viola [15] demonstrated the use of an information theoretic framework to register a surface model to a video image of a skull phantom. A video image of an object will be related to a 3D model of the object by a geometric transformation mapping model points to image points, and an imaging function describing lighting conditions, surface properties, imaging device characteristics and so on. In general, reflectance is a function of lighting direction, surface normal and viewing direction. If the light source can be assumed to be far from the object, its rays will be parallel. In addition if the camera is assumed to be far from the object, then the viewing direction at each point will be constant. Thus the observed intensity will vary with the surface normal direction. The problem of pose estimation can then be formulated as maximising the mutual information between the video intensities and the surface normal vectors of the model. This does not assume a specific lighting model, it only assumes that a relationship between the video intensities and the surface normals exists.

We have previously demonstrated a registration algorithm based on maximising the mutual information between video and rendered image intensities alone. We have studied several information theoretic methods for utilising the information from multiple video and rendered images which showed that a mean 3D error of 1.05 mm using five video views can be achieved [3].

1.2   Objectives

We present a novel tracking algorithm, which is used to maintain registration between multiple video cameras and a 3D surface model, through the use of the video image intensities and texture (colour) mapping. In addition we use an accurate gold standard to validate the accuracy of our algorithm. We performed five tracking experiments on simulated, phantom and volunteer data and tested the tracking over a range of motion that might be encountered during, for example, a neurosurgical or ENT procedure without head immobilization.

2   Methods

2.1   Coordinate Transformation

The matrix $\mathbf{G}$ in equation (1) represents a transformation from 3D scene coordinates to 2D video image pixels. In this paper we use stereo pairs of cameras. Let $i = 1, 2$ denote the camera number. Using these two cameras we acquire or simulate a sequence of video images. Let $j = 1 \ldots N$ denote the video image number. The matrix $\mathbf{G}$ will be different for each camera and for each video image. Therefore let $\mathbf{G}_{ij}$ be the transformation from 3D scene coordinates to 2D video image pixels for camera i and for video image j. The matrix $\mathbf{G}_{ij}$ can be represented as

$$\mathbf{G}_{ij} = \mathbf{P}_i \, \mathbf{T}_{ij} \, . \tag{2}$$

First we perform tracking experiments using a plastic skull phantom. In this case the 3D coordinate system is defined by the CT coordinate system. $\mathbf{T}_{ij}$ is a transformation from 3D CT coordinates to 3D camera coordinates, and $\mathbf{P}_i$ is a transformation from 3D camera coordinates into 2D image pixels. In addition we perform experiments using a volunteer who has been fitted with a locking dental registration device as described in Edwards et al. [5]. In volunteer based experiments $\mathbf{T}_{ij}$ is a transformation from MR coordinates to the camera coordinate system. The matrix $\mathbf{P}_i$ is calculated using a calibration process and is fixed throughout the tracking process. Consider a sequence of N images where $j = 1 \ldots N$ taken from camera i. Assume that for both cameras in the system $i = 1, 2$, the initial registration of 3D image coordinates to the video image pixels is known. This means that for $j = 1$, $\mathbf{T}_{i1}$ is known. The goal of the tracking is to find the rigid body transformation which when combined with the initial known registration matrix $\mathbf{T}_{i1}$ and camera calibration matrix $\mathbf{P}_i$, transforms 3D image points onto the corresponding 2D video image pixels throughout a sequence of video images. The desired rigid body transformation is represented by $\mathbf{R}_j$ where

$$\hat{\mathbf{T}}_{ij} = \mathbf{T}_{i1} \, \mathbf{R}_j \, . \tag{3}$$

$\hat{\mathbf{T}}_{ij}$ is the updated rigid body transform produced by our algorithm. The matrix $\mathbf{R}_j$ is determined by six parameters. These are t_x, t_y and t_z which represent translations with respect to the x, y and z axes respectively, and r_x, r_y and r_z which represent rotations about the x, y and z axes respectively. The matrix $\mathbf{R}_j$ is the output of the algorithm after each video frame, j, in the sequence. If the gold standard transformation $\mathbf{T}_{ij}$ is known then $\hat{\mathbf{T}}_{ij}$ should be approximately equal to $\mathbf{T}_{ij}$. Thus the tracking problem is to determine the six degrees of freedom t_x, t_y, t_z, r_x, r_y and r_z which updates the transformation from 3D model coordinates to 2D pixel coordinates for each video frame in a sequence.

2.2   Tracking Without Texture Mapping

The problem of finding the correct alignment for each video frame can be seen as a problem of re-registration. To find the correct registration our algorithm produces a rendering of the surface model and compares it to the video image using mutual information. Given a video image with intensities $a \in A$ and a rendered image with intensities $b \in B$, we can calculate the mutual information of A and B denoted by $I(A; B)$ using

$$I(A; B) = H(A) + H(B) - H(A, B) . \tag{4}$$

where H denotes the Shannon entropy [12]. Registration of one video image to a 3D image is performed by maximising $I(A; B)$ by varying the six transformation parameters $t_x \dots r_z$ and using a simple gradient ascent search strategy.

In some cases the registration of mono view video images can fail due to the symmetry of the surface or the lack of surface structure. Furthermore the registration of mono view video images is often poorly constrained along the optical axis of the video camera. We have previously shown that the use of stereo or multiple view video images can improve the accuracy, precision and robustness of the registration compared to the mono view case [3]. In our experiments images are always acquired in stereo pairs, and the transformation from one camera to the other is known. This means that we have two video images, denoted by A_1 and A_2, and we can produce the two corresponding rendered images, denoted by B_1 and B_2. Registration is performed by maximising an objective function which corresponds to the sum of the mutual information between each video image and the rendered image, i.e. $I(A_1; B_1) + I(A_2; B_2)$. As before the objective function is maximised using a simple gradient ascent search strategy.

2.3   Tracking With Texture Mapping

Texture mapping, or more specifically colour mapping [2] is a common computer graphics technique for adding realism to rendered images [6]. Each vertex in a surface model is given a 2D texture coordinate, which maps it to a position in a 2D texture image. The graphics pipeline then maps the texture image onto a surface patch of the 3D model. This can be seen in figure 1. The question arises as to how to map the video texture accurately to the surface model. As mentioned above, we start the tracking process with a known registration $\mathbf{G}_{i1} = \mathbf{P}_i \, \mathbf{T}_{i1}$. Using this equation, we take points in the surface model and project them onto 2D image pixels, and use these as the corresponding texture coordinates. The accuracy of the texture mapping is therefore determined by the accuracy of the initial registration.

Without texture mapping we were matching a rendering of a surface with a video image. This assumes that the rendering looks fairly similar to the video image. It also

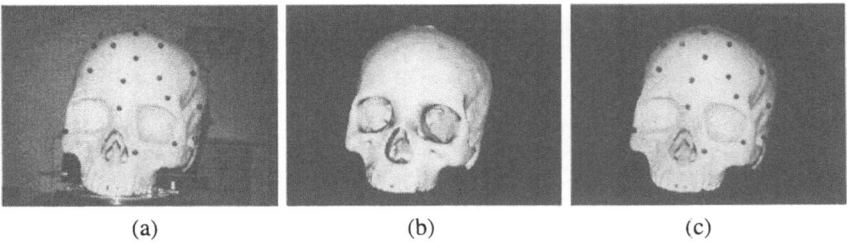

(a)   (b)   (c)

Fig. 1. Texture Mapping Example: (a) sample video image, (b) rendering of a registered model, (c) rendering of the same model with the video texture pasted onto the surface.

assumes that only one surface is being imaged and that this surface has constant reflectance. The algorithm is trying to match the component of diffuse reflection in the video image intensities. However, with texture mapping we can associate information from the video image directly with the 3D model. This means we now have additional knowledge about the surface texture of the 3D object. The algorithm can proceed as before, by producing a rendering, where the rendered image intensities are a projection of the texture map intensities, and matching this to subsequent frames in a video sequence. This can be seen as a region matching algorithm, with mutual information measuring the similarity of a surface patch in the current image, with its known appearance in the previous image.

3 Experiment Design

After registration to each video frame j, the parameters $t_x \ldots r_z$ produce an estimate $\hat{\mathbf{T}}_{ij}$ of the gold standard matrix $\mathbf{T}_{ij}$. To assess the error in the registration we measured the projection error in mm. The projection error is the mean of the Euclidean distance between a 3D point and the closest point on a line projected through the corresponding 2D point. In addition we measured the 3D error in mm, which is the mean of the Euclidean distance between a 3D point multiplied by the gold standard matrix $\mathbf{T}_{ij}$, and the same 3D point multiplied by the estimated rigid body matrix $\hat{\mathbf{T}}_{ij}$ [3]. Furthermore we can measure the 3D distance between video frames by measuring the mean of the Euclidean distance between a 3D point, multiplied by the gold standard matrix $\mathbf{T}_{ij}$, and the same point multiplied by the gold standard matrix of the frame before $\mathbf{T}_{ij-1}$. We can measure the accumulative 3D distance as the sum of the 3D distance over each frame of the video sequence.

3.1 Tracking Simulation

A CT scan (Philips TOMOSCAN SR 7000 $0.488 \times 0.488 \times 1.0$ mm, $512 \times 512 \times 142$ voxels) of a plastic skull phantom was acquired. Our skull phantom has 23, 5 mm aluminium ball bearings which have been painted black attached to it. Two video images were taken of the skull phantom, shown in figure 2(a) and (b), and a 3D surface model was extracted from the CT scan using VTK [13]. The initial registration can be calculated using six or more pairs of corresponding 2D and 3D points. The aluminium

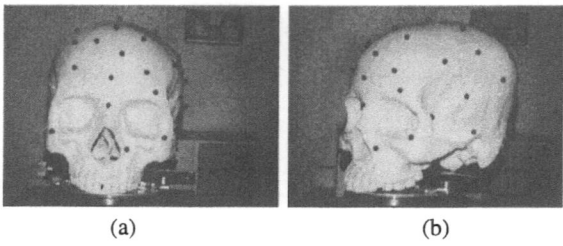

(a)   (b)

Fig. 2. Example images: (a) and (b) are the stereo pair used for the skull phantom experiments as described in section 3.1.

ball bearings can be accurately localised in the 3D image using an intensity weighted centre of gravity operator [1], and interactively localised in the 2D images. We used Tsai's [14] camera calibration method to calculate the matrices $\mathbf{P}_i$ and $\mathbf{T}_{i1}$ for the two cameras $i = 1, 2$. The two camera views were separated by 45 degrees. The video image texture was mapped onto the surface model by projecting the surface model points onto the texture image. We generated 100 pairs of simulated images. This was accomplished by changing the pose of the surface model with respect to each camera view and producing a corresponding pair of texture mapped renderings, ie. one rendering for each view. The change of the model pose between each frame was a rotation of one degree. The sequence was 10 rotations to the left, 10 up, 20 right, 20 down, 20 left, 10 up and 10 right. We added zero mean, Gaussian noise ($\sigma = 7$) to these simulated images. The value of σ was chosen to simulate video image noise. We then performed a 'mono view' tracking experiment by taking the sequence of simulated images for camera $i = 1$ and using the known initial registration $\mathbf{T}_{i1}$ to initialise the tracking algorithm. The algorithm then attempted to recover the transformations $\mathbf{R}_j$ for $j = 2 \ldots 100$. We repeated this experiment, performing a 'stereo view' tracking experiment by taking the sequence of images for both cameras $i = 1, 2$, and using our algorithm to recover the transformations $\mathbf{R}_j$ for $j = 2 \ldots 100$.

3.2   Tracking a Skull Phantom

We subsequently took a series of real video images of the same skull phantom. The skull phantom was placed on a goniometer and a sequence of 21 images was taken, where the skull was rotated by 2 degrees clockwise between each image. The 3D surface model was registered to the initial view, using the above method and the algorithm used to recover the rotating motion.

3.3   Tracking a Volunteer

We then tested the algorithm on images of a volunteer. An MRI scan ($1.016 \times 1.016 \times 1.250$ mm, $256 \times 256 \times 150$ voxels) was taken of the volunteer. This was corrected for scaling errors [9], and a skin surface extracted using VTK [13]. The volunteer was scanned whilst wearing a locking acrylic dental stent (LADS) [5]. A stereo pair of video cameras were fixed with respect to each other and calibrated using SVD [7], which produces the matrix $\mathbf{P}_i$ for each camera $i = 1, 2$ as mentioned in section 2.1.

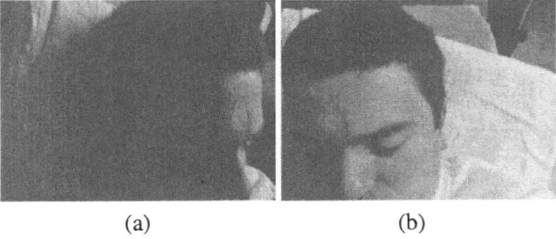

(a)   (b)

Fig. 3. Example images: (a) and (b) are the stereo pair used for volunteer experiments, as described in section 3.3.

A bivariate polynomial deformation field for each camera was calculated to correct for distortion effects. The translational separation of the two cameras was approximately 30 centimetres and the disparity between their optical axes was approximately 45 degrees. Using the LADS [5] we calculate the gold standard transformation $\mathbf{T}_{ij}$ for each camera $i = 1, 2$ and for each image $j = 1 \ldots 25$. We then performed a 'mono view' tracking experiment by taking the sequence of simulated images for camera $i = 2$ and using the known initial registration $\mathbf{T}_{i1}$ to initialise the tracking algorithm. The algorithm then attempted to recover the transformations $\mathbf{R}_j$ for $j = 2 \ldots 25$. Subsequently we repeated this experiment, performing a 'stereo view' tracking experiment by taking the sequence of images for both cameras $i = 1, 2$, and using our algorithm to recover the transformations $\mathbf{R}_j$ for $j = 2 \ldots 25$.

4 Results

Figure 4 (a) shows a graph of the results for the mono view simulation. The simulation did not include translations parallel to the optical axis of the camera so we would expect the mono tracking algorithm to work well. The mean projection error and mean 3D errors are 1.01 and 1.19 mm respectively for the 100 frames. Figure 4 (b) shows the results for the phantom tracking experiment. The sequence was a set of images, where the phantom had been rotated by 2 degrees between each video image. It can be seen that the tracking algorithm misses the first few frames, but then manages to recover approximately 2 degrees for the subsequent frames. The mean and standard deviation of the rotation estimates is 1.85 ± 0.76 mm. Figure 5 (a) shows the results for the mono view experiment on the volunteer. This graph shows that projection error and 3D error can be significantly different. Specifically the projection error can be reasonably low while the 3D error is high. A mono view experiment can fail to recover translations along the optical axis of the camera [3, 10]. Figure 5 (b) shows the 3D error plotted against the accumulative 3D distance (the sum of 3D distance over each frame of the video sequence), which shows that the camera has moved 140mm. Figure 6(a) shows that with stereo views, the tracking performance is much better. An example pair of images is shown in figure 3. It can be seen that of the two images, one is significantly lower in contrast than the other. Figure 6(b) shows the 3D error as a function of accumulative 3D distance moved. Table 1 summarises the performance of the mono and stereo view algorithms. The simulation experiment performed well for both mono and stereo views with a mean 3D error of 1.19 and 1.05 mm respectively over the whole of the 100 frames sequence. For the volunteer tracking experiment, it can be seen that the stereo algorithm performs significantly better. However after 14 frames, corresponding to 140 mm of accumulative 3D movement, the stereo algorithm fails to track successfully.

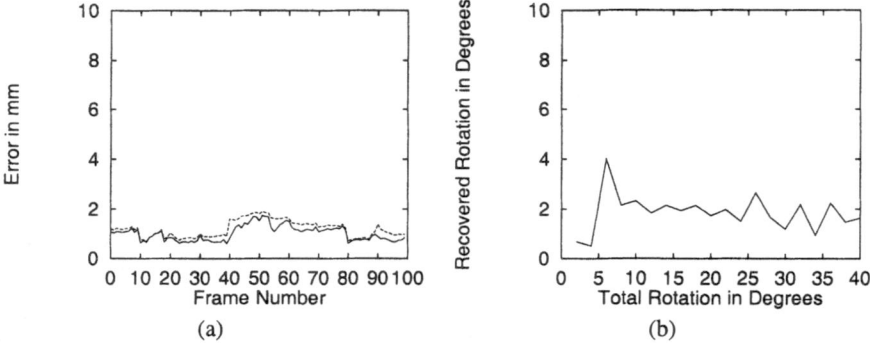

Fig. 4. 3D (dotted line) and projection (solid line) errors for (a) the mono view simulation and (b) the mono view phantom experiment. As described in sections 3.1 and 3.1 respectively.

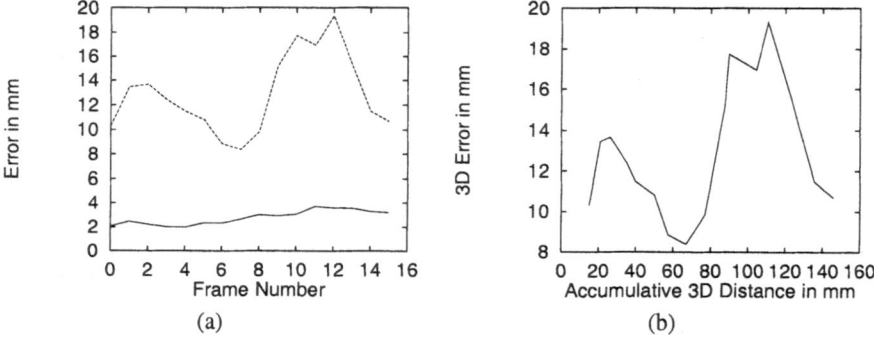

Fig. 5. (a) 3D error (dotted line) and projection error (solid line) for mono view, volunteer tracking experiment. (b) 3D error plotted against the accumulative 3D distance for the mono view volunteer tracking experiment. See section 3.3.

Table 1. A comparison of mono view and stereo view performance for (a) the simulation and (b) the volunteer experiments.

Case	Projection Error	3D Error
Mono	1.01	1.19
Stereo	0.83	1.05

(a)

Case	Projection Error	3D Error
Mono	2.75	13.03
Stereo	0.74	1.89

(b)

5 Conclusions

This paper has described a new tracking algorithm that uses texture mapping to register a pair of video images to a 3D surface model derived from MR/CT. We tested the algorithm with simulated data. This achieved registration with a mean 3D error of 1.05

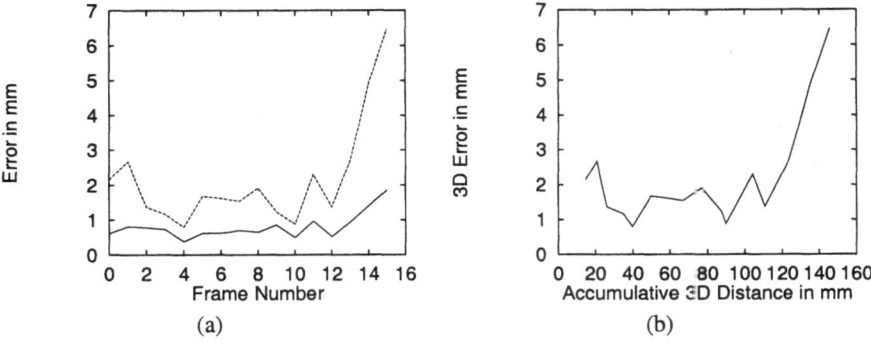

Fig. 6. (a) 3D Error (dotted line) and Projection Error (solid line) for stereo view, volunteer tracking experiment. (b) 3D Error plotted against the Accumulated 3D Distance for the stereo view volunteer tracking experiment. See section 3.3

mm for stereo views. This level of accuracy is largely determined by the step size of the gradient ascent algorithm, and so could be improved, but with increased computational cost. The mono tracking experiments with the phantom (section 3.1) and the volunteer (section 3.3) showed that tracking performance is poor if only one camera is used. However tracking was possible by using two camera views. We tested the tracking over a range of motion that might be encountered during for example a neurosurgical or ENT procedure without head immobilization. Future work will concentrate on improving robustness and assessing the effect of contrast, visible texture, surface area and surface curvature. In addition, this work uses a simple gradient ascent search method to maximise the mutual information. This could be improved by using predictive methods such as the Kalman filter.

Acknowledgements

MJC would like to thank the Engineering and Physical Sciences Research Council for funding his Ph.D. studentship, and also Jane Blackall, Graeme Penney and Daryl De-Cuhna at the Computational Imaging Science Group, for their assistance.

References

1. C. B. Bose and I. Amir. Design of fiducials for accurate registration using machine vision. *IEEE Transactions on Pattern Analysis And Machine Intelligence*, 12(12):1196–1200, 1990.
2. E. Catmull. Computer display of curved surfaces. In *Proceedings of the Conference on Computer Graphics, Pattern Recognition and Data Structures*, pages 11–17, New York, May 1975. IEEE Computer Society.
3. M. J. Clarkson, D. Rueckert, D. L. G. Hill, and D. J. Hawkes. Registration of multiple video images to pre-operative CT for image guided surgery. In *Proceedings of SPIE Medical Imaging 1999 - in press*, 1999.
4. A. C. F. Colchester, J. Zhao, S. K. Holton-Tainter, C. J. Henri, N. Maitland, P. T. E. Roberts, C. G. Harris, and R. J. Evans. Development and preliminary evaluation of VISLAN, a surgical planning and guidance system using intra-operative video imaging. *Medical Image Analysis*, 1(1):73–90, 1996.

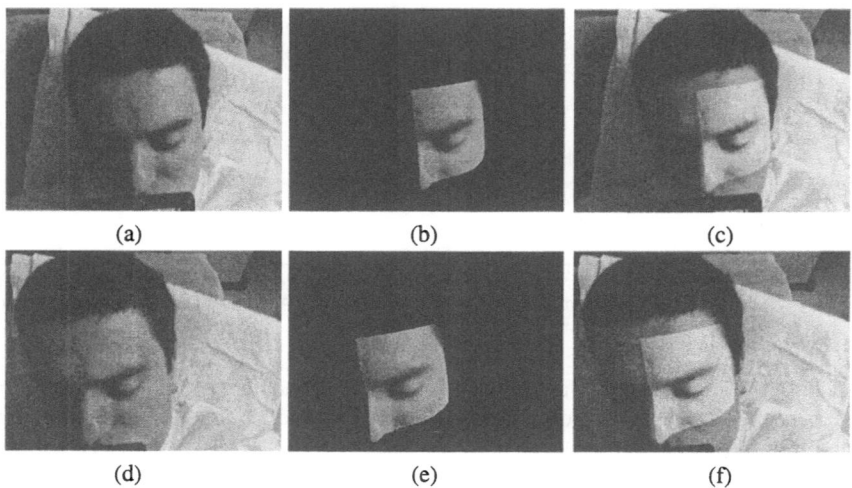

(a)   (b)   (c)

(d)   (e)   (f)

Fig. 7. Results of volunteer tracking experiment: (a) Video image 1 (b) Texture mapped model (c) Model registered and overlaid on video image, at the initial pose, before tracking. (d) Video image 12 (e) Texture mapped model at the tracked pose (f) Model registered and overlaid on video image at the tracked pose.

5. P. J. Edwards, A. P. King, D. J. Hawkes, O. Fleig, C. R. Maurer Jr., D. L. G. Hill, M. R. Fenlon, D. A. de Cunha, R. P. Gaston, S. Chandra, J. Mannss, A . J. Strong, M. J. Gleeson, and T. C. S. Cox. Stereo augmented reality in the surgical microscope. In *Proceedings MMVR.*, 1999.

6. J. Foley, A. van Dam, S. Feiner, and J. Hughs. *Computer Graphics 2nd Edition.* Addison Wesley, 1990.

7. R. C. Gonzalez and R. E. Woods. *Digital Image Processing.* Addison-Wesley Publishing Company, 1992.

8. R. B. Haralick, H. Joo, C-N. Lee, X. Zhuang, V. G. Vaidya, and M. B. Kim. Pose estimation from corresponding point data. *IEEE Transactions On Systems, Man, and Cybernetics*, 19(6):1426–1445, 1989.

9. D. L. G. Hill, C. R. Maurer Jr., C. Studholme, J. M. Fitzpatrick, and D. J. Hawkes. Correcting scaling errors in tomographic images using a nine degree of freedom registration algorithm. *Journal of Computer Assisted Tomography*, 22(2):317–323, 1998.

10. M. E. Leventon, W. M. Wells III, and W. E. L. Grimson. Multiple view 2D-3D Mutual Information registration. In *Image Understanding Workshop*, 1997.

11. T.Q. Phong, R. Horaud, and P. D. Tao. Object pose from 2D to 3D point and line correspondences. *International Journal Of Computer Vision*, 15:225–243, 1995.

12. F. M. Reza. *An Introduction To Information Theory.* McGraw Hill, 1961.

13. W. Schroeder, Martin K., B. Lorensen, L. Avila, R. Avila, and C. Law. *The Visualization Toolkit An Object-Oriented Approach to 3D Graphics.* Prentice-Hall, ISBN: 0-13-954694-4, 1997.

14. R.Y. Tsai. A versatile camera calibration technique for high-accuracy 3D machine vision metrology using off-the-shelf TV cameras and lenses. *IEEE Journal Of Robotics and Automation*, RA-3(4):323–344, 1987.

15. P. Viola and W. M. Wells III. Alignment by Maximization of Mutual Information. *International Journal of Computer Vision*, 24(2):137–154, 1997.

Brain Atlas Deformation in the Presence of Large Space-occupying Tumors

B. M. Dawant[1], S. L. Hartmann[2], and S. Gadamsety[1]

[1]Department of Electrical and Computer Engineering,
[2]Department of Biomedical Engineering,
Vanderbilt University, Nashville, Tennessee
{dawant, slh, srikanth}@vuse.vanderbilt.edu

Abstract. Brain atlases contain a wealth of information that could be used for radiation therapy or neurosurgical planning. So far, however, when large space occupying tumors and lesions drastically alter the shape of brain structures and substructures, atlas-based methods have been of limited use. In this work we present a new technique that permits warping a brain atlas onto image volumes in which large lesions are present. This technique involves several steps: a global registration to bring the two volumes into approximate correspondence, a local registration to warp the atlas onto the patient volume, the seeding of the warped atlas with a synthetic tumor, and the deformation of the seeded atlas. Global registration is performed using a mutual information criterion. The method we have used for atlas warping is derived from optical flow principles. Preliminary results obtained on real patient images are being presented. These results indicate that the method we propose can be used to automatically segment structures of interest in brains with gross deformation. Potential areas of application for this method include automatic labeling of critical structures for radiation therapy and presurgical planning.

Keywords: brain atlas, registration, deformation, segmentation

1 Introduction

In recent years, atlas-based methods have been proposed to segment automatically structures and substructures in medical images. These methods rely on the existence of a reference image volume (the atlas) in which structures of interest have been carefully segmented, possibly by hand. To segment a new image volume, a transformation that registers the atlas to this volume is first computed. This transformation is then used to project labeled structures from the atlas onto the image volume to be segmented. Medical image registration is a topic that has been studied by many researchers in the field over the years (see for instance Maintz [1] for a recent review article). But, the vast majority of these methods were developed to register multi-modal information (e.g. PET, CT, and MR) pertaining to a single subject. For this type of application, global transformation matrices involving rotation, translation, scaling, and possibly skew are sufficient. But, this type of transformation is unable to take into account non-linear differences between brain morphology and is thus inadequate for accurate atlas-based segmentation and labeling. A number of methods have been proposed that permit the computation of transformations with more degrees of freedom capable of warping one brain onto the other. Collins [2] has used a multi-resolution approach in which the overall non-linear transformation is composed of a set of local linear deformations obtained by maximizing the correlation of intensity and gradient features in the images to be registered. Bajcsy [3], [4] used an elastic model approach. Algorithms based on viscous fluid models were put forth by Christensen [5] and Bro-Nielsen [6]. Meyer [7] has proposed a technique based on thin-plate splines in which an optimizer is used to adjust the position of homologous control points in homologous data sets. Rueckert [8] uses a similar approach but with B-splines. Woods [9] relies on polynomials up to order five. Thirion [10] proposed a method called "demons" that is similar to an optical flow approach for small displacements and that trades the rigor of physical modeling for simplicity of implementation and speed of execution. These techniques have great potential for the creation of statistical atlases or for the comparison of morphological characteristics between populations. But, these methods have been limited to cases without gross anatomical abnormalities. Atlas-based methods have therefore not yet been used for applications such as radiation therapy or presurgical planning when tumors dramatically alter the morphology of the brain. In a recent paper [11], a method based on a biomechanical model of the brain has been proposed for atlas deformation in the presence of gross abnormalities. The proposed method consists of several steps. First, the tumor is shrunk to a small mass, resulting in an estimate of the brain before tumor growth. Tumor shrinking is modeled as a uniform contraction and brain deformation resulting from this contraction is computed using finite element methods. This results in a "normal" brain that can be registered to an atlas. After registration, the tumor is grown back to its original shape using the inverse of the procedure used for shrinking the tumor. We have the same goal as Kyriacou and Davatzikos, i.e., we want to be able to use the wealth of information provided by atlases for applications such as radiation therapy or surgical planning even when large tumors drastically alter brain morphology, but our approach is different. In particular, we do not rely on a biomechanical model of the brain and we do not need to shrink the tumor to be able to register the normal atlas with the pathological brain. In the remainder of this paper we describe our method, present results we have obtained on real patient data, and discuss ways by which our current method can be improved.

2. Methods

2.1 Data sets

Results presented in this study were obtained on two data sets acquired with a General Electric 1.5 Tesla Signa MR scanner using a spoiled gradient echo pulse sequence.

Each volume consists of 128 sagittal slices, and each slice has dimensions of 256 x 256 pixels. Voxel dimensions are .94 x .94 x 1.3 mm^3. Both the volumes have been obtained after injection of Gadolinium.

2.2 Atlas deformation

Our method involves the following steps. First, a similarity transformation (three rotation angles, three translation vectors, and three scaling factors) is computed to globally register the atlas and the patient volumes. The global transformation is computed using the MIRIT package developed at the Catholic University of Leuven [12]. Mutual information is used as the similarity criterion. Next, a highly non-linear transformation that brings the atlas and the patient volume in local correspondence is computed. The warped atlas is then "seeded" with a small structure centered approximately on the centroid of the tumor. Finally, the non-linear deformation algorithm is applied to the seeded warped atlas. In this step, the seeded tumor is grown until it reaches the size of the actual tumor and surrounding tissues in the atlas are displaced and deformed.

Local transformation: Thirion has presented the problem of image matching in terms of "demons" (by analogy with Maxwell's demons). This is a general framework in which object boundaries in one image are viewed as semi-permeable membranes. The other image, considered as a deformable grid, diffuses through these interfaces driven by the action of effectors (the demons) situated within the membranes. Various kinds of demons can be designed to apply this paradigm to specific applications. In the particular case of deformations based on voxel-by-voxel intensity similarity, the demons paradigm is similar to optical flow methods. It is an independent implementation of this approach [13] in which the displacement vector for each voxel is computed as follows that has been used in this study.

$$\vec{v}_{I_2 \to I_1} = \frac{(I_2 - I_1)\vec{\nabla}I_1}{\vec{\nabla}I_1^{\,2} + (I_2 - I_1)^2} \tag{1}$$

With I1 and I2 the intensity values of he images to be matched. In this approach, global smoothness of the displacement field is not enforced. Rather than using a global regularization method, a more local constraint imposing similar displacements for nearby pixels can be imposed by smoothing this field with, for instance, a Gaussian filter. The standard deviation of the Gaussian filter can also be used to change the characteristics of the matching transformation. The larger the standard deviation of the filter, the less elastic the transformation.

It should also be mentioned that large morphological differences between image volumes could render optical flow methods completely ineffective because the assumption of small displacement is violated. Two mechanisms have been used to make the algorithm more robust to large differences. First, the algorithm is applied in a hierarchical way. Second, a mechanism has been implemented that maintains compatibility between the forward and the reverse deformation fields. As proposed in [10], [15] this is done by computing the deformation field T12 (the deformation field warping image 1 onto image 2) and the deformation field T21 (the deformation field warping image 2 onto image 1) and distributing the residual R=T12 ° T21 onto these two fields. This construct, coupled with the smoothing of the field prevents its tearing as well as crossing over of neighborhood pixels. It also provides a way to obtain the inverse transformation.

Atlas seeding. As the results will show, after the first two steps (i.e, similarity transformation and atlas deformation), the atlas and the brain to segment are in correspondence except in regions that have been drastically deformed by the tumor. The tumor is then outlined manually in the patient volume and the inside of this contour is assigned an intensity value different from the surrounding tissues. The seed is created by eroding the tumor mask of the patient, and is placed into the atlas volume.

Seeded atlas deformation. Once the atlas volume has been seeded, the deformation algorithm described earlier is applied a second time. This time, the algorithm attempts to warp the seeded atlas onto the patient image. Because the atlas has been seeded with a small region with the same intensity value as the delineated tumor, the algorithm grows the tumor seed until it reaches the size of the tumor in the patient volume. Because the deformation field is regularized with a Gaussian filter, the displacement field generated by the growth of the tumor also displaces surrounding tissues. As discussed earlier, the size and the standard deviation of the Gaussian filter used to regularize the displacement field determine the characteristics of the warping transformation. A small standard deviation only imposes very local constraints, thus resulting in transformations that are more elastic than those obtained with larger standard deviations. Here we have used two values for the standards deviation of the Gaussian filter. One for the 3D warping of the original atlas to the patient volume (step two in our approach) and one for the 3D deformation of the seeded atlas. To warp the original atlas to the patient volume we have selected a relatively high sigma value (2.0). This value was obtained experimentally and it was found to be a good compromise between deforming the atlas and preserving its structural integrity. For larger values, the algorithm is unable to deform the atlas enough to register it accurately with the patient volume. Smaller values can lead to transformations that are completely inaccurate over areas affected by the tumor. Indeed, prior to seeding, the normal volume does not have any structure that corresponds to and could be warped onto the tumor. The algorithm could thus warp arbitrary structures in the atlas volume in an attempt to minimize intensity differences between the atlas and the patient volume. After seeding, the atlas and the patient volume have corresponding structures. The standard deviation of the smoothing filter can thus be reduced, which permits larger local deformation required to grow the tumor and displace surrounding tissues. For the data set used in this study a sigma of 0.5 was used for the 3D deformation of the seeded atlas. Again, this value was obtained experimentally.

3   Results

Figure 1 illustrates the results obtained after the first two steps. In each of these panels, the images on the right show one slice in a patient volume. The images on the left show the slice with the same index in the volume obtained after registering the atlas to the patient using a similarity transformation. The middle panels show the slice with the same index in the volume obtained by warping the volume on the left onto the volume on the right. The three top panels show one slice in the brain hemisphere without tumor; the three bottom panels show one slice in the hemisphere with a large space-occupying tumor.

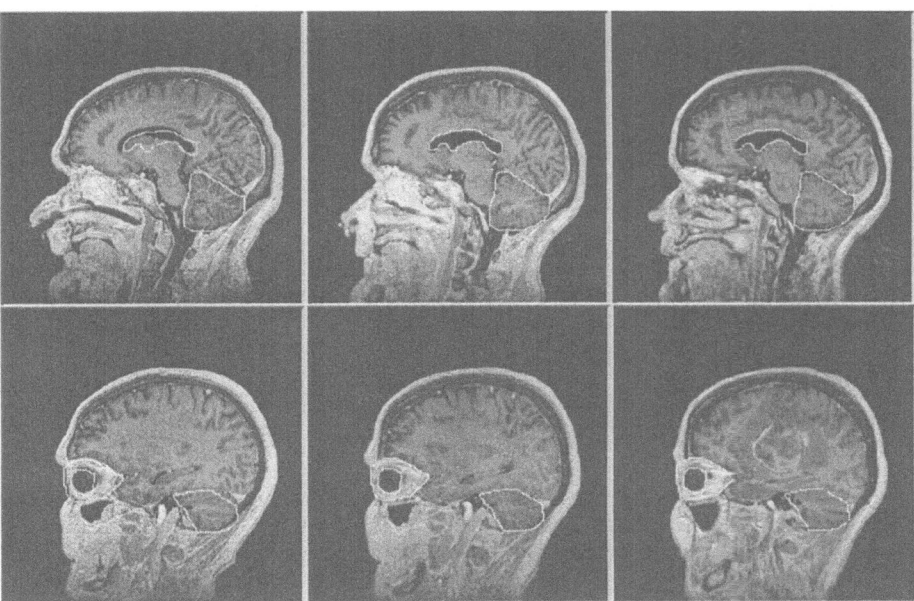

Fig. 1. Warping of the atlas to a patient volume. Right panels, patient volume. Left panels, global registration of the atlas to the patient volume. Middle panels, warping of the left volume onto the right volume. Top panels, hemisphere without tumor. Bottom panels, hemisphere with a large space-occupying tumor

Several important observations can be made from this figure. First of all, a nine degrees of freedom transformation is not sufficient to register the atlas to the patient volume. Contours have been drawn on the patient image (right panels) and echoed on the others. Note the registration inaccuracy around the ventricles, the cerebellum, and the eyes on the left panels. If a nine degrees of freedom transformation was sufficient, the contours drawn would also encircle precisely the regions of interest on the left panel images. Second, after warping (middle panels), structures that are far away from the tumor have been registered accurately, at least visually. A complete validation of this approach with quantitative validation on a number of structures of interest such as the optic nerve, optic chiasm, mamillary bodies, etc. has not yet been performed.

Equally important is the fact that the integrity of the structures in the atlas has not been compromised by the presence of the tumor in the patient volume. Figure 1 clearly shows that over the tumor region the atlas has simply not been deformed to make it similar to the volume with a tumor. This is a highly desirable behavior. Indeed, when a tumor is present in the patient volume, there is no similar structure in the atlas to which it could be matched. The algorithm could thus attempt to deform an arbitrary structure and match it to the tumor, thus resulting in a completely erroneous warping of the atlas.

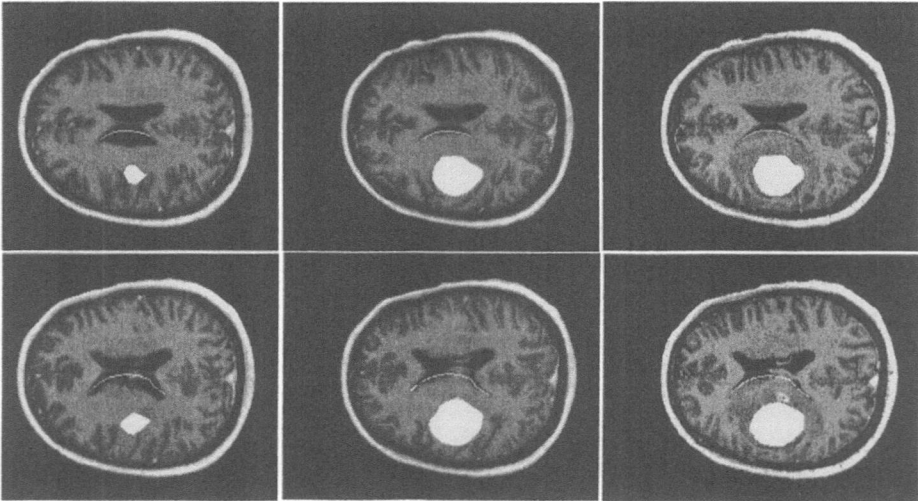

Fig. 2. Atlas seeding and deformation processes. Right, patient volume with manually delineated tumor. Left, warped atlas (same volume as left panel in figure 2) with tumor seed. Middle, seeded atlas after deformation. The top and bottom panels show different slice indexes.

Figure 2 illustrates the results obtained by seeding the atlas and warping the seeded atlas. The top and bottom panels of this figure show results on two different slices. The left panels in this figure are transverse slices in the volume obtained after deformation of the unseeded atlas. The right panels are transverse slices with the same index in the patient volume. The contour of the tumor has been delineated in the patient volume and the tumor has been assigned an arbitrary high value. The tumor region identified in the patient volume has been eroded to create the seed that has been placed in the warped atlas. The middle panels show the slices with the same indices in the volume obtained after warping the seeded atlas. Again, contours have been drawn on the patient volume (right panels) and copied on the other images. Prior to seed growing, the ventricles in the atlas kept their original shape. After seed growing, the ventricles and surrounding tissues such as the caudate have been displaced by the tumor. There is a good visual agreement between these contours and the actual structure boundary.

3   Discussion

This work is one of the first attempts at atlas deformation when the target volume contains large space-occupying lesions that drastically deform and displace normal anatomy. As opposed to our method, the approach proposed previously by Kyriacou and Davatzikos relies on biomechanical models. Their technique is based on a certain number of assumptions. First, white matter, gray matter, and cerebrospinal fluid regions should be known because the material constant in their model is different for each of these classes. Automatic segmentation of pathological image volumes may be challenging because the tumor and its edema may have intensity values similar to other tissue classes. More importantly, the tumor contraction algorithm used in their approach assumes the size of structures such as the ventricles prior to tumor growth to be known. Methods based on a-priori statistical information about ventricular shape and size have been proposed to address this problem but their effectiveness and accuracy has not yet been studied.

The method we propose does not require segmentation (except for the contours of the tumor in the patient volumes) and is not based on any explicit underlying mathematical model. This is both its strength and its potential weakness. It is its strength because the method is computationally simple and fast. The consistency of the deformation field is controlled by the smoothing filter and we have shown that by choosing values appropriately we can modify the behavior of the algorithm to obtain transformations that lead to accurate deformations both over normal and abnormal regions. The implicit assumption on which our approach is based is the local coherence of the deformation field, i.e., neighbor pixels are constrained to move in a similar way. The size of the smoothing filter defines the size of the neighborhood. The lack of an explicit underlying mathematical model is also the potential weakness of this approach. If the smoothing filter is not chosen correctly, the resulting transformation can be catastrophically wrong. It should also be noted, however, that, in our experience, both with normal volunteers [16] and with chronic alcoholics suffering from severe atrophy [17], the algorithm is robust with respect to the choice of the smoothing parameter.

Future work will involve improving the deformation algorithm by modeling structures of interest in the atlas volume. This will permit the automatic adaptation of the smoothing parameters according to the physical properties of these structures as well as guaranteeing the physical plausibility of the deformation field. Structures such as the optic nerve, optic chiasm, mamillary bodies, spinal cord, putamen, globus pallidus, etc. can indeed be labeled in the atlas and represented as 3D objects. The consistency of the deformation field could thus be imposed over these objects rather than on arbitrary neighborhoods, thus guaranteeing structural integrity in the deformed images.

Acknowledgements: This work was supported in part by NIH grant R01 AA 10583.

References

1. J.B. Maintz and M.A. Viergever, A survey of medical image registration. *Medical Image Analysis*, vol. 2, no. 1, Apr, 1998.
2. D.L. Collins, P. Neelin, T.M. Peters, and A.C. Evans, Automatic 3D intersubject registration of MR volumetric data in standardized Talairach space. *Journal of Computer Assisted Tomography*, vol. 18, no. 2, pp. 192-205, 1994.
3. R. Bajcsy and S. Kovacic, Multiresolution elastic matching. *Computer Vision, Graphics, and Image Processing*, vol. 46, pp. 1-21, 1989.
4. J.C. Gee, M. Reivich, and R. Bajcsy, Elastically deforming 3D atlas to match anatomical brain images. *Journal of Computer Assisted Tomography*, vol. 17 , no. 2, pp. 225-236, 1993.
5. G.E. Christensen, M.I. Miller, and M. Vannier, 3D brain mapping using a deformable neuroanatomy. *Phys Med Biol*, vol. 39, pp. 609-618, 1994.
6. M. Bro-Nielsen and C. Gramkow, Fast fluid registration of medical images. eds. K.H. Hohne and R. Kikinis. 1131, pp. 267-276, 1996. *Visualization in Biomedical Computing.* Hamburg, Germany.
7. C.R. Meyer, J.L. Boes, B. Kim, P. Bland, K.R. Zasadny, P.V. Kison, K. Koral, K.A. Frey, and R.L. Wahl, Demonstration of accuracy and clinical versatility of mutual information for automatic multimodality image fusion using affine and thin plate spline warped geometric deformations. *Medical Image Analysis*, vol. 3, pp. 195-206, 1997.
8. D. Rueckert, C. Hayes, C. Studholme, P. Summers, M. Leach, and D.J. Hawkes , Non-rigid registration of breast MR images using mutual information. *MICCAI Proceedings*, 1496, pp. 1144-1152, 1998.
9. R.P. Woods, S.T. Grafton, J.D.G. Watson, N.L. Sicotte, and J.C. Mazziotta, Automated image registration: II. Intersubject validation of linear and nonlinear models. *Journal of Computer Assisted Tomography*, vol. 22, no. 1, pp. 153-165, 1998.
10. J.-P. Thirion, Image matching as a diffusion process: an analogy with Maxwell's demons. *Medical Image Analysis*, vol. 2, no. 3, pp. 243-260, 1998.
11. S.K. Kyriacou and C. Davatzikos, A biomechanical model of soft tissue deformation, with applications to non-rigid registration of brain images with tumor pathology. *MICCAI Proceedings*, pp. 531-538, 1998.
12. F. Maes, A. Collignon, D. Vandermeulen, G. Marchal, and P. Suetens, Multi-modality image registration using information theory, MIRIT users manual, Version 97/08. *Internal report, Catholic University of Leuven*, 1997.
13. S.L. Hartmann, Automatic segmentation of medical images using optical flow based atlas deformation. *Master's Thesis, Department of Biomedical Engineering, Vanderbilt University*, 1998.
14. B. Horn and B. Schunck, Determining optical flow. *Artificial Intelligence*, vol. 17, pp. 185-203, 1981.
15. D.J. Burr, A dynamic model for image registration. *Computer Graphics and Image Processing*, vol. 15, pp. 102-112, 1981.
16. B.M. Dawant, J.-P. Thirion, F. Maes, D. Vandermeulen, and P. Demaerel, Automatic 3D segmentation of internal structures of the head in MR images using a combination of similarity and free form transformations. *SPIE Medical Imaging*, 1998.
17. S.L. Hartmann, M.H. Parks, H. Schlack, W.R. Riddle, R.R. Price, P.R. Martin, and B.M. Dawant, Automatic Computation of Brain and Cerebellum Volumes in Normal Subjects and Chronic Alcoholics. *IPMI Proceedings*, In Press, 1999.

Understanding the "Demon's Algorithm": 3D Non-rigid Registration by Gradient Descent

Xavier Pennec, Pascal Cachier, and Nicholas Ayache

INRIA Sophia - Epidaure Project
2004 Route des Lucioles BP 93
06902 Sophia Antipolis Cedex, France
{Xavier.Pennec, Pascal.Cachier, Nicholas.Ayache}@sophia.inria.fr
http://www-sop.inria.fr/epidaure/Epidaure-eng.html

Abstract. The "Demons Algorithm" in increasingly used for non-rigid registration of 3D medical images. However, if it is fast and usually accurate, the algorithm is based on intuitive ideas about image registration and it is difficult to predict when it will fail and why. We show in this paper that this algorithm can be considered as an approximation of a second order gradient descent on the sum of square of intensity differences criterion. We also reformulate Gaussian and physical model regularizations as minimization problems. Experimental results on synthetic and 3D Ultrasound images show that this formalization helps identifying the weak points of the algorithm and offers new research openings.

1 Introduction

Over recent years, a number of non-rigid registration techniques has been proposed. In 1981, Broit [Bro81] used the linear correlation as a measure of similarity between the two images to match. Bajcsy [BK89] differentiated this criterion and used a fixed fraction of its gradient as an external force to interact with a linear elasticity model.

Christensen [CJM97] shows that the linear elasticity, valid for small displacements, cannot guaranty the conservation of the topology of the objects as the displacements become larger: the Jacobian of the transformation can become negative. Thus, he proposed a viscous fluid model of transformations as it can handle larger displacement. This model is also linearized in practice.

Bro-Nielsen [BN96] started from the fluid model of Christensen and used the linearity of partial derivative equations to establish a regularization filter, several order of magnitude faster than the previous finite element method. He also justified his forces as the differential of the sum of square intensity differences criterion, but he still used a fixed fraction of this gradient, and show that Gaussian smoothing is an approximation of the linear elastic model.

Some authors [MMV98] tried to apply to non-rigid registration some criterions developed for rigid or affine matching using bloc-matching techniques. However, the evaluation of such a criterion imposes a minimal window size, thus limiting the resolution of these algorithm. Moreover, the regularization of the displacement field is usually implicit, i.e. only due to the integration of the criterion over the window, which means that there is no control on the quality of the solution transformation.

Recently, Thirion [Thi98] proposed to consider non rigid registration as a diffusion process. He introduced in the images entities (demons) that push according to local characteristics of the images in a similar way Maxwell did for solving the Gibbs paradox in thermodynamics. The forces he proposed were inspired from the optical flow equations. This algorithm is increasingly used in several teams as it it remarkably fast [BFC98,WGR$^+$99,PTSR98]. However, there is up to now no underlying theory that could predict when it fails and why.

In this paper, we investigate non-rigid registration as a minimization problem. In the next section, we differentiate the sum of square intensity differences criterion (SSD) and show that the demons forces are an approximation of a second order gradient descent on this criterion. In the third section, we investigate regularization and show that the Gaussian smoothing is a greedy optimization of the regularized criterion. The experiment section shows that really minimizing the SSD criterion can lead to improvement with respect to the original demons algorithm, but more importantly that regularization is the critical step for non-rigid registration.

2   Non-Rigid Registration by Gradient Descent

Simple transformations, like rigid or affine ones, can be represented by a small number of parameters (resp. 6 and 12 in 3D). When it comes to free-form deformations, we need to specify the coordinates $T(x)$ of each point x of the image after the transformation. Such a non-parametric transformation is usually represented by its displacement field $U(x) = T(x) - x$ (or $U = T - \text{Id}$).

Now, the goal of the registration is to find the transformation T that maps each point x of an image I to the "homologous" point $y = T(x)$ in image J. In this paper, we consider the registration of images from the same modality and we assume that they differ only by a geometric transformation and an independent Gaussian noise on the intensities. With these hypotheses, the well known SSD criterion is perfectly adapted for registration. Taking into account the fact that the image I deformed by T is $I \circ T^{(-1)}$ (and not $I \circ T$), we have:

$$SSD_I(T) = \int \left((T \star I)(x) - J(x) \right)^2 .dx = \int \left(I \circ T^{(-1)} - J \right)^2 \quad (1)$$

Known (or even unknown) intensity transformations are often better hypotheses even within mono-modal registration but they deserve other registration criterions. They will be investigated in a forthcoming study.

We note that the SSD criterion is not symmetric. Indeed, registering J on I leads to the criterion

$$SSD_J(T) = \int \left(I - J \circ T \right)^2 = \int \left(I \circ T^{(-1)} - J \right)^2 . |\nabla T^{(-1)}| \quad (2)$$

which has generally a minimum at a (hopefully slightly) different location.

2.1   Taylor Expansion of the SSD_J Criterion

Let T be the current estimation of the transformation and $(\nabla_J \circ T)(x)$(resp. $(\mathcal{H}_J \circ T)(x)$) be the transformed gradient (resp. Hessian) of the image J. A perturbation by a displacement field $u(x)$ gives the following Taylor expansion:

$$(J \circ (T + u))(x) = (J \circ T)(x) + (\nabla_J \circ T)^\mathsf{T}.u(x) + \tfrac{1}{2}u(x)^\mathsf{T}.(\mathcal{H}_J \circ T).u(x)$$

Thus, the Taylor expansion of the criterion is:

$$SSD_J(T + u) = SSD_J(T) + 2\int (J \circ T - I).(\nabla_J \circ T)^\mathsf{T}.u$$
$$+ \int ((\nabla_J \circ T)^\mathsf{T}.u)^2 + \int (J \circ T - I).u^\mathsf{T}.(\mathcal{H}_J \circ T).u + O(||u||^2)$$

where $||u||^2 = \int_x ||u(x)||^2.dx$ is the $\mathcal{L}_2$ norm of the small perturbation. As, by definition, $\int_x f(x)^\mathsf{T}.u(x).dx$ is the dot product of f and u in the space of square-integrable functions, we get by identification:

$$\nabla_{SSD_J}(T) = 2(J \circ T - I).(\nabla_J \circ T) \qquad (3)$$
$$\mathcal{H}_{SSD_J}(T) = 2(\nabla_J \circ T).(\nabla_J \circ T)^\mathsf{T} + 2(J \circ T - I).(\mathcal{H}_J \circ T) \qquad (4)$$

2.2   Second Order Gradient Descent on SSD_J

Let us now approximate the criterion by its tangential quadratic form at the current transformation T. We get the following first order approximation of the criterion gradient: $\nabla_{SSD_J}(T + u) \simeq \nabla_{SSD_J}(T) + H_{SSD_J}(T).u$

Assuming that the Hessian matrix of the criterion is positive definite, the minimum is obtained for a null gradient, i.e.: $u = -\mathcal{H}_{SSD_J}^{(-1)}(T).\nabla_{SSD_J}(T)$. This formula require to invert the Hessian matrix $\mathcal{H}_{SSD_J}(T)$ at each point x of the image. To speed up the process, we approximate this matrix by the closest scalar matrix (for the $\mathcal{L}_2$ norm on the matrix vector space):

$$\mathcal{H}_{SSD_J}(T) \simeq \frac{\mathrm{Tr}\,(\mathcal{H}_{SSD_J}(T))}{n}.\mathrm{Id} = \frac{||\nabla_J \circ T||^2 + (J \circ T - I).(\Delta_J \circ T)}{3}.\mathrm{Id}$$

where n is the space dimension (3 for us). Using this approximation, we get the following adjustment vector field:

$$u \simeq \frac{-3.(J \circ T - I).(\nabla_J \circ T)}{||\nabla_J \circ T||^2 + (J \circ T - I).(\Delta_J \circ T)} \qquad (5)$$

2.3   Second Order Gradient Descent on SSD_I

Let us now consider the criterion SSD_I (formula 1). We can follow the same calculi as above but replacing I by J and T with $T^{(-1)}$. Thus, the optimal adjustment field w is:

$$w \simeq \frac{-3.(I \circ T^{(-1)} - J).(\nabla_I \circ T^{(-1)})}{||\nabla_I \circ T^{(-1)}||^2 + (I \circ T^{(-1)} - J).(\Delta_I \circ T^{(-1)})}$$

Now, we can develop the expression $(T^{(-1)} + w)^{(-1)}$ using a first order Taylor expansion: $(T^{(-1)} + w)^{(-1)} = T \circ (\mathrm{Id} + w \circ T)^{(-1)} \simeq T \circ (\mathrm{Id} - w \circ T)$. Thus, $u' = -w \circ T$ is the optimal adjustment displacement field for SSD_I with this formulation:

$$\hat{T} = T \circ (\mathrm{Id} + u') \quad \text{with} \quad u' = \frac{3.(I - J \circ T).\nabla_I}{||\nabla_I||^2 + (I - J \circ T).\Delta_I} \quad (6)$$

2.4 The Demons Method

For monomodal registration of non-segmented images, Thirion [Thi98] proposed a force playing the same role as our adjustment displacement field. This force was inspired from the optical flow equations, but was renormalized to prevent instabilities for small image gradient values:

$$v = \frac{(I - J \circ T).\nabla_I}{||\nabla_I||^2 + \alpha.(I - J \circ T)^2} \quad (7)$$

2.5 Comparison

If we except the constant factor 3, absent from the demons equation, u' and v are almost equivalent. However, we get from the gradient descent an explicit and automatic normalization between the gradient norm and the intensities at the denominator: $\alpha = \Delta_I / (I - J \circ T)$ (Thirion used a constant value $\alpha = 1$).

Another important difference is that formula (6) is only valid when the Hessian matrix of the criterion is positive definite. With our approximation, this means $||\nabla_I||^2 + (I - J \circ T).\Delta_I > 0$. If this denominator becomes close to zero, we have to switch to another gradient descent method, such as Levenberg-Marquardt for instance. On the contrary, the demons forces (equ. 7) are always defined and even bounded for $\alpha > 0$ by $||v|| \leq 1/(2\sqrt{\alpha})$. However, nothing imposes that the SSD criterion decreases with such displacements.

3   Constraining the Transformation: Regularization

One of the main problem with free form deformations is that we can theoretically map all points of the same intensity to one point having this intensity in the other image. Of course, when repeated for all intensities, such a transformation perfectly minimizes the SSD criterion, but is also perfectly irregular. To regularize the transformation, there are two main methods: either rely on physical models, such as elastic and viscous fluid ones, or rely on regularization theory. We will see in the experimental part that the choice of the transformation constraints appears to be critical for doing measurements on the deformation field whereas it has little influence on the resampled image appearance.

3.1   Physical Models

Within physical models, elasticity was first used [BK89]. It is based on the *Green-St. Venant strain tensor*: $E = \frac{1}{2}(\nabla_T^\top.\nabla_T - \mathrm{Id}) = \frac{1}{2}(\nabla_U + \nabla_U^\top + \nabla_U^\top.\nabla_U)$. Then the St. Venant Kirchoff elastic energy is given by $W = \frac{\lambda}{2}(\mathrm{Tr}(E))^2 + \mu.\mathrm{Tr}(E^2)$, where λ and μ are Lamé coefficients describing the material. For linear elasticity, one simply neglects the quadratic term in the strain tensor, and one gets the following evolution equation: $f + \mu \Delta_U + (\lambda + \mu)\nabla(\nabla \cdot U) = 0$

When [CRM94] showed the invalidity of linear elasticity for large deformations, most efforts turned on viscous fluid models [CJM97,BN96]. This time, equations are based on the velocity v through the *rate of deformation tensor* $D = \frac{1}{2}(\nabla_v + \nabla_v^T)$. The energy is once again $W = \frac{\lambda}{2}(\mathrm{Tr}(D))^2 + \mu.\mathrm{Tr}(D^2)$ and we get the same evolution equation as before, but with the velocity field: $f + \mu \Delta_v + (\lambda + \mu)\nabla(\nabla \cdot v) = 0$

3.2   Gaussian Smoothing

The principle is to add a smoothness functional $\phi(T)$ to our criterion in order to disadvantage oscillatory solutions. Thus, ϕ should measure what remains of T after a high pass filter in the frequency domain [GJP93]. Let $K = k.\mathrm{Id}$ be an isotropic (i.e. radial basis) high-pass filter, $\tilde{K} = \tilde{k}.\mathrm{Id}$ its Fourier transform (also a high-pass filter) and $*$ the convolution operator. Thanks to Parseval theorem, the above properties of the smoothness kernel suggest functionals of the form:

$$\phi(T) = \frac{1}{2}\int \|K * T\|^2 dx = \frac{1}{2}\int \|\tilde{K}.\tilde{T}\|^2 = \frac{1}{2}\int \tilde{k}^2.\|\tilde{T}\|^2 d\omega$$

One can show that (for well formed kernel k), the gradient is: $\nabla_\phi(T) = (k*k)*T$. The Hessian matrix is more difficult to compute.

Ideally, we should add the gradient and Hessian matrix of the smoothing kernel to the gradient and Hessian matrix of our SSD criterion. In the original Demon's algorithm of [Thi98], Thirion prefers to use a greedy algorithm where he performs alternatively a gradient descent step on the SSD and a smoothing step. Let us consider the high-pass filter $k * k = (\delta - G_\sigma)/2$. Its gradient is $\nabla_\phi(T) = T - G_\sigma * T$, and a single step of a first order gradient descent gives:

$$T_{n+1} = T_n - \nabla_\phi(T_n) = G_\sigma * T_n$$

We note that smoothing the global displacement field U (or equivalently the global transformation T) could be considered as a rough simulation of an elastic model. By the way, [BN96] reported very similar results for these two methods. Following the same principle, we could consider the adjustment field u or v (equations 5,6,7) as an approximation of the velocity field: smoothing it with a Gaussian should be a rough simulation of a fluid model.

3.3   Comparison of Methods

Physical models are interesting because they model materials we are used to. However, the resolution of such models is often very complex and requires simplifications to be computationally tractable, such as the linearization of the strain tensor for elasticity of neglecting the pressure for fluids. Moreover computation times are usually high even if new implementations of fluid models are much faster [BN96]. Basically, the important point point seems to be that elastic equations are performing a regularization on the displacement field whereas fluid equations perform it on the velocity field.

On the other hand, Gaussian smoothing appears as a greedy optimization which is fast and easy to compute. Smoothing the global transformation (as in the original demons) could be considered as a rough simulation of an elastic model whereas smoothing the adjustment field simulates a rough fluid model.

4 Experiments

In Section 2, we saw the the demons are approximately minimizing the SSD criterion if the the Hessian matrix of this criterion is positive definite. To verify if minimizing the real criterion, we implemented a very simple version of the demons with a steepest descent instead of the newton like method: at each point of the image, we compute the gradient and look for the minimal difference of intensities along this line. Then we smooth the adjustment field (with standard deviation σ_{fl}), add it to the global transformation, and smooth the global transformation (with standard deviation σ_{el}).

4.1 Synthetic experiments

In this experiment, we want to register a small 2D disk on a "C". We made the experiment with the original demons method and our first order gradient descent simulating "elastic" ($\sigma_{el} \gg \sigma_{fl}$) and "fluid" ($\sigma_{el} \ll \sigma_{fl}$) deformations (Figure 1).

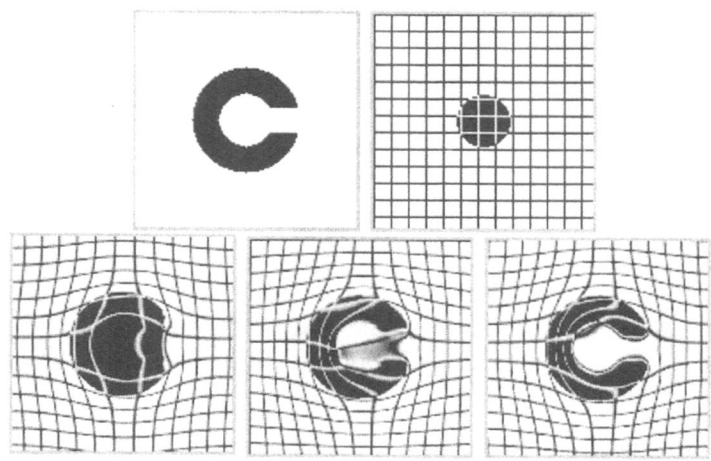

Fig. 1. Registration of a disk on a C. The grids are added after the registration to help visualizing the deformation. **Top:** reference image on the left, and image to register on the right. **Bottom:** from left to right, registration results with demons ($\sigma = 1.2$), with the new method simulating elastic deformations ($\sigma_{fl} = 0$, $\sigma_{el} = 1.2$) and with the new method simulating fluid deformations ($\sigma_{fl} = 3$, $\sigma_{el} = 0$).

Even using the same standard deviation for smoothing transformations, the demons (Figure 1, bottom left) and the minimization of the SSD criterion (bottom, middle) do not give the same results. This could be explained by demons forces where adding a high square intensity difference to a small gradient at the denominator lead to very small displacements. Smoothing is then sufficiently strong to prevent "white matter" to enter the interior of the "C". Thus, in this particular case, minimizing explicitly the SSD criterion gives better results.

There is surprisingly few differences between the structure of the "elastic" (Fig. 1, bottom middle) and the "fluid" (bottom right) deformations except in the interior of the "C". The "fluid" matches the edge much closer, but we can observe a singularity on the upper left part of the interior of the "C" (Jacobian going negative, visualized by an unexpected crossing of two grid lines). In fact, for such strong deformations, Gaussian smoothing is no more an approximation of physical models.

4.2   Registration of Ultrasound Images

In this experiment, we register two 3D US images from the European project ROBOSCOPE. A catheter was introduced in the brain of a (dead) pig and a balloon was inflated at different volumes to simulate the deformation that could happen during a tumor excision. Images presented in Figure (2) are 75x62x73 isotropic sub-images extracted from the original US images.

The result of the registration is visually correct both for the demons and for the new implementation. There is no significant difference on the difference image. Since we know that the deformation is physical and quite regular, we wanted to analyze the displacement field. We run the new implementation with $\sigma_{fl} = 3$ and $\sigma_{el} = 7$ whereas $\sigma(\simeq \sigma_{el})$ is limited to 2 in the original implementation of the demons. The visualization of the deformed grid on Figure (2) clearly shows that the new deformation field is much smoother.

To analyze the deformation field more carefully, we used the method developed in [RSDA99] to compute the Jacobian of the transformation that expresses the local volume variation due to the non-rigid transformation. We extracted an "edge surface" of this image of Jacobian and superimposed the results on the bottom of Figure (2). With the new method, we almost obtain the delineation of the balloon, except in the right part (the catheter in a fixed point and we segment on motion) and on the right lower part where the balloon is not visible in the images. More interestingly, the volumes measured inside our segmentation are respectively 0.982 and 0.875 cm^3 instead of 1.25 and 1 cm^3, which gives a ratio of 1.12 instead of 1.25. If this result is not perfect, it is encouraging. With the original demons, the deformation field is too noisy to measure something useful.

5   Discussion

Among non-rigid registration algorithms, the demon's method is fast but not well understood from a theoretical point of view. We showed in this article that the

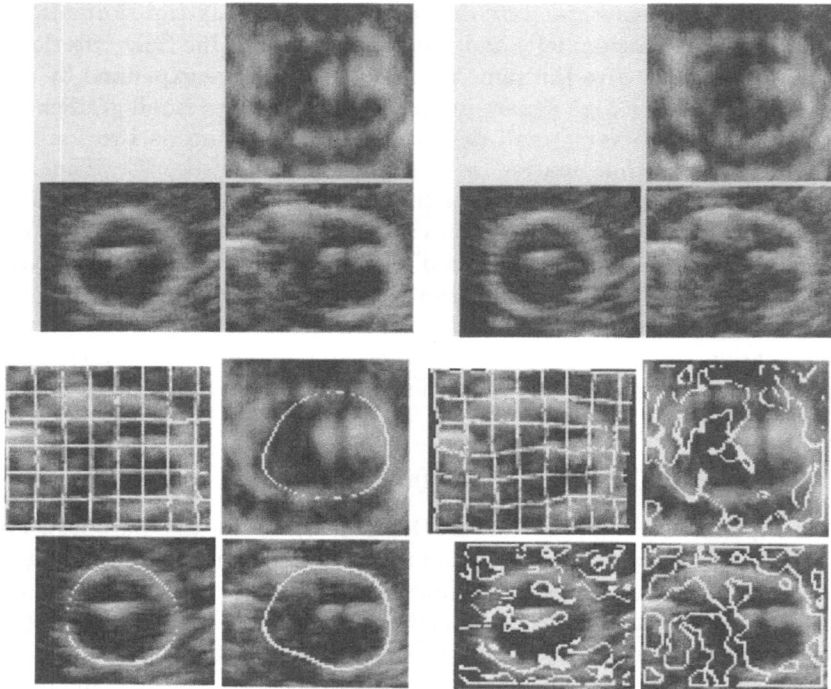

Fig. 2. Tracking deformations in 3D ultrasound images of a pig brain. Images were provided by Volker Paul, Fraunhofer (Institute) Society, Munich (Germany) as part of the EC-funded ROBOSCOPE project. **Top left:** three orthogonal views of the image to register (balloon volume: 1.25 cm^3). **Top right:** reference image (balloon volume: 1 cm^3). **Bottom:** "edges" of the Jacobian with new method (**left**) and with demons (**right**). We added on the upper left corner of each image triplet a slice (corresponding to the lower right image) after registration to visualize the corresponding deformation.

forces proposed by Thirion correspond to a second order gradient descent on the sum of square of intensity differences (SSD) criterion. Experiments showed that the real minimization of the SSD criterion could give a better results than the demons with synthetic data, but demons are performing well on real data. Both synthetic and real data experiments put into evidence that a good regularization is critical to obtain a useful deformation field.

The understanding of the demons algorithm and its weaknesses opens many new research avenues for non-rigid registration. Probably the most important one is regularization: the first work will be to minimize the criterion and the smoothing kernel in the same gradient descent step. The second work will be to look for families of smoothing kernels that better approximate physical models, the filtering methodology ensuring reasonable computation times.

Last but not least, the SSD criterion relies on imaging acquisition assumptions that are hardly verified in modalities such as US. We need to develop new criterions better adapted to the physics of the acquisition process. Then, the gradient descent scheme developed in this paper offers us a methodology to plug them into an operational registration algorithm.

Acknowledgments We would like to thank specially Volker Paul, Fraunhofer Institute Society, Munich (Germany) who provided us with the US images as part of the EC-funded ROBOSCOPE project HC 4018, a collaboration between The Fraunhofer Institute Society (Germany), Fokker Control System (Netherlands), Imperial College (UK), INRIA Sophia Antipolis (France), ISM Salzburg and Kretz Technik (Austria). Thanks also to Kretz and ISM for organizing / providing a high-end imaging system for these examinations. Many thanks also to David Rey, Alexandre Guimond and Jean-Philippe Thirion, for fruitful discussions and experiments on non rigid registration and analysis of the deformation field.

References

[BFC98]   I. Bricault, G. Ferretti, and P. Cinquin. Registration of real and ct-derived virtual bronchoscopic images to assist transbronchial biopsy. *Transactions in Medical Imaging*, 17(5):703–714, 1998.

[BK89]   R. Bajcsy and S. Kovačič. Multiresolution elastic matching. *Computer Vision, Graphics and Image Processing*, 46:1–21, 1989.

[BN96]   M. Bro-Nielsen. *Medical image registration and surgery simulation*. PhD thesis, IMM-DTU, 1996.

[Bro81]   C. Broit. Optimal registration of deformed images. Doctoral Dissertation, University of Pennsylvania, August 1981.

[CJM97]   G. E. Christensen, S. C. Joshi, and M. I. Miller. Volumetric transformation of brain anatomy. *IEEE Transactions on Medical Imaging*, 16(6):864–877, December 1997.

[CRM94]   G.E. Christensen, R.D. Rabitt, and M.I. Miller. 3d brain mapping using a deformable neuroanatomy. *Physics in Medicine and Biology*, 39:609–618, 1994.

[GJP93]   F. Girosi, M. Jones, and T. Poggio. Priors, stabilizers and basis functions: from regularization to radial, tensor and additive splines. A.I. Memo 1430, M.I.T., A.I. Laboratory, June 1993.

[MMV98]   J. B. A. Maintz, E. H. W. Meijering, and M. A. Viergever. General multimodal elastic registration based on mutual information. *Image Processing*, 1998.

[PTSR98]   S. Prima, J.-P. Thirion, G. Subsol, and N. Roberts. Automatic Analysis of Normal Brain Dissymmetry of Males and Females in MR Images. In *Proc. of MICCAI'98*, volume LNCS 1496, pages 770–779, 1998.

[RSDA99]   D. Rey, G. Subsol, H. Delingette, and N. Ayache. Automatic Detection and Segmentation of Evolving Processes in 3D Medical Images: Application to Multiple Sclerosis. In *Proc. of IPMI'99*, LNCS, Visegrád, Hungary, June 1999. Springer. To appear.

[Thi98]   J.-P. Thirion. Image matching as a diffusion process: an analogy with maxwell's demons. *Medical Image Analysis*, 2(3), 1998.

[WGR+99]   J. Webb, A. Guimond, N. Roberts, P. Eldridge an D. Chadwick, J. Meunier, and J.-P. Thirion. Automatic detection of hippocampal atrophy on magnetic resonnance images. *Magnetic Resonance Imaging*, 17, 1999. To appear.

Multi-variate Mutual Information for Registration

Jennifer L. Boes[1] and Charles R. Meyer[2]

[1] The University of Michigan, Department of Radiology
jboes@umich.edu
[2] The University of Michigan, Department of Radiology,
3307 Kresge III Research Bldg., Ann Arbor MI 48109-0553
cmeyer@umich.edu

Abstract. An extension of the mutual information metric to a three-variate cost function for driving the registration of a volume to pair of co-registered volumes is presented. While mutual information has typically been applied to pairs of variables, it is possible to compute multi-variate mutual information. The implementation of multi-variate mutual information is described. This metric is demonstrated using the problem of registering a deformed t2 slice of the visible male magnetic resonance data set to either a single t1 slice or a pair of co-registered t1 and proton density slices. Two-variable and three-variable metric registration results are compared. Adding the extra proton density information to the registration cost metric leads to faster optimization convergence and better final accuracy. Multi-variate mutual information has potential application in problems where the addition of more information can lead to solution convergence or improve accuracy.

1 Introduction

We present an extension of the mutual information metric (MI) into three variables to enable the registration of a volume with a pair of co-registered volumes. Mutual information (MI) is a metric proposed simultaneously by Collignon and Viola that works well as a cost function for registering data from different modalities [1, 2]. While mutual information is only one of a much larger set of metrics representing some kind of distance between two data sets, it has proven to work in a large number of situations. Since the early application of MI in registration, many researchers have explored its potential and limitations in this context. See for some examples [3-6]. This paper explores multi-variate computation of mutual information as a way to incorporate additional, potentially powerful information into the registration problem.

The difficulty in extending mutual information to multiple variables is the need to compute the underlying multi-dimensional probability density function (pdf). This, in general, is not an easy problem to solve. However, for this particular application, a simple brute force computation is sufficient to demonstrate the merit of the inclusion of additional evidence to solve the registration problem. The power of this extension of MI is demonstrated using simulated data based on an MRI from the visible male data.

2   Methods

This paper describes a simple experiment that illustrates the usefulness of multi-variate MI for registration. Existing software for MI-based registration was extended to provide for three-variate as well as two-variate MI. We ran experiments in both categories. The first category registered a slice with a known deformation back to a single slice using two-variate MI. The second category registered the same deformed slice back to a co-registered pair of slices using three-variate MI. The experiment was designed so that it would be possible to recover the exact non-affine warping applied to the deformed slice. Tests within the two categories were repeated multiple times with random starting points to provide for a robust analysis of results within and between categories.

2.1   Optimized Registration

The registrations were performed using the MIAMI Fuse software developed at the University of Michigan [7]. This software uses the Nelder-Mead Simplex optimizer to maximize the mutual information between a reference data set and the set to register [8]. Solution transforms can be either affine or warps, although for this experiment all solutions were warps. Parameters required are those controlling the stopping criteria of the optimizer. For this set of experiments we set the initial search bound of the optimizer to 4 voxels and set a stopping criteria of 0.5 voxel accuracy. The software runs multiple optimization cycles until the cost function changes by no more than 0.0001 for 3 out of 5 cycles. The number of cycles and corresponding MI are recorded to facilitate comparison of convergence.

2.2   Computation of 3D MI

The computation of mutual information for m variables, more than two, requires the estimation of the m-variate probability density function that is the basis for MI. As m grows large, this can be difficult to compute, due to problems estimating the underlying pdf of the variables. However, for small m like three in this set of experiments, this problem is still tractable [9]. We have chosen to implement multi-variate MI using a histogram estimation of the joint and single probability density functions. Fig. 1 shows a sample three-variate histogram. The mutual information is computed from the histogram as the sum over all gray levels trios of $P(g_a, g_b, g_c) log\{P(g_a, g_b, g_c)/P(g_a)P(g_b)P(g_c)\}$. Since the $P(g)$ values are computed from the 2-variate or 3-variate histograms with N samples as $H(g)/N$, this estimation depends on the selection of histogram binning. For this set of experiments, bin width for MI computation was separate and automatic for all two/three variables according to a formulation suggested by Freedman-Diaconis, $2(IQR)n^{-1/3}$, where IQR is the interquartile range of the data and n is the sample size [9]. This formula makes no assumptions about the shape of the probability density function.

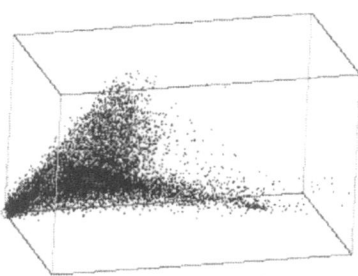

Fig. 1. Sample three-variate histogram for the estimation of the joint probability density of original slices–t1, proton density, t2–of the visible male MRI shown in Fig. 3

We can compare the two-variate and three-variate MI by graphing MI as a parameter of the transform changes. For example in Fig. 2, we use the original versions of the visible male MRIs shown in Fig. 3 and apply a thin-plate spline warp using five control points at the 4 vertices of a box and in the center of the box. The point in the center is moved in the x and y directions. The influence of this movement is shown by plotting MI in Fig. 2. Note that the additional information in the three-variate case yields a cost function with greater slope and better second derivatives near the solution.

2.3   Simulation Data Using Visible Male MRI

The simulation data is a trio of slices from the head of the visible male MRI data set (see http://www.nlm.nih.gov/research/visible/getting_data.html for more information on this data). Original 256x256 slices have been cropped to 167x219. Voxels are approximately 1mm x 1mm in size. The t1 and proton density images were left unchanged to use as a reference data pair (Fig 3a-b) while the t2 image was deformed with a known transform, a 5 point (16 degree of freedom) thin-plate spline (Fig 3c). The slices remained in integer format. Experiments registered the deformed t2 image back to either the t1 or the t1-density pair.

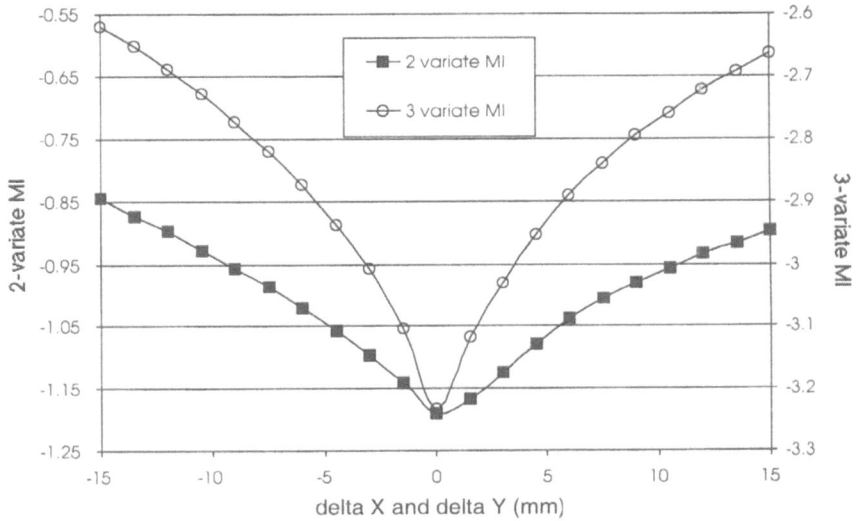

Fig. 2. Plot of two-variate and three-variate MI. Middle point of warp is being translated the same delta in x and y while outside 4 points of a box are held constant. The two graphs have been superimposed leaving vertical scales at the same units, but different range to promote visual comparison of the MI cost function progression. The lines shown are curves fit to the data points

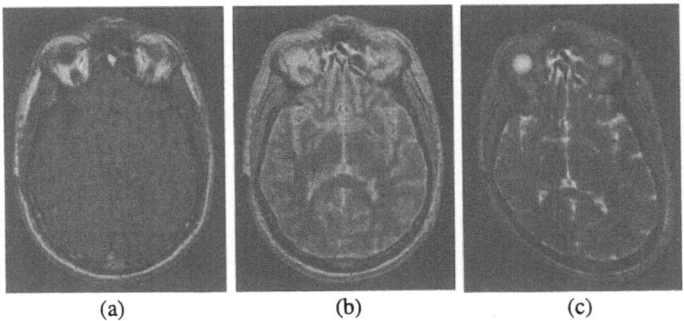

Fig. 3. Visible male MRI slice data for registration tests: (a) t1, (b) proton density, (c) warped t2

2.4   Registration Test and Analysis

Registrations in this experiment are based on the same feature set that was previously used to deform the image. This enables the recovery of the exact warp used to deform the slice initially. It also enables us to use the optimized locations of these points for analysis. A solution that removes the warp completely will optimize features to the exact original locations used to generate the warp. Good solutions yield points very near the original locations. The statistics of variation of these points from the mean and from the known solution, particularly the standard deviation σ, indicate the goodness of the solution.

3   Results

Twenty registrations were completed in each category, two-variate MI and three-variate MI. Results are summarized in Fig. 4 and 5 and Table 1. We expected that the three-variate case would converge more quickly and yield more accurate results for the same stopping criteria. We found that, indeed, the 3-variate MI yielded more accurate results (Fig. 4 and Table 1) with particularly good results at the feature in the center of the image, Feature 5, where the σ of the solutions improved considerably. Interior areas often lack strong texture or features to drive accurate registration, but the new information helps to overcome this. In addition, Fig. 5 illustrates that the three-variate optimization problem converged in much fewer optimization cycles than the two-variate case.

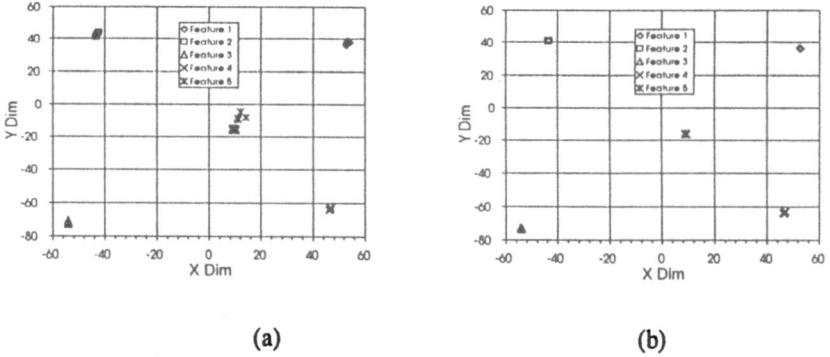

(a)   (b)

Fig. 4. Graphs of final location of feature points after optimization: (a) two-variate MI (t1 & t2), (b) three-variate MI (t1-pd & t2).

Table 1. Error analysis of two variate and three variate registration solutions. Shown are the average standard deviation from the mean final location for each feature as per Fig. 4 that was used in the registration. Results are reported in millimeters

	MI: t1 & t2 σ of final loc (mm)	MI: t1-pd & t2 σ of final loc (mm)
Feature 1	0.76	0.23
Feature 2	1.06	0.25
Feature 3	0.77	0.28
Feature 4	0.41	0.31
Feature 5	3.50	0.32
Ensemble	1.67	0.27

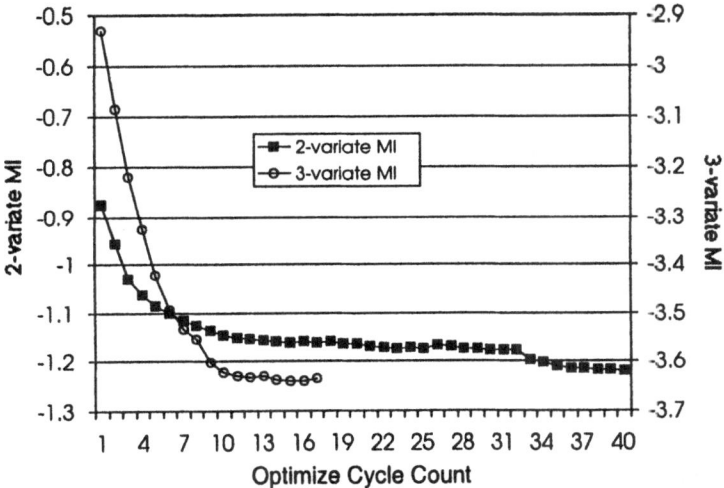

Fig. 5. Average mutual information at the conclusion of each optimization cycle. The two graphs have been superimposed leaving vertical scales at the same units, but different range to promote visual comparison of the MI progression. Numbers of cycles to solution varies with each run of the optimization algorithm. Average cycles for two-variate MI was 22 and average cycles for three-variate was 12.

4 Conclusions

We have presented a simple illustration of multi-variate MI as a cost function for driving the registration of a slice to a pair of co-registered slices. Although tests have been run on only one two-dimensional data set, the results indicate that this technique may be promising for registration problems in which additional information can either enable convergence or improve accuracy.

Acknowledgements

This work was supported in part by NIH Grants 2R01 CA59412-04A1 and 1R41 CA72351-01. Thank you to our reviewers for thoughtful feedback; our apologies for not being able to address all suggestions due to an impending move to England.

References

1. Collignon, A., Vandermeulen, D., Suetens, P., and Marchal, G. 3D multimodality medical image registration using feature space clustering. Presented at *CVRMed'95*, Nice, FR. In *Lecture Notes in Computer Science*, Vol. 905. Springer-Verlag (1995) 195-204
2. Viola, P. and Wells, W.M. Alignment by maximization of mutual information. Presented at *5th Int'l Conf on Computer Vision*, Cambridge, MA. In *Proceedings of the 5th Int'l Conf on Computer Vision*. IEEE (1995) 16-23S
3. Kim, B., Boes, J.L., Frey, K.A., and Meyer, C.R. Mutual information for automated multimodal image warping. Presented at *Visualization in Biomedical Computing*, Hamburg, Germany. In *Lecture Notes in Computer Science*, Vol. 1131. Springer-Verlag (1996) 349-354
4. Wells, W., Viola, P., Atsumi, H., Hakajima, S., and Kikinis, R.: Multimodal volume registration by maximization of mutual information. Medical Image Analysis 1:1 (1996) 35-51
5. Maes, F., Collignon, A., Vandermeulen, D., Marchal, G., and Suetens, P.: Multimodality image registration by maximization of mutual information. IEEE Transactions on Medical Imaging 16:2 (1997) 187-98
6. Hill, D.L., Maurer, C.R., Jr., Studholme, C., Fitzpatrick, J.M., and Hawkes, D.J.: Correcting scaling errors in tomographic images using a nine degree of freedom registration algorithm. Journal of Computer Assisted Tomography 22:2 (1998) 317-23
7. Meyer, C.R., Boes, J.L., Kim, B., Bland, P., Zasadny, K.R., Kison, P.V., Koral, K., Frey, K.A., and Wahl, R.L.: Demonstration of accuracy and clinical versatility of mutual information for automatic multimodality image fusion using affine and thin plate spline warped geometric deformations. Medical Image Analysis 1:3 (1997) 195-206
8. Press, W.H., Flannery, B.P., Teukolsky, S.A., and Vetterling, W.T.: Numerical recipes in C: the art of scientific computing. Cambridge University Press, Cambridge (1988)
9. Izenman, A.J.: Recent developments in nonparametric density estimation. Journal of the American Statistical Society 86:413 (1991) 205-224

Automatic Identification of a Particular Vertebra in the Spinal Column Using Surface-Based Registration

Jeannette L. Herring and Benoît M. Dawant

Department of Electrical and Computer Engineering,
Vanderbilt University, Nashville, TN 37235
jnet@vuse.vanderbilt.edu

Abstract. In this work, we register vertebral points collected in physical space to spinal column surfaces extracted from computed tomography images. The vertebral points are taken from a single vertebra to represent the region of surgical interest. The surface is automatically extracted using an iso-intensity-based algorithm and thus contains multiple vertebrae. This work introduces an enhancement to currently existing methods of intra-operative vertebral registration by allowing the portion of the spinal column surface that correctly matches a set of physical vertebral points to be automatically selected from several possible choices. We find the correct portion of the surface by registering the set of physical points to multiple surface areas, including all vertebral surfaces that potentially match the physical point set. We then compute the standard deviation of the surface error for the set of points registered to each vertebral surface that is a possible match, and the registration that corresponds to the lowest standard deviation designates the correct match. We have performed our current experiments on two plastic spine phantoms.

1 Introduction

Health problems associated with the lumbar region of the spine are prevalent, potentially debilitating, and often quite expensive to treat. In fact, more than 250,000 lumbar spine operations are performed annually in the United States at a cost of more than $6 billion per year [6]. Because of the prevalence of lumbar back problems, any improvement in surgical procedures can have a tremendous clinical impact. We are particularly interested in contributions provided by image-guided surgical techniques.

Improving the feasibility of image-guided back surgery by performing a real-time registration of vertebrae in different image modalities or in image and physical space is an active research area. Clinical studies have been done to show that the technique is a valid approach for the insertion of pedicle screws (for example, see [2] and [3]). Image-guided surgical techniques have also been used successfully to perform lumbar discectomies (for example, see [14]) and spinal biopsies (for example, see [16]).

In addition to the clinical studies that have been done in the area of image-guided vertebral surgery, several technical studies have been performed to investigate various methods of vertebral segmentation and registration. In particular, Lavallée and colleagues have done a substantial amount of work in this area. Their studies show that sub-millimetric registration accuracy can be achieved between points obtained intra-operatively (using an optically tracked ultrasound probe, a 3-D pointer, and projection x-ray images [8]) and surfaces extracted pre-operatively from CT images (using modified snake and spline techniques [10]). Points are registered to surfaces by minimizing the energy required to make projection lines from 2-D contours tangent to the 3-D surface when using x-ray images and by applying more traditional surface-based techniques when using 3-D methods of point collection [7,8]. Results reported so far using automatic or semi-automatic surface generation techniques have been achieved primarily on single isolated vertebrae [9].

An important premise of the clinical and technical studies is that the physical points must be collected from the correct vertebra; that is, from the vertebra that is involved in the surgical procedure or the registration trial. In clinical situations, this intra-operative identification of the correct vertebra can be a challenging task, especially for closed-back, minimally invasive procedures. It requires the surgeon to count vertebrae by feeling spinous processes through the skin, a procedure that is complicated by the presence of fatty tissues. Because this manual identification process introduces the possibility of error, it would be helpful to have a registration algorithm that could automatically locate the vertebra of interest.

Our research demonstrates that surface-based registration methods can be used to identify which vertebral surface in a CT image volume containing multiple vertebrae correctly matches a physical point set representing a single vertebra. To perform the surface-based registration, we use a method based upon the iterative closest point algorithm developed by Besl and McKay [1]. To segment the vertebral surface, we use the fully automatic marching cubes algorithm proposed by Lorensen and Cline [11]. Since each vertebra has a slightly different shape, measurements related to the quality of the registration results indicate which vertebral surface in the image volume best corresponds to the physical point set.

2   Methods

2.1 Image Acquisition

We have performed our experiments on two plastic phantoms of the spine. The first phantom, which we have designated Phantom I, is a life-size model of the entire spinal column. The second phantom, designated Phantom II, is a life-size model of the lumbar portion of the spinal column. Both phantoms are manufactured by the Carolina Biological Supply Company in Burlington, North Carolina.

CT scans of the two phantoms were obtained using a Philips Tomoscan AV scanner. For both phantoms, the image volume contains 70 slices with a slice thickness of 2 mm. Every slice has 512 x 512 voxels with voxel dimensions in millimeters of 0.625 x 0.625 x 2. Both CT image volumes used in this study were acquired as stacks of image slices with no inter-slice gap or slice overlap. The gantry tilt angle during image acquisition was zero. Phantom I was placed in the scanner to ensure that complete images of L1 and L2 were obtained, and Phantom II was placed in the scanner to ensure that complete images of L3, L4, and L5 were obtained.

2.2 Triangulated Surface Extraction

A triangle set representation of the surface of the spinal column was automatically extracted from each CT scan using an independently implemented version of the classic marching cubes method developed by Lorensen and Cline [11]. The number of triangles in the resulting mesh was reduced using the decimation algorithm from the commercially available Visualization Toolkit (VTK) [15].

The only parameter required by the marching cubes algorithm is an intensity value. This algorithm is well suited to the extraction of bone surfaces in CT images, since the intensity level of bone is generally an order of magnitude greater than the intensity levels of all other materials. Of course, the method results in the inclusion of overlapping parts of neighboring vertebrae, but the extraneous surface information does not appear to be a problem for the surface-based registration process we use.

Hounsfield numbers of the plastic phantoms range from approximately 600 to approximately 800, with Phantom II having a slightly higher Hounsfield number than Phantom I. The Hounsfield number of the air surrounding the phantom is −1024. There is an offset of 1024 introduced into the intensity values due to the method used to transfer the scans from the CT machine, resulting in average intensity values of about 1600 to 1800 for the plastic and 0 for the surrounding air. Thus, iso-surfaces were created for the phantom scans at the intermediate intensity values of 800 for Phantom I and 900 for Phantom II.

2.3 Surface Point Identification

The physical space coordinates of approximately 300 surface points were acquired for each vertebra using a three-dimensional spatial localizer (3DSL) consisting of a probe and an Optotrak 3020 system (Northern Digital, Ontario, Canada). These points were collected by sweeping the 3DSL over the vertebral surface, a method which allows hundreds of points to be acquired in a few seconds. The point collection process was performed by an engineering graduate student with advice from a general surgeon.

For each vertebra, the collected surface points represent the central laminar regions and the tip of the spinous process. In previous work, we have studied the sensitivity of surface-based registration to different regions of the posterior vertebral surface, and we have shown that points from the central laminar regions and the tip of the spinous process provide sufficient information for accurate surface-based registration [4].

2.4 Registration

We perform surface-based registration of physical points from each lumbar vertebra to the spinal column surfaces extracted from the CT scans of Phantom I and Phantom II. That is, we attempt to register physical points collected from vertebra L1 to surfaces corresponding to all five lumbar vertebrae, and we repeat the process for L2 through L5. Both spinal column surfaces contain multiple vertebrae, so our registration trials address the question of whether the vertebral surface that correctly matches our physical point set can be selected out of several choices.

To perform our registration trials, we use an independent implementation [12] of the iterative closest point algorithm of Besl and McKay [1]. The method is a two-step process. First, the closest point on one surface is computed for each point in a set of points representing the other surface. (In this study, the first surface is a triangle set representation of the surface in the CT image, and the point set representation of the second surface is a set of physical-space surface points.) Second, a transformation is determined by registering these two point sets. This process is iterated until some stopping criterion is satisfied. The method converges to a local minimum of the cost function, which is the root-mean-square (RMS) distance between the corresponding points at the last iteration. Because the physical-space surface points we record are the positions of the center of the ballpoint tip of the 3DSL, the recorded surface points are displaced from the actual surface by the radius of the tip. We use the method described by Maurer and colleagues to correct for this displacement [13].

Because of the possibility of convergence to a local minimum that is not the correct solution, the algorithm works best when it is initialized with rotations and translations that are close to the exact solution. In this work, the initial registration for correctly matched vertebral points and surfaces is computed by aligning the principal axes of the physical surface points and the CT image surface. This registration is translated along the spinal column to compute the initial position of the point set in relation to other (mis-matched) vertebral surfaces. We use a translation of plus or minus 30 mm per vertebra through which the correct position is displaced. This method of finding different initial positions along the spinal column should translate directly into clinical work: The principal axes transformation can be used to find the initial position of the chosen vertebra, and that position can then be translated up and down the spinal column to test whether the chosen vertebra is actually the correct one.

2.5 Error Computation

Our method of assessing registration error requires the comparison of registration results with a gold standard [4]. Since the work reported herein investigates mis-matched vertebral registrations, there is no associated gold standard. Thus, we report results in terms of surface error, which is computed as the RMS distance of the registered point set from the surface. It is important to distinguish surface error from registration error, since we have found that surface error is generally not a good predictor of registration error. However, our experiments show that surface error along with its standard deviation can provide a relative measure of how well the shape of the point set matches the shape of the surface. Our primary concern for this particular set of experiments is finding the closest match between the two shapes, so surface error and its standard deviation are appropriate error computation methods.

3   Results

Figure 1 shows the surface extracted from Phantom I. From top to bottom, the figure shows part of a thoracic vertebra, a complete thoracic vertebra, vertebrae L1 and L2 (which can be identified by the fiducial markers in the right central laminar regions),

L3, and part of L4. Note that the point sets we have chosen to use in our registration trials – the central laminar regions and the spinous process tips – have rather similar shapes, especially for neighboring vertebrae. The greatest visual variation tends to be in the transverse processes, which are not included in our physical point set. Also, note that the markers visible in Figure 1 are not used in this particular experiment; they are related to other registration trials we have conducted. A similar surface containing vertebrae L2 through L5 and part of the sacrum exists for Phantom II.

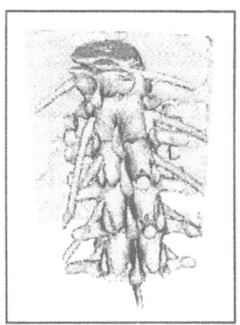

Fig. 1. Surface of spinal column extracted from CT scan of Phantom I. The surface contains parts of two thoracic vertebrae and four lumbar vertebrae.

Figure 2 shows the RMS surface errors obtained in our registration trials. Each bar represents the result of registering the physical point set designated by the legend to the vertebral surface shown along the x axis. Recall from the Methods section that the surface points are displaced from the actual surface by the radius of the ballpoint tip of the 3DSL, which is 0.5 mm. Our program to compute surface distance does not correct for this displacement, so the RMS surface error should be 0.5 mm in Figure 2 for a "perfect" fit.

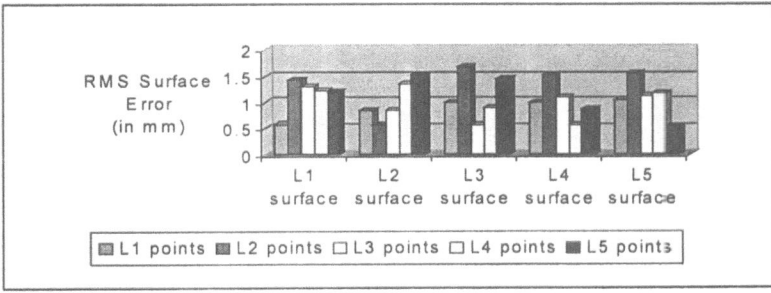

Fig. 2. RMS surface errors for physical point sets shown in the legend registered to vertebral surfaces shown along the x axis. All errors are in millimeters.

Without exception, Figure 2 shows that the correctly matched points and surfaces yield the lowest RMS surface errors. However, it is interesting to note that the RMS surface errors for mis-matched vertebrae are also consistently low, even when the two vertebrae being matched have quite different shapes, as is the case for L1 and L5 in this particular experiment. In fact, certain incorrect matches provide surface errors that are not dramatically higher than the errors generated by correct matches. For example, consider the results of registering points from L1, L2, and L3 to the surface of L2. The L2-to-L2 match has the lowest RMS surface error at 0.56 mm, but the L1-to-L2 and L3-to-L2 mis-matches both have surface errors of 0.85 mm, which is also a relatively low value.

The fact that RMS surface errors are relatively low for mis-matched points and surfaces suggests that this error may not be the best indicator of a vertebral mismatch. This observation led us to examine the standard deviation of surface error as a possible indicator. Figure 3 shows the standard deviation for each registration trial. As in Figure 2, each bar represents the registration result obtained for the physical point set designated by the legend and the vertebral surface shown along the x axis. As before, the correctly matched points and surfaces yield the lowest standard deviations in all cases. However, the spread is greater in this chart, suggesting that the standard deviation is a better predictor of a correct match than the RMS surface error.

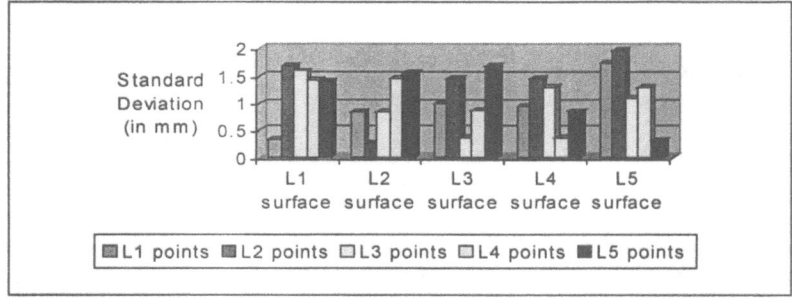

Fig. 3. Standard deviations of surface errors for physical point sets shown in the legend registered to vertebral surfaces shown along the x axis. All errors are in millimeters.

4 Discussion

It is not surprising that the correct match yields the lowest RMS surface error in Figure 2, but it is rather unexpected to find such small surface errors for mis-matched vertebrae. This finding is due to fact that the registration algorithm is designed to minimize distance between the point set and the surface, the very distance which also serves as our definition of surface error. In other words, because the behavior of the registration algorithm is controlled by point-to-surface distance, it will attempt to place the point set close to *some* surface (resulting in a relatively low RMS surface error), but there is no guarantee that the point set will be close to the *correct* surface.

As Figure 3 shows, a better predictor of a correct match is the standard deviation of surface error. Even though the registration algorithm attempts to place the entire set of registered points close to some surface, a mis-match between the point set shape and the surface shape results in less consistency among individual point-to-surface distances, or in other words, a larger standard deviation. For a correctly registered case, the excellent match between the shape of the point set and the shape of the surface results in a greater consistency among distances from the points to the surface, or in other words, a smaller standard deviation.

Whether or not the results we have obtained on phantom data can be verified on patient data remains to be tested. However, we have performed preliminary studies of the effectiveness of using an iso-intensity-based triangulation algorithm to segment vertebrae in patient data sets, and we have achieved satisfactory results [5]. We believe that shape differences among vertebrae in patient data sets will be at least as pronounced as differences among the phantom vertebrae we have used. Thus, it is likely that the observations we have made on these phantoms will apply to real data sets. We also note that there are other measures of comparison between point set and surface shapes that can be used if the standard deviation of the surface error proves to be insufficient. For example, additional experiments not included in this paper show that the use of physical points collected from the transverse processes and not used in registration can provide a clear distinction between matched and mis-matched vertebrae. In our trials using these supplementary points, correct matches have sub-millimetric RMS surface errors and incorrect matches have RMS surface errors of 4 to 6 mm.

It should be noted that knowledge of whether a correct match exists is required prior to surgical exposure of the physical points. For this reason, we are investigating the possibility of collecting the point set percutaneously from ultrasound images. Preliminary experiments suggest that registration results achieved using ultrasound point sets will be similar to those achieved using physical point sets.

5   Conclusion

Our experiments show that the standard deviation of surface error can be used to select the correct match between a set of vertebral surface points collected in physical space and a surface of the spinal column extracted from a CT scan of multiple vertebrae. The ability to make this determination automatically removes the need for manual identification of matching vertebrae in image and physical space. In the future, we will run similar experiments with patient scans and points collected via ultrasound. We will also test our findings on CT scans with larger slice spacings.

Acknowledgements

This work has been supported in part by an NDSEG fellowship awarded through the Office of Naval Research and by NIH grant 5R01-G752798-03. The authors gratefully acknowledge the many contributions of Alan Herline, M.D., who provided invaluable input from a surgeon's point of view, and Calvin Maurer, who provided the executable code for the registration algorithm. They would also like to express their appreciation to Diane Muratore, who helped collect the physical point sets, and Allen Jackson, who provided the CT scans used in our study.

Bibliography

1. Besl, P.J. and McKay, N.D., "A Method for Registration of 3-D Shapes." *IEEE Transactions on Pattern Analysis and Machine Intelligence* **14**, pp. 239-256, 1992.
2. Carl, A.L., Khanuja, H.S., Sachs, B.L., Gatto, C.A., vomLehn, J., Vosburgh, K., Schenck, J., Lorensen, W., Rohling, K., and Disler, D., "*In Vitro* Simulation: Early Results of Stereotaxy for Pedicle Screw Placement." *Spine* **22**, pp. 1160-1164, 1997.
3. Foley, K.T. and Smith, M.M., "Image-guided Spine Surgery." *Neurosurgery Clinics of North America* **7**, pp. 171-186, 1996.
4. Herring, J.L., Dawant, B.M., Maurer, C.R., Jr., Muratore, D.M., Galloway, R.L., Jr., and Fitzpatrick, J.M., "Surface-based Registration of CT Images to Physical Space for Image-guided Surgery of the Spine: A Sensitivity Study." *IEEE Transactions on Medical Imaging* **17**, pp. 743-752, 1998.
5. Herring, J.L., Maurer, C.R., Jr., and Dawant, B.M., "Sensitivity Analysis for Registration of Vertebrae in Ultrasound and Computed Tomography Images." *Proceedings of the SPIE Conference on Image Processing* (San Diego, California) **3338**, pp. 95-106, 1998.
6. Krause, T.M., "Case Management through a Multidisciplinary Spinal Evaluation." *Orthopaedic Nursing* **16**, pp. 46-50, 1997.
7. Lavallée, S. and Szeliski, R., "Recovering the Position and Orientation of Free-Form Objects from Image Contours Using 3D Distance Maps." *IEEE Transactions on Pattern Analysis and Machine Intelligence* **17**, pp. 378-390, 1995.
8. Lavallée, S., Szeliski, R., and Brunie, L. "Anatomy-Based Registration of Three-Dimensional Medical Images, Range image, X-Ray Projections, and Three-Dimensional Models Using Octree-Splines." In: *Computer-integrated Surgery: technology and clinical applications*, eds. R. Taylor, S. Lavallée, G. Burdea, and R. Mösges. Boston, Massachusetts: Academic Press, 1996. pp. 115-143.
9. Lavallée, S., Troccaz, J., Sautot, P., Mazier, B., Cinquin, P., Merloz, P., and Chirossel, J.-P. "Computer-Assisted Spinal Surgery Using Anatomy-Based Registration." In: *Computer-integrated Surgery: technology and clinical applications*, eds. R. Taylor, S. Lavallée, G. Burdea, and R. Mösges. Boston, Massachusetts: Academic Press, 1996. pp. 425-449.
10. Leitner, F., Marque, I., Lavallée, S., and Cinquin, P. "Dynamic Segmentation: Finding the Edge With Snake Splines." In: *Curves and Surfaces*, eds. P.J. Laurent, A. Le Méhauté, and L.L. Schumaker. Boston, Massachusetts: Academic Press, 1991. pp. 279-284.
11. Lorensen, W.E. and Cline, H.E., "Marching Cubes: A High Resolution 3D Surface Construction Algorithm." *Computer Graphics* (Anaheim, California) **21** [4], pp. 163-169, 1987.
12. Maurer, C.R., Jr., Aboutanos, G.B., Dawant, B.M., Maciunas, R.J., and Fitzpatrick, J.M., "A Method for Registration of 3-D Images Using Multiple Geometric Features." *IEEE Transactions on Medical Imaging* **15**, pp. 836-849, 1996.
13. Maurer, C.R., Jr., Maciunas, R.J., and Fitzpatrick, J.M., "Registration of Head CT Images to Physical Space Using a Weighted Combination of Points and Surfaces." *IEEE Transactions on Medical Imaging* **17**, pp. 753-761, 1998.
14. Mayer, H.M. and Brock, M., "Percutaneous endoscopic discectomy: surgical technique and preliminary results compared to microsurgical discectomy." *Journal of Neurosurgery* **78**, pp. 216-225, 1993.
15. Schroeder, W., Martin, K., and Lorensen, B. *The Visualization Toolkit*, Upper Saddle River, New Jersey: Prentice Hall PTR, 1998.
16. Stringham, D.R., Hadjipavlou, A., Dzioba, R.B., and Lander, P., "Percutaneous Transpedicular Biopsy of the Spine." *Spine* **19**, pp. 1985-1991, 1994.

Lecture Notes in Computer Science   1679

Edited by G. Goos, J. Hartmanis and J. van Leeuwen

Springer-Verlag Berlin Heidelberg GmbH

Chris Taylor Alan Colchester (Eds.)

Medical
Image Computing
and Computer-Assisted
Intervention – MICCAI'99

Second International Conference
Cambridge, UK, September 19-22, 1999
Proceedings

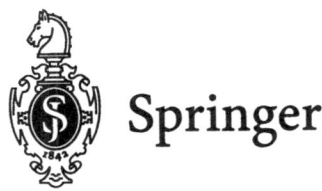

Springer

Series Editors

Gerhard Goos, Karlsruhe University, Germany
Juris Hartmanis, Cornell University, NY, USA
Jan van Leeuwen, Utrecht University, The Netherlands

Volume Editors

Chris Taylor
The University of Manchester
Oxford Road, Manchester M13 9PT, UK
E-mail: ctaylor@man.ac.uk

Alan Colchester
University of Kent
Canterbury, Kent CT2 7NT, UK
E-mail: a.colchester@ukc.ac.uk

Cataloging-in-Publication data applied for

Die Deutsche Bibliothek - CIP-Einheitsaufnahme

Medical image computing and computer assisted intervention : second
international conference ; proceedings / MICCAI '99, Cambridge, UK, September
19 - 22, 1999. Chris Taylor ; Alan Colchester (ed.). - Berlin ; Heidelberg ;
New York ; Barcelona ; Hong Kong ; London ; Milan ; Paris ; Singapore ; Tokyo :
Springer, 1999
(Lecture notes in computer science ; Vol. 1679)

CR Subject Classification (1998): I.5, I.3.5-8, I.2.9-10, I.4, J.3

ISSN 0302-9743

ISBN 978-3-540-66503-8   ISBN 978-3-540-48232-1 (eBook)
DOI 10.1007/978-3-540-48232-1

© Springer-Verlag Berlin Heidelberg 1999

Originally published by Springer-Verlag Berlin Heidelberg New York in 1999.

Typesetting: Camera-ready by author
SPIN: 10704282   06/3142 – 5 4 3 2 1 0   Printed on acid-free paper

Preface

This is the second MICCAI – the flagship international conference for medical image computing and computer-assisted intervention. MICCAI was created by merging three closely related and thriving conference series – VBC (Visualisation in Biomedical Computing), MRCAS (Medical Robotics and Computer Assisted Surgery) and CVRMed (Computer Vision, Virtual Reality and Robotics in Medicine) – to provide a single focus for the presentation of high-quality research in this important multi-disciplinary area. The first MICCAI was held in Boston, USA in October 1998. It attracted a large number of excellent submissions and was extremely well attended. The meeting went a long way towards meeting its ambitious objectives of bringing together the best theoretical and applied work in this rapidly emerging field, and encouraging constructive dialogue between computer scientists and clinicians.

We are delighted to report a similar level of interest in MICCAI'99. A total of 213 full-length papers were submitted, covering a broad range of topics. Of these, 133 were accepted for inclusion in the conference – 49 as oral presentations and 84 as posters. All the selected papers appear in these proceedings. Each paper was reviewed by four members of the Scientific Review Committee, selected for scientific or clinical expertise of relevance to the subject matter. Final decisions were made by the Programme Committee, following closely the advice of the reviewers. We are indebted to the members of the Scientific Review Committee for the time they devoted to the review process and for their well-informed and generally detailed feedback to authors.

The result is another volume of high-quality papers that we hope will contribute to the development of this important and exciting area. We are also indebted to the dedicated team of staff and students at Manchester who helped to put together the proceedings, particularly Angela Castledine, Alan Brett, Mike Rodgers, Danny Allen, Christine Beeston, Karen Davies, Tony Lacey, and Chris Wolstenholme. We were very pleased to welcome delegates to Cambridge and hope that you found MICCAI an enjoyable and stimulating experience. For readers unable to attend the conference, we hope that you will find this a valuable record of the scientific programme, and look forward to meeting you at MICCAI 2000, which will be held in Pittsburgh, USA.

September 1999   Chris Taylor and Alan Colchester

Conference Organising Committee

Second International Conference on
Medical Image Computing and Computer-Assisted Intervention
Cambridge, England
September 19–22, 1999

General Chair

Alan Colchester — University of Kent at Canterbury and Guy's Hospital, London, UK

Co-chairs

Mike Brady — University of Oxford, UK
Jun-Ichiro Toriwaki — University of Nagoya, Japan

Programme Chair

Chris Taylor (Chair) — University of Manchester, UK

Programme Committee

Nicholas Ayache — INRIA Sophia Antipolis, France
Richard D Bucholz — St Louis University School of Medicine, USA
Brian Davies — Imperial College, UK
Tony DiGioia — Shadyside Hospital, Pittsburgh, USA
James Scott Duncan — Yale University, USA
Guido Gerig — University of North Carolina, USA
David Hawkes — Guy's Hospital, UK
Max A Viergever — Utrecht University, Netherlands

Clinical Advisory Committee Chair

Tony DiGioia — Shadyside Hospital, Pittsburgh, USA

Tutorials

Guido Gerig — University of North Carolina, USA

Industrial Liaison

Nicholas Ayache	INRIA Sophia Antipolis, France
Mike Brady	University of Oxford, UK
Bart ter Haar Romeny	University of Utrecht, Netherlands
Jocelyne Troccaz	University of Grenoble, France
Nigel John (Coordinator)	University of Manchester, UK

Local Organising Committee

Richard Prager	University of Cambridge, UK
Andrew Gee	University of Cambridge, UK

Scientific Review Committee

James Anderson	Johns Hopkins School of Medicine, USA
Takehide Asano	Chiba University School of Medicine, Japan
Gerard A Ateshian	Columbia University, USA
Nicholas Ayache	INRIA Sophia Antipolis, France
Isabelle Bloch	Ecole Nationale Superieure des Telecommunications, France
Fred Bookstein	University of Michigan, USA
Mike Brady	University of Oxford, UK
Richard D Bucholz	St Louis University School of Medicine, USA
Steve Charles	University of Tenessee, USA
Philippe Cinquin	Institut Albert Bonniot, France
Ela Claridge	University of Birmingham, UK
Court Cutting	New York University, USA
Paolo Dario	ARTS Lab, Italy
Brian Davies	Imperial College, UK
Scott Delp	Stanford University, USA
Tony DiGioia	Shadyside Hospital, Pittsburgh, USA
Takeyoshi Dohi	University of Tokyo, Japan
James Scott Duncan	Yale University, USA
Norberto Ezquerra	Universidad Politecnica de Catalunya, Spain
Elliot Fishman	The Johns Hopkins Hospital, USA
J Michael Fitzpatrick	Vanderbilt University, USA
Henry Fuchs	University of North Carolina, USA
Toshio Fukuda	Nagoya University, Japan
Guido Gerig	University of North Carolina, USA
Sarah Gibson	Mitsubishi Electric Research Lab, USA
Eric L Grimson	MIT AI Lab, USA
Blake Hannaford	University of Washington, USA
Dave Hawkes	Guy's Hospital, UK
Derek Hill	Guy's Hospital, UK

Karl Heinz Hohne	University Hospital Eppendorf, Germany
Koji Ikuta	Nagoya University, Japan
Branislav Jaramaz	UPMC Shadyside, USA
Chris Johnson	University of Utah, USA
Ferenc Jolesz	Brigham and Women's Hospital, USA
Leo Joskowicz	Hebrew University of Jerusalem, Israel
Takeo Kanade	Carnegie Mellon University, USA
Lou Kavoussi	Brady Urological Institute, USA
Peter Kazanzides	Integrated Surgical Systems, USA
Ron Kikinis	Brigham and Women's Hospital, USA
Andres Kriete	University Clinic Giessen, Germany
Stephane Lavallee	PRAXIM, France
Heinz Lemke	Technical University Berlin, Germany
Robert J Maciunas	University of Rochester Medical Center, USA
Gregoire Malandain	INRIA, France
Jean-Francois Mangin	Service Hospitalier Frederic Joliot, France
Maurilio Marcacci	Laboratorio di Biomeccanica, Italy
Dwight Meglan	Mitsubishi Electric, USA
Dimitris Metaxas	University of Pennsylvania, USA
Chuck Meyer	University of Michigan, USA
Brent D Mittelstadt	Integrated Surgical Systems, USA
Heinrich Muller	Universitat Dortmund, Germany
Alison Noble	University of Oxford, UK
Lutz-P Nolte	M.E. Muller Institute, Switzerland
Wieslaw Nowinski	Kent Ridge Digital Labs, Singapore
Michael Peshkin	Northwestern University, USA
Stephen Pizer	University of North Carolina, USA
Rob Playter	Boston Dynamics Inc (BDI), USA
Jerry L Prince	Johns Hopkins University, USA
Klaus Radermacher	Helmholtz-Institut f. Biomedizinische Technik, Germany
Richard Robb	Mayo Clinic, USA
Jean-Marie Rocchisani	Hopital Avicenne, France
Joseph Rosen	Dartmouth-Hitchcock Medical Center, USA
Ichiro Sakuma	University of Tokyo, Japan
Tim Salcudean	University of British Columbia, Canada
Kenneth Salisbury	Intuitive Surgical, Inc, USA
Rick Satava	Yale Laproendoscopic Surgery Center, USA
Achim Schweikard	TU München, Germany
H Siegfried Stiehl	University of Hamburg, Germany
Paul Suetens	KU Leuven, Belgium
Gabor Szekely	Swiss Federal Institute of Technology, Switzerland
Mark A Talamini	Johns Hopkins University, USA
Russ Taylor	John Hopkins University, USA
Frank Tendick	University of California San Francisco, USA
Demetri Terzpoulos	University of Toronto, Canada

MICCAI Conference Series

MICCAI Board

Nicholas Ayache	INRIA Sofia Antipolis, France
Alan Colchester	University of Kent at Canterbury & Guy's Hospital, London, UK
Toni Digioia	Shadyside Hospital, Pittsburgh, USA
Takeyoshi Dohi	University of Tokyo, Japan
Jim Duncan	Yale University, USA
Eric Grimson	MIT Artificial Intelligence Laboratory, USA
Karl-Heinz Höhne	University of Hamburg, Germany
Ron Kikinis	Brigham and Women's Hospital, Boston, USA
Steve Pizer	University of North Carolina, USA
Richard Robb	Mayo Clinic, USA
Russ Taylor	Johns Hopkins Hospital, Baltimore, USA
Jocelyne Troccaz	University of Grenoble, France

Table of Contents

Data-Driven Segmentation

Segmentation Using Structural Models

Image Processing and Feature Detection

Surfaces and Shape

Measurement and Interpretation

Spatiotemporal and Diffusion Tensor Analysis

Registration and Fusion

Robotic Systems

Biomechanics and Simulation

3-D Deformable Registration of Medical Images Using a Statistical Atlas

Mei Chen, Takeo Kanade, Dean Pomerleau, Jeff Schneider

Robotics Institute, School of Computer Science, Carnegie Mellon University, Pittsburgh, PA 15213

{meichen, tk, pomerlea, schneide}@cs.cmu.edu

www.cs.cmu.edu/~meichen/registration.html

Abstract

Registration between 3-D images of human anatomies enables cross-subject diagnosis. However, innate differences in the appearance and location of anatomical structures between individuals make accurate registration difficult. We characterize such anatomical variations to achieve accurate registration.

We represent anatomical variations in the form of statistical models, and embed these statistics into a 3-D digital brain atlas which we use as a reference. When we register the statistical atlas with a particular subject, the embedded statistics function as prior knowledge to guide the deformation process. This method gives an overall voxel mis-classification rate of 2.9% on 40 test cases; this is a 34% error reduction over the performance of our previous algorithm without using anatomical knowledge.

1. Motivation

Registration between volumetric images of human bodies enables cross-subject diagnosis and post-treatment analysis. However, due to genetic and life-style factors, there are innate variations among individuals in the appearance and location of anatomical structures. Figure 1 displays cross-sections of T1-weighted magnetic resonance imaging (MRI) volumes of two non-pathological brains. The example structure, corpus callosum, has different intensity, shape, size, and location in these two brains. For registration algorithms that use only intensity or shape templates to achieve correspondence, results are typically poor due to these inherent variations.

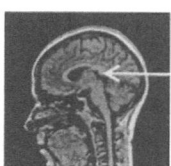
Corpus
Callosum
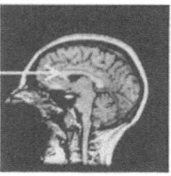

Figure 1. Innate variations between individuals.

Currently there exist many intensity correspondence based registration algorithms [1], [3], [5], [12]. Figure 2 shows a registration result using method [5]. The right image volume is deformed to register with the left image volume, and outlines of its anatomical structures are overlaid on the left image to illustrate the alignment. Note that there is significant misalignment between the deformed structures and the real structures. This is because the shape and density of anatomical structures in the two volumes are considerably different, and a method using intensity correspondence cannot address the difference.

Knowledge of anatomical variations provides information that can guide the registration process and improve accuracy. Characterization of such variations also facilitates quantitative study of anatomical differences between populations, as well as anomaly detection. We capture and model non-pathological anatomical differences between individuals, and use this knowledge to achieve accurate registration.

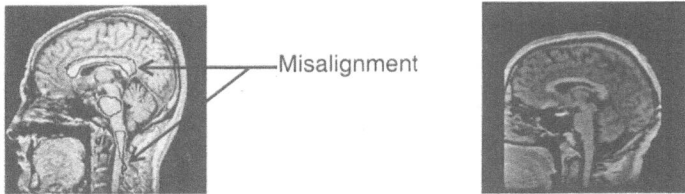

Figure 2. The right image volume is deformed to register with the left one. Outline of several deformed anatomical structures are overlaid on the real structures.

2. Problem Definition

We collected 105 T1-weighted MRI volumes of non-pathological brains, and use them as the training set for knowledge extraction. Examples from the training set are shown in the top row of Figure 3. Apart from the intrinsic differences between different people's brain structures, there are also extrinsic differences in image orientation, scale, resolution, and intensity.

In order to capture the anatomical variations in the training set, we compare each MRI volume to a common reference. Our reference is a 3-D digital atlas, which is a T1-weighted MRI of a non-pathological brain, accompanied by expert classification of its anatomical structures. Note that, this atlas is an example of a normal brain, not an average brain of a population. The method for comparison is an automatic 3-D deformable registration algorithm that was previously developed [12]. This method first eliminates the extrinsic variations between image volumes with preprocessing, then extracts the intrinsic anatomical variations by finding the deformable mapping between each image volume and the atlas.

The intrinsic variations are abstracted into a computational model. During registration, this model functions as prior knowledge to guide the registration process to tolerate anatomical variations, and to achieve higher accuracy.

3. Capturing Anatomical Variations

Different image acquisition processes result in variations in the 3-D orientation, position, resolution and intensity of image volumes in the training set. Differences in head size also add variation in the scales of the image volumes. These variations are extrinsic to the anatomical variabilities, and thus need to be removed before the intrinsic variations can be extracted.

3.1. Eliminating Extrinsic Variations

The registration algorithm employed for atlas-training set comparison [12] consists of a hierarchy of deformable models, of which the first level is a similarity transformation, which addresses the extrinsic geometric variations between different subject volumes via 3-D rotation, scaling, and translation. As a result, each subject volume in the training set has roughly the same orientation, size, and location as that of the atlas. The transformed subject volume is resampled to match the resolution of the atlas. A multi-level intensity equalization scheme is interwoven into the deformation hierarchy to adjust the differences in intensity distributions. The middle row in Figure 3 shows the result of having removed the extrinsic differences between the atlas and the training set.

3.2. Extracting Intrinsic Anatomical Variations

After the removal of extrinsic variations, intrinsic variations are apparent as the misalignment between anatomical structures in the subject volumes and the atlas. The employed registration algorithm captures this information by aligning the corresponding structures through 3-D deformation, and recording the 3-D displacement, as shown in the last row of Figure 3. Therefore, after aligning each subject's anatomical structures with those in the atlas, each atlas voxel is associated with two distributions: one is an intensity distribution of corresponding voxels in the subject volumes; the other is a geometric distribution of the 3-D displacement between the atlas voxel and the corresponding voxels in the subject volumes. The former contains density variations of anatomical structures over a population (density is reflected in image intensity), while the latter embodies geometrical variations of these structures, such as shape, size, and location.

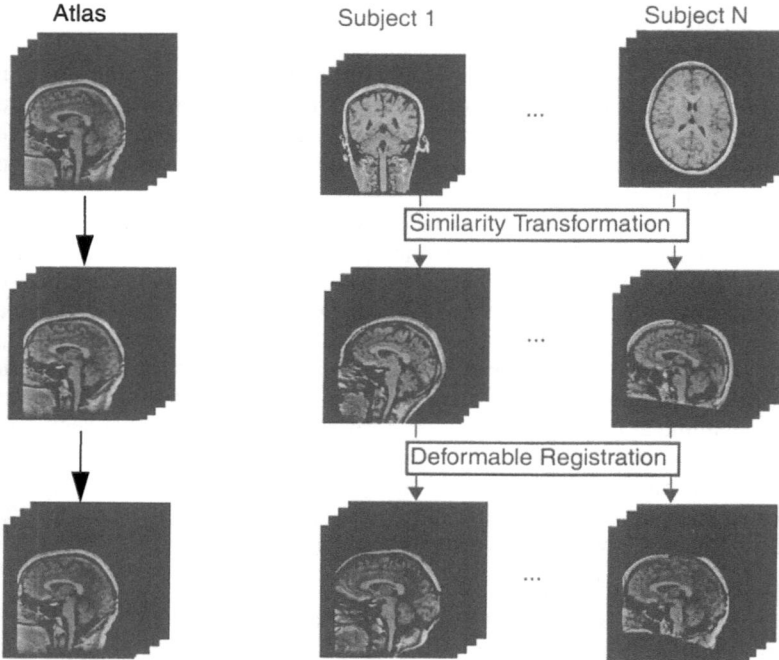

Figure 3. Remove extrinsic variations and extracting intrinsic variations.

4. Modeling Anatomical Variations

The purpose of capturing anatomical variations is to achieve accurate registration. We characterize these variations in a statistical manner, so as to employ them as prior knowledge in statistical models.

4.1. Modeling Density Variations

Once the training set is deformed to register with the atlas, each atlas voxel corresponds with its counterpart in each of the subject volumes. The histogram of their intensities captures tissue density variations in a population (Figure 4).

The intensity histogram at each atlas voxel is modeled as a 1-D Gaussian distribution, $P\langle dI|D\rangle$:

$$P\langle dI|D\rangle = \frac{1}{\sqrt{2\pi}\sigma}e^{-\frac{(dI-\mu)^2}{2\sigma^2}} \tag{1}$$

where $dI = I_s - I_a$, while I_s and I_a are corresponding voxel intensities in the subject

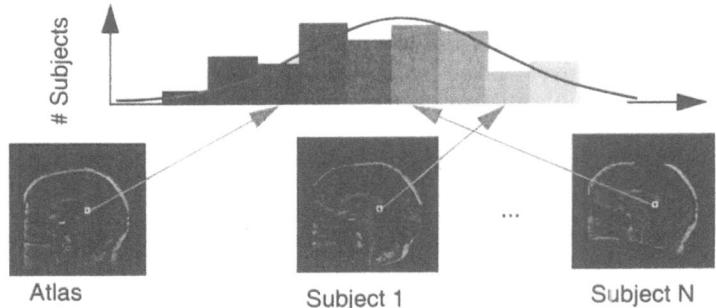

Figure 4. Model density variations at each atlas voxel as a 1-D distribution.

volume and the atlas. D is the 3-D deformation between them. μ is the mean intensity difference between the training set and the atlas at this voxel; σ^2 is the variance of the intensity difference distribution. dI has been adjusted for intensity variations caused by image acquisition processes.

4.2. Modeling Geometric Variations

After the training set is deformed to register with the atlas, the 3-D displacements between each atlas voxel and its counterparts in the training set embody the geometric variations between individuals. The distribution of the variations can be captured in a 3-D histogram. Figure 5 shows a 2-D illustration.

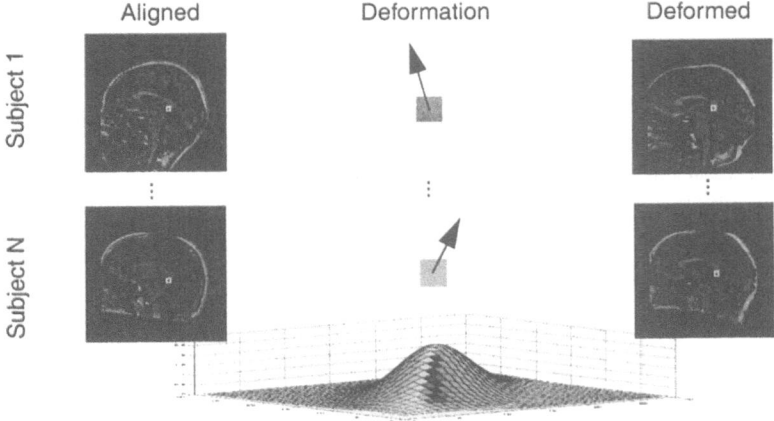

Figure 5. Model geometric variations at each atlas voxel as a 3-D distribution.

The 3-D histogram of displacements at each atlas voxel is modeled as a 3-D Gaussian distribution, $P(D)$:

$$P(D) = \frac{1}{\sqrt{(2\pi)^3 |\Phi|}} e^{-\frac{(\overrightarrow{\Delta\vartheta} - \bar{\omega})^T \Phi^{-1} (\overrightarrow{\Delta\vartheta} - \bar{\omega})}{2}} \qquad (2)$$

here $\overrightarrow{\Delta\vartheta}$ is the 3-D displacement between the atlas voxel and its counterparts in the training set, $\bar{\omega}$ is the mean 3-D displacement at this atlas voxel, and Φ is the 3x3 covariance matrix of the distribution. $\overrightarrow{\Delta\vartheta}$ has been adjusted for extrinsic variations.

4.3. A Statistical Atlas

The original atlas was one particular subject's brain MRI data, with each voxel's anatomical classification given; the above modeling associates each atlas voxel with a distribution of tissue density variations, and a distribution of geometric variations between
individuals. These distributions enrich the atlas into a statistical atlas that embodies the
knowledge of anatomical variations in a population. Figure 6 illustrates the concept.

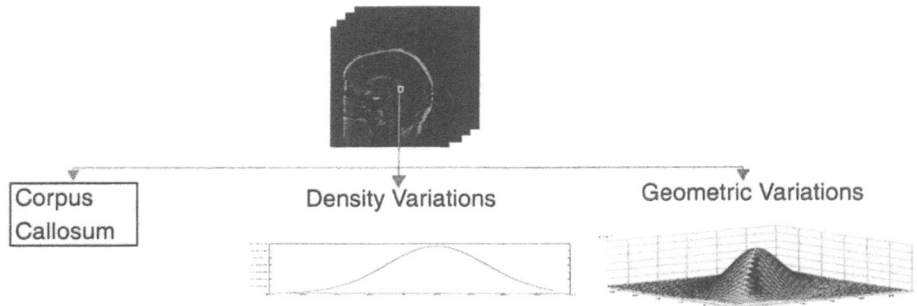

Figure 6. A statistical atlas.

5. Registration Using the Statistical Atlas

Using the statistical models as prior knowledge, the registration between a subject and
the atlas can be formulated as finding the deformation D that gives the highest posterior
probability $P\langle D|dI\rangle$. According to Bayes rule, $P\langle D|dI\rangle$ can be expressed as:

$$P(D|dI) = \frac{P(dI|D)P(D)}{P(dI)} \qquad (3)$$

Finding the highest $P\langle D|dI\rangle$ becomes maximizing the right hand side of equation (3).
Here $P(dI)$ is a constant for two given image volumes, and the numerator has the same
maximum as its logarithm. Substituting from equations (1) and (2) and taking logarithms we obtain:

$$\log P\langle D|dI\rangle = \log\frac{1}{\sqrt{2\pi}\sigma} - \frac{(dI-\mu)^2}{2\sigma^2} + \log\frac{1}{\sqrt{(2\pi)^3|\Phi|}} - \frac{(\vec{\Delta\vartheta} - \vec{\omega})^T\Phi^{-1}(\vec{\Delta\vartheta} - \vec{\omega})}{2}$$

hence maximizing $P\langle D|dI\rangle$ is equivalent to minimizing the term:

$$\frac{(dI-\mu)^2}{2\sigma^2} + \frac{(\vec{\Delta\vartheta} - \vec{\omega})^T\Phi^{-1}(\vec{\Delta\vartheta} - \vec{\omega})}{2} \qquad (4)$$

We use gradient descent to find the deformation that minimizes (4). The 3-D gradient,
∇, at each step of the descent is given by the first order derivative of (4):

$$\nabla = \frac{dI-\mu}{\sigma^2}\nabla I + \Phi^{-1}(\vec{\Delta\vartheta} - \vec{\omega}) \qquad (5)$$

where ∇I is the 3-D image gradient, which is a function of the voxel's position. Since
σ and Σ can have small values, The 3-D shift δD is then:

$$\delta D = -\lambda\nabla \qquad (6)$$

here λ *is a step size constant.* In this way, each voxel is guided to search for a counterpart so their match is most probable according to the statistics gathered from a popula-

tion. We apply 3-D Gaussian smoothing to the voxels' 3-D displacements after each iteration to smooth the deformation. This compensates for the fact that the dependence between the deformation of neighboring voxels is not modeled in the statistical atlas. This algorithm differs from the previously developed hierarchical deformable registration algorithm [12] in the measurement of the goodness of the voxel deformation flow. In this method, we maximize the posterior probability of the current deformation using statistics gathered from a population, whereas in the previous algorithm we minimize the intensity difference between spatially corresponding voxels in the atlas and the subject volume. Before undergoing deformation, both algorithms globally align the two image volumes to eliminate extrinsic variations[12].

6. Performance of Registration Using the Statistical Atlas

We evaluate the effectiveness of our model of anatomical variations by comparing registration using the statistical atlas, and registration using the original atlas.

6.1. Evaluation Metric

Since each voxel in the atlas is labelled with the anatomical structure that contains it, when we register the atlas with a subject, we can then assign the label to the corresponding voxel in the subject. This creates a *customized atlas* which contains classifications of the subject's anatomical features. Figure 7 illustrates this process. Given the *ground-truth* classification of the subject's anatomical structures, we can evaluate the quality of the registration by assessing the voxel classification accuracy. Currently we have 40 subjects' brain MRIs that have expert classification of one structure, the corpus callosum, in one plane, the mid-sagittal plane. They are not part of the training set, and are used as the test set. Our error metric is the ratio between the number of mislabelled voxels and the number of expert labelled voxels. Mislabelled voxels include those labelled as corpus callosum in the customized atlas but not by the expert, or vice versa.

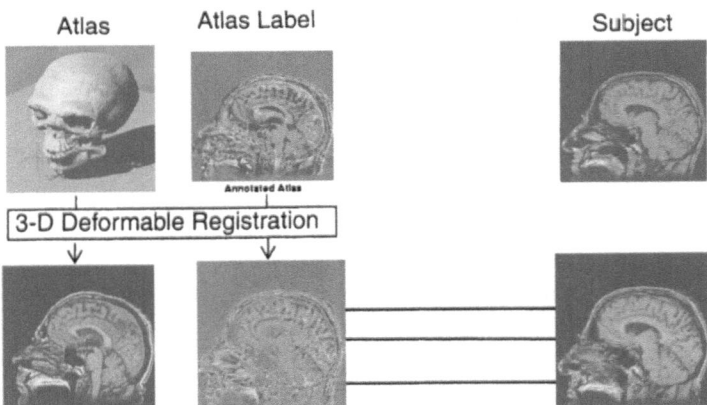

Figure 7. Classifying a subject's anatomical structures through registration with the atlas.

6.2. Registration Using the Intensity Statistics Model

First, we assess the effectiveness of the intensity statistics model alone with constant geometric prior probability. The maximization problem in equation (3) simplifies to $P\langle D|dI\rangle \propto P\langle dI|D\rangle$, and equation (5) becomes:

$$\nabla = \frac{dI - \mu}{\sigma^2}\nabla I$$

We apply this method to the test set, and compute the ratio of mislabelled voxels for all volumes. We find an overall mislabelled voxel ratio of 3.8%. This is a 14% error reduction over the algorithm with no knowledge guidance [12], which has 4.4% error.

6.3. Registration Guided by the Geometric Statistics Model

In this experiment, we assess the effectiveness of the geometric statistics model alone, with the intensity statistics assumed to be a constant. The optimum deformation maximizes $P(D)$. The 3-D gradient at each step is the second term in equation (5):

$$\nabla = \Phi^{-1}(\overrightarrow{\Delta\theta} - \vec{\omega})$$

however, ∇ alone is insufficient to determine the deformation because it ignores the images being registered. To combine the prior model prediction and the image gradient information, we use their inner product to obtain a 3-D deformation gradient $\tilde{\nabla}$:

$$\tilde{\nabla} = \left(\frac{\nabla}{\|\nabla\|} \bullet \frac{\nabla I}{\|\nabla I\|}\right)\nabla \qquad (7)$$

this balances the influence of the prior distribution and the fidelity to the image data. We apply this method to the test set, and it yields an overall mislabelled voxel ratio of 4.05%, which is an 8% error reduction

6.4. Registration Using the Statistical Atlas

The statistical atlas combines the strength of the intensity and geometric prior, as derived in equation (5). When applied to the test set, it has an overall mislabelled voxel ratio of 3.6%, which is a 23% error reduction over the algorithm with no knowledge guidance. Figure 8 shows an example of improved registration using the statistical atlas

No Knowledge Guidance   Use Statistical Atlas

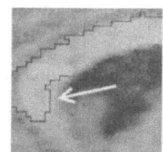   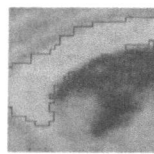

Figure 8. Comparison of registration results using the original and the statistical atlas.

7. Neighborhood Context

The voxel-based statistics models are efficient at modeling anatomical variations. In reality, however, the deformation of neighboring voxels are not independent. Figure 9 shows an example of the deformation flow overlaid on the image data. Note that the deformation flow is smooth and congruous locally. A more comprehensive model should consider the dependencies between the 3-D deformation of neighboring voxels.

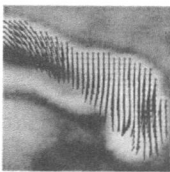

Figure 9 A close-up on the deformation flow overlaid on the image data. Note the local smoothness of the deformation.

Modeling neighborhood context can be a direct higher dimensional extension of the voxel-based statistics models. Consider a 3-D neighborhood of NxMxK centered at an atlas voxel; the intensity distribution of this neighborhood under a specific deformation D is modeled as an $\Re$ dimensional Gaussian distribution, where $\Re$ equals NxMxK:

$$P\langle \vec{dl}|D\rangle = \frac{1}{\sqrt{(2\pi)^{\Re}|\Sigma|}}e^{-\frac{(\vec{dl}-\hat{\mu})^T\Sigma^{-1}(\vec{dl}-\hat{\mu})}{2}} \qquad (8)$$

here $\vec{dl}$ is an $\Re \times 1$ vector of intensity differences between the corresponding neighborhoods in the subject volume and the atlas. $\hat{\mu}$ is the $\Re \times 1$ mean vector of the neighborhood intensity difference distribution; Σ is the $\Re \times \Re$ covariance matrix of the intensity difference distribution. $\vec{dl}$ has been adjusted for extrinsic intensity variations Similarly the geometric variations of a NxMxK neighborhood centered at each atlas voxel can be modeled as a $3\Re$ dimensional Gaussian distribution of the neighborhood's 3-D deformation:

$$P(D) = \frac{1}{\sqrt{(2\pi)^{3\Re}|\Psi|}}e^{-\frac{(\overrightarrow{\Delta\vartheta}-\bar{\omega})^T\Psi^{-1}(\overrightarrow{\Delta\vartheta}-\bar{\omega})}{2}} \qquad (9)$$

where $\bar{\omega}$ is the $3\Re \times 1$ mean vector of the neighborhood's 3-D deformation flow; Ψ is the $3\Re \times 3\Re$ covariance matrix of the geometric distribution; $\overrightarrow{\Delta\vartheta}$ is the $3\Re \times 1$ vectors of the neighborhood's 3-D displacement, and it has been adjusted for extrinsic geometrical variations. Note that the voxel-based statistics models are a special case of the neighborhood statistics models with a 1x1x1 neighborhood.

8. Registration Using Neighborhood Statistics

We follow the same deduction procedure as in Section 5 to achieve the deformation that maximizes the posterior probability $P\langle D|dl\rangle$ for a voxel neighborhood; the 3-D gradient of voxels in the neighborhood is:

$$\nabla = \Sigma^{-1}(\vec{dl}-\hat{\mu})\nabla I + \Psi^{-1}(\overrightarrow{\Delta\vartheta}-\bar{\omega}) \qquad (10)$$

Theoretically we can implement this algorithm in the same way as the voxel-based statistics models; however, the $\Re \times \Re$ intensity covariance matrix Σ has $(\Re(\Re+1))/2$ distinct entries, and the $3\Re \times 3\Re$ geometric covariance matrix Ψ has $(3\Re(3\Re+1))/2$ distinct entries. Our image volumes typically have more than 8 million voxels. Even if all entries in the covariance matrices can be stored as bytes, the covariance information for each 2x2x2 voxel neighborhood will require 336 MByte memory. Together with other memory requirements, the dimensionality of our image volumes makes this approach impractical.

To simplify the problem, we consider only the interaction between immediate neighbors. Instead of storing interactions between immediate neighbors, we compute them on the fly. We approximate the voxel-neighbor interaction using the *goodness* of its neighbors' current match according to their prior distributions. Using a weighted-window matching approach, the *goodness* is weighted by the distance between the voxel and the particular neighbor. Therefore, for a voxel neighborhood $\aleph$, the 3-D gradient determined by neighborhood statistics models is a direct extension of equation (5):

$$\nabla = \sum_{i,j,k} w_{ijk}\left(\frac{dI-\mu}{\sigma^2}\nabla I\right)_{ijk} + \sum_{i,j,k} w_{ijk}[\Phi^{-1}(\overrightarrow{\Delta\vartheta}-\bar{\omega})]_{ijk} \qquad ijk \in \aleph \quad (11)$$

8.1. Performance of Neighborhood Statistics Models

We evaluate the effectiveness of neighborhood statistics models in the same fashion as in Section 6. The size of the voxel neighborhood we used is 3x3x3.

Registration Guided by Neighborhood Intensity Statistics model: Using only the neighborhood intensity prior model, i.e., the first term in equation (11) achieves an overall error ratio of 3.18%. This is a 27.7% reduction over the algorithm with no knowledge guidance, and a 16% error reduction over registration guided by voxel-based intensity statistics.

Registration Guided by Neighborhood Geometric Statistics model: Using only the neighborhood geometric prior model, i.e., the second term in equation (11) gives an overall error ratio of 3.76%. This is a 14.6% reduction over the algorithm with no knowledge guidance, and a 7% error reduction over registration guided by voxel-based geometric statistics.

Registration Guided by Neighborhood Statistics models: Using both the neighborhood intensity and geometric prior distributions gives an overall mislabelled voxel ratio of 2.9%. This is a 34% error reduction over the algorithm with no knowledge guidance. and a 20.6% error reduction over registration guided by voxel-based statistics models. Figure 10 shows an example of improved registration using neighborhood statistics models.

Voxel Statistics   With Neighborhood Context

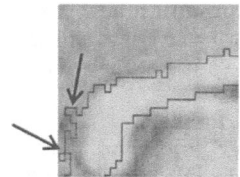   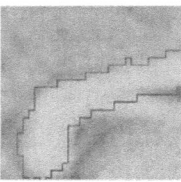

Figure 10. Compare results using voxel-based statistics and neighborhood statistics.

These experiments show that the neighborhood statistics models are significantly more effective than voxel-based statistics models. In the case of intensity statistics model, the neighborhood statistics model nearly doubled the error reduction of the voxel-based statistics model. The geometric statistics model did not seem to be as effective as the intensity statistics model. We attribute this to its higher dimensionality, which would require a larger training set for more accurate model extraction. We expect a complete implementation of the neighborhood statistics guided registration to yield an even greater improvement in performance.

9. Conclusion and Future Work

Inter-subject registration is made difficult due to inherent differences between individuals. Characterization of such anatomical variations can help improve registration performance. We extract the patterns of variations in the appearances of brain structures from a training set of 105 T1-weighted MRI. Registration guided by this prior knowledge achieves higher accuracy on a test set of 40 MRI volumes.

We capture the anatomical variations between individuals by registering the training set with a 3-D digital brain atlas, using a previously developed 3-D hierarchical deformable registration algorithm [12]. This associates each voxel in the atlas with multi-dimensional distributions of anatomical variations in density and geometry. We evaluate statistical properties of these distributions for a neighborhood of each atlas voxel, and embed these statistics into the brain atlas to build a statistical atlas.

Statistical models embedded in the atlas reflect anatomical variations of a population, and thus can function as prior knowledge. It can guide the registration process to tolerate non-pathological variations between individuals while retaining discrimination between different structures. When applied to the test set, the knowledge-guided registration gives an overall voxel mis-classification rate of 2.9%; this is a 34% improvement over the performance of the algorithm without knowledge guidance. Experiments have also shown that statistical models that incorporate local spatial congruity are more effective than single-voxel-based statistical models. Due to page limit, reviews of related work can be found in [16].

The statistical atlas was built upon results from a registration algorithm without knowledge guidance. Imprecisions in the results can affect the rigorousness of the statistical models. To improve model accuracy, we propose to build an initial statistical atlas from a small but accurately registered training set, then bootstrap it into a more reliable model. Besides guiding deformable registration, our computational model of anatomical variations can also facilitate quantitative investigation of anatomical differences between populations, and help detect abnormal variations due to pathology.

Acknowledgments

The authors are thankful to the Brigham and Women's Hospital of the Harvard Medical School for the brain atlas. We are grateful to Kate Fissell in the Carnegie Mellon Psychology Department, Dr. Daniel Rio in the National Institute of Health, and Dr. Matcheri Keshavan in the Western Psychiatric Institute and Clinic of the University of Pittsburgh Medical School, for the brain MRI data. We owe our gratitude to Marie Elm, John A. Hancock, Daniel Morris, and David laRose for their insightful comments.

References

[1] Christensen et al., "Individualizing Neuroanatomical Atlases Using A Massively Parallel Computer", *IEEE Computer*, pp. 32-38, January 1996.

[2] Evans et al., "Warping of Computerized 3D Atlas to Match Brain Image Volumes for Quantitative Neuroanatomical and Functional Analysis. *Proceedings of SPIE Medical Imaging*, vol. 1445, pp. 236-246.

[3] Vemuri et al., "An Efficient Motion Estimator with Applications to Medical Image Registration", *Medical Image Analysis*.

[4] Bajcsy and Kovacic, "Multiresolution Elastic Matching", *Computer Vision, Graphics, and Image Processing*, vol. 46, pp 1-21, 1989.

[5] Jean-Philippe Thirion, "Fast Non-Rigid Matching of 3D Medical Images", INRIA, Technical Report No. 2547, May, 1995.

[6] Szekely et al., "Segmentation of 2-D and 3-D objects from MRI volume data using constrained elastic deformations of flexible Fourier contour and surface models", *Medical Image Analysis*, vol. 1, No. 1, pp. 19-34.

[7] Bookstein, "Landmark methods for forms without landmarks: morphometrics of group differences in outline shape", *Medical Image Analysis*, vol. 1, No. 3, pp. 225-243.

[8] Martin et al., "Characterization of Neuropathological Shape Deformations", *IEEE Transactions on Pattern Analysis and Machine Intelligence*, vol. 20, No. 2, 1998.

[9] Guimond et al., "Automatic Computation of Average Brain Models", *Proceedings of the First International Conference on Medical Image Computing and Computer-Assisted Intervention*, pp. 631-640, 1998.

[10] Wang and Staib, "Elastic Model Based Non-rigid Registration Incorporating Statistical Shape Information", *Proceedings of the First International Conference on Medical Image Computing and Computer-Assisted Intervention*, pp. 1162-1173, 1998.

[11] Kapur et al., "Enhanced Spatial Priors for Segmentation of Magnetic Resonance Imagery", *Proceedings of the First International Conference on Medical Image Computing and Computer-Assisted Intervention*, pp. 457-468, 1998.

[12] Chen et al., "Anomaly Detection through Registration", *Pattern Recognition*, vol 32, pp. 113-128, 1999.

[13] Thompson et al., "High-Resolution Random Mesh Algorithms for Creating a Probabilistic 3-D Surface Atlas of the Human Brain", *NeuroImage*, vol 3, No. 1, pp. 19-34, February, 1996.

[14] Gee and Le Briquer, "An Empirical Model of Brain Shape", *Maximum Entropy and Bayesian Methods*, August 4-8, 1997.

[15] Joshi et al., "On the Geometry and Shape of Brain Sub-Manifolds", *International Journal of Pattern Recognition and Artificial Intelligence*, vol. 11, No. 8, pp. 1317-1343, 1997.

[16] Chen et al., "Probabilistic Registration of 3-D Medical Images", CMU-TR-99-16, July, 1999.

Probabilistic Brain Atlas Construction: Thin-Plate Spline Warping via Maximization of Mutual Information

C.R. Meyer, J.L. Boes, B. Kim, and P.H. Bland

Department of Radiology, University of Michigan,
3307 Kresge III Research, Ann Arbor, MI USA 48109-0553
cmeyer@umich.edu

The concepts of a probabilistic atlas are well known. The dispersions of the resulting atlas' spatial probability distributions depend not only on the intrinsic variation of structures between subjects, but also on the ability of the intersubject mapping method to compensate for gross spatial variations. We demonstrate an automatic method of registering patients to an atlas by maximization the mutual information between the atlas and the patient's gray scale data set. The global thin-plate spline (TPS) transformation for mapping each subject is computed by automatically optimizing the loci of 40 control points distributed within the atlas. The use of 40 control points, i.e. 3*40=120 degrees of freedom (DOF), is a compromise between viscous flow methods with huge DOF, and the 12 DOF affine mapping. We quantitatively compare the results between using a full affine transformation versus the MI-driven 40 control point thin-plate spline for the mean and standard deviation volume data sets computed over the gray scale volumes of 7 patients.

1. Introduction

For several years many noted groups have been both building probabilistic atlases of the human head as well as developing methods to further improve the classification specificity of such atlases. Evans, et al, developed early automatic techniques using affine transformations [1]. Since then the same group has developed a scale space incremental deformation method called ANIMAL and have pursued additional constraints [2] while applying such atlases to the detection of abnormalities such as multiple sclerosis [3] and epilepsy [4]. Thirion, et al, have pursued the registration of "crest lines" in the creation of atlases [5-9]. Christensen has demonstrated the ability to build atlases using viscous fluid flow models [10, 11], and Thompson has added additional free boundary surface constraints to the viscous flow deformation technique [12]. Our objective was to apply the global objective criterion of maximizing mutual information in developing an automatic method where the degrees of freedom (DOF) were sufficiently small so as to prevent unjustified local deformations, e.g. as in creating a tumor to match the patient's data using a tumorless model, but still had sufficient DOF and robustness to more accurately deform to fit a wider variation in patient geometries. The use of mutual information is attractive because the atlas matching technique is independent of modality or acquisition parameters as experienced in MRI. This middle ground approach yields a solution that requires only the use of current generation desktop workstations for reasonable case compute times.

In this paper we report on the quantitative and visual differences obtained by mapping 7 patients of significantly different brain anatomy into the geometry of the atlas using both the full affine, 12 DOF transform, and a 120 DOF thin-plate spline transform under automatic control.

2. Methods

The atlas was obtained from http://www.bic.mni.mcgill.ca/brainweb/), the web site of the McConnell Brain Imaging Centre, Montreal Neurological Institute, McGill University. The atlas was constructed under the direction of Alan Evans with funding from the International Consortium for Brain Mapping (ICBM). The ICBM atlas is a 1 mm cubic voxel MRI head scan that has been manually segmented. We modified our version of the atlas such that region 1 consists of cerebrospinal fluid, region 2 is gray matter, region 3 is white matter, and region 0 fills the remainder of the volume.

All patients were imaged using a GE 1.5 T MRI using a 3D T1-weighted, gradient recalled echo sequence with inversion recovery preparation which produces excellent gray/white matter contrast and B1-field uniformity (no subsequent B1-field correction was applied). For the registration method we used our "MIAMI Fuse" software package where the acronym stands for *m*utual *i*nformation for *a*utomatic *m*ultimodality *i*mage *fus*ion[13]. The subsampled ICBM atlas was chosen as the reference target into which to map the patient data volume. The atlas was decimated by using every third voxel in x and y, and every other voxel in z. Forty control point locations were spatially distributed in the atlas to yield relatively uniform distances between control points and provide local shape control near structures of large variability such as the ventral and dorsal horns of the ventricles.

To begin the mapping of the patient into the atlas, the user begins the process by identifying 4 control points in the patient's data volume that are approximately homologous to the first 4 control points in the atlas' set of 40. The method first optimizes a 7 degree-of-freedom (DOF) affine geometric fit (rotation, isotropic scaling, and translation computed from 4 control points) between the patient data and the ICBM model until the increase in mutual information between repeated optimization cycles is less than .0001 bit. The method continues by fitting a 12 DOF full affine model also using only 4 control points, followed a 120 DOF fit using 40 control points for a thin plate spline (TPS) warping model. At each DOF the same stopping criterion is used before proceeding to the next DOF level. The optimal solution at one DOF level is used as the initial starting condition for the next level by mapping the desired number of control points from the atlas into the patient data set using the previous, best solution. In this manner the patient MRI is first mapped onto the ICBM model using large scale, global controls while more local controls are applied last.

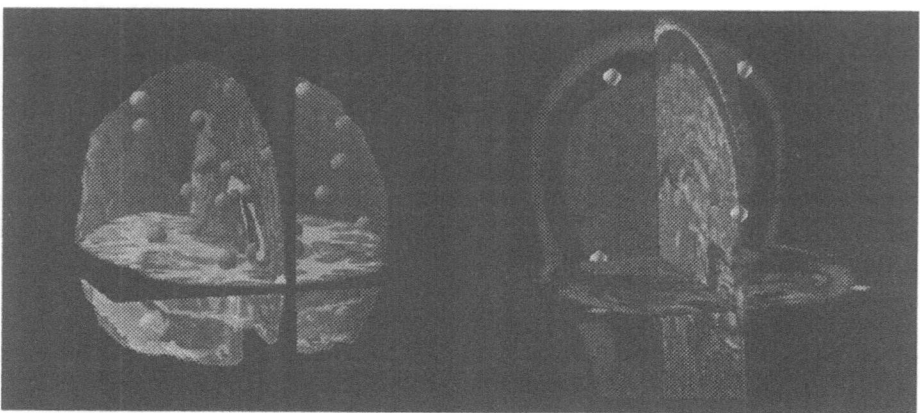

Fig. 1a: View of ICBM atlas with 40 control points distributed over volume. The first 4 control points are depicted in white.	Fig. 1b: View of typical patient data set with 4 approximate homologous control points placed in volume to roughly match the positions of the white markers in atlas

The optimizer used (to minimize the negative of mutual information) was the Nelder-Mead Simplex method commonly referred to as amoeba [14]. While not optimal in the number of iterations required to reach the solution vector in noiseless function optimization problems, the simplex method behaves very much like simulated annealing with its own computed cooling schedule, and is very robust against being trapped by local minima in noisy cost functions. The n-vector to be optimized consists of the coordinate positions of the control points in the patient data set where n equals three times the number of control points. Each optimization cycle is terminated when the requested movement of each of the control points in the patient volume set in any of the 3 cardinal coordinate directions is less than 0.1 mm.

After registration with the atlas, all patient data sets were gray scale amplitude normalized from the same white matter volume of interest. Next the mean and standard deviation gray scale volumes were computed for each of the two registration methods, full affine and 120 DOF TPS. Since these data sets were registered to a labeled atlas, we are able to easily dissect the distributions of gray scale values of these mappings for the specific labels, i.e. cerebrospinal fluid, gray matter, and white matter, and the overall combination.

3. Results

The following table reports the quantitative results for the combination of patients for the two different mapping methods.

Metrics on MRI Gray Scale Distributions Across Patients								
40 Point **TPS Warping**					For **Full Affine** Mapping			
Selected Volumes	CSF	Gray	White	Com-bined		CSF	Gray	White	Com-bined
	Computed Standard Deviation Volume								
mean	10.95	10.15	8.47	9.73		12.13	10.67	9.4	10.52
2.5%tile	3	3	2	3		3	3	2	2
97.5%tile	30	20	20	20		32	21	23	24
	Computed Coefficient of Variation Volume								
mean	0.47	0.30	0.18	0.29		0.48	0.31	0.21	0.31
2.5%tile	0.15	0.05	0.02	0.02		0.16	0.06	0.02	0.02
97.5%tile	0.95	0.66	0.52	0.75		1.00	0.72	0.60	0.80

Table 1.

More local effects can be observed by viewing both the mean and standard deviation volumes. Figures 2a and 2b show the same axial slice through the average volumes obtained by the two methods. Although the global objective function used for the mapping, i.e. mutual information, was computed only over the brain tissues of the atlas, Fig. 2 shows the average including extradural tissues so the reader can view the dural edges without clipping. Figures 3a and 3b show the same sagittal slice through the calculated standard deviation volume. The grayscale window-level was chosen such that white represents a standard deviation of 70 and black represents 0.

Additionally the graph in Fig. 4 depicts the improvement in the objective function, mutual information, and the average total number of optimization iterations required as the number of control points is varied between 4 and 40 points. The compute time using 40 control points was on the order of 11.5 hours on a 433 MHz Digital Equipment Corporation (DEC) single processor, Personal Alpha workstation running DEC UNIX 4.0.

4. Discussion

The first observation we make is that, similar to Collins [2], the global quantitative metrics understate the marked improvement that can be visualized in the images. Thus even though some small improvement in variance averaged over the atlas volume can be discerned between the two methods in Table 1, the automatic TPS

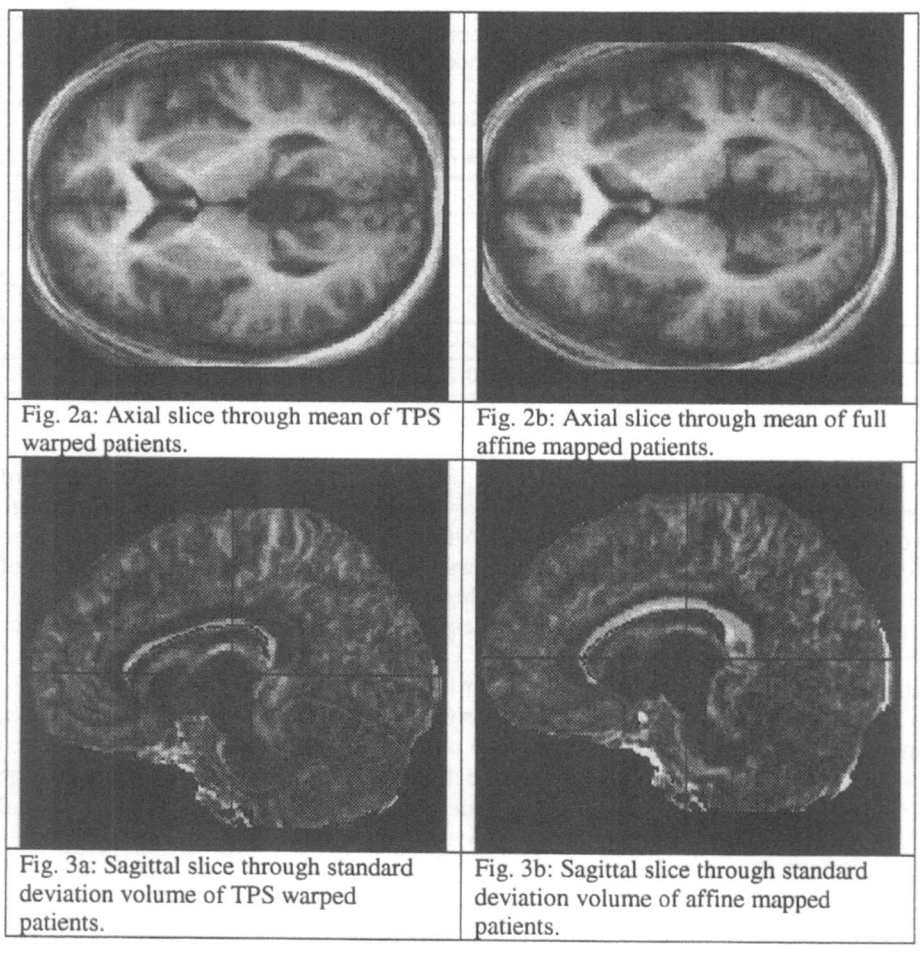

Fig. 2a: Axial slice through mean of TPS warped patients.

Fig. 2b: Axial slice through mean of full affine mapped patients.

Fig. 3a: Sagittal slice through standard deviation volume of TPS warped patients.

Fig. 3b: Sagittal slice through standard deviation volume of affine mapped patients.

warping results in an improved clarity of structures whether midbrain, or more peripheral. In Fig. 2a note the improved clarity of the putamen, globus pallidus, and caudate nuclei, as well as the regions near the vermis of the cerebellum, posterior ventricles, and lateral sulcus. In Fig. 3 the most striking difference is in the local standard deviation associated with the registration of the corpus callosum and ventricle; note the much thicker region of high standard deviation surrounding these midbrain regions as well as the edges of the thalamus and pons. Registration near the dura of the occipital cortex is noticeably improved as well.

From the following graph we observe that there are significant, easy gains in registration accuracy associated with small increases in degrees of freedom (DOF) beyond 12, i.e. 4 control points. Additionally we observe that the improvement in MI with increasing numbers of control points does not appear to be asymptotically approaching an upper threshold at 40 control points, which suggests that we can significantly increase, e.g. double, the number of control points and improve the resulting fit even further. Since the increase in iterations appears to be nearly linear with number of control points, the computational cost of using more control points should not be onerous.

In summary we have demonstrated an implementation of a method for automatically computing a human brain atlas using the mutual information (MI) maximization criterion where the variable degrees of freedom are specified by the number of control points used. The use of MI makes the registration of any MRI acquisition sequence trivial, and the use of limited, i.e. 120, degrees of freedom helps insure the unique mapping of similar structures across patients. The process is robust and typically requires no user intervention or repeated computational runs due to divergent registrations.

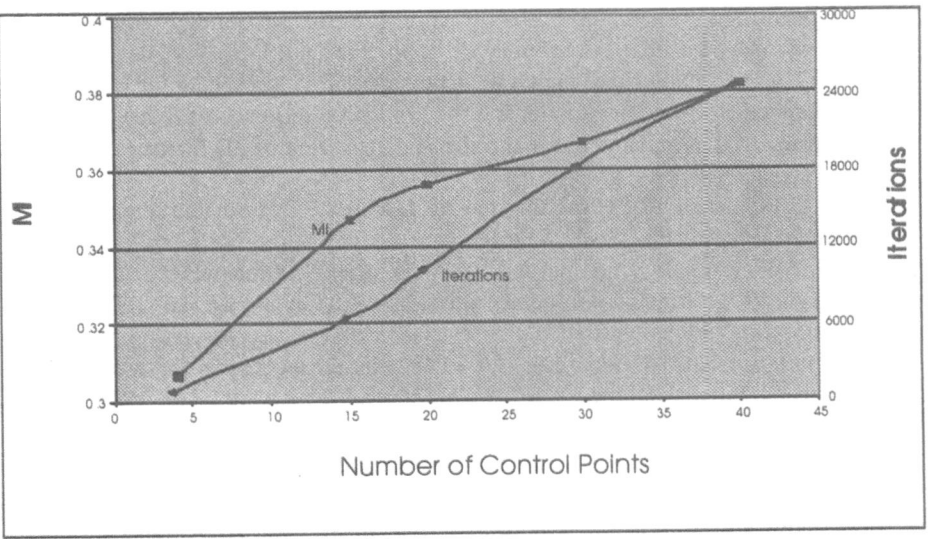

References

[1] D. L. Collins, T. M. Peters, and A. C. Evans, "An automated 3D non-linear image deformation procedure for determination of gross morphometric variability in human brain," , Rochester, MN, 1994.

[2] D. L. Collins, G. L. Goualher, R. Verugopal, A. Caramanos, A. C. Evans, and C. Barillot, "Cortical constraints for nonlinear cortical registration," presented at Visualization in Biomedical Computing, Hamburg, Germany, 1996.

[3] A. Zijdenbos, A. Evans, F. Riahi, J. Sled, J. Chui, and V. Kollokian, "Automatic quantification of multiple sclerosis lesion volume using stereotaxic space," presented at Visualization in Biomedical Computing, Hamburg, Germany, 1996.

[4] J. W. Lee, F. Dubeau, A. Bernasconi, D. MacDonald, A. Evans, and D. C. Reutens, "Morphometric analysis of the temporal lobe in temporal lobe epilepsy," *Epilepsia*, vol. 39, pp. 727-736, 1998.

[5] X. Pennec and J. Thirion, "A framework for uncertainty and validation of 3D registration methods based on points and frames," *Internat J Computer Vision*, vol. 25, pp. 203-229, 1997.

[6] G. Subsol, J.-P. Thirion, and N. Ayache, "Application of an automatically built 3D morphometric brain atlas: study of cerebral ventricle shape," presented at Visualization in Biomedical Computing, Hamburg, Germany, 1996.

[7] J. Thirion, "Image matching as a diffusion process: an analogy with Maxwell's demons," *Medical Image Analysis*, vol. 2, pp. 243-260, 1998.

[8] J.-P. Thirion, "Non-rigid matching using demons," presented at International Conference on Computer Vision and Pattern Recoginition (CVPR'96), 1996.

[9] J. Thirion, "The extremal mesh and the understanding of 3D Surfaces," , Seattle, 1994.

[10] G. E. Christensen, R. D. Rabbitt, and M. I. Miller, "Deformable templates using large deformation kinetics," *IEEE Image Proc*, vol. 5, pp. 1435-1447, 1996.

[11] M. I. Miller, G. E. Christensen, Y. Amit, and U. Grenander, "Mathematical textbook of deformable neuroanatomies.," *Proc. Natl. Acad. Sci. USA*, vol. 90, pp. 11944-8, 1993.

[12] P. Thompson and A. W. Toga, "A surface-based technique for warping three dimensional images of the brain," *IEEE TMI*, vol. 15, pp. 402-417, 1996.

[13] C. R. Meyer, J. L. Boes, B. Kim, P. Bland, K. R. Zasadny, P. V. Kison, K. Koral, K. A. Frey, and R. L. Wahl, "Demonstration of accuracy and clinical versatility of mutual information for automatic multimodality image fusion using affine and thin plate spline warped geometric deformations," *Medical Image Analysis*, vol. 3, pp. 195-206, 1997.

[14] W. H. Press, B. P. Flannery, S. A. Teukolsky, and W. T. Vetterling, *Numerical Recipes in C: The Art of Scientific Computing*. Cambridge: Cambridge University Press, 1988.

Out-of-Plane Non-linear Warping of a Slice into Volume

Boklye Kim[1], Jennifer L. Boes, Peyton H. Bland, Charles R. Meyer

Department of Radiology, University of Michigan Medical Center, Ann Arbor, Michigan, 48109-0553 USA

http://www.med.umich.edu/dipl/
[1]boklyek@umich.edu

This research was supported in part by DHHS NIH 2R01 CA59412-04A1

Abstract. Non-linear 3D warping is implemented for registration of a planar (2D) image into an anatomical reference volume space for accurate spatial mapping. The mutual information based automatic warping algorithm is expanded to include the 2D-to-3D mapping of slice images exhibiting localized out-of-plane geometric deformations. Presented in this work is demonstration and evaluation of the control point based 3D thin-plate-spline (TPS) function applied to the correction of local deformations in MR slice images. Automated 3D warping of a slice into an anatomical reference volume space is achieved by optimization of the mutual information cost function calculated from the gray values of the image pair, i.e., the reference volume and a slice. Accuracy in spatial mapping was assessed by using the simulated MR data sets in a standard anatomical coordinate system and locally induced deformations in a slice image with known TPS transformation parameters. The results indicate the sensitivity of the final optimization to DOF and selected control point locations.

1. Introduction

Recently, we have demonstrated the capability of retrospectively mapping a slice image into an anatomical reference volume from the same subject using a simple rigid body transformation of six degrees of freedom (DOF) [1]. The mapping is achieved by an automated registration routine driven by a cost metric calculated from the global mutual information of the two volume data [2, 3]. In practice, correction of 2D image deformations is often presented as a non-linear warping problem that is not limited to the imaging plane. Out-of-plane warp, typically encountered in multislice MRI data series, is the local field induced deformations induced by the gradient field or susceptibility effect, or localized out-of-plane motion artifacts [4, 5]. This research is focused on correcting the 3D warping artifacts localized in the brain regions that undergo physiological motion, i.e., brain stem, due to the cardiac cycle.

We have expanded the mutual information based automatic registration capability for correction of planar image data exhibiting geometric distortions that include out-of-plane and non-linear warping. The control point based thin-plate-spline (TPS) function is applied to the correction of the local deformations. The non-linear warping capability of TPS can be efficient for correcting local, 3D deformations [6, 7]. In regions distant from the control points, the solution becomes an affine (linear) transformation while its warping effects are limited to local regions. It is beneficial for this 2D-to-3D warping to respond to the 3D deformations locally and not affect other regions that require different solutions.

Initial homologous control points are obtained by the user marking the approximate locations in each data set. The degrees of freedom (DOF) in the solution is controlled by the number of homologous points used. Selecting one point more than the spatial dimension constrains the solution to the affine transformation while selecting additional points implements a general TPS warping solution. Since these control points drive the optimization, the number of variables to optimize is the product of the number of points and the number of spatial dimensions. The initial state vector contains the coordinates of the selected points that define the geometric mapping.

Presented in this paper are demonstration and evaluation of 3D warping of a slice image (2D) into a reference volume space. Accuracy of the spatial mapping was assessed by using simulated MR data sets in a standard anatomical coordinate system and local deformations induced by a known set of TPS transformation parameters.

2   Methods

A slice image taken out of the simulated volumetric brain MRI data from International Consortium of Brain Mapping (ICBM) was used to demonstrate the 3D non-linear warping of a slice image [8]. The localized out-of-plane warping artifact was induced to mimic the brain stem movement effect in slice images during the multislice single shot Echo-Planar imaging (EPI) acquisition [9, 10]. Slice images acquired from a volume containing non-stationary structures, i.e., squeezing of ventricles or brain stem movement, need nonlinear solutions to relocate the voxels to their actual positions at the time of the acquisition. For axial slices the brain stem motion would cause an out-of-plane systematic distortion, i.e., funnel effect. Use of a brain model and simulated local brain motion artifact provide the geometric truth for the warping solution.

2.1 Locally warped planar image

Out-of-plane warping was created by mapping eight control point sets in a pair of volumetric image data set using a TPS function. One point in the homologous control point set was displaced by 4 mm out of the image plane to induce the funnel effect. Figure 1 shows the local 3D funnel effect deformation in a slice image. The local out-of-plane warp is depicted by (a) the grid mesh and (b) superimposed on the slice image.

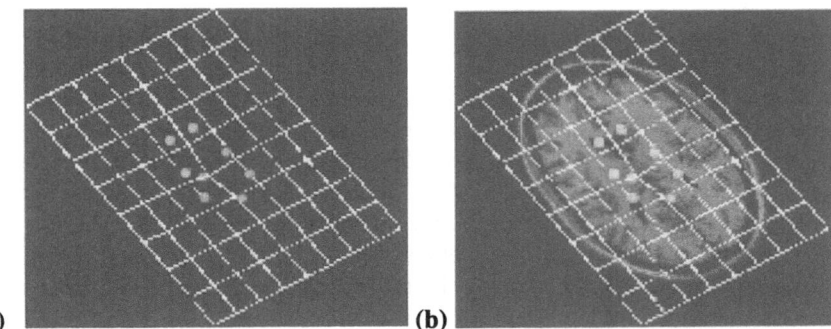

(a)   (b)

Fig.1. (a) An out-of-plane local warp, i.e., funnel effect, produced by the eight control point 3D TPS function with one homologous point (center) displaced out of the plane. (b) The planar image reconstructed from a T_1-weighted MRI volume using the warping function contains out-of-plane features.

2.2   Automated 3D unwarping of a slice into volume

The automated registration of a warped T_1-weighed MRI slice in Fig.1(b) into a reference volume space, T_2-weighted MRI volume data, was achieved by allowing the optimizer to move the control points in the homologous 3D space to positions that minimize the MI cost function calculated from the gray values of the image pair. The mutual information metric (MI = -mutual information) and Mutual Information Automated Multimodality Image Fusion (MIAMI Fuse) software were presented previously for spatial mapping of multimodal image data sets [2, 3, 11].

The registration process is an iterative method driven by MI cost metric and the Nelder-Mead downhill simplex optimization algorithm was implemented [12]. The optimization routine determines the transformation coefficients for a coordinate mapping using either affine or TPS warp transformation and performs trilinear interpolation to map gray scale values of the image voxels. The MI cost metric is computed from the voxel/pixel gray values in the reconstructed data set, therefore, the effect of the geometric mapping is manifested. The trilinear interpolation process uses the original data set for each iteration instead of using the previous interpolation to generate the successive data. This approach prevents round-off and other undesired interpolation effects such as smoothing from accumulating across iterations.

Each optimization cycle is initiated by a random perturbation of the initial transformation vector. During the iteration, the optimizer moves the control points by small increments in an orderly fashion within the given radial bound. At each configuration of the control points, the data sets are mapped, and the resulting MI is computed. The optimizer keeps a history of control point positions and MI values to allow it to move toward an optimal control point configuration. Each iteration was set to stop when movement of control points is < 0.01 mm and the optimization cycle was repeated till the ΔMI < 0.00001 for successive cycle.

3 Results

3.1. 2D-to-3D warping accuracy

The registration accuracy of a slice into the reference volume using the 3D TPS function with random displacement of the initial vector was evaluated. Figure 2 shows the resulting out-of-plane warp of the slice mapped into the anatomical volume space using TPS function defined by the coordinates of the final optimized vector. The slice exhibiting the local warp is reconstructed in the reference space (Fig. 2a) and superimposed on the reference volume data as displayed in a coronal view (Fig. 2b). The effect of the 3D unwarping the funnel effect artifact is demonstrated by the planar visualization of the selected slices from the final reconstructed volume data and the corresponding slices from the reference data in Fig. 2c and Fig.2d, respectively.

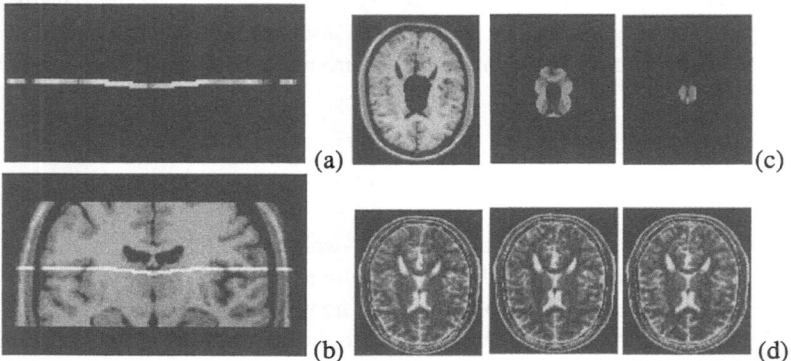

Fig. 2.   Pictorial presentation of the resulting 3D warping of a slice image into a volume. The acquired slice image reconstructed into the volume is indicated by the high intensity lines in coronal views (a) and (b). The planar axial images show the warping of a (c) slice with a 3D deformation reconstructed into a reference volume and (d) the corresponding reference images.

Table 1. The average and standard error (STE) of the final mapping error of the eight control points relative to the truth.

control points	average	STE
1	0.51063484	0.06689679
2	0.43713253	0.06933018
3	0.51385107	0.07932435
4	0.71478606	0.11352397
5	1.30181737	0.24647948
6	0.40896756	0.05031346
7	0.42290929	0.09483279
8	0.51820495	0.12233572

The averaged error of the solution was calculated for the final stopping positions of the eight control points over five optimizations with the initial search bound of 20 mm (=20 voxels). The error was assessed by computing the average and standard rms error (STE) of the control points with respect to the true solution as listed in Table 1. The averaged rms of the mapping coordinates and STE over all the points were 0.56±0.04.

3.2   2D-to-3D warping as a function of DOF

The mapping accuracy of the 3D TPS solutions for correction of the out-of-plane local warping in the slice image was evaluated as a function of number of control points. The registration was performed using sets of 4 to 10 control point points. The plot of MI cost metric versus number of control points in Fig. 3 displays the dependence of the final MI as a function of DOF. The plot indicates the optimal, i.e., minimum, MI with eight control points and increase in MI with the overshoot of DOF. For each number of control point set, the original eight homologous control points were mapped back into the reference space using the final transformation to determine the registration error. The transformed positions of the eight control points were used to compute the rms error of the coordinate displacement from the original eight points of the geometric truth. The plot of the average rms of the displacement over eight control points versus number of control points, Fig.4, demonstrates the geometric mapping as a function of DOF. Noteworthy is the sharp drop in MI values between the affine (four points) and warping starting at five points in Fig.3.

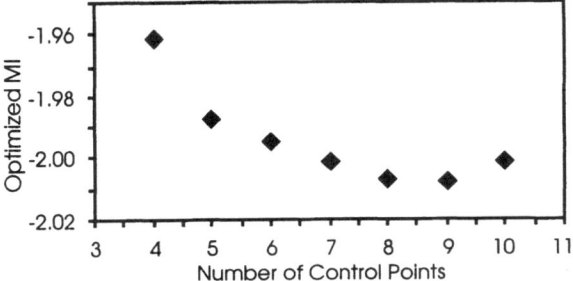

Fig.3. Plot of the final cost function versus number of control points.

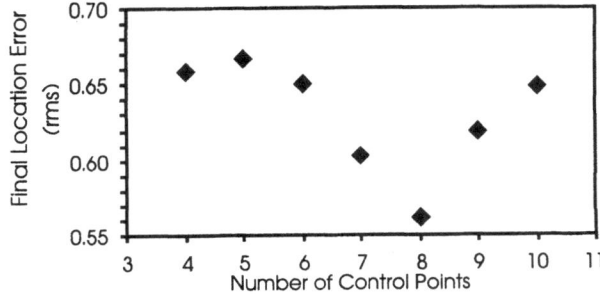

Fig.4. Plot of the final control point position rms error relative to the original positions.

3.3.   2D-to-3D warping as a function of control point selection

Performance of the non-linear 3D registration as a function of the initial control point selection was evaluated by the final optimized MI and mapping coordinates with respect to the true solution. The TPS warp was performed using eight control points with one point selected at a position different from the original location (point 8 in Table 1). The plots in Fig.5 and 6 show the behavior of TPS warping as a function of selected control point position. The plots were constructed by moving the displaced control point in a diagonal planar direction, i.e., toward (+15 mm) and away (-15 mm) from the center of the image. The rms of the final location error and optimized MI averaged over five optimizations are plotted versus the position of the displaced control point, as shown in Fig.5 and Fig.6, respectively.

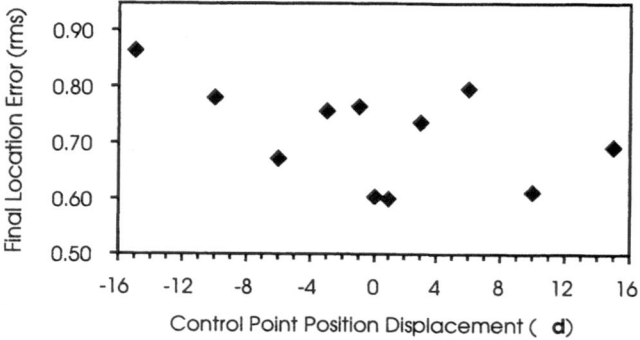

Fig. 5.   Plot of averaged rms of the final position errors versus control point displacement (**d**) along the diagonal planar direction. Negative and positive signs of **d** indicate direction "away from" and "toward" the center of the image, respectively, from the original position.

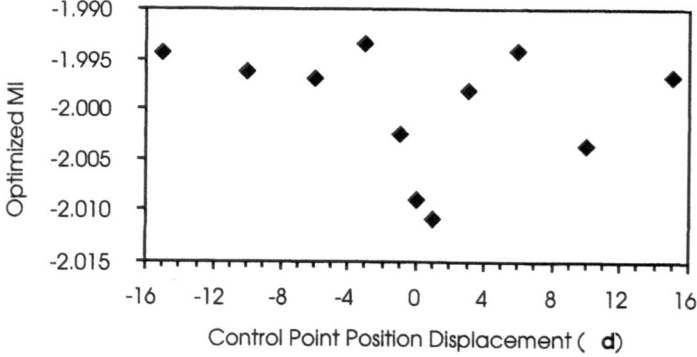

Fig.6.   Plot of averaged MI versus location of control point, 8 (Table 1), indicated by the displacement amount (**d**). The original location is indicated by **d**=0.

Table 2. Mapping error (rms) as a function of control point position.

d (mm)	average error	STE
-15	0.8667	0.1176
-10	0.7803	0.0883
-6	0.6728	0.0787
-3	0.7581	0.0907
-1	0.7669	0.0804
0	0.6035	0.0571
1	0.5993	0.0677
3	0.7351	0.0784
6	0.7980	0.0928
10	0.6128	0.0683
15	0.6923	0.1046

4 Discussion/Conclusions

Mapping of a 2D image into a 3D volume space to correct the out-of-plane non-linear deformations present in the 2D image has been demonstrated using the TPS warping function.   The test data sets provided the geometrical truth and sufficient spatial information content to drive the optimization to convergence.   With the known geometric deformation parameters defined by the control point driven TPS function, the warping of a slice image was evaluated as functions of number and of position of the selected control points. There is an accurate correlation in optimization pattern between the final MI cost metric and position error as a function of number of control points. A sharp decrease in final MI is observed between the affine solution and TPS of five control points in Fig.3. The corresponding spatial displacement error relative to the original control point positions, in Fig.4, may not represent the accurate mapping error for the case of affine transform and marks the limit to an affine solution for solving warping problems. At the other end of the series, the plots in Figs. 3 and 4 demonstrate that using more DOF than the true solution may result in less reliable registration at higher computational cost. Warping as a function of selected position of the control points was demonstrated in Fig.5 and Fig.6 with respect to the final spatial mapping and MI cost metric.   Both curves indicate the presence of local minima, i.e., at positions d = -6 and 10. The standard errors, at the local minima, though, are greater than the global minimum at the original spatial coordinate (d =0) as listed in Table 2. The significance of this work is the 2D-to-3D spatial warping capability by treating the slice image deformations as 3D warping problems without the need of exclusive conditionals.

Problem of non-linear 3D distortions are commonly encountered in MR images acquired using fast imaging sequences.   This work is focused on the effect of physiological brain motion, i.e. brain stem movement from the cardiac acceleration, as often observed in single shot EPI acquisition protocol [9, 10]. Such motion related artifacts pose problems for activation studies using functional MRI (fMRI) technique. Accurate geometric mapping is critical for accurate analysis of fMRI time series data since the activation detection is based on the differences in voxel intensities between the images from task-on and -off cycle assuming consistent voxel locations. In addition, fMRI is susceptible to spatial out-of-plane distortions from the field variation induced by the magnetic susceptibility as well as bulk head motion [5, 13]. This study demonstrates the feasibility of the 3D warping for accurate geometric mapping of multislice functional MR images that exhibit non-linear distortions.

References

1. Kim, B., *et al.*, Motion Correction in fMRI via Registration of Individual Slices into an Anatomical Volume. *Magn. Reson. Med.*, 1999, **41**(5): p 964-972.

2. Kim, B., *et al.*, Mutual information for automated unwarping of rat brain autoradiographs. *NeuroImage*, 1997. **5**(1): p. 31-40.

3. Meyer, C.R., *et al.*, Demonstration of accuracy and clinical versatility of mutual information for automatic multimodality image fusion using affine and thin plate spline warped geometric deformations. *Medical Image Analysis*, 1997. **3**: p. 195-206.

4. Jezzard, P. and R.S. Balaban, Correction of Geometric Distortion in Echo Planar Images from B0 Field Variations. *Magn. Reson. Med.*, 1995. **34**: p. 65-73.

5. Sumanaweera, T.S., *et al.*, MR Susceptibility Misregistration Correction. *IEEE Trans. Med. Img*, 1993. **12**(2): p. 251-9.

6. Bookstein, F.L., *Thin-plate Splines and the Atlas Problem for Biomedical Images*. 1991, Berlin: Springer.

7. Bookstein, F. and W.D.K.A. Green , A feature space for edgels in images with landmarks. *J of Math. Imag. and Vision*, 1993. **3**: p. 231-261.

8. Cocosco, C.A., *et al.*, BrainWeb: Online Interface to a 3D MRI Simulated Brain Database. *NeuroImage*, 1997. **5**(no.4, part 2/4): p. S425.

9. Maier, S.E., C.J. Hardy, and F.A. Jolesz, Brain and Cerebrospinal Fluid Motion: Real-Time Quantification with M-Mode MR Image. *Radiology*, 1994. **193**: p. 477-483.

10. Poncelet, B.P., *et al.*, Brain parenchyma motion: measurement with Cine Echo-planar MR imaging. *Radiology*, 1992. **185**: p. 645-651.

11. Collignon, A., *et al.* Automated multimodality image registration using information theory. *Pro. Computational Imaging and Vision*. 1995. Ile de Berder, FR: Kluwer Academic Publishers.

12. Press, W.H., *et al.*, *Numerical Recipies in C: The Art of Scientific Computing*. 1988, Cambridge: Cambridge Press. p. 305-309.

13. Weisskoff, R.M., *et al.*, Microscopic susceptibility variation and transverse relaxation: theory and experiment. *Magn. Reson. Med.*, 1994. **31**: p. 601-61-.

Tree Representation and Implicit Tree Matching for a Coarse to Fine Image Matching Algorithm

Julian Mattes[1] and Jacques Demongeot[1,2]

[1] TIMC-IMAG, Faculty of Medicine, 38 700 La Tronche, France
Julian.Mattes@imag.fr
[2] Chaire de Biomathématiques, Institut Universitaire de France
jacques.demongeot@mesr.fr

Abstract. In medical imaging arises the problem of matching two images of the same objects but after movements or slight deformations. We present a new method for a primitive global transformation and an improvement of a recent matching strategy which makes it more robust. The strategy consists of two steps. We consider the grey level function (modulo a normalization) as a probability density function. First, we apply a density based clustering method in order to obtain a tree which classifies the points on which the grey level function is defined. Secondly, we use the identification of the hierarchical representations of the two images to guide the image matching. The general transformation invariance properties of the representations permit to extract invariant image points. But in addition, we design a new robust coarse to fine identification of the trees which applies an implicit error measure in a prediction – correction scheme using thin plate splines to interpolate the transformation function in a finer way at each step. Therefore, we will find the correspondence between invariant points even if these have locally moved. The method's results for matching and motion analysis on real images will be discussed.

1 Introduction

The use of structural information in images for recognition tasks has been realized since the inception of machine vision ([14]). A graph structure is useful to represent information about topology and shape of and between extracted features in images and therefore to compare two images, but also, as we will show, to match images in which *local* movements appear (e.g., rigid transformations of *individual* objects in the image or images of deformable objects). For this, we have to construct the graph in such a way that its structure is kept even if deformations appear or features have moved and to use tree identification to find the correspondence between these features.

A grey level function $g : \mathbb{R}^n \to \mathbb{R}_{\geq 0}, n = 2$ or $n = 3$, associates to each physical point in the image scene (represented by $\mathbb{R}^n$) a value corresponding to its physical properties ($\in \mathbb{N}$ in the technical realization) and will be considered as given by the acquisition device. g is eventually smoothed and normalized, in order to have a continuous (or even derivable) density function. The present approach applies density based classification methods ([16], [5]) to the grey level function (considered as density function) in order to construct trees. These methods confine points in clusters at several levels if the points are in regions of (respective to the level) high density. We will call the resulting tree (section 2) a *confinement* (or *density) tree representation of the image*. If we choose the classification method proposed in [16] and [5] the resulting tree corresponds to the component tree defined in [4].

Matching is done now by identification of the two density trees corresponding to the two images. The idea behind this tree representation matching strategy is that the density tree will adapt itself to global and local movements in the image (Figure 1). Under reasonable conditions, we will demonstrate that the proposed representation is invariant with respect to an arbitrary *topological transformation* ϕ (for its definition see the proof in section 2). This allows us to define *characteristic* points (*candidates* for landmarks [2]) and to find corresponding point (i.e., landmark) pairs, associated to nodes in the tree, even if local movements appear. Moreover it allows us to detect if in one of the two images a cluster – intermediary node or leave in the tree – has been changed by noise effects (section 3). All this has a series of applications as detailed in section 4.

We proposed this approach recently in [11, 13], where we defined a cost function for a given association of the two tree structures and we minimized among possible associations in order to obtain the "best" association between the trees. Independently, a matching method based on the same hierarchical decomposition of the image in regions has been proposed in [7, 8]. The correspondence between the regions is established using a weighted combination of similarity criteria, such as the difference of regions' areas, contour lengths, or barycenters.

The present contribution lies in a new identification algorithm of hierarchical decompositions of images. The initialization step (to rediscover the composition of global translation, rotation, and scaling) is a new robust method based on gravity centers of image regions corresponding to the nodes of the tree. After, the method goes from coarse to fine using a prediction – correction scheme and a *local rigid* transformation is applied before the *thin plate spline interpolation* [2] of the topological transformation ϕ is refined *at each time* in order to apply an implicit error measure [1] to ever finer levels. The *prediction – correction scheme* enables us to avoid the association of not corresponding regions and to stop the matching process before it becomes noise sensitive.

We can remark that Leu and Huang [9] used a comparison of ordered trees to define a distance between objects for object recognition. However, a tree identification method, able to handle instabilities in the tree, was not proposed and the algorithm's suitability to match images where non-affine deformations appear was not investigated. Moreover, the tree construction approach does not use statistical methods, but is of geometrical nature based, in a segmented image, on a closed contour whereas simply edge detection is not sufficient.

A recent general overview of matching algorithms can be found in [10].

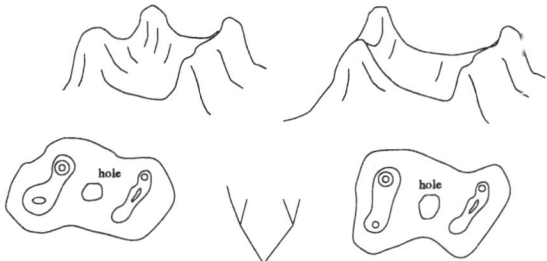

Fig. 1. *Illustration of the density based tree representation.*

The remainder of the paper is organized as follows. In section 2, we detail the construction of the confinement tree and its invariance property. In section 3, we show how to identify the hierarchical representations and we present some results on real images in section 4, before we conclude in section 5.

2   Construction and Invariance Properties of the Confinement Tree

Confronted with the classification task based on a density function we were led to a mathematical entity denoted confiner, appearing in a natural way when we consider level lines in a landscape. Given a density function $g : \mathbb{R}^n \to \mathbb{R}_{\geq 0}, n \in \mathbb{N}$, the *confiners* are defined as the maximal connected subsets (i.e., *components*, Gaal [3], p. 105) C_l of the level sets $L_l = \{x \in \mathbb{R}^n | g(x) \geq l\}, l \in \mathbb{R}_{\geq 0}$ (see Figure 1). In the classification domain we found these components first in a contribution by Wishart [16] and further investigations by Hartigan [5], where they are called *high density clusters*. Considering them taken on several levels $l_k, k = 1, ..., r$ (r from resolution) including the 0 level, they define obviously a tree (by "set inclusion") as illustrated in Figure 1. The tree is finite if g has a finite number of extrema. Let us call the level sequence $(l_k)_{k=0}^r$ with $l_0 = 0$ a *resolution* (of $\mathbb{R}_{\geq 0}$). Then, we call the corresponding tree *confinement* (or *density*) *tree* at resolution $(l_k)_{k=0}^r$ and if g is a grey level function ($n = 2, 3$) of an image I_g we use the term *confinement tree representation of* I_g. The confiners taken at level l_k are the nodes (intermediary nodes and leaves) of the tree at level k. We have chosen this classification method because of the invariance theorem and its consequences shown below. Curiously, this property has already been mentioned in the contributions of Wishart [16] and Hartigan [5] (without assuming the paradigm to hold and only in the case of an affine transformation) even if they did not address a matching problem.

In practice, we consider all grey levels of the image and we delete confiners with a *mass* (calculated as the sum of all normalized grey values associated to the pixels in the confiner) less than 1% of the mass of all confiners at this level. We choose the discrete $d4-distance$ for defining the connectivity between pixels.

Time to calculate the tree is $O(n + r)$, where n is the number of pixels and r is those of levels.

The following hypothesis is the foundation of the transformation invariance property of the investigated matching strategy [11, 8, 7, 13]. We can find similar hypotheses in Optical Flow research [6].

Medical Imaging Paradigm *Let $\phi : \mathbb{R}^n \to \mathbb{R}^n, n = 2$ or 3 be the transformation expressing movements of physical points in an image scene (rendered in the images A and B) which appear when passing from A to B, g_A the density associated to image A, g_B that associated to image B, and $X \in \mathbb{R}^n$. Then we can assume (apart from local noise effects):*
(i) *$g_A(X) = g_B(\phi(X))$ (strong version);*
(ii) *$\varphi(g_A(X)) = g_B(\phi(X))$ for some strictly monotonous function φ.*

Let us remark, that: (1) for the paradigm to hold, we should consider images covering the whole space in which movements appear (thus, 3D images in general) and that the paradigma is a realistic assumption in a larger context than in medical imaging but not in general; (2) if for two images A and B the detector (or detector location) has changed, we have to assume the general case; if we simplify and assume $g_A(X) = \alpha g_B(\phi(X)) + \beta$, we can calculate α and β a priori.

General Invariance Theorem *Let A, B, g_A, g_B, φ, and ϕ be defined as in the paradigm and let $(l_k)_{k=0}^r$ be a resolution of the grey level space. Then: if ϕ is a topological transformation, then, apart from noise effects, the confinement tree at resolution $(l_k)_{k=0}^r$ of image A and those at resolution $(\varphi(l_k))_{k=0}^r$ of image B are identical, moreover, the confiners of A are transformed into the confiners of B and reciprocally.*

Proof (i) The proof of the strong version (i.e., φ is the identity function) is based on the fact that (a) according to its definition (Gaal [3], pp. 186, 187) a *topological transformation* is a bijective and bicontinuous (i.e., ϕ and ϕ^{-1} are both continuous) application and (b) a component stays a component under a topological transformation ([3], Lemma IV.8.1). For details see [11].

(ii) For the general case, let us first suppose that ϕ is the identity function. We have $L_k^A := \{X | g_A(X) \geq l_k\} = \{X | \varphi(g_A(X)) \geq \varphi(l_k)\} = \{X | g_B(X) \geq \varphi(l_k)\} =: L_k^B$. The components of L_k^A are the nodes at level k in the confinement tree of A, the components of L_k^B are those of the B's tree, equally at level k. As $L_k^A = L_k^B$, this defines an isomorphism between the trees.

(iii) If ϕ is general and $h := g_B \circ \phi$, (ii) implies that there exists an isomorphism between the trees associated to h and to A, and from (i) an isomorphism between the trees associated to $h - B$. Then, trees of A and B are isomorph.

The importance of the theorem lies on the fact that the tree is invariant referred to local movements. This makes it more stable for matching than other well known hierarchical representations would be. In the presented formulation, the theorem is more general than previous versions [11, 8, 7, 13].

3   Implicit Tree Matching

Major innovations are developed in this section. Their motivation is to make
the strategy more robust with respect to previous publications [11, 8, 7, 13]. For
this aim, the new algorithm follows the *coarse to fine principle of implicit tree
matching* (below) and uses a *prediction – correction scheme*. Both innovations
are based on a classical implicit error measure [1] defined below, which us enables, together with the application of a local rigid transform at *each iteration
step k* (step (iii) below), to make fully use of proceeding coarse to fine in the
two hierarchical decompositions of the images. In order to use an implicit error
measure we need the correspondence between tree structure and image regions;
just the two (eventually weighted) trees are not sufficient. In this way "implicit
tree matching" differs from tree matching algorithms as presented in [17].

3.1   Implicit Error Measure

We call an *error-measure* between objects on two different images A, B *implicit*
or *transformation based* if it depends on a transformation $\phi_k : A \to B$ (at step
k) between the images A and B. A well known implicit matching algorithm is
ICP [1]. It uses the (implicit) error measure

$$\epsilon(C_A, C_B) = \frac{1}{|C_B|} \sum_{P_B \in C_B} d^2_{min}(P_B, C_A), d_{min}(P_B, C_A) = \min_{P_A \in C_A} ||P_A - P_B||, \quad (1)$$

where $|C_B|$ is the number of points in C_B, and where C_A (resp. (C_B)) is a set
of points in image A (resp. image B). C_A is the reference point set.

Coarse to Fine Principle of Implicit Tree Matching. (see Figure 2). Let
be given a selection order for A confiners (cf. subsection 3.2) and a transformation
function $\phi_k : A \to B$ obtained at iteration step $k - 1$. Iteration step k:
Substep (i) Find the corresponding confiner C_B^k in image B of the currently
    selected confiner C_A^k using the error measure $relPos_k(.,.)$ (see below).
Substep (ii) Match locally rigidly confiners C_A^k and C_B^k and so define points in
    B corresponding to sampled contour points of locally moved confiner C_A^k.
Substep (iii) Calculate the transformation function ϕ_{k+1} as the thin-plate
    spline interpolation [2] of the corresponding point pairs.
Substep (iv) Select the next A confiner C_A^{k+1}.
    Let us **remark** that substep (iii) can be omitted; in this case we have to
store the rigid transformation for confiners with not updated successors but we
avoid parameters due to interpolation.
    Euclidian Error Measure. Given a transformation $\phi_k : A \to B$ and the
current confiner C_A in image A, we have to find the corresponding confiner C_B
in B based on the transformed external contour $\phi_k(C_A)$ of *reference confiner*
C_A and on the contour C_B of C_B. We choose the confiner $C_{B_{min}}$ minimizing the
following error measure $relPos_k(.,.)$ based on $\epsilon(.,.)$ of equation (1):

$$relPos_k(C_A, C_B) = \epsilon(\phi_k(C_A), C_B) \frac{\max(A(C_A), A(C_B))}{\min(A(C_A), A(C_B))}, \quad (2)$$

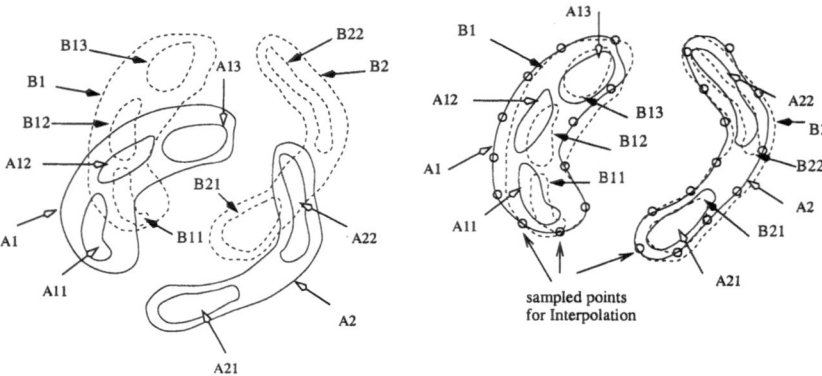

Fig. 2. *Coarse to Fine Principle of Implicit Tree Matching. On the left side we are able to find the coarse association (between A1 and B1, A2 and B2); but we are not able to find the fine association because relPos(A13, B12) < relPos(A13, B13). Therefore (right hand side), first, we match locally rigidly A1 with B1, we choose corresponding point pairs on the original and locally transformed contour of A1, we interpolate the transformation function and, finally, we transform A11, A12, and A13 using this function. After we repeat the procedure for A2, B2, A21, and A22. The A-confiners on the right have been translated and rotated around 25° with respect to the left hand side.*

where $A(\mathcal{C})$ denotes the area of confiner $\mathcal{C}$.

In order to associate to ϕ_k an error value, let denote by $\mathcal{G}(A)$ (resp. $\mathcal{G}(B)$) the set of gravity centers of clusters associated to the nodes of the tree corresponding to A (resp. B). We define:

$$\epsilon_{euclid}(\phi_k) = \epsilon(\phi_k(\mathcal{G}(A)), \mathcal{G}(B)) + \epsilon(\mathcal{G}(B), \phi_k(\mathcal{G}(A))). \qquad (3)$$

3.2 Matching Algorithm

Initialization. The initialization is based on the point sets $\mathcal{G}(A)$ and $\mathcal{G}(B)$ defined above. In practice, we take only the nodes appearing directly after bifurcations into account, in order to reduce search space. Our aim for initialization is to find the transformation ϕ_0 representing translation, rotation, and scaling (referred below as *semi-rigid* transformation) such that the error measure $\epsilon_{euclid}(\phi_0)$ is smallest. We proceed as proposed by Thirion for *extremal points* in [15]. Roughly spoken, for each given pair of points in $\mathcal{G}(A)$, we take a pair of points in $\mathcal{G}(B)$, we calculate the semi-rigid (or rigid) transformation S defined by the association of the two point pairs, we transform all points in A according to this transformation and determine the error $\epsilon_{euclid}(S)$. For a given pair of points in $\mathcal{G}(A)$ we can limit the number of possible corresponding points in $\mathcal{G}(B)$ using a preselection based on invariant features ([15]; in our case the features are, for instance, the normalized confiner mass, its area, etc.). Finally, we take the transformation associated to the two pairs of points minimizing the error.

It remains to apply the **coarse to fine principle** detailed hereafter.

Confiner Selection Order. First, we have to define in which order we select confiners in image A for which we look for corresponding confiners in B. We consider just confiners corresponding to a node directly after a bifurcation to update the interpolation function and we *update confiners* with the same father in order of increasing predicted error (see next step). We start with the confiners after the first bifurcation. After, we choose at each step the *bifurcating node* (cf. Figure 5) having the largest mass (section 2) among the bifurcating nodes with not updated children. The selected confiners are its children.

Predicted Identification. At iteration step k we choose for a given confiner C_A the confiner C_B minimizing $relPos_k(C_A, C_B)$ in equation (2).

Interpolation Point Pairs. We update $\phi_k \mapsto \phi_{k+1}^{temp}$ (i.e. the *corresponding points list* on which ϕ_k is based) at each time when we associated 2 confiners C_A and C_B according to the following interpolation point pair selection scheme illustrated in Figure 3. We match locally the confiners for which we detected a correspondence in order to obtain a semi-rigid transformation ϕ_{k+1}^{loc}. First, we remove that points from the corresponding point list that are in a tubular neighborhood (with thickness η) around the transformed confiner $\phi_{k+1}^{loc}(C_A)$. After, we sample points on the contour of C_A, apply ϕ_{k+1}^{loc} on them, put the so obtained point pairs in the corresponding point list and get ϕ_{k+1}^{temp}.

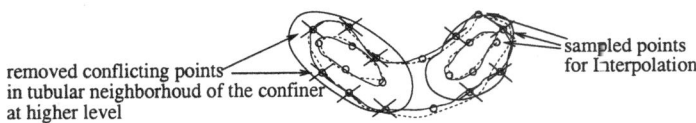

removed conflicting points
in tubular neighborhoud of the confiner
at higher level

sampled points
for Interpolation

Fig. 3. *Interpolation Point Pair Selection Scheme.*

Prediction – Correction Scheme. In the previous prediction step we obtained the temporary transformation ϕ_{k+1}^{temp}. This enabels us to define an *intrinsic criterion* to verify if the predicted association was correct:

If $(\epsilon_{euclid}(\phi_{k+1}^{temp}) \geq \epsilon_{euclid}(\phi_k)$ or another A confiner has been associated to C_B
) then { $\phi_{k+1} := \phi_k$;   /* reject identification */
} else $\phi_{k+1} := \phi_{k+1}^{temp}$;
We *stop* identification in a whole *subtree*, if we reject identification for the subtree root and all its children.

4   Applications

The first part of our new method, concerning global alignment of two 2D or 3D images, has a wide range of applications. Remember for instance, that we use such an alignment for reconstructing images from their 2D slides when their orientation has been lost during acquisition. Applications of the second part of our method include the study of the relative motion of grains in microscopic metallurgical images or of cells in microscopic biological images. On the other hand, we can also use our method to detect abnormalities in breast or brain images (with respect to reference images coming from the same patient at a former time or from an atlas), or to detect where in an image movements occur. In the first case this serves to detect a tumor and its location. In the second, the method helps us to apply optical flow or active contour techniques at the found place. A further interesting application of the proposed method is the comparison of two brain images resulting from functional MRI. Here occur small local deformations as well as global shifts. The aim is to locate positions where the brain activation (and therefore the intensity of the functional signal) changed.

Experimental Evaluation. Figure 4 and the middle row of Figure 5 illustrate the effectiveness of our (semi-)rigid matching algorithm initializating our coarse to fine algorithm. This second part is illustrated in the bottom row of Figure 5 which proves that very few confiners in a branch are sufficient for propagating the transformation allowing the correct association of confiners at heigher level. All experiments have been performed on a 450 MHz Intel Pentium III with less than 1s for calculation of the confinement tree as for the initialization step using a tree where confiners with a mass of less than 2.5% (with respect to their level) are deleted. See Figure 4 and 5 for first assessment, a more detailed evaluation can be found in [12].

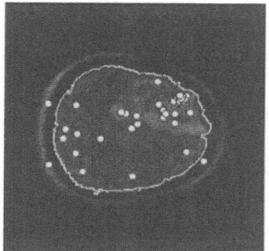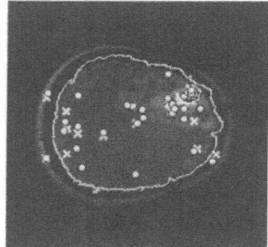

Fig. 4. *On the left: initial upper slide of a 256x256 brain image. The points represent the gravity centers of confiners corresponding to the nodes after bifurcations in the confinement tree. The line corresponds to the confiner covering the whole brain and is just displayed for visualization of the transformation. On the right: lower slide. The points and the line are the transformed points and line of the left picture. The crosses are the gravity centers of the right image. The transformation represents the composition of translation, rotation and scaling as found by the initialization step of our method described in section 3.2. We can notice that the global barycenter of the hole brain is perfectly preserved at a subpixel precision (0.7 pixel).*

5 Conclusion

We showed the use of a tree representation of the grey level function known in statistics (*density* or *confinement tree*) to define a hierarchical decomposition of an image in regions. This decomposition is first used for a new robust method

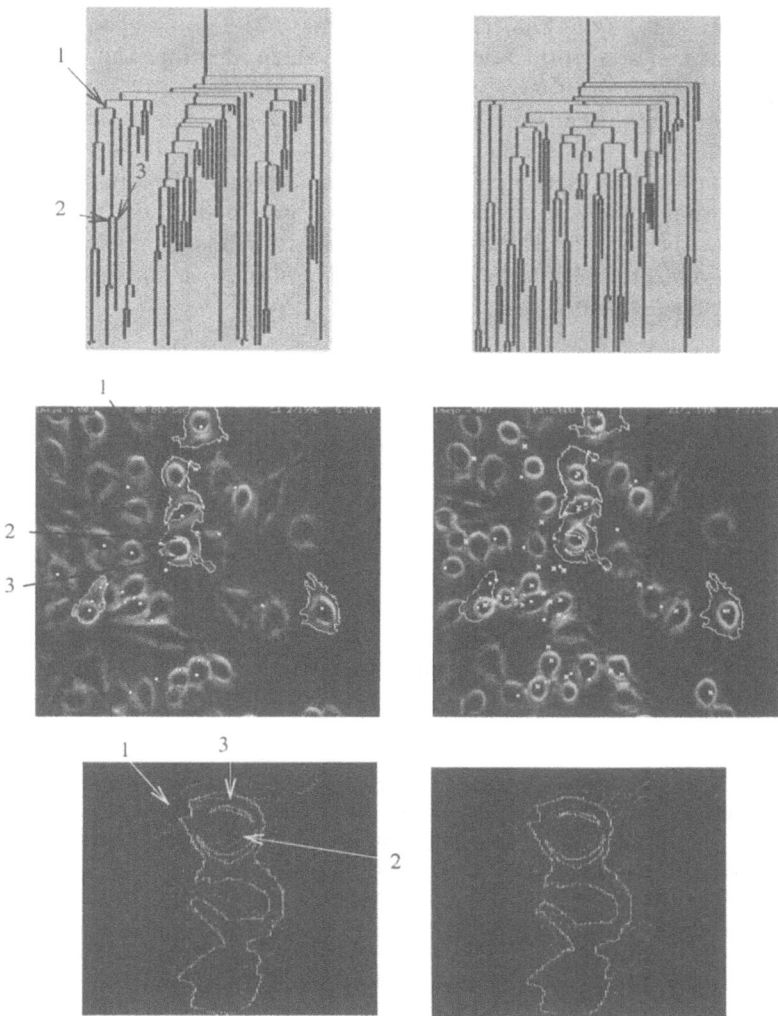

Fig. 5. *First column (top and middle): initial 512x480 image of cells (below) with its corresponding confinement tree. Second column (top and middle): same as in the first column for the moved image. Second row: it shows the result of the initialization step described in section 3.2. The white points in the picture on the left are the gravity centers of the confiners after the bifurcating nodes as described in section 3.2. These points and the lines are transformed and displayed on the right picture after transformation. The transformed points are still displayed as white points, the gravity centers of the right image are displayed as crosses. The lines marked by arrows are the external contours of the confiners of the nodes in the tree above marked with the same number. They are displayed also (as darker lines) in the bottom row together with the corresponding confiners in the moved image. The other lines in the middle row are just shown to better visualize the initial transformation. The bottom row is another illustration of our coarse to fine principle. After matching rigidlly the confiners at lower level (picture on the right), we can easily find the correspondence of the confiners at heigher level.*

for the alignment of two 2D (trivially to extend to 3D) image slides and after for a new coarse to fine identification algorithm which identifies the two image decompositions. With respect to previous versions of this second part, the method (a) avoids external parameters using an *intrinsic* criterion to determine when it is impossible to identify two regions and (b) is robust as it does just require that correspondence between several regions is identified. Especially, it would be possible that *no* local maximum in the first image has a corresponding local maximum in the second. Both, the new method for finding global and that for finding local transformations between two images improve matching and motion analysis of non segmented grey level images.

References

1. Besl, P.J., McKay N.D.: A method for registration of 3-D shapes. IEEE Trans. PAMI **14** (1992) 239-256
2. Bookstein, F.: Principal wraps: Thin-plate splines and the decomposition of deformations. IEEE Trans. PAMI **11** (1989) 567–585
3. Gaal, S.A.: Point set topology. Academic Press, New York, (1964)
4. Hanusse, P., Guillotaud, P.: Sémantique des images par analyse dendronique. In: AFCET, 8th RFIA, Vol. 2. Lyon (1992) 577–588
5. Hartigan, J.A.: Statistical theory in clustering. J. of Classification **2** (1985) 63–76
6. Horn, B., Shunck, B.G.: Determining optical flow. Art. Intel. **17** (1981) 185–203
7. Kok-Wiles, S.L.: Comparing mammogram pairs for the detection of mammographic lesions. PhD thesis, Brasenose College, University of Oxford, May 1998, (1998)
8. Kok-Wiles, S.L., Brady, J.M., Highnam, R.: Comparing mammogram pairs for the detection of lesions. In: Karssemeijer, N. (ed.): 4th Int. Workshop of Digital Mammography, Nijmegen, Netherlands, June 1998. Kluwer,Amsterdam, (1998)
9. Leu, J.G., Huang, I.N.: Planar shape matching based on binary tree shape representation. Pattern Recognition **21** (1988) 607–622
10. Maintz, J.B.A., Viergever, M.A.: A survey of medical image registration. Medical Image Analysis **2** (1998) 1–36
11. Mattes, J., Demongeot, J.: Dynamic confinement, classification, and imaging. In: 22nd Annual Conference of the Gesellschaft für Klassifikation e.V., Dresden, Germany, March 1998. Studies in Classification, Data Analysis, and Knowledge Organization. Springer-Verlag, Berlin Heidelberg New York (1999) 205–214
12. Mattes, J., Demongeot, J.: Statistical invariants and structures for image matching and representation. IEEE Trans. Medical Imaging (submitted)
13. Mattes, J., Richard, M., Demongeot, J.: Tree representation for image matching and object recognition. In: G. Bertrand, M. Couprie, L. Perroton (Eds.): DGCI'99. LNCS 1568 (1999) 298-309
14. Pavlidis, T.: Analysis of set patterns. Pattern Recognition **1** (1968)
15. Thirion, J.-P.: New feature points based on geometric invariants for 3D image registration. International Journal of Computer Vision **18** (1996) 121–137
16. Wishart, D.: Mode analysis: A generalization of the nearest neighbor which reduces chaining effects. In: Cole, A. J. (Ed.): Numerical Taxonomy. Academic Press, London (1969) 282–319
17. Zhang, K., Statman, R., Shasha, D.: On the editing distance between unordered labeled trees. Information Processing Letters **42** (1992) 133–139

Gray-Value Based Registration of CT and MR Images by Maximization of Local Correlation

J. Weese[1], P. Rösch[1], T. Netsch[1], T. Blaffert[1], and M. Quist[2]

[1] Philips Research Laboratories, Division Technical Systems,
Röntgenstraße 24–26, D-22335 Hamburg, Germany
[2] EVM Advanced Development, Philips Medical Systems Nederland B.V.,
Veenpluis 4-6, NL-5680 DA Best, The Netherlands

Abstract. For gray-value based multi-modality registration the similarity measure is essential. Excellent results have been obtained with mutual information for various modality combinations. In this contribution we consider local correlation as similarity measure for multi-modality registration. Using a software phantom it is analyzed why local correlation is suitable for this registration task whereas direct gray-value correlation itself is usually not. It is shown that registration with local correlation can be done using only a fraction of the image volume offering an opportunity to accelerate the algorithm. Within validation, registration of the phantom images, two simultaneously acquired dual contrast MR images, and a clinical CT-MR data set has been studied. For comparison, the data sets have also been registered with mutual information. The results show that not only mutual information, but also local correlation is suitable for gray-value based multi-modality registration.

1 Introduction

There are several clinical applications for which images from different modalities are required, because they provide complementary information. A typical example is the use of MR and CT images for radiation therapy planning. Another application is the combination of functional images with the underlying anatomy represented e.g. by an MR image. Different patient posture and positioning during image acquisition complicate the interpretation of the images, and various multi-modality registration algorithms have been developed therefore [1].

For gray-value based methods the similarity measure is essential. Correlation, for instance, relies on a linear relationship between the gray-values of the images to be registered. Such a linear relation cannot be expected for multi-modality data sets and gray-value correlation cannot be applied directly, therefore. To make correlation or the correlation coefficient suitable for CT-MR registration, several pre-processing techniques have been proposed. Studholme et al. [2] applied a non-linear remapping of the CT intensities. Maintz et al. [3] computed feature images with edges or ridges. Mutual information is much more suited for multi-modality registration, because it does not rely on a functional relationship between the gray-values. This distinguishes mutual information from other similarity measures. Multi-modality registration by maximization of mutual information has been proven to be very successful and excellent results have been obtained for various modality combinations (CT-MR, MR-PET etc.) [2, 4, 5].

In this contribution we consider the registration of CT and MR images by maximization of local correlation [6]. To compute local correlation, for each pixel in the reference image a neighborhood is defined, the correlation coefficient between this neighborhood and the corresponding neighborhood in the image to be registered is evaluated, and all resulting correlation coefficients are summed up. At the first glance, it is not obvious, why local correlation is suitable for multi-modality registration. In order to answer this question, a multi-modality data set has been simulated. Using this software phantom, the differences between correlation and local correlation are thoroughly discussed in the following section. In section 3 the experiments are described, which have been performed for validation. Apart from the software phantom, two simultaneously acquired MR images and a clinical CT-MR data set have been used. For comparison, the validation experiments have also been carried out using mutual information. The results are discussed in section 4. Section 5 contains the conclusions.

2   Local Correlation and Multi-Modality Registration

The starting point for the discussion of correlation and local correlation is a software phantom representing two images of different modality. This phantom is introduced in the first subsection. On the basis of this phantom the properties of correlation and local correlation are discussed in the second and third subsection.

2.1   Software Phantom

The software phantom represents a simple model of a multi-modality image set. It is based on the assumption that each type of tissue leads to a characteristic gray-value which depends on the physical effect used for imaging and the material parameters of the tissue. These gray-values are therefore different for different modalities and there is in general no functional relationship between the gray-values of multi-modality images.

The software phantom was generated with a segmentation editor based on the watershed algorithm of Vincent and Soille [7]. To enable interactive editing, markers can be placed which are handled as constraints within region merging. With this editor an MR image has been segmented into six different structures (skin, ventricles, eyes, cortex, background, rest), and two images of different modality have been simulated by assigning random gray-values to the segmented structures. The gray-values are listed in Tab. 1. A slice of each of the simulated multi-modality images is shown in Fig. 1.

Table 1. Gray-values assigned to the structures of the segmented MR image.

	skin	ventricles	cortex	eyes	background	rest
Image a	48	62	70	123	0	5
Image b	15	83	31	101	0	53

658   J. Weese et al.

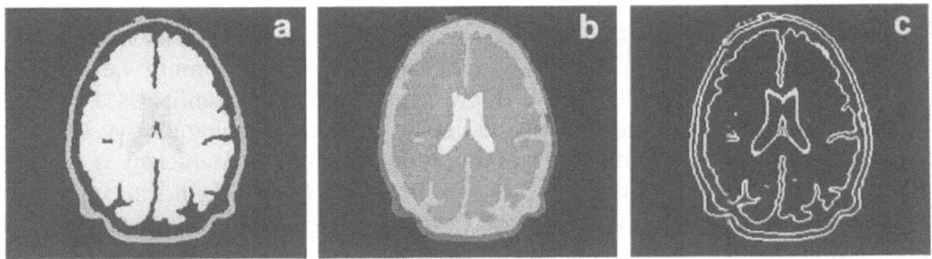

Figure 1. Simulated multi-modality images (a, b) and spatial distribution of the contributions to the local correlation for $r = 1$ (c).

2.2 Correlation

A possibility to register two images of the same modality is the minimization of the mean-square gray-value difference

$$D(\boldsymbol{\omega}, t) = \frac{1}{\#M} \sum_{i \in M} (I_1(i) - I_2(i))^2, \quad i = (i_x, i_y, i_z) \tag{1}$$

with respect to the translation t and the rotation $\boldsymbol{\omega}$ of a rigid transformation. In this equation, $I_1(i)$ denotes the reference image. The image $I_2(i)$ is registered and depends on the transformation parameters t and $\boldsymbol{\omega}$. The summation is performed over all pixels in the overlap region given by the set M.

This approach can be considered as a least-squares method. If the gray-values of the images differ by a gray-value scaling I_0 and a gray-value offset ΔI, the concept of least-squares methods suggests to insert these parameters into (1) and define the registration result by the minimum of

$$D'(\boldsymbol{\omega}, t) = \frac{1}{\#M} \sum_{i \in M} (I_1(i) - I_0 I_2(i) - \Delta I)^2 \tag{2}$$

with respect to the transformation parameters t and $\boldsymbol{\omega}$, the scaling I_0, and the offset ΔI. Minimization with respect to the latter two parameters leads to

$$D'(\boldsymbol{\omega}, t) = \frac{\sum\limits_{i \in M} (I_1(i) - \bar{I}_1)^2}{\#M} - \frac{\left(\sum\limits_{i \in M} (I_1(i) - \bar{I}_1)(I_2(i) - \bar{I}_2)\right)^2}{\#M \sum\limits_{i \in M} (I_2(i) - \bar{I}_2)^2} \tag{3}$$

with $\bar{I}_1$ and $\bar{I}_2$ denoting the average gray-values in the overlap region for the reference image and the image to be registered, respectively. The first term in this equation is the gray-value variance of the reference image $I_1(i)$ within the overlap region. The second term represents the reduction of the gray-value variance due to adaptation of the image $I_2(i)$. The ratio of both terms

$$C^2(\boldsymbol{\omega}, t) = \frac{\left(\sum\limits_{i \in M} (I_1(i) - \bar{I}_1)(I_2(i) - \bar{I}_2)\right)^2}{\sum\limits_{i \in M} (I_1(i) - \bar{I}_1)^2 \sum\limits_{i \in M} (I_2(i) - \bar{I}_2)^2} \tag{4}$$

is the square of the well-known correlation coefficient [8].

In the case of a linear relationship between the gray-values of the software phantom images, the quantity $D'(\omega, t)$ should take its global minimum value ($= 0$) and the square of the correlation coefficient its global maximum ($= 1$) if the images are registered. Because there is no linear relationship, the quantity $D'(\omega, t)$ has a larger value (354) and the square of the correlation coefficient is smaller (0.36). The maximum of the squared correlation coefficient found during registration (0.49) does no more correspond to a proper registration showing that the correlation coefficient is in general not suitable for multi-modality registration.

2.3   Local Correlation

To evaluate local correlation, for a pixel i in the reference image a spherical neighborhood $S_i = \left\{ l = (l_x, l_y, l_z) | (i_x - l_x)^2 + (i_y - l_y)^2 + (i_z - l_z)^2 \leq r^2 \right\}$ of radius r is defined and the squared correlation coefficient $C_i^2(\omega, t)$ between this neighborhood and the corresponding neighborhood in the other image is evaluated:

$$C_i^2(\omega, t) = \frac{\left(\sum\limits_{l \in S_i} \left(I_1(l) - \bar{I}_1(i) \right) \left(I_2(l) - \bar{I}_2(i) \right) \right)^2}{\sum\limits_{l \in S_i} \left(I_1(l) - \bar{I}_1(i) \right)^2 \sum\limits_{l \in S_i} \left(I_2(l) - \bar{I}_2(i) \right)^2} \tag{5}$$

with $\bar{I}_1(i)$ and $\bar{I}_2(i)$ denoting the average gray-value in the neighborhood S_i for the reference image and the image to be registered. In the case that one of the images has a constant gray-value within a neighborhood S_i, the contribution C_i^2 is set to zero to avoid undefined results. The local correlation $\mathrm{LC}^2(\omega, t)$ is obtained by summing up all contributions within the overlap region:

$$\mathrm{LC}^2(\omega, t) = \frac{1}{\#M} \sum\limits_{i \in M} C_i^2(\omega, t). \tag{6}$$

The essential difference between the correlation coefficient and local correlation refers to the relationship between the gray-values of the images to be registered. The correlation coefficient presumes a global linear relationship whereas local correlation assumes a linear relationship in a local neighborhood only. This linear relationship can be different in different regions of the image.

If the local correlation is applied to the software phantom, the contributions $C_i^2(\omega, t)$ can be divided into three categories:

1. One of the images has a constant gray-value within the neighborhood. In this case, the contribution $C_i^2(\omega, t)$ is zero and can be neglected.
2. Both images show only two different gray-values within the neighborhood S_i. In this case, the gray-values can be transformed into each other by a linear relationship. The better the structures within the neighborhood match, the larger becomes the contribution $C_i^2(\omega, t)$, therefore.

3. One of the images has at least two and the other one at least three different gray-values within the neighborhood S_i. In this case, it is usually not possible to map the gray-values onto each other assuming a linear relationship. Thus, the contribution $C_i^2(\omega, t)$ may not take its maximum value, if the images are registered optimally.

As there are only a few regions in the phantom images with three different structures next to each other, there are only few contributions of the last category. Local correlation is dominated by contributions of the second category, therefore. These contributions belong to neighborhoods with two different gray-values – i.e. a gray-value edge – in each image, and these contributions take their maximum values if respective edges are aligned. This is illustrated in Fig. 1c which shows the spatial distribution of the contributions to the local correlation. Contributions can clearly be found in the area of gray-value edges showing that local correlation essentially quantifies corresponding edges.

From the preceding discussion it is evident that all voxels for which the local gray-value variance is zero can be neglected. Because of noise, there will hardly be voxels in real images for which the local variance vanishes. Nevertheless, regions with almost no structures or gray-value edges contribute only little to the local correlation. All voxels with a local gray-value variance below some threshold can be neglected and only a fraction of the image volume is necessary for registration. This property can be used to accelerate registration.

3   Experiments and results

The validation results refer to three data sets. The first data set is the software phantom of Fig. 1. As both images originate from the same image, they are registered implicitly. The second data set is a set of MR images shown in Fig. 2. They have been acquired simultaneously with a multi-slice, dual contrast turbo spin echo sequence. Thus, the spatial correspondence is not disturbed and the images are registered, as well. The third data set is a clinical one. It consists of an MR and a CT image which are shown in Fig. 3. Information about resolution and the size of the voxel matrix of all images can be found in Tab. 2.

For the experiments, one of the two software phantom images (Fig. 1b) and one of the two dual contrast MR images (Fig. 3b) have been reformatted according to a rigid transformation with translation (10.3mm, 12.7mm, -3.5mm) and rotation (9.4°, 11.1°, -4.2°). For the CT-MR data set a registration has been carried out. Using these parameters, sets with 64 starting estimates have been generated by adding ±11.42mm and ±11.42° to the translations and rotations. Then, registration has been performed for each starting estimate using the multi-resolution algorithm of Studholme et al. [2]. As similarity measure local correlation ($r = 1$), local correlation ($r = 1$) with 10% of the image volume and mutual information have been used. Optimization was done using three isotropic resolutions of 4.0mm, 2.8mm and 2mm and a minimum step size of approximately 0.01mm and 0.01°. Finally, the mean rotations and translations as well as the corresponding standard deviations have been computed. For the CT-MR data set, 5 (local correlation with 10% of the image volume) and 11 (mutual information) results have been discarded in this final step, because optimization was obviously trapped in a local optimum. The results of all experiments are included in Tab. 3. Fig. 3c shows an overlay of the CT image edges onto the MR image after registration using local correlation.

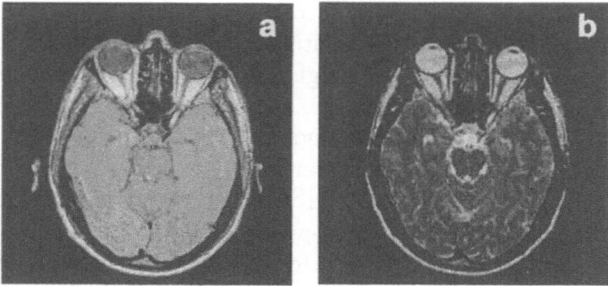

Fig. 2. Simultaneously acquired dual contrast MR images.

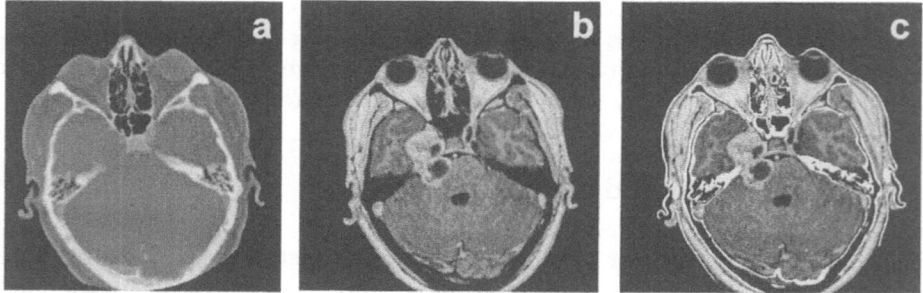

Fig. 3. Clinical data set. CT image (a), MR image (b) and overlay of the CT image edges onto the MR image after registration with local correlation (c).

Table 2. Dimension and voxel size of the images. For the clinical CT image the slice-to-slice distance is 1mm

	dimension (in voxels)	voxel size (in mm)
software phantom	$256 \times 256 \times 144$	$0.98 \times 0.98 \times 1.2$
dual contrast MR images	$256 \times 256 \times 64$	$0.90 \times 0.90 \times 3.0$
clinical CT image	$512 \times 512 \times 87$	$0.41 \times 0.41 \times 3.0$
clinical MR image	$256 \times 256 \times 128$	$0.78 \times 0.78 \times 1.5$

4 Discussion

The results for the software phantom and the dual contrast MR images show that with local correlation as well as with mutual information the registration result is almost independent of the starting estimate and that the "ground-truth" registration is recovered with high accuracy. Though the highest resolution used during optimization was 2mm, the accuracy of the translation and rotation parameters is 0.03mm and 0.01°, respectively. If only 10% of the image volume is used for registration with local correlation, the results are slightly degraded. In the case of the dual contrast MR images, the inaccuracies increase to 0.13mm and 0.05°. Nevertheless, the translation inaccuracy remains to be well below the voxel size used for registration and the rotation inaccuracy is very small.

Table 3. Registration results. Since optimization was obviously trapped in a local optimum, 5 ($LC_{10\%}^2$) and 11 (MI) registration results have been discarded for the clinical CT-MR data set.

	translations (in mm)			rotations (in °)		
	Software Phantom					
LC^2	10.30±0.01	12.69±0.01	-3.49±0.01	9.41±0.01	11.12=0.02	-4.19±0.01
$LC_{10\%}^2$	10.31±0.01	12.67±0.01	-3.50±0.02	9.40±0.01	11.11=0.03	-4.20±0.03
MI	10.30±0.00	12.70±0.00	-3.50±0.00	9.40±0.01	11.11=0.00	-4.20±0.00
	Dual Contrast MR images					
LC^2	10.30±0.01	12.71±0.01	-3.51±0.01	9.39±0.01	11.11=0.01	-4.20±0.01
$LC_{10\%}^2$	10.30±0.01	12.83±0.01	-3.47±0.01	9.35±0.01	11.11=0.01	-4.21±0.01
MI	10.29±0.01	12.71±0.01	-3.47±0.02	9.41±0.03	11.11=0.03	-4.20±0.02
	Clinical CT-MR data set					
LC^2	-3.49±0.02	-16.09±0.02	-31.00±0.01	6.92±0.02	-2.21±0.02	-5.13±0.01
$LC_{10\%}^2$	-3.46±0.01	-16.06±0.02	-30.69±0.01	6.81±0.01	-2.44±0.01	-5.11±0.01
MI	-3.33±0.07	-16.06±0.11	-30.74±0.12	6.79±0.13	-2.15±0.13	-5.00±0.09

In the case of the clinical data set, registration was only successful for all starting estimates when using local correlation and the entire image volume. When using only 10% of the image volume or mutual information, the capture range was slightly smaller and registration was trapped 5, respectively 11 times in local optima. The variations of the registration result for different starting estimates are larger for mutual information than for local correlation, though these variations are small and the registration result is nearly independent of the starting estimate. The deviations between the results for mutual information and local correlation have a magnitude of up to 0.26mm for the translations and 0.13° for the rotations. For local correlation using 10% of the image volume, the deviation for the rotations increases to 0.29°. Because mutual information has been used successfully for CT-MR registration, the small deviations are a strong indication that local correlation leads also to a proper registration. The good agreement of corresponding structures in the CT and MR image after registration (see Fig. 3c) confirms that local correlation is suitable for CT-MR registration.

5   Conclusions

Registration of CT and MR images using local correlation has been investigated. The differences between correlation and local correlation have been discussed, and it has been shown that local correlation quantifies corresponding edges in the images to be registered. There is, therefore, some analogy to the approach of Maintz et al. [3] where edges or ridges are extracted and registration is carried out on the basis of the feature images. An important difference is that registration with local correlation requires no explicit feature extraction. It can be applied directly to the gray-value images without sophisticated pre-processing. Since local correlation quantifies corresponding edges, image regions with almost no structures do not significantly contribute to the measure. Such image regions can easily be identified using a threshold for the local gray-value variance and can be excluded during registration. This technique allows to compensate a disadvantage related to the numerical evaluation of local correlation which is rather time consuming, because a neighborhood must be considered for each voxel.

Application to a software phantom and two MR images with different contrast led to accurate registration results being as good as the results obtained with mutual information. The good agreement between the registration results computed with local correlation and mutual information for a clinical CT-MR data set gave further evidence for the suitability of local correlation for multi-modality registration. The experiments showed also that registration based on local correlation can be done using only 10% of the image volume.

Acknowledgments

We would like to thank C. Studholme, D.L.G. Hill and D.J. Hawkes (UMDS, Guy's and St. Thomas' Hospitals, London) for the multi-resolution algorithm and our colleagues at the MR department (Philips Research Hamburg) for providing the dual contrast images.

References

1. Maintz, J. B. A., Viergever, M. A.: A survey of medical image registration. Med. Image Anal. **2** (1998) 1–36
2. Studholme, C., Hill, D.L.G., Hawkes, D.J.: Automated 3-D registration of MR and CT images of the head. Med. Image Anal. **1** (1996) 163–175
3. Maintz, J. B. A., van den Elsen, P. A., Viergever, M.A.: Comparison of edge-based and ridge-based registration of CT and MR brain images. Med. Image Anal. **1** (1996) 151–161
4. Wells III, W.M., Viola, P., Atsumi, H., Nakajima, S., Kikinis, R.: Multi-modal volume registration by maximization of mutual information. Med. Image Anal. **1** (1996) 35–51.
5. Maes, F., Collignon, A., Vandermeulen, D., Marchal, G., Suetens, P.: Multi-modality image registration by maximization of mutual information. IEEE Trans. Med. Imag. **16** (1997) 187–198.
6. Rösch, P., Blaffert, T., Weese, J.: Multi-modality registration using local correlation, accepted for CARS'99
7. Vincent, L., Soille, P.: Watersheds in digital spaces: an efficient algorithm based on immersion simulations. IEEE Trans. Pat. Anal. Mach. Int. **13** (1991) 583–598.
8. Buzug, T.M., Weese, J.: Voxel-based similarity measures for medical image registration in radiological diagnosis and image guided surgery. J. Comput. Inf. Tech. **6** (1998) 165–179.

Fully Automatic 3D/2D Subtracted Angiography Registration

E. Kerrien[1,2], M-O. Berger[1], E. Maurincomme[2], L. Launay[2] R. Vaillant[2], and
L. Picard[3]

[1] LORIA, BP 239, 54506 Vandoeuvre lès Nancy Cedex, France
[2] General Electric Medical Systems Europe, BP 34, 78533 Buc Cedex, France
[3] Therapeutic and diagnostic neuroradiology department, CHU, Hôpital
neurologique, 29, av. du Mal de Lattre de Tassigny, 54035 Nancy Cedex, France

Abstract. Today, 3-D angiography volumes are routinely generated from
rotational angiography sequences. In previous work [7], we have studied
the precision reached by registering such volumes with classical 2-D angiography images, inferring this matching only from the sensors of the
angiography machine. The error led by such a registration can be described as a 3-D rigid motion composed of a large translation and a
small rotation.
This paper describes the strategy we followed to correct this error. The
angiography image is compared in a two-step process to the Maximum
Intensity Projection (MIP) of the angiography volume. The first step
provides most of the translation by maximizing the cross-correlation. The
second step recovers the residual rigid-body motion, thanks to a modified
optical flow technique. A fine analysis of the equations encountered in
both steps allows for a speed-up of the calculations.
This algorithm was validated on 17 images of a phantom, and 5 patients. The residual error was determined by manually indicating points
of interest and was found to be around 1 mm.

1 Introduction

In interventional neuroradiology, it is very important for the neuroradiologist
to know, at any time, where the catheter lies within the patient's body, with
a millimetric precision. This information is deduced from Digital Subtracted
Angiography (DSA) images that he/she mentally links to pre-operative Magnetic
Resonance (MR) images, for example, thanks to his/her anatomical knowledge.

DSA images are the cornerstone of interventional neuroradiology. Lately, neu-
roradiologists have been using in clinical routine 3D X-ray angiography images
of the brain vasculature (3DXA). They have been proven to bring an actual
supplementary help to the physicians [2]. As a consequence, the registration of
DSA images with 3DXA volumes seems an extremely promising feature.

A registration between DSA images and a 3D modality is generally performed
using a stereotactic frame [13]. Nevertheless, many studies have been proposing alternative solutions. The closest subject to our work deals with DSA/MR

angiography (MRA) registration. Previous works made either use of external markers [11] and/or extract the skeletons of the vessels in both modalities [1, 3, 9], and matches the projection of the 3D skeleton with this extracted from the DSA image using various optimization schemes.

Widening our field of view, 3D/2D registration has also been used to register non-subtracted angiograms to CT acquisitions. Here again, salient features are segmented: crest lines [8], contours [4] for the images and the bone surface for the volume. The registration is reached when the surface is maximally tangent to the 2D features. However, similarity measures, very popular in 3D/3D matching studies (see [10] for a recent and complete review of research concerning medical image registration), recently appeared as a powerful alternative to the above segmentation-based methods [12].

2   Method

2.1   Definition of the problem

We showed in a previous work [7] that this registration problem could be formalized as follows:

- estimation of a distortion field in the DSA image: we described a calibration procedure of the angiography machine to solve that first aspect;
- estimation of a conic projection matrix, similar to those used to represent cameras in computer vision: we also showed that the intrinsic parameters of this matrix could be retrieved after a simple calibration of the angiography machine. Concerning the extrinsics, our study concluded on a good estimation of the rotation part, but quite a large imprecision on the translation.

The angiography machine, once it has been calibrated, provides an initial registration which differs from the expected matching ("perfect registration") by a rigid transformation (rotation+translation) in the 3D space. The residual rotation is small, whereas the translation can be considered as unknown.

2.2   Strategy

The type of images to be registered is important. Our algorithm is based on the comparison of a DSA image to a conic Maximum Intensity Projection of the 3DXA volume (MIP image). Both images are 512×512. Our strategy corresponds to the problem, as described above. First, the translation is retrieved while considering that there is no error made on the rotation. The optimal position is reached once the normalized centered cross-correlation between the DSA image and the MIP image is maximal.

This first step allows the assumption that the residual error is due to a small positioning error of the 3DXA volume in the proper space of the camera (corresponding to the projection matrix defining the registration).

In the second step, we consider that the MIP image (resulting from the first step) and the DSA image correspond to images of the same moving object, taken at times t and t' respectively. Then, observing the apparent motion between t and t' can give precious information about the small rigid-body transformation we are seeking. This information is extracted using a modified optical flow technique.

3 Algorithm

3.1 Maximization of the cross-correlation

The normalized centered cross-correlation between the DSA image, I_d, and the MIP image, I_m, is defined as:

$$\gamma = \frac{\sum_{(x,y)\in\mathcal{D}}(I_d(x,y) - \overline{I_d})(I_m(x,y) - \overline{I_m})}{\sqrt{\sum_{(x,y)\in\mathcal{D}}(I_d(x,y) - \overline{I_d})^2 \sum_{(x,y)\in\mathcal{D}}(I_m(x,y) - \overline{I_m})^2}}$$

where $\mathcal{D}$ is the common domain to both images and $\overline{I_d}, \overline{I_m}$ are the mean of images I_d and I_m respectively.

Let's consider that the projection matrix $\mathbf{M}$ represents the initial registration. The final matrix $\mathbf{M}'$ differs from $\mathbf{M}$ by the translation $\boldsymbol{D} = (D_x, D_y, D_z)$. Let's now consider a point P which projects on pixel (u, v) in the initial image (obtained by projecting the volume along $\mathbf{M}$) and on pixel (u', v') in the final image (obtained after translation). We have:

$$\mathbf{M}'P = (s'u', s'v', s')^t = \mathbf{M}P + \boldsymbol{D} = (su + D_x, sv + D_y, s + D_z)^t \qquad (1)$$

The initial matrix $\mathbf{M}$ is normalized thanks to Toscani's method [15]. We deduce:

$$\begin{cases} u' = \frac{s}{s+D_z}u + \frac{D_x}{s+D_z} \\ v' = \frac{s}{s+D_z}v + \frac{D_y}{s+D_z} \end{cases} \qquad (2)$$

This formula allows for an interpretation of vector $\boldsymbol{D}$: D_x and D_y involve a translation of the initial image, while D_z implies a zoom with respect to the upper left center of the image. As a result, this zoom entails a translation of the structures in the image. This dependency upon the parameters perturbs the optimization.

Now let's consider a movement composed of a translation (du, dv) parallel to the image plane and a zoom G with respect to the center of the image (u_c, v_c):

$$\begin{cases} u' = Gu + Gdu + (1 - G)u_c \\ v' = Gv + Gdv + (1 - G)v_c \end{cases} \qquad (3)$$

These more intuitive, independent, parameters du, dv and G better fit the optimization of cross-correlation; but they are not equivalent to vector $\boldsymbol{D}$. Indeed, in equation (2), s depends on the coordinates X, Y and Z of point P. Nevertheless, we assumed that s was constant over a volume, that is a 3DXA volume could be considered as reduced to a point. A 3DXA volume roughly occupies the volume of a sphere with a diameter of 15 cm. It is approximately located at half-distance between the focal spot of the camera and the image plane, within a system with a focal distance of approximately 1 meter. The approximation may seem rough but the matrices we obtain lead to a variation on s of about 1% over the whole 3DXA volume. This validates the hypothesis and we can determine a bijection between D and (du, dv, G) by identification of (2) and (3).

The optimization procedure with the parameters du, dv and G is as follows:

- exhaustive search at low resolution (64×64 pixels). The boundaries for the variation of the parameters are either constrained by the angiography machine characteristics (G) or satisfy a reasonable criterion: the images must overlap on at least one quarter of their surface. This resolution allows to keep the main arteries (diameter above 2 mm).
- pseudo-exhaustive search at maximal resolution. This technique has been described by Studholme et al. [14]. Lastly, we separate the optimization over (du, dv) and G: G's influence on the cost function is so small compared to du's and dv's that the optimization will not change its initial value.

3.2 Modified optical flow

Let's now assume we found the parameters (du, dv, G) which maximize the cross-correlation between the DSA image and the MIP image. Consequently, the initial matrix M is modified (see equation (1)) and the 3DXA volume is projected in order to generate a new MIP image. This image is close enough to the DSA image so that the velocity field may be computed using optical flow techniques.

Let's consider a point $P = (X, Y, Z)$ at time t and the point $P' = (X', Y', Z')$ reached at time t' by P after a small rigid displacement, composed of a rotation $\mathbf{R} = R_A R_B R_C$ (A, B and C are the rotation angles around the three basic vectors of the 3D space) and the translation $\mathbf{T} = (U, V, W)$:

$$P' = \mathbf{R}P + \mathbf{T}$$

That is, under the hypothesis that the rigid-body motion is small:

$$P' - P = \dot{P} = \mathbf{\Omega} \times P + \mathbf{T} \qquad \text{with } \mathbf{\Omega} = (A, B, C) \qquad (4)$$

Where the $\dot{}$ (dot) operator is the partial differentiation with respect to time $\frac{\partial}{\partial t}$. In the proper space of the camera, the point P projects on pixel (u, v),

$$u = \alpha X/Z \qquad \text{and} \qquad v = \alpha Y/Z \qquad (5)$$

where α stands for the ratio between the focal distance and the pixel size. From the derivation of (5) with respect to time, and combining with (4), it follows:

$$\begin{cases} \dot{u} = \alpha B - Cv - \frac{A}{\alpha}uv + \frac{B}{\alpha}u^2 + \frac{\alpha U - Wu}{Z} \\ \dot{v} = -\alpha A + Cu + \frac{B}{\alpha}uv - \frac{A}{\alpha}v^2 + \frac{\alpha V - Wv}{Z} \end{cases} \qquad (6)$$

This equation defines a transformation in the image plane, but for the $1/Z$ term. This is the classical problem one encounters who tries to retrieve the 3D motion from the apparent motion [5]: only 5 parameters out of 6 can be retrieved because of the undetermination on the depth of the object (given by Z) in the proper space of the camera. However, the MIP projection associates each pixel to one unique voxel. As a result, for each pixel, Z is uniquely set to the depth of the corresponding voxel. Thus, equation (6) completely relates the 6 motion parameters to the pixel coordinates.

Lastly, $\dot{u}$ and $\dot{v}$ remain to be dealt with. We follow the optical flow hypothesis, which assumes that the image intensity remains constant over time [6]:

$$\frac{dI}{dt} = \nabla I \bullet \begin{pmatrix} \dot{u} \\ \dot{v} \end{pmatrix} + \dot{I} = 0 \qquad (7)$$

This is not valid when comparing the DSA image to the MIP image: both images are obtained through very different means and, moreover, do not represent the same object (real object with regard to the result of a tomographic reconstruction). However, a mere normalization of both images provides images which are similar enough to satisfy this constraint.

Combining equation (6) (Z is set for each pixel as indicated above) and equation (7), we obtain for each pixel, two equations that the 6 motion parameters must obey. This leads us to an overdetermined system of equations with 6 unknowns, which is solved using a least squares technique (pseudo-inverse).

3.3   Speed-up

The two phases described above demand a large number of MIP projections. This is obvious in the optimization of the cross-correlation. Concerning the modified optical flow, results suffer from a long known disease: they are qualitatively good (we head towards the right direction) but quantitatively poor (the motion amplitude is underestimated). As a consequence, an iterative resolution of the residual motion through this technique was implemented: at the end of each iteration, the projection matrix is updated to take the newly found rigid-body transformation into account and the volume is reprojected ; this new MIP image is compared to the DSA image in the next iteration using equation (6). Therefore, we also need a large number of projections: one per iteration

Despite all our efforts, the generation of a MIP conic projection takes 1 second (3DXA volumes are 512^3). This constitutes a big handicap for our method, since it leads to an unacceptable calculation time: the exhaustive search at low resolution covers 32 values for du and dv, and 35 values for G. We must therefore perform $32 \times 32 \times 35 = 35840$ cross-correlation calculations, and, as a consequence, as many MIP projections. Given the time of 1 second per projection, this should take approximately 10 hours!

A finer analysis of the two basic equations (3) and (6) for our method, shows that they each define a 2D transformation in the image plane, if we know the motion parameters (du, dv and G for (3) and A, B, C, U, V and W for (6)). Thus, given a motion (either translation or small rigid motion), the new MIP image can be deduced from the old one with no need for an actual reprojection. This dramatically improves the calculation time.

4   Results

This algorithm allows for the implementation of a fully automatic 3D/2D angiography images registration in less than 90 seconds per DSA image (on a Sun UltraSparc workstation).

The gold standard for registration is usually provided by the use of a stereotactic frame. In our case, however, there is no established method to detect such a frame in 3DXA images: since the volume is reconstructed from subtracted images, the frame markers are not reconstructed The problem still remains with external markers.

Therefore, we adopted two ways of validating the result of a registration. First, the registration is visually assessed by comparing the original DSA image and the final MIP image. It allows us to state whether or not the registration succeeded, the more important information at this stage being whether or not the registration is usable for a neuroradiology intervention. Second, the error is manually estimated: given a biplane DSA sequence, each plane being registered with a 3DXA volume, we can point at salient features in the biplane images (bifurcations, marked curves, etc..) so as to reconstruct a point in the 3DXA volume. The error is the 3D distance between the reconstructed point and the effective location of the selected feature.

The algorithm has been tested on 17 images of a phantom and 5 biplane sequences of patients (that is, 10 DSA images). It always succeeded. The maximum 3D estimated error was 1.5 mm for the phantom images. However, the reconstructions of the phantom were all artifacted, lowering the quality of the registration.

Concerning the patient images, the maximum error found was 1 mm. We display on figure 1 two examples of registration performed with our algorithm (one per line): the first line shows an internal carotid artery with a previously treated aneurysm, the second line concerns an Arterio-Veinous Malformation (AVM) fed by the vertebral artery. The third line gives zoomed versions in order to better appreciate the quality of the registration.

5   Discussion

A strong filiation exists with studies on frameless DSA/MRA registration. External markers are difficult to design for angiograms. Furthermore, they have not proven to be accurate enough. Masutani [11] corrects such a registration by constraining the catheter to remain on the vessels skeleton extracted in MRA. All other methods [1,3,9] extract the vessels skeletons in both modality (DSA and MRA). The registration is considered to be attained when the projection of the 3D skeleton maximally superimposes the 2D skeleton.

All these skeleton-based methods have the same drawbacks. Liu [9] underlines that the projection of the centerline of the vessels in 3D does not correspond to the centerline in 2D. These techniques also generally require a test to reject some parts of the skeletons (parts which were detected in only one modality). In our opinion, the fundamental problems reside in the skeleton extraction itself.

670   E. Kerrien et al.

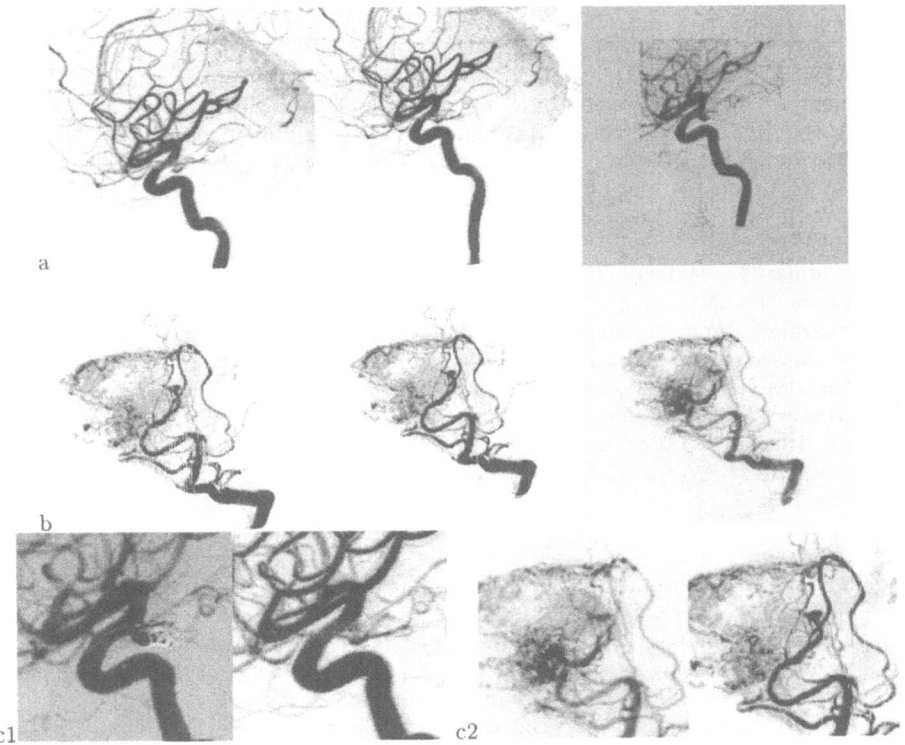

Fig. 1. Two examples of registration (a,b). Each line depicts a result on a DSA acquisition with 3 images: initial MIP image, MIP image at registration, DSA image. The third line shows a zoom of these results: (c1) left: DSA image, right: MIP image for example (a), (c2) same for (b). See the text for discussion of these examples.

Examples from figure 1 underline these difficulties. The image on figure 1a was acquired with a big zoom and a strong collimation (compare the DSA and MIP images). As a consequence, a lot of bifurcations, vessel superimpositions and tangencies are present (see zoom on figure 1c1) which is known to be a handicap for most segmentation methods. On the second example (figure 1b and 1c2), the AVM blush would clearly perturb the skeleton extraction, though it is the region of interest where we are looking for the best registration. Thus, our technique is well suited to the 3D/2D registration of complex vascular structures.

6   Conclusion

We presented in this paper a new algorithm which leads to a fully automatic 3D/2D subtracted angiography images registration. The initial conditions state that the DSA images are distortion-free, the intrinsics of the projection matrix are known and that a good initial guess can be made on the rotation: all of which are valid once the angiography machine has been properly calibrated [7].

References

1. Alperin N., Levin D., and Pelizzari C. "Retrospective registration of X-ray angiograms with MR images by using vessels as intrinsic landmarks" In *Journal of Magnetic Resonance Imaging*, volume 4, pages 139-144, 1994.
2. Anxionnat R., Bracard S., Macho J., Da Costa E., Vaillant R., Launay L., Trousset Y., Roméas R. and Picard L. "3D angiography: clinical interest and first applications in interventional radiology" *Journal of Neuroradiology*, vol. 25, pages 251-262, 1998.
3. Feldmar J., Malandain G., and Ayache N., Fernández-Vidal S. and Maurincomme E. "Matching a 3D MR angiography volume image and 2D X-Ray angiograms" In *First International Joint Conference on Computer Vision, Virtual Reality, and Robotics in Medicine and Medical Robotics and Computer Assisted Surgery*, volume 1205, pages 129-140, 1997.
4. Guéziec A., Kazanzides P., Williamson B., and Taylor R. H. "Anatomy-based registration of CT-scan and intraoperative X-ray images for guiding a surgical robot" In *IEEE Transactions on Medical Imaging*, volume 17, number 5, pages 715-728, 1998.
5. Gupta N. C., Kanal L. N. "3D motion estimation from motion field" In *Artificial Intelligence*, volume 78, pages 45-86, 1995.
6. Horn B. K. P., Schunck B. G. "Determining optical flow" In *Artificial Intelligence*, volume 17, pages 185-203, 1981.
7. Kerrien E., Vaillant R., Launay L., Berger M-O., Maurincomme E. and Picard L. "Machine precision assessment for 3D/2D digital subtracted angiography images registration" In *SPIE Medical Imaging*, volume 3338, pages 39-49, 1998.
8. Lavallée S., Szeliski R., and Burnie L. "Matching 3D Smooth Surfaces with their 2D projections Using 3D Distance Maps" In *SPIE Geometric Methods in Computer Vision*, volume 1570, pages 322-336, 1991.
9. Liu A., Bullitt E., Pizer S. M. "3D/2D registration via skeletal near projective invariance in tubular objects" In *Proceedings of MICCAI'98*, W.M. Wells, A. Colchester and S. Delp Eds, *Lecture Notes in Computer Science*, number 1496, pages 952-963, 1998.
10. Maintz J.B.A and Viergever M.A "A survey of medical image registration" In *Medical Image Analysis*, volume 2, number 1, pages 1-36, 1998.
11. Masutani Y., Furukawa C., Sonderegger M., Masamune K., Suzuki M., Dohi T., Yamane F., Iseki H., and Takakura K. "3D position visualization of catheter tip for intravascular neurosurgery using 3D structural description of vasculature" In *Computer Assisted Radiology*, pages 821-826, 1996.
12. Penney G. P., Weese J., Little J. A., Hill D. L. G, and Hawkes D. J. "A comparison of similarity measures for use in 2D-3D medical image registration" In *IEEE Transactions on Medical Imaging*, volume 17, number 4, pages 586-595, 1998.
13. Picard L., Maurincomme E., Söderman M., Feldmar J., Anxionnat R., Launay L., Ericson K., Malandain G., Bracard S., Kerrien E., Flodmark O. and Ayache N. "X-Ray angiography in stereotactic conditions: techniques and interest for interventional neuroradiology" In *Stereotactic and Functional Neurosurgery*, volume 68, pages 117-120, 1997.
14. Studholme C., Hill D., and Hawkes D. "Automated 3D registration of MR and CT images of the head" In *Medical Image Analysis*, volume 1, issue 2, March 1996.
15. Toscani, G. "Systèmes de calibration et perception du mouvement en vision artificielle" PhD thesis, Université de Paris-Sud, Orsay, 1987.

Multi-modal Medical Volumes Fusion by Surface Matching

Ayman M. Eldeib, Sameh M. Yamany and Aly A. Farag

Computer Vision and Image Processing Laboratory, University of Louisville,
Louisville, Kentucky 40292, USA, Email:ayman,yamany,farag@cvip.uofl.edu

Abstract. This paper presents a fast, six degrees of freedom registration technique to accurately locate the position and orientation of medical volumes (obtained from CT/MRI scans for the same patient) with respect to each other. The main contribution of this work is the use of a novel surface registration technique followed by a volume registration approach. The advantage of this combination is to have an accurate alignment and to reduce the time needed for registration. The surface registration uses a new surface representation scheme that captures the curvature information and codes it into 2-D images. Matching these images enables the recovery of the transformation parameters. For the multi-modal volume registration, the maximization of Mutual Information (MI) is used as a matching criterion and is enhanced by a new genetic based search technique. The results demonstrate that the new two-stage registration technique presented in this paper is robust in terms of speed and accuracy and allows for completely automatic registration of multimodality medical volumes.

1 Introduction

Medical imaging modalities produce different diagnostic information which complement each other. Skin and bone can be more easily extracted from Computed Tomography (CT) images than from Magnetic Resonance (MR) images. Also, in radiotherapy planning, CT data is used for dosage calculation, while soft tissues and tumor outlining is better segmented and extracted from the corresponding MR data. In many cases, other imaging modalities are needed for more diagnostic information, such as Magnetic Resonance Angiography (MRA) for extracting blood vessels, and Positron-Emission tomography (PET) for providing information on brain function. For our surgical planning system, navigation system and virtual neuroendoscope, we need all this information together. The objective of this work is to register data from multiple modalities into a single 3-D model using a high fidelity fusion method. Figure 1 shows a block diagram of the proposed system. This paper is organized as follows. Section 2 introduces the surface registration technique. Maximization of mutual information using genetic algorithms is described in Section 3. Results are discussed in Section 4 and conclusions are given in Section 5.

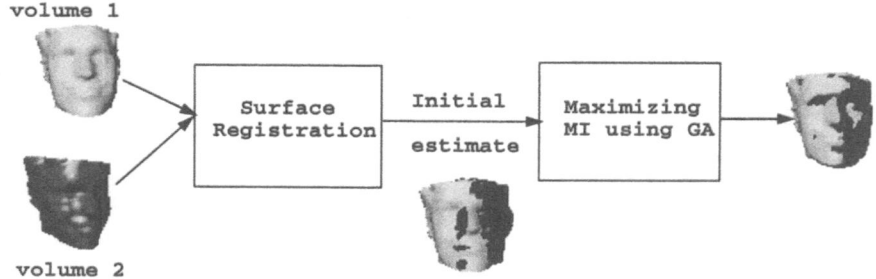

Fig. 1. *The block diagram of the proposed system. Two different volumes are fed into the system. Surface registration provides an estimate transformation between them. This result is further enhanced by maximizing the mutual information. A Genetic Algorithms technique is used in the search process.*

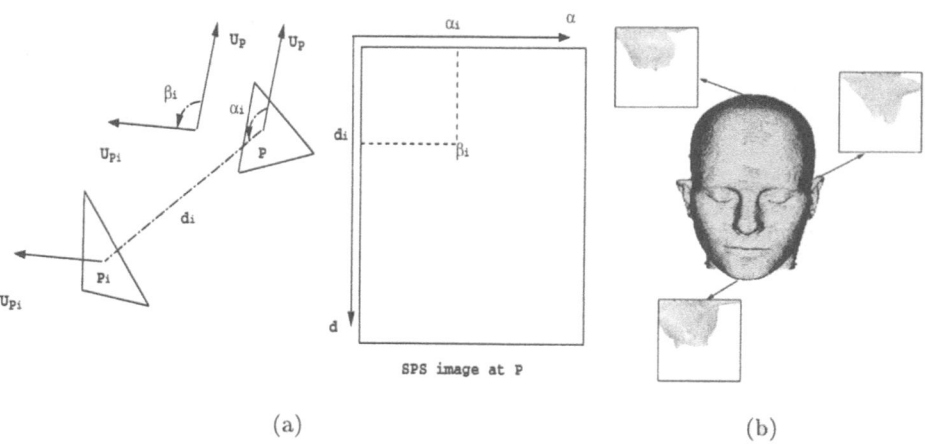

(a)   (b)

Fig. 2. *(a) For each important point on the surface an SPS image is obtained. This image encodes the angle difference between the normal at the point in focus and the normal at each other point on the surface. (b) Examples of SPS images taken at different important points locations. Notice how the image provides features the curvature information. The dark intensity in the image represents a high curvature seen from the point while the light intensity represents a low curvature. Also notice how different the image corresponding to a location is from images of other locations.*

2 Surface Registration Technique

In order for any surface registration algorithm to perform accurately and efficiently, an appropriate representation scheme for the surface is needed. Most of the surface representation schemes found in literature have adopted some form of shape parameterization especially for the purpose of object recognition. However, free-form surfaces, in general, may not have simple volumetric shapes that can be expressed in terms of parametric primitives. This paper presents a new concept, introduced in [1, 2], for 3-D free-form surface registration and object recognition using a new surface representation scheme. This representation scheme captures the 3-D curvature information of any free-form surface and encodes it into a 2-D image corresponding to a certain point on the surface. This image is unique for this point and is independent from the object translation or orientation in space. The process starts by identifying special points on the surface. These points are called *Important* points due to the information they carry. Then an image capturing the surface curvature information seen from each *important* point, is formed. We call this image the Surface Point Signature (SPS) because it is almost unique for each point on the surface. Surface registration is then performed by matching SPS images of different surfaces and hence finding corresponding points in each surface. For rigid registration, three point correspondences are sufficient to estimate the transformation parameters.

Definition 1. *A point P on a surface/curve S, is called* important *point, P_I, if and only if the absolute value of the curvature at this point is larger than a certain positive value (a threshold).*

$$A = \{P_I\} = \{P \in S| \quad |Curv(P)| > \epsilon, \epsilon > 0\} \tag{1}$$

As the *important* points are landmarks, one may expect that they are stable for the same object. However, due to scanning noise, their number and locations may vary. By adjusting the curvature threshold, a common subset can be found. Otherwise, the object has either suffered from non-rigid transformations or its visible surface has no landmarks.

Our approach for fast registration and recognition is to establish a "surface signature" for each of the obtained 3-D important points rather than just depending on the 3-D coordinates of the point.

The signature, computed at each important point, encodes the surface curvature seen from this point, thus giving it discriminating power. As shown in Figure 2 (a), for each important point $P \in A$ defined by its 3-D coordinates and the normal U_P at the patch where P is the center of gravity, each other point P_i on the surface can be related to P by two parameters: 1)The distance $d_i = ||P - P_i||$ and 2) the angle $\alpha_i = cos^{-1}\left(\frac{U_P \cdot (P - P_i)}{||P - P_i||}\right)$. This is a polar implementation of the SPS image, and it can be easily converted into Cartesian form. Also we can notice that there is a missing degree of freedom in this representation which is the cylindrical angular parameter. This parameter depends on the surface orientation which defies the purpose of having an orientation-independent representation scheme. The SPS generation is scale-dependent. However, this has a little effect on its use in multi-modal registration since the result is refined in the volume matching stage and also since there is no or only a small scale difference between the volumes in study. At each location in the image, we encode the angle $\beta_i = cos^{-1}(U_P \cdot U_{P_i})$. This represents the change in the normal at the surface point P_i relative to the normal at P. Due to the fact that we are ignoring the cylindrical angular degree, the same pixel in the SPS image can represent more than one 3-D point on the surface. This usually occurs when we have a surface of revolution around the axis represented by the normal at the point P. As all these points have the same d_i and α_i and lie on the circle that has a radius $d_i cos(\alpha_i)$ and is distant by $d_i sin(\alpha_i)$ from the point P along the axis U_P, we take the average of their angles β_i and encode it in the SPS corresponding pixel location.

Figure 2 (b) shows some SPS images taken at different important points on the skin model. We can see clearly how the images encode the curvature information of the object surface and each uniquely defines the location of the point on the surface.

The next step in the registration process is to match corresponding SPS images of two surfaces. The ultimate goal of the matching process is to find at least a three points correspondence in order to calculate the transformation parameters. The benefit of using the SPS images to find the correspondence is that we can now use image processing tools in the matching, hence reducing the time taken to find accurate transformation. One such tool is *Template Matching* in which a value defines how well a portion of an image matched a template.

The end result of the matching process is a list of groups of likely three point correspondences that satisfies the geometric consistency constraint. The list is sorted such that correspondences that are far apart are at the top of the list. A rigid transformation is calculated for each group of correspondences and a verification stage [3] is performed to obtain the best group. Detailed discussion concerning the SPS sensitivity and robustness can be found in [1].

3   Volume Registration Technique

Extracting skin from MR dataset using an automatic segmentation technique may produce an inaccurate 3-D skin model. In such a case, we start with the results (estimation of transformation parameters) of our surface registration as initial parameters for a volume registration as shown in Figure 1. We used the well-known maximization of Mutual Information (MI) as a matching criterion based on Genetic Algorithms (GA) as a search engine. The search is performed around the initial transformation parameters estimated by the surface registration technique. As a result, we need a fewer number of iterations than with volume registration that starts with random transformation parameters. MI is a basic concept from information theory, measuring the statistical dependence between two random variables or the amount of information that one variable contains about the other. The MI registration criterion used here states that the MI of corresponding voxel pairs is maximal if the two volumes are geometrically aligned [4]. No assumptions are made regarding the nature of the relation between the image intensities in either modality.

We refer to the two medical volumes to be registered as the reference volume R and the floating volume F. A voxel of the reference volume is denoted $R(x)$, where x is the coordinates vector of the voxel. A voxel of the floating volume is denoted similarly as $F(x)$. Given that T is a transformation matrix from the coordinate space of the reference volume to the floating volume, $F(T(x))$ is the floating volume voxel associated with the reference volume voxel $R(x)$. Note that in order to simplify the MI equation we will use T to denote both the transformation and its parameterization.

We seek an estimate of the transformation matrix that registers the reference volume R and floating volume F by maximizing their mutual information. The vector x is treated as a random variable over coordinate locations in the reference volume. Mutual information is defined in terms of entropy in the following way [5]:

$$I(R(x), F(T(x))) \equiv h(R(x)) + h(F(T(x))) - h(R(x), F(T(x))). \qquad (2)$$

where $h(R(x))$ and $h(F(T(x)))$ are the entropy of R and F, respectively. $h(R(x), F(T(x)))$ is the joint entropy. Entropy can be interpreted as a measure of uncertainty, variability, or complexity. The mutual information defined in equation (2) has three components. The first term on the right is the entropy in the reference volume, and is not a function of T . The second term is the entropy of the part of the floating volume into which the reference volume projects. It encourages transformations that project R into complex parts of F. The third term, the (negative) joint entropy of R and F, contributes when R and F are functionally related. Maximizing MI tends to find as much of the complexity that is in the separate volumes (maximizing the first two terms) as possible so that at the same time they explain each other well (minimizing the third term) [4, 5].

GA are adaptive, domain independent search procedures derived from the principles of natural population genetics. GA are briefly characterized by three main concepts: a Darwinian notion of fitness or strength which determines an individual's likelihood of affecting future generations through reproduction; a reproduction operation which selects individuals for recombination to their fitness or strength; and a recombination operation which creates new offspring based on the genetic structure of their parents. GA work with a coding of a parameter set, not the parameters themselves, and search from a population of points, not a single point [6]. Also, GA use payoff (objective function) information, not derivatives or other auxiliary knowledge, and employ probabilistic transition rules instead of deterministic ones. These four differences contribute to genetic algorithms' robustness and resulting advantage over other more commonly used search techniques. Our results demonstrate that MI, combined with a GA search, is a robust approach for multi-modal volume registration [7].

4   Results

We evaluated our results with experimental as well as with real datasets. For the experimental test, we implemented a tool which applies a certain rotation

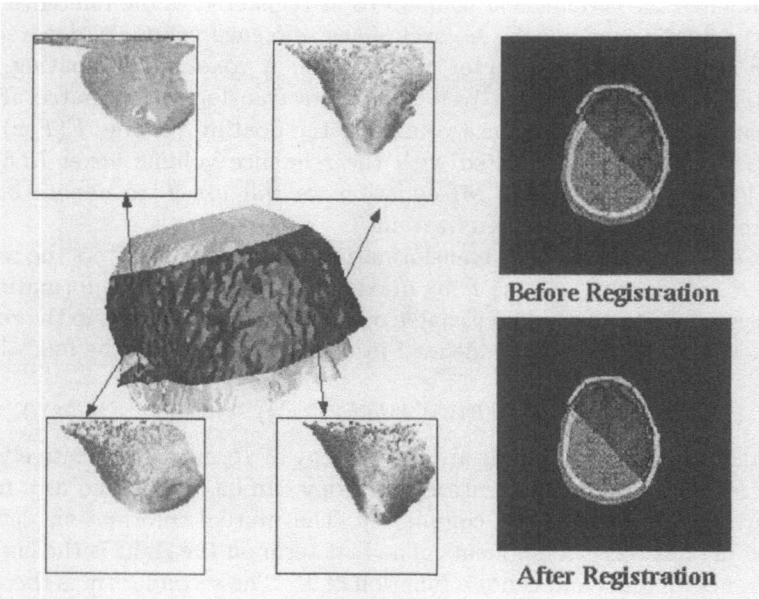

Before Registration

After Registration

Fig. 3. *Two different SPS samples. The upper two images are from the MR dataset; while the lower two are from the CT dataset. This figure shows similarity of the SPS images of each matched pair, although they are produced from two different datasets (CT and MR) with a different 3-D volume size (number of slices).*

and translation on a 3-D medical volume. We start with a 3-D volume V. Using our transformation tool, we produce a transformed volume V' with a known transformation matrix. Next, we apply our registration technique on the two volumes V and V' to obtain an estimate of the transformation matrix. Registration accuracy is measured by comparing the estimated results with the actual transformation parameters. We also evaluated the case of registering two different modalities, such as CT and MR, from the same patient (real datasets). To validate the results of the new technique, a ground truth was obtained by an exhaustive search performed on a 24-processors ONYX R10000 SGI machine. Registration accuracy is measured visually and/or by comparing the estimated results with the transformation parameters determined by the exhaustive search. Figures 3 and 4 show a sample of our results of CT/CT and CT/MR alignment. The SPS images shown in Figures 3 and 4 clearly show that each SPS image is unique at a certain point and is independent from 3-D volume translation or orientation in the space. A mathematical proof is presented in [1].

In comparing these results with conventional MI multi-modal registration techniques [7], it is found that using surface registration a priori to maximize the MI reduces the registration time while resulting in the same accuracy. The results are summarized in Table 1 and compared with the results of using a single-stage

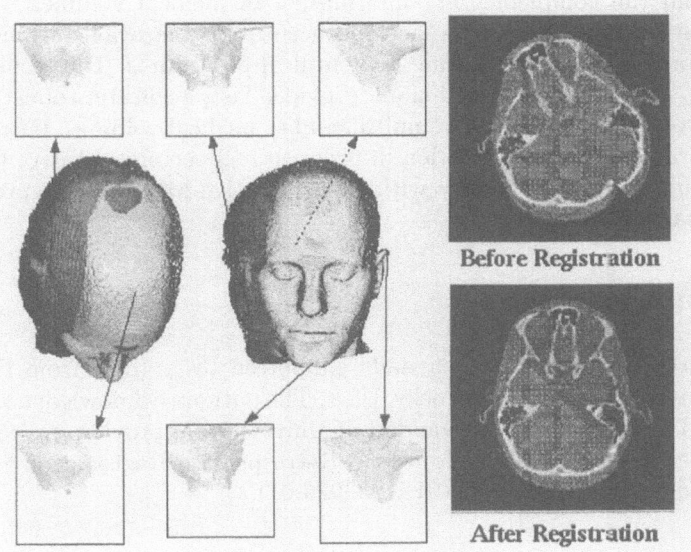

Fig. 4. Three different matched pairs of SPS images produced from a CT volume. This figure shows that the SPS images are independent from the 3-D volume translation or orientation in the space.

multi-modal volume registration technique presented in [7]. The new surface registration is also faster than existing approaches. The GA also contributes in the fast conversion. The time required for registration is approximately two to three minutes for high resolution volumes.

Table 1. Comparison between approximate times for single and dual stage volume registration

Case	No of slices	Dual-Stage				Single-Stage
		Surface Matching		Volume	Total time	MI-GA
		SPS Generation	SPS Matching	Matching	(sec)	(sec)
CT/CT	236	20 sec	30 sec	100 sec	15C	300
CT/MR	33/19	8 sec	20 sec	80 sec	10£	250

5   Conclusion and Future Work

Multi-modal medical volume registration is an important capability for finding the correct geometrical transformation that brings one volume in precise spatial correspondence with another. Multi-modal volume registration allows us to benefit from the complementary information in medical volumes from different modalities. Implementing a fast and accurate registration technique is one of the preprocessing stages during neursurgical procedures. The results demonstrate that our registration technique provides fast, accurate, robust and completely automatic registration of multimodality medical volumes. Future work is to incorporate volume deformation in order to register preoperative CT or MR volumes quickly and accurately with intraoperative MR volumes produced by an open-magnet system.

6   Acknowledgments

This research work has been partially supported by a grant from the Alliant Health System, Louisville, Kentucky, USA. The authors acknowledge Dr. J. Fitzpatrick and Dr. Jay West from Vanderbilt University for providing access to their multi-modal volume datasets from the Retrospective Registration Evaluation NIH Project (project number R01 NS33926-01).

References

1. S. M. Yamany and A. A. Farag, "Free form surface maching using surface signatures," *International Conference on Computer Vision and Pattern Recognition ICCV'99, Corfu, Greece, Sept. 20 - 25* , 1999.
2. S. M. Yamany, A. El-Bialy, and A. A. Farag, "Free form object recognition and registration using surface signatures," *IEEE International Conference on Image Processing - ICIP'99, Japan, Oct. 25 - 28* , 1999.
3. S. M. Yamany, M. N. Ahmed, and A. A. Farag, "A new genetic-based technique for matching 3d curves and surfaces," *Pattern Recognition (to appear)* , 1999.
4. F. Maes, A. Collignon, D. Vandermeulen, G. Marchal, and P. Suetens, "Multi-modality image registration by maximization of mutual information," *IEEE Transaction on Medical Imaging* 16(2), pp. 187–198, 1997.
5. W. M. Wells, P. Viola, H. Atsumi, S. Nakajima, and R. Kikinis, "Multi-model volume registration by maximization of mutual information," *Medical Image Analysis, Oxford University Press* 1(1), pp. 35–51, 1996.
6. D. E. Goldberg, *Genetic Algorithms in Search, Optimization and Machine Learning*, Addison-Welsey, 1989.
7. A. Eldeib, A. A. Farag, and T. Moriarty, "A fast genetic search algorithm for accurate multi-modal volume registration by maximization of mutual information," *Computer Assisted Radiology and Surgery - CARS'99, 13th International Congress and Exhibition, Paris, France, June 23 - 26* , 1999.

Medical Image Registration with Robust Multigrid Techniques

Pierre Hellier, Christian Barillot, Etienne Mémin, Patrick Pérez

IRISA, INRIA-CNRS unit, Campus de Beaulieu, F-35042 Rennes cedex, France.
e-mail : {phellier,barillot,memin,perez}@irisa.fr

Abstract. In this paper we describe a new method of medical image registration based on robust estimators. We propose a general hierarchical optimization framework which is both multiresolution and multigrid with an adaptative partition of the volume. The approach may easily be adapted to different similarity measures (optical flow, mutual information or correlation ratio for instance) and may therefore be used either for mono-modality or for multi-modality registration. Here, we concentrate on the estimation of the optical flow leading to a single-modality non-linear registration. We aim at registering two MRI volumes of two different subjects. Results on real data are presented and discussed. Since this work is in progress, we expect more attractive and extensive results for the time of the conference.
keywords Registration, atlas matching, incremental optical flow, multigrid minimization, robust estimators.

1 Introduction

1.1 Context

Since the development of modern imaging techniques (MRI, X-ray, PET, etc.), registration has become an important task in brain imaging. Nowadays surgeons must face not only the huge volume of data, but also the complementarity between the different images. As a matter of fact, these informations are not redundant but complementary, and should not be neglected for the health of the patient. Functional data must therefore be merged or compared with the use of an atlas. In order to build such an atlas, it is necessary to appraise the anatomical variability, what implies the registration of the anatomy of different subjects. We distinguish several registration applications:

- Registration of images of the same subject with the same modality. It is useful for surgeons, either to follow the development of a disease, or for operations (dynamic acquisition during the operation or validation of an operation).
- Registration of images of a same subject with different modalities. This problem arose with the development of different images, either anatomical (MR, X-ray) or functional (fMRI, PET, EEG, MEG). Merging these images is desirable so that no information is excluded from the diagnostic.

– Registration of brains of different subjects. Such a registration allows to build an anatomical atlas of the cortex. Atlases such as [13, 17] appear to be inadequate (legibility, capacity to evolve, difficulty of interpretation [8]). The major problem in building an atlas is the important variability of the human brain. To take it into account, a non-linear registration process is necessary.

1.2   Background

Medical image registration is a very productive field, from a bibliographical point of view. [11] present a complete review and classification of different registration procedures. Methods are usually classified using the following criterions: the nature and the dimension of the homologous structures to match, the domain of transformation (local or global), its type (rigid, affine, projective or "free form"), the similarity measure and the minimization scheme. We have selected a few methods that seem relevant to us:

The first method is Talairach's stereotactic referential [17]. The purpose is to enclose all the brains in the same box, which size and orientation are known. It uses a piecewise linear transformation. Many methods use geometric attributes that are extracted and then matched. They may be points [3], curves [15] or surfaces [16]. The extraction of these landmarks is of course a crucial problem (Is the extraction reliable? what is the number of landmarks that will invariably be present?), but the way these landmarks are matched -and the way the registration is computed throughout the volume- is also critical. Methods have been developed to overcome this problem: the TPS algorithm [3], spline transformations [16], or the ICP algorithm [15].

Other registration procedures are inspired by mechanical models, either elastic [1], or fluid [4]. Fluid models allow to reach, in theory, any displacements, but these methods are highly time-consuming.

Finally many registration procedures are "voxel-based" methods: Thirion [18] proposes the demon method, by reference to Maxwell's demons; Collins [5] estimates a locally affine transformation that maximizes the cross correlation of the image gradient.

1.3   Method

We propose in this paper a 3D method to estimate the optical flow, which is related to the work presented in [12]. The estimation of a dense displacement field leads to a non linear single modality registration. The problem is expressed in a Bayesian context as the minimization of a cost function. We introduce robust estimators in order to be less sensitive to the noise of acquisition (MRI data) and to preserve the discontinuities of the dense displacement field.

Finally the optimization procedure is multiresolution and multigrid, in order to accelerate the estimation and to improve its accuracy. We designed an adaptative partition of the volume in order to refine the estimation on the regions of interest and to avoid useless efforts. This minimization framework, including the multiresolution/multigrid plan and the robust estimators, is not limited to the estimation of the optical flow, but may be used as well for other similarity measures (mutual information, correlation ratio for example). We are focusing on different applications:

- Registration of MRI data of different subjects. The purpose is the automatic segmentation and labeling of the cortex and the possibility to exchange symbolic information from one brain to another.
- Registration of data from the same subject, for instance for fMRI acquisitions. The goal is to correct the movement of the head during the time of the protocol in order to ease the use and the interpretation of the data. In that case, only a global affine field will be sought.

2   Optical flow estimation

2.1   General formulation

The optical flow hypothesis, introduced by Horn et Schunck [9], assumes that the luminance of a physical point does not vary much between the two volumes to register. It gives: $f(s + dw_s, t_1) - f(s, t_2) = 0$ where s is a voxel of the volume, t_1 and t_2 are the index of the volumes (temporal index for a dynamic acquisition, index in a database for multi-subject registration), f is the luminance function and dw the expected $3D$ displacement field. Generally, a linear expansion of this equation is preferred : $\nabla f(s, t) \cdot dw_s + f_t(s, t) = 0$ where $\nabla f(s, t)$ stands for the spatial gradient of luminance and $f_t(s, t)$ the difference between the two volumes.

With the linearization, we are less sensitive to constant changes in the luminance due to the acquisition but only the projection of the displacement on the luminance gradient may be estimated. Furthermore, the linearization makes the estimation more sensitive to noise. For these reasons, it is necessary to introduce a prior regularization on the solution. Within a Bayesian framework [7], and using the MAP estimator, the problem is formulated as the minimization of the following cost function:

$$U(dw; f) = \sum_{s \in S} [\nabla f(s, t) \cdot dw_s + f_t(s, t)]^2 + \alpha \sum_{<s,r> \in C} ||dw_s - dw_r||^2 \qquad (1)$$

where S is the voxel lattice, C is the set of neighboring pairs (the 6 neighborhood system may be used for instance) and α controls the balance between the two energy terms. The first term represents the interaction between the field (unknown variables) and the data (given variables), whereas the second term expresses the smoothness constraint. The weakness of this formulation are known:

a. The optical flow constraint (OFC) is not valid in case of large displacements because of the linearization.
b. The OFC might not be valid in all the regions of the volume, because of the noise of acquisition, intensity non-uniformity in MRI data, occlusions.

c. The "real" field is not globally smooth and it probably contains discontinuities that might not be preserved because of the quadratic cost.

To cope with the (b) and (c) limitations, we replace the quadratic cost by robust functions. Furthermore, to face the problem (a), we use a multiresolution plan and a multigrid strategy to improve the minimization at each resolution level.

2.2   Robust estimators

Cost function (1) takes into account all the voxels and all the pairs of neighbors equally. This is not very robust, that's why we would like to reduce the importance of possible inconsistent data, or to avoid smoothing discontinuities of the field that must be preserved. Therefore, we introduce robust functions [10] and more precisely robust M-estimators [2]. An M-estimator ρ has the following properties:

a. ρ is increasing on $\mathbb{R}^+$. b. $\phi(u) \triangleq \rho(\sqrt{u})$ is strictly concave on $\mathbb{R}^+$. c. $\lim_{x \to \infty} \rho'(x) < \infty$.

(a) implies that ρ is a cost function. (b) implies that the graph of ρ is the inferior envelope of a set of parabolas. We have:

$$\exists \psi \in C^1([0, M], \mathbb{R}) \text{ such that } \forall u, \rho(u) = \min_{z \in [0,M]} \left(zu^2 + \psi(z)\right) \tag{2}$$

where $M \triangleq \lim_{u \to 0^+} \phi'(u)$. Furthermore one gets :

$$z^* \triangleq \arg \min_{z \in [0,M]} \left(zu^2 + \psi(z)\right) = \frac{\rho'(u)}{2u} = \phi'(u^2)$$

where $\frac{\rho'(u)}{2u} = \phi'(u^2)$ decreases from M to 0 according to (b) and (c).

The robustness of such an estimator is provided by the fact that the function ϕ' decreases. We introduce two robust estimators, the first one on the data term and the second one on the regularization term. According to (2), the cost function (1) can then be modified as:

$$U(\mathbf{dw}, \delta, \beta; f) = \sum_{s \in S} \delta_s \left(\boldsymbol{\nabla} f(s, t) \cdot \mathbf{dw}_s + f_t(s, t)\right)^2 + \psi_1(\delta_s)$$

$$+\alpha \sum_{<s,r> \in \mathcal{C}} \beta_{sr} \left(||\mathbf{dw}_s - \mathbf{dw}_r||\right)^2 + \psi_2(\beta_{sr}) \tag{3}$$

where δ_s and β_{sr} are auxiliary variables (acting as "weights") to be estimated. This cost function has the advantage to be quadratic with respect to $\mathbf{dw}$. When a discontinuity gets larger, the contribution of the pair of neighbors gets lower by the reduction of the associated weight β_{sr} ($\beta_{sr} = \phi_2'(||\mathbf{dw}_s - \mathbf{dw}_r||^2)$). In the same way, when the adequation of a data with the model is not correct, its contribution gets lower as the associated weight δ_s decreases ($\delta_s = \phi_1'([\boldsymbol{\nabla} f(s, t) \cdot \mathbf{dw}_s + f_t]^2)$).

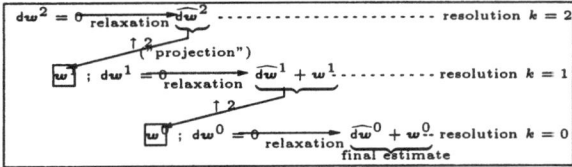

Fig. 1. Incremental estimation of the optical flow

2.3 Multiresolution and multigrid approaches

In case of large displacements, we use a classical incremental multiresolution procedure (see fig. 1). We construct a pyramid of volumes $\{f^k\}$ by successive Gaussian smoothing and subsampling in each direction. At coarsest level, displacements are reduced, and cost function (3) can be hopefully used. For the next resolution levels, only an incremental dw^k is estimated to refine estimate $\hat{w}^k$, obtained from the previous level. This is done using cost function (3) but with $\nabla f^k(s + \hat{w}^k_s, t_2)$ and $f^k(s + \hat{w}^k_s, t_2) - f^k(s, t_1)$ instead of $\nabla f^k(s, t)$ and $f^k_t(s, t)$.

Furthermore, at each level of resolution, we use a multigrid minimization (see Fig. 2). We aim at estimating an increment field not for one voxel, but for a group of voxels in order to have temporarily a larger system of neighborhood. The energy is consequently smoother, and has fewer local minima. As a matter of fact, the cost (3) is highly non convex, and we might be trapped into a local minimum. Moreover, this minimization strategy, where the starting point is provided by the previous result - which we hope to be a gross estimate of the desired solution -, improves the quality of the estimation and makes it possible to use a deterministic relaxation instead of a stochastic one.

The multigrid strategy consists in partitioning initially the volume into cubes of size 2^{3l} at the grid level l. The cost function (3) can then be expressed according to the partition and a 12-dimensions parametric model is estimated as an increment on each cube. The total field is therefore piecewise affine. The displacement increment estimated on a cube depends on the total displacement estimated on the neighborhood of this cube, what implies that the field will be continuous between the cubes, and we do not have a "block" effect.

When we change the grid level, we also change the partition of the volume by dividing, regularly or not, the previous partition. The criterion of subdivision may be either the measure of the way the model fits the data, or a prior knowledge such as the presence of an important anatomical structure where the estimation must be accurate (segmentation of the cortex, identification of the cortical sulci). Consequently, we can distinguish between the regions of interest, where the estimation must be precise, and the other regions where computation efforts are useless.

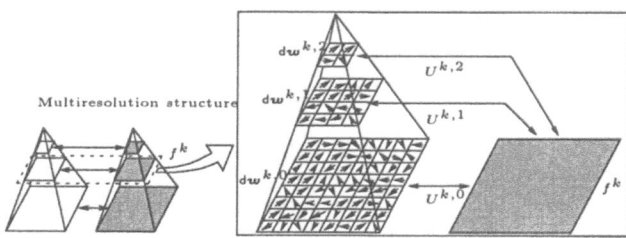

Fig. 2. Three-level multigrid relaxation at a given resolution level k

3 Results

Results of the $3D$ method are presented on figure 3. Two $3D$ MRI-T1 volumes of two different subjects are registered. The reconstructed volume -with trilinear interpolation- is presented, computed with the target volume and the final displacement field. We also present two volumes of difference, one before and the other after registration. The adaptative partition is also presented. We refine the estimation in the regions of interest (cortex) whereas we do not waste computation time on regions that do not necessitate too much attention.

The difference volumes are to be interpreted carefully, since we get the superposition of two errors: the first one is the registration error, the anatomical variability that we could not apprehend. The second error is due to the difference of acquisition of the two volumes, which implies that the two original histograms of the two volumes are different.

We notice that if some anatomical structures (ventricle, bulb) are correctly registered, errors remain, in particular for cortical sulci. As a matter of fact the variability is very high on these regions. It has been shown that this critical issue cannot be correctly solved with voxel-based methods [6].

The computation takes 1 hours on a Ultra Sparc 30 (300 Mhz). The volumes are $256 \times 256 \times 200$. We use 3 levels of resolution because the displacement amplitude may reach 30 voxels. We stop at the grid level 2 of the finest resolution, because below this grid level the estimation of 12 parameters is inconsistent. It should be noted that only 10 minutes are necessary to perform the estimation until the grid level 3 of the finest resolution (where the cubes are $7mm$ large), this means that almost 85% of the computation time is due to the last grid level.

4 Conclusion and perspectives

We have presented in this paper a new registration method based on a robust $3D$ estimation of the optical flow with promising results on real data. We use an efficient minimization framework, both multiresolution and multigrid with robust estimators. This optimization scheme is not limited to the estimation of the optical flow, but may as well be adapted to other similarity measures, leading to different registration applications. The adaptative partition of the volume improves the computation time but does not degrade the estimation in the regions of interest. We purchase different perspectives:

- The multigrid partition must be optimized so that no efforts are made in certain regions (outside the brain for instance) whereas the estimation is as accurate as possible in the regions of interest (cortex, cortical sulci).
- It could be desirable to correct the histograms -if it is nct a constant bias- of the two volumes [14], as the method is dependent on the optical flow hypotheses. But if the difference of the two histograms is affine, only one additional parameter needs to be estimated. This way to cope with the problem is certainly more correct than any histogram modification.
- We intend to extend this minimization procedure to multi-modality registration. To that purpose, the similarity measure in the cost function must be replaced by another (e.g. mutual information or correlation ratio).

References

1. R. Bajcsy, S. Kovacic. Multiresolution elastic matching. *CVGIP*, 46:1–21, 1989.
2. M. Black, A. Rangarajan. On the unification of line processes, outlier rejection, and robust statistics with application in early vision. *IJCV*, 19(1):57–91, 1996.
3. F. Bookstein. Principal warps: Thin plate splines and the decomposition of deformations. *IEEE PAMI*, 11(6):567–585, 1989.
4. G. Christensen, R. Rabbit, MI. Miller. Deformable templates using large deformation kinematics. *IEEE Trans. Image Processing*, 5(10):1435–1447, 1996.
5. L. Collins. *3D Model-based segmentation of individual brain structures from magnetic resonance imaging data*. PhD thesis, Mc Gill University, Montreal, 1994.
6. L. Collins, G. Le Goualher, R. Venugopal, A. Caramanos, A. Evans, C. Barillot. Cortical constraints for non-linear cortical registration. *Proc. Visu. in Biomed. Computing*, LNCS 1131, pages 307–316. Springer, September 1996.
7. S. Geman, D. Geman. Stochastic relaxation, gibbs distribution and the bayesian restauration of images. *IEEE PAMI*, (6):721–741, 1984.
8. B. Gibaud, S. Garlatti, C. Barillot, E. Faure. Computerised brain atlases vs. decision support systems : A methodological approach. *Artificial Intelligence in Medicine*, 14(1):83–100, 1998.
9. B. Horn, B. Schunck. Determining optical flow. Artif. Intell. 17:185–204, 1981.
10. P. Huber. *Robust statistics*. Wiley, 1981.
11. J. Maintz, MA. Viergever. A survey of medical image registration. *Medical Image Analysis*, 2(1):1–36, 1998.
12. E. Mémin, P. Pérez. Dense estimation and object-based segmentation of the optical flow with robust techniques. *IEEE Trans. Image Processing*, 7(5):703–719, 1998.
13. M. Ono, S. Kubik, C. Abernathey. *Atlas of the cerebral sulci*. Verlag, 1990.
14. J. Sled, A. Zijdenbos, A. Evans. A nonparametric method for automatic correction of intensity nonuniformity in MRI data. *IEEE TMI*, 17(1):87–97, 1998.
15. G. Subsol, JP. Thirion, N. Ayache. A general scheme for automatically building 3D anatomical atlases : Application to a skull atlas. INRIA RR 2586, 1995.
16. R. Szeliski, S. Lavallée. Matching 3D anatomical surfaces with non-rigid deformations using octree-splines. *SPIE geometric methods in computer vision*, 2031:306–315, 1993.
17. J. Talairach, P. Tournoux. *Co-planar stereotaxic atlas of the human brain*. Georg Thieme Verlag, 1988.
18. JP. Thirion. Image matching as a diffusion process: an analogy with Maxwell's demons. *Medical Image Analysis*, 2(3):243–260, 1998.

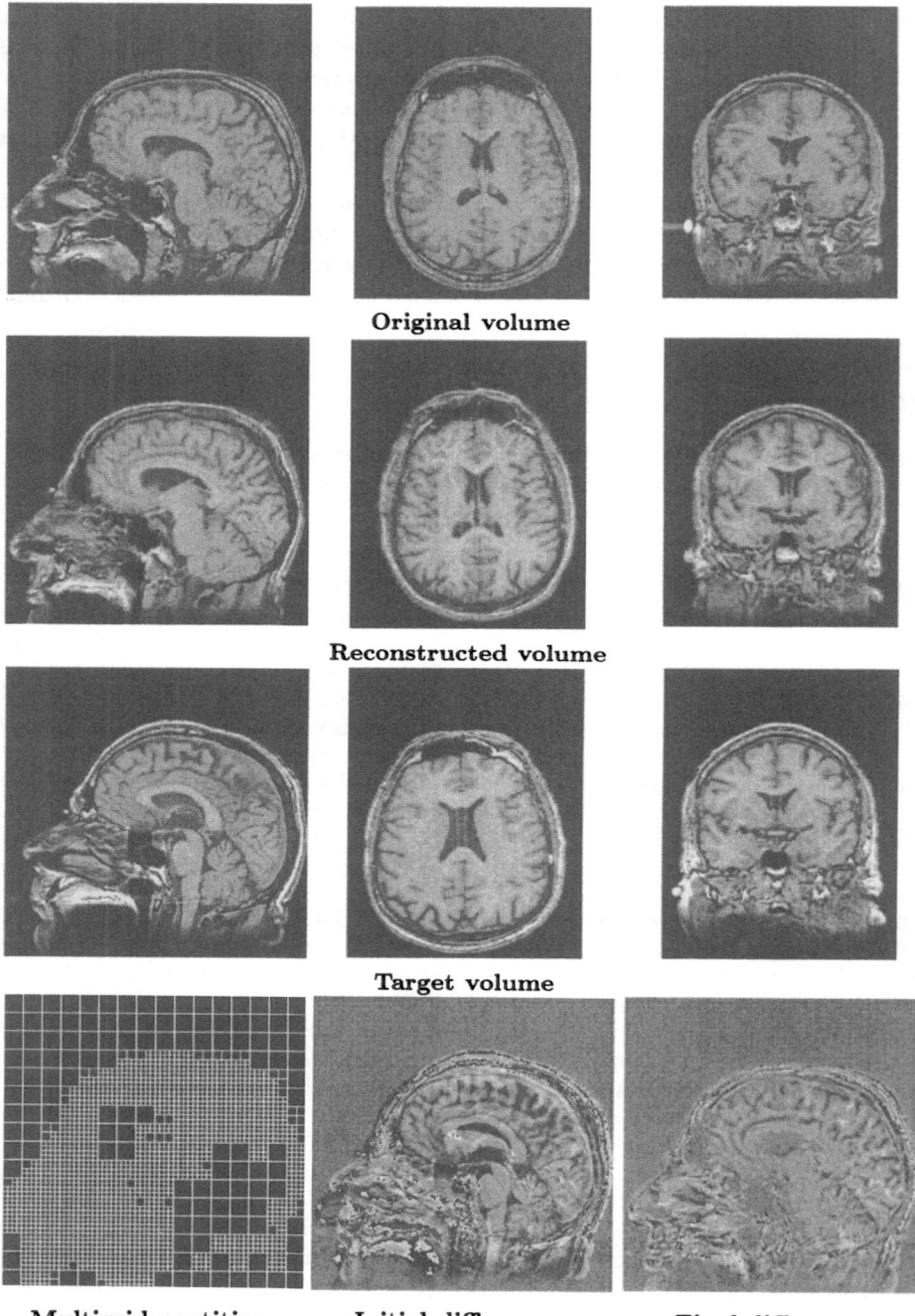

Fig. 3. Final results of the registration

Camera-Augmented Mobile C-arm (CAMC) Application: 3D Reconstruction Using a Low-Cost Mobile C-arm

N. Navab[1], M. Mitschke[2] and O. Schütz[2]

[1] Siemens Corporate Research, 755 College Road East, Princeton, NJ 08540, USA
[2] Siemens AG, Medical Engineering, Henkestr. 127, 91052 Erlangen, Germany
Nassir.Navab@scr.siemens.com,
{Matthias.Mitschke,Oliver.Schuetz}@med.siemens.de

Abstract. High-end X-ray C-arm gantries have recently been used for 3D reconstruction. Low-cost mobile C-arms enjoy the advantage of being readily available and are often used as interventional imaging device, but do not guarantee the reproducibility of their motion. The calibration and reconstruction process used for high-end C-arms cannot be applied to them. Camera-Augmented Mobile C-arm (CAMC) is the solution we propose. A CCD camera is attached to the (motorized) mobile C-arm in order to calibrate the C-arm's projection geometry on-line. The relationship between X-ray and camera projection geometry is characterized in an off-line calibration process. We propose the notion of Virtual Detector (VD), which enables us to describe both optical and X-ray geometry as pinhole cameras with fixed intrinsic parameters. We have conducted experiments in order to compare the results of CAMC calibration with the calibration method used for high-end C-arms and using an optical tracking system (Polaris from Northern Digital, Inc.).

1 Introduction

C-arm X-ray systems are used in many surgical procedures such as fluoroscopy-based orthopedic procedures. Even if a 3D CT reconstruction is computed off-line, often X-ray fluoroscopy is used as interventional image-guided modality. However, the success of the procedure depends on the ability of the surgeon to mentally recreate the spatio-temporal intraoperative situation from two-dimensional fluoroscopic X-ray images. In this work we would like to provide 3D reconstruction using the mobile C-arm itself. This eliminates the need for a pre-computed CT reconstruction. The same mobile C-arm is also used for intra-operative guidance. The registration between the 3D data and 2D fluoroscopic images is much easier since they are obtained with the same modality.

The major reason that mobile C-arm systems are still not used for 3D reconstruction is that, in general, they do not guarantee reproducible motion for consecutive examinations. The solution we propose to this problem is to compute the calibration data during the patient run. Markers opaque to X-ray which are

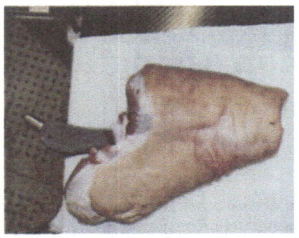
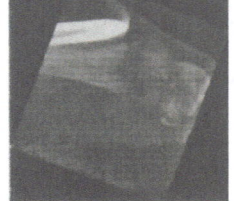
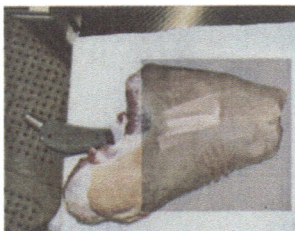

original optical image   3D reconstruction   result of overlay

Fig. 1. CAMC could enable the superimposition of X-ray on top of optical images

used in general for off-line calibration of C-arms cannot be used on-line, because they may interfere with the region of interest. Therefore we use optical markers which are transparent to X-ray in order to compute the motion of the mobile C-arm with the attached CCD camera. In this paper we present first results of 3D reconstruction using a Camera-Augmented Mobile C-arm (CAMC). This is only one of the possible advantages of using CCDs attached to a mobile C-arm. CAMC can also provide new possibilities for tracking, navigation and augmented reality. The optical camera can be used for registration between patient's optical and X-ray images. This would enable the system to combine X-ray and optical images and get images similar to Fig. 1. The "enhanced reality display" [5] and image overlay system for medical imaging [1] present excellent techniques for combining patient images with different medical imaging data. In both cases external sensors are brought in the operating room, and complicated registration and tracking procedures are necessary. The advantage of CAMC is that the registration is much easier since optical and X-ray system are rigidly attached. If equipped with a camera, the mobile C-arm which is often readily available in medical environment will be able to provide X-ray images, 3D reconstructed data, optical images and finally combined X-ray/optical images.

In this paper we present our first steps towards building such a Camera-Augmented Mobile C-arm system. We define the relationship between X-ray and CCD imaging geometry and use the attached CCD camera to characterize the motion of C-arm. We then present our first 3D reconstruction results using a mobile C-arm. We compare this result with the one obtained using X-ray phantoms (this would be ideal but it is not possible in real-time application) and using an external tracking sensor.

2   3D reconstruction from mobile C-arm[1]

In order to obtain the three-dimensional reconstruction the position of the C-arm mounted X-ray source and detector relative to the patient has to be measured. If the C-arm geometry is reproducible, the geometrical calibration can be done

---

[1] Here, we consider mobile C-arms equipped with a Solid State Detector with no distortion artifact. Distortion correction is necessary for traditional systems[4, 6].

off-line using X-ray phantoms [9, 2, 7] and the pose information can be used for the patient examination. However mobile C-arm systems do not guarantee reproducible motion for consecutive examinations.

Here, we propose to use a CCD camera attached to the C-arm in order to estimate the C-arm motion parameters and recover the X-ray projection geometry on-line. However the detector plane may also move relative to the X-ray source during the patient run. Therefore, we use a set of X-ray markers positioned on a plate directly in front of the X-ray source. These markers are designed and positioned in order to cover a small border of the X-ray image. In theory one can define a set of planar transformations that can be applied to the X-ray images before back-projection without affecting the 3D reconstruction results. We use the image of the marker plate to warp the X-ray image onto a virtual plane, we call the "virtual detector plane", before back-projection. By fixing this virtual plane, i.e. warping all X-ray images taken during the patient run such that the marker plate appears as it does on the virtual detector plane, one can fix the X-ray projection geometry relative to X-ray source. We then combine this information with C-arm motion computed using a CCD camera attached to the X-ray source in order to compute the full X-ray projection geometry during the patient run. This procedure provides a set of projection matrices, which can be used in order to back-project the X-ray image onto the voxel space for the 3D reconstruction process (see references for more details on back-projection and 3D reconstruction procedures [8, 3]).

2.1 X-ray and Camera Projection Geometry

The X-ray projection geometry as well as optical camera geometry is represented by P a 3×4 homogeneous matrix of projection. This matrix represents all the imaging geometry parameters which can be divided into two sets. The first set is called the extrinsic parameters. They define position and orientation of the imaging system in a world coordinate system. The second set is called the intrinsic parameters. They only depend on internal parameters of the imaging system. For the optical camera the intrinsic parameters could be defined as pixel size, image center, and principle distance or focal length. For a radiographic imaging system the intrinsic parameters could be defined as pixel size, image center, and source to detector distance. Note that the last two parameters are functions of relative position and orientation of source and detector. Both X-ray and optical imaging systems are modeled after a simple pinhole camera. A C-arm coordinate system is defined with its origin at the X-ray source. An optical camera coordinate system is defined with its origin at the optical center. We define the z-axis parallel to the normal dropping from X-ray source or the optical center for an optical camera onto the image plane. The x-axis and y-axis are parallel to the row and column vectors of the CCD for camera and 2D detector plane for X-ray imaging system.

2.2 Virtual Detector: connection between X-ray and optical camera projection models

For a CCD camera with fixed focal length it is reasonable to suppose that the intrinsic parameters remain fixed while acquiring a sequence of images. For X-ray images this is not the case. The intrinsic parameters of our C-arm imaging system are not constant over the image series. This is due to minor torsion of the C-arm caused by the weights of both X-ray source and detector. In order to be able to take the motion estimated from a CCD camera and apply it to X-ray geometry we need to fix the X-ray imaging intrinsic parameters. This is accomplished by a plate with a small number of X-ray opaque markers that is attached to the X-ray focus. These markers are projected onto the X-ray image close to the image borders. This bordering area is removed before the filtering and 3D reconstruction process. The marker plate is placed at a fixed position relative to the X-ray source. Therefore, its projection onto the image plane only depends on the intrinsic parameters of our X-ray imaging system.

Let us take two arbitrary X-ray images, I and I'. These two images correspond to two X-ray projection matrices P and P'. We can define a 2D-2D transformation H that maps the positions of each marker, $m_{i=1...k}$ (k = number of markers), on one X-ray image to its corresponding position on the other one, m_i'.

This planar transformation would actually warp one X-ray image onto an image plane at exactly same position and orientation relative to the X-ray source as the other X-ray image (detector) plane. We have:

$$m_i' = H m_i \, , \qquad i = 1 \ldots k \tag{1}$$

Instead of applying the transformation H to the image, we can simply multiply this transformation with the projection matrix P. Thereby we obtain a projection matrix $\tilde{P}$ with the extrinsic parameters of P, C-arm in the first position, and intrinsic parameters of P', relative position of X-ray source and detector plane, in the second position.

In this way, we take one of the X-ray images as a reference for fixing the relative position and orientation of X-ray source and detector plane, defining the *virtual detector*, and therefore fixing the intrinsic parameters, see Fig. 2. Now, we only need to compute the motion of the X-ray source, using the attached CCD camera, in order to recover all projection matrices.

2.3 Determination of X-ray projection matrices for a CAMC

Using the *virtual detector* described above allows us to treat our C-arm system as a pinhole camera with fixed intrinsic parameters. The motion of this C-arm imaging system (X-ray source with the virtual detector plane) for a whole image series will then be the same as the motion of a CCD camera attached to the X-ray source. Direct motion estimation from consecutive projection matrices as shown in [7] is more precise than motion estimation by decomposing these projection

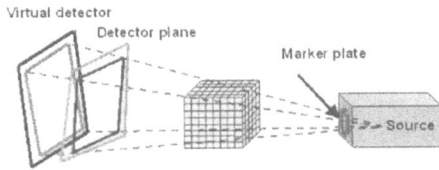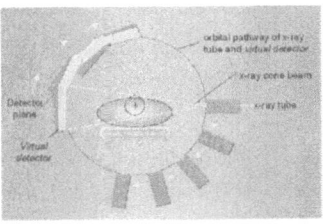

Fig. 2. Virtual Detector: The X-ray image can be first projected or back-projected onto a secondary plane, following the same X-ray projection geometry, and then back-projected onto the 3D voxel planes. The resulting 3D-2D mapping will theoretically remain unchanged (left). The intrinsic geometry of the C-arm remains unchanged for the whole patient examination when using the *virtual detector* (right).

matrices and computing the extrinsic parameters for each frame. We therefore propose a scenario in which we do not need to compute the intrinsic parameters of either our X-ray imaging system or the optical one. The scenario is divided into two steps:

1. *Off-line calibration*: One pair of images (X-ray and optical) is taken. The two projection matrices P_x (X-ray) and P_c (CCD camera) are used as reference for the transformation between X-ray and CCD camera coordinate systems. The image of the marker plate markers on the X-ray image defines the *virtual detector* for the on-line calibration.
2. *On-line calibration*: For each frame, the motion of the X-ray source relative to its position in the off-line calibration step is computed using optical cameras. This is done by computing the projection matrix for optical camera and estimating the motion without ever computing its intrinsic parameters: $([R, t] = f(P_c, P'_c))$, see [7] for more details on direct motion estimation. We then apply this motion to the reference X-ray projection matrix P_x, resulting in X-ray projection matrix $\tilde{P}'_x = P_x \cdot \begin{bmatrix} R & t \\ 0^T & 1 \end{bmatrix}$. This provides us with an X-ray projection matrix that projects 3D voxels onto our *virtual detector* plane for each frame. Using the marker plate (attached to the X-ray source) the planar transformation (2D-2D mapping) between the X-ray image and *virtual detector* H is computed (see sect. 2.2 for more details). The 3D-2D projection followed by the 2D-2D warping results in a new 3D-2D projection matrix $P'_x = H \cdot \tilde{P}'_x$. This projection matrix, for each frame, provides the final mapping between 3D voxels and 2D pixels on the corresponding X-ray image.

These projection matrices are used for 3D reconstruction from an unstable mobile C-arm. The results are described in the following section.

3   Experimental Results

This section describes experiments conducted in order to evaluate the performance of the proposed method. For the first experiment we use a motion platform

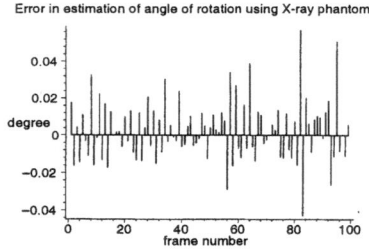 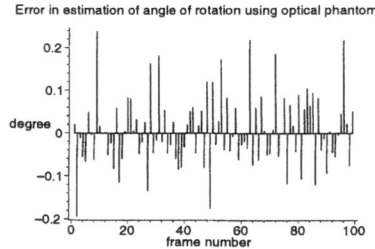

Fig. 3. Error in estimation of angle of rotation (in degrees) using X-ray (left) and optical (right) projection matrices versus ground truth of motion platform

with precise ground truth information. In this case, we evaluate the calibration result using both X-ray and optical phantoms with regard to the achieved accuracy of estimated rotation. Then a second experiment is conducted using a mobile C-arm with no available ground truth. The results of 3D reconstruction will be used for a qualitative evaluation. Questions we try to answer are: Can pose and motion of the C-arm be estimated using a CCD camera ? Is the achieved accuracy good enough for 3D reconstruction?

3.1 Motion platform

The goal of this first experiment is to quantitatively compare the accuracy of pose and motion estimation using optical and X-ray phantoms. We use the X-ray phantom and calibration process used in [7]. X-ray phantoms interfere with the patient's X-ray image and cannot be used for mobile C-arm systems in real application. However, this gives us the advantage of comparing our results with 3D reconstruction results which have been proved by physicians and successfully tested on patients already.

We first use a precise motion platform, providing the ground truth, for a comparative study of motion estimations using X-ray and CCD phantoms. The position and orientation of X-ray and optical phantom as well as the motion platform is known in the same coordinate system. We use a composite phantom which has two distinct but connected parts. One part is the X-ray ring phantom (see [7]), the other part is an optical phantom.

We take sets of 100 pairs of simultaneous X-ray and optical images. The motion consists of 99 steps of 1.8 degrees pure rotation around a fixed axis. For all consecutive pairs of X-ray as well as CCD images we compute the following estimation error measurement:

- *maximum rotational error*: angle of the residual rotation $\tilde{R}^T R$, between estimated rotation and the ground truth. This represents the maximum rotational error with regard to both estimation of angle of rotation and rotation axis
- *angle of rotation*: difference between the estimated angle of rotation and the ground truth given by the motion platform.

	angle of rotation (in deg.)		maximum rotation error (in deg.)	
	mean	std. dev.	mean	std. dev.
X-ray	0.012	0.010	0.083	0.060
optical camera	0.063	0.052	0.110	0.066

Table 1. Error in estimation of angle of rotation and maximum rotational error using X-ray and optical projection matrices versus ground truth of motion platform

The errors in the estimation of translational motion are negligible. We therefore compare different approaches only based on their success in estimation of dominant rotational motion.

Figure 3 depicts the absolute error in estimation of angle of rotation for both X-ray and optical phantoms for the fist experiment. Both Figure 3, and table 1 show that accuracy of the estimated rotation is better for X-ray projection matrices. However, these figures also show that both methods determine the rotation with high accuracy. Both methods determine the rotation with enough precision needed for 3D reconstruction.

3.2   Moving C-arm

In this experiment the C-arm is rotated 190 degrees around a reconstruction phantom (see Fig. 5(c)). Eighty five pairs of X-ray and optical images are taken during the C-arm motion. Additionally the 3D pose information of a marker plate attached to the X-ray tube is measured by an external optical tracking system (Polaris from Northern Digital). The C-arm is not able to provide the motion parameters with acceptable accuracy. Therefore, experimental results are primarily validated and compared with regard to the quality of the 3D reconstruction process.

In addition we also want to compare the results achieved with the optical phantom and the external tracking system in a quantitative way. For both methods, we compare the estimated motion between two consecutive image frames with respect to the estimated motion using the X-ray phantom, see [7] for more detail. The result of our experiment with motion platform, see sect. 3.1, lets us assume that this ground truth motion is estimated quite accurately. Both X-ray and optical phantom are physically attached and defined such that the C-arm motion is described in a common coordinate system. This is not the case for the external tracking system. In order not to add errors due to the extra necessary calibration between the two coordinate systems, we only compare the results of estimating the angle of rotation, which is independent of the choice of coordinate system.

Figures 5(a-c) show the experimental setup. The left image shows the C-arm, X-ray and optical phantom as well as the external tracking system. The close-up in the middle shows the CCD camera attached to the X-ray tube and the marker plate in front of the X-ray beam. The right image shows our reconstruction phantom. It consists of two cylindrical objects covered in an acrylic hull. Attached to it (not visualized in the picture) is a metal ring made from titanic alloy positioned inside an acrylic cover.

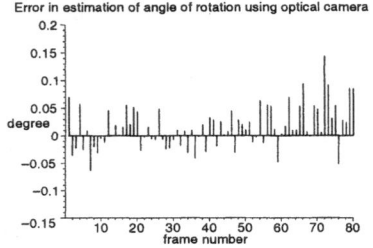
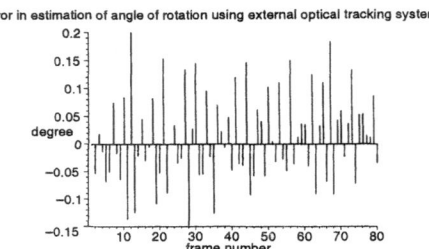

Fig. 4. Experimental results of estimation of C-arm motion: Error in estimation of angle of rotation using optical camera (left) and external tracking system (right) versus ground truth of X-ray projection matrices

rotation angle (in deg.)	mean	std. dev.
optical camera	0.031	0.027
external tracking system	0.065	0.047

Table 2. Experimental results of estimation of C-arm motion: Error in estimation of angle of rotation using optical camera and external tracking system versus ground truth of X-ray projection matrices

The X-ray and camera projection geometry are computed using an initial frame (in clinical applications this would be done off-line). The intrinsic geometry of this X-ray projection is used to define the *virtual detector* plane (see sect. 2.2).

Figures 5(d-f) show 3D reconstruction results using projection matrices obtained by the different calibration methods. These figures show the three orthogonal Maximum Intensity Projections (MIP) of the reconstructed volume. The differences are not dramatic and especially the amount of artifacts caused by the metallic part is very small for all three 3D reconstructions. Comparing the two new methods, the 3D reconstruction using the attached CCD camera matrices achieves better results than using the external tracking system. Figure 4 shows the absolute error in angle of rotation using CCD camera and external tracking system versus the assumed ground truth of X-ray projection matrices. The mean absolute error and standard deviation are smaller using optical projection matrices, see table 2. In average, the errors for this experiment are comparable to the errors of the experiment with the motion platform described in sect. 3.1.

Finally, Fig. 5(g) presents a 3D reconstruction of anatomical data. A part of a pig's spine has been reconstructed using our Camera-Augmented Mobile C-arm (CAMC). The reconstruction seems to be rich and precise enough to be used in interventional procedures. This must be fully tested and evaluated through clinical trials.

4 Conclusion and Future Work

In this paper, we propose to add optical cameras to a low-cost mobile C-arm. The optical system takes the responsibility of dynamically calibrating the C-arm motion during the patient run. The experimental results show that with this on-line calibration process one can recover the X-ray projection geometry and reconstruct the volume of interest. This integrated camera solution was compared to the use of an external tracking system for motion estimation and achieved better reconstruction result. Moreover, there is a need for on-line calibration of external sensor and X-ray imaging system which is not needed if the CCD camera is rigidly and permanently attached to the C-arm. The mobile C-arm is already being used in medical procedures. Therefore, Camera-Augmented Mobile C-arms have a great chance of getting easily accepted and used in clinical applications. The reconstruction results are quite satisfactory. Having shown the feasibility of our approach we will continue working on the design of a phantom that can be used in the clinical environment. This CAMC based reconstruction will reduce the need of pre-computation of the 3D geometry with another modality, and therefore reduces the complexity of on-line registration with X-ray fluoroscopic images. We also plan to use the optical images for real-time navigation and for real-time merging of patient's X-ray and optical images in the near future.

Acknowledgement: Authors would like to thank K. Wiesent and W. Seissler for providing the 3D reconstruction software. We would also like to thank A. Bani-Hashemi and R. Graumann for useful discussion during the progress of this work. This work was accomplished thanks to partial support from Bayerische Forschungsstiftung.

References

1. M. Blackwell et al. An image overlay system for medical data visualization. In *First International Conference on Medical Image Computing and Computer-Assisted Intervention (MICCAI)*, pages 232–240, 1998.
2. R. Koppe et al. 3d vessel reconstruction based on rotational angiography. In *Computer Assitsted Radiology*, pages 101–107. Springer, June 1995.
3. R. Fahrig, A. J. Fox, and D. W. Holdsworth. Characterization of a c-arm mounted xrii for 3d image reconstruction during interventional neuroradiology. pages 351–360. Proc. SPIE 2708, 1996.
4. R. Fahrig, M. Moreau, and D. W. Holdsworth. Three-dimensional computer tomographic reconstruction using a c-arm mounted xrii: Correction of image intensifier distortion. *Medical Physics*, 24:1097–1106, 1997.
5. W. E. L. Grimson et al. Clinical experience with a high precision image-guided neurosurgery system. In *MICCAI'98*, pages 63–73, Cambridge, MA, USA, 1998.
6. E. Gronenschild. The accuracy and reproducibility of a global method to correct for geometric image distortion in the x-ray imaging chain. *Medical Physics*, 24:1875–1888, 1997.
7. N. Navab, A. Bani-Hashemi, M. S. Nadar, K. Wiesent, P. Durlak, T. Brunner, K. Barth, and R. Graumann. 3D reconstruction from projection matrices in a c-arm based 3d-angiography system. In *MICCAI'98*, pages 1305–1306, Cambridge, MA, USA, 1998.
8. D. L. Parker. Optimal short scan convolution reconstruction for fanbeam ct. *Medical Physics*, 9(2):254–257, March/April 1982.
9. A. Rougée, A. C. Picard, Y. Trousset, and C. Ponchut. Geometrical calibration of x-ray imaging chains for three-dimensional reconstruction. *Computerized medical Imaging and Graphics*, 17(4/5):295–300, 1993.

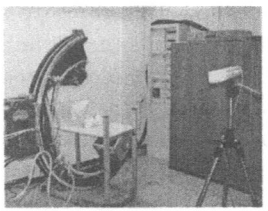 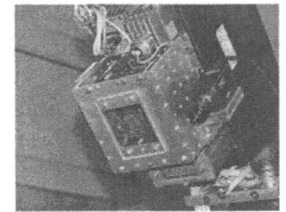 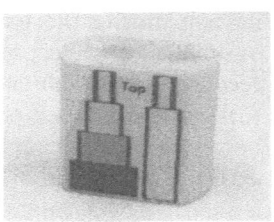

(a) Experimental setup   (b) Camera and marker plate   (c) Reconstr. phantom

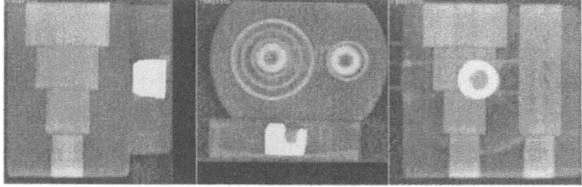

(d) 3D reconstruction using X-ray phantom

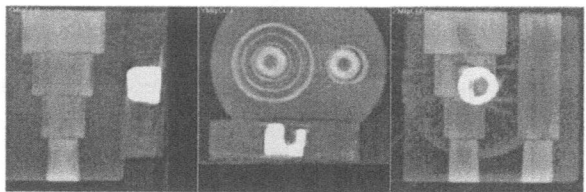

(e) 3D reconstruction using optical phantom

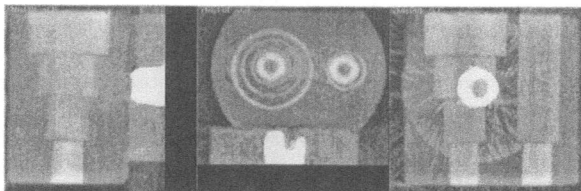

(f) 3D reconstruction using external tracking system

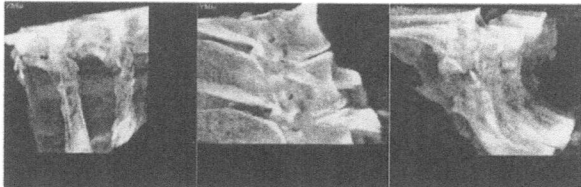

(g) 3D reconstruction of a part of a pig's spine

Fig. 5. Experimental setup (a,b), reconstruction phantom (c), and 3D reconstruction results (d,e,f,g)

Image Analysis of Nailfold Capillary Patterns from Video Sequences

P.D. Allen[1], C.J. Taylor[1], A. L. Herrick[2], and T. Moore[2]

[1] Wolfson Image Analysis Unit,
Imaging Science and Biomedical Engineering,
University of Manchester,
Manchester M13 9PT, U.K.
pa@sv1.smb.man.ac.uk
http://www.wiau.man.ac.uk
[2] University of Manchester, Rheumatic Diseases Centre,
Hope Hospital, Salford M6 8HD, UK.

Abstract. Video capillaroscopy is a widely used technique to assess the condition of the blood capillaries in the nailfold of patients suffering from reduced peripheral circulation (Raynaud's phenomenon). This approach is complicated by the fact that gaps in the flow of blood can render capillaries incomplete in any single video frame. This paper describes a computer based system in which sequences of video frames are registered and combined to provide a composite image for analysis. We show that the images can be registered to an accuracy of approximately 2 μm, and that temporally variable features can be enhanced significantly by subtracting one standard deviation from the mean value for each pixel position in the video sequence.

1 Introduction

Among the symptoms produced by the connective tissue disease Scleroderma is a reduction in peripheral circulation exacerbated by exposure to cold (Raynaud's phenomenon). Extreme conditions can lead to amputation of fingers and toes and so improvement of the circulation in patients with Scleroderma is a major concern to clinicians. Trials aimed at this require an objective method of assessing the condition of the peripheral vasculature and quantifying changes caused by treatments under test.

One technique that has been explored is direct visualisation of the blood capillaries in the skin at the base of the finger nail (nailfold). Here the tiny vessels that link the arterial and venous system can be seen using an optical microscope (see figure 1). In previous work [1], a video camera has been coupled to the microscope, and the condition of the capillary network has been assessed by measuring certain key capillary loop dimensions from single video frames. Gaps in the flow of red blood cells through the capillary loops (the capillary wall itself is transparent) mean that not all of the capillary network is visible at any one instant. Thus it would be preferable to integrate the information from a sequence of successive video frames. Also, measuring the capillary dimensions by hand is tedious and therefore error prone.

This work forms part of an on going project to develop a computer based system for the analysis of nailfold capillary patterns in which the capillary dimensions will be measured automatically.

2   Video Frame Registration

The video information recorded by the clinicians is recorded in the form of a series of overlapping scenes. This is achieved by holding the finger as still as possible under the microscope for about 20 seconds or so, then moving the finger laterally on to the next scene, maintaining an overlap of one or more capillary loops. Two magnifications are used, ×200 and ×600. The low magnification images are used to give a general overview of the capillary structure, whilst the high magnification images are used for capillary dimension measurement. At the lower magnification, the region of the capillary network of interest is covered in three scenes. The aim of the system being developed is to register and combine the video frames from this material to form a single panoramic video mosaic showing the whole capillary network under study. Capillaries of interest identified in this mosaic can then be measured from their corresponding image in the ×600 material.

For a sequence of video frames to be combined the small relative motions between finger and microscope during a sequence must be detected and corrected for, and in this application we require this process to be automatic. Accurate frame registration requires that the blood capillaries are separated from other elements in the image such as video noise or lens dust. Segmenting curvilinear structures such as blood vessels is a common problem in medical imaging [2]. The solution employed here is to apply a linear feature detector previously developed to detect line patterns in X-Ray mammograms [3]. The output of this process is a binary image containing a skeletal representation of the capillary structure where the capillaries are reduced to lines one pixel thick. From these binary images the transformation from one image to the next can be found. The extremely narrow depth of field inherent in optical microscopy means that changes in scale or perspective distortions are impossible. Thus the transformation from one frame to the next can be completely described by a combination of 2D translation and rotation. There are a variety of approaches to such an image registration problem [4]. Here the translation between two successive frames can be found from the skeletal representations using a Hough transform method. Each of the skeletal pixels from image A is matched with every skeletal pixel from image B. Each match represents a possible translation if rotation is known. If these matches are used to vote in a translation space, a peak emerges at the point representing the translation for which the largest number of pixels in the two images agree. If the two images are miss-aligned by a rotation as well as translation, the size of the peak in the translation image will be smaller than if there had been no rotation. Thus if the translation space is created for a number of possible rotations, the one which yields the highest peak corresponds to the correct, or at least best, rotation.

2.1 Robustness

The nature of the images in a video sequence can vary greatly from one patient to the next for two basic reasons. The first is the variation in image content caused by different capillary morphologies. In most healthy subjects the nailfold capillaries are in the form of long thin vertical loops arranged in roughly parallel horizontal rows (see figure 1), whereas the capillary loops of scleroderma patients tend to be enlarged and the regular row structure can become completely distorted (see figure 2). There can also be a complete absence of recognisable capillary loops in some places known as avascular regions.

The second source of image variability is caused by the condition of the skin. Viewing the nailfold capillaries with an optical microscope relies on the overlying skin being transparent, but one of the effects of scleroderma is to thicken the skin and this can reduce its transparency considerably.

Thus, designing a system that can successfully register and combine video frames corresponding to a single patient is no guarantee that it will work on any other patient, and so the system must be tested on as wide a set of patients as possible. The registration algorithms of the system being developed have been tested on the data of 25 patients so far. The 25 were chosen to include as wide a range of morphologies and image qualities as possible, and the results for two of the patients are shown in figures 1 and 2. The registration appears to be successful in all of the 25 cases even when, as in the case of overlapping scenes, the mutual information is relatively low.

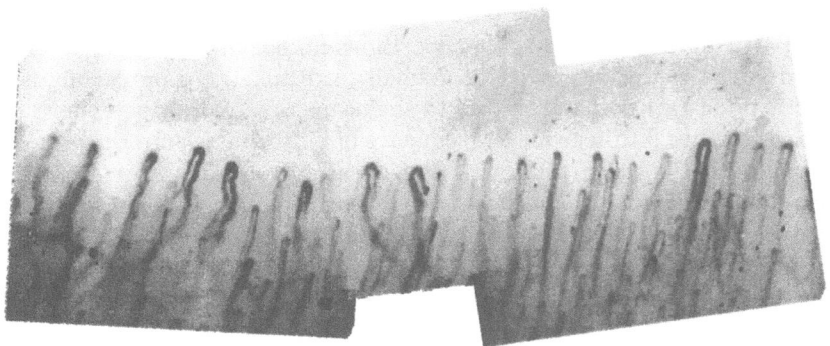

Fig. 1. *Nailfold capillary structure at ×200 magnification. This subject (patient B in table 1) has scleroderma, but the capillary structure in this case exhibits the regular pattern of long thin loops typical of most healthy patients. The image shown is a composite of 48 video frames, 16 in each of the three overlapping scenes.*

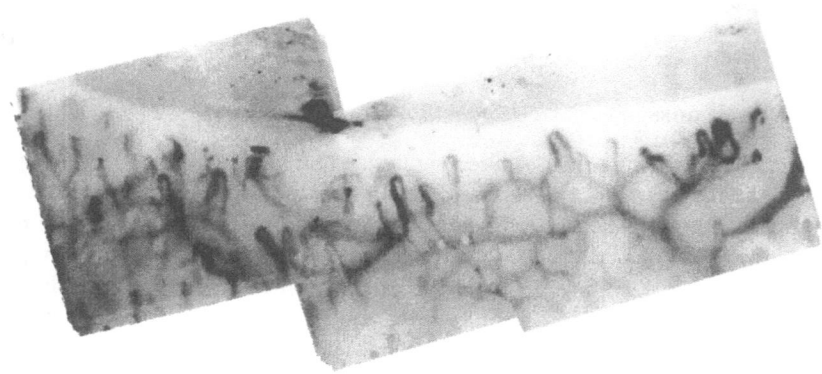

Fig. 2. *Nailfold capillary structure at ×200 magnification. This subject (patient A in table 1) has diffuse scleroderma and exhibits distortion of the capillary loop pattern when compared with the more usual regular row structure visible in figure 1. The image shown is a composite of 48 video frames, 16 in each of the three overlapping scenes.*

2.2   Registration accuracy

To test the registration accuracy of the system a temporally stable feature is required in the scene which belongs to the tissue of the finger and hence reflects the motion of the capillary network through the sequence. In some of the patients (about 50%), small dark specks about 6 pixels in diameter can be seen in the video frames. Examination of the moving video sequence reveals that some of these are specks of dust on the lens, but others belong to the finger's skin tissue, and are therefore ideal for testing registration accuracy.

Basically, a number of these dark specks are identified in each of the frames from a particular sequence and their positions noted. In each case the position recorded is the center of gravity of a small (6×6 pixel) region calculated as a geometric point rather than rounded to the nearest pixel position. The transformation vectors used to register the sequence of video frames are then applied to these points. If the registration was perfect, all of the points corresponding to the same image feature would be transformed to the same point. Instead, due to miss registrations, a cluster of points results and the spread in this cluster is a measure of registration accuracy.

Out of the 25 patient data sets examined so far, a set of four were chosen which exhibited point features suitable for testing registration accuracy and the results are shown in table 1. For each patient there are one or more suitable scenes and each scene consists of either eight or sixteen video frames. Within each scene the number of usable image features, or points, will also vary and here the figures given are averaged over all the points used in the scene.

For each chosen feature a cluster of points (one for each video frame) will appear in the composite scene after registration. The average deviation from their geometric center in X and Y (horizontal and vertical) is quoted as the registration

Table 1. *Estimates of image registration accuracy based on selected stable point like image features associated with skin tissue. The scene is simply the number of the scene used, N_F is the number of video frames in that scene, and N_P is the number of image points or features used for testing registrations accuracy. After image registration, clusters of points appear in th composite image corresponding to each of the selected features, and the standard deviation in X and Y from the mean position is taken to be the registration error. The X and Y errors (pixels) quoted are the average over all selected features in the scene, and the equivalent values for image combination without registration are shown for comparison.*

Patient	Scene	N_F	N_P	Registered		Unregistered	
				X error	Y error	X error	Y error
A	2	16	3	0.64 ± 0.07	0.7 ± 0.2	7.13 ± 0.08	10.46 ± 0.1
	3	16	4	1.9 ± 0.4	1.9 ± 0.3	6.56 ± 0.05	17.80 ± 0.08
B	1	16	13	0.91 ± 0.08	1.54 ± 0.08	3.77 ± 0.09	7.13 ± 0.13
	2	16	7	1.3 ± 0.1	1.22 ± 0.09	2.97 ± 0.2	6.43 ± 0.07
	3	16	6	1.1 ± 0.1	1.7 ± 0.2	5.12 ± 0.1	9.3 ± 0.1
C	3	8	6	1.0 ± 0.1	1.4 ± 0.1	1.45 ± 0.1	4.3 ± 0.06
D	2	8	3	1.4 ± 0.2	1.2 ± 0.2	3.57 ± 0.2	4.29 ± 0.08

error. The reason that X and Y errors are determined separately rather than a simple scalar distance from the point cluster centroid is due to nature of the information in the nailfold images. For images in which the capillaries appear as long thin vertical loops there is less information from which to determine the Y displacement, and so a greater registration error in the Y axis may result. For example, the capillary loops of patient B in table 1 can be seen in figure 1. Here, most of the capillaries are long thin loops and the results do indicate a greater registration error in the Y direction for scene 1 and 3.

The last two columns of table 1 show the registration errors derived if the points are not transformed according to the registration vectors. In other words these figures represent the spread we would expect in the position of the points belonging to a particular image feature if the video frames were simply combined without any attempt at registration. They show that there tends to be more vertical motion than horizontal. Here, vertical corresponds to the direction the finger is pointing and the larger displacements observed in this direction are simply a consequence of the way the finger is physically constrained during the microscopy session. This means that the greatest displacements between video frames will tend to be in the same direction as the capillary loops in subjects such as patient B, and so how much of the extra registration error in the Y direction in this case is due to the nature of the image, and how much is due simply to the fact that most of the movement was in this direction anyway, is difficult to assess.

At the moment there are only a small number of patients exhibiting suitable features to test registration accuracy and larger numbers will be utilised to obtain a more definitive assessment of the system's performance. From the data analysed so far we can say that the registration errors are less than two pixels in either X or Y. Since we expect the registration accuracy to be dependent on the capillary structure it is less meaningful to quote averages over a number of patients than to focus on the worst cases. In the current manual system the capillary dimensions are measured from single video frames and so the limiting factor is the image resolution i.e. any dimension measured is known to ± 1 pixel (corresponding to approximately 2 μm). However, the noise levels in a single frame is considerably higher than in a composite scene and this will reduce the accuracy to which a feature's dimensions can be measured. Also of course, temporal variability may result in a feature being completely absent in a particular scene. The registration accuracy exhibited so far is therefore acceptable.

2.3   Combining Images

Once a sequence of video frames has been registered with respect to the capillary network, the information from the set of images has to be combined in such a way as to make maximum use of the available information. The most obvious approach is to take the mean of the image set. This is the most desirable way of enhancing stable image features, as the random noise present in the individual images is averaged out. However, if we consider the case of a capillary in which the column of red blood cells contains visible gaps, at any given point on the capillary the intensity of the image will vary with time as the 'lumps' of blood flow through. If an average of the sequence is taken, this variation between light (background) and dark (blood cells) will result in an average value in between and so the contrast between capillary and background will be lower than it was in a single frame. Thus, the complete capillary becomes visible, but contrast is lost. Another commonly used approach is to select the minimum value for each pixel from the sequence. This improves signal contrast, but involves no noise averaging, so it is not obvious that the visibility of the results will be any better than taking the mean. We propose a third alternative, which is to subtract some multiple of the standard deviation from the mean. The idea is to estimate a value representative of the minimum over the sequence but less susceptible to noise.

If the contrast between a capillary and the surrounding tissue in a composite scene can be quantified, then the relative merits of the image combination techniques described above can be assessed. If we consider the difference between the intensity of the capillary and the surrounding tissue as the signal, then the contrast can be quantified as the signal to noise ratio. To define the signal to noise ratio mathematically we must make assumptions about the average grey level intensities of blood and background tissue, and what the noise will be on these values. These can be estimated from the nail-fold images encountered in this study. The other important variables to consider are the fraction of time F_S that a particular pixel's grey level intensity corresponds to blood, and the number of images in the sequence N. F_S can also be thought of as a measure of the capillary's temporal variability - a low F_S would correspond to a capillary in which the gaps in the flow of blood were large compared to the length of the column of red blood cells, and visa versa.

There is insufficient space in this paper to go through the resulting derivations [5], however, figure 3 shows the predicted relationship between signal to noise ratio and F_S for the mean image, minimum projection, and $\mu - n\sigma$, when the number of frames in the sequence N is 100. The best results are obtained from $\mu - n\sigma$, but the optimum value of n is a function of F_S.

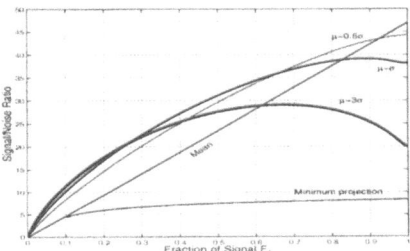

Fig. 3. Signal to noise ratio as a function of feature variability F_S.

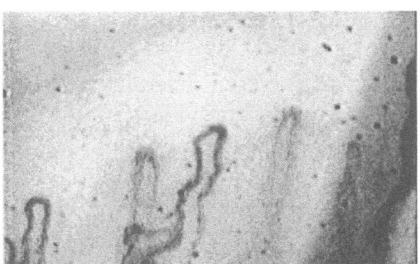

Fig. 4. *Single video frame of nailfold capillaries at ×600 magnification.*

3   Applying Image Combination Techniques to Data

The discussion in section 2.3 is partly illustrated in figures 4 to 6. Figure 4 shows a single frame from a sequence of 20, the central capillary in this scene displays large gaps in the flow of blood and so the capillaries appearance was variable with time.

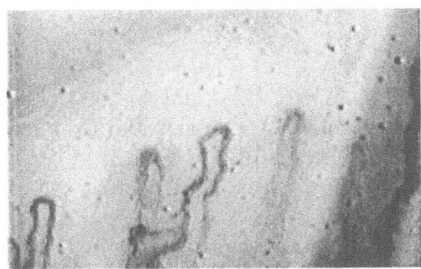

Fig. 5. *The mean pixel values of the registered video frame sequence.*

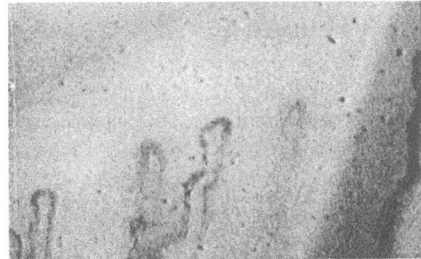

Fig. 6. *The mean image minus one standard deviation.*

Figure 5 shows the result of taking the mean of the image sequence. The central capillary loop now appears complete and the noise in the scene has been reduced. The capillary loops either side of the central loop still appear relatively indistinct - this is because they are slightly deeper in the skin than the others. With the reduction in noise, the texture of the skin obscuring them is just becoming apparent. Figure 6 shows the result of subtracting one standard deviation from the mean image. The contrast of the central capillary has been enhanced but there has been a slight increase in the noise levels of the surrounding temporally stable background.

4 Conclusions

So far this system has only been tested on 25 patient data sets, but the indications are that the video frame registration is robust and acceptably accurate.

The signal to noise ratio estimates in figure 3 show that for the noise and contrast levels found in nailfold images, the best signal to noise ratio is achieved by using $\mu - n\sigma$, where the value of n is a function of the degree of temporal variability F_S. If the contrast between blood cells and surrounding tissue and the noise level σ is known and can be assumed to be constant, then the value of F_S can be derived at each pixel position from the equations on which figure 3 was based. However, the blood/background contrast varies from one patient to the next. The extent of this variation and whether this will render evaluation of F_S impracticable requires further study. However, figure 3 suggests that subtracting between a half and one standard deviation gives an improved signal to noise ratio over the mean for most values of F_S. Also the set of images in section 3 show that using $\mu - \sigma$ improves the contrast of the variable capillary without noticeable degradation of stable ones. Thus, in the absence of a reliable estimate of F_S, $\mu - \sigma$ would seem to be the best option for image combination of the nailfold images encountered in this study.

These results are also of general application to problems requiring temporal or spatially varying data to be compounded.

References

1. M. Bukhari, A.L. Herrick, T. Moore, J. Manning, and M. I. V. Jayson. Increased Nailfold Capillary Dimensions in Primary Raynaud's Phenomenon and Systemic Sclerosis. *British Journal of Rheumatology*, 35:1127–1131, 1996.
2. R. Kutka and S. Stier. Extraction of Line Properties Based on Direction Fields. *IEEE Trans. Med. Imag*, 15(1):51–58, February 1996.
3. R. Zwiggelar, T. Parr, and C. Taylor. Finding Oriented Line Patterns in Digital Mammographic Images. In *Proc. of 7th BMVC Edinburgh*, 1996.
4. L. G. Brown. A Survey of Image Registration Techniques. *ACM Computing Surveys*, 24(4):321–376, December 1992.
5. P. D. Allen, C. J. Taylor, A.L. Herrick, and T. Moore. Enhancement of Temporally Variable Features in Nailfold Capillary Patterns. In *British Machine Vision Conference*, volume 2, pages 535–544, 1998.

Modeling Spectral Changes to Visualize Embedded Volume Structures for Medical Image Data

H.J. Noordmans[1], H.T.M. van der Voort[2], M.A. Viergever[1]

[1] Image Sciences Institute E.01.334, P.O. Box 85500, University Hospital Utrecht, 3508 GA Utrecht, The Netherlands, herke@isi.uu.nl, http://www.isi.uu.nl/People/Herke/herke.html.
[2] Scientific Volume Imaging BV, Alexanderlaan 14, 1213 XS Hilversum, The Netherlands, info@svi.nl, http://www.svi.nl/.

Abstract. When a volume structure is embedded in another volume structure, it is difficult to see the inner structure without destroying the view on the outer structure. We present a solution by letting the volume structures scatter light with a different wavelengths. The outer volume structure only absorbs light scattered by the structure itself and does not absorb the light scattered by the inner structure, by which the inner structure is visible without destroying the view on the outer structure. Examples are shown of vascular imaging and CT imaging.

1 Introduction

The increasing number of image modalities, their increasing quality and the progress in image segmentation algorithms increase the number of volume structures one wants to combine in a volume rendering. This can be done by giving each structure a distinct color and opacity. However it becomes more complicated to show a structure which is embedded in another volume structure. One can think of seeing the organs inside the skin of the surrounding abdomen for laprascopy or to see the veins surrounding the brain in order to avoid them in neurosurgery. It is possible to cut a virtual hole in the outer structure[1] or to decrease its opacity, but a disadvantage is loosing surface information of a part or the total outer structure. If one still wants to see surface detail, for example for navigation, the visualization problem is more difficult. A simple option is to render the two structures separately and combine them at display. Possibilities are taking the square root of their squared intensities[2], putting them in a separate RGB channel[2], or averaging the RGB colors. The result may be satisfying, but the question remains whether there exists a less ambiguous and less ad-hoc way of visualizing an embedded volume structure.

2 Spectral approach

In our search for such a 'ideal' method, we started by looking at nature. In the real world, a light source emits light that illuminates an object. The light is

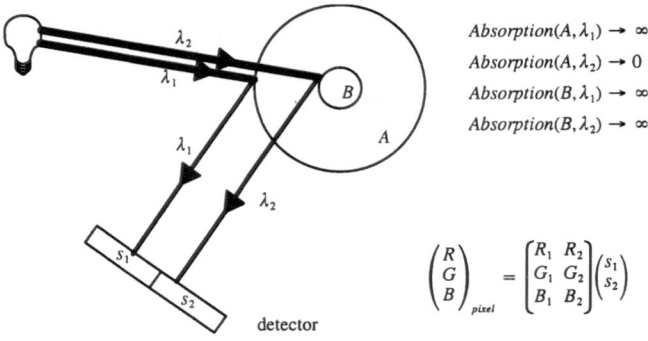

Fig. 1. Schematic layout spectral volume rendering.

absorbed, reflected and scattered by the object before it reaches our eye. The light has a spectrum (light has a color not an object!) which changes in the absorption, reflecting, scattering process. This 'changed' spectrum is seen by our eyes. The human eye can be considered as a detector which, by its cones, converts the spectrum into a kind of RGB signal. In our volume renderer we simulate the same principle (Simulated Fluorescence Process[3]). We simulate a light source emitting an illumination spectrum. We assume that a voxel contains an amount of material with specific scatter and absorbing properties. The value of the voxel determines the amount, a label the type of material. The illumination spectrum excites the material which on its turn emits a part of it. A part of the light is absorbed and a part passes the voxel to illuminate other voxels. The emitted spectrum of the materials is seen by a detector which contains a kind of spectrum analyzer. The result is a sequence of numbers which is mapped by a matrix to an RGB value.

Returning to our problem, to visualize object B inside object A (Fig. 1), we assume that the illumination spectrum consists of two main wavelength bands, characterized by λ_1 and λ_2. Object A has material with strong absorption bands around λ_1 but with almost no absorption around λ_2. Object B absorbs spectral bands both around λ_1 and λ_2. Object A only scatters the spectral band around λ_1, while object B only scatters the spectral band around λ_2. The detector sees both wavelength bands and converts them to an RGB value. The result is that we see surface detail of object A while seeing object B through it.

2.1   Theoretical background

Although the spectral volume renderer can be reduced to a more common RGBα volume renderer [4], [5], [6], the main difference is the more physically realistic basis which underlies our renderer. Whereas in an RGBα renderer rays are traced

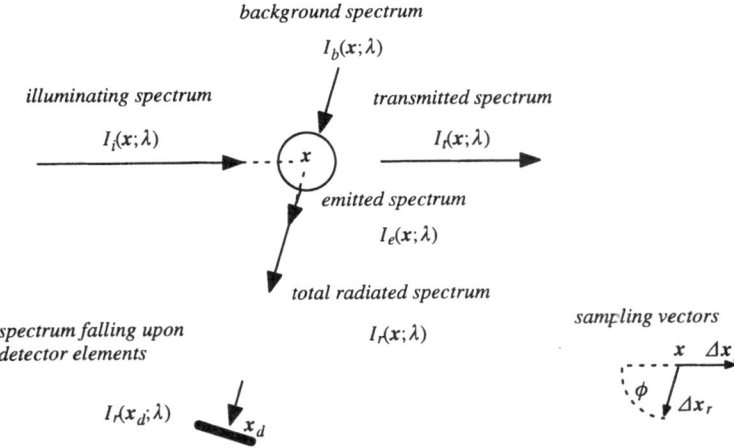

Fig. 2. Spectra involved in light/matter interaction process.

through an RGBα volume (where each voxel is described by a RGB triplet and opacity α), we simulate how light from a light source interacts with materials inside a voxel. Each segmented object or image modality is assumed to consist of one type of material m. By letting the material types have different absorbing and scattering properties, objects have a different opacity and color.

There are many physical ways how light can interact with a material. The material can reflect it perfectly (e.g. metal sphere), absorb some of the incident energy (e.g. convert it into heat), scatter it elastically (no energy loss, Rayleigh scattering), or inelastically (energy loss, e.g. phosphoresce, fluorescence). This process is angle and wavelength dependent. As we are not trying to simulate nature, but only want to improve volume rendering such that we have a better understanding of the volume data, we omit the (in our eyes disturbing) angular dependence. We also restrict ourselves to low-albedo scattering, i.e. light is only scattered once and not multiple times, as we want sharp locking shadows and not diffuse ones. The advantage of low-albedo scattering is that the scattering process can be divided into a illumination and radiation phase[7].

Putting it mathematically, the spectral changes which occur in the illumination phase can be written as (Fig. 2):

$$I_t(\vec{x}, \lambda) = I_i(\vec{x}, \lambda) \cdot \left(1 - \sum_{m=1}^{M} \rho(\vec{x}, m) A(m, \lambda)\right), \qquad (1)$$

$$I_i(\vec{x} + \Delta\vec{x_i}, \lambda) = I_t(\vec{x}, \lambda),$$

where $\rho(\vec{x}, m)$ describes the density of material type m at voxel position $\vec{x}$, and $A(m, \lambda)$ the spectral absorption of material type m. The second part of Eq. 1 describes how the transmitted spectrum $I_t(\vec{x}, \lambda)$ acts as the illumination spectrum $I_i(\vec{x}, \lambda)$ for the next sampling position.

In the radiation phase, we have similar equations:

$$I_r(\vec{x}, \lambda) = I_e(\vec{x}, \lambda) + I_b(\vec{x}, \lambda) \cdot \left(1 - \sum_{m=1}^{M} \rho(\vec{x}, m) A(m, \lambda) \right), \quad (2)$$

$$I_b(\vec{x} + \Delta \vec{x_r}, \lambda) = I_r(\vec{x}, \lambda).$$

The difference is that materials now add energy during the ray tracing process. Note that for an efficient implementation the equation should be rewritten in a front to back manner in order to use adaptive ray termination[4].

To incorporate different kinds of scattering processes the emitted spectrum is also a function of the incident spectrum:

$$I_e(\vec{x}, \lambda) = \sum_{m=1}^{M} \rho(\vec{x}, m) E(m, \lambda, I_i).$$

The final spectrum emerging from the data volume falls upon a set of detectors which converts the spectra into an RGB signal:

$$\begin{pmatrix} R \\ G \\ B \end{pmatrix} = \begin{pmatrix} \int_{\lambda=-\infty}^{\infty} I_r(x_d) s_R(\lambda) d\lambda \\ \int_{\lambda=-\infty}^{\infty} I_r(x_d) s_G(\lambda) d\lambda \\ \int_{\lambda=-\infty}^{\infty} I_r(x_d) s_B(\lambda) d\lambda \end{pmatrix}, \quad (3)$$

where $s_R(\lambda)$, $s_G(\lambda)$, and $s_B(\lambda)$ are the sensitive spectra of respectively the red, green and blue element. This RGB value defines the final color of the view pixel. Note that this is a major difference of our method compared to other methods: that the color of an object is not fully determined by the material itself, but also by the illumination source and the light detector.

Although Eqs 1 to 3 allow you to simulate the light interacting with real materials, we chose for 'ideal' materials which scatter only a specific band of the spectrum in order to speed up the rendering process. To have all degrees of freedom, each material should be associated with one spectral band λ_m.

To get the behavior to selectively let pass light by embedded objects (Fig. 1), but not change the color of objects, we looked how materials could influence the volume rendering process. Looking at Fig. 2, we see that there are three instances at which materials influence the light spectrum: (a) Materials may absorb some of the spectral components during illumination, (b) materials may change the spectrum in the scattering process itself, and (c) materials may absorb some of the spectral components of light emitted by other materials. We investigated three types of scattering processes:

- *Achromatic scattering.* As each wavelength is scattered with the same efficiency, the emitted photon has the same wavelength as the incident photon. An example is a perfectly reflecting sphere.
- *Elastically scattering.* The emitted photon has the same wavelength as the incident photon, but the materials do not equally scatter all wavelengths.

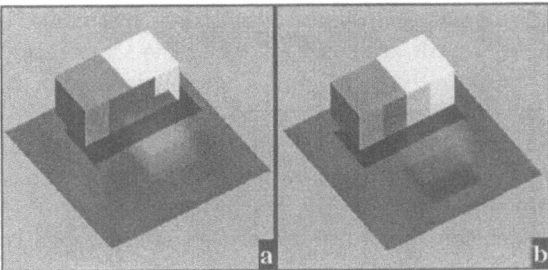

Fig. 3. Neutral transmittance. **a** Violation, the red block with chromatic absorption makes the transmitted light red. The purple and yellow block can no longer be distinguished in the shadow; **b** Agreement, the red block with achromatic absorption does not change the color of the transmitted light, the purple and yellow block can still be distinguished in the shadow. Note that there are two light sources: one from above, and one from the front.

- *Inelastically scattering.* As energy is lost in the inelastic scattering process, the emitted photon has a longer wavelength that the incident photon. Also, not all wavelengths are scattered equally.

When considering absorbing characteristics, we distinguish two types:

- *Achromatic absorption.* All spectral components are absorbed to the same extend. The overall absorption may vary from material to material.
- *Chromatic absorption.* One spectral component may be more absorbed than another. The absorption is wavelength dependent.

We combine the three scattering processes and the two absorption types into six material models. We examine them one by one on the following requirements: (a) potential of object discrimination by color, (b) visibility of interactive tools, (c) ability to render unsegmented images, and (d) neutral transmittance. Objects have a neutral transmittance when they do not influence the color of another object seen or illuminated through them (Fig. 3), permitting clear object identification. In this examination, we assume a white light source, i.e. a source radiating a uniform spectrum.

1. *Achromatic scattering with achromatic absorption.* For achromatic scattering, the shape of the light spectrum does not change in the scattering process. As materials differ only in their scattering efficiency and as the absorption is achromatic, discrimination among different volume objects is only possible with different transparencies, but not with colors.
2. *Achromatic scattering with chromatic absorption.* The chromatic absorption inevitably influences the illuminating light spectrum, with the effect that semi-transparent objects change the color of other objects (Fig. 3). Also, within one material there is a gradual change in color of light passing through. Both effects are a violation of the principle of neutral transmittance.

3. *Elastic scattering with achromatic absorption.* In this model the absorption spectra of the materials are constant. Only the scattering process influences the shape of the radiated spectrum. The perceived color is determined only by the volume object and there is no color interference by other volume objects. The principle of neutral transmittance is satisfied.

4. *Elastic scattering with chromatic absorption.* The light spectrum scattered by a material is influenced by the scattering efficiency of the material itself, and by all absorption spectra of materials the light spectrum has traversed. Similarly to model 2, the chromatic absorption violates the principle of neutral transmittance. The violation does not occur under specific conditions: If the spectral range of the emitted spectra is limited, and if the media do not change the shape of these spectra. Then the media can attenuate these spectra without changing their shape, thereby satisfying the principle of neutral transmittance. The advantage of wavelength dependent media is that media can be chosen in such a way that they selectively pass light scattered by other materials. An object of one material might absorb light scattered by the material itself, but passes light scattered by materials of an inside object (Fig. 1). This is particularly useful to bring to the front otherwise occluded interactive tools.

5. *Inelastically scattering with achromatic absorption.* As the absorption is achromatic, materials cannot selectively suppress light scattered by other materials. The visualization possibilities are similar to those of model 3.

6. *Inelastically scattering with chromatic absorption.* Due to the chromatic absorption, the visualization properties are similar to those of model 4. However, there are additional visualization possibilities, because the emitted spectrum has spectral components not present in the incident spectrum. Assuming that the materials emit a spectrum with no overlap with the incident spectrum, media may have an absorption value for the incident spectrum that differs from the absorption value for the emitted spectrum. This gives a separate control of the illumination depth and the view depth (Fig. 4bc). The example given in Fig. 4, where the volume image consists of one material, is representative for unsegmented images. Therefore, the availability of different absorption constants provides flexibility in analyzing, in particular, unprocessed images.

Considering the six models, we can draw the following conclusions. Achromatic scattering should not be used as a physical basis for the light/matter interaction model of a volume renderer, because colored absorption, then needed to color an object, does not satisfy the requirement of neutral transmittance. Elastic scattering provides a far better basis because objects can get an individual color. In addition, by using different absorption values for light scattered by different materials, embedded objects can be made visible without disturbing the view on the surface structure of surrounding objects. Inelastic scattering provides an even better basis as it also gives the option to use absorption values in the viewing phase that are different from the illumination phase. This creates the possibility to view the illumination distribution (Fig. 4c), or to view the volume and surface

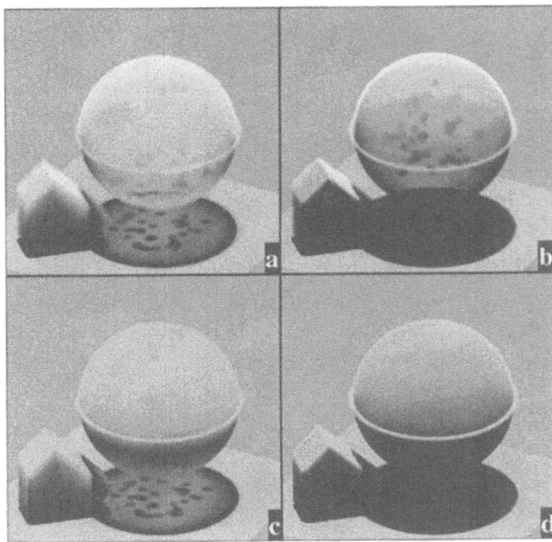

Fig. 4. Visual capabilities of inelastic scattering with chromatic absorption. The emitted light has a longer wavelength than the incident light, therefore the illumination absorption A_{ill} and radiation absorption A_{rad} can have different values: **a** Both A_{ill} and A_{rad} have a low value, giving a clear view on the volume structure and shadow. **b** $A_{ill} \gg A_{rad}$, the surface structure is visible through the sharp shadows created in the illumination phase. The volume structure is visible because the view-depth is large, the sphere does not occlude the table. **c** $A_{ill} \ll A_{rad}$, the volume structure is visible through shadows, but also the surface structure through the short view-depth. These absorption settings enable a close look on the light distribution. **d** Both A_{ill} and A_{rad} have a high value, light is almost totally absorbed and only surface structures are visible.

structure at the same time (Fig. 4b). From the 6 material models, model 6, inelastic scattering with chromatic absorption offers the largest visualization flexibility.

3   Applications

The following two examples have been reproduced from [8]. We did not reproduce the visualizations of fMRI data.

3.1   Vascular tree

As a first example (reproduced from [8]), we visualize the veins inside and outside the brain segmented from a MR angiogram recorded with gadolinium (Fig. 5). We visualized the structures as separate entities (a and b), and combined (c). To see the inner veins we tried a hole (d), transparent brain (e), taking square

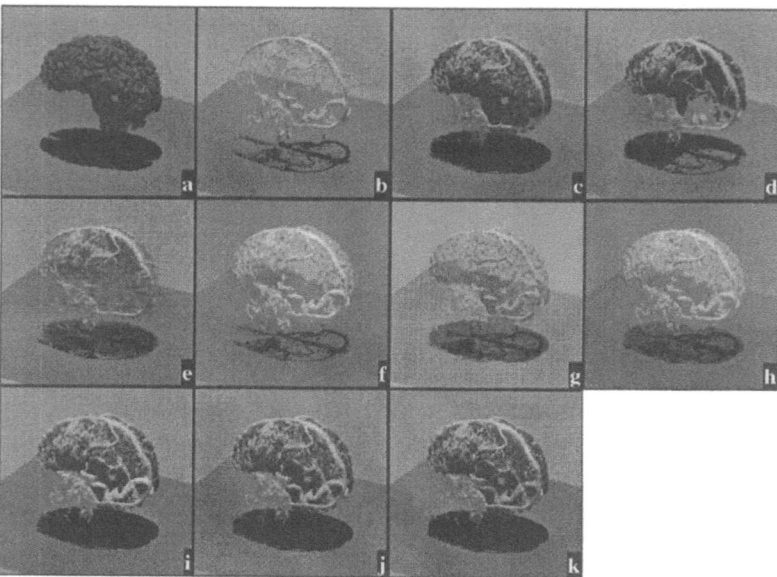

Fig. 5. Options to visualize veins in relation to the brain. (T1 weighted MR scan with gadolinium as contrast agent). **a** View on the cortex. **b** View on the veins. **c** Default way to visualize veins on a cortex. The embedded and background veins are occluded by the brain. **d** Artificially removing a part of the brain reveals embedded veins, but deteriorates the view on the cortex. **e** Making the brain transparent reveals embedded veins, but deteriorates the view on the cortex. **f** Square root squared intensities, grey result. **g** Averaging RGB values, table and background shine through. **h** Fig. a placed in red channel, b in red and blue channel; erroneous colors of table and background. **i-k** Spectral approach, the brain is transparent for light scattered by the veins, not for light scattered by the brain itself. From **i** to **k**, the brain absorbs the light scattered by the veins more and more. Note that the embedded or 'occluded' veins are white while the unoccluded veins have cyan color. See also http://www.isi.uu.nl/people/herke/neuro/vascular/vascular.html.

root of the squared intensities (f), adding (g), or taking a separate channel (h). Our spectral approach is shown in (i), (j) and (k), the difference between the individual images is that the brain absorbs the light of the inner and background veins more and more.

3.2 CT: Skin/bone and artificial objects

Another application of spectral rendering is given in Fig. 6, where the task was to visualize the relation between skin and skull of a patient with Morbus Crouzon. In a normal renderer, it would only be possible to render the skin and skull as separate entities and not in one view (Fig. 6a-c). Spectral rendering gives the *option to view the skull inside the skin* without degrading the view on the skin (Fig. 6d,e).

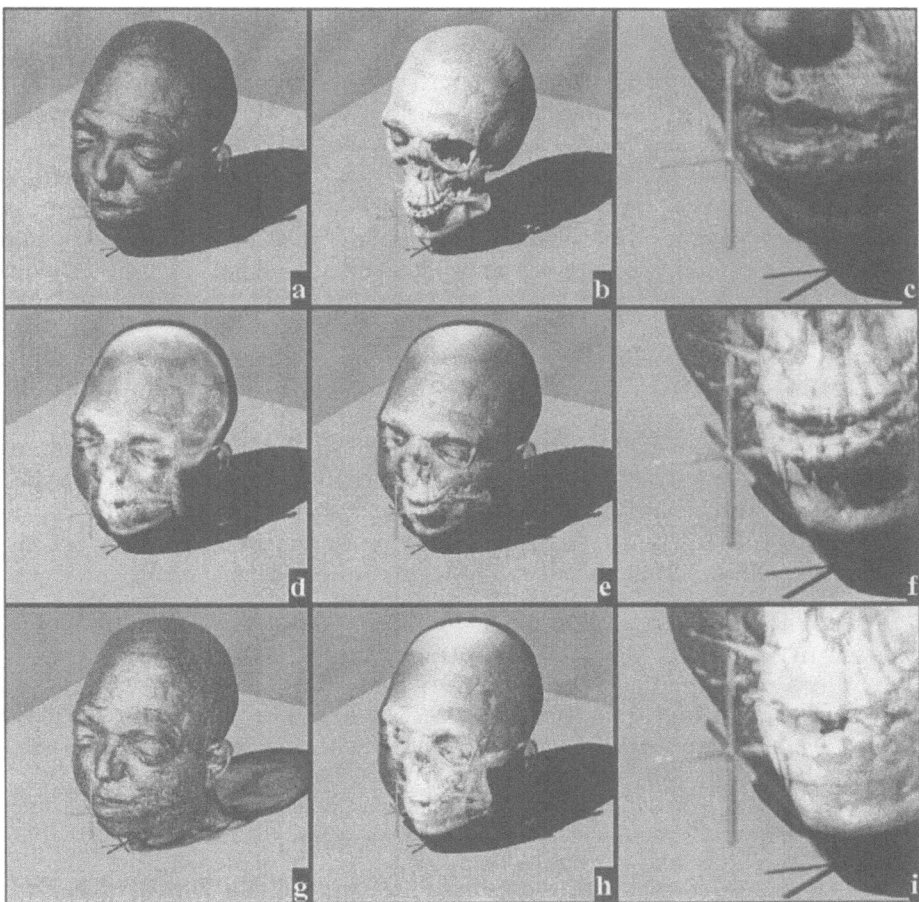

Fig. 6. Volume renderings of a segmented skin and skull from a patient with Morbus Crouzon and a 3D cursor. The image modality is CT, size 320x320x229. The skin, skull scatter different wavelengths: **a-c** Normal rendering, the absorption is similar for all wavelengths. **d-i** The skin is transparent for light scattered by the skull and 3D cursor. **g-i** Special scattering process (inelastic): the absorption in the radiation phase differs from the absorption in the illumination phase. Data courtesy University Hospital Utrecht, the Netherlands. See also http://www.isi.uu.nl/people/herke/neuro/ct/ct.html.

Spectral rendering can also be used for interactive analysis. By moving a 3D cursor which is visible through the skin, but not through the skull, one can interactively estimate the thickness of the skin (Fig. 6f). This is accomplished by letting the 3D cursor scatter the same spectral band as the skull. Another application of spectral rendering may be to highlight interactive tools, for example, when a 3D cursor is obscured by surrounding media and the user has lost sight of the cursor.

The bottom row of Fig. 6 shows some visualizations where the restriction of having an absorption value that is constant for both the illumination and the radiation phase has been removed. When there is no absorption during the illumination phase, the skin gets illuminated uniformly (Fig. 6gh). There are no shadows by which every cavity can be inspected in detail. We believe that a slightly less absorption in the illumination phase than in the radiation phase, gives the best compromise between showing all detail and having a good shadow cue (Fig. 6i).

4   Conclusions

We proposed a feasible, physical realistic method to visualize volume structures inside other volume structures by modeling the changes in the illumination spectrum when it interacts with the material inside a voxel. Advantages over existing methods are: (1) still getting a visual hint which structures are inside, (2) easy integration with artificial objects, and (3) user selectable shadowing.

References

1. J. Burtscher, C.Kremser, M. Seiwald, M. Wagner, F. Aichner, K. Twerdy, and S. Felber, "Three Dimensional Computer Assisted MR-Imaging for Neurosurgical Planning", Proc SPIE 3031, 1997, 85-91.
2. J.H. Kim, K.M. Yeon, M.C. Han, D.H. Lee, and H.I. Cho, "Enhanced visualization of MR angiogram with modified MIP and 3D image fusion", Proc SPIE 3031, 1997, 31-36.
3. H.T.M. van der Voort, H.J. Noordmans, J.M. Messerli and A.W.M. Smeulders, "Physically realistic volume visualization for interactive analysis", Fourth Eurographics on rendering, 1993, 295-306.
4. M. Levoy, "A hybrid ray tracer for rendering polygon and volume data", IEEE Computer Graphics and Applications 10, 1990, 33-40.
5. R.A. Drebin, L. Carpenter, P. Hanrahan, "Volume rendering", Computer Graphics (SIGGRAPH '88 Proc) 22(4), 1988, 65-74.
6. P. Sabella, "A rendering algorithm for visualizing 3D scalar fields. Computer Graphics (SIGGRAPH '88 Proc) 22(4), 1988, 51-58.
7. J.T. Kajiya, and B.P. von Herzen, "Ray tracing volume densities", Computer Graphics (SIGGRAPH '84 Proc) 18(3), 1984, 165-174.
8. H.J. Noordmans, H.T.M. van der Voort, G.J.M. Rutten, M.A. Viergever, "Physically realistic visualization of embedded volume structures for medical image data", in SPIE Medical Imaging 1999, Image Display 3658, eds. S.K. Mun, Y. Kim, 1999, 613-620.

Non-planar Reslicing for Freehand 3D Ultrasound

Andrew Gee[1], Richard Prager[1], and Laurence Berman[2]

[1] Department of Engineering, University of Cambridge, UK
[2] Department of Radiology, University of Cambridge, UK

Abstract. Any-plane slicing is a visualisation technique common to many medical imaging modalities, including 3D ultrasound. The acquired data is resampled on a user-specified plane and rendered, usually after some interpolation, on a standard graphics display. In this paper, we motivate and develop *non-planar* reslicing for freehand 3D ultrasound: the data is resampled not on a flat plane, but a curved surface, which is then unrolled for display on a flat screen. We show how to implement non-planar reslicing in a *sequential* manner, so the reslice image can be constructed directly from the raw B-scans and positions, without going through an intermediate voxel array stage. Care is taken to ensure that distances measured along lines in the non-planar reslice image are the same as the distances measured along the corresponding curves in 3D space. The resulting tool has interesting clinical applications, made accessible through an effective Graphical User Interface (GUI), which allows the user to specify the required reslice surface rapidly and intuitively. The GUI, and some of the applications, are illustrated in this paper.

1   Introduction

Conventional diagnostic ultrasound imaging is performed with a hand-held probe which transmits ultrasound pulses into the body and receives the echoes. The magnitude and timing of the echoes are used to create a 2D greyscale image (B-scan) of a cross-section of the body in the scan plane.

Using a technique called **freehand 3D ultrasound imaging** [9, 13], it is possible to construct 3D data sets from a series of 2D B-scans — see Figure 1. A conventional 3D freehand examination can be broken into three stages: scanning, reconstruction and visualisation. Before scanning, some sort of position sensor is attached to the probe. This is typically the receiver of an electromagnetic position sensor [1, 2, 5–8, 10, 11, 14], as illustrated in Figure 1, although alternatives include acoustic spark gaps [3], mechanical arms [4] and optical sensors [15]. Measurements from the position sensor are used to determine the positions and orientations of the B-scans with respect to a fixed datum, usually the transmitter of the electromagnetic position sensor. In the next stage, the set of acquired B-scans and their relative positions are used to fill a regular voxel array. Finally, this voxel array is visualised using, for example, any-plane slicing, volume rendering or surface rendering (after segmentation).

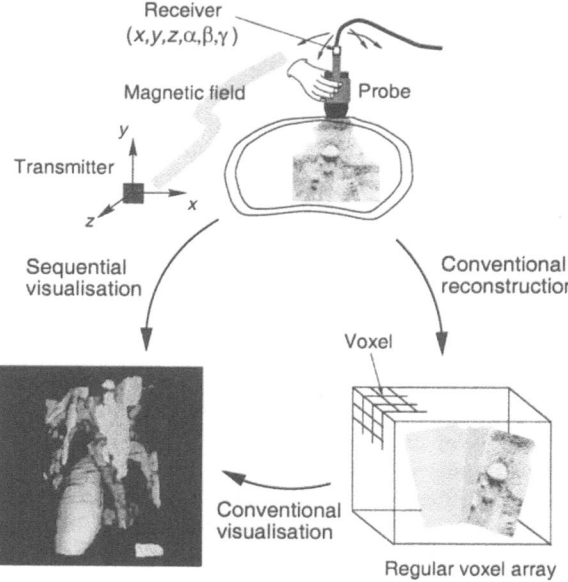

Fig. 1. Freehand 3D ultrasound imaging. The conventional approach is a three-stage process, involving scanning, reconstruction and visualisation. The alternative, sequential approach allows visualisation directly from the raw B-scans and positions. The figure illustrates an examination of a gall bladder.

Recently, we have proposed an alternative approach to freehand 3D ultrasound, which bypasses the voxel array stage. In **sequential** freehand 3D ultrasound, the data is visualised and analysed directly from the raw B-scans and positions — see Figure 1. Any-plane slicing, panoramic imaging, volume estimation and surface rendering can be performed without the use of an intermediate voxel representation [5–7, 14]: all of these facilities are implemented in the Stradx freehand 3D ultrasound system[1]. The sequential approach offers several advantages:

- When reslicing, the data is resampled only once, from the B-scan pixels to the slice pixels. The conventional approach requires two resampling stages, from the B-scan pixels to the voxel array, then from the voxel array to the slice pixels. Since resampling usually involves data approximation, more accurate visualisation is possible by avoiding one resampling process.
- Reslicing can be performed at the full resolution of the B-scan pixels without the significant memory overhead of a high resolution voxel array.
- Visualisation and data analysis can be performed in real time, as the data is being acquired, since the sequential visualisation and volume measurement

---

[1] Available at http://svr-www.eng.cam.ac.uk/~rwp/stradx/.

algorithms reference each B-scan only once, in the order in which they are acquired.

- Segmentation (for volume measurement and surface rendering) is performed on the B-scans themselves, instead of parallel slices through the voxel array. The B-scans are high resolution and exhibit no reconstruction artifacts, making them relatively easy to interpret for manual or assisted segmentation. The same cannot be said of slices through the voxel array.

In this paper, we consider a visualisation technique called **non-planar reslicing**. This is similar to any-plane slicing, except the data is extracted along a simple curved surface instead of the usual flat plane. In Section 2, we describe how non-planar reslicing can be performed in the sequential framework, providing full implementation details. In Section 3, we show how the reslice surface can be specified using a simple, intuitive Graphical User Interface (GUI), such that the desired view is arrived at rapidly. In this section, we also illustrate several valuable *in-vivo* applications. Finally, we draw some conclusions in Section 4.

2   Non-planar reslicing

Figure 2 illustrates the idea behind non-planar reslicing. A **developable** (unrollable) surface is specified by the user and its intersection with the 3D ultrasound data is computed, so that the surface can be 'painted' with the data it intersects. The painted surface is then unrolled for display on a flat screen.

The particular class of developable surface considered here is defined by a plane π with unit normal $\mathbf{n}$ and the plane curve $\mathbf{c}(s)$ lying in π — see Figure 2. The surface is swept out by the set of **rulings** $\mathcal{R}$ which are all of length $2r$, are all parallel to $\mathbf{n}$ and intersect $\mathbf{c}(s)$ at their midpoints. In the non-planar reslice image, we will refer to the unrolled plane curve and rulings as $\mathbf{c}'(s)$ and $\mathcal{R}'$ respectively.

In designing the reslicing algorithm, there are two issues of paramount importance:

1. Distances should be preserved, so that distances measured along lines in the non-planar reslice image are the same as the distances measured along the corresponding curves in 3D space.
2. The surface will intersect the B-scans along a set of curves, and some sort of interpolation will be required to produce a continuous reslice image. To be compatible with the sequential approach, the interpolation scheme should reference each B-scan only once, in the order in which they are acquired.

The starting point is the curve $\mathbf{c}(s)$ and the distance r, which are both specified by the user as described in Section 3. It is sensible to ensure that the scale of the reslice image (in mm/pixel) is the same as the scale of the original B-scans, so that the two types of image can be directly compared. The B-scan scaling can be deduced from the settings of the ultrasound machine or by a separate calibration process [8]. Using the same scaling, we can deduce the

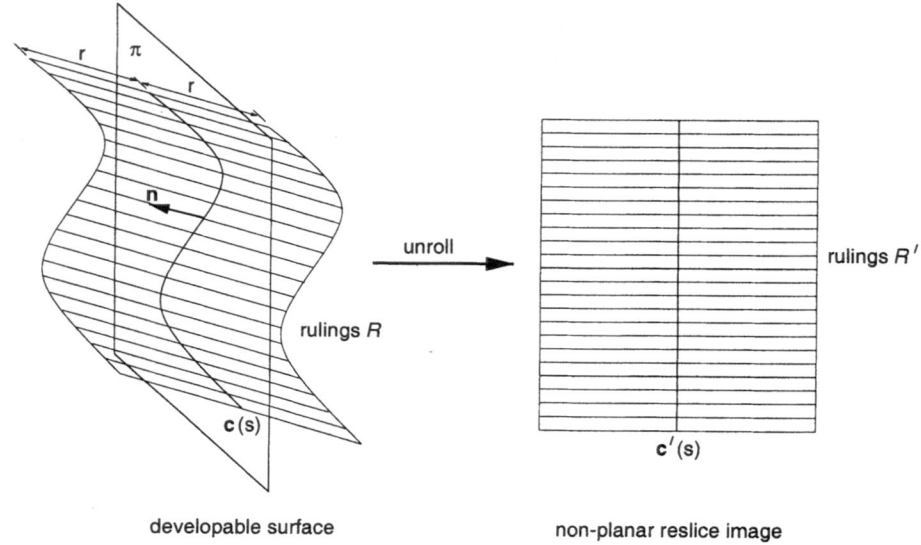

Fig. 2. Non-planar reslicing. The non-planar reslice image shows the intersection of the 3D data with a special class of developable surface, unrolled for display on a flat screen.

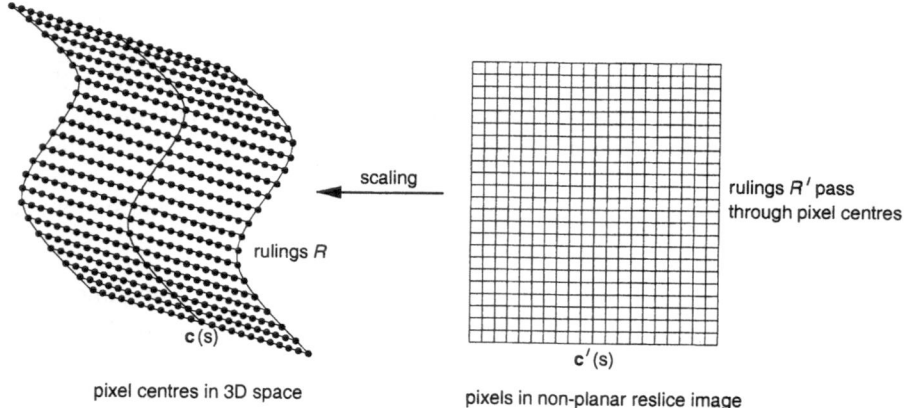

Fig. 3. Pixel mapping. Using the known B-scan scaling, the centres of the individual pixels in the non-planar reslice image can be located in 3D space.

length of the unrolled curve $\mathbf{c}'(s)$ in pixels, which gives us the height of the reslice image. We can also use the scaling and r to deduce the width of the reslice image in pixels.

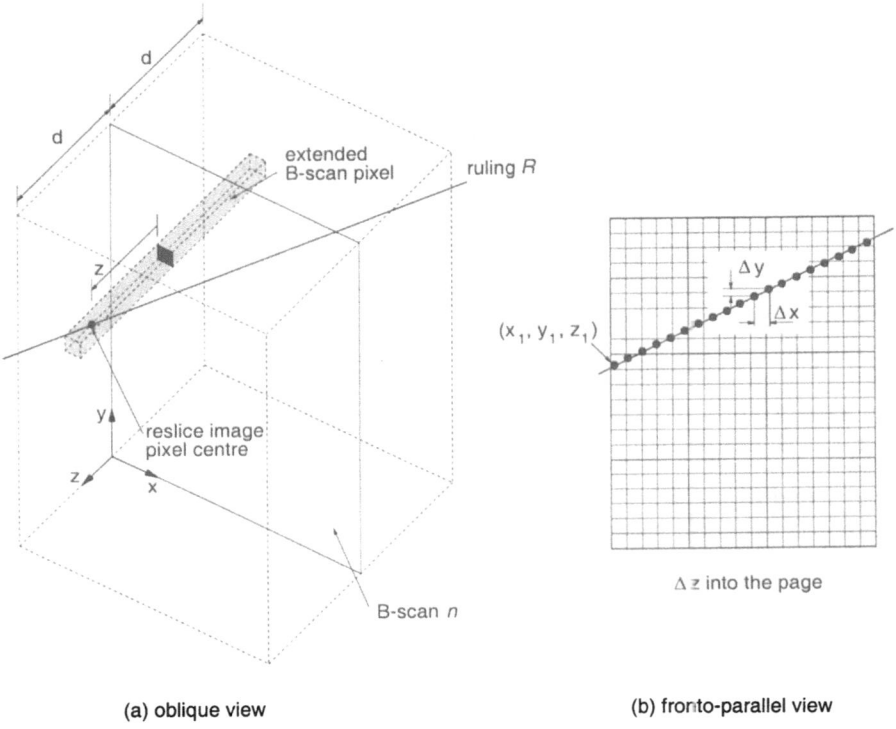

(a) oblique view   (b) fronto-parallel view

Fig. 4. Efficient sequential interpolation. The range of influence of B-scan n is defined by a box extending a distance d on either side of the B-scan, as shown in (a). Each reslice image pixel centre is tested for intersection with the box. If there is an intersection, the reslice image pixel is rendered with the intensity of the extended B-scan pixel it intersects, at a depth of $|z|$. In this way, the intensity will be updated if a subsequent B-scan lies closer to the reslice image pixel centre. The intersections can be calculated efficiently using an incremental algorithm, as shown in (b).

The reslicing algorithm works with the set of rulings $\mathcal{R}'$ passing through the pixel centres in the reslice image. Using the known scaling once more, we can deduce the corresponding rulings $\mathcal{R}$ in 3D space. We can also translate individual pixel centres in the reslice image to particular locations along the rulings $\mathcal{R}$ — see Figure 3. Having located each reslice pixel in 3D space, we can finally shade each pixel according to the intensity of the nearest B-scan pixel. It is desirable to introduce one user-defined parameter at this stage, namely the maximum distance d allowable between the reslice pixel and the nearest B-scan pixel. In this way, areas of the surface which are a long way away from any recorded data will be left blank, instead of interpolated with misleading data.

Note that the line joining the reslice pixel to the nearest B-scan pixel will always be normal to the plane of the B-scan. This observation allows us to implement the interpolation scheme in an efficient, sequential manner. Consider the box defined by the two polygons a distance d either side of the nth B-scan — see Figure 4(a). This box defines the maximum range of influence of the pixels in B-scan n. Now consider the intersection of one of the rulings $\mathcal{R}$ with the box. Each extended B-scan pixel containing one of the reslice image pixel centres is a candidate for shading the reslice image pixel, since it is the closest pixel on B-scan n and lies within the distance limit d. The only circumstance that could change the shading of the reslice image pixel is if a pixel from another B-scan is closer. Therefore, we render the reslice image pixel with the intensity of the extended B-scan pixel it intersects, *but at a depth* $|z|$, where $|z|$ is the distance from the reslice image pixel centre to the B-scan plane. By exploiting the graphics z-buffer in this way, we are able to perform the interpolation efficiently in a sequential manner: should a pixel in a future B-scan be closer, the reslice image pixel will be rendered again at a shallower depth, overwriting the old value. The non-planar reslice image is therefore constructed as follows:

> find rulings R and 3D locations of reslice image pixel centres;
> for each B-scan n
>   for each ruling in R
>   find any intersections of reslice image pixel centres with extended B-scan pixels;
>   render the reslice image pixel with the intensity of the intersected B-scan pixel, at a depth $|z|$;

The fronto-parallel view in Figure 4(b) reveals how the intersection tests can be performed efficiently. For each ruling in $\mathcal{R}$, we locate only the first intersection (x_1, y_1, z_1) to sub-pixel accuracy, and the increments Δx, Δy and Δz. We then repeatedly add the increments to (x_1, y_1, z_1) to find subsequent intersections, rounding down the x and y values to locate the intersected B-scan pixels.

Note that the interpolation scheme is well motivated by the physics of ultrasound acquisition. Since real ultrasound beams have a finite thickness, often as much as 10 mm [12], data in any particular B-scan is affected by structures a certain distance on either side of the B-scan plane. The notion of an extended B-scan pixel, as defined in Figure 4, is therefore justified. Good practice would be to set the distance limit d to half the width of the ultrasound beam.

3   Defining the reslice surface

If the non-planar reslice tool is to be useful, we need to develop a straightforward way for the user to specify the curve $\mathbf{c}(s)$ and the width r. In practice, $\mathbf{c}(s)$ will correspond to some curved anatomical structure that the user wishes to unroll.

The first stage is to find the plane π in which $\mathbf{c}(s)$ lies. This can be achieved using a standard any-plane slicing tool, such as the one already implemented in earlier versions of the Stradx freehand 3D ultrasound system [5–7]. The plane is defined by a line in one B-scan and a point in another, so that the resulting planar reslice reveals the key curved structure. The user can then draw along the structure to define $\mathbf{c}(s)$.

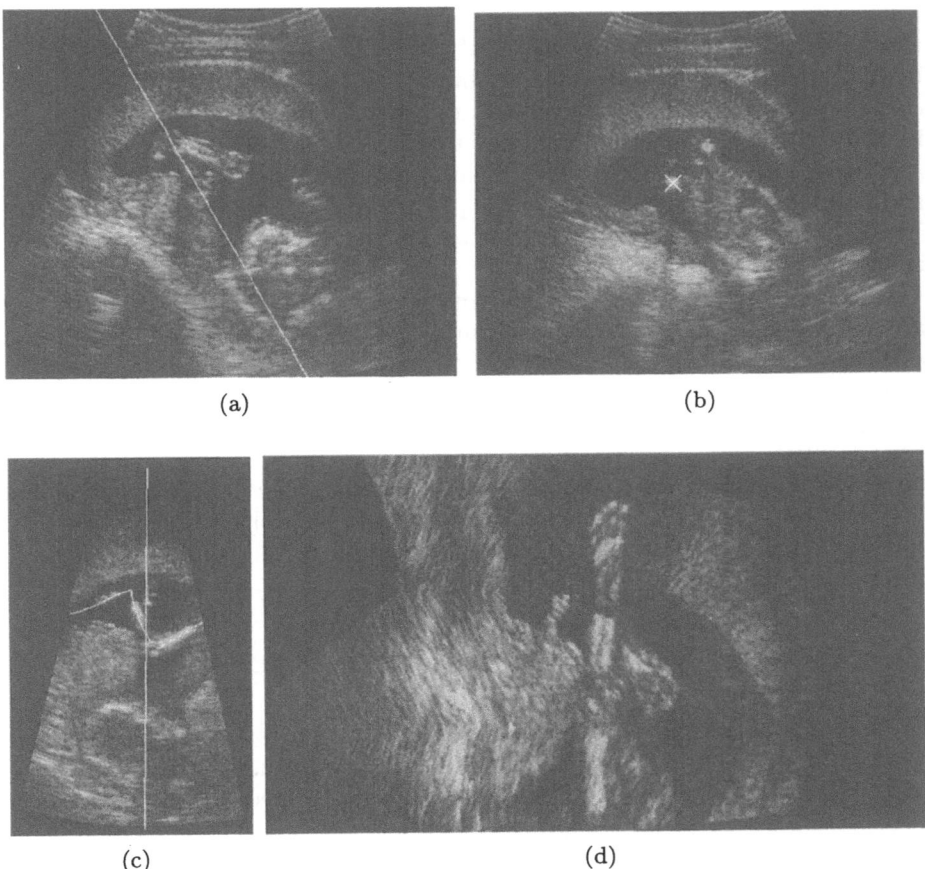

(a)   (b)

(c)   (d)

Fig. 5. Visualisation of a 16-week foetus' left leg. (a) and (b) show two B-scans from the recorded sequence. (c) is a planar reslice of the data, passing through the diagonal line in image (a) and the cross in (b). The planar reslice (c) shows the foetus' left leg in profile: the vertical line corresponds to the B-scan (a). (d) is a non-planar reslice, defined by the curve drawn by the user in (c). The non-planar reslice shows an unrolled, frontal view of the leg, including all five toes.

Consider the example in Figure 5, which illustrates an examination of a 16-week foetus. The goal is to obtain a frontal view of the entire left leg, including all the toes: since the leg is bent at the knee and ankle, a non-planar reslice is necessary. The user starts by finding the plane π passing through the hip, knee and ankle. This is achieved by scanning through the B-scans until one is found which shows some of the fibula and tibia, as in Figure 5(a). The user draws a line down the middle of the two bones. To fully define the plane, the user now scans through the B-scans, following the femur up towards the hip, and marks a point near the top of the femur, as in Figure 5(b). The resulting planar reslice image, revealing the entire leg in profile, is shown in Figure 5(c). The user then draws along the leg to specify $c(s)$. The non-planar reslice can now be constructed, using some default value of r, as in Figure 5(d). The user can change r by simply resizing the non-planar reslice window, while a slider at the bottom of the window controls the interpolation limit d. Note how all five toes are clearly visible in the non-planar reslice, ruling out one of the more common foetal abnormalities. Since lengths are preserved in the non-planar reslice, it is straightforward to measure the hip-to-toe distance along the unrolled leg, which is approximately 75mm.

A further application is illustrated in Figure 6: here, the goal is to construct a frontal view of a 22-week foetus' unrolled spine. The first step is to select a B-scan through the thorax, as in Figure 6(a), and draw a line between the vertebrae. The plane π is fully defined by another point on the midline of the spine, marked by the user on a B-scan through the neck, as in Figure 6(b). The resulting planar reslice in Figure 6(c) shows the full length of the spine in profile. The user then draws along the spine to specify $c(s)$. The non-planar reslice in Figure 6(d) shows a frontal view of the entire length of the unrolled spine, including some of the rib cage. The length of the spine, from neck to coccyx, is approximately 117mm.

4   Conclusions

The non-planar reslice tool is a valuable addition to the portfolio of visualisation techniques for freehand 3D ultrasound. It can be implemented in a sequential manner, allowing reslices to be constructed without the need for an intermediate voxel array. The sequential implementation described in this paper takes care to preserve distances, so the clinician can easily measure the lengths of curved anatomical structures. Two interesting applications in obstetrics have been illustrated. There are many other potential applications: the body is full of curved structures that would benefit from being visualised as a whole.

References

1. P. R. Detmer, G. Bashein, T. Hodges, K. W. Beach, E. P. Filer, D. H. Burns, and D.E. Strandness Jr. 3D ultrasonic image feature localization based on magnetic scanhead tracking: in vitro calibration and validation. *Ultrasound in Medicine and Biology*, 20(9):923–936, 1994.
2. S. W. Hughes, T. J. D'Arcy, D. J. Maxwell, W. Chiu, A. Milner, J. E. Saunders, and R. J. Sheppard. Volume estimation from multiplanar 2D ultrasound images using a remote electromagnetic position and orientation sensor. *Ultrasound in Medicine and Biology*, 22(5):561–572, 1996.

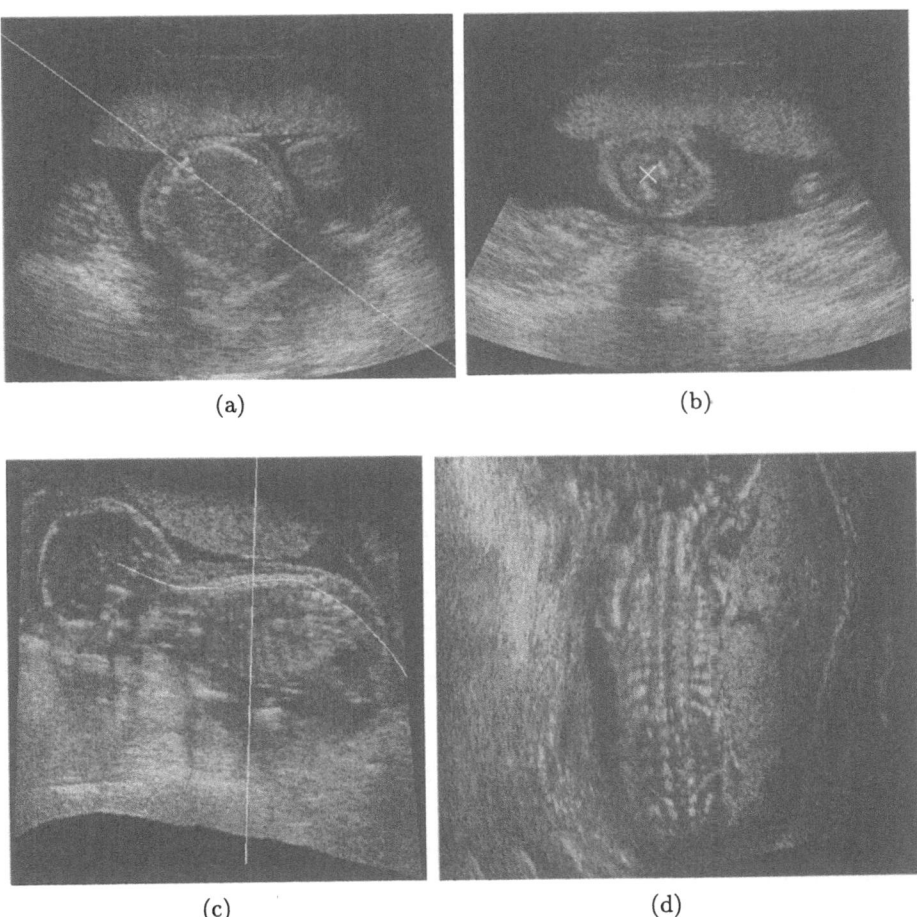

(a)   (b)

(c)   (d)

Fig. 6. Visualisation of a 22-week foetus' spine. (a) and (b) show two B-scans from the recorded sequence. (c) is a planar reslice of the data, passing through the diagonal line in image (a) and the cross in (b). The planar reslice (c) shows the foetus' spine in profile: the vertical line corresponds to the B-scan (a). (d) is a non-planar reslice, defined by the curve drawn by the user in (c). The non-planar reslice shows an unrolled, frontal view of the spine, from neck (top) to coccyx (bottom).

3. D. L. King, D. L. King Jr., and M. Y. Shao. Evaluation of in vitro measurement accuracy of a three-dimensional ultrasound scanner. *Journal of Ultrasound in Medicine*, 10:77–82, 1991.

4. R. Ohbuchi, D. Chen, and H. Fuchs. Incremental volume reconstruction and rendering for 3D ultrasound imaging. In R. A. Robb, editor, *Proceedings of Visualization in Biomedical Computing*, SPIE 1808, pages 312–323. International Society of Optical Engineering, Bellingham, WA, USA, 1992.

5. R. W. Prager, A. H. Gee, and L. Berman. 3D ultrasound without voxels. In *Proceedings of Medical Image Understanding and Analysis*, pages 93–96, Leeds, UK, 1998.

6. R. W. Prager, A. H. Gee, and L. Berman. Real-time tools for freehand 3D ultrasound. In *Medical Image Computing and Computer-Assisted Intervention — MICCAI'98*, pages 1016–1023, Cambridge, MA, USA, 1998. LNCS 1496, Springer.

7. R. W. Prager, A. H. Gee, and L. Berman. Stradx: real-time acquisition and visualization of freehand three-dimensional ultrasound. *Medical Image Analysis*, 3(2):129–140, 1999.

8. R. W. Prager, R. N. Rohling, A. H. Gee, and L. Berman. Rapid calibration for 3-D freehand ultrasound. *Ultrasound in Medicine and Biology*, 24(6):855–869, 1998.

9. R. N. Rankin, A. Fenster, D. B. Downey, P. L. Munk, M. F. Levin, and A. D. Vellet. Three-dimensional sonographic reconstruction: techniques and diagnostic applications. *American Journal of Roentgenology*, 161(4):695–702, 1993.

10. R. N. Rohling, A. H. Gee, and L. Berman. Three-dimensional spatial compounding of ultrasound images. *Medical Image Analysis*, 1(3):177–193, 1997.

11. R. N. Rohling, A. H. Gee, and L. Berman. Automatic registration of 3-D ultrasound images. *Ultrasound in Medicine and Biology*, 24(6):841–854, 1998.

12. M. L. Skolnick. Estimation of ultrasound beam width in the elevation (section thickness) plane. *Radiology*, 180(1):286–288, 1991.

13. H. Steiner, A. Staudach, D. Spitzer, and H. Schaffer. Three-dimensional ultrasound in obstetrics and gynaecology: technique, possibilities and limitations. *Human Reproduction*, 9(9):1773–1778, 1994.

14. G. M. Treece, R. W. Prager, A. H. Gee, and L. Berman. Fast surface and volume estimation from non-parallel cross-sections, for freehand 3-D ultrasound. *Medical Image Analysis*, 3(2):141–173, 1999.

15. J. W. Trobaugh, D. J. Trobaugh, and W. D. Richard. Three-dimensional imaging with stereotactic ultrasonography. *Computerized Medical Imaging and Graphics*, 18(5):315–323, 1994.

The Perception of Transparency in Medical Images

Reza Kasrai[1,2], Frederick A.A. Kingdom[2], and Terry M. Peters[1,3]

[1] McConnell Brain Imaging Ctr., Montreal Neurological Inst., Canada H3A 2B4
[2] McGill Vision Research Unit, Royal Victoria Hospital, Montreal, Canada, H3A 1A1
[3] Imaging Research Labs., Robarts Research Institute, London, Canada, N6A 5K8
rkasrai@bic.mni.mcgill.ca, fred@jiffy.vision.mcgill.ca,
tpeters@irus.rri.on.ca

Abstract. Many of the tasks performed by clinicians during surgical planning or diagnosis rely on the visualization of medical images. When information from multiple modalities is integrated, some images must be seen through others. In these cases, surfaces or volumetric images are rendered semi-opaque, or transparent. It is necessary, therefore, to understand the nature of transparency perception in human visual system. A set of experiments is presented which begins to look at the role of stereoscopy, spatial frequency, and multiple layers in the perception of transparent achromatic surfaces. An adjustment technique has been developed for the measurement of observer performance, and a physical and algebraic model for the perception of multiple transparent surfaces is described. The results show good agreement with the models developed.

1 Introduction

With the continual increase in the speed of relatively affordable computers, and the rise in the number of their applications to medicine, the question of how well computers and algorithms perform is being replaced by one examining the nature of the interaction of humans with machines. Although computers are now involved in various aspects of medicine, in many cases the output of algorithms is in the form of images. These images are subsequently used by clinicians for the purpose of diagnosis or surgical planning. It stands to reason then, that when users make decisions about surgical procedures or courses of treatment based on images, that these images convey not only the correct information, but that they represent it in a manner that an observer can best understand.

Recent visualization systems allow the registration and integration of images from many different imaging modalities, in order to provide the maximum amount of information to the clinician. 2-dimensional (2D) sections of volumetric anatomical data (e.g. MRI, CT) are typically overlaid with the corresponding functional or chemical (EEG, PET, fMRI, MRS) images, such that the structural image can be 'seen through' the functional image. From the same volumetric data, surfaces corresponding to structures of interest are segmented out. In many cases, a surface is enclosed within, or is transected by, another surface, such as when viewing a thalamotomy lesion target (typically the *vim*–one of the thalamic nuclei) through the wall of the thalamus [1], or when visualizing virtual radiofrequency lesions enveloping a target structure (Figure 1)[1]. In all these situations, the surface or reconstructed slices simulated to be closer to the observer are rendered as semi-opaque, or transparent[2]. An early example of multi-modality integration of 3D data, is shown in Figure 3, where a volume rendering of the distal hemisphere is overlaid by a co-registered digital subtraction angiogram (DSA) of the proximal hemisphere.

While the number of such rendering algorithms is ever increasing, little or no work is dedicated to the rigorous psychophysical study of the nature of the interaction of the human visual system with the images generated. Clearly, given the complexity and richness of medical images, especially those integrating multiple imaging modalities, this is not a simple task. Nevertheless, an extensive literature exists in the realm of psychophysics, exploring different aspects of human visual perception, which provides the beginnings of a course of investigation.

The aim of this paper is to begin to bridge the gap between the fields of computer graphics, medical image visualization, and human vision research, using the techniques of experimental psychology, by introducing a series of experiments focusing on specific aspects of the perception of transparency. The purpose of these studies is twofold: to understand how and to what degree of accuracy properties of transparent surfaces (reflectance, opacity, color, texture, etc.) and opaque surfaces seen through transparent ones are encoded, and subsequently to apply these results to medical images, in order to optimize and facilitate the transmission of relevant information to clinical users, especially in the context of image-guided neurosurgery.

2 Related Work

2.1 Vision Literature

Work on the perception of transparency began in earnest following the first in a series of papers by Metelli [3, 4]. He developed an algebraic formulation based on Talbot's law of color fusion, $z = \alpha x + (1 - \alpha)y$, where $0 \leq \alpha \leq 1$ is the linear mixing proportion of the achromatic colors x and y, as measured by their reflectances, resulting in the color z. This formulation is similar to the "blending" function used in computer graphics [6], whence the term alpha-blending. By analogy, the color of a pixel p, which is the combination of a background surface $\mathbf{A}$, seen through a transparent surface $\mathbf{P}$, is given by $p = ta + (1 - t)r$, where a is the reflectance of surface $\mathbf{A}$, and $t, r \in [0, 1]$ the transmittance and reflectance of surface $\mathbf{P}$. The assumption here is that the absolute values of r and t can be somehow calculated or encoded by the visual system given the four reflectance

---

[1] In this case, the surface was segmented out of a volumetrically defined digital atlas of the human brain.

[2] The term transparent, as opposed to translucent, is used to imply that the image is *not distorted* by the overlying surface. Transparency is also the term conventionally used in vision literature.

values, a, b, p, and q, and also that both the background and transparent surfaces are illuminated identically.

Although matching tasks with stimuli generated using this model have produced very good results in human observers [4], limiting the values of t and r to between 0 and 1 has been shown to be too restrictive [7], leading to a modified set of equations based on luminances rather than reflectances [8, 9]. This modification allows for the possibility of inhomogeneous illumination:

$$P = taI + (1 - t)rI' = tA + (1 - t)rhI = tA + F,   \tag{1}$$

where P and A are now luminances (e.g. in cd/m^2), I and I' the (non-equal) illumination components for the two surfaces with ratio h, such that $I' = hI$. The second term is collapsed into an overall additive component F, since with four known luminances (A, B, P, Q) and two equations, only two unknowns, t and F, can be extracted, and the product rhI cannot be disambiguated without additional assumptions or *a priori* knowledge.

2.2 Imaging Literature

In a review of the cues relevant to the visualization of medical images, Kundel [10] wrote, "No matter what the task or the image, as long as an observer is needed to read out the information, performance is the final arbiter of the goodness of the image." This implies that regardless of what may be considered a set of important features in a medical image for a given task (high contrast, texture, lighting, etc.), human performance, measured if possible against some known gold standard or truth, must be the determining measure, since it is after all the human system for which the images are generated.

Even though the latter may be considered a truism, very few developers of visualization software actually set out to evaluate rigorously the sensitivity and accuracy of a given rendering technique. More typically, validation is described in terms of clinical utility as reported anecdotally by a clinician, or in the context of a limited number of cases where a diagnosis is confirmed by biopsy or at surgery [11, 12]. Part of the problem may lie in the complexity or non-specificity of the task, in that no algorithm or software can be made optimal for all tasks, or range of tasks. In addition, it is often difficult to find a large number of sufficiently similar clinical cases where the 'true' diagnosis is known. As a result, compromises are made, or the software is designed with enough flexibility that users can choose a rendering method or a segmentation algorithm which they believe suits the task [13]. It is nonetheless possible to conduct meticulous studies to show the superiority of one human-machine system over another using well-developed statistical methods, such as receiver operating characteristic curves [14] or simple analysis of variances.

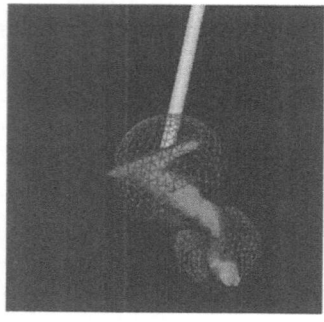

Fig. 1. Simulated spherical rf lesions encompassing the *vim* nucleus of the human thalamus.

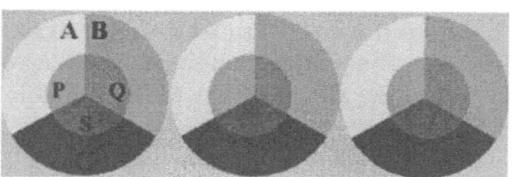

Fig. 2. Stereo transparecy stimuli arranged for crossed-eye viewing. Crossing the right pair produces a positive disparity (in front) percept, and the left pair gives the negative (behind) percept.

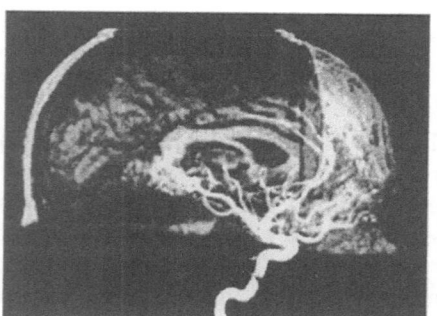

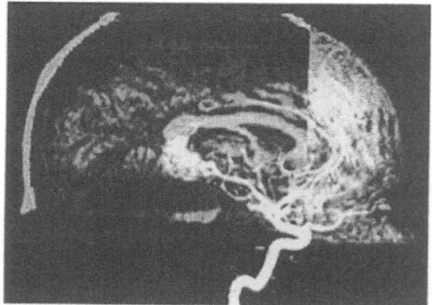

Fig. 3. Volume-rendered MRI with overlaid DSA, arranged for crossed-eye viewing [2].

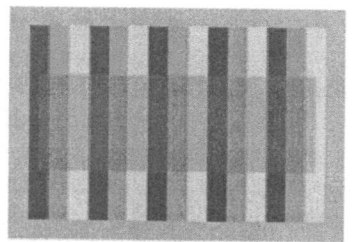

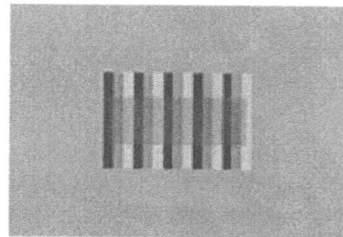

Fig. 4. Spatial frequency stimuli.

3   Methods

3.1   General

All experiments were performed using an SGI (Silicon Graphics Inc., Mountain View, CA, USA) O2 workstation (150 MHz R10000 Processor) on a 17" monitor displaying 1280x1024 pixels at a vertical refresh rate of 72 Hz. The luminance output of the monitor was measured using a single channel optometer with photometric detector (Model S370, United Detector Technology), and calibrated such that desired luminances between 0 and $\approx$40 cd/m^2 could be reliably reproduced. Stereoscopic image pairs (maximum size of 9 x 9 cm^2 each) were viewed through a custom-built 8-mirror stereoscope with a principle ray path of 45 cm, for a maximum visual angle of 11.4°. Subjects adjusted the luminance of test patches using the arrow keys on a standard keyboard, and pressed a separate key to end the trial once they were satisfied with their adjustment. Responses were recorded to a text file for later analysis.

3.2   Generation of stimuli

Transparency in Stereo. A six-luminance stimulus, originally described by Gerbino (unpublished results; personal communication, 1999), was generated (Figure 2). The stimulus consisted of two concentric circles each divided into three equal overlapping sectors, producing an illusory transparent layer on a tri-partite background, such that the sectors with luminances P, Q, and S were 'on top' of the luminances A, B, and C. The layer luminances P and Q were calculated according to the luminance transparency model (Equation 1). The subjects' task in all conditions was to adjust the luminance S (set to a random value at the beginning of each trial) such that the transparent layer formed a contiguous disk with uniform transmissive and reflective characteristics on the tri-partite background. For each trial a stereo-pair was presented so that the inner circle simulating a transparent layer was disparate with respect to the outer circle. Three different conditions were produced under which the disparity was less than, equal to, or greater than zero, such that the layer was stereoscopically defined as being respectively behind, coplanar with, and in front of the background circle. Subjects' adjustments of the luminance S were compared to the theoretically expected luminance, $S = tC + F$, as calculated according to the model. The luminance of the area surrounding the stimulus was fixed at an intensity of half the maximum luminance produced by the display (i.e, 20 cd/m^2). Values of A, B, C, and F were generated randomly, along with five different values of t (0.1, 0.3, 0.5, 0.7, 0.9) with the constraints that $\{A, B, C\} \neq$ 20 cd/m^2 (surround color), and $\{A, B, C, P, Q, S\} < 40$ cd/m^2 (the maximum luminance output). A set of 40 different stimuli were produced and presented for the three disparity conditions.

Transparency and Spatial Frequency. A stimulus consisting of a variegated background overlaid with an illusory horizontal transparent strip was generated using the same combination of six luminances (Figure 4). The spatial frequency content of the stimulus was manipulated either by changing the size of the stimulus or by changing the viewing distance.

Multiple Surface Transparency. Following by analogy from the single layer transparency model of Equation 1, a model for two layer transparency was devised, allowing for different illuminations of each layer. The optic array corresponding to the model is shown in Figure 5. If layer 1 (t_1, r_1) is above layer 2 (t_2, r_2), the contributions from each layer sum to give the theoretical luminance,

$$Z = t_2 t_1 aI + t_2(1 - t_1)r_1 I' + (1 - t_2)r_2 I'', \qquad (2)$$

or more simply,

$$Z = t_2 t_1 A + t_2 F' + F'', \qquad (3)$$

where F' and F'' are defined as before for simplification. It can be easily shown that if layer 1 is on top of layer 2, the indices are simply reversed, such that,

$$Z = t_1 t_2 A + t_1 F'' + F'. \qquad (4)$$

This implies that, in the absence of any binocular cues, for given values of t_1, t_2, F', and F'', Z can take two different values, depending on the depth order of the layers. Z is uniquely defined, however, when disparity information is available in stereo pairs. A square (**A**) was overlaid with two orthogonal transparent strips, simulated to have different transmissive and reflective properties, such that the region of overlap (**Z**) was a square patch in the center of the square (Figure 6). The two strips were presented in stereo depth relative to the background square, such that one of the strips (t_1, r_1) was between the background square and the other strip (t_2, r_2). The depth order of the strips was randomized. The subjects were to adjust the luminance Z of the central patch such that it was consistent with the properties of both strips, including their relative depth.

4 Results

Figure 7 shows the lines of best fit to the data under the three disparity conditions for one subject (RK). The correlation coefficients (r^2) for the no disparity, the positive disparity, and negative disparity conditions were 0.94, 0.95, and 0.85, respectively. In addition, the root-mean-square (RMS) residuals for each condition were calculated. For the no disparity, the positive disparity, and negative disparity conditions, respectively, the RMS residuals were 1.49, 1.45, and 2.37 cd/m^2 with standard deviations of 1.51, 1.42, and 2.38 cd/m^2. RMS residuals as a function of spatial frequency for two subjects (RK, FK) are shown in Figure 8. Each point on the graph represents the RMS residual for a set of 40 trials. Figure 9 shows the regression parameters for the set of 40 double-transparency adjustments by one subject (RK).

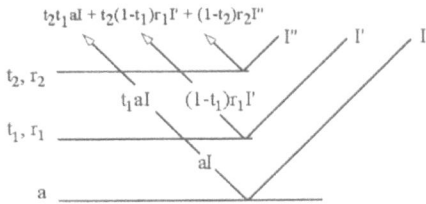

Fig. 5. Optic array for two transparent layers.

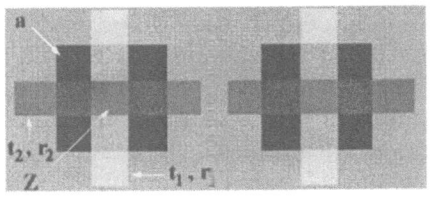

Fig. 6. Double transparency stimulus (stereo-pair).

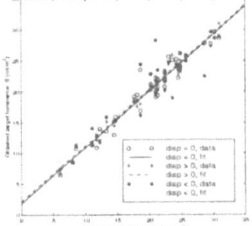

Fig. 7. Results for stereo transparency conditions.

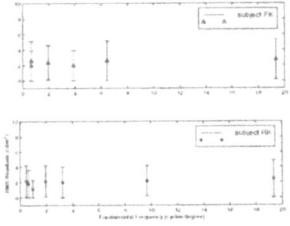

Fig. 8. Root-mean-square residuals (with standard deviation error bars) for spatial frequency experiments.

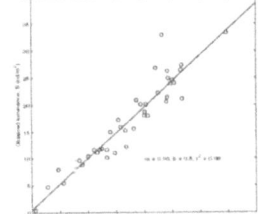

Fig. 9. Regression through double-transparency data.

5 Conclusions

Even though the results presented here are preliminary, we may derive a number of significant ideas. The stereo transparency correlation coefficients show that the model accounts for better than 94% of the variance in the data under ecologically valid conditions (flush and in-front disparities). A transparent surface, on the other hand, would not be expected to be visible through an opaque one–a condition which is simulated when negative disparity stimuli are presented. As a result, the RMS residual is higher than the other two conditions and the correlation coefficient lower. This effect is corroborated by observers of early multiple modality renderings, where rivalrous depth cues (occlusion/transparency and binocular disparity) produce competing or uncomfortable percepts. Above all, the zero- and positive-disparity results are a validation of the luminance transparency model. The measurement technique described is quite simple, considering only six distinct luminances are used. As such it may be modified such that stimuli which incorporate more of the complexity of medical images are employed in similar studies. The results showing subjects' performance as a function of spatial frequency content show no definitive trends. Although one might conclude from the figures that spatial frequency plays no role in transparency perception, the effects at higher frequencies remain to be seen. Clearly as the resolution limit of the eye is approached, one would expect a degradation in performance. Unfortunately the resolution of the display was a limiting factor at the viewing distances utilized in these experiments. Studies exploring these higher frequencies are already underway, since it would be interesting to measure whether 'transparency acuity' follows a trend similar to the contrast sensitivity function. In addition, if a maximum sensitivity in transparency adjustments within a particular frequency band can be found, it might correspond to an ideal surface texel (texture element) size. The double layer results show good agreement with the model, indicating the optic array of Figure 5 is a reasonable one, not only for two transparent layers, but perhaps extending to multiple layers.

References

1. P. St-Jean, A. F. Sadikot, L. Collins, D. Clonda, R. Kasrai, A. C. Evans, and T. M. Peters, Automated atlas integration and interactive three-dimensional visualization tools for planning and guidance in functional neurosurgery, *IEEE Trans Med Imaging*, vol. 17, pp. 672-80, 1998.
2. D. L. Collins, Volumetric Rendering of Medical Data, *Ph.D. Thesis*, Montreal, Canada: McGill University, 1990.
3. F. Metelli, The perception of transparency, *Sci Am*, vol. 230, pp. 90-8, 1974.
4. F. Metelli, O. Da Pos, and A. Cavedon, Balanced and unbalanced, complete and partial transparency, *Percept Psychophys*, vol. 38, pp. 354-66, 1985.
5. M. D'Zmura, P. Colantoni, K. Knoblauch, and B. Laget, Color transparency, *Perception*, vol. 26, pp. 471-92, 1997.
6. M. Woo, J. Neider, and T. Davis, in *OpenGL programming guide: the official guide to learning OpenGL, version 1.1:* Addison-Wesley Developers Press, 1997, pp. 213-26.
7. J. Beck, K. Prazdny, and R. Ivry, The perception of transparency with achromatic colors, *Percept Psychophys*, vol. 35, pp. 407-22, 1984.
8. W. Gerbino, C. I. Stultiens, J. M. Troost, and C. M. de Weert, Transparent layer constancy, *J Exp Psychol Hum Percept Perform*, vol. 16, pp. 3-20, 1990.
9. W. Gerbino, Achromatic Transparency, in *Lightness, Brightness, and Transparency*, A. L. Gilchrist, Ed.: Lawrence Erlbaum Associates, 1994, pp. 215-255.
10. H. L. Kundel, Visual cues in the interpretation of medical images, *J Clin Neurophysiol*, vol. 7, pp. 472-83, 1990.
11. R. A. Robb, S. Aharon, and B. M. Cameron, Patient-specific anatomic models from three dimensional medical image data for clinical applications in surgery and endoscopy, *J Digit Imaging*, vol. 10, pp. 31-5, 1997.
12. P. Kay, R. Robb, R. Myers, and B. King, Creation and validation of patient specific anatomical models for prostate surgery planning using virtual reality, presented at *Visualization in Biomedical Computing, 4th International Conference*, Berlin, Germany, 1996.
13. G. D. Rubin, M. D. Dake, S. Napel, R. B. Jeffrey, Jr., C. H. McDonnell, F. G. Sommer, L. Wexler, and D. M. Williams, Spiral CT of renal artery stenosis: comparison of three-dimensional rendering techniques, *Radiology*, vol. 190, pp. 181-9, 1994.
14. C. E. Metz, ROC methodology in radiologic imaging, *Invest Radiol*, vol. 21, pp. 720-33, 1986.

Localisation of Subdural EEG Electrode Bundles in an Interactive Volume Rendering Framework

H.J. Noordmans[1], C.W.M. van Veelen[2], M. A. Viergever[1]

[1] Image Sciences Institute E.01.334, [2] Dept. Neurosurgery G03.124, University Hospital Utrecht, P.O. Box 85500, 3508 GA Utrecht, The Netherlands, herke@isi.uu.nl, http://www.isi.uu.nl.

Abstract. When the focus of epilepsy is so deep that skin EEG electrodes do not give enough accuracy in calculating the position of the focus, it may be decided to surgically implant EEG electrodes inside the patient's head. To localise these electrodes, a high resolution 3D CT scan is made of the patient's head. As manual tracking of the electrodes slice by slice is tedious and erroneous, a virtual reality environment has been created to give the radiologist a view from inside patient's skull. With the help of a high quality but fast volume renderer, the radiologist can get an overview of the electrode bundles and can interactively characterise the bundle of interest. For the localisation of the lead markers, we compared manual placement, centre of gravity and Gaussian image matching. For the interpolation, we compared line and NURBS interpolation with the optional restriction of equal segment size or zero curvature at the end of the bundle. It appeared that the electrodes could be characterised with high accuracy, that manual positioning equally performed as centre of gravity methods, and that NURBS interpolation with equal segment size outperformed line interpolation and NURBS interpolation without the equal segment restriction.

1   Introduction

For patients with local epilepsy, it is sometimes difficult to determine the exact location of the focus of epilepsy. The first option is to put EEG electrodes on the skin of the patient's head, but when the focus lies deeper in the brain, the accuracy in determining the focus[1] is often limited. In such cases, it can be decided to operatively implant EEG electrodes inside the patient's head (2,5, Fig. 1). Then often two bundles, called depth bundles, are inserted with a hollow needle into the head of the hippocampi. Other bundles are inserted through a bore hole and shifted over the brain cortex, the subdural bundles. The electrodes are embedded in plastic and make contact with the surrounding tissue at locations where isolation has been removed. A depth bundle contains six contacts, a subdural bundle seven. The subdural bundles have three lead markers to localise the bundles in an X-ray scan; the depth bundles do not have these markers.

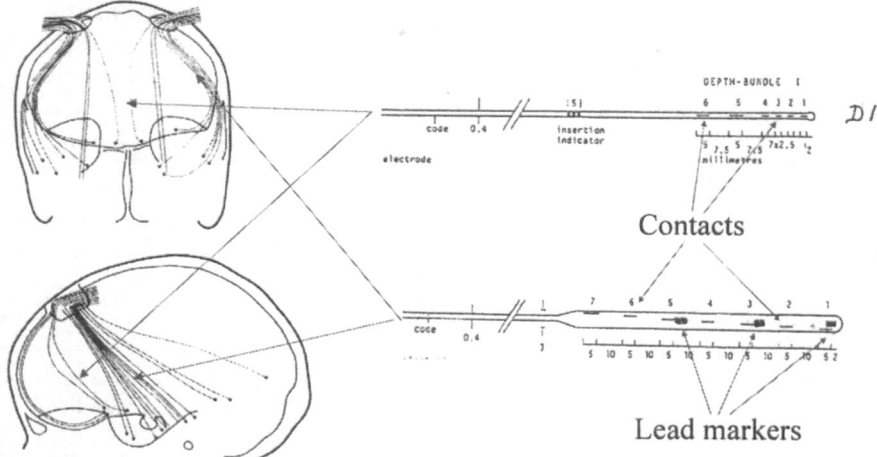

Fig. 1. Technical drawing of the implanted EEG electrode bundles.

Apart from the surgical procedure and the characterisation of the depth bundles, the biggest problem is to recognise the subdural bundles on an X-ray scan. Although a high resolution 3D X-ray scan is made of the patient's head and the individual lead markers can be distinguished from each other, it is often difficult to determine from X-ray slices which lead markers belong to the same bundle 2 (Fig. 2). Problems are that bundles are inserted from the same bore hole and therefore often cross in the patient's head. Also, bundles are sometimes so close to the skull that they seem to vanish.

We try to solve these problems by giving the user a 3D view from the inside of the patient's skull (Fig. 3). Thanks to the overview, the user has less difficulty to recognise the individual electrode bundles and to interpret the information from the scanned slices. If the rendering quality is high enough, it is also easier to visually connect separate parts of the electrode bundles than by looking at individual slices.

We use volume rendering to generate the 3D view. We chose for that option instead of using fast graphics on specialised hardware (e.g. OpenGL), as we did not accept possible errors introduced by converting the volume data to graphical surface patches. This erroneous 'segmentation' step is avoided in volume rendering, by which the image quality is higher and the user can visually check his segmentation results with the original data.

For the problem of localising the electrode bundles, we developed a 3D interactive system consisting of a high qualitative, but fast volume renderer combined with interactive tools enabling the user to accurately characterise surgically implanted EEG electrodes. The user indicates a subdural bundle by placing artificial blobs in the neighbourhood of lead markers. The computer refines the positions of the artificial blobs and fits a curve through the three positions. The final curve is showed, eventually together with the interpolated EEG contacts. The user then accepts the result or adapts his initial guess.

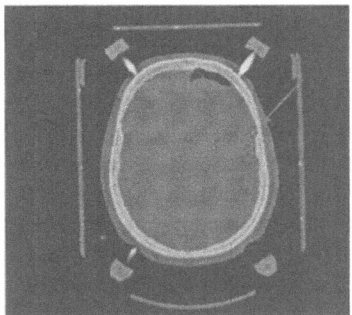

Fig. 2. CT slice showing the two depth electrode bundles and three subdural EEG bundles next to the skull.

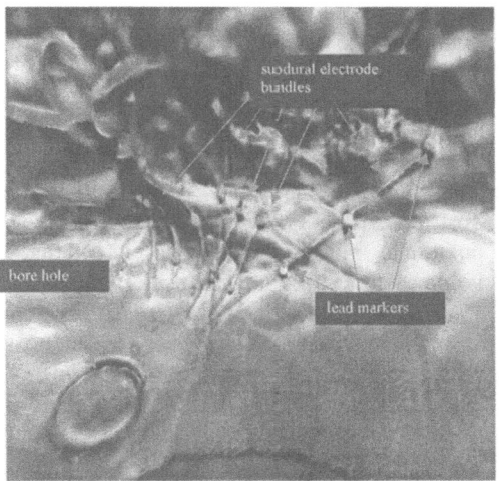

Fig. 3. Volume rendering of EEG electrode bundles implanted inside the skull of a patient with epilepsy. Through a bore hole in the skull, the electrode bundles are pushed over the cortex. Each bundle contains 7 contacts (not visible) and three lead markers (purple blobs). The user moves one magenta and two yellow artificial blobs to the lead markers to indicate which bundle he/she wants to characterise.

A 3D CT scan is made of the head of the patient. Matrix size 512x512x90, FOV 300 mm, slice thickness 1.5mm (Philips Tomoscan SR7000). The data is read on a SGI workstation with four R10000 processors running at 194 MHz, and 1GB of memory. After cropping the data to remove the stereotactic frame mounted on the head (remaining matrix approximately 300x400x90), the data is thresholded to segment the skull, the electrode bundles and the lead markers. A second threshold is used to segment the more intense lead markers.

The original data set and the two segmentations are combined in a volume rendering to show the user the original data. We use Phong shading to enhance surface detail 6, a semi-transparent skull to illuminate the inner side of the skull, and a table with a shadow as a projection of the data set. To get a fast initial visual response, the renderer uses optimisation schemes like adaptive ray termination, template based viewing, adaptive progressive refinement, presence sampling, blur prevention, local volume update, and view movement 3,7. The result is a first update within a second and a final update in 10 seconds.

An overview of the system is given in Fig. 4. In the window with name para_0, the user gets an overview of the entire data set (parallel projection). The windows persp_0 and persp_1 give the user a look inside the head of the patient (perspective projection). The subdural bundles are visible as ridges on the skull, the depth bundles appear as antennas in the emptied skull. The magenta dots denote the lead markers. The window plane_0 shows an arbitrarily formatted slice. By dragging the mouse inside a parallel, perspective view or plane, the user can interactively change the view position or direction. The user can move the perspective viewpoint by using the step buttons in the perspective view control panel.

After selecting the appropriate viewpoints, the measurement starts by creating three artificial blobs: A cyan blob to denote the lead marker at the end of an electrode bundle, and two yellow blobs for the other two lead markers. The user moves the blobs in the neighbourhood of the desired lead markers by selecting them through any of the view or planes, and dragging them with the mouse. The computer matches the positions of the blobs to the real marker positions and fits a curve to the three positions. The final curve and the calculated contacts are combined with the original volume rendering to let the user qualitatively validate the result.

The artificial objects are visualised as voxel objects instead of graphics as a hybrid volume renderer would be more difficult to implement, computational complex, and would easily create artefacts at subvoxel scale (e.g. does a graphic intersect the data at the visual correct position?). We therefore voxelize all artificial objects and draw them in a geometry volume. An additional label volume specifies their colour. An additional advantage of voxelized objects is that is relatively easy to identify the artificial objects the user has selected through a view. Starting from the position where the user presses a mouse button, a search is performed in the view direction to find the first artificial object. This is implemented by tracing rays through a so-called identification volume, which is derived from the voxel representations of the artificial objects.

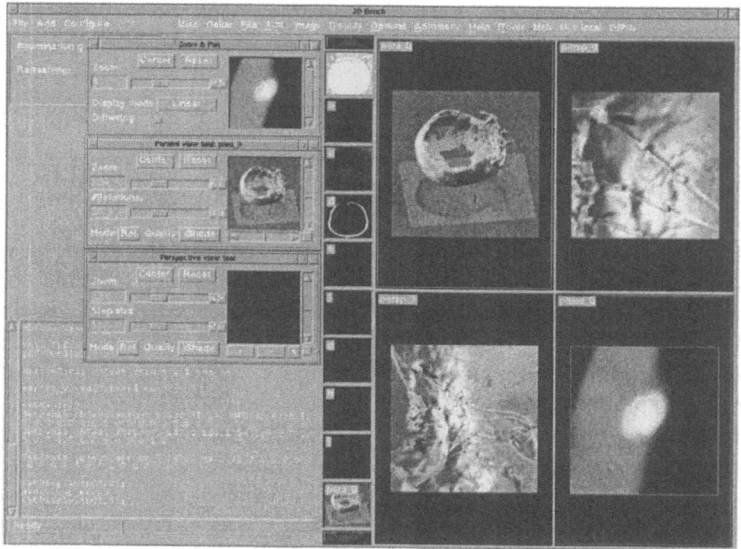

Fig. 4. Overview of the EEG bundle localisation system. Windows: para_0, fast overview using parallel projection; persp_0, persp_1, two perspective projections from inside; plane_0, arbitrarily orientable slice. The windows zoom tool, plane tool and perspective view tool are display, respectively view control panels. The left-bottom panel shows the command line C-interpreter.

1.1   Localisation techniques

To improve the accuracy and robustness in localising the lead markers, the computer refines the position indicated by the user. We looked at three refinement techniques:
Centre of gravity. The final lead marker position is calculated by averaging over the marker co-ordinates $\mathbf{x}$ in a local environment around the user-specified region V,

$$\mathbf{m} = \frac{\int_V \mathbf{x} f(I(\mathbf{x}) > 0) d\mathbf{x}}{\int_V f(I(\mathbf{x}) > 0) d\mathbf{x}}, \qquad (1)$$

with $I(\mathbf{x})$ the image values and $f()$ the indicator function.
Intensity weighted centre of gravity. The image co-ordinates are weighted by the image intensity:

$$\mathbf{m} = \frac{\int_V \mathbf{x} I(\mathbf{x}) d\mathbf{x}}{\int_V I(\mathbf{x}) d\mathbf{x}}. \qquad (2)$$

Weighted image matching with a Gaussian profile 8. Starting from the initial guess, the computer changes a parameter vector $\mathbf{p}$ to optimise the match between the Gaussian intensity model and image data:

$$\varepsilon = \frac{\int_V (I(\mathbf{x}) - F(\mathbf{p};\mathbf{x}))^2 G(\mathbf{p};\mathbf{x}) d\mathbf{x}}{\int_V G(\mathbf{p};\mathbf{x}) d\mathbf{x}}, \qquad (3)$$

with parameter vector $\mathbf{p} = (\mathbf{x}, a, \sigma)$, Gaussian profile $F(\mathbf{p};\mathbf{x}) = ae^{-\frac{|\mathbf{x}|^2}{2\sigma^2}}$, and weight function $G(\mathbf{p};\mathbf{x}) = e^{-\frac{|\mathbf{x}|^2}{2\rho^2\sigma^2}}$.

1.2   Interpolating curve

To determine the positions of the EEG contacts from the lead marker positions, we investigated two techniques:
    Line interpolation. Fig. 5a. Draw two lines, one from the first to second marker, and one from the second to third marker.
    Second degree NURBS interpolation 4. Fig. 5b. Generally, none of the n-derivatives of the NURBS is specified. As the electrode bundle has a free end, it is sensible to specify a zero 2nd derivative at that end. We also know that the arclength between marker 1 and 2 and the arclength between marker 2 and 3 should be 30 mm, thus equal. As the knot vector contains one free parameter, we can change it such to make the calculated arclengths equal. We therefore looked at four interpolation options: (1) free arclengths + no zero curvature restriction, (2) equal arclengths + no zero curvature restriction, (3) free arclengths + zero curvature restriction, and (4) equal arclengths + zero curvature restriction.

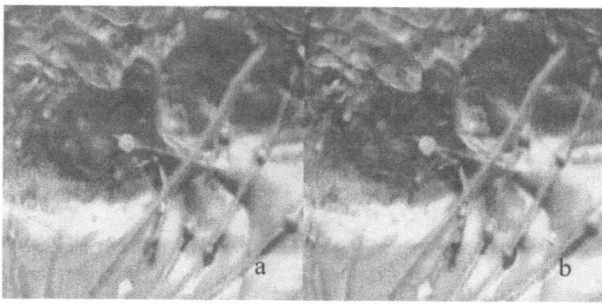

Fig. 5. Line interpolation (a) versus curve interpolation (b).

2   Evaluation

We tested the system on four patients with epilepsy. The numbers of implanted subdural bundles were 3, 3, 7, and 13; 26 in total. We evaluated the measurement qualitatively by comparing the interpolating curve with the original electrode bundle. We evaluated the measurement quantitatively by comparing the measured arclength between the first and second marker, and the arclength between the second and third marker to the value of 30 mm expected from the technical specifications.

3   Results

Qualitative. The complete procedure is illustrated in Fig. 6. At the start of the procedure, where no EEG bundles are characterised yet, the user has a good view on the inside of the skull and the imprints of the EEG bundles on the CT scan (a). After localising the subdural EEG bundles, the interpolating NURBS are shown (green) together with the interpolated contact positions (red) (b). After the depth electrode is tracked, its measurements are reconstructed as red rods (c). Finally, the results are merged with a CT-registered 3D T1 MRI scan (d).

Quantitative validation. After manual placement, the computer refines the location of the artificial blobs by one of the three techniques mentioned above. Then the computer fits a line or curve and measures the arclengths. The arclengths after each measurement are summarised in Table 1. Each time, the first row shows the mean and standard deviation for the segment between the end marker and the second marker. The second row shows the mean and standard deviation for the segment between the second and third marker.

We saw that, when looking qualitatively at the results, line interpolation gave larger errors than curve interpolations (Fig. 5). Regarding curve interpolation, the largest errors occurred when the end segment was strongly bent and the interpolating curve had a slightly lower curvature (images not shown). The calculated contact was then estimated to be 1 or 2 mm from the real contact position.

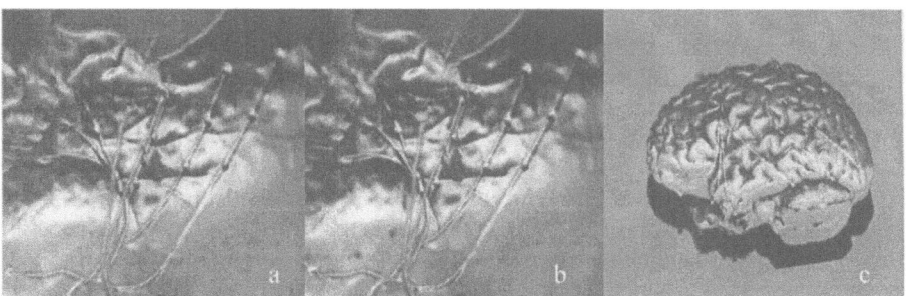

Fig. 6. Overview of the electrode characterisation process: **a** Initial view showing the electrode bundles and lead markers (purple). **b** Result after bundle characterisation: Interpolated NURBS splines (green) and contact positions (red). **c** Bundles visualised on segmented brain from a registered 3D T1 MRI scan.

Table 1. Mean and standard deviation of measured segment lengths (mm).

	Manual		Centre of gravity		Intensity weighted centre of gravity		Gaussian image matching	
Line	28.7	1.5	28.8	1.4	28.8	1.4	28.7	1.5
interpolation	29.9	0.9	29.9	1.0	29.9	1.0	29.9	0.6
Curve 1	29.1	1.3	29.2	1.2	29.1	1.2	29.1	1.3
	30.3	0.8	30.3	0.9	30.3	0.8	30.3	0.6
Curve 2	30.2	0.7	30.2	0.7	30.2	0.7	30.2	0.5
	30.2	0.7	30.2	0.7	30.2	0.7	30.2	0.5
Curve 3	28.9	1.4	28.9	1.3	28.9	1.3	28.9	1.4
	30.4	0.8	30.4	0.8	30.4	0.8	30.4	0.6
Curve 4	30.2	0.7	30.2	0.7	30.2	0.7	30.1	0.5
	30.2	0.7	30.2	0.7	30.2	0.7	30.1	0.5

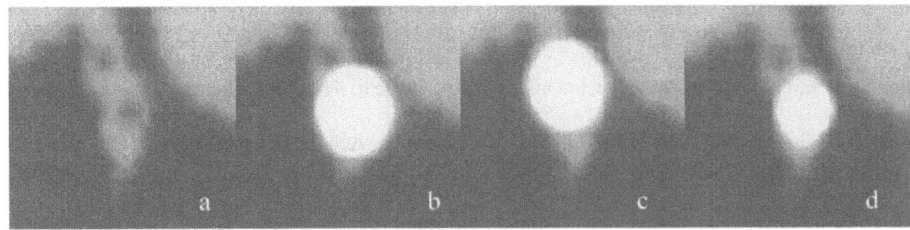

Fig. 7. Errors in marker localisation when markers are close. **a** Two lead markers at 2 mm distance. **b** Artificial blob after manual adjustment. **c** Refinement with centre of gravity technique; The second marker disturbs the proper calculation of the centre. **d** Refinement after match with Gaussian.

From Table 1, the following conclusions can be drawn: (1) The end segment of an electrode bundle has a significantly shorter line length than the second segment; this means that the end of the bundle is always more bent than the second segment. (2) Manual placement is not significantly less accurate than automatic refinement procedures. This, because the user has the disposal of an interactive slice, which he/she can zoom in on the actual marker of interest. The slice enables the user to accurately position the artificial blob over the actual marker. (3) Refining the position by matching the marker with a Gaussian is slightly more accurate than the other techniques. The reason is that in some cases the gravity techniques fail when two markers are so close that the centre is found between the two markers (Fig. 7.). Gaussian image matching has less trouble in such cases, as the weight function effectively reduces the disturbing influences of a neighbouring spot 8. (4) Imposing zero curvature at the end of the bundle does not significantly increase the accuracy, but does not decrease it either. Imposing equal arclengths does increase the accuracy.

In summary, the best technique would be Gaussian image matching of marker positions followed by NURBS fitting with equal length and zero curvature restriction. Less difficult to implement but still giving good results, would be manual placement followed by NURBS fitting with equal length restriction.

4   Conclusions

A practically useful method has been presented to characterise surgically implanted EEG electrode bundles. The volume rendering method is fast and gives high quality feedback to accurately locate the lead markers and interpret the interpolating curve. The results showed that manual placement of artificial objects to denote the marker positions is equally accurate as calculating the position centre of gravity techniques, but less accurate than Gaussian image matching. A NURBS interpolating curve with the restriction of equal segment size outperformed line interpolation and NURBS interpolation without the equal segment restriction.

References

1. B.J. Roth, D. Ko, I. von Albertini-Carletti, D. Scaffidi and S. Sato Dipole localization in patients with epilepsy using the realistically shaped head model. Electroencephalography and clinical Neurophysiology 102, 1997, 159-166.
2. L.C. Meiners, The role of MR in drug-resistant epilepsy with special emphasis on mesial temporal sclerosis. PhD Thesis University of Utrecht, The Netherlands. Chapter 4 and 12, 1997.
3. K.J. Zuiderveld, A.H.J. Koning, M.A. Viergever, Acceleration of ray-casting using 3D distance transforms. Visualization in Biomedical Computing 1992, Proc. SPIE 1808, 1992, 324-335.
4. L. Piegl, W. Tiller, The NURBS book. Springer Verlag, Berlin, Second Edition, chapter 9.2.2, 1997.
5. C.W.M. van Veelen, R.M. Chr. Debets, A.C. van Huffelen, W. van Emde Boas, C.D. Binnie, B. Chir, W. Storm van Leeuwen, D.N. Velis, A. van Dieren, Combined Use of Subdural and Intracerebral Electrodes in Preoperative Evaluation of Epilepsy, Neurosurgery 26(1), 1990, 93-101.
6. B.T. Phong, Illumination for computer generated pictures. Comm ACM 18(6), 1975, 311-317.
7. H.J. Noordmans, A.W.M. Smeulders, H.T.M. van der Voort, Fast volume render techniques for interactive analysis. The Visual Computer 13, 1997, 345-358.
8. H.J. Noordmans, A.W.M. Smeulders, Detection and characterisation of isolated and overlapping spots, Computer Vision and Image Understanding 70(1), 1998, 23-35.

System of Modeling and Visualization of Domain of the Heart Excitation

Dmitry Belov

Grodno State University, 22, Ozheshko Street, 230023 Grodno, Belarus
belov@grsu.grodno.by

Abstract. The mathematical aspects of the problem of the reconstruction of domain of the heart excitation from the body surface potentials are investigated. We propose modeling algorithms allowing to reduce endless set of solutions of the problem. These algorithms take into account local and global time restrictions of the function whose support is equal to the domain. As a result a new model of cardiogenerator is developed. This model operates within the framework of classical model of excitation spreading as a multidipole generator. At the same time our generator provides stable solution of the problem in contrast to multidipole one. In final the system of modeling and visualization of domain of the heart excitation is developed. The clinical tests have shown efficiency of applying of the system for the myocardial infarction diagnostics.

1 Introduction

The problem of identification of cardiogenerator characteristics from the potentials given on the body surface is called the inverse problem of the electrocardiography. For example, in [7] the problem of identification of characteristics of the potential field on the ventricular surface is investigated. In [3] the problem of identification of electrostatics volume sources inside heart is researched. Let us consider the problem of construction of domain of the heart excitation from the body surface potentials. This problem will be called Ω-problem. From the mathematical point of view the domain of the heart excitation is a support of volume function of the electrostatics sources inside heart, i.e. domain of non-zero values of the function. The fundamental meaning of the problem has been emphasized in [5]. Observing in any time the domain of the heart excitation cardiologist can diagnose various cardiac irregularities. It is known [4], that the problem of determination of the volume function of the electrostatics sources from the surface potentials has non-unique solution. Therefore Ω-problem has non-unique solution as well. Thus the important problem of restriction of the set of solutions of Ω-problem arises.

Going over to the general mathematical aspects of Ω-problem we consider the operator equation of first kind:

$$A(\vec{r}, \vec{s}, t)p(\vec{r}, t) = u_\delta(\vec{s}, t), \tag{1}$$

where $t \in [0, T]$ is time, $p(\vec{r}, t)$ is unknown volume function of electrostatics sources with domain of definition $P(t)$, $A(\vec{r}, \vec{s}, t)$ is unknown and non-linear operator, $u_\delta(\vec{s}, t)$ is potentials given on the body surface $U(t)$ with error $\delta > 0$. Support $P'(t)$ of the $p(\vec{r}, t)$ is unknown but for any time $P'(t) \subset P(t)$ and

$$\int_{P'(t)} p(\vec{r}, t) dr = \int_{P(t)} p(\vec{r}, t) dr = 0 \tag{2}$$

We suppose functions $p(\vec{r}, t)$ and $u(\vec{s}, t)$ belong to the Hilbert spaces H_p and $H_u = L_2(U(t))$ respectively. Thus Ω-problem is a problem of determination of $P'(t)$. Obviously we can solve this problem after the construction of the solution of the equation (1). In electrocardiography any solution of (1) is called equivalent cardiogenerator, because it generates the same body surface potentials as desired one. It is wide known multipole [2, 3] and multidipole [2, 3] equivalent generators. Let us suppose that the body is infinitely wide homogeneous medium, then equation (1) transforms to the equation:

$$\frac{1}{4\pi\sigma} \int_{P(t)} \frac{p(\vec{r}, t)}{\|\vec{r} - \vec{s}\|_{R_3}} dv = u(\vec{s}, t), \tag{3}$$

where σ is a specific conductivity of the medium.

For the reconstruction of $P'(t)$ we will reject from $P(t)$ points such that $|p_\Omega(\vec{r}, t)| \leq \tau$, where τ is a threshold and $p_\Omega(\vec{r}, t)$ is a solution of regularized according to Tikhonov [6] equation (3) solved by Voevodin method [6]. The result subset of $P(t)$ will approximate $P'(t)$.

The Tikhonov regularization method is based on the fundamental idea of the restriction of the domain of definition of the integral operator in (3), i.e. restriction of the solutions set of (3). Moreover in our case this restriction is determined by definition of the Hilbert space of function $p(\vec{r}, t)$. So taking into account biophysics phenomena of heart work we construct Hilbert space of function $p(\vec{r}, t)$ in which all functions have equal support, and we can identify unique solution of Ω-problem. Thus if equation (3) has non-unique solution then Ω-problem can have unique solution. This fact is very important for electrocardiography applications.

2   Methods of the Restriction of Solutions Set of Ω-problem

Let for given t the following restriction is true:

$$P(t) = \bigcup_{i=1}^{k} P_i(t), \quad \bigcap_{i=1}^{k} P_i(t) = \emptyset, \ k \geq 1, \ \forall i : \int_{P_i(t)} p(\vec{r}, t) dr = 0 \tag{4}$$

It is easy to prove, that functional space $W_{2+}^1(P(t))$ with the norm

$$\|f(\vec{r})\| = \sqrt{\int_{P(t)} (f^2(\vec{r}) + f'^2(\vec{r}))dr + \frac{1}{\varepsilon}\sum_{i=1}^{k}\left(\int_{P_i(t)} f(\vec{r})dr\right)^2} \qquad (5)$$

is Hilbert space [1], where $f(\vec{r}) \in W_{2+}^1(P(t))$ and $f'(\vec{r})$ is generalized derivative of first order [1]. It follows, that if $p(\vec{r}, t)$ belongs to $W_{2+}^1(P(t))$ then the method of construction of $P'(t)$ stated above is true and solving Ω-problem we take into account restriction (4). In the norm (5) the last member is a penalty.

In computer experiments we reconstruct positions (Ω-problem) and tracks (Ω'-problem) of two moving charges having equal values and different signs from the potentials given on a containing circle, where $\delta = 1.0e - 4$. Obviously in this case corresponding equation (3) has non-unique solution. On the fig.1,2 dots correspond to the knots of grid belonging to $P(t)$, squares correspond to solutions of the Ω'-problem, circles correspond to current positions of the charges.

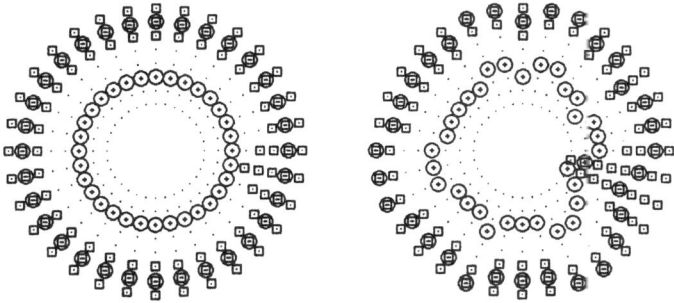

Fig.1. Two solutions of Ω'-problem. We have assumed that $p(\vec{r}, t) \in W_2^1(P(t))$.

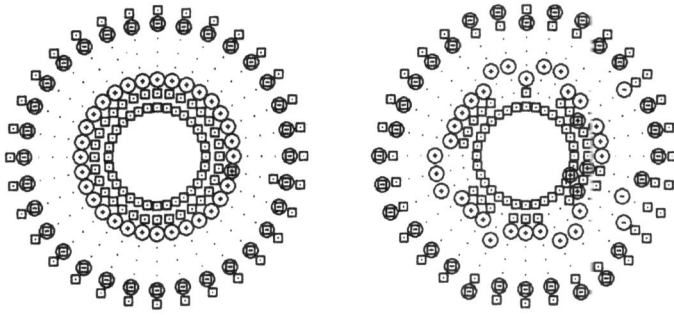

Fig.2. Two solutions of Ω'-problem. We have assumed that $p(\vec{r}, t) \in W_{2+}^1(P(t))$.

One can see on fig.1,2 that use of constructed space $W_{2+}^1(P(t))$ allows to reconstruct track of positive charge in contrast to use of Sobolev space $W_2^1(P(t))$ [1]. In [9] the results of computer experiments on reconstruction of positions and tracks of dipole on the plain are presented.

Let for the time segment $[0, T]$ the following condition is true:

$$G \supset G' = \bigcup_{t=0}^{T} P'(t) \, , \forall \vec{r} \in G' \int_{0}^{T} p^2(\vec{r}, t)dt = \int_{t(\vec{r})}^{t(\vec{r})+\Delta t} p^2(\vec{r}, t)dt, \qquad (6)$$

where G and G' are connected sets, and $P'(0)$ and G are known. Obviously the condition specifies 3D object that are continuously changing its form and position in the course of time. For the construction a sequence of $\{P(t_i)\}$ taking into account (6) we propose the following algorithm:

1. $P(t_0) = P'(0)$, $G_d = \emptyset$
2. Let $P(t_i)$ is known, then if $M^{\alpha}[p, P(t_i)] \leq \tau_s$ then $P(t_{i+1}) = P(t_i)$, $G_d = G_d \cup P(t_i)$. Otherwise, $P(t_{i+1}) = P_{\Omega}(t_{i-1})$ and while for $P(t_{i+1})$ inequality $M^{\alpha}[p, P(t_{i+1})] > \tau_s$ will be valid we add to $P(t_{i+1})$ points from G, that are neighbors of points from $P(t_{i+1})$ and do not belong to $G_d/P_{\Omega}(t_{i-1})$. Here $M^{\alpha}[p, P(t_i)]$ is regularization functional [6] and τ_s is a threshold.

Choosing neighbor points randomly we get algorithm of random search of $\{P(t_i)\}$.

3   The Structure of the Equivalent Generator of the Heart

Solving electrocardiography Ω-problem we have:

1. $P'(t)$ is domain of the heart excitation, i.e. support of $p(\vec{r}, t)$.
2. $U(t)$ is a geometric model of the body surface.
3. $P_{\Omega}(t)$ is model of domain of the heart excitation for the given t, i.e. solution of Ω-problem.
4. $P(t)$ is a set containing domain of the heart excitation for given t.
5. In (4) each $P_i(t)$ is preferable direction of the excitation for the given $t \in [0, T]$. Obviously if restriction (4) is true then restriction (2) is true as well. Is follows restriction (4) specifies the state of classical excitation model for given t. Today it is known preferable direction of the excitation for the main parts of the heart [2].
6. In (6) G is a geometric model of the heart, $P'(0)$ is a geometric model of sinus knot. Thus restrictions (4) and (6) specify classical model of excitation spreading inside heart.
7. Time segment $[0, T]$ is excitation period.

Thus we developed equivalent generator of the heart, that operates within the framework of classical model of excitation spreading as a multidipole generator. At the same time using regularization technics our generator provides stable solution of the Ω-problem in contrast to multidipole one.

For the development of system of modeling and visualization of domain of the heart excitation we assume:

1. Body surface model $U(t)$ is time fixed truncated cylinder U (fig.3). This analytical model permits to use surface integral in regularization functional [6] and therefore reduces time and space of computations.

2. Heart model $P(t) = G$ is time fixed logical combination P of ellipsoids (fig.3).

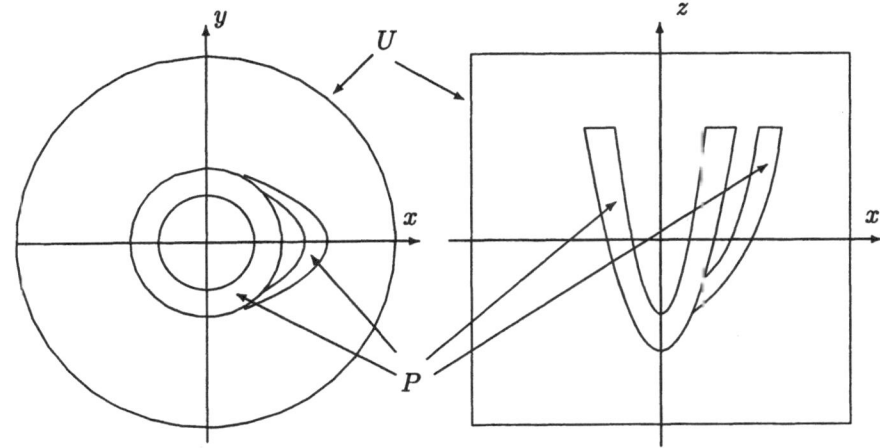

Fig.3. Geometric model of heart and body surface.

3. For the approximation of function $u_\delta(\vec{s}, t)$ on U vectorcardiographic (VCG) data is used.

4. In (4) we assume that $k = 1$, i.e. we take into account restriction (2).

5. We do not take into account restriction (6).

4   System of Modeling and Visualization of Domain of the Heart Excitation

Let us consider main stages of the system operation:

Preparation: It is regularization of equation (3) and preparation by Voevodin scheme. The results of the stage is saved in the preparation bank. This stage take into account H_u, H_p, U and P.

Solution: Using data from the preparation bank the system numerically solves the equation (3) for the different value of potentials. The solution is resulted on 3D grid and further is saved in solutions bank.

Construction and visualization of the layer-model: Layer-model of 3D object given on 3D grid is effective alternative for the voxel model, where one needs to identify form and position of the objects only. Geometric properties of the layer-model allow to develop fast visualization algorithms [10]. Let us present our investigation object as a set of generalized vertical cylinders standing bottom on top. Each cylinder, corresponding to the determined contour of the object in layer is approximated with the simple polyhedron. These polyhedrons will be called layers. A set of such layers will be called a layer-model. This approach is considered for computer tomography applications in [8], but for visualization authors suggested scan-line algorithm. Obviously it is sufficient to know only the respective polygon and the height of the respective layer for the description of a polyhedron. Let L be a number of layers. Further, if an object of the given set of objects has a maximum number of vertices, then it will be called a maximum object. Let N be a number of vertices of the maximum polygon, then the $O(LN)$ space is sufficient for the presentation of the layer-model. It is easy to prove that elimination of hidden-surface for layer-model runs in optimal $O(logL + LNlogN)$ time.

Let us consider general sequence of the system operation:

Preparation of the equation (3) $\Rightarrow$ Preparation data bank $\Rightarrow$ Obtaining of the vectorcardiographic (VCG) data $\Rightarrow$ Approximation body surface potentials by VCG $\Rightarrow$ Solution of the equation (3) $\Rightarrow$ Construction of the layer-model $\Rightarrow$ Visualization of the layer-model.

5   Clinical Experiments

System of modeling and visualization of domain of the heart excitation is being used in cardiology department of Grodno region clinical hospital. The system provides 2D and 3D visualization of the excitation process in ventricle of a heart.

On fig.4 the model of domain of the heart excitation of healthy man for the time of the ventricle excitation is presented. On fig.5,6 for the same time the models of domains of the heart excitation of myocardial infarction patients are shown. One can see that for the same threshold value volume of the excitation domain on fig.5,6 is less than one on fig.4. This fact says about partial affection of the conductor cells for sick men. Different configuration of the domains on fig.5,6 says about affection in different parts of the ventricles.

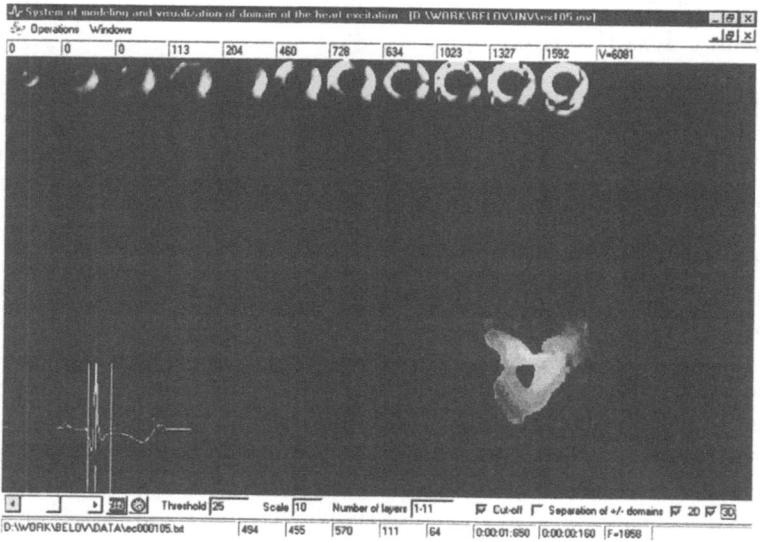

Fig.4. Excitation domain in ventricles zone for the healthy man.

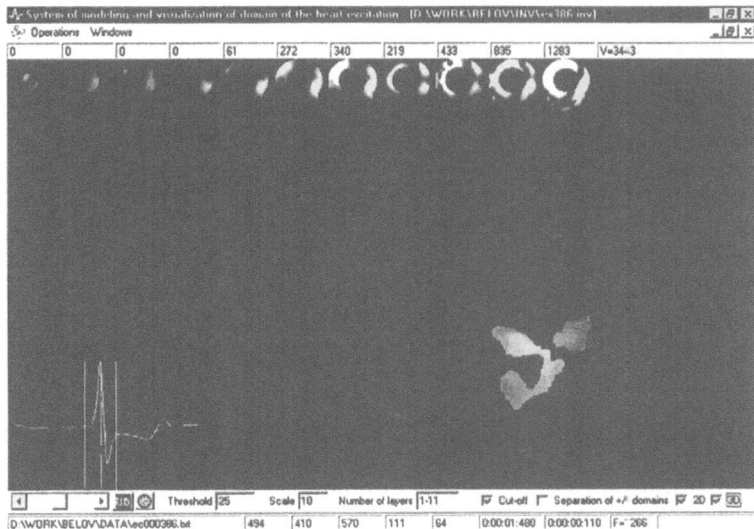

Fig.5. Excitation domain in ventricles zone for the sick man.

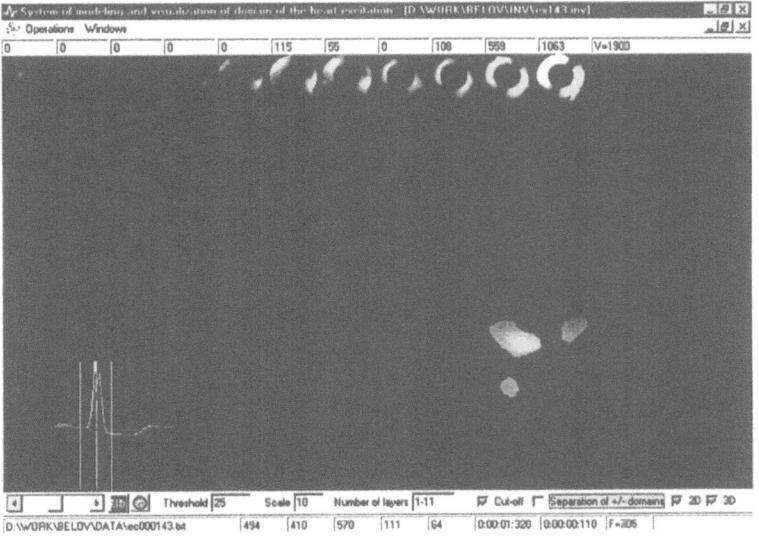

Fig.6. Excitation domain in ventricles zone for the sick man.

During of the test period (nine month) the 40 patients with myocardial infarction have been investigated. For all patients cardiologist determined correct diagnosis using our system. Thus developed system allows to determine visually part of the ventricles in which the break of the excitation spreading occurs. In addition cardiologist can estimate volume and distribution of the excitation domains. This results permit to use the system for the diagnostics and educational process.

6 Future Goals

The results of the paper can be developed to the following directions:

1. Use of the genetics algorithms solving Ω-problem taking into account time segment restriction (6). This can permit to reconstruct desired domain more accuracy.

2. Advance of the system on the base of the non-truncation variants of the restrictions (4), (6). This can permit to diagnose cardiac irregularities more accuracy.

7 Conclusions

The new model of cardiogenerator is developed. This model operates within the framework of classical model of excitation spreading as a multidipole generator. At the same time our generator provides stable construction of domain of the heart excitation from the body surface potentials (Ω-problem) in contrast to multidipole one. The system of modeling and visualization of excitation process in ventricle of the heart is developed and clinical approved.

References

1. Lusternik, L.A., Sobolev, V.I.: Elements of Functional Analysis, Moskwa, Nauka, (1965)

2. The Theoretical Basis of Electrocardiology, ed. by Nelson, C.V., Geselowitz, D.B., Clarendon Press, Oxford, (1976)

3. Titomir, L.I.: Electric Generator of the Heart, Moskwa, Nauka, (1980)

4. Sezginer, A.: The Inverse Source Problems of Magnetostatics and Electrostatics. J. Inverse Problems, **3** (1987) L87-L91

5. Geselowitz, D.B.: To Electrocardiogram Theory, J. IEEE Transactions, Vol.77, **6** (1989) 34-55

6. Tikhonov, A.N., Goncharsky, A.V., Stepanov, V.V., Yagola, A.G.: Numerical Methods for the Solution of Ill-posed Problems, Moskwa, Nauka, (1990)

7. Greensite, F.: A New Method for Regularization of the Inverse Problem of Electrocardiography, J. Mathematical Biosciences, Vol.111, **1** (1992) 131-154

8. Ivanov, V.P., Batrakov, A.S.: Three-Dimensional Computer Graphics, Moskwa, Radio i svjazj, (1995)

9. Belov, D.I., Sadykhov, R.H.: Computer Simulation of the Inverse Problem of Electrocardiography, Proceedings of the 22 Annual International Computer Software and Applications Conference (IEEE COMPSAC'98) , Vienna, (1998) 563-567

10. Belov, D.I., Sadykhov, R.H.: New Approach to Hidden-surface Elimination of 3D Medical Images. Int. J. Machine Graphics and Vision, Vol.7, **4** (1998) 831-840

A 3d Puzzle for Learning Anatomy

Bernhard Preim[1], Felix Ritter[2], Oliver Deussen[2]

[1] MeVis gGmbH, Universitätsallee 29, 28359 Bremen, Germany
[2] Otto-von-Guericke-University of Magdeburg Dept. of Computer Science, Inst. for
Simulation and Graphics, Universitätsplatz 2, 39106 Magdeburg, Germany
email: bernhard@mevis.de, {deussen, fritter}@isg.cs.uni-magdeburg.de

Abstract. We present a new metaphor for learning anatomy - the 3d
puzzle. With this metaphor students learn anatomic relations by assembling a geometric model themselves. For this purpose, a 3d model is
enriched with docking positions which allow objects to be connected together. As complex 3d interactions are required to compose 3d objects,
sophisticated 3d visualization- and interaction techniques are included.
Among these techniques are shadow generation, 3d input devices, snapping mechanisms and collision detection.
The puzzle, similar to a computer game, can be operated at different levels. To simplify the task, a subset of the geometry, e.g. the skeleton, can
be correctly assembled initially. Moreover, textual information concerning the region of objects is provided, along with snapping mechanisms
to support the user. With this approach we expect to motivate students
to explore the spatial relations between parts of the human body.
Keywords: Anatomic atlas, metaphors for anatomy education, depth-
cues, 3d interaction, two-handed interaction

1 Introduction

The study of anatomy requires a deep understanding of the complex spatial relations inside the human body. With interactive 3d computer graphics, based on
high resolution geometric models, these spatial relations may be explored. To
exploit this potential, dedicated 3d interaction- and visualization techniques as
well as convincing metaphors have to be developed. To date, most of the available systems for learning anatomy are based on the atlas-metaphor: Students
explore geometric models and related textual information in a way inspired by
a (printed) atlas. The leading example is the Voxel-Man [2]; another more recent system is the Zoom Illustrator [8]. The atlas metaphor does not lend itself
to the development of 3d interaction techniques. Nevertheless 3d interaction is
provided to a certain extent. The Voxel-Man allows the user to rotate geometric
models, to place cutting planes and to cut holes. However, students are often
unaware of these possibilities.

Therefore it is particularly useful to structure the user interface on the basis of
a spatial metaphor and to provide tasks which necessarily include 3d interaction.
In this paper, we introduce the metaphor of a 3d puzzle for learning systems in
medicine: users compose geometric models from anatomic objects themselves.
This idea arose out of an empirical evaluation of the Zoom Illustrator with 12

medical doctors and students of medicine [6]. As part of a study of the usefulness of the available features, we asked what features they would like to see included in the system. Several students expressed a desire for more powerful 3d interaction.

To enable students to compose geometric models themselves, is a challenging task. Students must be able to sort geometric objects, to compose subsets before composing the whole model. Interaction- and visualization techniques which communicate depth relations play a key role in the usefulness of such a system.

2 Metaphors for the Composition of 3d Models

Interactive systems, especially new and unfamiliar applications, should be based on metaphors which help developers to structure the design and help users to handle the system. Metaphors should have their origin in daily life or in the work environment of the intended users.

The Construction-kit Metaphor. This wide-spread metaphor is used mainly in advanced CAD-systems. The design of cars, for example, is based on various CAD-models from different sources which are assembled into virtual prototypes using sophisticated 3d interaction techniques. An interesting variant was developed in the VLEGO-project [4]. Users take primitives, like LEGO-bricks, and combine them at discrete, predefined positions and angles. Dedicated 3d widgets are provided for all 3d interaction tasks: composition, separation, picking and copying. These 3d widgets can be handled with a 3d input device and for some interaction tasks a two-handed interaction is suggested.

The Metaphor of a 3d Puzzle. The construction kit-metaphor is well-known, and the 3d interaction techniques designed in the context of this metaphor are desirable for learning anatomy. However, building blocks in construction kits are not unique. In the learning context, we have unique parts which can be assembled in only one correct manner. Therefore a metaphor is required for the composition of complex models from unique elements.

A 3d puzzle is a familiar concept for this task and consequently the puzzle metaphor is more appropriate. This raises a question: which aspects of a 3d puzzle can and should (from a user's point of view) be realized? Moreover, we have to decide what we can offer over and above mimicking the metaphor. In a puzzle, a set of elementary objects should be composed. The shape of these objects gives an indication as to which parts belong together. When puzzling with dozens or even hundreds of objects several deposits (e.g. tables) are used to sort and compose subsets. Obviously, when puzzling one uses both hands and has all DOF of spatial interaction. In a puzzle, photos are provided to show how the final composed image (or 3d model) looks. These images motivate users and help them to perform the composition. Our design is guided by the metaphor of a 3d puzzle but differs in two major respects to real puzzles:

- Our system should support learning rather than provide entertainment.
- A computer system is restricted as to what can be achieved in real time but offers additional possibilities in that the computer "knows" how the model should be assembled.

To support learning, we have incorporated textual information about the objects of the puzzle. Objects have names, belong to regions and organ systems (e.g. an eye muscle) and have textual explanations as to their shape This information may be exploited in order to place objects in the right position. Since the system "knows" how the model is composed snapping mechanisms may be activated.

3   Interaction Tasks with a 3D Puzzle

In this section we describe the tasks which need to be accomplished in order to realize the metaphor of a 3d puzzle. Actually, there are two kinds of users:

- *authors* who prepare models (segment the model or refine an existing structure, define docking positions and assign related textual information) and
- *students* who use the information space provided by the author for the puzzle.

In this paper we restrict ourselves to describing how students explore the information space and assume that it is carefully defined by an author. For students some typical interaction tasks include:

Sort objects. The student must be able to create and manage subsets of the total set of objects. These subsets should be placed in separate viewers which can be named by the user. Within these viewers, 3d interaction is required to enable users to explore this subset. As not all viewers are visible at the same time, an overview about existing viewers is crucial.

Recognition of 3d objects. Two factors are crucial for the identification of objects: to be able to see an object from all viewing angles and to be able to inspect textual information as to spatial relations (e.g. name, description of shape). From our experience [7] we hypothesize that visual and textual information mutually reinforce one another in their effect upon the viewer.

Selection of 3d objects. The selection of 3d objects is the prerequisite for 3d interaction. Picking, typing the object name and the choice from a list of names are possible interaction techniques for this task.

Transformation of 3d objects. The transformation task includes translating and rotating 3d objects. As the objects are not deformable, transformations like shearing are irrelevant.

Camera control. In all viewers pan-and-zoom functionality is required to be able to recognize the shape of individual objects.

Docking of objects. The final goal of exploring, selecting and transforming a set of 3d objects is to assemble objects at the "right" docking positions. Less obvious is that objects sometimes have to be separated. For instance, if objects in deeper layers must be assembled first but have been forgotten, objects in the outer areas may have to be decomposed to allow objects to be placed inside.

4   Visualization of and Interaction with 3d data

A 3d puzzle requires precise interaction in 3d and thus the simulation of depth-cues and 3d interaction techniques similar to those in the real world. Humans perceive depth-relations particularly from the following depth-cues [10]:

- shadow,
- occlusion of objects,
- partial occlusion of semi-transparent objects,
- perspective foreshortening, and
- stereoscopic viewing.

Some of these depth-cues, such as occlusion and perspective foreshortening, are part of standard renderers and are implemented in hardware. Shadow generation is usually not supported. In an evaluation, Wanger et al. [9] demonstrated that shadow cast on a groundplane is the most important depth-cue for distance estimation and shape recognition. Therefore we developed a shadow viewer which enables the shadow projection on a groundplane. On graphics workstations with hardware-based alphablending, the display of semi-translucent objects and stereoscopic viewing is also feasible in real-time.

Interaction with 3d Data On the base of a comprehensible rendition of objects, 3d interaction is possible. The design of 3d interaction techniques must take into account how humans interact in the real world. The following aspects are essential for interaction in the real world:

Collision. When one object touches another, it is moved away or will be deformed. Under no circumstances can one object be moved through another without deformation.

Tactile feedback. When we grasp an object we perceive tactile feedback which enables us to adapt the pressure to the material and weight of the object.

Two-handed interaction. People tend to use both hands if they manipulate 3d objects. In medicine, two-handed interaction has been successfully applied e.g. for pre-operative planning in neurosurgery (see Hinckley in [1]). Hinckley argues that for the interaction tasks involved (e.g. defining cross-sections with cutting planes), the most intuitive handling can be achieved with two-handed 3d interaction where the dominant hand (usually the right hand) does fine-positioning relative to the non-dominant hand.

We regard collision detection as the most important aspect of 3d interaction. However, this is a challenging task if complex non-convex objects are involved. Fortunately, software for this purpose is now available. The system V-COLLIDE [3] accomplishes this task in a robust manner. Tactile feedback requires special hardware, such as data gloves or joysticks with force feedback. To avoid the overhead with an unfamiliar input-device, we have not integrated this technique.

5   The Realization of a 3d-Puzzle

The 3d puzzle incorporates the visualization and interaction techniques described in Section 4. In addition, some techniques from technical and medical illustration have been added to further improve the understanding of spatial relations. Our prototype is based on polygonal models (30.000 to 60.000 polygons segmented into 40 to 60 objects) acquired from Viewpoint Datalabs. The software is written in C++ using Open Inventor and Open GL.

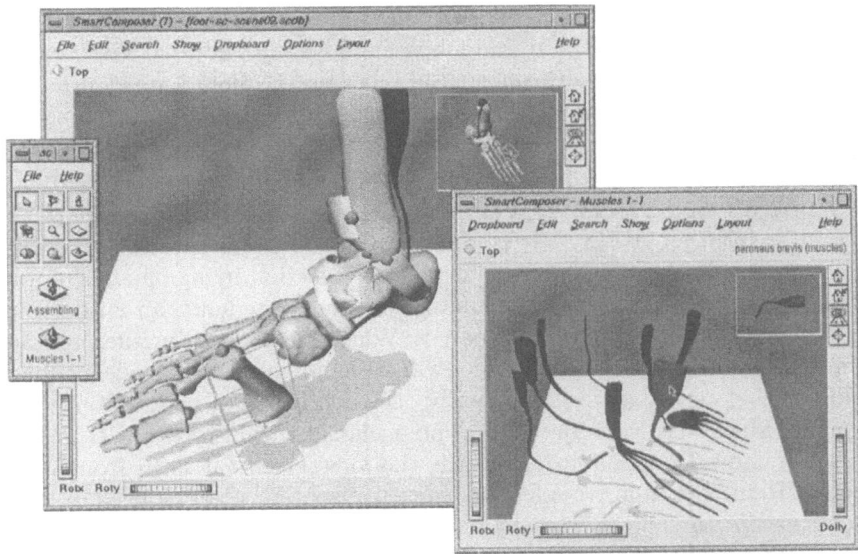

Fig. 1. In the left view sinews and bones are composed, while in the right view muscles are randomly scattered. The small panel on the left provides an overview on all viewers.

The puzzle starts with three views: the *final view* where the whole model is displayed, the *construction view* in which the user composes the model (starting from scratch or a subset of the model), and a *random view* in which objects which do not belong to the construction view are randomly scattered. The initial position of the objects is adjusted such that they do not overlap (see Fig. 1).

5.1   Realization of the Interaction Tasks

Sort objects. For the management of the objects, subsets can be created and attached to an unlimited number of 3d viewers. For this purpose a multiple selection of objects is possible. In addition, all objects in a region or an organ-system might be selected. The command "create view" opens a new viewer and moves all selected objects to this viewer while the relative position of the objects is preserved. An overview with icons for all viewers is presented to enable switching between the viewers (recall Fig. 1). While the final view is read-only, objects can be exchanged between the other views by drag-and-drop (objects may be dropped either in the viewers or the corresponding icon in the overview).

   Recognition of objects. To enable the recognition of objects, we developed a shadow viewer with a light groundplane. This plane is scaled such that all objects cast a shadow on it, even if the camera is rotated (the plane remains fix as it is used only for orientation). To further enhance the recognizability of an object, we provide a detailed view, like an inset in technical illustrations. If an object is selected it is presented in this view slightly enlarged without any object occluding it. It is rotated automatically to faciliate recognition.

In technical illustrations, exploded views are provided to improve the recognizability of objects. This technique is employed in the final view to enable users to become familiar with the spatial relations. Exploded views are realized by scaling down all objects at their original positions, thus leaving empty space. Stereorendering is realized as an extension of the Silicon Graphics X-Server and requires the use of shutter glasses to perceive the rendition as a stereo image.

Selection of objects. Selection by picking with a pointing-device is the interaction inspired by the real 3d puzzle. Picking is useful but limited to objects which are visible and recognizable. Therefore, selection by name and from a list are also provided. As typing long anatomic names is tedious, an auto-complete mechanism is employed to expand names. When one of these textual interaction techniques is used, the selected object will be highlighted to provide feedback. If the object belongs to a viewer currently occluded it is sent to the front to make it visible. Moreover, the object might be occluded within its view. If this is the case, it is moved continuously towards the viewer until it is in front of other objects. To further improve selection, semi-transparency can be used, so that all objects except the one selected by name are semi-translucent.

Transforming objects. For the transformation of 3d objects, manipulators (the trackball and the handlebox) from Open Inventor are used. These widgets can be operated with a 2d mouse. However, with a standard 2d mouse users tend to decompose 3d translations and rotations in sequential 2d translations. It is more effective to use several DOF simultaneously as in the real world. For this purpose a 3d space mouse is employed. Collision detection prevents objects from being moved through others. When objects collide they are highlighted for a moment to provide visual feedback. If the user continues to attempt to move an object through another one, an acoustic signal is initiated and textual output is provided in the status line We incorporated the above-mentioned software V-COLLIDE for collision detection. With a variety of acceleration techniques, including hierarchical decomposition of geometric models and bounding box tests, it is reasonably fast. V-COLLIDE provides an interface which allows us to control precisely for which objects the test is carried out.

Camera control. The virtual camera can be manipulated with the widgets provided by Open Inventor. Wheel-widgets make it possible to change azimuth- and declination angle and to zoom in and out. Camera control can be realized by two-handed interaction intuitively by simultaneously rotating and zooming.

Composing and separating objects. The composition is the most challenging task. Objects are composed correctly if the docking points (represented as spheres) touch each other. To ease this task, a snap-mechanism is included (see Fig. 2). With snapping enabled, objects snap together if their distance is below a threshold and no other docking point is in the vicinity. If docking points are very close to each other snapping does not help. In this case, the user may select the docking position to which the selected object should be attached. Once an object is correctly attached it is prevented that these objects are separated inadvertently. With a quick movement, however, separation is possible. Reverse snapping makes it difficult to attach an object to a wrong docking position.

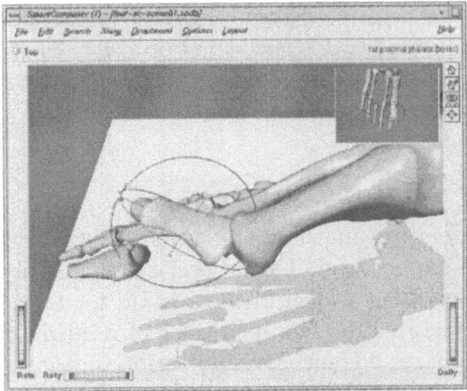

Fig. 2. A bone has been snapped at one docking point. The transformation is now restricted to the rotation to correctly orient this bone.

5.2   Two-handed Interaction

The 3d puzzle supports the simultaneous use of two input devices. The optimal configuration is a 3d mouse for 3d interaction and a 2d mouse for other interactions (selection from lists and the menu). For this purpose two cursors are provided; a 3d cursor for 3d interaction in addition to the usual cursor. People use their dominant hand (DH) for interaction with menus and dialogue boxes. Therefore the 2d mouse is usually operated with the DH while the 3d mouse is used with the non-dominant hand (NDH). The 3d mouse is mainly used for the orientation of the camera and the 3d objetcs - orientation tasks which are carried out with the NDH also in the real world. The use of two input devices prevents the user from distractive movements from the 3d viewers to other components of the user interface and vice versa. This separation of concerns is inspired by Leblanc [5]. Informal tests indicate that users have superior performance with this equipment compared to the standard pointing device.

5.3   Adapting the Level of Complexity

A learning system should be operable at different levels. Usually interactive systems should be as easy to operate as possible. However, with the 3d puzzle it should take some time to succeed because the time spent on solving this task is probably related to the learning success. On the other hand, users might become frustrated if it is too difficult to succeed. There are two strategies to adapt the level: to "scale" the task to be solved, and to provide support for solving the task. The easiest way to use the system is to watch the model being assembled in an animation, so the user has no task at all. The composition can be restricted to objects of certain categories (e.g. bones) and regions (e.g. eye muscles). The composition can be performed at two levels. At the beginners level, objects are rotated correctly when they are dropped to the construction view. The task is thus restricted to the correct translation of the object. The display of textual information for a selected object (e.g. Musculus procerus, eye muscle) and the mechanisms for snapping and reverse snapping (recall Section 5.1) provide support for the puzzle.

6 Summary

We presented a system for anatomy education based on the metaphor of a 3d puzzle. With this metaphor users have a precise task involving spatial relations. The puzzling task provides a level of motivation for learning which is hard to achieve with other metaphors. The metaphor of a 3d puzzle guided our design and led us to incorporate advanced visualization and interaction techniques to enable students to compose 3d models. Different levels are provided to acommodate users with different capabilities. The development of our system has been accompanied by informal usability tests which yielded promising results. We intend to perform a rigorous usability test. In particular, the use of two-handed interaction, the snapping mechanisms and the different levels will be evaluated. With regard to the interaction, tactile feedback offers great promise as an addition to collision detection.

References

1. Hinckley, K. (1997): Haptic Issues for Virtual Manipulation, PhD-thesis, University of Virginia
2. Höhne, K.-H., B. Pflesser, A. Pommert et al. (1996): "A Virtual Body Model for Surgical Education and Rehearsal", Computer - Innovative Technology for Professionals, January, 25-31
3. Hudson, T.C., M.C. Lin, J. Cohen, S. Gottschalk and D. Manocha (1997): "V-COLLIDE: Accelerated Collision Detection with VRML", Proc. of VRML
4. Kiyokawa, K., H. Takemura, Y. Katayama, H. Iwasa and N. Yokoya (1997): "VLEGO: A Simple Two-handed Modeling Environment Based On Toy Block", In Proc. of VRST '97, 27-34, ACM, New York
5. LeBlanc, A., P. Kalra, N. Magenat-Thalmann and D. Thalmann (1991): "Sculpting with the 'ball and mouse' metaphor", Proc. of Graphics Interface, 152-159
6. Pitt, I., B. Preim and S. Schlechtweg (1999): "Evaluation of Interaction Techniques for the Exploration of Complex Spatial Phenomena", Proc. of Softwareergonomie '99, 275-286
7. Preim, B. (1998): Interaktive Illustrationen und Animationen zur Erklärung komplexer räumlicher Zusammenhänge, PhD-thesis, Otto-von-Guericke-University of Magdeburg
8. Preim, B., A. Ritter and Th. Strothotte (1996): "Illustrating Anatomic Models - A Semi-Interactive Approach", Proc. of Visualization in Biomedical Computing, Springer publishing company, Lecture Notes in Computer Science, Vol. 1131, 23-32
9. Wanger, L., J. Ferwerda and D. Greenberg (1992): "Perceiving Spatial Relationships in Computer-Generated Images", IEEE Computer Graphics and Applications, Volume 12 (3), 44-58
10. Zhai, S., W. Buxton and P. Milgram (1996): "The partial occlusion effect: utilizing semi-transparency in 3D human computer interaction", ACM Transactions on HCI, Vol. 3 (3), 254-284

3D Functional Database of Subcortical Structures for Surgical Guidance in Image Guided Stereotactic Neurosurgery

K.W. Finnis[1], Y.P. Starreveld[1,2], A.G. Parrent[2], A.F. Sadikot[3], and T.M. Peters[1]

[1] John P. Roberts Research Institute, University of Western Ontario,
Box 5015, 100 Perth Drive, London ON N6A 5K8, Canada
[2] London Health Sciences Center, London, ON Canada
[3] Montreal Neurological Institute, Montréal, QC, Canada
kfinnis@irus.rri.on.ca

Abstract. Current techniques for deep brain stereotactic neurosurgery require identification of targets by preoperative imaging localization. Many critical structures targeted in this way (the thalamic nuclei) are functionally distinct but not discernable on magnetic resonance images. These structures are also surrounded by critical brain areas which must not be damaged by the surgical procedure. These factors make accurate localization of lesion targets crucial. Digitized anatomical atlases derived from histochemically stained brain specimens registered to patient MRI datasets aid in delineating targets but accuracy of registration within-homogeneous anatomy remains questionable. To address this problem, we have designed a searchable and expandable database of functional organization for the sensorimotor thalamus, internal capsule, and internal pallidum from a population of patients (n=40). Data were obtained through microcellular recording, microstimulation, and macrostimulation mapping performed during stereotactic thalamotomies and pallidotomies. After registration of the database into standard stereotactic space, clustering of like physiological responses was noted in the internal capsule and sensorimotor thalamus and an articulated joint-based organization was observed in the internal pallidum. Furthermore, a clear delineation of the kinesthetic-paresthetic functional border was observed within the thalamus. When registered to a patient MRI within our image guided visualization platform, the database provides a visual representation of deep brain functional organization facilitating physiological exploration and preoperative planning.

1 Introduction

1.1 Surgical Procedure and Target Localization

The main surgical procedure for Parkinson's Disease (PD) involves stereotactic localization and lesioning of discreet areas within the midbrain. For over 50 years now, stereotactic thalamotomy for relief of contralateral tremor has been the primary surgical treatment for parkinsonian tremor [1][2]. In this procedure, the Ventralis intermedius (Vim) nucleus of the thalamus is lesioned via leukotome lesioning or radiofrequency thermocoagulation. Lesioning of this motor nucleus eliminates the excessive and abnormal activity associated with it in the parkinsonian state and as a result, tremor is alleviated. Pallidotomy, or lesioning of the globus pallidus internus(GPi), was first performed 40 years ago with a resurgence in interest over the last 10 years. Lesioning the GPi has proven to greatly reduce contralateral limb rigidity and the accompanying dyskinesias associated with PD[1][2][3]. Currently, the posteroventral aspect of the GPi and the Vim nucleus of the thalamus constitute the desired targets for pallidotomy and thalamotomy respectively at both the Montreal Neurological Institute (MNI) and the London Health Sciences Center (LHSC).

Target localization is based upon preoperative magnetic resonance imaging. A stereotactic head frame equipped with fiducial markers filled with copper sulfate solution is rigidly affixed to the patient's skull prior to scanning. The fiducial markers are visible on the resulting MRI images and provide the neurosurgeon with a reference for calculation of a frame-to-MRI coordinate transformation. An arc system mounted on top of the frame provides a means of attaching and orienting surgical tools during the procedure while a small hole drilled through the skull provides access to the calculated target structure coordinates. Since this is an arc-centered system, once the depth of the surgical tool is locked into position, trajectory angles may change while the tip of the tool remains on target.

The benefits of electrophysiological confirmation for radiographical localization have been demonstrated in the past by several investigators [1][4][5]. Electrophysiological exploration helps localize the target by locating characteristic firing patterns. Surgeons may also appreciate and adjust for the inherent distortion found in the patient MRI due to field inhomogeneities using the results of exploration. As described below, three different electrophysiological methods are employed during this procedure: microcellular recording (LHSC), microstimulation (LHSC), and macrostimulation (LHSC, MNI). Each method is used to locate and map the specific somatotopic organization within deep brain anatomy.

1.2 Microcellular Recording

Mapping deep brain structures with microcellular recording electrodes identifies neurons that produce characteristic firing patterns in response to specific stimuli. Kinesthetic neurons are cells which respond to movement around articulated joints and are detected by sharp excitation or inhibition of firing rates in the presence of joint movement. Only those joints which exist within the somatotopic domain of that kinesthetic neuron evoke cell firing[5][6]. Tactile neurons are cells which are activated by light touch to skin within their receptive field. When the receptive field of a tactile neuron is touched, rapid cell firing of that neuron is produced. Typically, a neurosurgeon introduces a recording electrode into the thalamus or GPi to record neuronal firing patterns both deep and superficial to the target coordinate along each trajectory. In the case of a thalamotomy, kinesthetic neurons are detected throughout the Vim until the functional border between the Vim and the Ventral caudal (Vc) sensory nucleus, is traversed. When kinesthetic neurons are encountered along a trajectory, electrode depth and the stimuli which evoked the neuronal response are catalogued by the surgeon in the surgical log. Since thalamic nuclei are somatotopically organized[4][6], every data point collected aids the surgeon in mentally reconstructing the somatotopic organization contained within that nucleus, and in establishing the functional borders which separate them. During a pallidotomy, microcellular recording is performed in much the same way although pure sensory neurons are not present in this area of the brain. The somatotopic organization of the GPi has previously been described, based on a small patient sample, as kinesthetic joint-based with only partial somatotopy observable[7].

A distinct benefit of using microcellular recording is its ability to precisely locate tremor cells[8]. Tremor cells, a term coined by Guiot et al. in the early sixties, refer to neurons which fire in synchrony with patient tremor, typically in the range of 3 to 5 Hz in PD. Subsequent macrostimulation within regions containing tremor cells usually abates or arrests all signs of physiologic tremor contralaterally.

1.3   Microstimulation

By introducing a small electrical current within a discreet area of brain, neuronal membranes will depolarize beyond threshold resulting in cell excitation. When microstimulation supplies enough current to reach neuronal threshold and excite a small pool of neurons, the effects of stimulation are immediately demonstrated by the fully aware patient, usually in the form of paresthesias or muscle contractions. During thalamotomies, it has been demonstrated that microstimulation within the Vim do not induce muscle contractions, although on rare occasions, a sensation of movement within stationary limbs may be induced[4]. Responses are reported by patients immediately after the sensory Vc nucleus of the thalamus is stimulated at suprathreshold levels. The Vc receives afferents primarily from the spinothalamic tract relaying information pertaining to temperature, vibration, superficial sensation and pain pathways. Typical patient descriptions after stimulation within the Vc nucleus include tingling, electrical, or pins and needles and may range from a localized pleasant numbness to occasional sharp pain or burning sensations. Direct control over stimulation current by the surgeon enables determination of neuronal thresholds and control of the extent of stimulation influence within the brain tissue. All verbal responses provided by the patient are entered into the surgical log with microelectrode depth and amount of current which evoked the response. Microstimulation confirms the functional border between the Vim nucleus (no response) and its caudal neighbor the Vc nucleus (induced paresthesia) in the sagittal plane parallel to the probe trajectory. Microstimulation is incorporated into the pallidotomy procedure to test for proximity of the optic tract and in establishing the border between the internal capsule and the GPi. Patients experience visual phenomena such as homonymous scotoma or phosphenes during optic tract stimulation and demonstrate contractions of muscles during capsular stimulation.

1.4   Macrostimulation

Macrostimulation introduces higher voltages into the brain through the nonin-
sulated tip of the stimulation electrode. Macrostimulation commonly ranges in
frequency from 60 to 200H with the surgeon in control of the voltage introduced
into the brain (usually between 0.25 and 4V). Application of increasing voltage
includes more neurons in the activated pool and obvious patient responses may
be elicited. Macrostimulation is the method of choice at the MNI for mapping
both motor responses obtained in the internal capsule for use as physiological
landmarks and for evoking paresthetic responses within the Vc. Macrostimulation is also quite effective in demonstrating reversible lesions within an area
of the Vim. When high frequency stimulation is applied to a pool of tremor
cells, for example, these neurons cease firing and tremor arrest occurs within
the body parts localized in that somatotopic area[9]. Once stimulation subsides,
physiological function returns to prior levels.

1.5   Anatomical Atlases

In order to facilitate identification of invisible anatomical targets, stereotactic anatomical maps created from stained sections of postmortem brains are
often consulted. The Schaltenbrand Wahren atlas[10] is based on stained postmortem brain slices which clearly display thalamic nuclear borders and surrounding structures. This atlas presents slices in sagittal, coronal, and axial planes and
is frequently used in preoperative planning. Several groups, including the MNI,
have digitized the Schaltenbrand Wahren atlas for superposition over patient
MRI to aid in surgical planning and for intraoperative guidance[11][12]. While
this has proven to be a beneficial addition to the surgical environment, several
caveats should be addressed. Each series of brain slices contained within the
Schaltenbrand Wahren atlas were created from separate cadaver brain hemispheres. Digitizing and concatenating a slice series into a 3D volume will create
an atlas representative of a single individual brain and not the general population. Varying interslice distances contained in the Schaltenbrand atlas results
in the digitized atlas displaying jagged edges when viewed in planes orthogonal to the original slice. A smoothing operation is usually performed on the 3D
volume. Due to intrinsic limitations within the anatomical atlases themselves,
nonlinear registration and superposition over patient MRI provide only a close
approximation of target loci.

1.6   Goals and Clinical Motivation

It is impossible to explore and map the functional organization of large portions of midbrain during a single stereotactic procedure. Surgeons must mentally reconstruct somatotopic organization sometimes based on as few as one
exploratory trajectory alone within a single plane. In order to fully appreciate
the functional organization within deep brain structures, complete functional

maps would have to be created from whole individual brains. As this is not feasible, we must compromise by constructing a map of midbrain function based on multiple brains. It was our goal to combine intraoperatively derived functional data from a large population of movement disorder patients for compilation into a database of function with the following attributes. It must

- be capable of nonlinearly warping to match any patient MRI volume compensating for anatomical variability in three-dimensions;
- be fully searchable via an interactive database search engine;
- contain detailed somatotopic information relevant to Parkinson's Disease and movement disorder neurosurgery;
- possess compatibility with the image guided visualization platform currently under development at the RRI;
- allow integration of new patient data and new anatomical structures into the database with minimal user intervention, and
- present data in a manner interpreted easily by any user.

A functional database satisfying these criteria has the potential to facilitate preoperative planning of electrode trajectories and act as a somatotopic reference during the surgical procedure.

2   Method

2.1   Data Collection

All surgical procedures included in this study consisted of patients receiving left or right pallidotomies or thalamotomies involving mechanical lesion, leukotome (MNI)[11], RF lesioning (LHSC) or deep brain stimulator insertion (MNI, LHSC). Patients ranged from 25 to 75 years of age and included both Parkinson's Disease patients and essential tremor patients. In order to create a database of function representative of a specific population, certain patient exclusion criteria were necessary. Patients in the study did not have space occupying brain masses prior to or at time of surgery or other pathologies which might distort somatotopy. The inherent plasticity of the brain allows reorganization when afferent information is suddenly removed. Any patients with a physical condition that might alter the functional organization of their brain, such as an amputation or congenital anomaly, were also excluded. Patient verbal response provides a large proportion of data included in this atlas. Those patients deemed not fully coherent or totally aware of the procedure they were experiencing were excluded. Patients undergoing treatment for tremor resulting from other pathological origin such as trauma induced tremor, or multiple sclerosis were also excluded.

2.2   Standardizing Physiological Responses

A protocol was developed to encode for all possible sensory or motor responses elicited at different stimulation voltages or locations. After designing a subdivided model based on Tasker's anatomical model for physiological data[4], anatomical numbers can be assigned to discreet areas of the body. To encode for sensory responses, we developed a list of response codes which could successfully describe every response produced by the 40 patients using stimulation and microcellular recording. All patients and each exploratory trajectory performed for that patient were assigned an identification number for inclusion into a tag code containing all pertinent information. All tag codes are of the format: patientID#_trajectory#_method_bodyside_bodypart#_responsecode

For example, patient 12 felt a weak tingling sensation at the tip of his third digit, left hand during macrostimulation at 0.25V on trajectory 1. This response would be encoded as: 012_1_0.25V_L_66_PTw . This coding method was designed so an experienced user could tell at a glance, after searching the database, the patient origin of the data tag, which physiological method was used at what parameters, the side of the body eliciting the response, area of the body, and the evoked response. Tag codes of this nature make it possible to design highly flexible database search engines which search for any field or combination of fields within the tag code. In order to plot these codes onto the appropriate anatomical area of the patient MRI in three-dimensional space, images must be registered to the coordinate system defined by the stereotactic head frame. Registration may be performed manually by identifying the frame-based fiducial markers within 10 axial images then calculating a rigid transformation from MRI space to frame space or automatically using the frame finder aspect of our visualization platform.

When all codes for a particular patient are tagged to their respective MRI at appropriate coordinates, they are transformed into standard stereotactic space and added to the collective somatotopy. Interpatient similarities may then be analyzed.

2.3   Nonlinear Warp Algorithm

Nonlinear transformation matrices for each patient were calculated which accurately describe the warp from native MRI patient space to our high resolution reference brain in standard stereotactic space. This nonlinear transformation matrix was calculated for each patient using ANIMAL (Automatic Nonlinear Image Matching and Anatomical Labelling)[13], a nonlinear deformation algorithm that requires no user intervention or identification of homologous landmarks. Registration of the patient to the reference brain is accomplished by ANIMAL in two optimization steps: a linear component through automatic estimation of the best affine transformation matrix between the two volumes, and a nonlinear component, achieved through a hierarchial multi-scale, multi- resolution strategy. The end result is a nonlinear transformation matrix which maps the anatomy of the patient brain onto the anatomy of the reference brain. Each unique transformation matrix was used to resample the original patient data codes tagged onto their respective MRI s into reference brain stereotactic space. Inversion of a patient's nonlinear transformation and subsequent resampling of the functional atlas with this inverted matrix will transform all database codes into that patient's native MRI space.

2.4   Searchable Database

The usefulness of the database was maximized by permitting searches through every code for any combination of tag fields. A search engine was written using a scripting language, Python, that is compatible with the source code of the vtk/Python based image guided neurosurgical program under development at the RRI. We have incorporated an interactive query facility into this visualization platform to allow direct access to database entries. A digitized and segmented image of the anatomical model with point-and-click functionality linked to the database allow data codes pertinent to anatomy selected by the user to be extracted.

3   Results

We show here the results of some representative database searches displayed over the reference brain which provides information pertinent to PD surgery for surgical planning or intraoperative guidance. Since statistical significance of an atlas of this nature will increase with the number of patients added, most examples are taken from the left thalamotomy database currently containing the most patients. Functional data contained within the database is quite specific and encompasses a small area of midbrain. Prior to lesioning in a thalamotomy case, a neurosurgeon attempts to detect tremor cells located in the kinesthetic area of the thalamus using microelectrode recording. When tremor cells are detected within the suspected Vim region and the surrounding area sufficiently mapped, a lesion protocol is determined. Figure 1 shows a clustering of tremor cells in reference brain space that were detected in thalamotomy patients during microcellular recording. Once these data points are nonlinearly warped to a patient preoperative MRI, the surgeon may use these data as a predictor of tremor cell location and plan trajectories accordingly.

A functional border between kinesthetic cells detected via microcellular recording and sensory cells detected through microstimulation was observed (Figure 2, left). In agreement with the literature, kinesthetic cells lie anteriorly and slightly superior to the sensory neurons within the predicted Vc region. Note the delineation of a functional border where the two data types meet and slightly overlap. The asterisk indicates a trajectory which was determined intraoperatively as too posterior. Subsequent exploration within that patient was moved anteriorly based on the functional information provided by that trajectory.

We have gathered electrophysiological data bilaterally for the GPi. All neurons detected within the GPi were kinesthetic however a greater number of data codes have to be collected before displaying a clustered visualization. Outside of the GPi, clustering was noted around the optic tract located deep to the inferior GPi border (Figure 2, right). Responses surrounding the optic tract were from three patients who experienced visual phenomena in the form of flashing white lights during microstimulation.

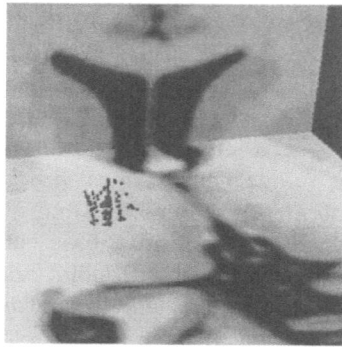

Fig. 1. Tremor cells (red spheres) located through microcellular recording during 12 different left thalamotomies.

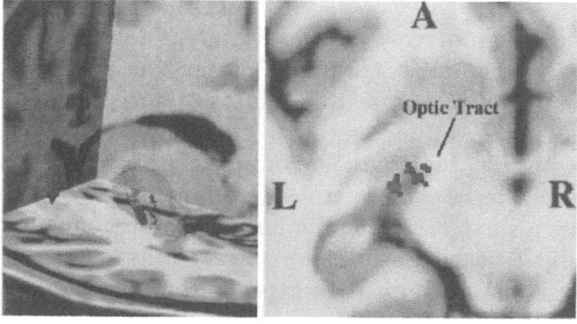

Fig. 2. Left:Functional border between Vim area (light blue spheres) and the Vc sensory area (red spheres). Surface rendered thalamus also shown in green. Right: Axial plane showing locations where microstimulation evoked visual phenomena during 7 different left pallidotomies. L=left, R=right, A=anterior

4 Discussion

Functional data superimposed within patient MRIs will have many applications. Preoperative planning will be facilitated through comparison of predicted lesion targets obtained through MRI localization with data provided by the database. Studies have shown that due to anatomical variability, the site of actual lesions can vary up to 5mm from the original MRI based target site[1]. A functional atlas with nonlinear warping capabilities will accommodate the large variation of anatomical structures throughout a population and greatly assist target localization. Intraoperatively, patient responses evoked through electrophysiological exploration may be compared directly with the functional database as they occur. Direct consultation and comparison with the database will help the surgeon confirm location of the electrode tip within that patient's anatomy.

A probability database like this has the advantage that data points may easily be validated when added through simple comparison with existing points. All data, archived or current, are obtained through actual physiological mapping of human brain, and once coded require no further analysis prior to inclusion into the database. Following the addition of archived electrophysiological data from previous patients, a series of validations will be performed. Intraoperative validation will assess its predictive value during surgical guidance. Comparative studies will be possible for contrasting the functional organization displayed by the database with print atlases of function like Emmers and Tasker's physiological maps[14]. Data will be analyzed to elucidate the medial to lateral representation of the human body within thalamic nuclei at the finest resolution possible. Results of this analysis will be compared and contrasted with Hassler's map of thalamic homuncular organization[15]. Further elucidation of joint-based somatotopy observed within the pallidum will also be investigated. Plans for inclusion of other surgically relevant structures, the subthalamic nuclei for example, will be realized when data becomes available.

Ultimately, clustered population data representing one response type for a discrete area of the body will be displayed as a 3D fuzzy region of probability within the reference brain. This probability region will indicate an area of anatomy that, when explored electrophysiologically, would likely produce a specific response. The strength of prediction will be dependent on the amount of data the region represents and how tightly the population responses cluster around the centroid of the fuzzy region.

In addition, this database could prove useful for surgical training once fully integrated into RRI's surgical guidance program. Full three-dimensional appreciation of a very complex structure like a homunculus can be difficult to visualize from standard textbook images. Surgical residents would be provided with a unique and novel representation of three-dimensional somatotopic organization to increase their understanding of functional stereotactic procedures.

5 Conclusions

We have developed a robust and novel method to display intraoperatively derived functional data from a large population of patients within the space of one standard brain. Our method demonstrates delineation of functional borders within the thalamus and identifies high probability tremor areas. The resulting database contains all physiological responses recorded during 40 stereotactic procedures after standardization with comprehensive anatomical models and response codes. Nonlinearly warping data into native patient MRI space using the inverse nonlinear transform permits simultaneous display of physiological maps from several stereotactic procedures on different patients within the space of a patient's MRI data-set. Displaying physiological responses in this fashion allows real time comparison of the functional atlas with responses obtained during intraoperative stimulation and can facilitate preoperative planning.

References

1. Iacono R.P., Henderson J.M., Lonser R.R.: Combined stereotactic thalamotomy and posteroventral pallidotomy for Parkinson's Disease. *Journal of Image Guided Neurosurgery* **1**:133-140, 1995
2. Speelman J.D., Bosch D.A.: Resurgence of functional neurosurgery for Parkinson's Disease: A historical perspective. *Movement Disorders* **13(3)**:582-588, 1998
3. Narabayashi H.: Pallidotomy revisited. Analysis of posteroventral pallidotomy. *Stereotactic and Functional Neurosurgery* **69(1-4 Pt.2)**:54-61, 1997
4. Tasker R.R., Organ L.W., Hawrylyshyn P.A.: *The Thalamus and Midbrain of Man*, C.C. Thomas Publisher, Springfield, Illinois, USA. 1982
5. Keller T.M., Tcheng T.K., Burkhard P.R. Richard H., Tamas L.B.: Stereotactically guided thalamotomy for treatment of parkinsonian tremor isolated to the lower extremity. *Journal of Neurosurgery* **89**:314-316, 1998
6. Honda S., Seike M., Nishimura H., Kurisaka M., Mori K.: The distribution fields of sensory neurons in the human thalamus. *Stereotactic and Functional Neurosurgery* **67**:218-230, 1996-97
7. Lozano A., Hutchinson W., Kiss Z., Tasker R., Davis K., Dostrovsky J.: Methods for microelectrode-guided posteroventral pallidotomy. *Journal ofNeurosurgery* **84(2)**:194-202, 1996
8. Guiot G., Hardy J., Albe-Fessard D.: Delimitation precise des structures sous-corticales et identification des noyaux thalamiques chez l'homme par l'electorphysiologie stereotaxique. *Neurochirugia* **5**:1-18, 1962
9. Benabid A.L., Benazzouz A., Hoffmann D., Limousin P., Krack P., Pollak P.: Long-term electrical inhibition of deep brain targets in movement disorders. *Movement Disorders* **13(Suppl3)**:119-125, 1998
10. Schaltenbrand G., Wahren W.: *Atlas for Stereotaxy of the Human Brain*. Stuttgart: Georg Thieme Verlag. 1977
11. St-Jean P., Sadikot A.F., Collins L., Clonda D., Kasrai R., Evans A.C.: Automated atlas integration and interactive three-dimensional visualization tools for planning and guidance in functional neurosurgery. *IEEE Transactions on Medical Imaging* **17(5)**:672-680, 1998
12. Nowinski W.L., Fang A., Nguyen B.T., Raphel J.K., Jagannathan L., Raghavan R., Bryan R.N., Miller G.A.: Multiple brain atlas database and atlas-based neuroimaging system. *Computer Aided Surgery* **2**:42-66, 1997
13. Collins D.L., Holmes C.J., Peters T.M., Evans A.C.: Automatic 3-D model-based neuroanatomical segmentation. *Human Brain Mapping* **3**:190-208, 1995
14. Emmers R., Tasker R.R. *The Human Somesthetic Thalamus*. Raven Press, New York, 1975
15. Hassler R.: Architectonic organization of the thalamic nuclei.: *In* G. Schaltenbrand, A.E. Walker(eds): *Stereotaxy of the Human Brain*. Stuttgart: Thieme, 1982

Automated Registration of Ultrasound with CT Images: Application to Computer Assisted Prostate Radiotherapy and Orthopedics

Gelu Ionescu, PhD., Stéphane Lavallée, PhD., Jacques Demongeot, MD., PhD.

TIMC Laboratory, University Joseph Fourier, Grenoble France
gelu.ionescu@imag.fr

Abstract. Ultrasound (US) imaging could potentially play a major role in the field of Computer Assisted Surgery (CAS). For doctors and surgeons to make full use of CAS tools in planning and executing surgical operations, they also need user-friendly automatic software based on fast, precise and reliable registration algorithms. The main goal of this paper is to take advantage of the segmentation/registration duality to extract the relevant information from US images. This information will allow the precise and automatic registration of anatomical structures contained in the pre-operative model and of intra-operative data contained in US images. The result of registration will be further used to guide a computer-assisted intervention such as orthopedics or radiotherapy.

1 Introduction

Among the various imaging techniques available, $2D$ echography is becoming more and more important, both for the diagnostic purposes and registration in CAS applications. In this paper, we will consider the latter case, with the specific instance of Computer Assisted Orthopedics Applications [1, 2] and patient positioning in prostate radiotherapy [3]. In spite of the problems inherent to US imaging such as low signal-to-noise ratio and the fact that the images depend on the angle and the texture of the target anatomy, this modality has become very popular among practitioners mainly because of its safety, low cost and non-invasiveness.

Since external radiotherapy makes use of the properties of $X - rays$ to destroy live tissue, the precise localization of the tumor is extremely important in order to avoid the destruction of neighboring healthy tissues. As described in details in [4], in the context of isocentric technique applied to radiotherapy, the procedure for repositioning must ensure that the center of the tumor localized by the practitioner in the pre-operative model, coincides with the center of rotation of the radiation device. For the intra-operative data acquisition, we are interested particularly in the transpubic way to realize the US examination of the prostate. The goal of the registration is to realize an automatic orientation of the external $X - ray$ beams according to a predetermined dosimetry plan. The results presented here were obtained on patients. In orthopedic applications, a high precision is also required in order to respect the planning established by the surgeon. Our aim is either to place a screw in a pedicle vertebra [2], or to insert percutaneously screws in the sacro-iliac bone [1,5]. In both cases, the goal is to realize a minimally invasive operation. To demonstrate the feasibility of the method, we worked, for the first application, on a plastic vertebra immersed in water, for the second application tests were performed on a cadaver.

In this paper, we present an automatic, reliable and precise method that can be used in soft tissues (e.g. abdominal cavity) as well as in hard tissues (e.g. bone, cartilage). The medical imagings we focus mainly on, are computed tomography (CT) and US imaging. The former is used to build the pre-operative $3D$ model and the latter to acquire the $3D$ intra-operative data volume.

2   Related Work

The general problem of registration between a set of $3D$ data points and a $3D$ model was treated in [6,7]. In this paper, we consider a $3D$ model made from a set of CT slices. This approach has been discussed in [2,5] for various applications. The methods known in the literature is based on the segmentation of the surface S of an anatomical structure on CT images. This is followed by a manual segmentation of pieces of contours corresponding to this same structure on US images. Each US image being located in the intra-operative reference frame by using an external optical localization device, one obtains an image of points belonging to the surface of the reference structure. The rigid registration of $3D$ points with the surface S starting from an initial position is described in various papers [7–9]. Unfortunately none of the existing segmentation procedure of US images is automatic, precise and robust. Here we propose a method featuring these characteristics [10].

Grey-level Approach. The most obvious method, as often used in registration, would be to register directly CT images with US images without going through segmentation. For images originating from the same modality, one could use methods based on maximization of correlation, confinement tree [11]. For images of different nature, optimization based on mutual information could be used [12]. For a given initial registration T_0, for each US image in a given position, one can calculate the slice corresponding to the echographical plane in the volume of CT images but the calculation of reformatted slices is very time consuming [10]. For this reason an approach based on the use of contours seemed preferable.

Contour Approach. As a starting point, the $3D$ model is assumed to be both segmented and labeled. To achieve this it is of course possible to use semi-interactive procedures since the model is constructed before the operation. In general, one segments contours on $2D$ slices. These are then interpolated to create a homogeneous $3D$ surface using the shape-based interpolation algorithm described in [13,10]. Although many registration/$3D$ labeling procedures are described in the literature, those based on elastic registration of a model (Atlas like) seem the most promising ones [14]. The segmentation/registration duality was discussed previously in different context. Hamadeh [15] proposed to register the $3D$ model of a segmented vertebra on CT images with intra-operative $X - ray$ of the same vertebra. Mangin [16] proposed a two-step registration of Positron Emission Tomography and CT images of the brain while recently Geraud [17] proposed a progressive approach using Atlas-type models to segment the Magnetic Resonance images of the brain. Our approach, as in the above cited works, is based on the segmentation/registration duality, its specificities are that we rely on US imaging and that we propose an original mechanism for segmentation, guided by the model. As in the method based on gray-levels, we propose to generate pseudo US images, however, we strictly limit ourselves to the contours of structures segmented in the model. This is equivalent to considering only the specular reflection and to neglect all other phenomena. This approach is detailed in the following sections.

3   Methods

The method we have proposed consists of three stages, the first consists of a low-level segmentation of a sequence of US images. The second stage exploits the *segmentation/registration* duality to extract relevant contours obtained in the previous step. The last step consists of the final rigid registration of these relevant contours and the pre-operative model.

3.1   Intra-operative Data Acquisition

Images are taken from an US imager. The US probe is localized in $3D$ space by an optical localizer. The US image is calibrated according to a technique described in [10]. In this way, the position of an image pixel is known in $3D$ space with a precision in the range of localizer accuracy (about $1\,mm$).

3.2   Low-level Segmentation

By low-level segmentation, we mean classical image segmentation techniques based mainly on linear filtering or mathematical morphology. At the end of this stage, the images are generally over-segmented (presence of false positives) [18] and the contours are not labeled. In this work, we choose the watershed as the segmentation technique. The main advantages of watershed segmentation relative to methods based on filtering [19] are the following: the watershed always contains some segments placed correctly on the real contours, the resulting contours are closed, detection of multiple junctions is very insensitive to noise and the algorithm is based on the modulus of the gradient $\|\nabla I\|$ of the image (the direction of the gradient is ignored).

To eliminate undesirable effects produced by the speckle on the complexity of the watershed, the original image is filtered by a recursive Canny-Deriche filter [20]. The width of this filter is chosen in an empirical way but it remains unchanged for the processing of the whole sequence of images. Furthermore, we observed that the filter width does not change significantly from one patient to the next. For the test-patient used for the prostatic application, the parameter for the Canny-Deriche filter is $\alpha = 0.2$. The result of this first step presented in Fig. 1.e shows two false watershed segments going through the bladder/prostate structure and the right iliac bone. One notes immediately that the prostate is well isolated which demonstrates that the use of watershed is completely realistic. At this stage, the processing is specific to the structure that needs to be detected.

3.3   High-level Segmentation

At this stage, we assume the availability of a set of M initial attitudes $T_i (i = 1, M)$, relating the echographical data and the CT model. Each initial attitude T_i is applied to each of the N echo slices. One then obtains M possible intersections between each echo plane and the dense cluster of points representing the surface of the model. In order to increase the resolution for the exploration of the volume of the model, to each initial attitude T_i, one associates six additional transformations $\Delta T_j (j = 0, 6)$ which slightly displace the image plane as presented in Fig. 2.a. In this scenario, we voluntarily neglected the displacements inside the image plane since these could be compensated by the $2D/2D$ elastic registration described in this section.

For each combination $(T_i, \Delta T_j)$, we keep the model points which lie within the thickness of the US beam ($\simeq 2\,mm$). We then perform an elastic multi-level $2D/2D$ registration between the simulated echo slice and the real echo slice. As described hereinafter, we minimize an expression of the form:

$$\varepsilon = \sum_{i=1}^{N} dist_{2D} \left(Q_j, T_p(P_i) \right)_{i=1,M} \tag{1}$$

where P_i is the set of N simulated echo points, Q_j is the set of M real echo points and T_p is the elastic $2D$ transformation relative to the parameter vector p we are looking for.

In order to give to the registration process the necessary elasticity, we associate to the image a regular network, the nodes of which can be individually adjusted. A displacement vector $(V_x, V_y)^\tau$ is associated to each node as presented in Fig. 2.b. The global transformation T_p we are looking for is parameterized by the vector p:

$$p = \left(\alpha, t_x, t_y; (V_x, V_y)^\tau_{0,0}, \cdots, (V_x, V_y)^\tau_{i,j}, \cdots, (V_x, V_y)^\tau_{I_x, I_y} \right)^\tau \tag{2}$$

where τ means transposition, (I_x, I_y) is the network dimension, $(\alpha, t_x, t_y)^\tau$ is the purely rigid component and $\left((V_x, V_y)^\tau_{0,0}, \cdots, (V_x, V_y)^\tau_{i,j}, \cdots, (V_x, V_y)^\tau_{I_x, I_y} \right)^\tau$ is the purely elastic component of the transformation T_p. To determine the vector

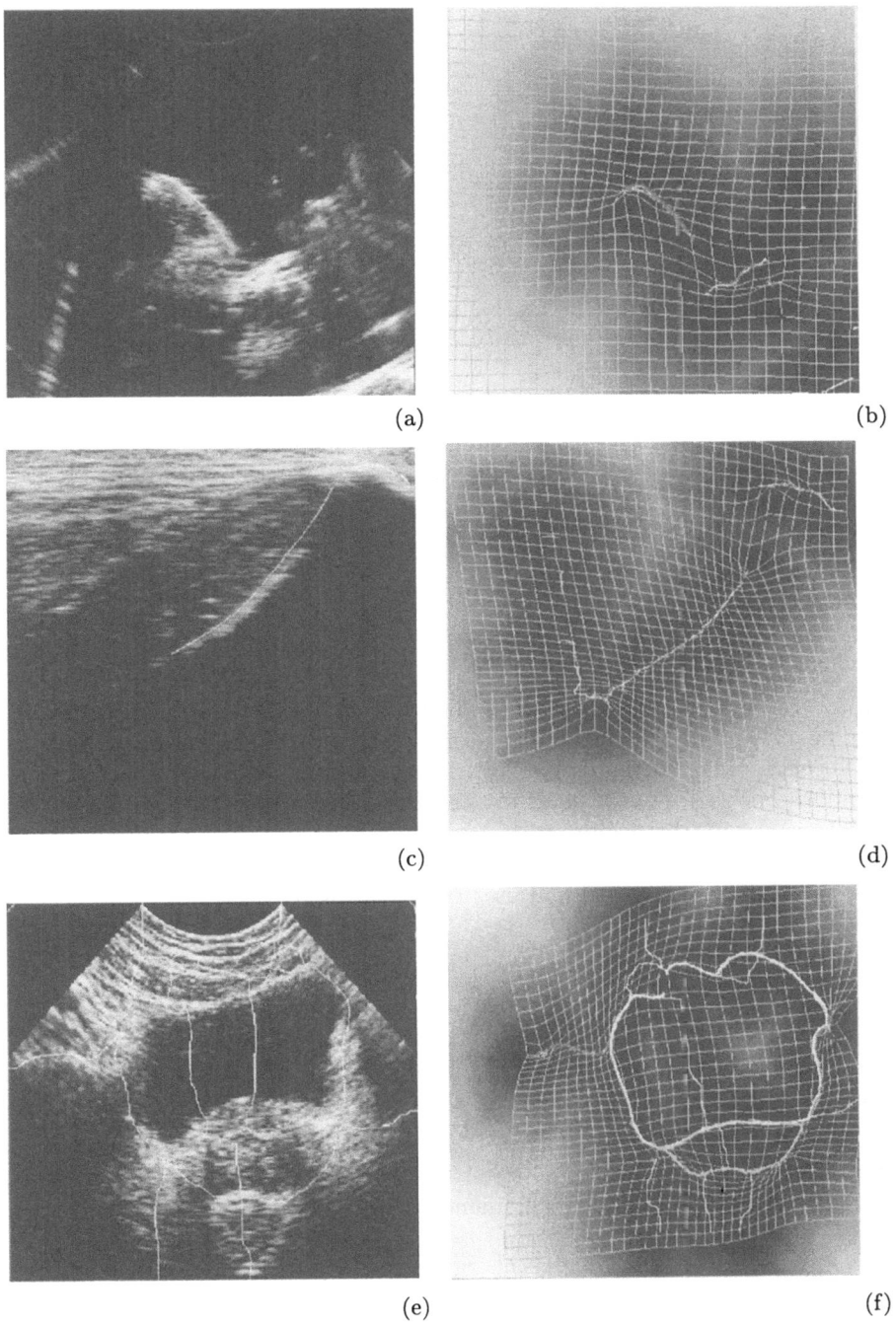

Fig. 1. Typical US images (left) and $2D/2D$ elastic registration (right). (a-b) Vertebra. (c-d) Sacro-iliac region. (e-f) Bladder and prostate.

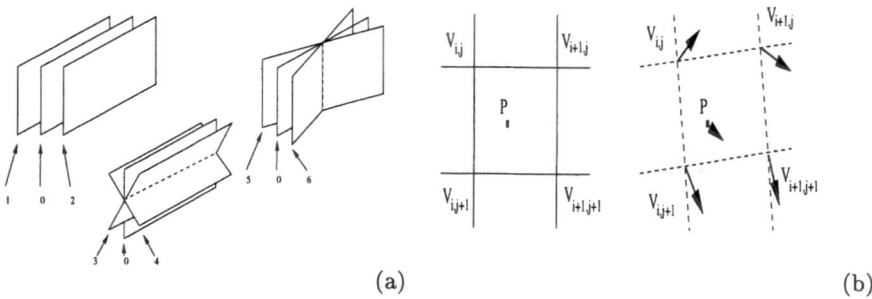

(a)   (b)

Fig. 2. (a) Additional transformations associated to initial attitude T_i. (b) Elastic $2D$ transformation.

p, we have developed a nonlinear iterative optimization algorithm based on the minimization of the following objective function:

$$\varepsilon = \frac{1}{N}\sum_{i=1}^{N}\|Q_j - T_p(P_i)\|^2 + \rho_1 \frac{1}{I_x \times I_y}\sum_{(i,j)=[0,0]}^{[I_x,I_y]}\|V_{i,j}\|^2 +$$

$$\rho_2 \frac{1}{I_x \times I_y}\left(\sum_{(i,j)=[0,0]}^{(I_x,I_y]}\|V_{i+1,j} - V_{i,j}\|^2 + \sum_{(i,j)=[0,0]}^{[I_x,I_y)}\|V_{i,j,1} - V_{i,j}\|^2\right) \quad (3)$$

where the first term represents the distance from the transformed point P_i to the nearest point Q_j, the second term regularizes the dimension of the vectors $V_{i,j}$ associated with the (i,j) network node and the third term regularizes the similarity of vectors associated with neighboring nodes.

To speed up the computation of distances, we use the $2D$ chamfer distance map for the set of real points Q_j. The minimization method used is based on the calculation of gradient and uses the following iterative mechanism:

$$p_k^{t+1} = p_k^t - \lambda\nabla\varepsilon_k \quad (4)$$

$$\delta p_k = -\lambda\nabla\varepsilon_k \quad (5)$$

where λ is a dimension less scale factor and $\nabla\varepsilon_k$ is the gradient of the objective function expressed in (3) relative to the component k of the vector p.

Convergence Criteria. The criteria for stopping the iterative procedure are related to the energy and the gradient:

1. $\frac{\varepsilon_{t+1}^2 - \varepsilon_t^2}{\varepsilon_t^2} \le T_1$; the relative energy gain between two successive successful iterations must be below a reasonable threshold T_1.
2. $N_{iterations}$; after $N_{iterations}$ successive unsuccessful iterations.
3. (I_x, I_y); after the convergence using the previously defined criteria, the network resolution can be increased and the minimization starts again.

Retaining the Best $(T_i, \Delta T_j)$ Combination. In the case of hard tissues, the choice of the best $(T_i, \Delta T_j)$ combination relies on a likelihood principle. Consequently, we construct an objective discriminating function based on the first term of (3) and on the number of points P_i of the model. Among many possibilities, the solution retained is based on the Student test t in order to compare variances. We have adopted the solution proposed in [21] where the original data are transformed in the absolute values of the deviation of each distance relative to the average value using the relation:

$$t = (\overline{x}_1 - \overline{x}_2)s\sqrt{\frac{1}{n_1} - \frac{1}{n_2}} \tag{6}$$

$$s = \left((n_1 - 1)s_1^2 + (n_2 - 1)s_2^2\right) / (n_1 + n_2 - 2) \tag{7}$$

where $n_{1,2}$ is the sample size, $\overline{x}_{1,2}$ is the sample mean value, $s_{1,2}$ is the sample variance and s is the global variance. The value $t_{k,l}$ obtained from expression (6) is used as a dissimilarity measure for the couple $[(T, \Delta T)_k, (T, \Delta T)_l]$. A symmetric matrix $T = [t_{k,l}]; k, l \in [1, N \cdot M]$ is then constructed. An objective function $f_t(l) = \sum_{k=1}^{N \cdot M} t_{k,l}$ is obtained by summing over the columns of the matrix T. The decision mechanism is based on minimizing $f_t(l)$. Consequently, the optimal $(T, \Delta T)_{opt}$ combination corresponds to the relation $(f_t)_{opt} = \min_{l=1,N \cdot M} f_t(l)$.

In the case of soft tissues, one cannot defend the use of maximum likelihood as an objective discriminatory function. For instance it is very easy to register elastically two transversal slices through the bladder. Taking into account the preceding observation, we propose a solution adapted to all soft tissues based on two criteria, a quantitative one followed by a qualitative one: 1. Establish a measure that determines how well the points of the model fit the intra-operative data. To achieve this, we compute a distance map based on the new coordinates of the deformed model points taken after the $2D/2D$ elastic registration. From this distance map, we obtain the distance of each intra-operative data point relative to the model. The average value of all these distances, $\overline{d}_{i,j}$, defines the objective measure characterizing the $(T_i, \Delta T_j)$ combination. The best combination being the one with an uniform distribution of the points of the deformed model as compared with intra-operative data. With a minimization procedure one obtains $(T, \Delta T)_{opt} = \min_{l=1,N \cdot M} (\overline{d}_{i,j})_l$. 2. In problematic situations when none of the $(T_i, \Delta T_j)$ combinations represent a realistic situation (the model points are not well-distributed) this image will be marked and eliminated from the final $3D/3D$ registration process. The decision criteria are the following: the model points must cover at least 50 % of the data and in the case of the prostate, this area must necessarily cover the base of the bladder. After the choice of the best $(T, \Delta T)_{opt}$ combination, another step of $2D/2D$ elastic registration will be necessary. This time, intra-operative data are represented by the watershed while pre-operative model is represented by the set of anatomic structure of the region of interest (i.e. the bone, the bladder and the prostate). The results are presented in Fig. 1.

3.4   Rigid Registration

Choice of Segments. For this step, we had to choose between two possibilities: isolate all segments of the watershed pointed by the model or retain the new coordinates of the points of the model. To show that both possibilities are realistic, we used the first one in orthopedic applications and the second one in radiotherapy applications.

A final $3D/3D$ registration step is necessary to match the points previously extracted and labeled on US images with the surface of the CT model. For that purpose, one could use elastic registration [22], but both the prostate (for radiotherapy) and the bones (for orthopedics) are considered as rigid bodies. Therefore, standard $3D$ surface registration techniques were used to estimate the transformation between CT model and the patient coordinate system in the local region of interest [23].

4   Results

In order to validate our technique, we compared the final results obtained after the rigid $3D/3D$ registration with either those obtained from a manual segmentation of the prostate or, in the case of the orthopedic application, with manual digitalization of the bone surface with a finger probe localized in $3D$ space. All numerical results are presented in the following table where we display the errors obtained both on rotations $\varepsilon_{\max}^{\alpha}$ expressed in degrees and on translations $\varepsilon_{\max}^{t}$ expressed in mm. In the last column, the same results are presented in terms of Rodriguez's rotation and translation.

	$\varepsilon_{\max}^{\alpha}[\deg]$	$\varepsilon_{\max}^{t}[mm]$	$Rodriguez$
prostate	$(-1.23, 1.30, 0.75)$	$(0.19, -0.67, -2.58)$	$(2.67°, 2.07mm)$
vertebra	$(1.90, 2.05, -0.98)$	$(-0.15, -0.52, 0.87)$	$(1.23°, 1.70mm)$
bassin	$(-2.93, 1.13, -1.83)$	$(-0.39, 0.12, -1.02)$	$(1.14°, 1.91mm)$

In Fig. 3, we present the repositioning of a typical US image in $3D$ space of the CT per-operative model. Fig. 3.a displays the superposition of the model on the spinal process of the vertebra, Fig. 3.b presents a superposition with the US image representing the sacrum and Fig. 3.c displays an US image of the bladder and the prostate.

5   Conclusion

In this paper, we have presented automatic and robust algorithms necessary for registration between a $3D$ CT model and a set of $2.5D$ US images. Essentially, these algorithms use methods of low-level segmentation as described in paragraph §3.2 and high-level segmentation by labeling as described in §3.3. To emphasize the generality of our approach, each application has been analyzed in the following framework: description of clinical objectives, presentation of specific pre-processing, labeling by elastic $2D/2D$ registration, choice of segments

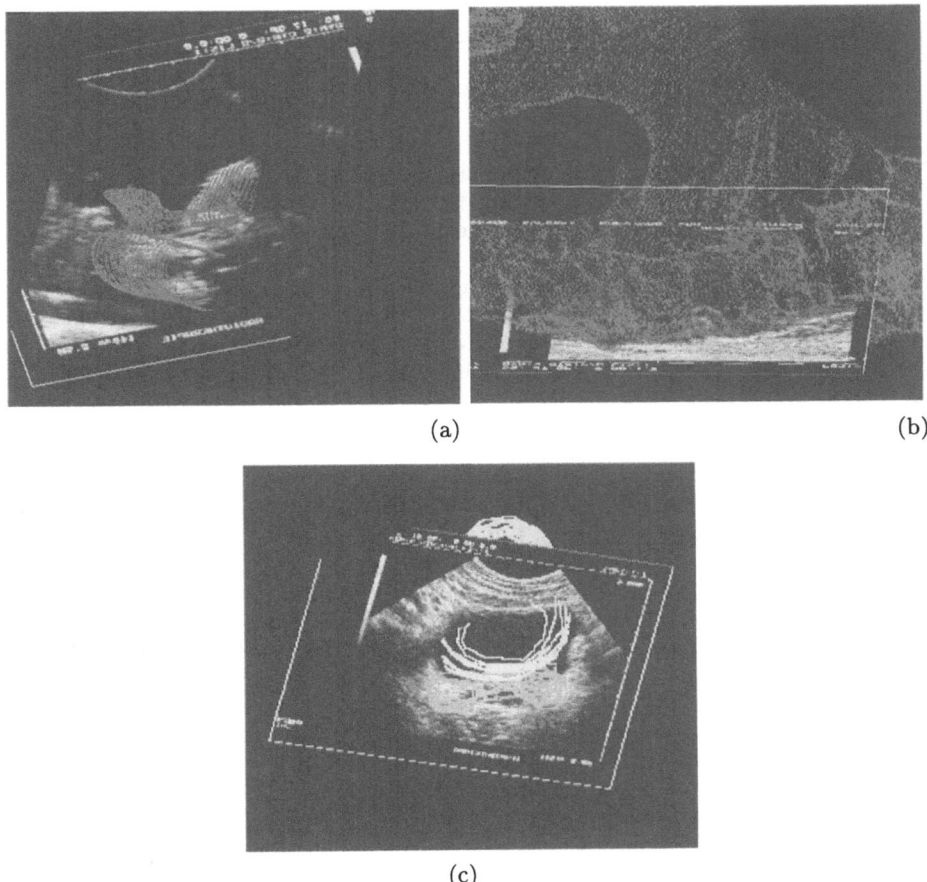

(a)   (b)

(c)

Fig. 3. Results: (a) Vertebra registration. (b) Sacrum registration. (c) Bladder and prostate registration

and presentation of results. In all this work, we paid special attention to the precision and we could demonstrate that the maximum errors are about $2\,mm$ and 2^{0} which is compatible with most of applications. While the orthopedic application chosen clearly deals with high-risk regions, in the case of the prostate, the risk is to irradiate healthy organs. Considering the important risks inherent to an intervention on the spine or in the sacral region, we have tested our method *in vitro*. The preliminary results obtained in the automatization of the segmentation process are very encouraging. It is clear that the result of a minimization procedure generally used in matching depends strongly on the precision of the initial attitude T_0, this also affects the global computing time. To improve on this, we hope to find a procedure that estimates an initial attitude T_0 as close as possible to the final attitude for each application. We plan also to correct the US images, in term of the velocity of US. This will influence the precision of the results specially in the radiotheray applications. This method is generic and it could be easily applied to other organs such as liver and kidney.

References

1. Tonetti J. et al, Percutaneous iliosacral screw placement using image guided techniques, *CORR special issue*, pp. 103-110, 1998.
2. Merloz P. et al, Pedicle screw placement using image guided techniques, *CORR special issue*, pp. 39-48, 1998.
3. Troccaz J. et al, Conformal external radiotherapy pf prostatic carcinoma: requirements and experimental results, *Radiother. Oncol.*, no. 29, pp. 176-183, 1993.
4. Vassal P., Fusion d'images multi-modales pour la radioth. conformationnelle: appli. au repos. du patient, *Ph.D. Thesis TIMC-IMAG, Grenoble University*, 1998.
5. Carrat L.et al, Treatment of pelvic ring fractures: percutaneous computer assisted iliosacral screwing, *MICCAI'98-Proceedings*, pp. 84-91, 1998.
6. Lavallée S. et al, Computer integrated surgery and therapy, *C. Roux and J.L. Coatrieux ed., Contemp. Persp. in 3D Biomed. Im. IOS Press*, pp. 239-310, 1997.
7. Maintz A. and Viergever M.A., A survey of medical image registration, *Medical Image Analysis*, vol. 2, no. 1, pp. 1-36, 1998.
8. Pelizzari C.A. et al, Accurate 3D registration of CT, PET and/or MR images of brain, *L. Comput. Assist. Tomo.*, no. 13, pp. 20-26,1989.
9. Lavallée S. et al, Matching 3D smooth surf. with their 2D proj. using 3D dist. maps, *SPIE vol. 1570 Geom. Models in Computer Vision - San Diego*, pp 322-336, 1991.
10. Ionescu G., Segm. et recalage d'images échographiques par utilisation de conaissances physio. et morpho., *Ph.D. Thesis TIMC-IMAG, Grenoble University*, 1998.
11. Mattes J. and Demongeot J., Dynamic confinement, classification and imaging, *New techn. of classific., Lecture Notes in Comput. Sci., Springer Verlag*, 1998.
12. Wells W.M. et al, Multimodal volume registration by minimisation of mutual information, *Medical Robotics and CAS Wiley New York*, pp 55-62, 1995.
13. Grevera G.J. and Udupa J.K., Shape-based interpolation of multidimensional greylevel images, *IEEE Trans. Medical Imaging*, vol. 15, no. 6, pp. 881-891, Dec. 1996.
14. Bittar E., Modèles déformables surfaciques, implicites et volumiques, pour l'imagerie médicale, *Ph.D. Thesis TIMC-IMAG, Grenoble University*, 1998.
15. Hamadeh A., Une approche unifiée pour la segm. el la mise en corresp. 3D/2D d'images multi-modales, *Ph.D. Thesis TIMC-IMAG, Grenoble University*, 1997.
16. Mangin J., Mise en correspondance d'images médicales 3D multi-modalités pour la corrélation anatomo-fonctionnelle cérébrale, *Ph.D. Thesis ENST Paris*, 1995.
17. Géraud T., Segmentation des structures internes du cerveau en IRM 3D, *Ph.D. Thesis TLCOM Paris*, 1998.
18. Maes F., Segmentation and registration of multimodal medical images, *Ph.D. Thesis ISBN 90-5682-135-0 D/1998/7515/37*, 1998.
19. Najman L. and Schmitt M., Geodesic saliency of watershed contours and hierarchical segmentation, *IEEE Trans. PAMI*, vol. 18, no. 12, pp. 1163-1173, Dec. 1996.
20. Deriche R., Fast algorithms for low-level vision, *IEEE Trans. PAMI*, vol. 12, no. 1, pp. 78-87, Jan. 1990.
21. Manly B., Statistical methods, *Chapman and Hall*, 1989.
22. Szeliski R. et al, Matching 3-D anatomical surfaces with non-rigid deformations using octree-splines, *Intern. Journ. of Comp. Vis.*, 18(2), pp. 171-186, 1996.
23. Lavallée S. et al, Recovering the pos. and orient. of free-form obj. from image contours using 3D dist. maps, *IEEE Trans. PAMI*, vol. 17, no. 4, pp. 378-390, 1995.

A Robust 3-D Reconstruction System for Human Jaw Modeling

Sameh M. Yamany[1] and Aly A. Farag[1]
David Tasman[2], and Allan G. Farman[2]

[1] Computer Vision and Image Processing Laboratory, University of Louisville
[2] School of Dentistry, University of Louisville,
Louisville, KY 40292, USA.
farag@cvip.uofl.edu

Abstract. This paper presents a model-based vision system for dentistry that will assist in diagnosis, treatment planning and surgical simulation. Dentistry requires the accurate 3-D representation of the teeth and jaws for diagnostic and treatment purposes. The proposed integrated computer vision system reconstructs a 3-D model of the patient's dental occlusion using an intra-oral video camera. A modified shape from shading (SFS) technique, using perspective projection and camera calibration, extracts the 3-D information from a sequence of 2-D images of the jaw. Data fusion and 3-D registration techniques develop the complete jaw model. Triangulization is then performed, and a solid 3-D model is obtained via rapid prototyping. The system performance is investigated using ground truth data, and the results show sub-millimeter reconstruction accuracy. The system is shown to be robust in terms of speed and accuracy compared to current practices.

1 Introduction

Dentistry requires the accurate 3-D representation of the teeth and jaws for diagnostic and treatment purposes. For example, orthodontic treatment involves the application, over time, of force systems to teeth to correct malocclusion. In order to evaluate tooth movement progress, the orthodontist monitors this movement with visual inspection, intra-oral measurements, fabrication of plastic models (casts), photographs, and radiographs; this process is both costly and time consuming. Moreover, repeated acquisition of radiographs may result in untoward effects. Obtaining a cast of the jaw is a complex operation for the dentist, an unpleasant experience for the patient, and may not provide all the necessary details of the jaw.

Oral and maxillofacial radiology can provide the dentist with abundant 3-D information of the jaw. Current and evolving methods include computed tomography (CT) [1], tomosynthesis, tuned-aperture CT (TACT), and localized, or "cone-beam," computed tomography [2]. While oral and maxillofacial radiology is now widely accepted as a routine technique for dental examinations, the equipment is rather expensive and the resolution is frequently too low for

3-D modeling of dental structures. Furthermore, the radiation dose required to enhance both contrast and spatial resolution can be unacceptably high.

Recently, efforts have focused on computerized diagnosis in dentistry[3]. Usually, most of the 3-D systems for dental applications found in the literature rely on first obtaining an intermediate solid model of the jaw (cast or teeth imprints) and then capturing the 3-D information from that model. User interaction is needed in such systems to determine the 3-D coordinates of fiducial reference points on a dental cast. Other systems measuring the 3-D coordinates have been developed using either mechanical contact or a traveling light principle [4]. Generally, such systems are either not accurate or are time and labor intensive.

The authors have been involved for the last five years in a project to develop a system for dentistry to go beyond traditional approaches in diagnosis, treatment planning, surgical simulation, and prosthetic replacements. Specific objectives are as follows: (i) to design a data acquisition system that can obtain sequences of calibrated video images of the upper/lower jaw using small intra-oral cameras with respect to a common reference in 3-D space; (ii) to develop methods for accurate 3-D reconstruction from the acquired sequence of intra-oral images. This involves using a new algorithm for shape from shading (SFS) that incorporates the camera parameters; (iii) to develop a robust algorithm for the fusion of data acquired from multiple views, including the implementation of an accurate and fast 3-D data registration; (iv) to develop a specific object segmentation and recognition system to separate and to recognize individual 3-D tooth information for further analysis and simulations; and (v) to develop algorithms to study and to simulate tooth movement based on the finite element method and deformable model approaches. This research will have an immense value in various dental practices including implants, tooth alignment, and craniofacial surgery. The research will also have wide applications in dental education and training.

This paper describes the project's first phase concerning the development of a 3-D model of the jaw, not from a cast, but from the actual human jaw. The work reported here is original and novel in the following aspects: (1) data acquisition is performed directly on the human jaw using a small off-the-shelf solid state camera, (2) the acquisition time is relatively short and is less discomforting to the patient compared to current practices, (3) the acquired digital model can be stored with the patient data and retrieved on demand, (4) these models can also be transmitted over a communication network to remote sites for further assistance in diagnosis and treatment planning, and (5) dental measurements and virtual restoration can be performed and analyzed. This work also involves three important areas in the computer vision and medical imaging fields, namely: shape recovery, data fusion, and surface registration.

2   System Overview

As shown in Fig 1, our approach to reconstruct the human jaw consists of the following stages. The first stage is data acquisition. A small intra-oral Acu-

Cam(Dentsply/New Image, Canaga Park, California) CCD camera with built-in laser light, is calibrated and then placed inside the oral cavity. The camera acquires a set of overlapping images $\{I_j \mid j = 1, 2, .., J\}$ for different parts of the jaw such that $\bigcup_{j=1}^{J} I_j$ covers the whole jaw. The images are preprocessed to reduce noise, sharpen edges, and remove specularity. Specularity removal was done using an approach similar to the Tong and Funt technique [5]. J sets of points are then computed with a modified SFS algorithm, which accounts for the camera perspective projection. To obtain accurate metric measurements, range data is obtained using a five link digitizer arm. These data consist of some reference points on the jaw. Fusion of the range data and the SFS output provides accurate metric information that can be used later for orthodontic measurements and implant planning. A fast registration technique is required to merge the resulting 3-D points to obtain a complete 3-D description of the jaw [6]. The final stage is to transform this model into patches of free form surfaces using a triangulization technique. This step enables the development of a 3-D solid model via rapid prototyping. Further processing on the digital model includes tooth separation, force analysis, implant planning, and surgical simulation.

3   Shape from Shading using Perspective Projection and Camera Calibration

Among the tools used in shape extraction from single view is the shape from shading (SFS) technique. The surface orientation at a point M on a surface S is determined by the unit vector perpendicular to the plane tangent to S at M. Most of the research done in SFS assumes orthographic projection from which the elemental change in the depth Z at an image point (x, y) can be expressed as $\delta z \approx \frac{\partial Z}{\partial x} \delta x + \frac{\partial Z}{\partial y} \delta y$. The partial derivatives are called surface gradients (p, q). The surface normal to a surface patch is related to the gradient by $\mathbf{n} = (p, q, 1)$. By assuming that surface patches are homogeneous and uniformly lit by distant light sources, the brightness $E(x, y)$ seen at the image plane often depends only on the orientation of the surface. This dependence of brightness on surface orientation can be represented as a function $R(\cdot)$ defined on the Gaussian sphere. Thus, we can formulate the shape from shading problem as finding a solution to the brightness equation: $E(x, y) = R(p, q, \mathbf{L})$, where $R(p, q, \mathbf{L})$ is the surface reflectance map and $\mathbf{L}$ is the illuminant direction. Many algorithms were developed to estimate the illuminant direction [7]. Because the laser light beam is built in the CCD camera, we assume that this will be the only source of light inside the mouth cavity and that the illuminant direction is known beforehand. However, the assumption of orthographic projection is not adequate as the camera is very close to the object. We propose to calibrate the CCD camera and use the perspective projection matrix to enhance the SFS algorithm and to obtain a metric representation of the teeth and gum surfaces. The perspective projection equation is as follows:

$$s\mathbf{m} = \mathbf{B}\mathbf{M} + \mathbf{b} \qquad \qquad or, \qquad \qquad (1)$$

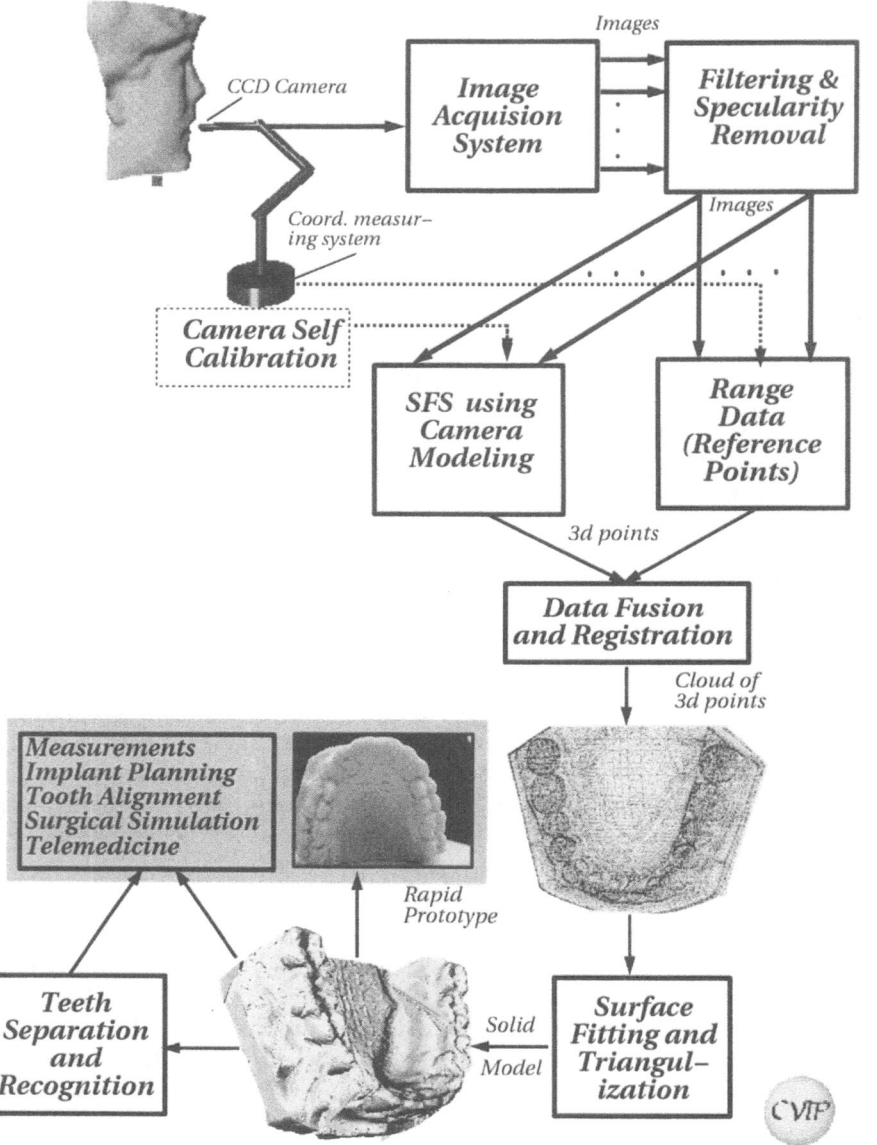

Fig. 1. *The process starts by capturing a sequence of video images using a small intra-Oral CCD camera. These images are preprocessed to remove specularity. Reference points are obtained using the CMM system. SFS is applied to the images. The range data are fused to the SFS output and then registration takes place. A cloud of points representing the jaw is obtained and, by triangulization, a solid digital model is formed. This model is reproduced using a rapid prototype machine. Further analysis and orthodontics application can be performed on the digital model.*

$$\mathbf{M} = \mathbf{B}^{-1}(s\mathbf{m} - \mathbf{b}) = f(s(x, y)) \tag{2}$$

where $\mathbf{B}$ is a 3×3 matrix and $\mathbf{b}$ is a translation vector. The matrix $[\mathbf{Bb}]$ is called the perspective projection matrix. The function $f(s(x, y))$ maps $\mathbf{M}$ to a point $\mathbf{m}$ in the image. The normal to the surface at $\mathbf{M}$ is defined to be the cross product of the two gradient vectors $\mathbf{p} = \frac{df(s(x,y))}{dx}, \mathbf{q} = \frac{df(s(x,y))}{dy}$. The surface reflectance $R(.)$ becomes a function of the scalar s defined in equation[1] as follows,

$$R(s) = \frac{(\mathbf{p} \times \mathbf{q}) \cdot \mathbf{L}}{|\mathbf{p} \times \mathbf{q}||\mathbf{L}|} \tag{3}$$

The new formulation of the SFS problem becomes finding the scalar s that solves the new brightness equation $g(s) = E(x, y) - R(s) = 0$. This can be solved using a Taylors series expansion and applying the Jacoby iterative method [8] where at the nth iteration, for each point (x, y) in the image, $s_{x,y}^n$ is as follows:

$$s_{x,y}^n = s_{x,y}^{n-1} + \frac{-g(s_{x,y}^{n-1})}{\frac{d}{ds_{x,y}}g(s_{x,y}^{n-1})} \quad \text{where,} \tag{4}$$

$$\frac{d}{ds_{x,y}}g(s_{x,y}^{n-1}) = -\frac{d\mathbf{N}}{ds_{x,y}} \cdot \frac{\mathbf{L}}{|\mathbf{L}|} \tag{5}$$

$$\frac{d\mathbf{N}}{ds_{x,y}} = \frac{d\mathbf{v}}{ds_{x,y}} \frac{1}{\sqrt{\mathbf{v}^t\mathbf{v}}} - \frac{\mathbf{v}}{\sqrt{(\mathbf{v}^t\mathbf{v})^3}} \left(\mathbf{v}^t \frac{d\mathbf{v}}{ds_{x,y}}\right) \tag{6}$$

$$\frac{d\mathbf{v}}{ds_{x,y}} = \mathbf{B}^{-1}\mathbf{m} \times \mathbf{B}^{-1}(0, s_{x,y-1}, 0)^t + \mathbf{B}^{-1}(s_{x-1,y}, 0, 0)^t \times \mathbf{B}^{-1}\mathbf{m} \tag{7}$$

where $\mathbf{v} = \mathbf{p} \times \mathbf{q}$.

Even though camera parameters are used in the SFS implementation, accurate metric information cannot be deduced from the resulting shape because only one image is used. Additional information is needed to complement the SFS output and to incorporate the metric measurements.

4   Fusion of SFS and range data

The most important information for reconstructing an accurate 3-D visible surface, missing in SFS, is the metric measurement. SFS also suffers from the discontinuities due to highly textured surfaces and different albedo. The integration of the dense depth map obtained from the SFS with sparse depth measurements obtained from a coordinate measurement machine (CMM) for the reconstruction of 3-D surfaces with accurate metric measurements has two advantages [9]. First, it helps in removing the ambiguity of the 3-D visible surface discontinuities produced by shape from shading. Second, it complements the missing metric information in the SFS. The integration process, as depicted in Fig 2, includes the following. First, the error difference in the available depth measurements between the two sensory data are calculated. Next, a surface that fits this error

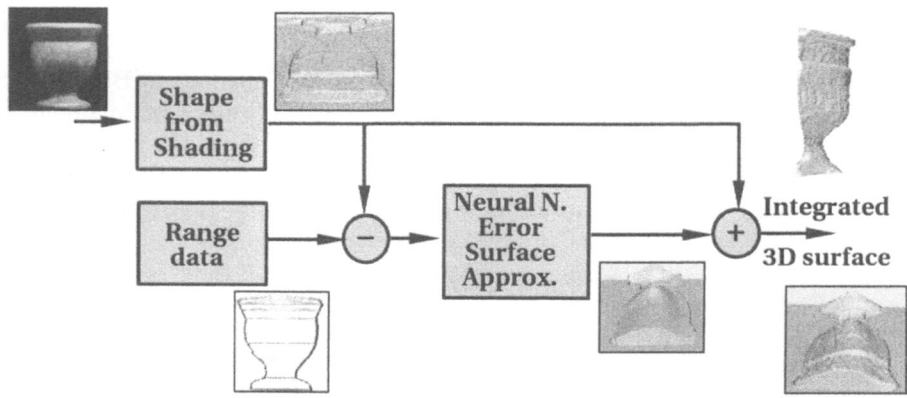

Fig. 2. *Functional block diagram of the integration process of SFS and range data. The surface approximation process uses neural networks. An example of using this system on the image of a vase is demonstrated.*

difference is approximated. Finally, the approximated surface is used to correct the SFS.

We used a multi-layer network for the surface approximation. The x- and y-coordinates of the data points are inputs to the network, while the error in the depth value at the point (x, y) is the desired response. The learning algorithm used is the error Kalman-filter learning technique because of its fast weights computation. The error difference between the SFS and the range measurements and their x-y coordinates are used to form the training set. The input to the network is the x-y coordinates and the output is the error difference at that coordinate. After training, the neural network provides the approximated smooth surface that contains information about the errors in the SFS at the locations with no range data. This approximated surface is then added to the SFS. The result is the 3-D surface reconstruction containing accurate metric information about the visible surface of the sensed 3-D object. An example performed on the image of a vase is shown in Fig 2.

The output of the fusion algorithm to each image is a set of 3-D points describing the teeth surface in this segment. However, there is no relation between the 3-D points of a segment and the following segment. Thus we needed a fast and accurate 3-D registration technique to link the 3-D points of all the segments to produce one set of 3-D points describing the whole jaw surface. Yamany et. al.[6, 10] introduced a new 3-D registration technique using the Grid Closest Point (GCP) transform and Genetic Algorithms (GA). This technique was faster and more accurate than the existing techniques found in the literature.

5   Validation

To validate the SFS and data fusion methods and to determine the accuracy of
the proposed system and the required resolution, we used a ground truth dense
depth map registered with intensity images obtained from a laser range scanner.
Although laser scanners have accuracy limitation, their output can be considered
as ground truth since they are now widely accepted in the dentistry practices.
The RMS error between the integrated surface and the ground truth is used as a
measure of the system performance. Two different types of surfaces, a sphere as
a smooth surface and a free-form surface (see Mostafa et al. [9] for more details),
are investigated. Figure 3 shows the results of this analysis. The RMS error for
the smooth surface is smaller compared to that of the free-form surface. This is
an expected result because the surface approximation process tends to smooth
the surface where range data are not available, producing a large RMS error
in the case of free-form surfaces. The results show that a higher sampling rate
increases the accuracy in the case of free-form surfaces, yet this will increase the
time to acquire the data. However, the sampling rate has minimal effect in the
case of smooth surfaces. The results and the above analysis show that the system
can achieve sub-millimeter accuracy with a small number of reference points.

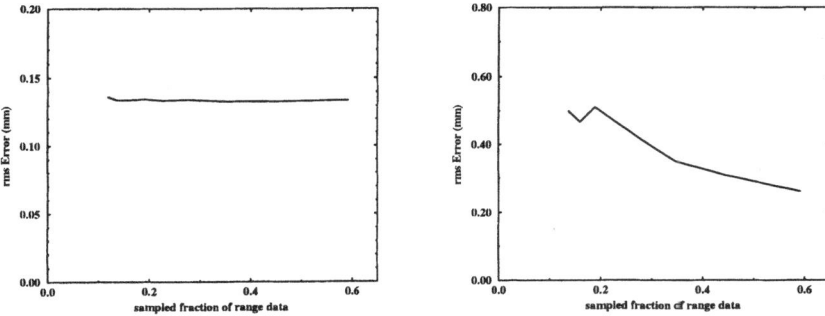

Fig. 3. *The RMS error between the integrated surface and the ground truth is used as
a measure of the system performance. Two different types of surfaces:(left) a sphere as
a smooth surface and (right) a free-form surface are investigated.*

6   Results and Discussions

Intra-Oral cameras are quickly becoming standard equipment used by many
dental practitioners[11]. In our experiments, we used an intra-oral CCD camera, AcuCam (Dentsply/ New Image Inc.). The experiments were conducted

on different pediatric subjects at the Orthodontics Department, University of Louisville,KY. After calibrating the camera, a sequence of images capturing segments of the jaw are obtained. The process of taking the images was relatively fast, taking about 4 to 5 minutes to cover the upper/lower jaw. The images were taken carefully to cover all visible surfaces of the teeth. With the CMM system (with a resolution of 0.23 mm, and sampling rate of 1,000 points/second), reference points were calculated for each image. Figure 4(a) shows an example of two images taken of a patient's tooth. The complete tooth surface is covered in these two images. Figure 4(b) shows the outputs of the SFS stage. Using the range data shown as cross signs in Fig 4(a) and applying the fusion algorithm results in the corrected surfaces shown in Fig 4(c). The registration procedure on these two data sets provides the complete surface model of the tooth as shown in Fig 4(d). A smooth version of the whole jaw model is shown in Fig 4(e). This model contains all required metric information, and can be used to measure any orthodontic parameter and can be reproduced with the same original scale. More results of applying the reconstruction algorithms on another subject are shown in Fig 4(f,g,h). The resulting jaw models have sub-millimeter accuracy and are faithful enough to show all the information about the patient's actual jaw in a metric space. Both the time and convenience for the patient must be considered when comparing these results with those from scanning a cast. Further processing was performed on the digital jaw model, and Fig 4(i) shows the result of the teeth segmentation and identification stage.

7   Conclusions and Future Extensions

The 3-D reconstruction of the human jaw has tremendous applications. The model can be stored along with the patient data and can be retrieved on demand. The model can also be used in telemedicine were it is transmitted over a communication network to different remote dentists for further assistance in diagnosis. Dental measurements and virtual restoration could be performed and analyzed. This work enables many orthodontics and dental imaging research projects, applied directly to the jaw and not to a cast, using computer vision and medical imaging tools. The paper describes the results of the first phase in a project aimed to enhance current dental imaging practices.

The next phase includes the analysis and simulation of dental operations including tooth alignment, implant planing, restoration, and measurement of distances and orientation of teeth with respect to each other. Similar work was performed by Alcaniz et al.[12]. However, their analysis was done on the tooth contours and not on the actual 3-D model of the tooth . Also, the arch-wire model does not account for the 3-D displacements of the tooth.

8   Acknowledgment

This work was supported in part by grants from the Whitaker Foundation,and the NSF (ECS-9505674) institutions.

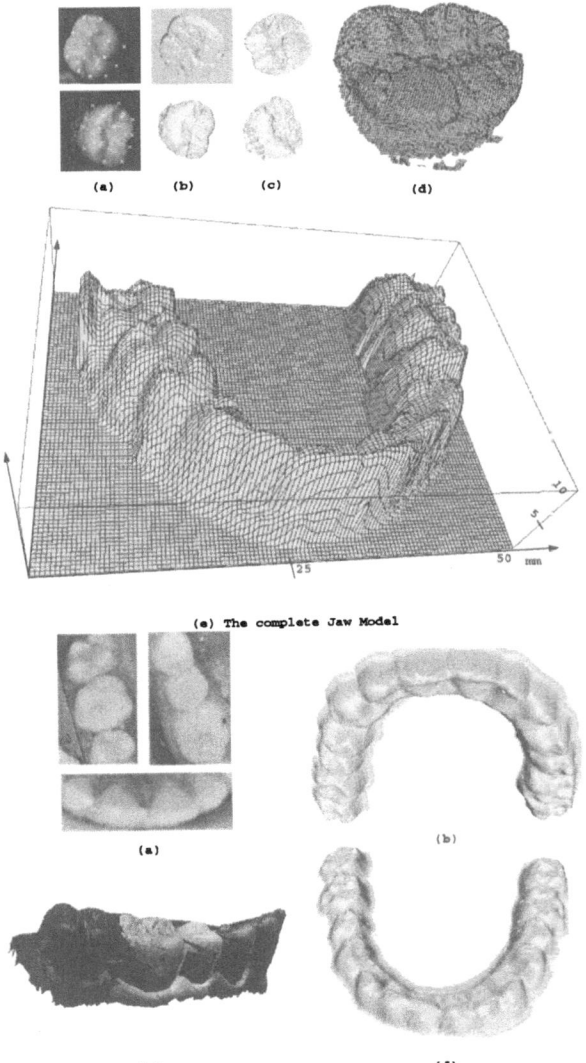

(a)   (b)   (c)   (d)

(e) The complete Jaw Model

(a)   (b)

(c)   (d)

Fig. 4. *(a) Intra-oral intensity images from one patient with range data marked as cross signs. (b) 3-D visible surfaces obtained from the SFS. (c) The final surfaces obtained from the integration process. (d) A visible surface mesh obtained from registering the two views in (c). (e) A smoothed version of the whole jaw model. (f) Some intensity images taken from another patient. (g-h) The upper and lower digital jaw models of this patient. (i) The result of the teeth segmentation and identification stage.*

References

1. P. van der Stelt and S. M. Dunn, "3d-imaging in dental radiography," in *Advances in Maxillofacial Imaging*, A. G. Farman, ed., pp. 367–372, Elsevier Science B. V., 1997.

2. R. L. Webber, R. A. Horton, D. A. Tyndall, and J. B. Ludlow, "Tuned-aperature computed tomography (tact). theory and application for three-dimensional; dento-alveolar imaging," *Dentomaxillofac. Radiol.* **26**, pp. 51–62, 1997.
3. D. Laurendeau and D. Possart, "A computer-vision technique for the aquisition and processing of 3-d profiles of dental imprints: An application in orthodontics," *IEEE Transactions on Medical Imaging* **10**, pp. 453–461, Sep 1991.
4. A. A. Goshtasby, S. Nambala, W. G. deRijk, and S. D. Campbell, "A system for digital reconstruction of gypsum dental casts," *IEEE transactions on Medical Imaging* **16**, pp. 664–674, Oct 1997.
5. F. Tong and B. V. Funt, "Removing specularity from color images for shape from shading," in *Computer Vision and Shape Recognition*, A. Krzyzak, T. Kasvand, and C. Y. Suen, eds., vol. 14 of *Computer Science*, pp. 275–290, World Scientific, 1989.
6. S. M. Yamany, M. N. Ahmed, and A. A. Farag, "A new genetic-based technique for matching 3d curves and surfaces," *Pattern Recognition (to appear)* , 1999.
7. A. Pentland, *Extract Shape From Shading*, Academic Press, MIT Media Lab, 2nd ed., 1988.
8. P. S. Tsai and M. Shah, "A fast linear shape from shading," *IEEE Conference on Computer Vision and Pattern Recognition* , pp. 734–736, July 1992.
9. M. G.-H. Mostafa, S. M. Yamany, and A. A. Farag, "Integrating shape from shading and range data using neural networks," *Proc. IEEE Int. Conf. Comp. Visi. Patt. Recog. (CVPR)* , June 1999. Fort Collins, Colorado.
10. S. M. Yamany, M. N. Ahmed, and A. A. Farag, "Novel surface registration using the grid closest point (gcp) transform," *Proc. IEEE International Confenrence on Image Processing, Chicago* **3**, pp. 809–813, October 1998.
11. L. A. Johnson, "A systematic evaluation of intraoral cameras," *Journal of the California Dental Association* **22**, pp. 34–47, November 1994.
12. M. Alcaniz, C. Montserrat, V. Grau, F. Chinesta, A. Ramon, and S. Albalat, "An advanced system for the simulation and planning of orthodontic treatment," *Medical Image Analysis* **2**, pp. 37–60, March 1998.

Level-Set Surface Segmentation and Fast Cortical Range Image Tracking for Computing Intrasurgical Deformations

M.A. Audette[1], K. Siddiqi[2], and T.M. Peters[3]

[1] Montreal Neurological Institute (McGill University), Montreal, Canada
maudette@nil.mni.mcgill.ca
[2] McGill Center for Intelligent Machines (McGill University), Montreal, Canada
siddiqi@cim.mcgill.ca
[3] The John P. Robarts Research Institute, London, Ontario, Canada
tpeters@irus.rri.on.ca

Abstract. We propose a method for estimating intrasurgical brain shift for image-guided surgery. This method consists of five stages: the identification of relevant anatomical surfaces within the MRI/CT volume, range-sensing of the skin and cortex in the OR, rigid registration of the skin range image with its MRI/CT homologue, non-rigid motion tracking over time of cortical range images, and lastly, interpolation of this surface displacement information over the whole brain volume via a realistically valued finite element model of the head. This papers focuses on the anatomical surface identification and cortical range surface tracking problems. The surface identification scheme implements a recent algorithm which imbeds 3D surface segmentation as the level-set of a 4D moving front. A by-product of this stage is a Euclidean distance and closest point map which is later exploited to speed up the rigid and non-rigid surface registration. The range-sensor uses both laser-based triangulation and defocusing techniques to produce a 2D range profile, and is linearly swept across the skin or cortical surface to produce a 3D range image. The surface registration technique is of the iterative closest point type, where each iteration benefits from looking up, rather than searching for, explicit closest point pairs. These explicit point pairs in turn are used in conjunction with a closed-form SVD-based rigid transformation computation and with fast recursive splines to make each rigid and non-rigid registration iteration essentially instantaneous. Our method is validated with a novel deformable brain-shaped phantom, made of Polyvinyl Alcohol Cryogel.

1 Introduction

Image-guided surgery is a technique whereby a model of a patient's head, typically featuring skin, cortex and lesion surfaces, is constructed from a set of segmented MRI/CT images and is then registered with the patient's head in the OR, using a locating device. The usefulness of this technology hinges on the

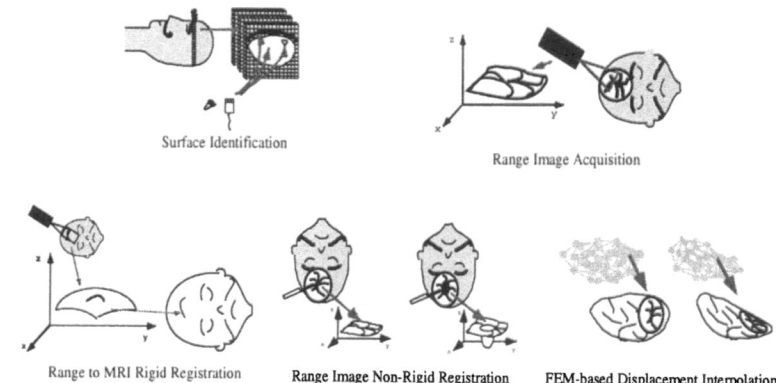

Surface Identification

Range Image Acquisition

Range to MRI Rigid Registration   Range Image Non-Rigid Registration   FEM-based Displacement Interpolation

Fig. 1. Brain shift estimation framework

accuracy of the transformation between the image and patient spaces. However, this transformation becomes less accurate as the brain shifts during surgery.

To alleviate this problem, we propose a method for estimating brain shift which is characterized by the following stages (see figure 1):

- semi-automatic identification (segmentation) of relevant anatomical surfaces within the MRI/CT volume;
- range-sensing of the skin and cortex in the OR;
- rigid registration of the skin range image with its MRI/CT homologue, which will serve as a baseline for the next stage;
- non-rigid motion tracking, over time, of the cortical range image;
- and lastly, interpolation of the resulting surface displacement over the whole brain volume, assuming null displacement at the base of the skull, via a realistic finite element model (FEM).

Our discussion here focuses on identification of anatomical surfaces by level-set segmentation, range-sensing of visible anatomical surfaces, and cortical motion estimation. We also describe a novel phantom design, whose material properties and shape are very good approximations of those of the human brain. This phantom will be used to validate our research on intrasurgical motion estimation.

Intrasurgical brain shift has been documented by Maurer [13] and by Skrinjar [19], who attribute it to the effect of gravity, to a gradual seepage of CSF, to cerebral blood volume manipulation, and to the effect of certain drugs. Existing techniques for dealing with brain shift include intraoperative MR scanners [13] and intraoperative ultrasound [7]. Miga [14] and Škrinjar [19] have independently developed FEM-based solutions in the same spirit as ours, although we emphasize the estimation of a dense surface displacement function, which is then interpolated over the brain volume (assuming null displacement at the base of the head), whereas their work focuses on the physical modelling which most realistically performs this interpolation or generically models this phenomenon.

Our goal is to first demonstrate the proof of concept of a technique integrating surface displacement estimation and finite-element modelling, with a highly accurate range-sensor and a brain-shaped phantom made of a well-characterized elastic material. A method based on surface displacement estimation and finite-element modelling is extremely compelling from a strictly economic standpoint, as the combination of range-sensor and FEM software is significantly cheaper than ultrasound or intraoperative MR. Moreover, our method also benefits from the speed, ease-of-use, and accuracy of range-sensors and state-of-the-art physical models. Also, our method does not preclude the integration of resection information, provided by a tracked hand-held probe [17] for example. Lastly, a surface displacement-FEM framework, minus the range-sensor, constitutes the foundation of a realistic patient-specific *surgical simulation* system, at the cost of a haptic feedback device, some optimization of the FEM computation for this environment, and modelling of surgical tools.

This paper is organized as follows. After the introduction, a presentation of our materials and methods is given in § 2, namely level-set segmentation of the skin and cortex (§ 2.1), range-sensing of the same two surfaces in the OR (§ 2.2), cortical motion estimation (§ 2.3), and an elastic brain phantom (§ 2.4). The results appear in § 3, and we discuss the results and future directions in § 4.

2   Materials and Methods

2.1   Level-set Surface Segmentation

The skin and cortex surface identification technique is an implementation of a recent algorithm, known as a *surface evolution* model, which imbeds 3D surface segmentation as the zero level-set of a 4D hypersurface Ψ, as illustrated in figure 2(a) for the problem of lesser dimensionality, namely identifying 2D contours. This approach possesses certain advantages over physically-based models, in particular its capacity to capture a large variety of topologies and a relative insensitivity to initial conditions [12].

In general, a surface evolution model is initialized by a user-defined surface completely inside (or outside) the desired anatomical boundary. The front then moves in a strictly outward (inward) manner as the zero level set of the evolving hypersuface [23]:

$$\frac{\partial \Psi}{\partial t} = \phi(x,y,z)\|\nabla\Psi\|(H + \nu) + \nabla\phi \cdot \nabla\Psi , \qquad (1)$$

where mean curvature H of the front is given by $div(\nabla\Psi/\|\nabla\Psi\|)$.

The model features a diffusive term $\|\nabla\Psi\|H$ which tends to smooth out the front, a hyperbolic term $\|\nabla\Psi\|\nu$ which pushes the front forward while preserving discontinuities, and two image terms: a speed function ϕ which slows down the front near strong gradients, and a so-called "doublet" term $\nabla\phi \cdot \nabla\Psi$ which prevents the front from overshooting these gradients. This model has been further

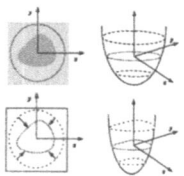 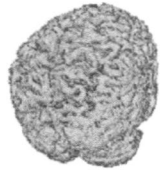 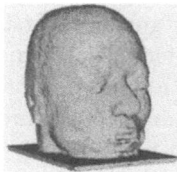

Fig. 2. Level-set segmentation: (a) imbedding of 2D contour estimation in 3D; (b) 3D surface of the cortex (seen from behind the occipital lobe), obtained with an outward-moving front initialized with 18 small spheres in the white matter (c) 3D surface of the skin, identified with an inward-moving front initialized at the scan perimeter.

generalized in [18]. The image cofactor ϕ is expressed as

$$\phi = \frac{1}{1 + \|\nabla \tilde{I}(x, y, z)\|^n} ,   (2)$$

where $\tilde{I}(x, y, z)$ is the *anisotropically* filtered equivalent of the original volume $I(x, y, z)$ and $n = 2$ or 3. We filter anisotropically, prior to computing gradients, because we will eventually *register* the result of the segmentation operation with a skin or cortex range image, and want to prevent unwanted blurring across relevant anatomical surfaces. This preprocessing is actually implemented within a level-set framework, namely by inputing the raw MRI/CT volume (as opposed to a distance map defined over the same volume) to a surface evolution model, but with only the diffusive term computation enabled [8]. Moreover, anatomical information can be taken into account by considering the result of an *Artificial Neural Network* (ANN) voxel classifier [10], in defining the image cofactor, for example to prevent an outward front from getting snagged at the grey matter-white matter boundary. Also, to reduce the complexity of computing a 4D, rather than 3D, function, we adopt the *narrow band* approach proposed by Adelsteinsson [1], which restricts the computation of the evolution equation near the evolving 3D surface.

A distance map is computed from the final surface by the fast marching level-set method [16], which estimates the arrival time $T(x, y, z)$ of a monotically advancing front by expressing an evolution equation of the type $\Psi_t + \phi(x, y, z)\|\nabla\Psi\| = 0$ as the Eikonal relation $\|\nabla T\|\phi = 1$. By using a constant unit speed ($\phi = 1$), this arrival time function corresponds to a *sub-pixel Euclidean distance map* [9]. Moreover, the propagative nature of the algorithm can be exploited to reveal *which surface point is closest to a given voxel* (i.e.: which surface point possesses the shortest arrival time). The relevance of this map is emphasized in § 2.3.

Lastly, not only is this segmentation technique useful in identifying the cortex and skin for the purpose of registration, we can further exploit it to label the nodes of our patient-specific finite-element model, according to tissue type, by combining the nodes initially circumscribed by the analytical user-defined surface with those traversed by the moving front. With this application in mind, we can also segment the external surface of tumours and ventricles.

2.2   Range-sensing

The three-dimensional coordinates of the visible surfaces of the skin and evolving cortex are computed by a commercial range-sensor made by Vitana Corp. (Ottawa, Canada), which uses both laser-based *triangulation* and *defocusing* techniques to estimate range [22]. Laser-based range-sensing is the industrial standard for quickly and accurately acquiring dense, quantitative information on 3D shape, used for example in robotic navigation, industrial quality control, and welding automation.

Triangulation involves projecting a thin ray of laser light onto an object, capturing the reflected light by a charge-coupled device (CCD), and inferring depth from the trigonometric relationship relating the pixel position of the reflected point, the position of the laser source and the CCD. Defocusing is implemented by allowing the laser light to pass through a mask featuring *two* holes, at a predetermined distance d apart, rather than one. The CCD sees two laser profiles instead of one, and range is determined by measuring the space (in each pixel column) between the two images. The sensor has .5mm pixel accuracy, based on a depth of field of 135mm and field of view of 10-12cm. During its linear travel, our program acquires 256 laser profiles at a constant rate, when the positioner is known to move at a constant speed. The *equal spacing* of our samples, resulting from the CCD being regular (in the i-k pixel coordinates, not in x-z spatial coordinates) and from constant-rate acquisition along the y-axis, is exploited later on in the registration process.

2.3   Surface Displacement Estimation

We estimate cortical surface deformation by first establishing a baseline for this movement, then by registering the initial cortical range image with its homologue identified in the MRI volume, and finally by tracking non-rigid cortical surface motion between time t_n and time t_{n+1}. Currently, we work with a brain-shaped phantom which does not possess a skin or a bone layer, and obtain this movement baseline by manually providing a rough alignment (based on the four corners of the range image domain) between the initial range and MRI surfaces of this phantom, and by refining it with a rigid-body registration to initial range data. The rigid-body refinement, at t_0, and all subsequent non-rigid stages of cortical registration are implemented with an *iterative closest point* (ICP) technique [5, 11]. This technique provides a much denser displacement map than a feature-based technique, which is important to best quantify non-rigid surface motion, which in turn is fundamentally underdetermined.

Our iterative registration technique bears some comparison to that of Lavallée and Szeliski [11], in that a distance map is precomputed for the MRI volume from the identified cortical surface, thereby accelerating the computation of distances between closest-point pairs, rather than imposing an expensive search for them. Because the Lavallée method produces only distances between closest point pairs, but does not provide information about which particular point is closest, it must resort to a search method, such as Levenberg-Marquardt, to determine the optimal transformation. In contrast, closed-form methods for computing transformation parameters all require *explicit* point-pairs, not distances between them. As emphasized in § 2.1, we make use of the fast marching level-set method to produce a dense map of both *closest point labels and the distances to them*, allowing us to do away with a search for closest points as well as producing explicit point pairs which can take advantage of closed-form transformation algorithms, thereby making each iteration of our ICP technique essentially instantaneous. We currently use Arun's SVD [3] technique to compute the rigid transformation between the two sets of points.

The non-rigid registration stage uses the same ICP matching technique to produce a smoothed displacement vector function. The expression of the deformation over a 2D domain is a consequence of our explicit displacement information being available only on an open surface, below and outside of which we defer to a realistically valued finite-element model to estimate volumetric movement. Furthermore, in characterizing non-rigid surface movement, we can exploit the regularity of the range domain by using Unser's extremely efficient *recursive splines* [21]. The justification for emphasizing computational efficiency here is two-pronged: *clinical acceptability* and the inherent *temporal underdetermination* in estimating non-rigid motion. We adopt a *smoothing spline* approach, whose first stage is a convolution with a smoothing kernel [1]

$$S_\lambda^n(Z) = 1/\left(B_1^n(Z) + \lambda(-Z + 2 - Z^{-1})^{\frac{n+1}{2}}\right), \qquad (3)$$

where $B_1^n(Z)$ is the *indirect B-spline transform* given by Unser [21], n is the order of the spline fitting (we use a linear fit: $n = 1$) and λ is the regularization parameter of the smoothing. This stage produces B-spline coefficients and is followed by a convolution with the indirect transform $B_1^n(Z)$ to yield the smoothed output. The filters can simply be cascaded to implement smoothing in 2D. In order to make the non-rigid motion estimation well-behaved, the smoothing parameter λ is initially set very high, and is gradually lowered as the process iterates, progressively resolving finer-level motion detail. Just as for the rigid ICP stage, each iteration of the non-rigid surface motion estimation is essentially instantaneous.

2.4   Elastic Brain Phantom

For the purpose of reproducing non-rigid cortical movement, we have implemented a brain-shaped phantom with elastic material properties. We use a jello mold in the shape of the brain (obtained from the Anatomical Products Online website [2]), into which we pour *PolyVinyl Alcohol Cryogel* (PVA-C), as illustrated in figure 3(a). The latter is a relatively *viscous liquid*, which upon freezing and thawing, becomes an *elastic solid* [6] as shown in figure 3(b). Furthermore, PVA-C can sustain several freeze-thaw cycles to acquire more rigidity, and the PVA concentration can also be manipulated to that effect, producing a Young's

---

[1] *Note: Z here relates to the Z-transform, not to be confused with the depth axis of the range-sensor.*

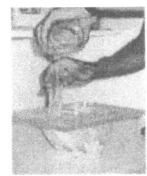
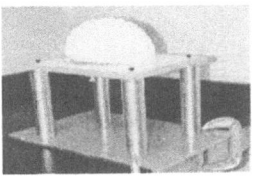

Fig. 3. Elastic PVA-C brain phantom: (a) liquid stage (b) final result after freezing and thawing.

modulus E in the .1 to .7 MPa spectrum [20]. This is comparable to values published in the literature for gray and white matter material properties [24]. This phantom features a moving assembly consisting of a small disk and rod of plexiglass, imbedded within the elastic material, as well as some glass beads used to validate the surface displacement/FEM approach to volumetric motion estimation. The position of the moving assembly can be modified by means of some set screws, drawing the embedded disk toward its support plate and triggering a compression of the elastic material.

3 Results and Discussion

Our segmentation implementation produces the expected results, as apparent in figure 2. The only new finding we report is the consideration of voxel classification results in making the image cofactor account for prior anatomical information. One of the main contributions of this paper, namely that the level-set framework leads to a very efficient iterative surface registration, is simply a fortuitous by-product of our segmentation design choice.

Our tests indicate that our implementation of an iterative closest point registration efficiently produces results comparable to other ICP techniques, as shown in figures 4 and 5 for rigid and non-rigid registration respectively. The algorithm, given a good starting point, does indeed converge to a very good pose estimation. The results of figure 4 are based on an initial alignment carried out by choosing four points on the level-set surface which roughly correspond to the corners of the range image, to which an arbitrary vertical distance of 15 pixels, or roughly 13.5mm was added.

In order to assess non-rigid surface tracking, we turn the set screws under the support plate of our elastic phantom, triggering a deformation of up to 15mm at the top, and image the cortical surface with our range-sensor, while maintaining the support plate fixed with respect to the range-sensor/positioner reference (see figure 3(b)). We then compare the results of a strictly rigid transformation computation with a sequence of rigid and non-rigid ICP registrations. Each option uses the same rough initial alignment based on the corners of the range domain. This comparison is currently based on visual inspection of how the original MRI level-set surface, subject to the inverse of the range-to-MRI transformation, aligns with the range data of the deformed cortical surface, and on

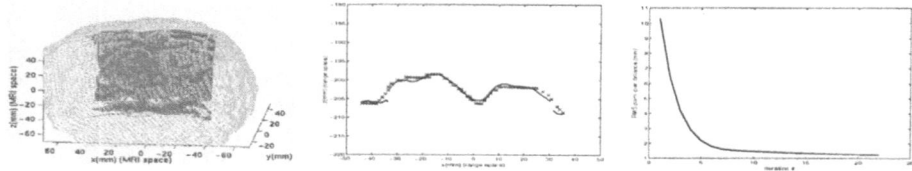

Fig. 4. Typical rigid registration results: (a) transformed range image overlaid on MRI level-set surface (both decimated by a factor of 2 for readability), in MRI space; (b) single range profile ($j = 192$ or $y = 79.592$) with projections of closest MRI points on $y = 79.592$ plane, in range space; (c) RMS point-pair distance plotted against ICP iteration number.

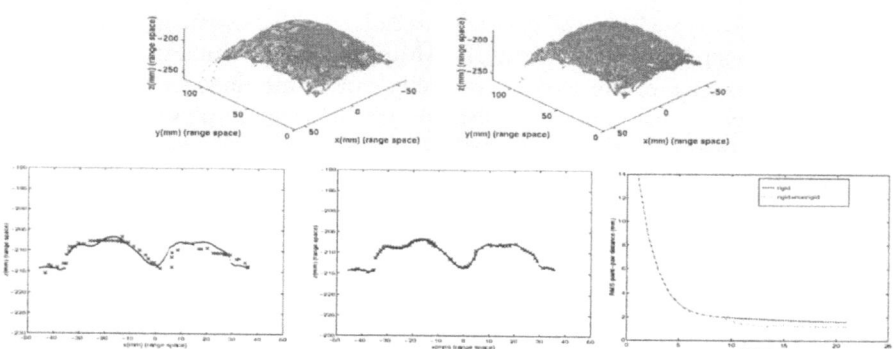

Fig. 5. Typical non-rigid registration results: (a) MRI level-set surface rigidly registered to the range image of the deformed phantom, in range space (both decimated by a factor of 2); (b) MRI level-set surface non-rigidly registered to the range image of the deformed phantom (both decimated by a factor of 2); (c) slice through (a), at $y = 79.592$; (d) slice through (b), at $y = 79.592$; (e) evolution of RMS point-pair distance with ICP iteration.

the two plots of the RMS distance between point-pairs against iteration number. The abrupt improvement of RMS distance on the second curve indicates the onset of the non-rigid stage, with an earlier rigid stage termination than the rigid-body stage illustrated by the first curve.

The RMS point-pair distance which appears in figures 4 may in fact overestimate the registration error between the two surfaces, due to the range data being much denser than the overlapping MRI-voxels which constitute the homologous patch of the level-set surface (65536 vs. 5782 points). In other words, because the ICP range-to-level set matches can be *many-to-one*, the point-pair distance has a large component which lies in the plane normal to the vector along the shortest path between the two surfaces which emanates from each level-set surface voxel. Furthermore, if the displacement vectors between the original (many-to-one) closest point pairs are used to determine the non-rigid spline-based transformation, we find that they distort the displacement map by inflating the components normal to the shortest path at each point between the two surfaces. We obtain better results by considering only the displacements of *mutually* closest (i.e.: one-to-one) pairs, which can be determined fairly easily from the original set of point pairs, and by iteratively propagating this displacement information everywhere else (this appears in figure 5).

Future registration work includes a *calibration* procedure which will relate points in range-sensor space to points in a global coordinate system in the OR, in a manner similar to Comeau's technique for relating the position of ultrasound data to a global OR reference [7]. This will serve as a good initial alignment for our rigid-body ICP range-MRI skin registration stage. Further work will address the sensitivity of ICP-type methods to initial alignment [5]. Finally, a validation of the surface tracking/FEM framework, by tracking glass beads imbedded in the brain phantom, is also planned.

4   Conclusion

This paper proposes a novel means of estimating intrasurgical deformations, based on level-set segmentation, range-sensing of the skin and cortex, fast rigid and non-rigid surface registration, and finite-element based estimation of volumetric displacement. We have emphasized some of the machine vision issues in this approach, in particular how the level-set framework can be exploited to yield computational speedups in the surface registration. The use of recursive splines is also a factor in our algorithmic efficiency. We have also presented a new brain-shaped elastic phantom with which non-rigid cortical movement can be enacted and our method can be validated.

5   Acknowledgements

The authors wish to thank Frank Ferrie and Sylvain Bouix of McGill, and Ken Chu and Kathleen Surry of Robarts for their help with this research. This work was supported by the National Science and Engineering Research Council of Canada NSERC grant OGP0155058, and the Medical Resarch Council of Canada MRC grant MT11540.

References

1. D. Adelsteinsson & J.A. Sethian, A Fast Level Set Method for Propagating Interfaces, *J. Computational Physics*, No. 118, pp. 269-277, 1995.
2. Anatomical Products Online: *www.anatomical.com/catalogs/product/21013brainmold.html*, 1998.
3. K.S. Arun et al., Least-squares Fitting of Two 3-D Point Sets, *IEEE Trans. Pattern Analysis & Machine Intelligence*, Vol. 9, No. 5, pp. 698-700, May 1987.
4. M.A. Audette, F.P. Ferrie & T.M. Peters, An Algorithmic Overview of Surface Registration Techniques for Medical Imaging, *Medical Image Analysis*, submitted.

5. P.J. Besl & N.D. McKay, A Method for Registration of 3-D Shapes, *IEEE Trans. Pattern Analysis & Machine Intelligence*, Vol.14, No.2, pp. 239-256, 1992.
6. K.C. Chu & B.K. Rutt, Polyvinyl Alcohol Cryogel: An Ideal Phantom Material for MR Studies of Arterial Flow and Elasticity, *Magnetic Resonance in Medicine*, No. 37, pp. 314-319, 1997.
7. R.M. Comeau, A.F. Sadikot, A. Fenster & T.M. Peters, Intraoperative Ultrasound for Guidance and Tissue Shift Correction in Image-guided Neurosurgery, *Medical Physics*, submitted, 1999.
8. B.B. Kimia & K. Siddiqi, Geometric Heat Equation and Nonlinear Diffusion of Shapes and Images, *Computer Vision and Image Understanding*, Vol. 64, No. 3, pp. 305-322, Nov. 1996.
9. R. Kimmel, N. Kiryati, and A.M. Bruckstein. Sub-pixel Distance Maps and Weighted Distance Transforms, *J. Mathematical Imaging and Vision*, No. 6, pp. 223-233, 1996.
10. V. Kollokian, *Performance Analysis of Automatic Techniques for Tissue Classification in MRI of the Human Brain*, Master's thesis, Concordia University, Montreal, Canada, November 1996.
11. S. Lavallée & R. Szeliski, Recovering the Position and Orientation of Free-form Objects from Image Contours Using 3D Distance Maps, *IEEE Trans. Pattern Analysis & Machine Intelligence*, Vol. 17, no. 4, pp. 378-390, 1995.
12. R. Malladi, J.A. Sethian & B.C Vemuri, Shape Modeling with Front Propagation: A Level Set Approach, *IEEE Trans. Pattern Analysis & Machine Intelligence*, Vol. 17, No. 2, Feb. 1995.
13. C.R. Maurer et al., Measurement of Intraoperative Brain Deformation Using a 1.5 Tesla Interventional MR System: Preliminary Results, *IEEE Trans. Medical Imaging*, Vol. 17, No. 5, pp. 817-825, Oct. 1998.
14. M. I. Miga et al., A 3D Brain Deformation Model Experiencing Comparable Surgical Loads, Proc. 19th Int. Conf. IEEE EMBS, pp. 773-776, 1997.
15. H. Murase & S.K. Nayar, Visual Learning and Recognition of 3-D Objects from Appearance, *Int. J. Computer Vision*, No. 14, pp. 5-24, 1995.
16. J.A. Sethian, Fast Marching Level Set Method for Monotonically Advancing Fronts, *Proc. Nat. Acad. Sci. USA*, Vol. 93, pp. 1591-1595, Feb. 1996.
17. M. Sinasac & T.M. Peters, Use of 3-D Deformable Surface Models for Intraoperative Visualization and Quantification of Cerebral Tissue Resection, *Medical Physics*, Vol. 24, No. 7, p. 1211, July 1997.
18. Kaleem Siddiqi et al., Area and Length-Minimizing Flows for Shape Segmentation, *IEEE Transactions on Image Processing*, Vol. 7, No. 3, pp. 433-443, 1998.
19. O. Škrinjar, D. Spencer & J. Duncan, Brain Shift Modeling for Use in Neurosurgery, *Medical Image Computing and Computer-Assisted Intervention- MICCAI'98*, pp. 641-649, 1998.
20. K. Surry, *www.irus.rri.on.ca/~kath*, 1999.
21. M. Unser, A. Aldroubi, & M. Eden, B-Spline Signal Processing: Part I- Theory, *IEEE Trans. Signal Proc.*, Vol. 41, No. 2, pp 821-833, Feb. 1993.
22. Vitana Corporation, *ShapeGrabber Reference Manual*, 1997.
23. A. Yezzi Jr. et al., A Geometric Snake Model for Segmentation of Medical Imagery, *IEEE Trans. Medical Imaging*, Vol. 16, No. 2, pp. 199-209, Apr. 1997.
24. C. Zhou, T.B. Khalil, & A.I. King, A New Model Comparing Impact Responses of the Homogeneous and Inhomogeneous Human Brain, *Society of Automotive Engineers, Inc. report #952714*, 1995.

A Single Image Registration Method for CT Guided Interventions

Robert C. Susil[1], James H. Anderson[2], Russell H. Taylor[3]

Department of Biomedical Engineering[1], Department of Radiology[2]
Department of Computer Science[3], The Johns Hopkins University
3400 N. Charles Street, Baltimore, Maryland 21218
rht@cs.jhu.edu

Abstract. Minimally invasive image guided interventions are an attractive option for localized therapy delivery and diagnostic biopsy. We have developed a method for CT guided needle placement, based upon the Brown-Roberts-Wells frame, which requires no immobilization or fiducial implantation. A localization module, placed on a needle holding robotic end effector, allows for localization of the effector in the image space using a single CT image. In a theoretical analysis, we show that this registration method has attractive sensitivity and error attenuation properties. Experimentally, the average error in needle tip location over 63 trials was 470 μm; 95% of the errors were below 1.0mm. This method is a fast, accurate, and easily implemented registration method for cross sectional image guided stereotaxis.

1 Objective

1.1 Motivation

Recent advances have identified a variety of novel anticancer therapeutic agents and targets. However, significant obstacles still hinder the effective *delivery* of these therapies to target tumor sites [1]. As cancer is expected to surpass cardiovascular disease as the major cause of death in the United States within five years [2], effective solutions to these delivery problems are warranted.

One solution to this delivery problem is to physically place therapeutic agents in or near the tumor site. However, for neural or visceral tumors, the physical delivery of therapy to the tumor is inherently a stereotactic problem. Therefore, effective image guided methods are needed to facilitate the accurate placement of therapy. In addition, these same methods can be applied to tumor biopsy for diagnostic tests.

Computed Tomography is a popular diagnostic imaging modality that is often used for the visualization of tumors. While CT provides high resolution cross sections of the anatomy, few techniques exist which can easily integrate this information with percutaneous therapy delivery to soft tissues. Extensive past efforts have been made to use CT images for guidance during biopsy and therapy for intracranial lesions [3] However, these methods largely involve the fixation of a stereotactic frame to the patient's skull, a significantly invasive procedure. For procedures involving soft tissue, such as within in the abdominal cavity, attaching a stereotactic frame is not feasible. Therefore, it would be preferable to have a method for CT guided tissue biopsy and therapy delivery which could obviate the need to physically attach a stereotactic frame to the patient.

1.2 Solution method

We have applied a localization method that allows for the guidance of stereotactic procedures using single CT image slices. Instead of attaching a frame to the patient, a localization module, based on the Brown-Roberts-Wells frame [4, 5], is attached to a needle holding robotic end effector (Figure 1). Due to the localization module's fiducial pattern, a single cross sectional image allows us to determine the pose of the needle in the image space. Instead of determining the position of the lesion in some external reference frame, we simply find the biopsy needle in the image coordinate system, along with the anatomy. Therefore, in a single image slice that intersects the target lesion and our needle localization module, we have enough information to determine the necessary kinematics to guide the needle to the target.

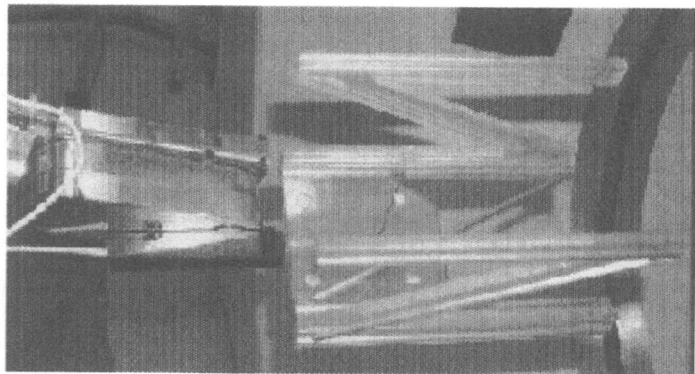

FIGURE 1: Localization module attached to the end effector. When inserted into the image field of view, a cross section of each of the nine aluminum fiducial bars appears in the CT image, allowing for registration.

1.3 Current Aims

Our final goal is complete automation of the needle placement, using a robotic arm, once the target is identified by the physician. However, the currently reported work focuses on the development and testing of the needle localization module itself. First, we show that the localization motif is theoretically robust over a range of poses, having both sensitivity to small positional changes and relative insensitivity to measurement errors. Subsequently, we compare our ability to determine the needle pose using single CT image slices with an independent multiple slice pose determination method, which we show to be an accurate ground truth. For 63 CT images, the average net displacement error at the needle tip (located 10 cm from the center of the needle holder) was 630 μm and 95 % of the errors were under 1.0 mm. This localization scheme, which still can be improved upon with minor modifications, is therefore shown to be both simple and accurate.

1.4 Prior Work and Present Contribution

Percutaneous procedures require one to determine the position of an internal target without direct visualization. Most often, this involves registration of an image data set, in which the target is identified, with physical space. This procedure, stereotaxy, was founded by Clarke and Horsley in 1906 [6]. Most techniques have been based upon an rigid frame which is attached to the patient, providing a common coordinate system through which the image and physical spaces can be related [3]. While stereotactic procedures were initially advanced using two-dimensional imaging modalities, the advent of Computed Tomography in the 1970's greatly accelerated development and application. Instead of projecting three-dimensional structures into two-dimensions, this modality provides a series of 2D image slices, allowing for true three-dimensional reconstruction.

The Brown-Roberts-Wells (BRW) frame was first introduced in 1979 [4]. The frame, consisting of three N shaped motifs attached to the patient's skull, represented a major advance in CT localization. Previous frames were constrained to remain strictly perpendicular to the image plane, providing little flexibility [3]. However, the BRW frame was more versatile in that the position and orientation of the frame was fully encoded within each image slice, allowing for rotations and tilting of the frame relative to the image plane[4]. Therefore, the position of any point can easily be found in both the frame and the image space coordinate systems.

We have applied this fiducial motif with several additions. Primarily, instead of fixing the frame to the patient, we have placed the frame on our end effector. Therefore, while we are still able to find the relation between the patient's anatomy and the end effector with a singe CT slice, the procedure is markedly less invasive. Moreover, in previous applications, the base ring of the N-frame fiducials remained *nearly* parallel to the image plane.[7-9]. However, because the frame is now placed on the mobile end effector (Figure 1), we need to ensure that this localization scheme is robust over a range of operating points. Therefore, we perform a theoretical analysis, examining both sensitivity to small positional changes and attenuation of measurement errors. In addition, we experimentally compare this single image registration method with an independent multislice registration method.

Many techniques have been developed which integrate robotic guidance of end effectors with image based stereotactic procedures using a variety of registration techniques. For example, Lavallee et al. implemented a system for image guided intracranial needle placement using biplaner x-ray [10]. In another neurosurgical system, Kwoh et al. develop a surgical plan using multiple CT image slices, register by docking their robot with the patient's stereotactic head frame, and then place the needle without CT surveillance[11]. Glauser et al. also use a stereotactic head frame to register the robot and image space, but are able to perform needle placement under active CT surveillance to confirm the position of their end effector [12]. Similarly, Masamune et al. perform needle placement within the CT scanner and register using a stereotactic head frame [13]. More recently, Bzostek et al. have developed a technique for stereotactic procedures, under biplanar fluoroscopy, in order to access mobile organs (e.g. the kidneys) [14, 15].

Similarly, our technique is designed to facilitate end effector placement within the CT scanner. However, while previous techniques have relied on techniques that only register the robot space once, we are able to perform our registration with every image slice. Primarily, the technique is simple, requiring no extensive calibration routine. Moreover, it allows for immediate confirmation of the end effector position with each slice and therefore, the system is robust and well suited for dynamic and error prone situations.

1.5 Target Application Example

Although the applications of this localization scheme are numerous, an obvious application is for percutaneous tissue biopsy within the abdominal cavity. First, the patient is placed in the CT scanner and a complete set of images in the area of interest is collected. Next, upon recognition of a tumor mass, the physician selects a biopsy target and a skin entry site from the image set. The robot, with biopsy needle end effector and localization module, is positioned such that the localization module is within the imager field of view. Next, a single image is taken, containing both the biopsy target and a cross section of the localization module. From this one image, the necessary translation and rotation to reach the target is determined and subsequently executed by the robot. The robot, or an attendant surgeon, can then drive the biopsy needle. Because the patient remains within the scanner, a single image will confirm that the needle has reached the target site. The biopsy is then taken, completing the procedure quickly and with minimal invasiveness. We emphasize that this system, with minor material modifications, can easily be extended to use with MRI.

2   Methods

2.1 Description of registration method

In order to register the biopsy needle to the image space, we need to find a set of three corresponding points in both the needle holder coordinate system, H, and the image coordinate system, I. These three points define a coordinate system P. By finding the position and orientation of P in the image, $_P^I T$, and the holder space, $_P^H T$, we can then determine the pose of the holder in the image coordinate system, $_H^I T = _P^I T (_P^H T)^{-1}$. Having previously performed the calibration of the needle holder, H, and the needle, N, coordinate systems, $_N^H T$, we can find $_N^I T$, the pose of the biopsy needle in the image space.

In order to find the set of three corresponding points in both the image and holder coordinate systems using only one CT image, we use the Brown-Roberts-Wells frame.[4]

2.2 Description of Holder

The localization module of the needle holder is illustrated in Figure 1. The module is *designed to easily attach to a needle driver end effector* [16, 17] using four screws. The basic structural element of the module is the 'N' shaped fiducial motif (Figure 2a). This motif is repeated three times, forming a 'U' shaped module with one fiducial motif as a base and the other two fiducial motifs as sides (Figure 1).

The fiducial lines in each motif are made of 0.25 inch diameter aluminum rod inlaid in acrylic. In our prototype, $L_1 = 8$ inches and $L_2 = 4$ inches (Figure 2a). We define a

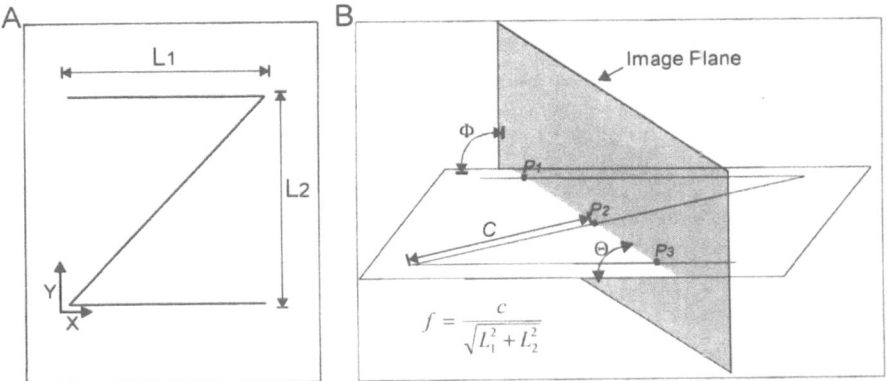

FIGURE 2: Panel A: Dimensioning and coordinate system conventions for the fiducial motifs. **Panel B**: One fiducial motif intersected by the image plane. p_1, p_2, and p_3 are the three fiducial bar points of intersection with the image plane. f, ϕ, and θ define the orientation of the image plane relative to the fiducial motif (f=fraction of distance along diagonal fiducial where intersection occurs).

holder coordinate system, H, with an origin at the center of the 'U' shaped module and an orientation coincident with that of the base plate fiducial motif (Figure 2a).

2.3 Single image registration method

A CT image of each fiducial motif produces a cross section of the three bars, yielding three ellipses in the image. By finding the centroids of these ellipses we can locate the centers of the three bars where they intersect the image plane. Using these three points, ${}^I p_1$, ${}^I p_2$, and ${}^I p_3$, we can determine the position of one corresponding point, cp_n, in both the holder space, ${}^H cp_n$, and the image space, ${}^I cp_n$.

We can describe the relationship between the fiducial motif and the image plane with three parameters: f, the fraction of the distance along the diagonal fiducial where the intersection occurs; ϕ, the angle between the fiducial motif plane and the image plane; and θ, the angle between the parallel fiducial bars and the line of intersection (Figure 2b).

The distances $|{}^{FM}p_1 - {}^{FM}p_2|$ and $|{}^{FM}p_3 - {}^{FM}p_2|$, expressed as a function of f, ϕ, and θ, are:

$$\left| {}^{FM}p_1 - {}^{FM}p_2 \right| = \csc(\theta)L_2(1-f) \tag{1}$$

$$\left| {}^{FM}p_3 - {}^{FM}p_2 \right| = \csc(\theta)L_2(f) \tag{2}$$

The ratio of these distances is:

$$\frac{\left| {}^{FM}p_1 - {}^{FM}p_2 \right|}{\left| {}^{FM}p_3 - {}^{FM}p_2 \right|} = \frac{1}{f} - 1 \tag{3}$$

This ratio is only a function of f, the fraction of the distance along the diagonal fiducial where the intersection occurs. Because the transformation from the fiducial motif coordinate system to the image space is a rigid body transformation, we can determine the point where the image plane intersects the diagonal bar, $^{FM}p_2$, by finding the ratio of the distances between points $^{I}p_1$, $^{I}p_2$, and $^{I}p_3$. From a previous calibration of our holder, we know the transformation for this point, $^{FM}p_2$, to the holder coordinate system, $^{H}_{FM}T$. Therefore, we know the position of this intersection in both the image space, $^{I}p_2$, and the holder space, $^{H}p_2$, providing one of the three corresponding points, cp_1. We repeat this method for the two remaining fiducial motifs, generating all three corresponding points, cp_1, cp_2, and cp_3.

2.4 Error analysis

With the set of three points generated by the intersection of each of the three fiducial motifs and the image plane, we could do more than determine one corresponding point in the image and holder coordinate systems. Namely, we could also determine the angle θ (Figure 2b). However, we have very little accuracy in determining this angle. When operating about $\theta = 90^{o}$, the sensitivity of our assessment of θ ($\partial \theta_{measured} / \partial \theta_{actual}$) is zero. In contrast, determination of the corresponding point has much more attractive error properties, which we demonstrate here.

To robustly determine the corresponding points, the localization method must have two properties. First, the assessment of $^{H}cp_n$ should be relatively insensitive to small measurement errors in $|^{I}p_1 - {}^{I}p_2|$ and $|^{I}p_3 - {}^{I}p_2|$. These sensitivities to measurement error are:

$$\frac{\partial c}{\partial \left| {}^{I}p_1 - {}^{I}p_2 \right|_{measured}} = -f\sqrt{1 + \left(\frac{L_1}{L_2}\right)^2} \sin(\theta) \tag{4}$$

$$\frac{\partial c}{\partial \left| {}^{I}p_3 - {}^{I}p_2 \right|_{measured}} = (1-f)\sqrt{1 + \left(\frac{L_1}{L_2}\right)^2} \sin(\theta) \tag{5}$$

Near the operating point ($\theta = 90^{o}$ and $f=0.5$), the magnitudes of the sensitivities are 0.71. As θ decreases, the system becomes less sensitive to measurement errors. The worst case measurement error sensitivity is 1.41. However, we can improve these values by decreasing the L_1/L_2 ratio (see Future Work).

Second, the measured parameters, $|^{I}p_1 - {}^{I}p_2|$ and $|^{I}p_3 - {}^{I}p_2|$, must be sensitive to small changes in c, the distance from the image plane intersection with the diagonal fiducial to the fiducial motif origin (i.e. $c = f\sqrt{L_1^2 + L_2^2}$) (Figure 2b). This sensitivity is:

$$\frac{\partial \left| {}^{I}p_1 - {}^{I}p_2 \right|}{\partial c} = -\csc(\theta) \Bigg/ \sqrt{1 + \left(\frac{L_1}{L_2}\right)^2} \tag{6}$$

$$\frac{\partial \left| {}^{I}p_3 - {}^{I}p_2 \right|}{\partial c} = \csc(\theta) \Bigg/ \sqrt{1 + \left(\frac{L_1}{L_2}\right)^2} \tag{7}$$

At the operating point of $\theta = 90^o$, the magnitudes of the sensitivities are 0.71, which is the worst case for the system. As θ decreases, the sensitivity increases. Also, as was the case previously, we can improve the sensitivity by decreasing the L_1/L_2 ratio (see Future Work).

In summary, we find that the system has relatively good error characteristics. The worst case sensitivity to measurement error is 1.41 and the worst case sensitivity of the system is 0.71 (for L_1/L_2=1).

2.5 Multislice registration method

In order to determine the accuracy of the single slice registration method, we need to determine the ground truth pose of the holder in the image space. To do this, we performed a multislice registration of the holder. By using several image slices, we can find a series of points along each fiducial bar in the image coordinate system. By performing a least squares line fit, we can very accurately determine the pose of the holder in the image space.

The accuracy of this registration method was assessed by comparing the calculated transformations between the three fiducial motif coordinate systems which compose the localization module. As these transformations are determined by the geometry of the module (Figure 1), they are invariant. Over the six image sets studied, the calculated transformations had an average variation of 0.066° and 120 μm. Therefore, we are confident in using this multislice registration method as our ground truth.

3   Results

3.1 Experiment Design

To determine the accuracy of our single slice localization method, we compared the single slice determination of the needle pose, ${}_{N}^{I}T_{SS}$, with the multislice ground truth determination of needle pose, ${}_{N}^{I}T_{MS}$. An average of 13 images were obtained with the holder in each of 5 different poses (a total of 63 images). All images were obtained in a GE Genesis CT Scanner. Image slices were 5 mm thick and the image pixels were 0.7 mm by 0.7 mm.

3.2 Results

Error is defined as the difference between the multislice determined ground truth and the single slice determined pose. Components include angular error of holder pose and offset error of holder pose. From these two components, net displacement error at the needle tip, 10 cm from the center of the holder, was found. The average angular error was 0.32°, the average displacement offset error was 380μm, and the average displacement error at the needle tip was 630 μm. Figure 3 presents the displacement error probability density function with a best-fit gamma distribution (λ =2.95 and α =0.16). 95 % of the needle tip displacement errors were below 1.0 mm and the maximum error seen in the 63 images was 1.45 mm.

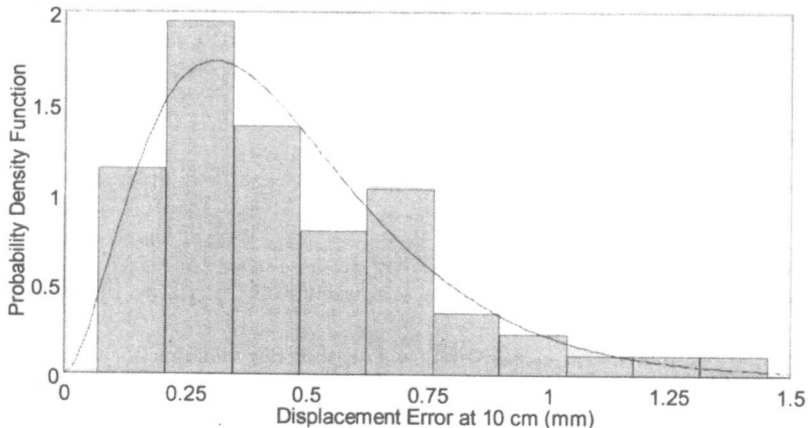

FIGURE 3: Experimental data and the best fit, by maximum likelihood, gamma distribution (λ=2.95 and α=0.16). 95% of the errors are found below 1.0 mm.

4   Discussion

We have developed a system, based upon the Brown-Roberts-Wells frame, that allows for accurate determination of end effector pose using a single CT image. While this study was carried out entirely under CT, the same methods can be applied to other cross sectional imaging modalities, namely, MRI.

Most notably, we find that the localization frame provides accurate registration over a range of operating points. In previous work, it was found that the Brown-Roberts-Wells was accurate enough to be applied in neurosurgical interventions [6-8] However, these applications employed a narrow operating range with the stereotactic base ring nearly parallel to the scan plane. Here, because the frame is attached to the robotic end-effector, we have a very large operating range. Even over this large range, both our theoretical and experimental error analysis show that the system is accurate and reliable.

We emphasize several positive features of this system. First, it is minimally invasive. There is no need to attach any fiducial frames or markers to the patient, making it ideal for soft tissue interventions where attachment of a stereotactic frame is not practical.

Second, it allows for real time confirmation of needle position relative to the anatomy. Because the whole system is integrated within the CT scanner, images can be taken at any point, such as for positive confirmation of needle placement within a lesion. Finally, the system is relatively simple in that it requires no external reference frames. All registration is done based upon single CT images. While work remains to be done in order to integrate this system with a robotic actuator and on-line target selection, our localization module is a significant first step in developing a versatile, integrated image guided stereotactic system.

5   Future Work

Although we achieved a good level of accuracy in the present study, there are several ways in which our system can be more robust.

5.1 Multiple resolution fiducial motifs

As discussed in the Methods section, the localization system's sensitivity is dependent upon minimizing the ratio L_1/L_2 (Figure 2 and Equations 4-7). That is, the steeper the diagonal fiducial bar, the better. In the present study, $L_1/L_2=2$. While this may not seem optimal, a high L_1/L_2 ratio gives us a larger range of valid image slices. In order for the localization module to work, all three fiducial motifs, therefore all nine fiducial bars, must intersect the image plane. While a low L_1/L_2 ratio yields better sensitivity, it also shortens the localization module, resulting in only a few valid image slices. Therefore, we must reach a balance between a low ratio for good sensitivity and a higher ratio for a larger number of valid images.

In order to obtain both of these benefits, we could place multiple fiducial motifs on each of the three planes. This would appear as several diagonal fiducial bars, one with a small slope and several with large slopes, on each plane. The high L_1/L_2 ratio motif (i.e. small slope) could provide an initial pose estimate while a smaller L/L_2 ratio motif (i.e. larger slope) could then provide more accurate pose determination.

5.2 Centroid Finding Method

In the present work, we used a simple centroid finding routine in order to find the centers of our fiducial bars in the CT image. The images were thresholded and binarized, removing all data except for the locations of the aluminum fiducial bars. To find the centroids, the centers of mass of the binarized 'blobs' were computed.

A more sophisticated routine, such as fitting an ellipse to the boundary of the aluminum bars, would surely yield increased centroid finding accuracy.

5.3 Reconfiguration of fiducial motifs

In order to find the transformation from the holder coordinate system to the image space, $_H^I T$, we find three corresponding points in both the holder and image coordinate systems. Upon examining our data, we find that the accuracy in determining the holder orientation is dependent upon the distance between these three points. That is, a set of points that are widely separated will produce a more accurate orientation than a set of closely placed points. In order to demonstrate this, we plot the angular error versus the shortest 'moment arm' of the three points (Figure 4). The moment arm is defined as the perpendicular distance from one point to the line connecting the other two points. We find that there is a significant dependence of angular error on the shortest moment arm (p value of 0.02).

With a simple reconfiguration of the localization module (i.e. reversing the base plate orientation) we can ensure that the smallest possible moment arm is 67 mm. This is a significant increase over the present configuration, where the shortest moment arms vary from 15 mm to 47 mm. With an increase in distance between corresponding points, we can expect an increase in angular accuracy.

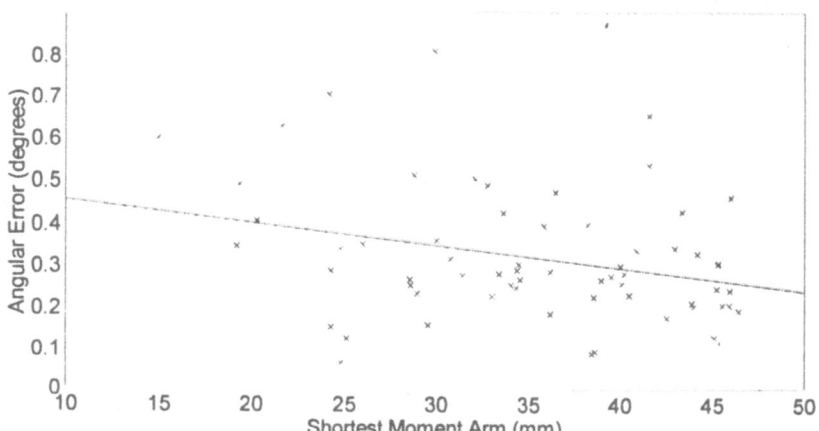

FIGURE 4: Angular error is a function of the shortest 'moment arm'. The p value for the linear regression is 0.02. With minor modification of our localization module, we can increase the shortest possible moment arm to 67 mm.

5.4 Adaptation/Extension to MRI

We note that with minor changes in materials, our localization system can be easily extended for applications using magnetic resonance imaging. With fast spin echo MRI, which allows for rapid image acquisition (e.g. 'MR fluoroscopy'), both the patient's anatomy and our end effector could be followed in real time, allowing for accurate and interactive effector guidance in a variety of percutaneous procedures.

References

1. Jain, R.K., *The Next Forntier of Molecular Medicine: Delivery of Therapeutics.* Nature, 1997(4): p. 655-657.
2. Klausner, R.D., *The Nation's Investment in Cancer Research: A Budget Proposal for Fiscal Year 1999*, . 1997, National Cancer Institute.
3. Galloway, R.L., *Stereotactic Frame Systems and Intraoperative Localization Devices,* in *Interactive Image-guided Neurosurgery,* R.J. Maciunas, Editor. 1993, American Association of Neurological Surgeons. p. 9-16.
4. Brown, R.A., *A stereotactic head frame for use with CT body scanners.* Invest. Radiol., 1979. 14: p. 300-304.

808   R. C. Susil et al.

5. Brown, R.A., T.S. Roberts, and A.G. Osborne, *Stereotaxic frame and computer software for CT-directed neurosurgical localization.* Invest. Radiol., 1980. **15**: p. 308-312.
6. Clarke, R.H. and c. al., *On the intrinsic fibers of the cerebellum, its nuclei, and its efferent tracks.* Brain, 1905. **28**: p. 12-29.
7. Goerss, S., et al., *A computed tomographic stereotactic adaptation system.* Neurosurgery, 1982. **10**: p. 375-379.
8. Leksell, L. and B. Jernberg, *Stereotaxis and tomography: a technical note.* Acta Neurochir., 1980. **52**: p. 1-7.
9. Mundinger, F., *CT-stereotactic biopsy of brain tumors,* in *Tumors of the Central Nervous System in Infancy and Childhood,* D. Goth, P. Gutjahr, and C. Langmaid, Editors. 1982, Springer-Verlag: New York. p. 234-246.
10. Lavallee, S., et al., *Image-Guided Operating Robot: A Clinical Application in Stereotactic Neurosurgery,* in *Computer-Integrated Surgery,* R.H. Taylor, et al., Editors. 1996, MIT Press: Cambridge, Mass. p. 343-352.
11. Kwoh, Y.S., Hou. J., and E.A. Jonckheere, et. al., *A robot with improved absolute positioning accuracy for CT guided stereotactic brain surgery.* IEEE Trans Biomed Eng, 1988. **35**(2): p. 153-161.
12. Glauser, D., et al. *Neurosurgical Robot Minerva, First Results and Current Developments.* in *Proc. 2nd Int. Symp. on Medical Robotics and Computer Assisted Surgery.* 1995. Baltimore, Maryland: MRCAS '95 Symposium, C/O Center for Orthop Res, Shadyside Hospital, Pittsburgh, Pa.
13. Masamune, K., et al. *A newly developed stereotactic robot with detachable driver for neurosurgery.* in *Proc. 2nd Int. Symp. on Medical Robotics and Computer Assisted Surgery (MRCAS).* 1995. Baltimore, Md.: MRCAS '95 Symposium, C/O Center for Orthop Res, Shadyside Hospital, Pittsburgh, Pa.
14. Bzostek, A., et al. *An automated system for precise percutaneous access of the renal collecting system.* in *Proceedings the First Joint Conference of CVRMed and MRCAS.* 1997. Grenoble, France.
15. Schreiner, S., et al. *A system for percutaneous delivery of treatment with a fluoroscopically-guided robot.* in *Joint Conf. of Computer Vision, Virtual Reality, and Robotics in Medicine and Medical Robotics and Computer Surgery.* 1997. Grenoble.
16. Stoianovici, D., et al. *An efficient needle injection technique and radiological guidance method for percutaneous procedures.* in *First Joint Conference: CRVMed II & MRCAS III, March.* 1997. Grenoble, France.
17. Stoianovici, D., et al. *A Modular Surgical Robotic System for Image-Guided Percutaneous Procedures.* in *Medical Image Computing and Computer-Assisted Interventions (MICCAI-98).* 1998. Cambridge, Mass: Springer.

An Integrated Visualization System for Surgical Planning and Guidance Using Image Fusion and Interventional Imaging

David T. Gering[1], Arya Nabavi[2], Ron Kikinis[2], W. Eric L. Grimson[1], Noby Hata[2], Peter Everett[2], and Ferenc Jolesz[2] and William M. Wells[1,2]

[1] MIT AI Laboratory, Cambridge MA, USA
gering@ai.mit.edu
http://www.ai.mit.edu/people/gering
[2] Brigham and Women's Hospital, Harvard Medical School, Boston MA, USA

Abstract. We present a software package which uniquely integrates several facets of image-guided medicine into a single portable, extendable environment. It provides capabilities for automatic registration, semi-automatic segmentation, 3D surface model generation, 3D visualization, and quantitative analysis of various medical scans. We describe its system architecture, wide range of applications, and novel integration with an interventional Magnetic Resonance (MR) scanner to augment intra-operative imaging with pre-operative data. Analysis previously reserved for pre-operative data can now be applied to exploring the anatomical changes as the surgery progresses. Surgical instruments are tracked and used to drive the location of reformatted slices. Real-time scans are visualized as slices in the same 3D view along with the pre-operative slices and surface models. The system has been applied in over 20 neurosurgical cases at Brigham and Women's Hospital, and continues to be routinely used for 1-3 cases per week. [1]

1 Introduction

Image-guided surgery systems facilitate surgical planning and analysis by aligning various data sets with information on morphology (MR, CT, MR angiography), cortical function (fMRI), or metabolic activity (PET, SPECT). Systems for surgical guidance additionally provide a means of estabishing a correspondance between the fused, pre-operative data and the patient as positioned on the operating table.

1.1 Limitations of Conventional Image-Guided Surgery

The accuracy provided by frame-based and frameless stereotaxy decreases as surgery progresses. The positions of anatomical structures change as the brain

---

[1] Ron Kikinis and Ferenc Jolesz received partial support from NIH grants P41 RR13218-01, P01 CA67165-03, and R01 RR11747-01A. Eric Grimson received partial support from NSF grant IIS-9610249.

swells when the skull is opened, cerebrospinal fluid (CSF) egresses, or tumor tissue is removed. Greater dynamics accompany the resection of larger or deeper tumors.

Intra-operative imaging is being developed to address these concerns and also to detect unexpected complications during surgery such as hemorrhage. Interventional imaging is typically performed with X-ray fluoroscopy or ultrasound [2]. More recently, technological developments have led to high-resolution, high-contrast 3D interventional imaging, such as interventional CT [8], and MRI [12]. Compared to the other named interventional imaging modalities, an open MR system provides the advantages of high soft-tissue contrast, a lack of radiation exposure to patient and surgeon, a clear definition of resection boundaries, and continuous access to the operative field [7].

1.2   Augmenting Interventional MRI with the 3D Slicer

In order to amplify the benefits of interventional MRI, we propose augmenting the scanning component with computer software that maximizes the interactivity of an image-guided therapy system through focusing on the following five areas:

Image Resolution — Some anatomical structures are difficult to distinguish on interventional MR images, but are clearer on conventional, diagnostic MRI that benefit from a higher magnetic field and longer imaging times.

Imaging Time — For surgical guidance to be interactive, images must be acquired quickly enough to be utilized without disrupting or slowing down the procedure. Fast imaging techniques are being developed, but in general, faster imaging brings lower image quality.

Multi-modal Fusion — Functional and metabolic data that is acquired pre-operatively could deliver increased benefit if integrated with intra-operative, anatomical information.

Faster Localization — Interventional MR provides the capability of planning approach trajectories by maneuvering a tracked wand and collecting images at the rate of 6-20 seconds per image. While this is valuable, an ideal interactive system needs an update rate of 10 frames per second.

3D Visualization — Interventional images are presently two-dimensional — requiring the surgeon to mentally map the 2D images seen on a computer screen to the 3D operating field.

The 3D Slicer is a software package that addresses the aforementioned areas. Image resolution, imaging time, and localization are improved by performing real-time re-slicing of both pre-operative and intra-operative data sets, and displaying them for simultaneous review. Multi-modal information is incorporated through automatic registration. The 3D Slicer features a computer graphics display that offers the flexibility to see the situation from viewpoints not physically possible. It has the ability to "fly through" virtual data to facilitate the understanding of complex situations, and aid in avoiding damage to healthy tissue.

After testing basic concepts in a clinical trial described in [5], the system was redesigned from scratch. The important developments we report here are the lessons learned in engineering of the system into an effective and frequently-used surgical tool, and the experiences of using the system in a variety of applications.

2   System Architecture

2.1   Development Platforms

We developed the 3D Slicer on top of the OpenGL graphics library using the Visualization Toolkit (VTK) [13] for processing, and the Tcl/Tk scripting language for the user interface. VTK provides a set of objects written in C++ that can be chained together to form a data-processing pipeline. Pipelined processing maximizes interactivity because the output of each stage is stored in memory, and any update from user-interface controls triggers a change at a minimal depth into the pipeline. We added several classes to VTK by deriving them from existing, documented classes, which results in well-defined inputs and outputs. Appropriately coded classes handle multiple data types and multi-threading. We run the 3D Slicer on PCs running Windows and Sun workstations running Solaris.

2.2   Visualization

Reformatting: We visualize volume data (3D array of voxels) through Multi-Plane Reformatting (MPR). A reformatted image is derived by arbitrarily orienting a plane in 3D space, and assigning values to each 2D pixel of the plane by interpolating the 3D voxels of the volume data intersected by the plane. We reformat up to three slices at once with independent orientations, in real time. Slices can be arbitrarily oblique, or orthogonal and oriented relative to either the coordinate frame of the scanner or the tracked pointing device. Some radiological applications insist on minimum interpolation, and so we provided additional orientation options that generate orthogonal slices relative to the data itself rather than the coordinate frame it has been registered to.

Multiple Volumes on the Same Slice: Each reformatted slice may be generated from any of the available data sets. For example, one slice could be reformatted from preoperative SPGR, a second slice could be reformatted from preoperative T2-weighted MRI, and a third slice could display the images that are being scanned in real time. We extended reformatting to slice through both anatomical and functional volumes of data simultaneously. Each slice is the composite of a background layer, foreground layer, and label layer. The background image is typically gray-scaled anatomical data, and the optional foreground can be colored, functional information. The foreground layer is overlaid on the background layer with an adjustable opacity to form the image that is displayed on the slice. As for the third layer, the output of image segmentation is a label map where each voxel is assigned an integer label according to the segmented structure it belongs to. The boundaries of each of these structures can optionally be drawn in color on the image.

Display Windows: There is an image-processing pipeline for each slice that takes 3D volume data as input, computes a fast reformat using integer math to create 2D data, converts from scalar values to screen colors, overlays the foreground layer on the background layer, and draws cursors and annotation. The output images are displayed in 2D image windows (one for each slice) and texture-mapped onto graphics planes that are correctly positioned in 3D space and rendered in a 3D view. We found that users often need to vary their focus between the 2D images and the 3D rendering. We provided three different methods in attempting to create a convenient interface for all users. First, there is a foveal view in the form of a 2D window that provides a magnified version of the area around the cursor. Second, each 2D image may be zoomed independently. Third, the display mode may be set to show a huge 3D view, a large 3D view and the three 256x256 2D images, or all 4 windows set to size 512x512.

Surface Models: Surface models of key anatomical structures can be visualized in the 3D view along with the reformatted slices. Our surgical colleagues like to see a portion of the skin as a landmark, so we allow for the slice planes to selectively clip away the skin model to reveal other unclipped models beneath, such as a tumor or physiologically critical structures like blood vessels, as well as the respective image planes. In cases where the tumor is near the eloquent cortex, such as centers of speech or motor processing, functional models are included to illustrate their proximity to tumor tissue. These models display the 3D structure of a detected correlation of functional response. Each model is colored differently (and consistently between cases), and rendered with adjustable opacity (Figure 1). We also support applications that require varying a model's color along its surface to visualize a property, such as bladder wall thickness, for example.

Trajectory Assistance: In addition to slices and models, the locator (a tracked wand or surgical instrument) is also rendered as a cylinder in 3D space at its correct location and orientation. The software can also provide means for assisted trajectory planning and guidance. Once a low-contrast target is identified using near real-time imaging, it is sometimes difficult to quickly find it again. This can be simply avoided by marking the probe's position with a bright red sphere on the 3D display, so the location can be easily returned to.

Trajectory assistance is achieved through marking the point of entry with one sphere, and the target tissue with another sphere, and rendering a cylinder between the two points. Thus the surgeon has only to align the rendered locator with the target in a video-game-like exercise to find the planned approach.

2.3 Multi-Modal Registration

The 3D Slicer supports rigid, manual registration by allowing the user to specify which volume to move, and then intuitively translate and rotate that data set by clicking and dragging on the images in the 2D windows. The reference volume can be displayed as the background layer of the slices, and the registered volume can be displayed translucently as the foreground layer. Furthermore, with one button click, the result of manual registration can be used as an initial pose for automatic registration by maximization of mutual information [16]. This method is of general utility, and other implementations of it have performed well in an NIH-sponsored test [6]. The registration capability is implemented as a separate process that communicates with the 3D Slicer through the use of MRML files as described below.

2.4   Volume Editor

Volumetric data can be semi-automatically segmented using the 3D Slicer's suite of editing tools. Effects such as thresholding, morphological operations, island-removal (erasing small groupings of similar pixels), measuring the size of islands, cropping, and free-hand drawing of polygons, lines, or points can be applied to the data on a 3D or slice-by-slice basis. We found it very helpful to users to allow the slice-by-slice editing to be administered on either axial, coronal, or sagittal slices merely by clicking on the appropriate slice. Each effect may be applied to either the *original* volume, or a *working* volume. Multiple editing effects may be applied to the working volume, and when finished, the working volume may be merged with a *composite* volume to overlay smaller structures onto larger ones.

For example, we segment skin automatically from an MR scan by applying a threshold at the first trough of the histogram (where the noise and signal lobes overlap) and storing the binary output in the working volume. We then remove islands in the working volume, and finish with an erosion and dilation to smooth the edges, as was performed in the making of Figure 1. This working volume is then copied to the composite volume. Next, segmentation of the brain can be performed in the working volume, and all non-zero voxels of the working volume can overwrite the composite volume to form a combination of skin and brain. A strength of our system is that effects can be visualized by overlaying the working volume translucently on the original volume and explored in the 3D view.

Through a modular architecture that exploits C++ inheritance, other researchers can easily add new segmentation tools to this suite.

2.5   Model Generation

The output of the segmentation process is a set of label maps, where pixels take on values corresponding to tissue type. The bounding surfaces of the label maps are extracted and represented as a collection of triangles using marching cubes. Decimation reduces the number of triangles to a quantity that can be more quickly rendered with little observable loss in detail [14]. For example, a typical brain surface is reduced from approximately 500,000 triangles to 150,000.

We found it helpful to have the 3D Slicer call a separate process to generate the models so that sets of many models could be performed as a batch job in the background while the user continues to use the 3D Slicer for other tasks. Model generation can be run on another machine with more memory and the user is emailed when the job is complete so the models can be viewed in the 3D Slicer.

2.6   Measurements

The 3D Slicer facilitates several types of quantitative measurements that may be made in 3D space. One can click on a particular surface model to measure its surface area or volume. Markers can be positioned on the surface models and slice planes by clicking on the 3D view, and then the distances or angles between markers can be measured.

2.7   Image-Guided Surgery

We integrated the 3D Slicer with the interventional MR system (Signa SP, GE Medical Systems, Milwaukee, WI) to form a computerized surgical assistant. The location of the imaging plane can be specified with an optical tracking system (Image Guided Technologies, Boulder, CO), which we will refer to as the *locator*. Light-emitting diodes affixed to a locator are tracked by 3 CCD cameras that are attached to a rail above the operating field. The spatial relationship of the instrument relative to the scanner is reported as both a position and an orientation with an update rate of approximately 10 Hz.

The Signa SP console and the Signa SP imaging workstation have a network connection with a TCP/IP interface by which we added a visualization workstation (Ultra 30, Sun Microsystems, Mountain View, CA) running the 3D Slicer. The 3D Slicer connects through a socket to a server we created on the SP imaging workstation. Whenever the locator's position or orientation updates, or a new image is scanned, the server sends the new data. The server is concurrent so that when the 3D Slicer opens a connection to it, the server spawns a child process to perform the actual serving, and the parent server goes to sleep. This way, if the server crashes, the 3D Slicer merely reconnects to the sleeping parent, and the surgery can continue uninterrupted.

The visualization workstation contains two Sun Creator3D graphics accelerator cards. One drives the 20 inch display placed in the control area of the surgical suite. The other card outputs only the 3D view and no control panels. Its signal is converted to NTSC TV and displayed on an LCD panel in the scanner gantry.

2.8   Medical Reality Modelling Language

Visualizing medical data involves combining various data sets collected in various geometric locations into a single scene, and exploring the scene interactively. A scene is created from a variety of volume data sets, surface models derived from those volumes, and transformations derived from 3D registrations of both the volumes and models. We have found that the proper coordination of these items is easiest to obtain by the use of a hierarchical modeling paradigm as exemplified by the modeling systems and languages of graphics and CAD/CAM.

Toward this end, we created a novel file format: the Medical Reality Modeling Language (MRML). MRML files are not a copy of the data in another format. Instead, a MRML file describes where the data is stored so the data can remain in its original format and location. Second, a MRML file describes how to position the data sets relative to each other in 3D space. Third, a MRML file describes how to display the data by specifying parameters for rendering and coloring.

A scene is represented in MRML as a tree-like graph where volumes, models, the coordinate transforms between them, and other items are the nodes in the graph. Each node has attributes for specifying its data. Transforms along each branch are concatenated to form a composite transform applied to the leaf node.

3 Results

To evaluate the performance and utility of the 3D Slicer, we have applied it in a variety of applications including guiding biopsies and craniotomies in the operating room, offering diagnostic visualization and surgical planning in the clinic, and facilitating research into brain shift and volumetric studies in the lab. While extensive details of the applications and their procedures will be reported in medical specialty venues, we include illustrative summaries here.

3.1 Pre-operative Planning

Outside of the operating room, the 3D Slicer is routinely relied upon as a standalone tool for analysis and planning. A vitally important component of neurosurgical planning is plotting an approach trajectory that avoids critical structures such as the blood vessels and the motor cortex. Tumors can either infiltrate functional tissue or push it aside, and a tumor that intricately invades eloquent cortex can be considered inoperable for the sake of preserving the quality of life rather than longevity. In the case shown in Figure 1, a functional MRI exam was registered to an anatomical exam. Surface models of the skin and tumor were constructed from the anatomical exam, and models of the motor cortex, and areas for auditory verb generation and visual verb generation were constructed from the fMRI. The same three slices that are visible in the 3D view are displayed as cross-sections at the bottom. The volumetric form of the fMRI results are overlaid in color on the grayscale, anatomical images.

This patient had a tumor in Broca's area on the left side of the brain where 96% of speech is generally processed. The functional MRI exam was administered to ascertain whether the tumor tissue had infiltrated the eloquent cortex. The 3D Slicer's integrated 3D view clearly demonstrated that the speech activity migrated to the right side, proving the operability of this lesion. It is interesting to note that although the 3D Slicer was scheduled for use only in pre-operative planning for this patient, the surgeon came out of the operating room halfway through the surgery to view the 3D Slicer again.

3.2 Surgical Guidance

After several clinical trials during development, we have used the 3D Slicer as a navigational tool in 22 cases between January and May of 1999. This initial feasibility phase proved the 3D Slicer to be a stable and reliable application. As we apply the 3D Slicer on a routine basis, a clinical evaluation of its influence on surgical decision making and resection control is being conducted.

The 3D Slicer is set-up and tested for about 5 minutes before the patient enters the MR. After the patient is positioned within the interventional MRI, an initial 3D volume is acquired. For cases in which pre-operative data sets have been fused, a second rigid registration using mutual information relates the pre-operative data sets to this new volume in order to align them with the coordinate frame of the interventional MR scanner.

The surgeon points at his intended craniotomy at various angles. As the tracked pointer moves within the surgical field, it is rendered in the 3D view, and the reformatted slice planes follow its position, sweeping through the volumes. The surgeon verifies, and in one case to date, alters, the planned approach by visualizing it on the display relative to all the surface models of critical structures. Reformatted images can be automatically generated along this path with the click of one button. A single 2D view cannot reveal all hazards, but when two slices are reformatted in the plane of the locator, yet perpendicular to each other, multiple hazards in 3D space may be seen simultaneously.

Cerebrospinal fluid leakage as well as tumor removal itself causes brain shift. Subsequent acquisitions at various times during the surgery allow adjustments to intraoperative changes. According to the magnitude of the intraoperative changes these acquisitions are carried through (on average 3-5 times during the case) as demanded by the surgeon. The Surgeon sees the location of the pointer's tip on the display, giving him a direct correlation of his visual impression of the tissue and the MR definition of the tissue. This is especially useful for areas that appear normal to the eye but display abnormal signal intensities in the applied sequences (T1 or T2). The Slicer's capability of displaying intraoperative T1 and T2 imaging as well as preoperative multi-modal information allows the comparative evaluation and the subsequent modification of the surgical tactic. The surgeon can observe the changes in position of anatomy on the intra-operative images, while also benefitting from the higher resolution, higher constrast, functional information, and administered contrast agents of the pre-operative images. Since model deformation has yet to achieve a sufficiently dependable accuracy for surgeons, we may stop using pre-operative models once resection is well underway.

The 3D Slicer's validity for planning and guiding resection is highlighted by the histopathology and location of the clinical cases for which it was used. Ten tumors were low-grade gliomas, for which total resection is correlated with a prolonged survival time and presumably even with total cure. Of these, six were located in the patients' dominant left hemisphere, three in the immediate vicinity of the motor cortex, and two close to speech areas. In these cases, precise margin definition is of utmost importance. Visually differentiating tissue in these tumors can be difficult to impossible, whereas T2-weighted images give a good estimate of the tumor extent. The display of these images allows a more careful control of total tumor resection. Of the remaining seven cases with high-grade (astrocytoma III and glioblastoma multiforme) tumors, four were adjacent to the motor cortex, thus making updated navigation a valuable tool to define the surgical goal and prevent morbidity.

3.3 Volumetric Analysis and Studies of Dynamics

The 3D Slicer is used outside of surgery for quantitative studies that require making measurements on source images and 3D models simultaneously. Applications to date include modeling the female pelvic floor for studying incontinence [3], measurements of muscle mass, and orthopedic range of motion studies.

The open MR presents unprecedented opportunities for scientifically studying the dynamics that accompany intervention. We are using the 3D Slicer to analyze brain shift [11] in an effort to eventually reach a level of understanding that includes predictive power. Then image-guided surgical techniques currently used in the open MR could be transferred to conventional operating rooms.

4 Discussion

Aside from the ongoing benefits reaped from its applications, the 3D Slicer itself contributes to the field of image-guided surgery in the following four ways.

1.) Highly Integrated Analysis and Visualization — Image-guided surgery systems strive to achieve one or more of the following:

- Data analysis
- Surgical planning
- Surgical guidance
- Surgical guidance with intra-operative updates

Several existing software packages, such as ANALYZE [9], MEDx [15], and MNI [10], present a more extensive collection of tools for data analysis and planning, but do not support surgical guidance. Systems have been developed to facilitate surgical guidance tracking [4], but they feature leaner support for analysis and planning, and they are not designed to incorporate intra-operative updates. Interleaving the results of several of the currently available systems can be cumbersome and time-consuming — making it impractical for clinical applications.

Our system is uniquely valuable in its integration of all of these facets into a single environment. Such cohesion is required for seamless integration of pre-operative and intra-operative data. Feedback from clinical users of the 3D Slicer suggest that they most appreciate its ability to help them navigate a complicated assembly of information.

2.) Integration with interventional MR —

The 3D Slicer is the first software system to augment an open-MR scanner with a full array of pre-operative data. The analysis previously reserved for pre-operative data [9] can now be applied to exploring anatomical changes that occur as surgery progresses.

3.) Medical Reality Modeling Language —
MRML conveniently describing 3D scenes composed of a heterogeneous mixture of scanned volumes, 3D surface models, and the coordinate transforms that express the geometric relationships between them.

4.) Freely Available, Open-Source Software —
We have made the 3D Slicer freely available as a tool to clinicians and scientists [1]. It has a modular, easily extendable design for other researchers to expand its value in a rapidly evolving field.

References

1. Brigham & Women's Hospital and Harvard Medical School. *Surgical Planning Lab.* http://www.splweb.bwh.harvard.edu:8000.
2. R.D. Bucholtz, D.D. Yah, J. Trobaugh, L.L. McDurmont, C.D. Sturm, C. Baumann, J.M. Henderson, A. Levy, and P. Kessman. The correction of stereotactic inaccuracy caused by brain shift using an interaoperative ultrasound device. In *Proceedings First Joint CVRMED/MRCAS*, Grenoble France, March 1997.
3. J. Fielding, H. Dumanli, A. Schreyer, S. Okuda, D. Gering, K. Zou, R. Kikinis, and F. Jolesz. MR based three-dimensional modeling of the normal female pelvic floor with quantification of muscle mass. *American Journal of Roentgenology*, In Press, 1999.
4. W.E.L. Grimson, M. Leventon, G. Ettinger, A. Chabrerie, F. Ozlen, S. Nakajima, H. Atsumi, R. Kikinis, and P. Black. Clinical experience with a high precision image-guided neurousurgery system. Boston, November 1998. Springer-Verlag.
5. N. Hata, T. Dohi, R. Kikinis, F.A. Jolesz, and W.M. Wells III. Computer assisted intra-operative MR-guided therapy: Pre and intra-operative image registraion, enhanced three-dimensional display, deformable registration. In *7th Annual meeting of Japan Society of Computer Aided Surgery*, pages 119–120, 1997.
6. J. Fitzpatrick J. West. Comparison and evaluation of retrospective intermodality brain image registration techniques. *Journal of Computer Assisted Tomography*, 21:554–566, 1997.
7. F.A. Jolesz. Image-guided procedures and the operating room of the future. *Radiology*, 204:601–612, May 1997.
8. L.D. Lunsford, R. Parrish, and L. Albright. Intraoperative imaging with a therapeutic computed tomographic scanner. *Neurosurgery*, 15:559–561, 1984.
9. Mayo Clinic. *ANALYZE Software.* http://www.mayo.edu/bir/analyze/ANALYZE_Main.html.
10. MNI. *MNI Software.* http://www.bic.mni.mcgill.ca/software/.
11. A. Nabavi, D. Gering, R. Pergolizzi, N. Hata, R. Kikinis, F. Jolesz, and P. Black. Shift happens. Submitted for publication.
12. J.F. Schenk, F.A. Jolesz, P.B. Roemer, et al. Superconducting open-configuration MR imaging system for image-guided therapy. *Radiology*, 195:305–814, 1995.
13. W. Schroeder, K. Martin, and W. Lorensen. *The Visualization Toolkit: An Object-Oriented Approach to 3-D Graphics.* Prentice Hall, NJ, 1996.
14. W. Schroeder, J. Zarge, and W. Lorensen. Decimation of triangle meshes. *Computer Graphics*, 1992.
15. Sensor. *MEDx Software.* http://www.sensor.com/medx_info/medx_docs.html.
16. W.M. Wells III, P.A. Viola, H. Atsumi, S. Nakajima, and R. Kikinis. Multimodalvolume registration by maximization of mutual information. *Medical Image Analysis*, 1(1):35–51, 1996.

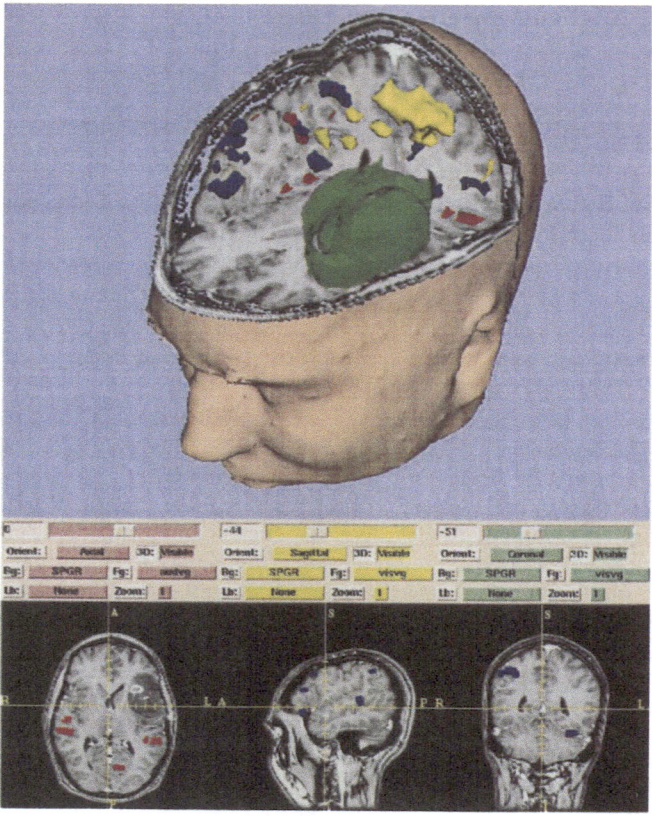

Fig. 1. Surface models of skin, tumor (green), motor cortex (yellow), auditory verb generation (red), and visual verb generation (blue), are integrated with slices.

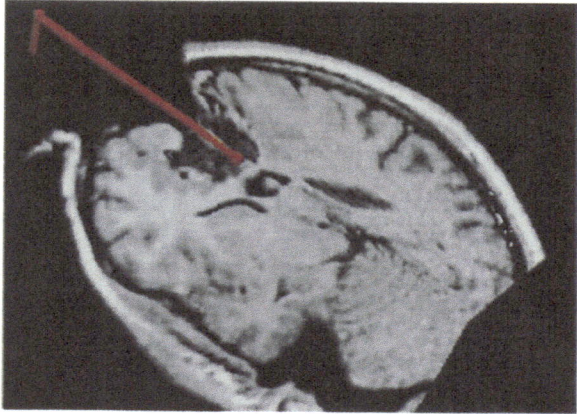

Fig. 2. The surgeon leads a probe through the surgical cavity to check for tumor remnants while observing the 2 orthogonal reformatted images.

Exploiting 2-D to 3-D Intra-operative Image Registration for Qualitative Evaluations and Post-operative Simulations

André Guéziec[1]*, Kenong Wu[2], Bill Williamson[2], Peter Kazanzides[2], Robert Van Vorhis[2], and Alan Kalvin[3]

[1] Multigen-Paradigm, 550 S. Winchester Bd., Suite 500, San Jose, CA 95128
[2] Integrated Surgical Systems, 1850 Research Park Drive, Davis, CA 95616
[3] IBM T.J. Watson Research Center, 30 Sawmill River Road, Hawthorne, NY 10532, USA

Abstract. This paper addresses a key issue of providing clinicians with visual information to validate the accuracy of 2D/3D registration for robot-assisted total hip replacement (THR) surgery. In practice, clinicians rely on post-operative X-rays to assess the accuracy of implant placement. Motivated by this, we simulate a set of post-operative X-ray images by superimposing the implant positioned pre-operatively onto the intra-operatively collected and calibrated images of the femur, through a transformation computed by the 2D/3D registration. With these images, a judgment on the registration accuracy can be made. In addition, this paper introduces methods for superimposing pre-operative data on intra-operative X-ray images that were not corrected for distortion, by applying the same image distortion to the data. This paper also introduces a new framework for incorporating surface normals in the objective function for registration. A comparison between marker-based and image-based registration is conducted.
Keywords: Simulation of post-operative X-ray images, Anatomy- and Image-Based Registration, Total Hip Replacement Surgery, ROBODOC[R], CT, X-ray Fluoroscopy

1 Introduction

In this paper, we address a key issue of providing clinicians with visual information for determination of accuracy of the image-based registration for robot-assisted surgery. Although numerous registration approaches have been presented, the topic of registration validation has scarcely been addressed in the literature. This is vital however for the acceptance of image-based registration and image guidance of therapy in practice.

This work is part of a joint study with Integrated Surgical System (ISS), of Davis, CA, to extend the ROBODOC[R] system [1]. Used for Total Hip Replacement (THR) surgery, the surgical robot of the ROBODOC[R] system accurately mills the cavity for the femoral implant. The robot trajectory is planned using the ORTHODOC[R] software, based upon a CT-scan of the hip and a CAD model of an appropriate femoral implant. To register the surgical robot to its planned trajectory, the basic clinical protocol uses two or

---

* A. Guéziec is also a consultant in Medical Imaging based in the Silicon Valley. E-mail: gueziec@computer.org. This work was done while the first author was with IBM.

three metallic markers. These markers are surgically inserted in the femur [2, 3]. They are pre-operatively imaged with CT and located by the ORTHODOC^R software. Intra-operatively, they are located by the robot. With their positions in both CT and robot co-ordinate systems, a transformation between these two coordinate systems can be easily computed. This *marker-based* registration produces very reliable results and has been performed on more than 4,000 patients. However, marker insertion requires an additional surgery and sometimes causes discomfort for patients. We note that a CT-to-robot registration for robotic THR based on a proprietary technology (DIGIMATCH^{TM}) without using markers was developed at ISS and used in clinics recently. The approach reported in this paper was developed independently and is different from DIGIMATCH^{TM}.

One of our goals is to study the feasibility of substituting external marker-based registration with X-ray image-based registration [1]. After a registration is performed, the following question is always raised: Is the computed transformation accurate enough to guide surgery? If the answer is yes, the surgeon will execute the robot surgery. Otherwise, another registration must be performed. Our approach is aimed at providing surgeons with simulated post-operative X-ray images to assess registration accuracy.

In this paper, we introduce new developments of a method for registering CT-scan images acquired pre-operatively to intra-operative X-ray images [4]. This registration allows us to accurately associate a surgical plan with the current pose of the surgical robot and the patient inside the operating room. To do this, we first extract the surface model of the femur from the CT image. Then, we acquire a few X-ray images from different points of view intra-operatively and compute projection lines for all images. Finally, we compute the transformation between CT space and robot space by matching the projection lines to the contours of the femur surface. Since the registration accuracy depends critically on this matching process, we introduce in Section 3 a new improvement: we refine the matches by exploiting the correlation between surface normals measured from surface models and surface normals estimated from 2-D X-rays using projection lines.

In Section 5, using an X-ray camera calibrated with respect to physical space and a registration of pre-operative data to physical space, we can effectively integrate various parts of the pre-operative data onto intra-operative X-ray images, as if the data had been part of the scene captured by the X-ray camera. This can be performed accurately, with or without correcting images for distortion, depending on which images the clinician is more comfortable with. In this way, we can, for instance, simulate post-operative X-rays.

2   X-Ray Camera Calibration[4]

We have attempted to work with X-ray images that reflect the data that can realistically be acquired during intra-operative X-ray fluoroscopy. The characteristics of these images are as follows: limited field of view (typically 6 inches and sometimes 9), geometric distortion, and in particular, occlusion of anatomical structures by various metal-

---

[1] In addition to external markers, anatomical features, such as bone surfaces, can also be used for registration, which is usually called *anatomy-based* registration. The *image-based* registration in this paper is a particular type of anatomy-based registration.

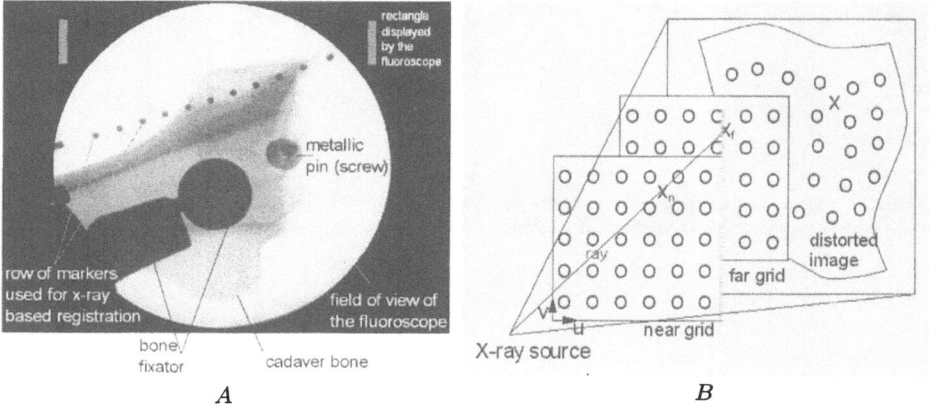

Fig. 1. A: Characteristics of typical X-ray images in this study: limited field of view, geometric distortion and occlusion (dots are used for calibration). B: Multi-grid calibration method. Any image pixel X can be associated to two locations X_f and X_n on the grids, specifying a ray in three-dimensional space.

lic instruments (see Fig. 1-A). Assuming that direct digital acquisition of X-rays will at some point supersede image intensifiers, intra-operative X-ray image quality should improve significantly, and the results of this paper correspond to a worst-case X-ray image quality.

The goal of camera calibration (X-ray, or other) is to determine a set of geometric parameters characterizing how a three-dimensional scene was projected onto the image. A perspective projection provides a suitable model for an X-ray camera. In addition, intra-operative X-rays are typically corrupted with two main types of distortion : "pincushion" distortion, and "S-shaped" distortion caused by interactions with stray magnetic fields during the image intensification process. This distortion must be compensated for before determining perspective projection parameters. Conventional methods would operate in two steps, by first correcting for the distortion and then determining the projection parameters using distortion-corrected images. Generally, both steps are accomplished by imaging grids of markers, whose position and orientation are precisely known with respect to the coordinate system that is relevant for calibration [5–11].

The method that we retained combines distortion correction and geometric calibration in a single step, and extends the methods by Martins *et al.* [12] and by Champleboux *et al.* [13]: for each pixel of a digitized X-ray image, we determine directly the equation of a ray in three dimensional space that projected to that pixel. Knowledge of two points along the ray is sufficient for determining a ray. As illustrated in Fig. 1-B, the method works by imaging two grids, a "near" grid and a "far" grid, and observing the distorted grid points on the X-ray image. The grids are preferably observed by capturing separate images, and can even be "virtual", by moving a linear probe and collecting multiple images [4]. Knowing the correspondence between observed and physical grid points, for each pixel X of the distorted image, it is possible to match it with a location on both grids (X_n on the near grid and X_f on the far grid) by interpolation (preferably using thin-plate spline functions: we refer to [4] for a mathematical formulation). Both locations X_n and X_f in three-dimensions specify the ray that was sought for.

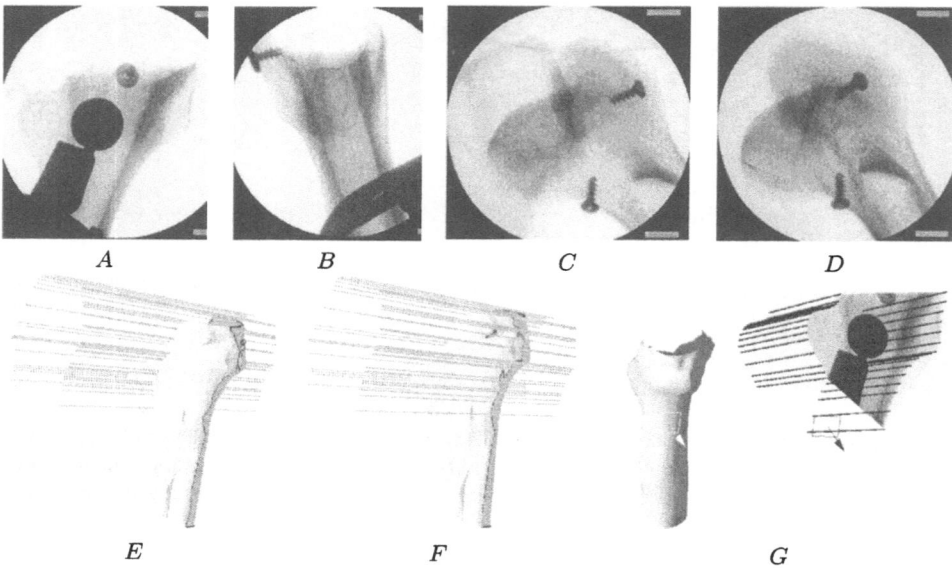

A B C D

E F G

Fig. 2. A,B,C,D: four fluoroscopic views used for marker-less 2-D to 3-D image-based registration. E,F: Pre-operative proximal femur model before (E) and after (F) registration to three-dimensional X-ray paths (straight lines) starting from the intra-operative X-ray source and going through bone contours in the X-ray images. The dark three-dimensional curves on the femur models are silhouette curves (depending on the position). G: pre-operative model in registered position with a distortion corrected X-ray image. Two X-ray paths taken consecutively along the bone contour define a normal vector shown in black. At the location where the (continuation of) an X-ray path is tangent to the bone surface, the surface normal (shown in white) should be aligned with the black normal vector.

3   2-D TO 3-D Registration using Normals

The new framework for handling normals that we are proposing could potentially be incorporated in other 2-D to 3-D registration methods [14–18].

The principle of the method that we built upon is as follows [4]: when the pre-operative femur model is perfectly registered with respect to physical space (surgical robot and X-ray images), X-ray paths (see Figs. 2) corresponding to the bone contours in the two-dimensional X-ray images and determined using image calibration information are tangent to (grazing) the surface of the femur model. Since the femur model is expected to be mis-registered in the beginning of the process, X-ray paths are a-priori not grazing (but intersecting, or "missing" the femur model altogether), and the registration process determines a rigid transformation optimizing the position and orientation of the surface model such that as many X-ray paths as possible become tangent to the surface. Figure 2 shows an experimental registration result: the position of the pre-operative bone model is gradually optimized until a large majority of the X-ray paths become tangent to it. The dark three-dimensional curves on the femur model of Figs. 2-E,F are silhouette curves. Silhouette curves, or "apparent contours", are an important component of this registration method: the method attempts to bring each X-ray path in contact with a silhouette curve. Given a center of perspective projection determined by calibration, silhouette curves are such that rays emanating from the center of perspective and tangent to the surface meet the surface on a silhouette curve.

To determine the rotation and translation that minimizes the sum of weighted squared distances between the silhouette curve points and the X-ray paths, we use the following formulation:

$$\min_{\mathbf{Q},\mathbf{t}} \sum_{i=1}^{m} d_i^2 = \min_{\mathbf{Q},\mathbf{t}} \sum_{i=1}^{m} \|\mathbf{V_i}(\mathbf{c_i} - (\mathbf{Q}\mathbf{p_i} + \mathbf{t}))\|^2, \mathbf{V_i} = \begin{bmatrix} 0 & -v_3 & v_2 \\ v_3 & 0 & -v_1 \\ -v_2 & v_1 & 0 \end{bmatrix} \quad (1)$$

where $\mathbf{p_i}$ are silhouette curve points (on the three-dimensional bone surface), $\mathbf{v_i}$ are the unit direction vectors of the lines, $\mathbf{c_i}$ are the positions of the center of perspectives corresponding to the lines (in this way, several views with several centers of perspective can be accommodated simultaneously), d_i distances between straight lines and silhouette curve points, and $\mathbf{Q}$ and $\mathbf{t}$ are the unknown rotation matrix and translation vector. We use the Cayley rotation parameterization, which states that if $\mathbf{U}$ is a skew symmetric matrix obtained from a vector $\mathbf{u}$, then the matrix $\mathbf{Q} = (\mathbf{I} - \mathbf{U})(\mathbf{I} + \mathbf{U})^{-1}$ is a rotational matrix. The advantage of this form is that for small rotations, $\mathbf{Q} \sim \mathbf{I} - 2\mathbf{U}$. The problem becomes:

$$\min_{\mathbf{u},\mathbf{t}} \sum_{i} \|\mathbf{V_i}(\mathbf{p_i} - \mathbf{c_i} + 2\mathbf{P_i}\mathbf{u} + \mathbf{t})\|^2 \quad (2)$$

where $\mathbf{P_i}$ is a skew symmetric matrix derived from $\mathbf{p_i}$. Following Kumar et al. (1994) [19], we use the Tukey weighting function to scale each distance error, allowing the registration to operate in a fashion that is robust to outliers (incorrectly matched pairs: line, point). After some additional computations detailed in [4], we obtain a linear system that we solve for the desired transformations.

This formulation, and the registration accuracy, depend upon an algorithm to discover meaningful (lines, surface points) correspondences (although the robust formulation automatically ignores some erroneous correspondences). One strategy is to find the closest silhouette curve point from each straight line. In [4] the closest point was found by first decomposing each three-dimensional silhouette curve as a hierarchy of nested polygonal segments, each associated with a volume bounding the corresponding silhouette curve portion. Using this hierarchical description, a closest point can be queried in time proportional to the logarithm of the number of vertices in a silhouette curve.

In this paper we propose a general framework to improve the (lines, surface points) correspondences using information on normals. As illustrated in Fig 2-G, two X-ray paths taken consecutively along the bone contour define a normal vector. At the location where (the continuation of) an X-ray path is tangent to the bone surface, the surface normal should be aligned with the normal to the X-ray path. This allows us to define constraints on the silhouette curve points that can be matched to the X-ray path, by considering matches for which the angle between the above-defined normals does not exceed a maximum value.

One method for incorporating surface normals in a projective registration process is described in Feldmar et al. [16]. Feldmar et al. develop an iterative closest point approach, wherein the distance is a (weighted) compromise between a three-dimensional

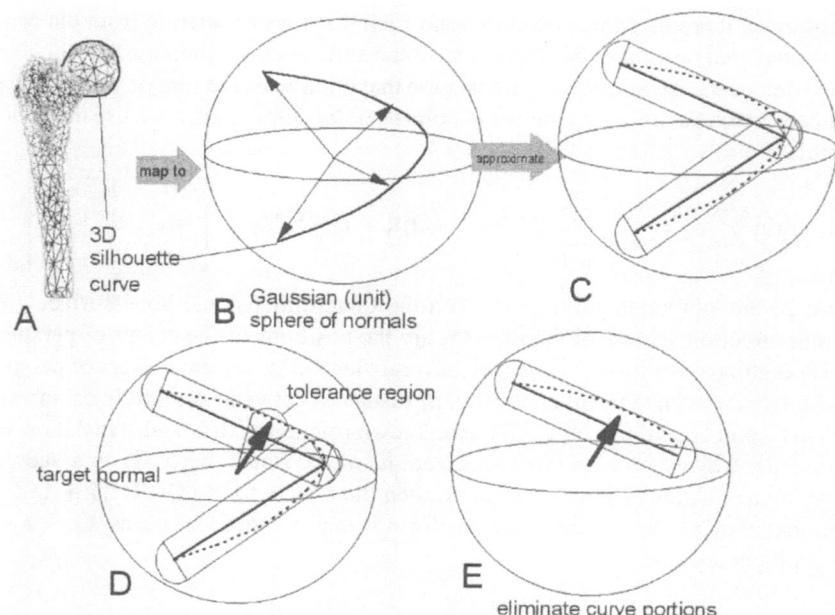

Fig. 3. A 3-D silhouette curve extracted from a surface model in (A) is mapped to the Gaussian sphere of normals in (B), is approximated by line segments in (C), keeping accurate bounding volumes. Curve portions whose bounding volumes do not intersect the target normal (D) are unlikely matches and thus eliminated during the search for the closest point.

distance and difference in normal orientation. Although this method succeeds in using surface normal information, since both position and normal terms are (squared, and then) added, one can compensate for the other: there is no difference between an erroneous positional match but correct normal match, a correct positional match but erroneous normal match or an incorrect match of both.

The approach we advocate is quite different and novel. The idea is to continue looking for a closest point in a usual (Cartesian) sense but also impose some constraints on the difference in normal orientations at the same time, essentially pruning out irrelevant curve portions. This is justified as follows: using the closest point is particularly relevant when we get very close to the ideal registration, since the exact match is a closest point with zero distance (modulo feature detection and calibration accuracy). Conversely, using normal orientation is better justified at the early stages of the registration to avoid local minima. We have observed for our data that although the normal orientation is generally correct, there is some question about its accuracy relative to the positional accuracy.

The algorithm used to implement the normal constraints can be better understood by examining Fig. 3. A silhouette curve (A) is mapped in (B) to the Gaussian sphere (unit sphere centered at the origin of Cartesian space) of normals by connecting the vertex normals of the surface model corresponding to the vertices of the silhouette curve. A hierarchical description of this mapped curve is built (C) in parallel to the hierarchical description in Cartesian space depicted above. For each X-ray path, a target normal (D) is determined as explained above and illustrated in Fig 2-C, with an associated tolerance region. Since the hierarchical description has segments with bounding areas, if a given bounding area (defined by a cylinder capped with two half spheres) does not intersect the tolerance region of the target normal (E), this means that this normal cannot possibly occur along the corresponding portion of silhouette curve, and thus the entire portion should not be considered for finding a closest point.

The algorithm explores the hierarchical curve description and decides to examine further a branch of the hierarchy (corresponding to a curve portion) only if the test on normals described above is passed. The rest of the algorithm is the same as before. Utilizing this new method has improved results in all the practical cases that we encountered as described next.

4   Quantitative Evaluation of the Registration

We used implanted fiducials on a cadaver bone and ROBODOC[R]to obtain precise and reliable transformations that can be compared to the image-based method. We CT-scanned the cadaver bone, then brought it to the operating room and fixated it to the robot. We then captured sets of X-ray fluoroscopy images and calibrated them geometrically with respect to the robot. We registered a CT-based model of the bone to the X-ray images. The results were compared with the marker-based technique. Starting with the registered position computed using the markers, we perturbed it with various rigid transformations, whose rotational axis was chosen using a random vector generator and whose rotation magnitude was fixed to three and five degrees. The translational component of the transformation was computed so as to leave the centroid of the markers invariant by the perturbation (any suitable point inside the bone could have been used), and simulate an initial position that could potentially occur in practice. The registration was completed in about 6 seconds on a UNIX workstation.

In clinical practice, orthopedic surgeons commonly examine the placement accuracy in terms of implant positions. We examined the registration accuracy by comparing the registered implant positions in the robot coordinate system. Specifically, we compared the displacements at the implant origin and tip as well as the rotation angle around the Z axis of the implant coordinate system. This comparison is illustrated in Fig. 4. The implant coordinate system is shown in Fig. 4-A. The positions in the robot space transformed by the marker-based and image-based registrations are shown in Fig. 4-B. d_0 and d_t are the displacements at the implant origin and tip, respectively.

Table 1 shows the comparison results. The average and maximum of absolute displacements at the implant tip and origin are 0.49mm and 1.053mm, respectively. The average and maximum of the Z rotation errors are 2.64 and 4.55 degrees, respectively. According to our experience with surgeons, the requirements for displacement errors are approximately 1.5mm, and approximately 3 degrees for the rotation about the Z axis. [2]. Thus, assuming that the marker-based results are the gold standard for registra-

---

[2] These criteria are derived by evaluating post-operative X-ray films. The exact values vary slightly among surgeons, and are difficult to evaluate. Note that we treat the marker-based registration results as the ideal results since we do not know the ideal answers.

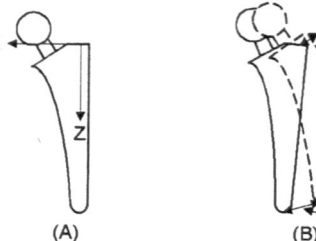

Fig. 4. Comparing implant positions. (a) Implant coordinate axes. (b) Implant positions in robot space: the implant transformed using the marker-based registration result is shown using a solid line while the implant transformed using the image-based registration result is shown using a dashed line.

	displacements and rotation in the implant coordinate system						
	Origin displacement			Tip displacement			Rotation
Perturbation	x	y	z	x	y	z	around Z
rotation 3 degrees 1	0.975891	0.015485	0.565460	0.855482	0.414210	0.565020	1.979850
rotation 3 degrees 2	0.830098	-0.489192	0.163470	0.534467	-0.114655	0.162864	3.128288
rotation 3 degrees 3	0.982567	-0.221832	0.271217	0.687081	0.115406	0.270682	2.688964
rotation 3 degrees 4	0.819053	-0.357789	0.247661	0.620627	0.021679	0.247200	2.796623
rotation 3 degrees 5	0.941361	0.243733	0.672319	1.052943	0.678233	0.671715	0.976155
rotation 5 degrees 1	0.810275	0.411480	-0.833420	0.658433	0.429188	-0.833468	-0.097202
rotation 5 degrees 2	0.848678	-0.348916	0.222854	0.628410	0.015002	0.222230	2.846277
rotation 5 degrees 3	1.003069	-0.685573	-0.152810	0.351603	-0.509426	-0.154009	4.449264
rotation 5 degrees 4	0.843969	-0.381169	0.258526	0.573869	-0.006363	0.258017	2.872721
rotation 5 degrees 5	1.009851	-0.774564	-0.165820	0.432842	-0.600543	-0.166881	4.553174

Table 1. Registration results measured with respect to the implant: displacements in millimeters at the implant origin and tip, and rotation in degrees with respect to the implant's main axis.

tion, the accuracy in displacement achieves the clinical requirements in all cases while the rotational accuracy achieves the requirements in seven out of ten cases.

The reason for obtaining less accurate Z rotation parameters is the following. Since the shape of the femur is extremely elongated in the Z direction, the rotation change around the Z axis is much more sensitive to the same amount of distance mismatching than around the X and Y axes. This is also the reason why the normal constraints improve the registration accuracy. There are a few ways that the Z rotation accuracy can be improved. For example, we can choose better views for X-ray acquisition (different surgical approaches allow collection of different views), start with a better initial estimate, obtain more accurate femur surface models or give additional weight to particular measurements in the objective function.

In real situations where the image-based registration is actually performed, markers are not used. To evaluate the accuracy of registration, pre-operatively planned data must be transformed into the robot space with the computed registration and compared to the relevant data measured in the robot space. This subject is discussed next.

5   Fusing Pre-Operative Three-Dimensional Models With Intra-Operative Images: Qualitative Evaluation

Let us suppose that we wish to show in one or several of the captured X-ray images, the position that the implant would have after surgery, assuming that the registration coordinates as determined in Section 3 are used to position and orient the robot with respect to the surgical plan. In this way, the surgeon will be able to see the clinical equivalent of post-operative X-ray images before the operation was actually executed. The following discussion applies as well if we wish to superimpose other three-dimensional shapes, such as a pre-operative femur bone model, or a model of a marker (screw) for marker-based registration.

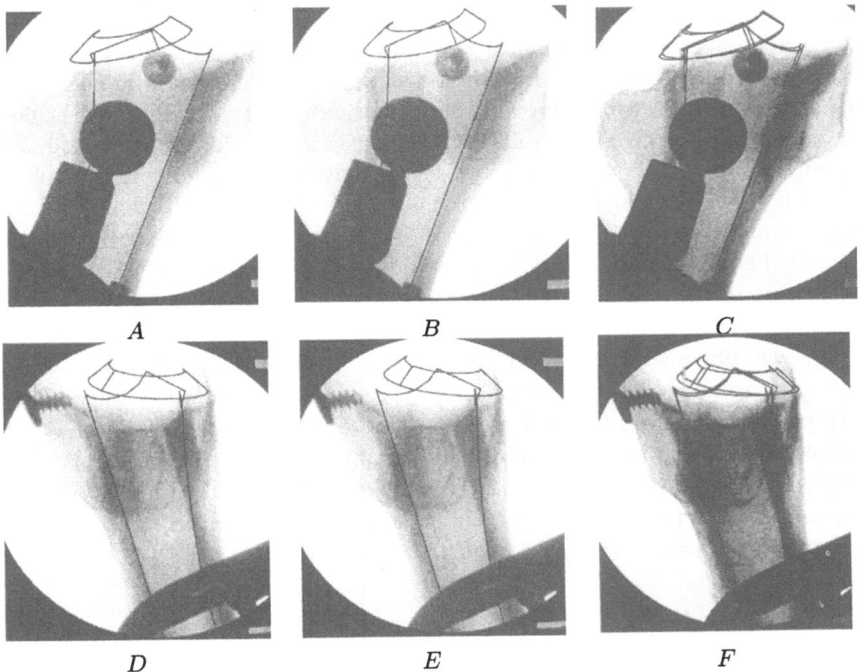

Fig. 5. A: fusion of X-ray and implant data using the marker-based registration. B: using the anatomy-based registration. D, E: idem on a second intra-operative X-ray image, captured with a 60 degree rotation with respect to the previous image. C, F: comparing (superimposing) the marker-based registration with the image-based registration. The error in implant position is 1mm or less (see Table 1). All images are corrected for distortion.

For a given X-ray image, using calibration information, we first determine a center of perspective (for instance, by finding a "best" point of intersection of several X-ray paths using Eqn 2, wherein all p_i are at the origin and the resulting t gives the center of perspective), and use it to compute silhouette curves of the implant model as explained in Section 3 (for more detail, see [4]). Then, the method works independently of whether we wish to produce distortion-corrected images or distorted images: for each pixel of the X-ray image (original image pixels, or rectified image pixels) we determine an X-ray path knowing the pixel coordinates and the center of perspective. We then compute the distance from each X-ray path to the implant as discussed in Section 3. Finally, we convert the computed distances to gray-scale values. Various methods can be used to do this. To produce the images of Fig. 5 the following mapping was used: if the distance was less than 0.05 mm, a gray-scale value of 0 was used, otherwise, if the distance was less than 0.1 mm, a gray-scale value of 30 was used, otherwise, if the distance was less than 0.2 mm, a gray-scale value of 60 was used, and otherwise, no change to the existing gray-scale value was done. This simple method allowed to avoid "aliasing" in the implant outline. One advantage of using distances to silhouette curves is that the resulting projection of the implant shows only the projected silhouette, which is sufficient to precisely indicate the position of the implant, but does not obscure any of the anatomy (see Fig. 5).

In Figure 6-A,E we show the pre-operative shapes that were used for fusion purposes. The implant was pre-operatively positioned accurately inside the CT data using the ORTHODOC^R software. The implant model is shown projected inside (fused with) two distortion-corrected intra-operative X-ray images in Fig. 5. In Figs. 5-A,D, the implant model was registered using the marker-based method (current pin-based clinical protocol). In Figs. 5-B,E we use an image-based registration (without markers) obtained as in Section 3. Using Fig 5 we can reproduce a classical surgical planning method of superimposing acetate implant models onto film X-rays generally taken at right angles. Hence the images of Fig 5 should be easily interpretable by clinicians. In Figs. 5-C,F we superimpose the implant using both the marker-based and image-based registration. The difference in implant placement is no larger than 1mm, as reported in Table 1.

Fig.6 was obtained without correcting images for distortion. In Fig. 6-F, we superimpose the proximal marker onto a distorted X-ray image using the same registration transform as in Fig. 5-A. Fig. 6-A indicates that the pre-operative and intra-operative pin do not overlap exactly (the pin model, however, is longer than the physical pin): This confirms that the measured error is larger at the markers than at the implant. The error at the markers was measured in [20]. In Figs. 6-G,H, we also project the pre-operative femur model used for image-based (marker-less) registration.

6   Conclusion

Calibrated intra-operative X-rays can be used for registration and more. This paper described how to produce simulated post-operative X-rays. These images are particularly valuable because they are computed *after* the registration process: their validity is not subjected to a successful registration, but only to (1) the reliability and correct calibration of robotic devices executing the surgical plan. (As reported in [2, 3] these are particularly reliable devices and processes.), and (2) the assumption that an incorrect registration cannot entirely compensate for an incorrect image calibration (for instance some inaccurate overlaps of the anatomy should be identifiable in fused images).

As illustrated in Fig. 5, we can thus provide post-operative simulations of the outcome of surgery before executing it. Furthermore, the simulations are presented in a standard clinical fashion, and are straightforward for a surgeon to interpret. Such images may help a surgeon decide to accept or reject a surgical plan or registration before any execution of the plan and thus may help prevent errors.

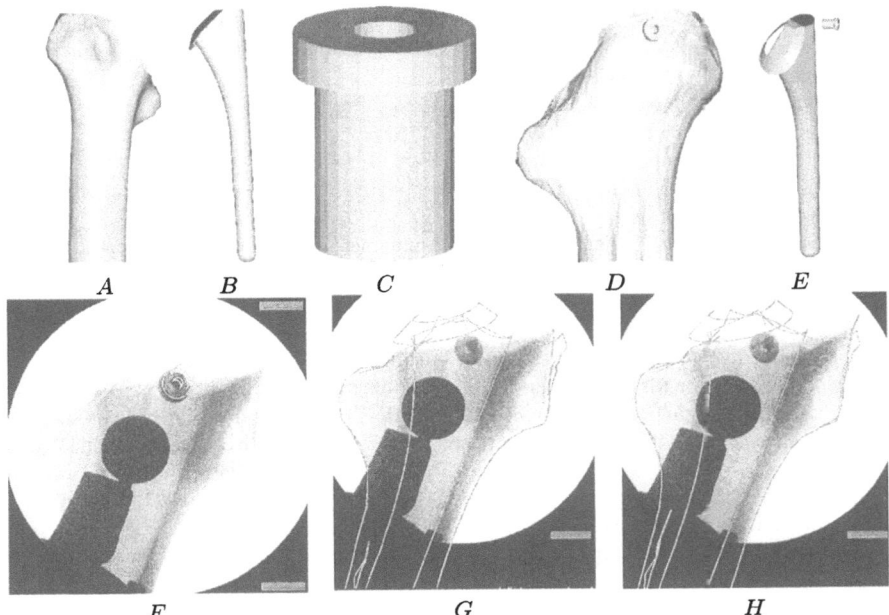

Fig. 6. A-E: Pre-operative model. A: CT-based proximal femur model B: implant CAD model (Depuy AML). C: simplified CAD model of fiducial pin (8 mm diameter by 10 mm). D: Femur and pin model registered in CT space. E: implant and pin model registered in CT space. F,G, and H are distorted images: the projection of shapes is distorted according to the image distortion model F: Superimposing the proximal pin (anatomy-based registration); the pin model is longer than the physical pin. G. H: superimposing femur and implant models. G: marker-based registration. H: anatomy-based registration.

By observing the simulated post-operative X-rays of total hip replacement surgery and studying the reported quantitative results, we are led to conclude that X-ray-to-CT registration using anatomical features provides comparable results to marker-based registration.

Acknowledgments: This work was partially funded by a Cooperative Agreement No. 70NANB5H1088 from the NIST Advanced Technology Program (ATP).

References

1. R.H. Taylor, L. Joskowicz, B. Williamson, A. Gueziec, A. Kalvin, P. Kazanzides, R. Van Vorhis, R. Kumar, A. Bzostek, A. Sahay, M. Boerner, and A. Lahmer. Computer-integrated revision total hip replacement surgery: Concept and preliminary results. *Medical Image Analysis*, 1999. to appear.
2. R.H. Taylor, H.A. Paul, P. Kazanzides, B.D. Mittelstadt, W. Hanson, J.F. Zuhars, B. Williamson, B.L. Musits, E. Glassman, and W.L. Bargar. An image-directed robotic system for precise orthopaedic surgery. *IEEE Transactions on Robotics and Automation*, 10(3):261–275, 1994.
3. B.D. Mittelstadt, P. Kazanzides, J. Zuhars, B. Williamson, P. Cain, F. Smith, and W.L. Bargar. The evolution of a surgical robot from prototype to human clinical use. In R.H. Taylor *et al*, editor, *Computer-Integrated Surgery*, pages 397–407. MIT Press, 1996.

4. A. Guéziec, P. Kazanzides, B. Williamson, and R.H. Taylor. Anatomy-based registration of ct-scan and intraoperative x-ray images for guiding a surgical robot. *IEEE Transactions on Medical Imaging*, 17(5):715–728, oct 1998.

5. S. Rudin, D.R. Bednarek, and W. Wong. Accurate characterization of image intensifier distortion. *Medical Physics*, 18(6), 1991. 1145-1151.

6. J.M. Boone, J.A. Seibert, W.A. Barrett, and E.A. Blood. Analysis and correction of imperfections in the image intensifier-TV-digitizer imaging chain. *Medical Physics*, 18(2), 1991. 236-242.

7. L. Launay, C. Picard, E. Maurincomme, R. Anxionnat, P. Bouchet, and L. Picard. Quantitative evaluation of an algorithm for correcting geometrical distortions in dsa images: Applications to stereotaxy. In Murray H. Loew, editor, *Medical Imaging: Image Processing*, volume 2434. SPIE, March 1995.

8. S. Schreiner, J. Funda, A.C. Barnes, and J.H. Anderson. Accuracy assessment of a clinical biplane fluoroscope for three dimensional measurements and targeting. In K.M. Hanson, editor, *Medical Imaging: Image Display*, volume 3031, pages 160–166. SPIE, February 1997.

9. K.R Hoffmann, B.B Williams, J. Esthappan, S.Y.J Chen, J.D. Carroll, H. Harauchi, V. Doerr, G.N. Kay, A. Eberhardt, and M. Overland. Determination of 3D positions of pacemaker leads from biplane angiographic sequences. *Medical Physics*, 24(12), 1997. 1854-62.

10. J. Weese, T.M. Buzug, C. Lorenz, and C. Fassnacht. An approach to 2D/3D registration of a vertebra in 2D x-ray fluoroscopies with 3D CT images. In *Computer Vision and Virtual Reality in Medicine II – Medical Robotics and Computer Assisted Surgery III*, volume 1205 of *Lecture Notes in Computer Sciences*, pages 119–128. Springer, 1997.

11. L. Tockus, L. Joskowicz, A. Simkin, and C. Milgrom. Computer-aided image-guided bone fracture surgery: Modeling, visualization, and preoperative planning. In *MICCAI'98*, Boston, MA, October 1998.

12. H. A. Martins, J. R. Birk, and R.B. Kelley. Camera models based on data from two calibration planes. *Computer Graphics and Image Processing*, 17:173–180, 1981.

13. G. Champleboux, S. Lavallée, P. Sautot, and P. Cinquin. Accurate calibration of cameras and range imaging sensors: the npbs method. In *International Conference on Robotics and Automation*, pages 1552–1557, Nice, 1992. IEEE.

14. S. Lavallee, R. Szeliski, and L. Brunie. Matching 3-D smooth surfaces with their 2-D projections using 3-D distance maps. In *Geometric Methods in Computer Vision*, volume 1570, pages 322–336, San Diego, July 25–26 1991. SPIE.

15. B. Lee. *Stereo Matching of Skull Landmarks*. PhD thesis, Stanford University, 1991.

16. F. Betting, J. Feldmar, N. Ayache, and F. Devernay. A new framework for fusing stereo images with volumetric medical images. In N. Ayache, editor, *Computer Vision, Virtual Reality and Robotics in Medicine*, volume 905 of *Lecture Notes in Computer Science*, pages 30–39, Nice, April 1995. Springer Verlag.

17. A. Hamadeh, P. Sautot, S. Lavallée, and P. Cinquin. Towards automatic registration between ct and x-ray images cooperation between 3D/2D registration and 2D edge detection. In *Proc. 2nd Int. Symp. on Medical Robotics and Computer Assisted Surgery*, pages 39–46, Baltimore, MD, November 1995.

18. A. Liu, E. Bullitt, and S. Pizer. Surgical instrument guidance using synthesized anatomical structures. In *Computer Vision and Virtual Reality in Medicine II – Medical Robotics and Computer Assisted Surgery III*, volume 1205 of *Lecture Notes in Computer Sciences*, pages 99–108. Springer, 1997.

19. R. Kumar and A.R. Hanson. Robust methods for estimating pose and a sensitivity analysis. *CVGIP-IU*, 60(3):313–342, 1994.

20. A. Guéziec. Registering intra-operative x-rays images with pre-operative data to simulate post-operative x-ray images. In *2nd Israeli Symposium on Computer-Aided Surgery, Medical Robotics and Medical Imaging*, May 1999.

LOCALITE – A Frameless Neuronavigation System for Interventional Magnetic Resonance Imaging Systems

K. Kansy[1], P. Wisskirchen[1], U. Behrens[1], Th. Berlage[1], G. Grunst[1],
M. Jahnke[1], R. Ratering[1], H.-J. Schwarzmaier[1,2], and F. Ulrich[2]

[1] GMD - German National Research Center for Information Technology,
Project VEP, D-53754 Sankt Augustin, Germany
Email: kansy@gmd.de; http://fit.gmd.de/hci/projects/vep/vep.html
[2] Department of Neurosurgery, Klinikum, Krefeld, Germany

Abstract. LOCALITE is a frameless neuronavigation system that particularly addresses a problem with current interventional magnetic resonance imaging (iMRI) systems: non-interactive response time in the interactive scan mode and poor image quality with fast scanning sequences.

LOCALITE calculates image planes selected via a handheld localizer from pre- or intra-operative volume data sets. This approach provides a really interactive localizer device with high quality images. The volume data are generated after the patient has been brought into the operating room and fixed within the iMRI. Images are part of an enhanced reality scenario containing only the salient visual information for the intra-operative task rather than letting the surgeon drown in lots of images. First studies show that LOCALITE enables the surgeon to use the iMRI system intuitively and much faster.

1 Introduction

With minimally invasive interventions, the surgeon's direct view is often extremely restricted. Recent progress in computerised imaging techniques such as magnetic resonance imaging (MRI) has provided pre- and intra-operative images which are exploited to obtain information about the interior of the body. This has increased the use of minimally invasive techniques, e.g., in brain surgery [1]. Image-guided procedures [2] replace open operations. In this situation, only image-based information is used for planning and guidance.

Usually, pre-operative imaging information is employed for diagnosis and planning of the intervention. Here, an accurate transfer of the plan to the patient in the operating room must be guaranteed. Guiding systems have been developed to connect pre-operative images and planning data with the operating room facilities, i.e., to register data, device, and patient. Troccaz et al. [3] give a survey on active, semi-active, and passive guiding systems. In active guiding systems, a computer controls the position and handling of the surgical device; in passive systems, the surgeon controls the surgical devices, the actual position and orientation of which has to be tracked and related to the images and the plan. To guarantee precise registration between the planning data and the patient in the operating room, frame-based stereotaxy has been used where the frame provides good reference points. Today, high precision registration can be achieved by frameless stereotaxy usually based on optical tracking [4] [5]. However, the whole effort is rendered obsolete if the target tissue moves during the intervention. This applies to brain surgery where significant brain shift is reported [5].

The problem of intra-operative motion can be overcome by interventional imaging devices like the interventional magnetic resonance imaging (iMRI) [6]. iMRI systems with instrument trackers can provide real-time images of arbitrary planes through a defined point (e.g., instrument tip). The instrument tip can be controlled during its way along the planned trajectory towards the target tissue to notice deviations from the planned situation and to adapt the intervention accordingly.

However, the iMRI systems currently available have shortcomings. In the interactive mode, they deliver only single 2D planes which do not give the surgeon sufficient context and orientation for efficiently finding the planned access path and the target. The online slices are generated with a delay of about 7 seconds which prohibits efficient interactive work. Last but not least, the image quality of real-time images is inadequate for the recognition of critical details.

To bring iMRI really into practical use, we need:

- high quality real-time images of the patient for an efficient finding and detailed recognition of the target, e.g., a tumour;
- images of the device and the actual situation around the device tip in real-time, i.e., 1/5 sec or better;
- a cognitively adequate, intuitive guiding scene which gives the surgeon efficient intra-operative guidance in performing the planned intervention;
- to register data, device, and patient;
- a solution of the brain shift problem.

In this paper we describe a frameless neuronavigation system, LOCALITE, which tackles these issues and offers some practical solutions. The requirements for LOCALITE have been set up after a careful on-site study of surgeons and radiologists at work with an existing iMRI. A major concern was to look into the cognitive aspects of a neurosurgical intervention to identify just the information and images the surgeon needs for the task on hand. The aim is to put the surgeon into the picture rather than let him drown in a multitude of images.

2   Problems tackled by LOCALITE

The LOCALITE system is designed as an enabling system which supports a *surgeon to master a high tech* system in an intuitive way [7]. In this chapter we will discuss some of the problems tackled by LOCALITE.

834   K. Kansy et al.

2.1 Orientation problem

In the pre-operative stage, a full volume of the region of interest (the brain) is scanned with a MRI and analysed to find and locate a tumour. In an interactive mode, the iMRI produces single slices, i.e., 2D information, only. The slice position and orientation are determined using an interactive handpiece which is connected to the interventional device, e.g., a needle or catheter.

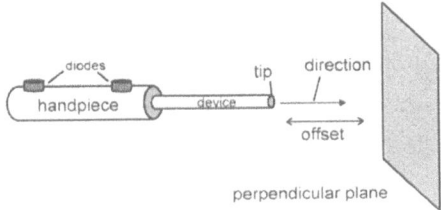

Fig. 1. Schematic figure of a handpiece for the Flashpoint system.

On-site cognitive studies revealed that the surgeon often looses the exact spatial orientation of this angulated slice with respect to the pre-operative volume data, i.e., he does not know how to move the handpiece to get to the intended position. This problem is aggravated by the time delay of several seconds which occurs between the positioning of the handpiece and the display of the respective image on the iMRI monitor. Even with a visualisation of the planning data in the context of the volume, it is a complicated, time consuming, and tedious task to position the device towards the planned entry point and to obtain the precise orientation along the planned path.

To provide the surgeon with optimal visualisations, we started with real-time volume visualization [8] [9] enhanced with real-time fusion of planning data and interactively selected planes. However, we found that complete information is not necessarily helpful but may even be distracting for the surgeon. Therefore during the phase of positioning and aligning the device, the LOCALITE system does not show the volume but only a MRI plane orthogonal to the planned access path in combination with markers for the entry and target point and a phantom device (Fig. 2 left). A further abstraction lead to the scene in (Fig. 2 right).

The visualization is further simplified by looking at the scene in the direction of the access path, such that the target is just behind the entry point (Fig. 5). In this simple scenario, finding the entry point is as simple as moving the locator device to the given entry marker. Alignment is achieved by angulating the device about the fixed entry point until it is perpendicular to the plane and degenerates to a dot (Fig. 5 right). This simple procedure can be performed in one minute whereas the previous procedure could take up to one hour.

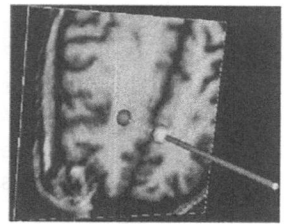
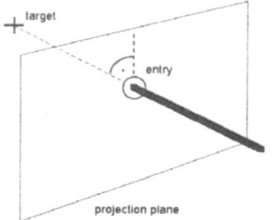

Fig. 2. Navigation scene. Left: MRI plane through the target, coloured markers at planned entry and target points, and a phantom device. Right: abstract scene used for navigation (see section 3.3-4

2.2   Interactivity

During the delicate process of precision surgery, the surgeon needs precise spatial feed-back in real-time to perform his job. However, it takes the iMRI several seconds to generate a single slice and to display the image on the iMRI monitor. Interactive work is significantly disturbed by this delay. From studies of interactive computer systems we know that a feedback cycle must finish within fractions of a second to allow efficient work, e.g., with positioning devices like mice.

LOCALITE achieves true interactivity by calculating any plane selected via the handheld device from a pre-registered volume data set rather than relaying on the inherent capability of the iMRI to obtain a real-time image of the patient. Calculating a plane from a volume is done by interpolating cell values in the volume to get the value of each cell on the selected plane. This operation is a standard function of visualisation packages (e.g., see vtkProbeFilter in [10]) which are available on standard PCs. The calculation can be done in fractions of a second which is sufficiently fast for our purposes. The probing can be further sped up by using texturing hardware [11] [8] available for high-end PC and SGI workstations. We are using this texturing hardware when displaying and manipulating volume data sets in real-time. The production system has been taylored to use only slices which can be handled efficiently on standard PCs.

2.3   Image quality

It is critical for the surgeon to have a clear view of the tumour and its spatial relation with the surrounding tissues. Although this is true for all surgical interventions, it is of special importance for brain surgery where the unwanted removal of even small parts of the brain may have disastrous consequences. Therefore, the current quality of the real-time images is not sufficient. LOCALITE provides the high image quality obtained from the pre- operative 3D-data sets during the whole procedure. Fig. 3 shows a real-time slice from the iMRI and the corresponding calculated plane from a volume scanned during the same session.

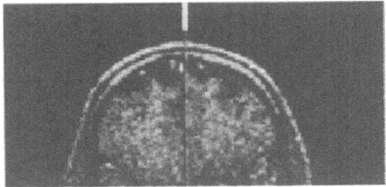 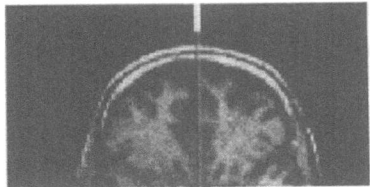

Fig. 3. Slice from a typical real-time scan (2D FSPGR, 3 sec.) (left) and the corresponding calculated image from a volume (3D SPGR) (right) both obtained on a 0.5T SIGNA SP of General Electric Medical Systems, Milwaukee, WI, USA.

2.4   Registration

In its current version, LOCALITE is dependent on a fixed patient position. A change of the patient's position between the acquisition of the volume data and the navigation process will invalidate the volume data. This, however, is not a insurmountable problem because the scanning procedure can be repeated intra-operatively if required within about 5 minutes.

With this simple trick, the delicate registration problem can be overcome for the cost of an acceptable interrupt time. On the negative side, the surgeon has to be aware that the calculated images shown are potentially outdated. Only the real-time planes of the iMRI are true online images of the patient. Therefore, LOCALITE has chosen to show both images, the calculated and the scanned plane, side by side for permanent comparison (Fig. 3). It is the surgeon's responsibility to observe both images and to demand new volumes when the patient might have moved, e.g., after skull opening, or before critical decisions, e.g., treatment of the tumour.

The acquisition of a new volume will also invalidate the planning and positioning data which are associated with a volume to support the navigation. However, the navigation as described in section 2.1 can be finished with the initial volume.

3   Operating the LOCALITE system

3.1   Intra-operative volume scan

After the patient has been brought to the operating room, a volume scan of the respective body part is taken.

3.2   Planning: marking of target and entry

The surgeon/radiologist will inspect the volume on the display to identify the target. He may select any slice or any 3D volume view in real-time. When the target has been localized, a red marker will be put on that position. Then the optimal access path will be selected and a yellow marker will identify the entry point (Fig. 4). The surgeon/radiologist will inspect the access path and may reposition target and entry.

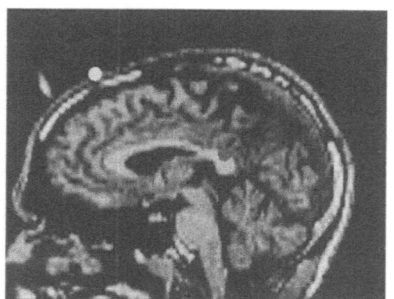 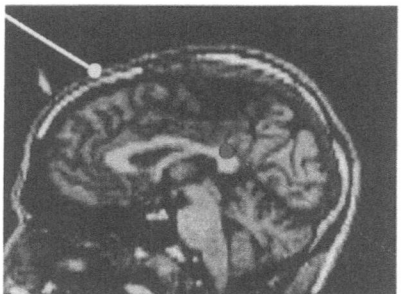

Fig. 4. Slice view of the brain with two balls identifying target and entry point (left); slice overlaid with device in correctly aligned position (right).

3.3   Navigation to the entry

Next, the locator device is activated. The SIGNA SP of General Electric Medical Systems is equipped with a Flashpoint locator system where the position and orientation of a handpiece with two or three LEDs (Fig. 1) are measured via cameras. The handpiece can carry the surgical device.

The LOCALITE system presents the surgeon with a guiding scene showing an abstract plane, the entry point on this plane and the current position of the device (Fig. 5 left). This scene is controlled by the Flashpoint locator system in a way that the phantom device always shows the correct 3D position and orientation of the locator device on the plane. The surgeon's task is now to move the real device until the tip of the phantom device points to the entry designated by a circle (Fig. 5 middle). Thus, the guiding scene allows him to easily identify the entry position on the patient's body. The result will be verified by comparing the real-time images of the iMRI at the final position with the simulated images of the same slice.

The skull will be opened by a trepanation at this point. A specially designed holder is then fixed in the trepanation aperture. The tip of the surgical device, e.g., a sheath or hollow needle, will then be fixed in this holder. Thus, the position of the tip is fixed at the entry point while the special construction of the holder *still permits angulation of the device*. The guiding scene should show the tip of the device pointing to the entry (Fig. 5 middle).

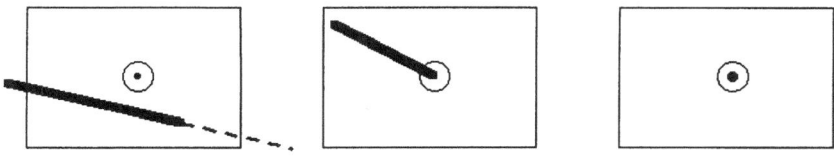

Fig. 5. Interactive positioning and alignment of the surgical device.

3.4   Angulating the device towards the target

Having fixed the tip, the instrument has now to be oriented such that it points precisely to the target. The guiding scene has been constructed as a plane orthogonal to the access path, i.e., the target is straight below the entry. Therefore, the orientation can be achieved effectively just by moving the device's tail until its projection degenerates to a point (Fig. 5 right). Then, the device is fixed with respect to its angulation.

The result will be verified by comparing the real-time images of the iMRI with the simulated images of the same slice (Fig. 3).

As the patient may have moved a little bit during the trepanation process, the surgeon has to consult the real-time images whether the position chosen with the possibly outdated planning data is still correct. He can perform slight corrections using the real-time images or ask for a fresh volume scan which will take some 5 minutes.

3.5   Surgical intervention

If the position of the device is considered to be correct, the device can be introduced under control of both, high quality images probed from the last volume data and low quality real-time images. Any image plane can be selected and continuously be moved through volume and patient to show any desired view of the access path defined by the device.

4   Methodology: Scene-Based Design

The interface of the LOCALITE system has been designed using a methodology we call scene-based design [12]. In this methodology, a 3D-target scene is shown from different viewpoints depending on different activities of the user. Each viewpoint not only represents a particular camera view point to look at the scene, but also a set of visualisation parameters affecting, for example, the transparency of different structures.

In this way, for each viewpoint, the minimal information presentation is achieved providing the optimal information condensation at a particular stage. For example, the LOCALITE interface is divided into several stages: planning,

Flashpoint navigation, and real-time simulation. These stages are controlled via buttons on the right side of the window (Fig. 6). Each stage has an associated viewpoint controlling the information visible for this stage.

Of course, the selection and design of viewpoints and the scene in general must be based on a detailed analysis of the tasks to be performed. Only rapid prototyping ensures that the design matches the new procedure which is possibly different with a new system than the original state.

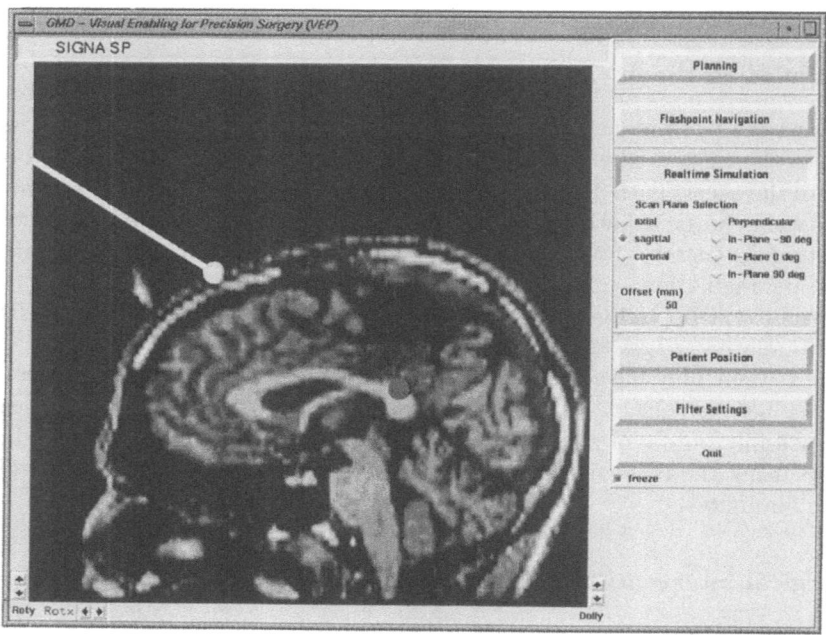

Fig. 6. User interface of the LOCALITE system.

5 Discussion

Minimally invasive procedures are of increasing importance because of their benefits for the patient and their cost effectiveness. However, many of these techniques lack direct visual control, which is provided by an open operation. Therefore image-guided interventions have been developed, based, for example, on iMRI techniques [2].

The current systems, however, are still lacking appropriate navigation facilities because, for example, conventional neuronavigation devices cannot be used in the magnetic environment.

Furthermore, the image information provided intra-operatively is substantially different from the images provided by pre-operatively performed routine scans. Because the latter are also used for therapy planning [13], this situation is even more unsatisfying.

We have seen in our field studies that the visual information provided by the iMRI System used for this study (GE SIGNA SP, Milwaukee, Wisconsin, USA) may result in a substantial loss of the surgeon's spatial orientation. This is predominantly due to the unintuitive presentation of the time-delayed angulated 2D image of a quality insufficient to provide the desired structural information.

Some authors [2], [14] report attempts to improve this unsatisfying situation. Most of this work, however is directed towards an improved presentation of the complex pre- and intra-operative data material, e.g., the development of new surface renderers [9] in combination with an optimised planning software.

The key idea of LOCALITE, however, is to omit all information not required for the current stage. Thus, the system allows the surgeon to concentrate on the essential information only. During certain phases of the navigation, even the MR images themselves are omitted and, instead, LOCALITE focuses on the spatial orientation of the interventional device using the iMRI guidance coordinates. This approach is new to our knowledge.

The neuronavigation as described in sections 3.1-4 has been extensively tested in place. Even personnel unskilled in neuronavigation such as, e.g., a technical assistant, is able to position an interventional device (e.g., biopsy needle) within 2 minutes, while experienced neurosurgeons previously needed one hour and more when using the genuine iMRI features only.

A main limitation at the present time is the need of maintaining the patient in a fixed position. If the patient moves or brain shift occurs, an additional intra-operative acquisition of a new volume is necessary. This invalidates the planning data related to the first volume and takes time and, therefore, is an obstacle for an efficient intervention. Given that intra-operative moves of patient or brain will be limited to slight changes in most cases [5], we are expecting that an intervention can be finished with the initial volume alone. The real-time images may give sufficient information about changes which can be meaningful interpreted with respect to the volume data.

Another approaches to compensate for movements of the patient and the brain are real-time tracking and registration techniques. However, tracking of external landmarks is not sufficient as the critical brain shift cannot be detected. We are working on incorporating real-time volume registration algorithms [15] which are especially optimised for slight movements typical for brain surgery. Volume registration would allow the planning data to be retained for new volume data sets without forcing the surgeon to reset them interactively.

6   Conclusion

LOCALITE is a simple but efficient approach for solving some problems related with neurosurgical interventions in iMRI systems. It gives the surgeon important orientation clues during navigation which improves the security and significantly reduces the navigation time.

The system is operational at Klinikum Krefeld, Germany, as an add-on for the iMRI system SIGNA SP of General Electric Medical Systems with a Flashpoint locator system.

References

1. Antonio De Salles, Robert Lufkin (eds) (1997) *Minimally Invasive Therapy of the Brain*. Thieme, New York, Stuttgart
2. Ferenc A Jolesz (1997) Image-guided procedures and the operating room of the future. *Radiology* 204:601-612
3. Jocelyne Troccaz, Michael Peshkin, and Brian Davies (1998) Guiding systems for computer-assisted surgery: introducing synergistic devices and discussing the different approaches. *Medical Image Analysis* 2(2) pp. 101-119
4. E Grimson et al. (1998) Clinical Experience with a High Precision Image- Guided Neurosurgery System. In: Wells WM, Colchester A (eds) *Medical Image Computing and Computer-Assisted Intervention - MICCAI '98*. Springer-Verlag Berlin (1998) pp. 63-73
5. D G T Thomas et al. (1997) Clinical Experiences with the EasyGuide Navigation System. In: Lemke HU, Vannier MW, Inamura K (eds) *Proceedings CAR '97*. Elsevier Science, Amsterdam, pp. 757-760. ISBN 0-444-82756-0
6. Nobuhiko Hata et al. (1998) Computer-Assisted Intra-Operative Magnetic Resonance Imaging Monitoring of Interstitial Laser Therapy in The Brain: A Case Report. *J of Biomedical Optics* 3(3) pp.304-311
7. Uwe Behrens et al. (1998) Enabling Systems for Neurosurgery. In: Lemke HU, Vannier MW, Inamura K, Farman A (eds) *Proceedings CAR '98*. Elsevier Science, Amsterdam, pp. 589-593. ISBN 0444829733
8. Ralf Ratering (1998) *Texturbasiertes Volumen-Rendering medizinischer Bilddaten*. Diplomarbeit Universität Bonn
9. Uwe Behrens, Ralf Ratering (1998) Adding Shadows to a Texture-Based Volume Renderer. *Procs IEEE Symp on Volume Visualisation 1998*, pp. 39-46
10. Will Schroeder, Ken Martin, Bill Lorensen (1998) *The Visualization Toolkit*. 2nd ed. Prentice-Hall, London. ISBN 0-13-954694-4.
11. Brian Cabral, Nancy Cam, Jim Foran (1994) Accelerated volume rendering and tomographic reconstruction using texture mapping hardware. In: Arie Kaufmann, Wolfgang Krger (eds) *1994 Symposium on Volume Visualization*. ACM SIG-GRAPH, (October 94) pp. 91-98. ISBN 0-89791-741-3
12. Thomas Berlage, Gernoth Grunst, Klaus Kansy (1999) Grundlagen chirurgischer Enabling-Systeme und ihre informationstechnische Umsetzung. to appear
13. Hans-Joachim Schwarzmaier, Ilya V. Yaroslavsky, Anna N. Yaroslavsky, Volkhard Fiedler, Frank Ulrich, Thomas Kahn (1998) Treatment Planning for MRI- Guided Laser-Induced Interstitial Thermotherapy of Brain Tumors - The Role of Blood Perfusion. *JMRI* 8(1) pp.121-127
14. M Breeuwer et al. (1998) The EASI Project-Improving the Effectiveness and Quality of Image-Guided Surgery. *IEEE Trans Inf Techn in Biomedicine* 2(3) pp. 156-168
15. Manja Fieberg (1999) *Registrierung zwei- und dreidimensionaler multimodaler medizinischer Bilder angewendet für Ultraschall- und Magnetresonanzbilder*. Diplomarbeit Universität Bonn

Design and Evaluation of a System for Microscope-Assisted Guided Interventions (MAGI)

Philip J. Edwards[1], Andrew P. King[1], Calvin R. Maurer, Jr.[1], Darryl A. de Cunha[1], David J. Hawkes[1], Derek L. G. Hill[1], Ron P. Gaston[1], Michael R. Fenlon[2], Subhash Chandra[3], Anthony J. Strong[4], Christopher L. Chandler[4], Aurelia Richards[5], and Michael J. Gleeson[5]

[1] Computational Imaging Science Group (CISG), Radiological Sciences, KCL, Guy's Hospital, London, UK.
[2] Department of Prosthetic Dentistry, Guy's Hospital, London, UK.
[3] Leica, USA.
[4] Neurosurgery Dept., King's College Hospital, London, UK.
[5] ENT surgery dept., Guy's Hospital, London, UK.

Abstract. The problem of providing surgical navigation using image overlays on the operative scene can be split into four main tasks - calibration of the optical system; registration of preoperative images to the patient; tracking of the display system and patient and display using a suitable visualisation scheme.
To achieve a convincing result in the magnified view through the operating microscope high alignment accuracy is required. We have simulated our entire system to establish the major sources of error. We have improved each of the stages involved. The microscope calibration process has been automated. We have introduced bone-implanted markers for registration and incorporated a locking acrylic dental stent (LADS) for patient tracking and/or registration.
These improvements have significantly increased the alignment accuracy of our overlays. LADS repositioning on volunteers showed a mean target registration error of 0.7mm. Phantom accuracy is 0.3-0.5mm and clinical overlay errors were 0.5-1.0mm on the bone fiducials and 0.5-4mm on target structures. We have improved the graphical representation of the stereo overlays. The resulting system provides 3D surgical navigation for microscope-assisted guided interventions (MAGI).

1 Introduction

In conventional image-guided surgery a 3D representation of the patient is generated, usually from MR or CT images, prior to surgery. At surgery correspondence between this representation and the patient is established by registration. A computer displays the location in this representation of a pointer held within the surgical field. Use of such a system relies on the surgeon looking away from the surgical scene to the computer workstation. This is not ideal as it requires mental reorientation between the surgical view and the workstation display.

A solution that we are pursuing is to overlay 3D projections derived from the preoperative images, into the binocular optics of a surgical microscope, accurately aligned with the surgical scene. The microscope optics are of high quality and provide an ideal device for incorporation of an augmented reality display. Proof of principle has been presented [1] and was inspired by the earlier work of Kelly and Roberts [2, 3]. To exploit fully the potential of this technology in microsurgery it has become clear that registration between overlay and surgical scene must be as accurate as possible.

In the following sections we describe the equipment and methods of calibration, registration, tracking and visualisation. An error analysis of the system is given along with the results of volunteer, phantom and clinical experiments.

2   Method

2.1   Equipment

A Leica M695 or M500 binocular operating microscope with an interface to record focus and zoom settings is adapted by incorporating two purpose built monochrome VGA 640x480 displays. These project overlay images into the left and right views via beam-splitters. A video camera system records the combined overlays and microscope views. Changes in the position of the microscope are tracked using an array of 13 infra-red emitting diodes (IREDs) mounted on a bracket which is rigidly attached to the microscope assembly. The 3D IRED coordinates are measured using an Optotrak localiser (Northern Digital Inc.).

For registration we use fiducials that are based on the bone-implanted marker designs of Maurer et al [4]. A post is screwed into the skull. Attached to this post is either an imaging marker or a physical locator, the centres of which coincide.

Changes in patient position are determined by tracking the position of 6 IREDs fixed to the custom built locking acrylic dental stent (LADS). The LADS assembly also contains 10 fiducials which are the same as those implanted in the bone and may be used for registration.

The main user interface and preoperative image display system runs on a Sun sparcstation. This communicates with an Intergraph graphics PC which provides the two overlay images injected into each eyepiece of the microscope.

2.2   Calibration

In order to produce good alignment of the overlays with the real world, accurate calibration of the microscope optics is necessary. We assume a pinhole camera model and neglect distortion, which we have measured to be only 1-2% at the extreme edge of the field-of-view.

We employ an automated calibration method which uses the calibration object shown in Figure 1(a). This object is fitted with a set of IREDs and tracked whilst the calibration images are acquired by a camera mounted inside the microscope. The calibration object has a known pattern of circular markings which are automatically detected and matched. A calibration image is shown in Figure 1(b). The matching information is combined with the tracking data to produce a set of corresponding 3D and 2D points, which can be used to calibrate the microscope optics. For each calibration, a number of images are acquired from different relative positions of the microscope and calibration object. This increases the number of point correspondences used in the calibration; reduces any random errors in tracking the microscope; and provides a better spread of calibration points along the optical axis. The Tsai calibration algorithm[5] is used to obtain estimates of the camera parameters. This procedure is carried out separately for both eye-pieces of the microscope.

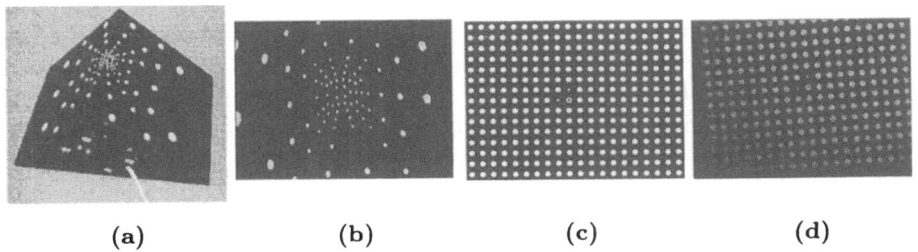

| (a) | (b) | (c) | (d) |

Fig. 1. The calibration object and 2D calibration pattern: (a) perspective view of the calibration object showing the IREDs used for tracking, (b) an image of the calibration object acquired by the microscope camera, (c) the 2D calibration pattern, (d) an image of the 2D calibration pattern acquired by the microscope camera

We calibrate over the range of variable zoom and focus parameters. This is achieved by modelling the variation in the values of the camera parameters as bivariate polynomial functions of zoom and focus[6, 7].

Currently there are two modes of operation of the MAGI system: variable zoom and focus calibrations are useful when a range of zoom and focus settings will be used in a single procedure, whereas fixed zoom and focus calibrations are used when we have prior knowledge of the required zoom and focus settings.

Alignment of the coordinate systems of the microscope camera and the image injectors is achieved by injecting an image of a calibration pattern into each microscope eye-piece, and automatically matching it with the known model. The pattern used is shown in Figure 1(c) and an image acquired through the microscope camera is shown in Figure 1(d). The circles in the calibration pattern can be accurately localised using a centre of gravity operator, so the 2D overlay calibration mapping can be done with sub-pixel accuracy.

2.3   Image-to-Physical Registration and Patient Tracking

For registration, the application accuracy for skin markers or anatomical landmarks is typically about 3 mm or worse [8], whereas bone-implanted markers inserted prior to preoperative imaging give a clinical accuracy of ~0.7mm[4]. We have produced markers based on this system. We can mark the physical caps with a tracked pointer to an accuracy of ~0.2mm. The image markers can be found repeatably to an accuracy of ~0.4mm in MRI images of voxel size 1x1x1.5mm. Taking a gradient echo MRI scan we get typical fiducial registration errors of 0.7-1.2mm due to imager distortion.

A tracker needs to be rigidly attached to the skull to track movement of the patient. In conventional systems the head is immobilised in a Mayfield or similar clamp to which a tracker is fixed. Since we are interested in both ENT and neurosurgical applications a more convenient tracking system is required. We have designed a locking acrylic dental stent (LADS) which attaches to the patient's upper teeth. This enables much freer movement of the patient's head.

Dental appliances such as occlusal splints and bite blocks have been proposed for use as positional reference devices [9, 10]. For our purposes the standard occlusal splint was redesigned to maximise retention and stability with the aim of improved repeatability of placement. The main occlusal block is clamped with titanium screws to left and right locking wings. It is possible that the need to insert markers into the skull can be avoided by attaching the fiducials to the LADS. For this purpose we have designed a set of extended arm pieces to which imaging and physical locators can be attached. The LADS is shown in figure 2.

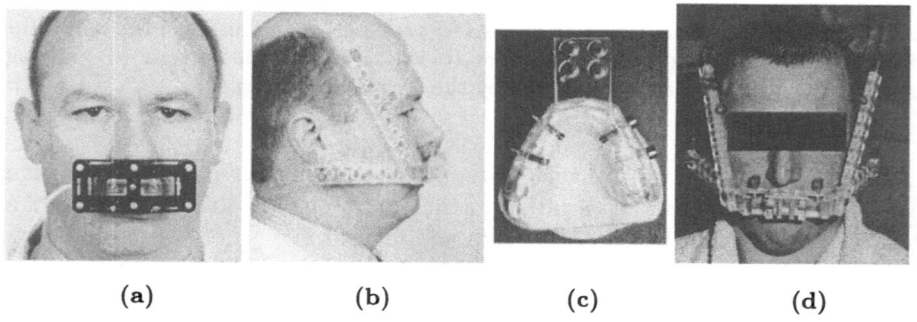

(a)   (b)   (c)   (d)

Fig. 2. Registration methods. The locking acrylic dental stent (LADS) construction, showing (a) the optical tracker attachment, (b) the image and physical fiducial frame, (c) the acrylic stent with locking screws and (d) a patient with both the LADS marker frame and bon-implanted fiducials.

To assess the suitability of the LADS for registration we need to measure how accurately the stent can be relocated in the same position. For this purpose we have scanned four volunteers with the LADS device in place. Multiple scans are taken and the LADS is removed and replaced between each scan. The scans are registered to each other using the fiducials on the LADS frame. This transformation is compared with that obtained by fully automated registration of each pair of MR images by maximisation of Normalised Mutual Information

[11]. The transformations incorporate 3 extra degrees of freedom to compensate for scaling inaccuracy along the axes of the MR scanner.

2.4 Visualisation

Accurate calibration of each eye should give the correct stereo disparity for overlaid objects. For true 3D image guidance it is necessary to provide correct 3D perception of the position of overlaid objects. To this end we have conducted, both in a laboratory and through the microscope itself, a number of vision experiments to establish the optimum parameters for 3D stereo perception through transparent surfaces. Preliminary results show that the overlay should be carefully controlled and provide maximum colour separation from the surgical scene. The detail should include identifiable regions with different spatial frequencies. A reasonable approximation to this is provided by a wireframe representation.

2.5 Error Analysis

We have undertaken a numerical simulation of the MAGI system, which enables the levels of the various noise sources to be varied individually and their effect on the overall system error observed. The simulation is achieved by taking a typical configuration of IREDs, fiducials and calibration points and adding Gaussian noise of a similar size to the relevant measurement error - Optotrak IRED tracking, fiducial identification in the images and calibration marker localisation in the camera image. All the necessary processing (calibration, registration and rigid body tracking of each object) is performed using both noisy and exact values the comparison of these two gives us the simulated error. This was repeated 1000 times to produce the error statistics, with a set of 500 random points within the surgical field being used to compute target errors. The values of interest are calibration error, error in the 3D location of virtual structures, and the corresponding 2D overlay error after projection onto the image plane.

2.6 Phantom Experiments and Initial Clinical Evaluation

The entire system has been tested on a phantom and in the operating theatre. Overlay accuracy is assessed by identifying corresponding real and virtual structures in grabbed images. This gives a 2D overlay error which has a corresponding 3D error in mm at the focal plane.

3 Results

3.1 Simulation Results

The sources of error in the MAGI system can be split into three categories: error in localising the circular markings in the calibration images; error in localising the bone-implanted imaging markers in the preoperative image; and tracking error. For each of these we estimate typical error values. For localising the calibration object marks with a centre of gravity operator we estimate an error of 1 pixel RMS. For a typical CT and MRI slice thickness and in-plane resolution, and using a centre-of-gravity operator to obtain sub-voxel accuracy in the preoperative image, we estimate the imaging marker localisation error to be 0.4mm RMS (neglecting MR distortion). Finally, careful experiments have confirmed that the Optotrak tracks individual IREDs to an accuracy of 0.2mm RMS.

Table 1. The effects of individual error sources on the overall system error. Tracking errors are broken down by tracked object. A final system error is predicted. Typical error values are used for the three error sources: 1 pixel RMS for calibration mark localisation; 0.4mm RMS for imaging marker localisation; and 0.2mm RMS for tracking.

Error Source	Calibration Error (mm at focal plane)	3D Alignment Error (mm)	2D Overlay Error (mm at focal plane)
Calibration marks	0.014	-	0.014
Imaging markers	-	1.1	0.55
Tracking	0.29	1.2	0.71
Calibration object	0.060	-	0.060
Microscope	0.28	0.43	0.45
LADS	-	0.86	0.41
Pointer	-	0.69	0.30
Combined system error	0.26	1.6	0.91

Using these estimates, Table 1 shows the relative importance of the 3 error sources. Whilst errors in localising the imaging markers are significant, tracking errors are the most important error source. For this reason these are broken down further. Four objects are tracked in the current system configuration: the calibration object, the localisation pointer, the LADS and the microscope. Using the estimated tracking error of 0.2mm RMS, Table 1 shows the relative importance of errors in tracking each of these four objects. As can be seen, microscope tracking is the most important factor in the final 2D overlay error. This is because it contributes both to the calibration error and the intraoperative errors. Also, the area of interest (i.e. the surgical scene) is relatively far from the microscope, so rotational errors will have a greater effect. Tracking of the patient (LADS) and the localisation pointer also have a significant effect, in particular on the 3D alignment error. Combining all of these error sources, and using the same estimated typical error values, we get an estimate of the final overall accuracy of the MAGI system. The total error prediction is 0.91mm at the focal plane of the microscope for a typical intraoperative marker configuration. This figure is reduced to 0.6mm for the idealised phantom marker positions.

Calibration of Zoom and Focus The simulation suggests that the error of the automatic fixed zoom and focus calibration technique is approximately 0.26mm. This is consistent with observed calibration accuracies. Further errors will be introduced from the modelling of the perspective projection parameters with zoom and focus. After this modelling the average calibration error over all possible zoom and focus values is 0.3-0.4mm. The error rises for minimum zoom and far focus due to inadequate modelling with the bivariate polynomial in this region. At these settings a fixed zoom and focus calibration is used.

3.2   LADS Relocation Accuracy

All image pairs for a given volunteer were registered using the LADS fiducials and the automated method [11]. The target registration error (TRE) was computed as the Euclidean distance between all voxels within the head transformed with the automated registration and that derived from the LADS fiducials. Table 2 gives the results. The mean TRE over all datasets was 0.7 mm with a maximum TRE over all the data of 3.64 mm. Registration accuracy is best around the oral and nasal region, where the error produced by the relocation of the LADS assembly is comparable to that using the bone-implanted markers.

Table 2. LADS target registration accuracy for four volunteers

Volunteer	mean TRE		max TRE
	mean	stddev	
A	0.69	0.22	1.82
B	0.57	0.18	1.44
C	1.14	0.38	3.64
D	0.60	0.17	2.19
Combined	0.70	0.30	3.64

3.3   Phantom and Clinical Results

Incomplete versions of the system have been evaluated on 6 patients. The full system with stereo graphics for the overlays and the latest version of the LADS has been used on two patients described below. Overlays on the phantom have been measured to have errors of 0.3-0.5mm, slightly less than the predicted 0.6mm error.

The first patient underwent removal of a petrous apex cyst. Since the patient had bilateral cysts a trans-labyrinth approach was not appropriate. A more anterior approach was used in order to preserve hearing. The LADS and bone fiducials were both used. One fiducial was marked at the start and end of the procedure, giving a positional error of 1.4mm. This is a small change indicating that the LADS was stable over the 8 hours of the operation. The alignment of

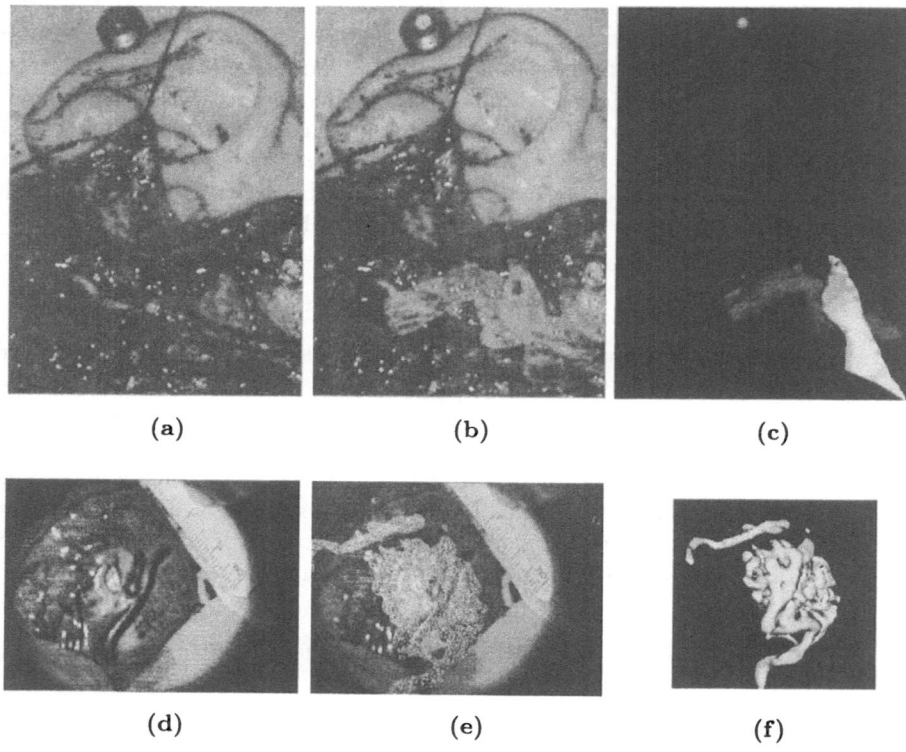

(a)   (b)   (c)

(d)   (e)   (f)

Fig. 3. Clinical results for petrous apex cyst patient (**a**) the microscope view, (**b**) the same view with overlay of zygomatic arch, carotid artery and bone pin and (**c**) a rendering from a similar viewpoint; results for a patient with an AVM showing (**d**) the microscope view, (**e**) the same view with overlay of the AVM and (**f**) a rendering from a similar viewpoint.

the overlays was visually accurate (see figure 3) to 0.5-1.0mm on the registration pins and better than 1mm for the zygomatic arch.

To our knowledge this is the first operation guided by microscope overlays providing good 3D overlay perception by stereo. The feedback from the surgeon was very positive. He remarked that the system had improved confidence in this unusual approach. The cyst was removed and the patient's hearing preserved.

For the second patient only the LADS was used for registration. The patient had a small arteriovenous malformation (AVM) in the parietal lobe between the motor and sensory strips. The system was used to provide an overlay of the lesion before craniotomy and influenced the craniotomy site chosen. The surgeon remarked that this had been helpful. The overlay on the microscope view of the brain surface is shown in figure 3. We estimate the displacement to be 3-4mm, the brain surface having sagged in the 40 minutes since the dura was opened.

Such deformation has been observed as a common occurrence in neurosurgical procedures [12, 13].

For the results above a fixed zoom and focus calibration at maximum focal length and minimum zoom was used to give the easiest depth perception.

4 Discussion

It became clear in early clinical evaluations of the initial system [1] that improved accuracy in the operating theatre was essential. We have achieved this through investigation of errors and a number of improvements to the system.

Automated calibration has provided us with a microscope calibration accuracy of 0.3-0.4mm for the practical range of zoom and focus values. An error simulation of the entire system has been implemented which can be used to experiment with alternative configurations. An overall system error of 1.6mm in 3D and 0.91mm in the 2D overlays is predicted. As a result of experiments with the simulation we intend to add IREDs to the microscope frame, and also possibly the LADS tracker, with greater separation to reduce the tracking error. To reduce registration error we have incorporated bone-implanted fiducials.

For patient tracking we introduce the locking acrylic dental stent (LADS). This is an extremely versatile tracker which allows free movement of the head within the line-of-sight of the Optotrak and enables image guidance in operations for which a head clamp is unacceptable. This is an important advancement which makes the MAGI system applicable to many more procedures. The LADS may also be a good registration device. Volunteer experiments are very encouraging and clinical accuracy will be measured in forthcoming cases. As well as providing a non-invasive registration system the physical fiducial localisation can take place without the patient, which saves valuable time in the operating theatre.

For visualisation we have incorporated high speed graphics cards with wireframe rendering to improve stereo perception. Experiments are underway to establish the ideal visual parameters for perception of the virtual structures beneath the operative surface. This has been achieved through the microscope on a skull phantom, with structures being easily perceived in the correct position by the majority of people.

Phantom results showed accuracy of 0.3-0.5mm and initial clinical results had errors of 0.5-4mm on target structures. We will be continuing clinical trials of the system in which the accuracy of the registration and the overlays as well as the perception of depth will be assessed. The aim is to enable the surgeon to see structures beneath the operative surface as though the tissue were transparent. Initial results using the improved accuracy and visualisation capabilities of MAGI have been very encouraging.

Acknowledgements

We would like to thank Leica and the EPSRC for funding this project through the DTI's MedLINK programme (project P108). We are also grateful to the radiology, radiography and theatre staff at Guy's and King's hospitals for their cooperation and to Prof. Rolf Hauser of the ENT surgery dept., Kantonsspital, Basel, Switzerland for advice on the development of the LADS device during his stay at Guy's hospital in 1997.

References

1. P. J. Edwards, D. J. Hawkes, D. L. G. Hill, D. Jewell, R Spink, A. J. Strong, and M. J. Gleeson. Augmentation of reality in the stereo operating microscope for otolaryngology and neurosurgical guidance. *Computer Assisted Surgery (formerly Journal of Image Guided Surgery)*, 1(3):172–178, 1995.
2. P. J. Kelly, G.J. Alker, and S. Goerss. Computer-assisted stereotactic laser microsurgery for the treatment of intracranial neoplasms. *Neurosurgery*, 10:324–331, 1982.
3. D. W. Roberts, J. W. Strohbehn, J.F. Hatch, W. Murray, and H. Kettenberger. A frameless stereotaxic integration of computerized tomographic imaging and the operating microscope. *Journal of Neurosurgery*, 65:545–549, 1986.
4. C. Maurer, M. J. Fitzpatrick, M. Y. Wang, R. L. Galloway, R. J. Maciunas, and G. S. Allen. Registration of head volume images using implantable fiducial markers. *IEEE Transactions on Medical Imaging*, 16(4):447–461, 1997.
5. R. Y. Tsai. A versatile camera calibration technique for high-accuracy 3d machine vision metrology using off-the-shelf tv cameras and lenses. *IEEE Journal of Robotics and Automation*, 3(4):323–344, 1987.
6. R. G. Wilsson. *Modelling and Calibration of Automated Zoom Lenses*. PhD thesis, The Robotics Institute, Carnegie Mellon University, 1994.
7. O. J. Fleig, P. J. Edwards, S. Chandra, H. Stüttler, and D.J. Hawkes. Automated microscope calibration for image guided surgery. In *Proceedings of Computer-Assisted Radiology and Surgery 1998*. Elsevier, Amsterdam, 1998.
8. J. P. Wadley, N.L. Dorward, M. Breeuwer, F.A. Gerritsen, N.D. Kitchen, and D. G. T. Thomas. Neuronavigation in 210 cases: further development of applications and full integration into contemporary neurosurgical practice. In *Proceedings of Computer-Assisted Radiology and Surgery 1998*, pages 635–640. Elsevier, Amsterdam, 1998.
9. M. A. Howard, M. B. Dobbs, T. M. Siminson, W. E. LaVelle, and M. A. Granner. A non-invasive reattachable skull fiducial marker system. *Journal of Neurosurgery*, 83:372–376, 1995.
10. R. Hauser, B. Westermann, and R. Probst. Non-invasive tracking of patients' head movements during computer-assisted intranasal microscopic surgery. *Laryngoscope*, 211:491–499, 1997.
11. C Studholme, D.L.G. Hill, and D.J. Hawkes. Automated 3-D registration of MR and CT images of the head. *Medical Image Analysis*, 1(2):163–175, 1996.
12. D. L. G. Hill, C. R. Maurer, R. J. Maciunas, J. M. Barwise, J. A. Fitzpatrick, and M. Y. Wang. Measurement of intraoperative brain surface deformation under a craniotomy. *Neurosurgery*, 43(3):514–528, 1998.
13. D. W. Roberts, A. Hartov, F. E. Kennedy, M. I. Miga, and K. D. Paulsen. Intraoperative brain shift and deformation: A quantitative analysis of cortical displacement in 28 cases. *Neurosurgery*, 43(4):749–760, 1998.

Percutaneous Posterior Stabilization of the Spine

N. Glossop[1], R. Hu[2], D.Young[2], G. Dix[2], and S. DuPlessis[2]

[1] Traxtal Technologies, 5116 Bissonnet St., Suite 324,Bellaire, Texas, USA 77401
email: neil@traxtal.com http://www.traxtal.com
[2] Division of Orthopaedic and Neurosurgery, Foothills Hospital, University of
Calgary, Calgary, Alberta Canada

Abstract. We have demonstrated the use of computer assisted techniques for performing posterior spine stabilization in a series of *in-vitro* studies. The techniques are still under development but have undergone early laboratory verification. Registration is the biggest limitation of conventional IGS systems when attempting to use them for percutaneous implantation of pedicle screws. This can be overcome by palpating structures beneath the skin or by implanting special tracked fiducial arrays attached prior to CT-scanning. Visualization of the posterior elements and placement of bone graft can be performed using a combination of endoscopic and IGS techniques, and pedicle screws placed using percutaneous approaches. Assembly of the stabilization construct is performed by subcutaneously threading the rods onto top-loading screws. Four cadaver studies have shown good results and demonstrated the possibilities and difficulties of registration, pedicle screw placement, and construct assembly using the minimally invasive techniques.

1 Introduction

The placement of posterior pedicle screws has been made safer and more accurate through the use of image guided surgery (IGS) workstations. Radiation exposure to the surgeon from intraoperative fluoroscopy has also been reduced but there has been little improvement in morbidity or patient recovery time despite the added equipment. This is primarily because the surgical exposure is essentially unchanged. In some cases the exposure may be even larger, especially if tissues are aggressively retracted in order to obtain access to potential registration locations. Use of IGS equipment also increases the time spent performing the surgical procedure.

Computer assisted techniques initially appear to be ideal for assisting with accurate *percutaneous* screw placement. Unfortunately, the need to register (or "match") the system to the underlying anatomy makes this more difficult. Registration in the spine for IGS systems is normally performed by touching carefully selected anatomical landmarks over each vertebral body, or by randomly selecting 20-40 surface points on the vertebra, or a combination of these methods. Unlike cranial surgery, skin fiducials placed on the back move too much after the scan to make external registration reliable.

Techniques suitable for assisting with registration for percutaneous pedicle screw placement include fluoroscopy, intraoperative ultrasound, intraoperative CT and interventional MRI. All these techniques have limitations, however.

Image guided fluoroscopic methods can be used either in either a purely 2D manner with graphic image overlay as demonstrated by Hofstetter et al. [1], or in conjunction with 2D to 3D matching techniques. The first approach has the advantage of automatic registration, since images are taken while the spine is being dynamically referenced. Intraoperative navigation however, must be performed on the stored fluoroscopic images, which may suffer from poor image quality compared to that available from CT based IGS systems. In addition, these systems require careful calibration and correction of distortions in the images and of the fluoroscope's support structure itself. The second approach, 2D-3D registration [2], is also potentially automatic but is still computationally expensive, especially when using poor quality fluoroscope images. Ultrasound to 3D registration algorithms [3] also suffer from difficulties with distortions and may require manual intervention. Intraoperative CT and MR [4] are still extremely costly, and cumbersome to work with.

Our own work has used two simpler approaches that show promise, namely percutaneous matching and tracked fiducial arrays. These techniques also have disadvantages but are simple to apply.

In this paper we report recent developments in percutaneous image guided spine stabilization, particularly in the registration techniques required to perform the procedure closed.

2   Materials and Methods

2.1   Techniques

The operative procedures required for percutaneous image guided spine stabilization differ significantly from conventional image guided spine surgery as well as the non computer-assisted approach. Both the order and the actions performed are different. Some additional steps are required, and a preoperative CT is mandatory. Not all aspects of a full decompression/stabilization are possible using these techniques, but a significant subset of spinal procedures are potentially treatable.

Several studies were performed to demonstrate aspects of the procedure. Many of these are described below. This work was conducted using the SCOUT IGS workstation (SNS, Mississagua, Ontario, Canada) although almost any system could have been used.

Dynamic Referencing Dynamic referencing of vertebral bodies in image guided spine surgery is required to compensate for vertebral body motion. Normally, a clamp is attached to the spinous process of the segment. An optically tracked dynamic reference body (DRB) is then attached to this clamp enabling the location and orientation of the vertebra to be monitored. While it is possible to percutaneously attach a clamp to the vertebra, a solution that we have employed is a small locking screw (Traxtal Technologies, Bellaire, Texas) placed into the spinous process or the facet. Such a device can be inserted through the skin and locked onto the bone surface. It is necessary to target the placement of the pin using fluoroscopy, which also is used to confirm the vertebral level.

Registration We used two methods of registering. The first (see Glossop et al. [5]) is a percutaneous matching technique. Stab incisions were made posterolaterally, and locations along the transverse processes and medial pars were selected for a paired point matching. Surface fitting was then used to assist and improve this initial registration. Although difficult at first, it was possible to obtain good registrations through tactile feedback alone, especially if 3D reconstructions of the vertebra are available for the surgeon to view on the computer during the process.

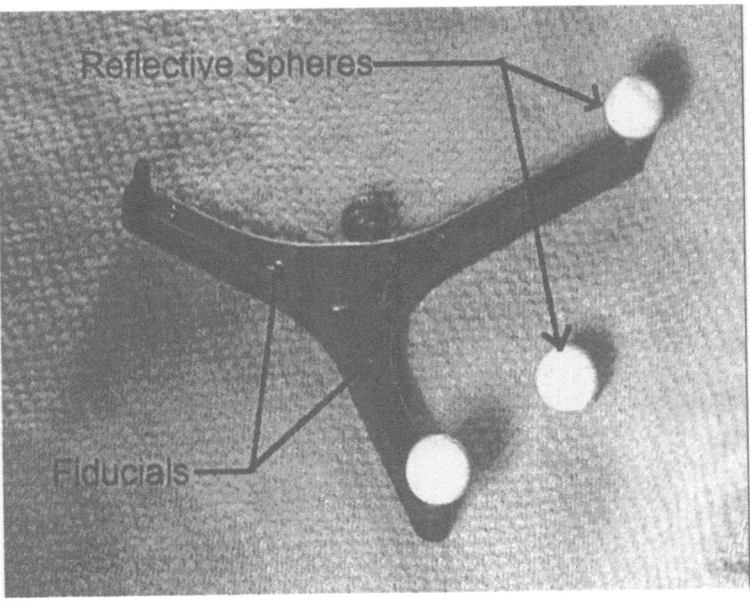

Fig. 1. The radiolucent trackable fiducial array/DRB used in these studies (Traxtal).

The second registration method used is reminiscent of traditional frame-based neurosurgery. Arrays of radiolucent, trackable fiducial carriers were attached to the vertebrae of interest using locking screws prior to the scan. The carriers (also described in [5]) contained fiducials that were imaged and selected as registration points on the preoperative scan. By using a carrier that also functions as a passive DRB with the Polaris position sensor (Northern Digital, Waterloo, Ont., Canada), it was possible to register the carrier - and the vertebra - semi-automatically, since the patient-space positions of the fiducials are accurately known *a priori* from the carrier's construction. We wrote software to perform the matching and to generate a valid registration file for the SCOUT system to use. All that was required was to locate and save the fiducial coordinates in image-space prior to surgery and execute this program. The fiducials never had to be touched with a probe as in our original technique [6].

Pedicle screw and graft placement After registration, channels can be made in the pedicles in the conventional manner, using an optically tracked pedicle awl to puncture the cortex, followed by a pedicle probe to create the hole. Although a tracked drill guide was available, we were more comfortable with hand instruments that provided more tactile feedback. K-wires can be inserted into the holes and paths confirmed with fluoroscopy before proceeding. A tracked screwdriver was not used to follow the progress of the screw into the hole although this can be done if required.

We were able to place bone grafts through direct visualization of posterior spinal elements through an endoscope. Although it is not necessary to register to visualize the anatomy in this manner, a tracked endoscope and probe were sometimes used. This enabled the positions of the instruments to be displayed on the IGS workstation.

Construct Assembly Top-loading pedicle screw systems are generally required for the system to work easily. Rods are threaded beneath the subcutaneous facia and secured using the screws.

Corrections of kyphosis etc. may best be performed using image-guided techniques to manipulate the vertebrae into an "ideal" location, but so far this has not been attempted, and would require significant changes to the software of the IGS system.

2.2   Studies

We have performed parts of the described techniques on four cadaver specimens with good success. We have still to evaluate the absolute accuracy to which the procedures have been performed, but the qualitative results have been very successful.

The first study examined the feasibility of percutaneous endoscopic navigation and visualization in the spine. An endoscope was inserted using a posterolateral approach and used to visualize the spinal anatomy.

The next two studies considered the possibility of registration using the paired point/surface fitting technique detailed above. The surgical approach used the concepts of the paraspinal posterolateral approach to access the transverse processes and most medial aspects of the pars in order to register the vertebral body. This enabled us to use the workstation to target the pedicles and implant screws percutaneously directly into the vertebra.

Finally, a combined study sought to evaluate the possibility of performing a complete procedure. Vertebrae were registered using both techniques detailed above and screws placed in the pedicles and pelvis. Rods were then threaded through the incisions and secured using a top loading fixation system.

3   Results and Discussion

We have been able to demonstrate percutaneous registrations using bony landmarks is an effective technique, with 4/6 screws being placed successfully in the cadavers. One miss was identified (from the videotape made during the procedure) to have been caused by a movement of the DRB after registration and prior to making the pedicular tunnel. It should have been detected while the surface of the vertebra was being checked with the probe, but this step was accidentally skipped for this side of the segment.

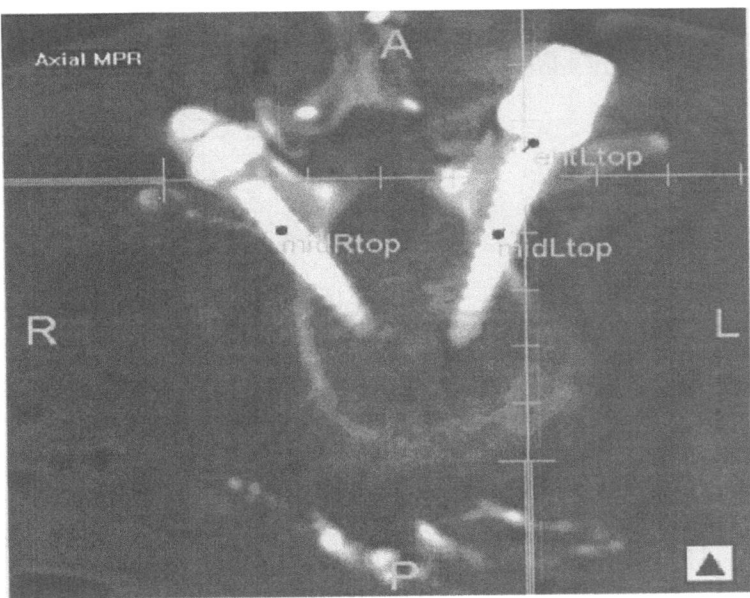

Fig. 2. Screw placed into the L2 body using the trackable fiducial array

The second misplacement was actually perfectly placed in the pedicle of the segment beneath the intended target. This could have been avoided by pre-planning the screw path. Although offered in the software, we did not elect to pre-plan the screw's path because the excellent real-time feedback offered by the workstation during conventional IGS cases was always sufficient. In the percutaneous approach where there is little relative motion between vertebral levels (as in the cadaver study), simple surface checking will not reveal "off-by-one" errors of this nature and it is easy to become confused.

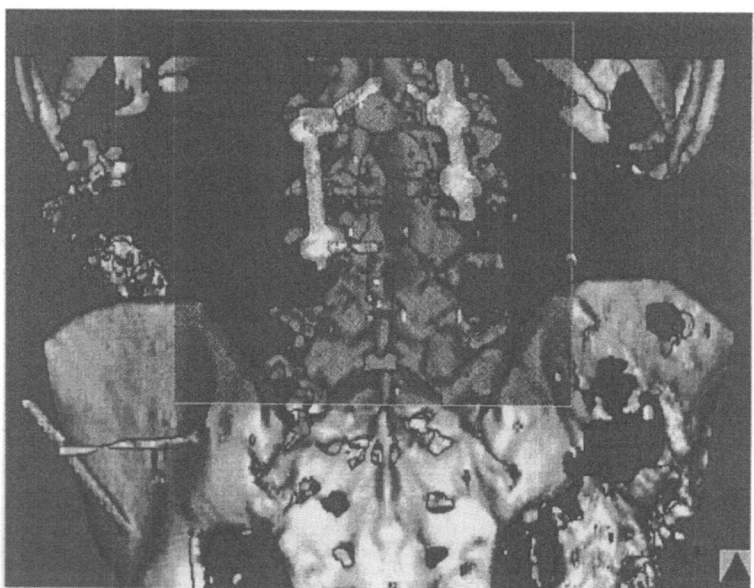

Fig. 3. Three dimensional reconstruction showing the misplaced screw in L3.

This miss alludes to another potential problem with percutaneous registration, namely inadvertent multi-segment or different-segment registration. It is always recommended to perform separate registrations on each level undergoing screw placement. The lack of direct visual confirmation of the location and level makes it extremely easy to accidentally perform all or part of the registration on an adjacent vertebra than the one intended. It is almost impossible to tell from the surface of the skin when the incorrect level is being accessed.

Registration based on trackable fiducial carriers was more successful, with 7/7 screws being correctly targeted in the pelvis and spine. It eliminates the need to register during surgery but does require an extra surgical intervention before the scan to insert the pins for the tracker. Two iliosacral screws, an anterior column screw and 4 pedicle screws were placed using the technique.

This type of registration is potentially extremely accurate, since matching errors introduced by inaccurately touching the registration landmark are eliminated. In addition, no errors attributable to the position sensor and probe are introduced during registration.

Both solutions have been shown to be able to cope with the requirements of registration. The trackable fiducial carrier was felt to be qualitatively more accurate and convenient for the surgeon, with more rigorous accuracy studies currently underway. The additional surgery that is required for implantation of the carrier may be justified if it can be shown that there is improved morbidity and recovery time for the stabilization procedure. Work in the open MRI scanner indicates that this is indeed the case [4]. We are currently working to improve the logistics of this procedure to make it more acceptable for the patient. The current procedure is probably acceptable in its current form for pelvic ring disruptions, where an external fixator is often applied as part of the resuscitation effort prior to the CT scan.

While it will be some time before percutaneous posterior spine stabilization becomes realistic in all situations, there is a large subset of surgical candidates for whom such a procedure is beginning to be practical using these techniques. The new methodology clearly demonstrates the reduced the morbidity that percutaneous stabilization might attain.

4   Conclusion

Despite the progress that has been made, we urge caution. The results are preliminary and it will be some time before instrumentation and procedures are developed enough to perform percutaneous posterior stabilization on a routine basis. Indications for this intervention currently include no prior surgery with short 2-3 segment runs. We also recommend the larger vertebrae, with L4-L5 ideal. Constraints on the current instrumentation also suggest that thin patients would also be most amenable to these techniques. In all cases, verification using fluoroscopy is and will continue to be indicated.

References

1. Hoffstetter, R., Slomczykowski, Bourquin, I., and Nolte, L.-P., Fluoroscopy Based Surgical Navigation - Concept and Clinical Applications. in *CAR'97 : Computer Assisted Radiology and Surgery*, Proceedings of the 11th International Symposium and Exhibition, Lemke, H. Vannier, M., and Inamura, K., eds., Elsevier (1997) pp. 956-960.
2. Liu, A., Bullitt, E., and Pizer, S., 3D/2D Registration Via Skeletal Near Projective Invariance in Tubular Objects. In *Medical Imaging and Computer Assisted Intervention - MICCAI'98*, Wells, W., Colchester, A., and Delp, S. eds., Lecture notes in computer science 1496, Springer (1998) pp. 952-963
3. Carrat, L., Tonetti, J., Lavalee, S., Merloz, P., Pittet, L., and Chirossel, J-P, Treatment of Pelvic Ring Fractures: Percutaneous Computer Assisted Ilioscral Screwing. In *Medical Imaging and Computer Assisted Intervention - MICCAI'98*, Wells, W., Colchester, A., and Delp, S. eds., Lecture notes in computer science 1496, Springer (1998) pp. 84-91

4. Verheyden, P., Katscher, S., Schultz, Th., Schmidt, F., and Josten, Ch., The Open MRI for Real Time Guidance and Monitoring in Less Invasive Spine Surgery - A new Perspective? In *CARS'99: Computer Assisted Radiology and Surgery*, Proceedings of the 13th International Symposium and Exhibition, H. Lemke et *al.* eds., Elsevier (1999) pp. 607-611
5. Glossop, N., Hu, R., Dix, G., and Behairy, Y., Alternate Registration Methods for Image Guided Spine Surgery. In *CARS'99 : Computer Assisted Radiology and Surgery*, Proceedings of the 13th International Symposium and Exhibition, H. Lemke et *al.* eds., Elsevier (1999) pp. 746-750
6. Hu, R., Glossop, N., Steaven, D., and J. Randle, Accuracy of Image Guided Placement of Iliosacral Lag Screws. In *CVRMed-MRCAS'97*, Proceedings of the First Joint Conference on Computer Vision, Virtual Reality and Robotics in Medicine, and Medical Robotics and Computer-Assisted Surgery, Troccaz, J., Grimsom, E., and R. Moesges, eds., Lecture notes in computer science 1205, Springer (1997) pp. 592-596

Image-Based Planning and Validation of C1-C2 Transarticular Screw Fixation Using Personalized Drill Guides

Kirsten Martens[1], Kris Verstreken[1], Johan Van Cleynenbreugel[1],
Karel Van Brussel[3], Jan Goffin[2], Guy Marchal[1], Paul Suetens[1]

[1] Laboratory for Medical Image Computing (ESAT and Radiology) K.U.Leuven,
[2] Department of Neurosurgery,
University Hospitals of Leuven, Herestraat 49, B-3000 Leuven, Belgium
[3] Department of Biomechanics and Engineering Design, Celestijnenlaan 200A,
B-3001 Heverlee, Belgium
Kirsten.Martens@uz.kuleuven.ac.be

Abstract. Posterior transarticular spine fusion is a surgical procedure used to stabilize the cervical bodies C1 and C2. Currently, spine screws are used most frequently, according to the procedure of Magerl. As the anatomy is rather complex and the view is limited, this procedure has a high risk factor. Thus we present and validate a planning system for cervical screw insertion based on preoperative CT imaging. It allows a neurosurgeon to interactively determine the desired position of the cervical screws, based on appropriate and in real-time calculated reslices through the preoperative CT data. Guided by this information, a personalized mechanical drill guide is produced. The system is validated by five cadaver experiments. Based on the preoperative planning, screws are inserted through the drill guide. A semi-automatic technique is used to extract the screw locations from the postoperative images. The deviations of the axes of the planned and the inserted screws are determined in this way. We have observed that the drill guides are not yet stable enough to cope with the drilling forces that they are subjected to. As a result, they tend to displace. However, most of the inserted screws were judged to be adequately placed. No vascular compromise nor invasion of the spinal canal was observed.

Keywords Image-based surgery, C1-C2 instability, personalized drill guides

1 Introduction

Posterior transarticular screw fixation of the spinal segment C1-C2 has gained an increasing popularity. This technique was introduced by Magerl and Seemann [1] and has been widely used for atlantoaxial instability [2,3]. This instability poses special stabilization challenges compared with the remainder of the cervical spine. The unique architecture of the atlantoaxial complex (Figure 1a and 1b), with its horizontal articular surfaces, ligamentous connections and distinctive vertebral anatomy, allows not only flexion, extension and lateral bending, but also significant axial rotation [4]. C1-C2 transarticular screw fixation has become popular because it achieves greater biomechanical stability and superior fixation of atlantoaxial rotation [5] compared with the standard fusion techniques described by Gallie [6] or Brooks and Jenkins [7]. The success of this technique has been demonstrated in a number of clinical series [2, 3, 5, 9–11]. However, despite of the reported success rates ranging from 87 to 100 %, the variable anatomy of the atlantoaxial complex often limits the use of the transarticular screw technique. The technique is potentially dangerous because the screw path is close to important structures. The following complications associated with this procedure have been reported: malpositioning of screws, pseudoarthrosis, implant failure, dural tear, neurologic deficit and vascular compromise causing brain stem infarction and death [12, 3, 13]. Consequences of injuries of the vertebral artery range from occult arteriovenous fistula to frank arterial compromise [12, 14]. When inserting the screw the surgeon uses his or her anatomic knowledge to align the drill in the proper direction. A significant error may be induced by only a slight deviation of the direction. To check the correct placement of the screw in the pedicle, fluoroscopy is used. However, the vertebral artery, which is particularly at risk at the isthmus of C2, can not be visualized, neither directly, nor by fluoroscopy.

In order to enhance the surgeon's confidence in placing the screws, we have developed a novel technique that combines preoperative computer tomography with the use of a personalized mechanical drill guide produced by stereolithography. After a description of the system and the method, a first validation on five cadavers is presented. Quantitative and qualitative results are shown. At the time of writing 3 more cadavers and 2 real patients are in the planning stage.

2   Surgery Planning and Support

2.1   About the Planning System and Steps

The planning system for endosseous oral implants [15] has been adapted for planning the insertion of C1-C2 transarticular screws. In short, the user is working in a virtual environment wherein all objects are located. This scenery is viewed by multiple cameras from random viewing positions and with various viewing angles and zoom factors [15]. All objects present can be manipulated by the user to suit his or her viewing needs. The major modification made to the existing system was the incorporation of the possibility to make 2D reslices perpendicular to and containing the inserted screws. This is an indispensable feature for assessing the correct placement of the screws in 3 dimensions, especially within the joint itself.

A stepwise account of the planning procedure is now given. Insertion of the virtual screw is done as follows. A screw, represented as a cylinder with a central axis, is defined using two points named origin and end point. The cylinder has a transparent safety zone around it that indicates a distance of 2 mm. Using the CT-derived surface model of the vertebrae, the surgeon indicates the starting

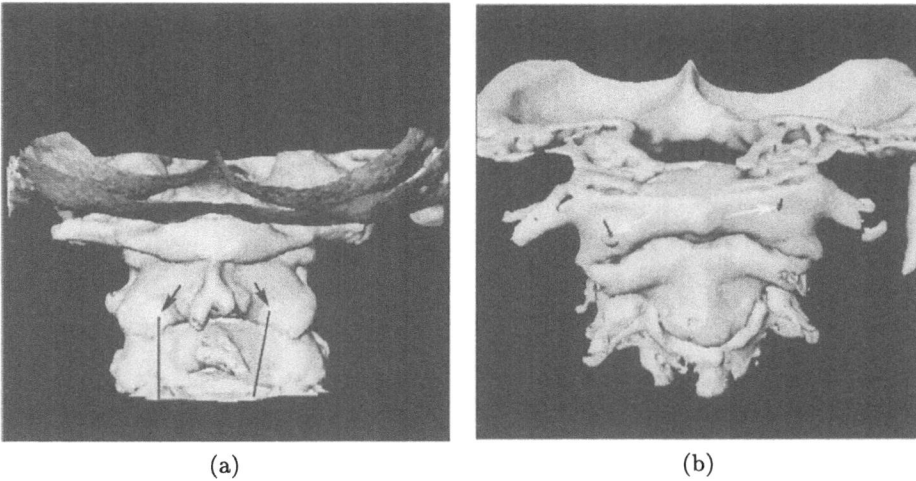

(a)   (b)

Fig. 1. *(a) Full posterior view of the C1-C2 complex and skull base, with arrows indicating the entry points (origins) of the transarticular screws at C2 (b) Full anterior view of the C1-C2 complex and skull base, with arrows indicating the exit points (end points) of the transarticular screws at the anterior cortical bone of C1*

point for the drill and the desired end point (Figure 1a and 1b). At this point the surgeon can attach a set of planes to the central axis of the screw (Figure 2a and 2b). Each of these planes shows a slice through the CT data set. Thus the axis is used as a guidance path for a camera, whose view is shown in a separate window. By default, this camera is aimed at the slice perpendicular to the axis and it is moved along it by means of the thumbwheel located in the lower left corner of the window (Figure 2a). This view is especially useful to assess the correct positioning of the screw within the narrow isthmus. The camera can also be switched to a view containing the screw. This is used to check the correct upward angle of the inserted screw (Figure 2b). Once the screw is inserted, its angulation can still be adjusted and its dimensions adapted to obtain the optimal fixation of the vertebrae (Figure 3a). This procedure is then repeated for the contralateral screw. The design process thus consists of a loop where 2D and 3D are alternatively or simultaneously checked and adjusted.

2.2   Personalized drill guide

In order to enhance the precision and the safety of the screw insertion, a mechanical drill guide is derived from the planned trajectories of the screws (Figure 3b). The aim is to have a patient dependent drill guide that exactly fits to the posterior part of vertebra C2, incorporating drill holes indicating the correct position and orientation for the screws [16,17]. The reason the drill guide does not fit on vertebra C1, is the possible change in relation between C1 and C2. They do not behave as one rigid body and so their relative position might be different at the time of CT scan and at the time of actual surgery. The drill guide can

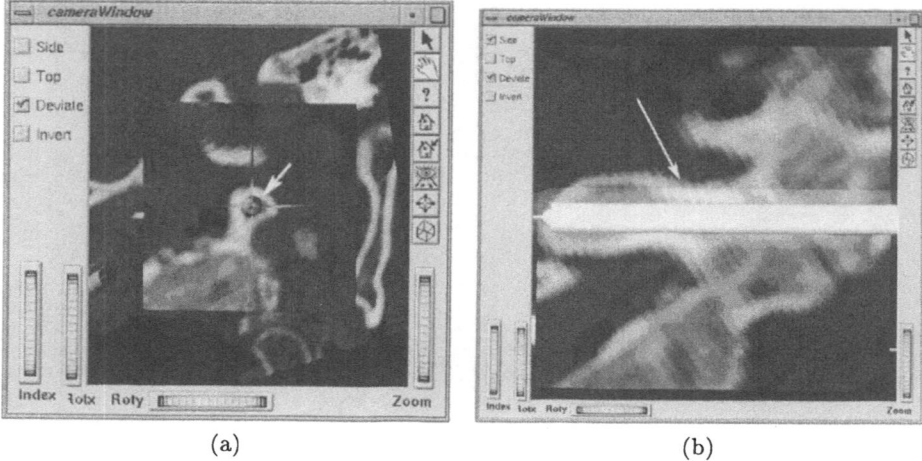

(a)   (b)

Fig. 2. *(a) Reslice through the CT data, orthogonal to the inserted screw with arrow indicating the screw transversing the isthmus of C2 (b) Reslice through the CT data, containing the screw with arrow indicating the level at which Figure 1a was resliced*

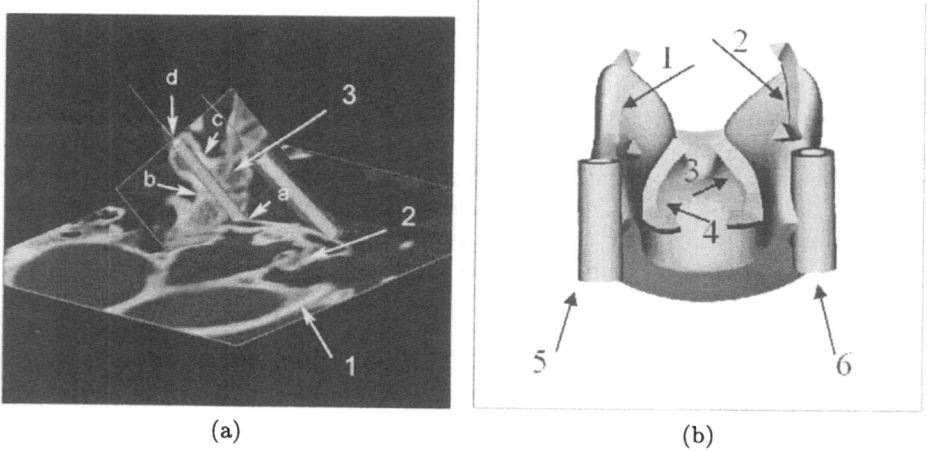

(a)   (b)

Fig. 3. *(a) Single viewpoint containing one transverse slice, two planned screws and a reslice through one of the axes; 1 = skull base, 2 = vertebra C1, 3 = vertebra C2; a = origin of the screw, b = joint between C1 and C2 that has to be stabilized, c = smallest diameter through which the screw needs to travel, d = end point of the screw (b) Full frontal view of the personalized mechanical drill guide. 1 to 4: connection interfaces ("knife-edges") between the drill guide and the vertebra; 5 and 6: right and left drill hole*

only be placed on the posterior part of C2 in one unique way. A CAD/CAM program uses the shape of the vertebra and the 3D information of the planned drill paths to design the drill guide. Shape and trajectories are available from the planning. The drill guide then is produced by stereolithography. We have opted not to use fully computer assisted spine surgery [18–20] because of the three major advantages a mechanical drill guide has to offer. First of all, only a low investment is required since no expensive computer equipment and 3D optical tracking hardware is needed in the operating room. Furthermore, the drill guide does not significantly increase the complexity of the surgery. And lastly, no preoperative referencing is needed, since the position of the drill guide upon the posterior part of the vertebra is unique. Of course there is a downside to this approach. At the time of operation the trajectories are fully fixed, no deviation from the planning is possible in the operating theater. Computer assisted surgery is much more flexible and allows continuous adjustment of the planning.

3 Validation

Five cadavers were CT scanned. Based on the planning, personalized drill guides were made. After insertion using these drill guides, postoperative CT scans were acquired under the same imaging conditions as for the preoperative images.The screws are made of Ti, so they generate very little metallic streak artifact. The postoperative images therefore show very little distortion. In order to be able to view the planned screw superposed correctly upon the inserted one, the pre- and postoperative images have to be registered. This is achieved by using a technique, previously described [21]. Visualizing the planning on the result already leads to a qualitative assessment of the insertion (Figure 4a and 4b). To get quantitative results the following procedure was devised. In the postoperative images both screws were segmented by thresholding. This results in a voxel cloud of which the center of gravity is found. The principal axis through this center is found by analyzing eigenvalues and eigenvectors associated with the voxel cloud. At this point we can mathematically compare the axis of the planned screw with the one derived from the inserted screw. Since we know only the coordinates of the origin and endpoint of the planned screws, it is evident we should only find the corresponding points in the inserted screws and compare the coordinates. In order to do this, we look up the z coordinate of the planned screws and calculate in the same z plane the x and y coordinates of the inserted screws. The planned coordinates are then subtracted from the calculated ones to obtain Δx and Δy. The coordinate system is defined as follows. The z axis runs caudocranial, the y axis anteroposterior and the x axis from left to right. Another way of comparing the plan and its execution, is to assess the angles between them when projected onto sagittal, coronal and transverse planes. In addition to that the angle between the two axis directions was computed. The results of the measurements can be found in Table 1. Finally we have asked the neurosurgeon to qualitatively judge each resultant insertion, by placing it into either of four categories: clinically good, clinically acceptable, clinically unacceptable and clinically bad.

4 Results and discussion

Table 1 presents the comparison between the planned and the inserted screws. The first part of the table lists the differences between x and y coordinates of planned and inserted screws on the left and right hand side. Looking at the

Table 1. *Comparison of planned screws versus inserted screws. The first part of the table lists the absolute differences (in mm) between (x, y) coordinates of origin and end point in planned and inserted screws. The second part of the table lists the angles (in degrees) between planned and inserted screws.*
L = left, R = right; μ = mean, σ = standard deviation; subscripts o and e denote origin and end point respectively.

Cadaver	Absolute Differences				Angles			
	Δx_o	Δy_o	Δx_e	Δy_e	Total	Sagittal	Coronal	Transverse
1L	0.75	2.13	0.07	0.23	2.37	2.04	1.23	1.92
1R	1.36	2.85	0.30	1.17	4.26	3.79	2.55	2.90
2L	0.46	8.96	0.26	14.79	4.84	4.58	1.36	2.63
2R	0.07	1.62	2.23	11.75	9.03	8.47	5.35	3.86
3L	0.22	7.12	0.26	1.43	5.11	5.10	1.10	0.05
3R	1.36	7.16	1.10	5.75	5.93	5.91	0.78	0.58
4L	2.20	5.20	0.39	4.38	2.64	0.43	5.01	3.11
4R	2.83	2.12	1.29	2.30	2.04	0.01	4.11	2.32
5L	1.64	6.92	0.34	7.09	8.07	8.04	4.44	0.69
5R	1.84	3.48	0.01	4.93	7.17	6.92	4.73	1.99
μ (ex. 2)	1.52	4.62	0.47	3.41	4.70	4.03	2.99	1.70
σ (ex. 2)	0.81	2.24	0.47	2.47	2.27	2.98	1.78	1.13

numbers, one cadaver clearly stands out. Indeed, cadaver number two seems to have extremely large values for Δy, especially with respect to the end points. However, this can be entirely attributed to human error. During the insertion of the screws into the C1-C2 complex of cadaver number 2, it was observed by the neurosurgeon that the personalized drill guide did not fit at all, contrary to the other cadavers. Since this problem was not encountered with one of the other cadavers, a mere switch of drill guides did not take place. The only plausible explanation for this fact, is that probably the wrong cadaver was set up for the operation. Its results thus were excluded from all computations, as they are not relevant. When we compare the mean of the absolute differences in Table 1, it is obvious that Δx on average is smaller than Δy. However a plausible explanation can be offered for this observation. When the drill guide is used, the direction of the drilling forces coincides with the y direction almost perfectly. This results in a displacement of the template in that direction. Looking at the standard deviations of the differences, one will observe that the standard deviations of Δy are much larger than those of Δx. This is probably due to the fact that the tendency of the drill guide to shift is much larger in the y direction.

The second part of Table 1 lists the different angular deviations that have been computed.It is obvious that the angular deviations in the sagittal and coronal plane on average are larger than in the transverse plane. Hence, we conclude that the shift not only occurs in the y direction, but also in the z direction (as seen in the sagittal projection). This would corroborate our assumption that the drill guide slides away from its optimal posterior position as a consequence of the drilling force being exerted. The qualitative assessment of the screw insertion yielded following results. Of the relevant insertions i.e. all except cadaver 2, two screws from a total of eight were judged to be clinically unacceptable. In both cases there was a deviation of the screw axis that can only be attributed to a displacement of the drill guide. However, in none of the cases the screw

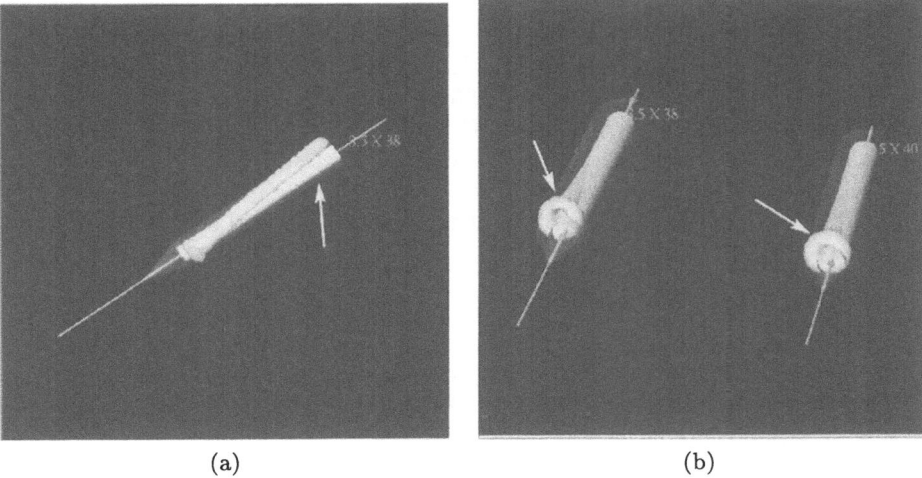

(a)   (b)

Fig. 4. *(a) Sagittal view of the right hand screw in cadaver 5 superposed upon the planned screw. The arrow indicates the displacement error that prompted the rejection of this insertion. (b) View of both screws in cadaver 1 superposed upon the planned screws. They were judged to be very well placed. The arrows indicate the very small deviation which exists between the inserted and the planned screws.*

invaded the spinal canal, nor was there any evidence of vascular compromise. Both screws were rejected only because their trajectory deviated too far from the ideal one (Figure 4a). Three screws were clinically well placed, three were clinically acceptable. In cadaver number 1 both screws were very well placed. This can be seen in Figure 4b.

5   Conclusion and future developments

As was already stated [22] we can certainly conclude that the use of computer assistance may help in placing C1-C2 transarticular screws. It certainly can assist navigation within C2. However, as we have observed, the drill guide's positioning is not yet stable enough to cope with the forces exerted during drilling. This instability can lead to unacceptable deviations from the optimal screw placement as a slight error in direction may result in a significant error in the position of the tip of the screw. The next 3 cadavers that are scheduled for the operation will have the advantage of being treated with a slightly different drill guide. Having a better contact with the spinous process of C2, this one is designed to have greater stability in the direction of the drilling force. As for the surgeon, this preoperative planning system allows him/her to rehearse the screw insertion in a more life-like way than by studying only the 2D CT images. It requires a minor time investment on his/her part, but this increases significantly the level of safety and tranquility associated with the procedure.

Acknowledgments

The work discussed here belongs, partly to the EU-funded *Stereotactic Laser-Neurosurgery* project (nr. BMH4-CT96-0716), and partly to the EU-funded Brite Euram III *PISA* project (nr. BRPR CT97 0378). Partners in the latter are Materialise NV, Belgium; Philips Medical Systems BV, the Netherlands: ICS-AD; DePuy International Ltd, UK; Ceka NV, Belgium; K.U. Leuven, Belgium: ESAT/Radiology & Div. Biomechanics; University of Leeds, UK: Research School of Medicine.

References

1. Magerl F, Seeman PS. *Stable Posterior Fusion of the Atlas and Axis by Transarticular Screw Fixation.* In Kehr P. Weidner A (eds). Cervical Spine. Vienna, Springer Verlag 322 - 317, 1987
2. Grob D, Jeanneret B, Aebi M, et al. *Atlanto-axial Fusion with Transarticular Screw Fixation.* J. Bone Joint Surg [Br] 1991; 73: 972 - 976
3. Stillerman CB, Wilson JA. *Atlanto-axial Stabilization with Posterior Transarticular Screw Fixation: Technical Description and Report of 22 Cases.* Neurosurgery 1993; 32: 948 - 955
4. Panjabi CG, Dvorak J, Duranceau J, et al. *Three-dimensional Movements of the Upper Spine.* Spine 1988; 13: 726 - 730
5. Wilke HJ, Fischer K, Kuger A, Magerl F, Claes L, Wörsdörfer O. *In Vitro Investigations of Internal Fixation Systems of the Upper Cervical Spine. II: Stability of Posterior Atlanto-axial Fixation Techniques.* Eur Spine J 1992; 1: 191 - 199
6. Gallie WE. *Fractures and Dislocations of the Upper Cervical Spine.* Am J Surg 1939; 46: 495 - 499
7. Brooks AL, Jenkins EW. *Atlanto-axial Arthrodesis by the Wedge Compression Method.* J Bone Joint Surg [Am] 1978; 60: 279 - 284
8. Grob D, Dvorak J, Panjabi M. *Posterior Occipitocervial Fusion. A Preliminary Report of a New Technique.* Spine 1991; 16(Suppl): S17 - S20
9. Madawi AA, Casey ATH, Solanki GA, Tuite G, VEres R, Crockard HA. *Radiological and Anatomical Evaluation of the Atlantoaxial Transarticular Screw Fixation Technique.* J Neurosurg 1997; 86: 961 - 968
10. Sasso RC, Jeanneret B, Fischer K. *Occipitocervical Fusion with Posterior Plate and Screw Instrumentation. A Long-term Follow-up Study.* Spine 1994; 19: 2364 - 2368
11. Jeanneret B, Magerl F. *Primary Posterior Fusion C1-2 in Odontoid Fractures: Indications, Technique and Results of Transarticular Screw Fixation.* J Spinal Disord 1992; 5: 464 - 475
12. Apfelbaum RI. *Screw Fixation of the Upper Cervical Spine: Indications and Techniques.* Contemp Neurosurg 1994; 16: 1 - 8
13. Smith MD, Phillips WA, Hensinger RN. *Complications of Fusion to the Upper Cervical Spine.* Spine 1991; 16: 702 - 705
14. Coric D, Branch CL Jr, Wilson JA, Robinson JC. *Arteriovenous Fistula as a Complication of C1-C2 Transarticular Screw Fixation: Case Report and Review of the Literature.* J Neurosurg 1996; 85: 340 - 343
15. Verstreken K, Van Cleynenbreugel J, Martens K, Marchal G, van Steenberghe D, Suetens P. *An Image-Guided Planning System for Endosseous Oral Implants.* IEEE Transactions on Medical Imaging 1998; 17: 842 - 852
16. Van Brussel K, Vander Sloten J, Van Audekercke R, Swaelens B, Vanden Berghe L, Fabry G. *A Medical Image Based Template for Pedicle Screw Insertion.* Conference Proceedings CARS'98, volume II: 347 - 354
17. Goffin J, Van Brussel K, Vander Sloten J, Van Audekercke R, Smet M-H, Marchal G, Van Craen W, Swaelens B, Verstreken K. *3D-CT Based, Personalized Drill Guide for Posterior Transarticular Screw Fixation at C1-C2: Technical Note.* Neuro-Orthopedics 1999; 25: 47 - 56
18. Merloz P, Tonetti J, et al. *Computer Assisted Spine Surgery.* Clinical Orthopaedics and Related Research 1997; 337: 86 - 96
19. Schwarzenbach O, Berlemann U, et al. *Accuracy of Computer-Assisted Pedicle Screw Placement. An In Vivo Computed Tomography Analysis.* Spine 1997; 22: 452 - 458
20. Berlemann U, Monin D, Arm E, Nolte L-P, Ozdoba C. *Planning and Insertion of Pedicle Screws with Computer Assistance.* Journal of Spinal Disorders 1997; 10: 117 - 124
21. Maes F, Collignon A, Vandermeulen D, Marchal G, Suetens P. *Multimodality image registration by maximization of mutual information,* IEEE Transactions on Medical Imaging 1997; 16: 187-198
22. Gebhard JS, Schimmer RC, Jeanneret B. *Safety and Accuracy of Transarticular Screw Fixation C1-C2 Using an Aiming Device. An Anatomic Study.* Spine 1998; 23: 2185 - 2189

POP: Preoperative Planning and Simulation Software for Total Hip Replacement Surgery

Constantinos Nikou[1], Branislav Jaramaz[1,2], Anthony M. DiGioia III[1,2], Mike Blackwell[1], Merle E. Romesberg[1], and Mallory M. Green[1]

[1] Center for Medical Robotics and Computer Assisted Surgery,
Carnegie Mellon University, Pittsburgh, PA
{costa,mkb,merle,morgang}@ri.cmu.edu   http://www.mrcas.ri.cmu.edu
[2] Center for Orthopaedic Research, UPMC Shadyside Hospital, Pittsburgh, PA
{branko, digioia}@cs.cmu.edu   http://www.cor ssh.edu

Abstract. Proper implant placement during total hip replacement (THR) surgery has been shown to reduce short and long term complication including dislocations, accelerated wear, and loosening of the implants. Correct implant orientation is the most important factor in preventing impingement, which is a major cause of dislocation and wear following total hip replacement surgery. However, proper implant orientation is also dependent upon patient-specific factors such as pelvic anatomy bone coverage and level of femoral osteotomy, and can affect leg lengths and offsets. This paper describes a preoperative planner for THR that enables the surgeon to determine the optimal placement of the femoral and acetabular components for THR taking all of these factors into account. Coupled with a computer-assisted clinical system for precise implant positioning, this approach could significantly improve patient outcomes and lower costs.

1 Introduction

Primary total hip replacement surgery is one of the most successful surgical procedures performed today. Dislocation following total hip replacement (THR) surgery represents a significant cause of early failure, incurring additional medical costs and patient distress in 1 to 5% of cases [1, 2]. Joint replacement can also result in leg length discrepancies which cause problems such as increased stress on the hip joint, abnormal gait, loss in muscle strength, and implant loosening [3, 4].

Proper placement of the acetabular and femoral components can lessen the risk of these postoperative complications. One significant cause of dislocation is impingement of prosthetic components, in which the implant neck hits the rim of the acetabular liner and levers the head out of the socket. This impingement can lead not only to dislocation, but also to accelerated wear of the implants (leading further to instability and implant loosening via bone resorption). Another dislocation mechanism is bone-to-bone impingement, where the femoral head is levered out of the socket with a bone-on-bone collision acting as a fulcrum

[5]. Placement of the implant components relative to their associated bony structures and relative to one another will determine the envelope of impingement-free range of motion. Proper femoral component choice and placement can also help minimize the leg length inequalities that may result after THR.

Traditional methods of planning typically involve matching only implant size to the anatomy using preoperative radiographs and acetate implant templates. These methods can only provide alignment information relative to the radiographic plane, which is often not representative of the functional orientation of the pelvis or femur. Without full three-dimensional location information for the implants and bones, the envelope of impingement-free motion cannot be calculated.

We have developed a comprehensive preoperative planner (POP) for total hip replacement surgery that includes a joint simulator with real-time range of motion analysis. This planner allows the surgeon to preoperatively determine the desired position and orientation of both the acetabular and femoral implants relative to the patient's anatomy. Once these positions and orientations are established, real-time data describing range of motion limited by implant-to-implant and bone-to-bone impingement is available. Because the data is presented in real time, the surgeon can fine-tune the placement of the implants in order to maximize patient range of motion while monitoring other factors such as leg length and offset, implant surface coverage, and the amount of removed bone.

2 Methods

The planning process begins with a preoperative CT scan of the patient. This CT data is used throughout the planning process for visualization purposes. From this data, triangular surface models of the pelvis and femur are constructed with an alternate software package. The datapoints in those surfaces remain in CT coordinates.

2.1 Setup Stage

In the Setup Stage, information about the upcoming surgical case is requested. This data includes the surgeon's name, which side of the pelvis is being operated on (left or right hip), and the surgeon's approach. This data is used both for future calculation and for optimizing the user interface controls. The relevant patient data volumes (such as CT volumes and surface models) and an implant database are also associated with the current case in this stage.

2.2 Pelvic Landmark Stage

The next stage defines the transform from CT coordinates to a pelvic coordinate system, defined by four points on the pelvis: the left and right anterior iliac spine points and the left and right pubis symphysis points. The iliac spine points and

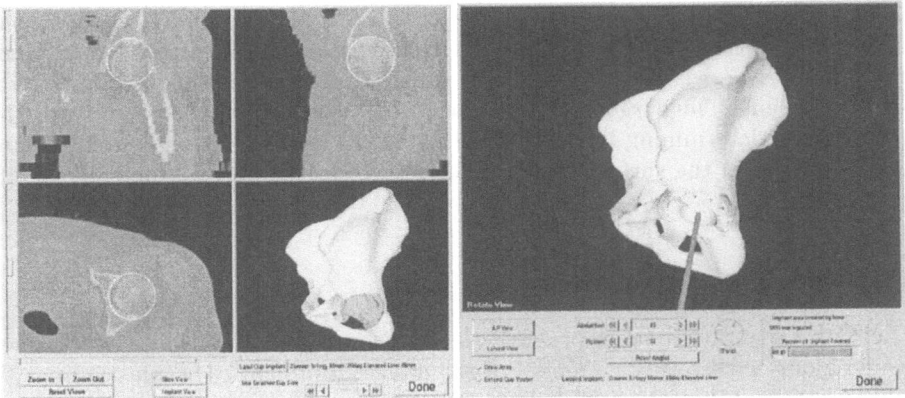

Fig. 1. Acetabular component position and orientation stages.

the median of the pubis points define an anterior plane of the pelvis. The pelvic coordinate system lies in this plane, centered at the median of the spine points.

At first, the four pelvic landmark points are chosen automatically by the planner. Their locations are presented to the surgeon in a combined CT/surface model interface in succession. Coronal, sagittal, and transverse CT slices through each landmark point are presented to the surgeon. The point is marked with cross-hairs on the CT slices as well as by a small sphere on the surface model. This allows the surgeon to view the cross-sections as well as the whole pelvis. The surgeon can change the position of the point with a mouse by clicking on the desired CT slice point or the surface model. Once the surgeon has determined the location of all four points, the points are used to define the anterior pelvic plane and the pelvic coordinate system.

2.3   Cup Find Stage

The Cup Find stage presents the surgeon with a surface model of the pelvis. By clicking on a smooth point within the acetabulum, the software can automatically detect the acetabular rim and other points within the acetabulum. These rim points are fit to a plane, which provides an estimate for the orientation of the natural acetabular opening. This orientation is then used as a starting point for placement of the acetabular implant. The size and location of the acetabulum are determined by fitting the points on the surface of the natural cup to a sphere.

2.4   Cup Position Stage

Once the location and size of the natural cup is established, POP can then recommend the most appropriately sized implant from the implants available in the database. The surgeon is presented with data similar to the Pelvic Landmark stage. This time, however, the cup size and position are marked in the CT slices with a circle. The surgeon can arbitrarily size this circle, or he can fix the circle's size to that of a selected implant. The surgeon can therefore try different implant sizes and styles to determine which implant is the most appropriate for the patient. The surgeon can also use this view to plan the reaming of the acetabulum, determining the level of bone removal required for the given implant size. A sphere in the surface model reflects the selected position and size of the implant cup.

2.5 Cup Orientation Stage

The Cup Orientation stage presents the surgeon again with the pelvic surface model along with a surface model of the selected implant. The plastic liner (if relevant) is also displayed. The surgeon is also presented with controls allowing him or her to modify the abduction, flexion (both relative to the pelvic frame), and the twist around the axis of the cup. The surgeon can also orient the cup by dragging the cup's axis about in the window containing the displayed surface model. Bone coverage surface area and percentages are displayed and updated in real time.

2.6 Femoral Landmark Stage

In order to plan femoral component placement, a femoral coordinate system must be established. Given the cup location as a starting point, the surgeon locates the femoral head with a similar interface. Once the surgeon accepts the femoral head location, POP then automatically finds other femoral landmark points. These points are the posterior lesser trochanter point, the posterior lateral and medial condyle points, and two points marking the central axis of the femoral canal. The surgeon again refines the location of these points, and moves to the next stage. These points define a femoral coordinate frame parallel to both the mechanical axis of the femur and the plane containing the points on the lesser trochanter and the condyles.

2.7 Femoral Component Placement Stage

Finally, the surgeon plans the position and orientation of the femoral component. POP uses relevant information about the chosen acetabular component (e.g. compatible head diameter) along with femoral information (e.g. average thickness of the femur) to choose an appropriate femoral stem/head combination. The femoral landmarks are then used by POP to provide an initial guess for position and orientation of the femoral stem within the bone. The stem is initially placed to match the version of the native femoral neck, aligning its long axis with the axis of the femoral canal. The surgeon is again presented with the three-slice view of the CT along with the surface model. This time, however, *the projection of the femoral stem in each slice is shown in the CT views, and a surface model of the femoral stem is shown along with the femoral surface,*

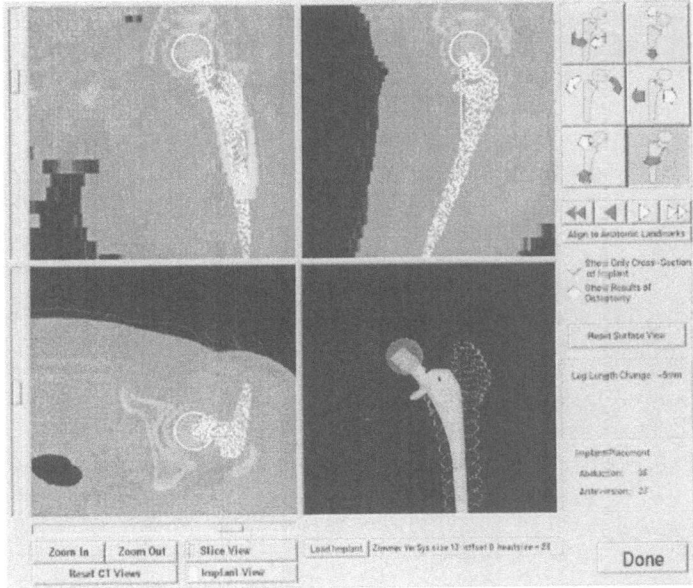

Fig. 2. Femoral component placement stage.

which is represented by a point cloud. The surgeon has the option for displaying the femur after the recommended osteotomy associated with the current femoral stem.

The surgeon can re-position the stem with the mouse by clicking on the CT slices or by using buttons that are attached to incremental movements of the stem in 6 degrees of freedom. The CT views of the stem can also be set to display only the proper cross-section of the femoral stem in each plane, allowing the surgeon to determine proper fit of the implant. The surgeon can choose different implants from the implant database, and all information will be updated in real time, including osteotomy calculations, and leg length and offset changes.

2.8   Range of Motion Analysis Stage

The final stage, (known as ROM, for Range of Motion) allows the surgeon to check motion limits for arbitrary sets of commonly accepted leg motion. In the ROM stage, the surgeon can determine the allowable envelope of motion for any given placement of implant components, and see the effects of changes in placement in real time. The ROM analysis software here has the same capabilities as in previously published work [7], and has the added feature of bone impingement checking. Bone collision detection is implemented using a point-to-point proximity checking algorithm. For each point in the femoral model at a given position, ROM calculates the distance from that point to all points on the pelvic surface

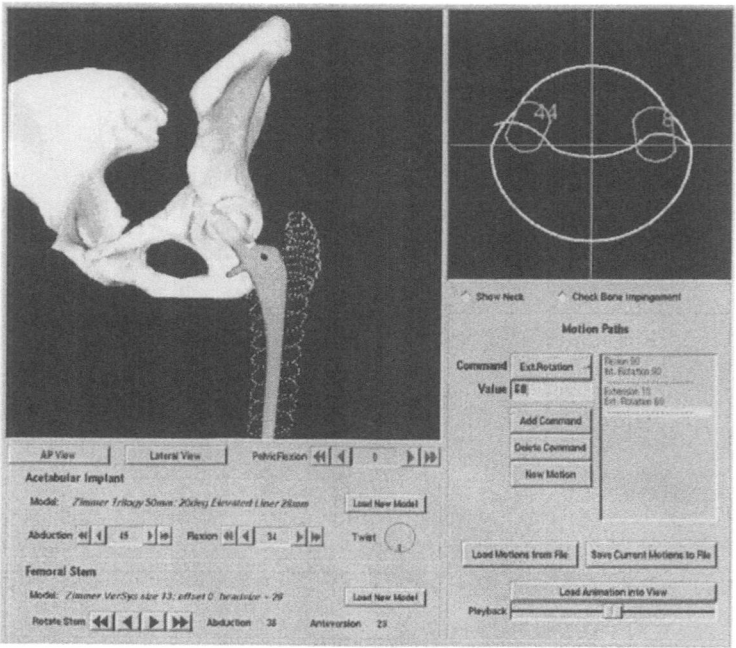

Fig. 3. POP screenshot during ROM simulation stage. In the upper left is a rendered model of the anatomy and implants in their planned orientation. Points of impingement are marked on the models and animations of simulated motions can be viewed. To the upper right is a plot describing impingement limits.

model that lie at a similar distance to the center of the joint. If any of these distances falls below the resolution of the models, then collision is reported. This method of collision detection is fast enough for real-time calculation while providing a conservative estimate for bony impingement. Therefore, testing remains interactive even while determining bone impingement limits, and the surgeon can see instant results of changes in implant cup and liner orientation, femoral stem version, and varied pelvic flexion.

3 Results

POP has been used in its current and previous forms for over 50 HipNav cases. Detection of bony impingement is a new feature of the range of motion simulator, and it has proven to be a valuable capability. Without bony impingement checking, incorrect conclusions about range of motion change are possible. To illustrate the effects of simulation, we list the results of a typical case below.

With bone impingement disabled during the planning of one case, the acetabular implant cup was oriented to match the natural opening of the acetabulum (at 45°abduction/34°flexion). The femoral implant neck was placed with

874   C. Nikou et al.

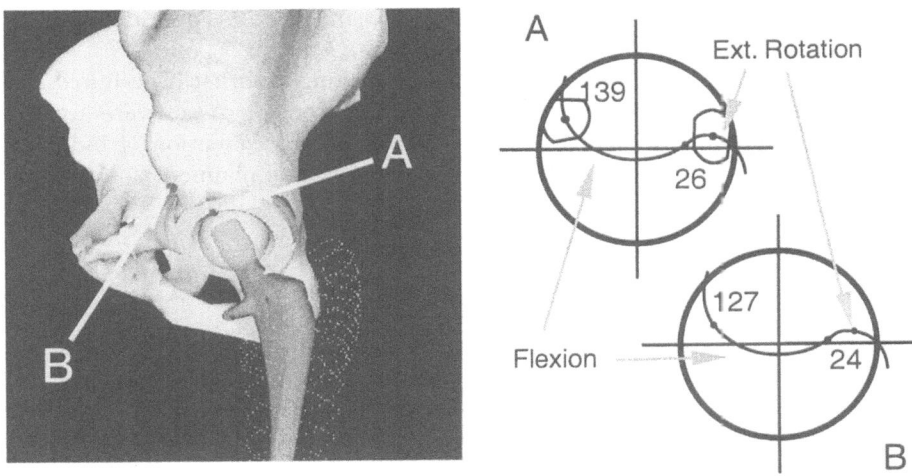

Fig. 4. POP display along with ROM plots for implant (A) vs. bone (B) impingement. The points of impingement on the surface model are impingements during leg flexion. Limits for flexion are 130° and 112° and limits for external rotation after extension are 39° and 36° for implant and bone impingement respectively

37° abduction, 13° anteversion, and a 0 mm functional leg length change. Disregarding bone impingement, the maximal flexion of the femur from neutral position was 130°, and after 10 degrees of extension from neutral position, maximal external rotation was 39°. However, once bone impingement checking was enabled, both the anterior and posterior motion limits were decreased. Possible maximal flexion before bone-to-bone impingement was reduced to 112°, and maximal external rotation after extension was reduced to 36° (Figure 4). Results such as this strengthen previous theories [6] that position of the prosthetic joint components relative to the pelvis within the patient cannot be ignored.

4   Discussion and Future Work

POP allows the surgeon to see the effects of implant component placement prior to the surgery, giving the surgeon the chance to optimally plan the procedure. Range of motion analysis and calculation of leg length and offset changes should prove invaluable feature of the system. Though POP is currently being used with the HipNav system, the utility of POP as either a patient-specific planning tool or an educational program is enough to warrant its use without coupling it with an image-guided surgical system.

Though POP has been used with many cases, its use has been limited to one surgeon. Future success of the system will require some optimization of the user-interface, and that is best achieved by getting feedback from a wider user base. Use of this system by a number of surgeons will provide this feedback and allow proper studies of patient outcomes for planned cases, provided that the plans can be implemented accurately during surgery.

Future development of POP may include planning for other procedures, such as periacetabular osteotomies and total knee replacement. A software architecture for preoperative planning can be realized, allowing creation of individual planners for separate surgical procedures and creation of planners that are more general, supporting many types of surgery.

References

1. Cobb, T. K., Morrey B. F., Ilstrup D. M.: The elevated-rim acetabular liner in total hip arthroplasty: Relationship to postoperative dislocation. The Journal of Bone and Joint Surgery, Vol 78-A, No. 1, January 1996, 80-86.
2. McCollum, D. E. and Gray, W. J.: Dislocation after total hip arthroplasty (causes and prevention). Clinical Orthopaedics and Related Research 261 (1990): 159-170.
3. Hiokka, V., T. Paavilainen, T. Lindholm, T. S., Turula, K. B., and Ylikoski, M.: Measurement and Restoration of Equality in Length of the Lower Limbs in Total Hip Replacement. Journal of Skeletal Radiology (1987) 16: 442-446.
4. Woolson, S. T.: Leg Length Equalization During Total Hip Replacement. Orthopedics, January 1990, 13(1): 17-21.
5. Amstutz, H. C. and Markolf, K. L.: Design features in total hip replacement. In Harris W.H. (ed.): Proceedings of the Second Open Scientific Meeting of the Hip Society, New York, C.V. Mosby, 1974.
6. DiGioia et al.: Image Guided Navigation System to Measure Intraoperatively Acetabular Implant Alignment. Clinical Orthopaedics and Related Research 355 (1998): 8-23.
7. Nikou, C., Jaramaz, B., and DiGioia, A.M.: Range of Motion After Total Hip Arthroplasty: Simulation of Non-axisymmetric Implants. Proceedings of the First International Conference on Medical Image Computing and Computer-Assisted Intervention (MICCAI '98), October 1998: 701-709.

CupAlign: Computer-Assisted Postoperative Radiographic Measurement of Acetabular Components Following Total Hip Arthroplasty

Branislav Jaramaz[1,2], Constantinos Nikou[2], Timothy J. Levison[1],
Anthony M. DiGioia III[1,2], and Richard S. LaBarca[2]

[1] Center for Orthopaedic Research, UPMC Shadyside Hospital, Pittsburgh, PA
{branko, levison, digioia}@cs.cmu.edu   http://www.cor.ssh.edu
[2] Center for Medical Robotics and Computer Assisted Surgery,
Carnegie Mellon University, Pittsburgh, PA
{costa,rlabarca}@ri.cmu.edu   http://www.mrcas.ri.cmu.edu

Abstract. Clinical problems following total hip replacement surgery, such as dislocation and implant wear, remain as significant clinical problems with many contributing factors. Although it is intuitive to surgeons that acetabular component alignment is one important factor, large clinical series have produced conflicting results with respect to cup alignment as a risk factor in predisposing to dislocation. One reason is that postoperative measurements of alignment are limited to single or biplanar radiographic measurements. However, the radiographic measurements are limited only to radiographic alignment and may not accurately detail true anatomic orientation of the cup. In this paper, software designed to accurately measure radiographic alignment is described. Postoperative measurements using this system are compared to the actual intraoperative measurements of cup orientation determined by the HipNav^{TM}image-guided surgical system to assess the accuracy of radiographic evaluation of cup orientation.

1 Introduction

Orientation of implant system components during total hip replacement (THR) surgery is a key factor in success of the procedure. Implant dislocation following THR ranges between 1 and 5% [1, 2] and represents a significant cause of early failure, incurring additional costs to the total surgery expenses. The causes of dislocation are related to factors such as surgical approach, soft tissue tension, and prosthetic design. One possible dislocation mechanism is the impingement of prosthetic components, in which the implant neck hits the rim of the acetabular liner and levers the head out of the socket[3]. In addition to dislocation, implant impingement causes excessive wear of the cup liner and creation of debris, a contributor to implant loosening via bone resorption. Proper alignment of implant components, which is patient and implant specific, reduces the incidence of impingement and reduces the risk of associated complications.

Previous studies have tried to correlate acetabular implant position to dislocation rates. Some researchers have proposed a "safe zone" of cup placement that may lead to minimize the risk of dislocation [4]. Other large clinical studies found no relationship between dislocation and implant placement [5].

Planar radiographs are inexpensive, widely available, and have superior resolution compared with other imaging techniques, and are therefore a preferred tool for post-operative evaluation. This study presents "CupAlign", a new methodology for computer-assisted measurement of cup orientation from radiographs after total hip replacement surgery, and compares its postoperative measurements with intraoperative measurements collected with an image-guided surgical navigation system. The HipNav^{TM}system [6] provides surgeons with the tools to place the cup precisely within the pelvis and measure its position relative to the pelvic anterior plane (i.e. the plane containing the two anterior iliac spine points and the anterior pubis symphysis points) which is generally oriented vertically when the patient is standing. The HipNav^{TM}measurement of true anatomic alignment is used in this study to evaluate the results obtained by radiographic techniques for postoperative measurement of cup alignment.

2   Methods

During all surgeries in this study, the acetabular cup was placed in the position selected in the preoperative plan using the HipNav^{TM}image-guided system. Postoperatively, AP radiographs were taken at one and three months. Digitized radiographs are analyzed to reconstruct the position of the cup based on its projected shape using a computer-assisted procedure described below. The measurements are compared to the ones made with the HipNav^{TM}system, in which the cup orientation is precisely measured intraoperatively, and expressed relative to the pelvic anterior plane.

2.1   Computer-assisted measurement procedure

After the radiograph is taken, it is digitized using a flatbed scanner. The digital image is loaded by the cup alignment measurement software (CupAlign). CupAlign allows a surgeon or technician to digitally mark landmarks on the radiographic image using a simple interface (Figure 1).

The first step determines the center of the x-ray beam relative to the radiograph. Metal markers are placed on the patient prior to imaging. The markers denote the central axis of the beam. The distance of the film to the x-ray source is entered to CupAlign as well. This defines the exact position of the x-ray source relative to the radiographic film. With this position, the proper projected images of arbitrary objects in the x-ray beam can be determined.

Next, the transverse plane is defined using standard radiographic landmarks of the pelvis, such as the "teardrops". This gives an estimate of rotation of the patient pelvis in the radiographic plane. With that rotation estimate, an object's

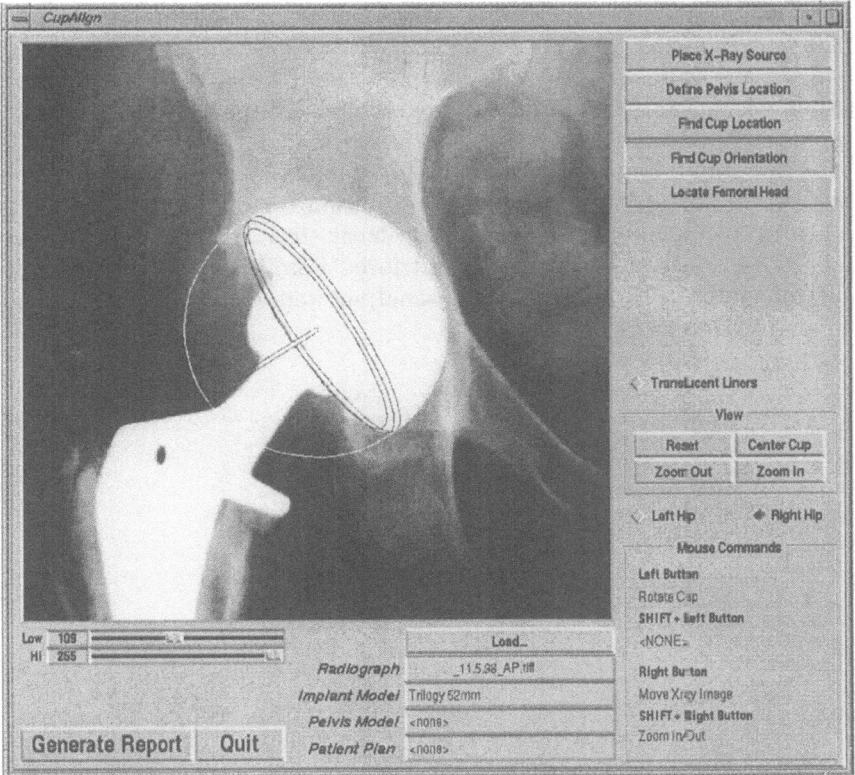

Fig. 1. CupAlign screenshot.

position relative to the pelvis can be determined, provided the position relative to the radiograph is known.

Since the cup diameter is known, we can then manipulate the position of a virtual sphere with the cup's diameter in radiograph space. CupAlign calculates the projected image of the sphere, and overlays that image on the digitized radiograph (Figure 2). Once the size and shape of the sphere's projection matches the cup on the radiograph, the position of the virtual sphere in radiographic space is the same as the position of the cup during the x-ray imaging.

Once the position of the cup center in space is determined, the user can rotate a model of the cup (from CAD data) about its center until the calculated projection of its characteristic features matches the image in the radiograph (Figure 2). When there is a match, the orientation of the cup relative to the radiograph during the imaging is known. Because we know the position and orientation of the pelvis relative to the radiograph as well, we can determine the cup position in the estimated pelvic reference frame.

Once all components are located, CupAlign reports a listing of the relevant data in a text file that can be easily parsed by other software packages. The report includes information describing pelvic abduction relative to the radiograph, x-ray source location relative to the radiograph, and cup position and orientation relative to the estimated position of the pelvis.

For this study, CupAlign was used to determine the postoperative alignment of the cup in 22 HipNav^{TM} cases. One technician performed the measurements in all cases to eliminate cross-user measurement error. In order to determine the reliability of orientation information retrieved from standard radiography, the results of the postoperative CupAlign analysis were compared with the actual intraoperative measurements.

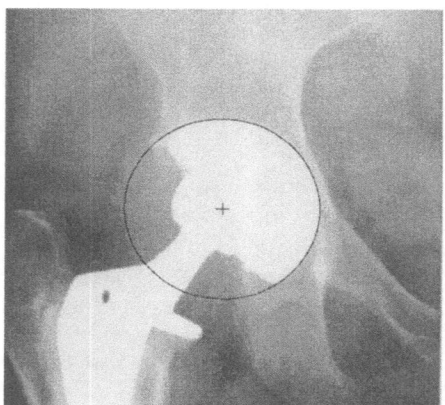 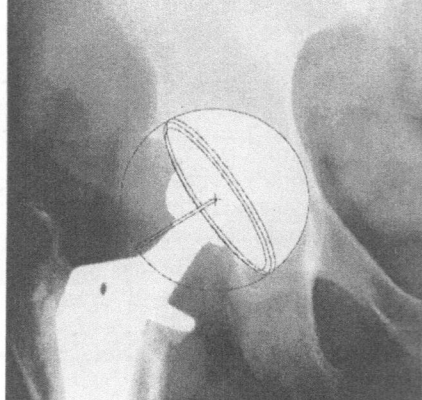

Fig. 2. Placement of the cup in CupAlign. First the position is determined by projecting a sphere with the same size as the cup onto the x-ray film plane and manipulating the location of the sphere (a). The orientation is then determined by matching a projection of a CAD model of the cup's distinguishing features on the image(b).

3   Results

Twenty-two of the initial 45 HipNav^{TM} cases had data including one and three month radiographs available for study. CupAlign was used to determine the postoperative alignment of the cup in all cases. One technician performed the measurements in all cases to eliminate cross-user measurement error.

Figure 3 displays the inter-radiograph position variation. For each case, the X-value of the data point on the graph represents the change in cup flexion, and the Y-value represents the change in cup abduction. The mean changes in abduction and flexion were -.1°and -1.1°, with standard deviations of .96°and 3.85°, respectively.

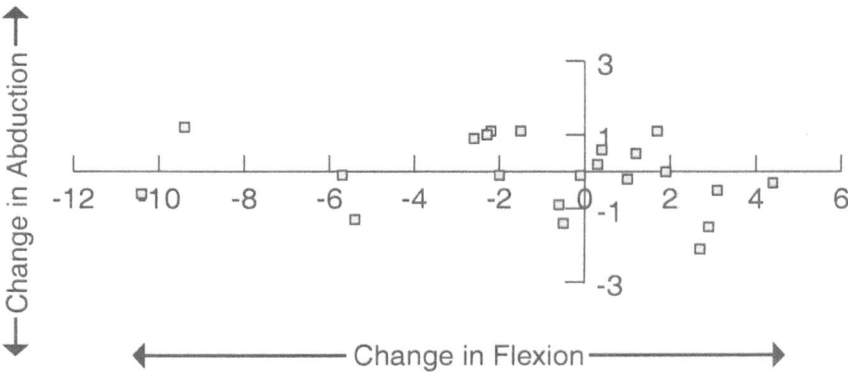

Fig. 3. Change in cup orientation measurement (in degrees) between radiographs taken at one and three months.

The variations between intraoperative and radiographic measurements for both the one and three month groups are presented in Figure 4. (The values in the graph are intraoperative values minus the postoperative values). For the one-month radiographs, the mean change in abduction from the final intraoperative measurement to the CupAlign measurement was 1.2°, with a standard deviation of 3.0°. The flexion change mean was 7.4°with a standard deviation of 9.4°. Similar results were found when analyzing the three-month radiographs. The abduction changes had a mean of 1.2°with a standard deviation of 2.8°. The flexion changed an average of 6.5°with a standard deviation of 8.8°.

4   Discussion and Future Work

The minimal change in cup abduction between radiograph measurements is evidence to the repeatability and relative accuracy of abduction measurements with this technique. The variation in cup flexion can be attributed to slight differences in the orientation of the pelvis (flexion and anteversion) relative to the x-ray film from the one month to three month radiographs. Because projection matching is a manual process, human error is also a factor in all measurements.

However, there was a significant variation between intraoperative and all postoperative radiographic measurements for the evaluated cases. Intraoperative measurement of cup orientation with the HipNav™system is expressed relative to the pelvic anterior plane, which represents standing neutral pelvic flexion. The variations of cup positions (especially cup flexion) from neutral position are mostly attributed to patient-to-patient differences in pelvic position during imaging. Therefore, without additional controls and measurements of the relative orientation of the pelvis, radiographic measurements are not a reliable method to evaluate cup orientation, especially anteversion alignment. Improvements can be achieved by carefully aligning the neutral plane of the pelvis at the time the radiographs are acquired, or by developing improved techniques for radiographic

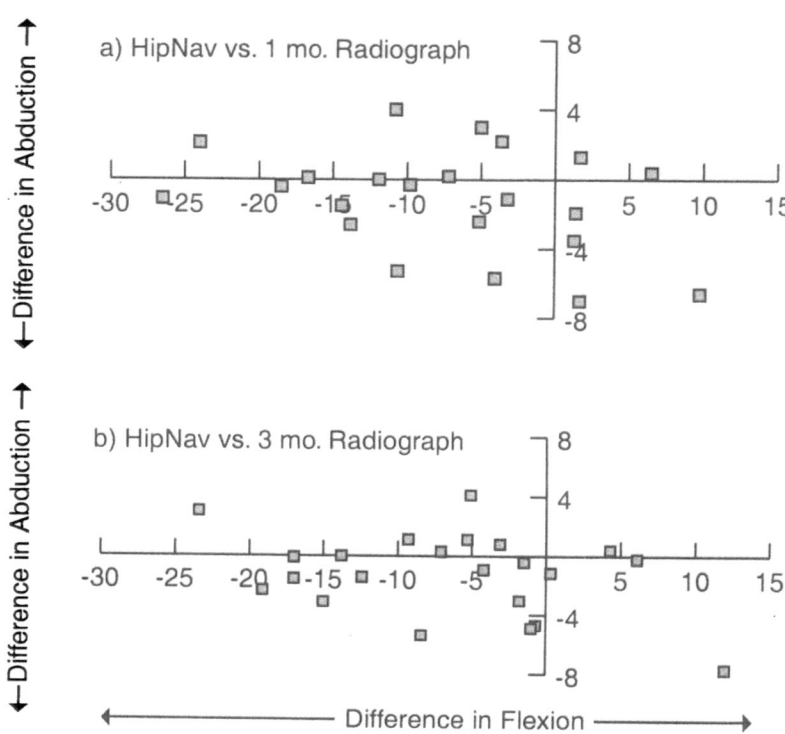

Fig. 4. Difference in cup orientation (in degrees) between intraoperative and postoperative measurements for (a) radiographs one month after surgery and (b) radiographs three months after surgery.

interpretation of pelvic orientation. Because we measure the cup flexion as well as the more traditional measure of cup anteversion, we can get an estimate of pelvic flexion for each patient, an initial step in understanding functional positions of the pelvis.

In future research, the location of the femoral component head and stem could be calculated in a similar fashion in future versions of CupAlign. Knowledge of postoperative femoral head location relative to the center of the cup liner could be used to estimate wear of the polyethylene liner. Future studies will also address measurement of pelvic position during x-ray acquisition (via automated 2D to 3D registration of the pelvis to the radiographic reference frame) and validity of radiographic landmarks.

References

1. Cobb, T. K., Morrey B. F., Ilstrup D. M.: The elevated-rim acetabular liner in total hip arthroplasty: Relationship to postoperative dislocation. The Journal of Bone and Joint Surgery, Vol 78-A, No. 1, January 1996, 80-86.

2. McCollum, D. E. and Gray, W. J.: Dislocation after total hip arthroplasty (causes and prevention). Clinical Orthopaedics and Related Research 261 (1990): 159-170.
3. Amstutz, H. C. and Markolf, K. L.: Design features in total hip replacement. In Harris W.H. (ed.): Proceedings of the Second Open Scientific Meeting of the Hip Society, New York, C.V. Mosby, 1974.
4. Lewinnek, G. E., Lewis, J. L., Tarr R., Compere, C. L., Zimmerman, J. R.: Dislocation after total hip-replacement arthroplasties. J. Bone Joint Surg.: 217-220, Vol 60-A, No. 2, March 1978. Clinical Orthopedics and Related Research 354 (1998): 70-81.
5. Paterno, S. A., Lachiewicz, M. D., and Kelley, S. S: The Influence of Patient-Related Factors and the Position of the Acetabular Component on the Rate of Dislocation After Total Hip Replacement. The Journal of Bone and Joint Surgery, Vol 78-A, No. 8, August 1997, 1202-1210.
6. DiGioia et al.: Image Guided Navigation System to Measure Intraoperatively Acetabular Implant Alignment. Clinical Orthopaedics and Related Research 355 (1998): 8-23.

Computer - Aided Implant Dentistry
— An Early Report —

Wolfgang Birkfellner[1]*, Peter Solar[2], André Gahleitner[2,3], Klaus Huber[1],
Franz Kainberger[3], Joachim Kettenbach[4], Peter Homolka[1], Markus Diemling[1],
Georg Watzek[2], and Helmar Bergmann[1,5]

[1] Department of Biomedical Engineering and Physics, General Hospital Vienna
[2] Department of Oral Surgery, Dental School
[3] Department of Diagnostic Radiology, Division of Osteoradiology,
General Hospital Vienna
[4] Department of Diagnostic Radiology, Division of Angiography and
Interventional Radiology, General Hospital Vienna
[5] Ludwig-Boltzmann Institute of Nuclear Medicine
All: University of Vienna, Austria

Abstract. Computer–aided implant dentistry (CAID), the direct translation of preoperative prosthetic planning to the operating theater by means of image guidance technologies, is a novel application of computer aided surgery (CAS). This work deals with the application of a modular software system for computer-aided interventions to CAID. The system is based on AVW-2.5, a software library dedicated to biomedical image processing, and a custom interface for communication with an optical tracker. A specific CAID toolset was also manufactured. We assessed the performance of two different point-based registration algorithms for this specific application of computer-aided preprosthetic surgery on several jaw models. The fiducial localization error (FLE) achievable with our system was found to be 0.7 mm, the fiducial registration error (FRE) accounted for 0.7 mm, and the target registration error TRE (the overall navigation accuracy) was found to be 1.3 mm. Since these results compare well to the resolution of the high-resolution computed tomography scan used we consider the precision of our system to be sufficient. Future enhancements of our system include the implementation of a medical augmented reality display system and the customization of the software package for exploration of other clinical applications of CAS.

1   Introduction

Implant dentistry is an established therapy for partially and completely edentulous patients. Esthetic, phonetic and functional outcome, the long-term stability of the implant, and the decrease in alveolar ridge atrophy depend on the optimum placement of the implant in the jawbone. A number of techniques are

---

* e-mail: Wolfgang.Birkfellner@univie.ac.at

aimed at transferring the preoperative planning data obtained from high resolution computed tomography (HRCT, Dental CT) [5, 15] to the operating room. A straightforward approach is to produce a template of the patients jawbone with drillguides, a so-called splint [5]. The splint can be adapted in such a manner that the preoperative prosthetic planning matches the position of the drillguides. This approach, however, has some severe drawbacks. In completely edentulous patients the severe atrophy of the alveolar ridges renders a reproducable fixation of the splint difficult; this is confirmed by our clinical experience with earlier applications of computer-aided surgery (CAS) and registration techniques based on dental molds [10, 16]. Furthermore the distance of the drill tip to critical structures such as the inferior alveolar nerve, the floor of the nasal cavity, or the maxillary sinus cannot be determined exactly during surgery, and interactive decision making based on the intraoperative situation is not possible. Therefore the authors in [10] and [13] have used a commercial CAS system (ARTMA Virtual Patient System, ARTMA Medizintechnik Vienna, Austria) for implantology. These experiments utilized electromagnetic trackers which exhibit erratic behavior in metallic environments [2]; furthermore, a patient-to-CT registration protocol requiring a slice thickness of 3 mm was used. Therefore the accuracy reported was in the vicinity of 3 mm. Visualisation was done on frontal and lateral cephalograms and the original CT-scan. Taking into account the small dimensions of the oral cavity, a more accurate solution had to be found.

In a further step these techniques were refined by adding an optical tracker to the ARTMA system [16]. While the precision of implant drill positioning improved significantly, refining the registration protocol to meet the high accuracy requirements in computer-aided implant dentistry (CAID) was still essential to enhance the clinical applicability of this method. Furthermore, advanced visualization techniques like oblique reformatting, perspective volume rendering, segmentation of anatomical structures like the mandibular canal [14], image fusion of Dental CT with dental magnetic resonance (Dental MR) images [6], and augmented reality visualisation techniques were desired features for visualisation in complicated indications for endosteal implantology.

We therefore decided to develop a programming shell providing a graphical front end to a powerful library for medical image processing; routines for communication with an optical tracker system were added. The modular structure of the system allows for the rapid development of specialized research prototype navigation systems for a wide range of indications. This work deals with the features of VISIT, a first application of this system to CAID.

2   Materials and Methods

2.1   Visualization Hard- and Software

The graphical user interface was developed under Tcl/Tk 8.0p2 (Scriptics Corp., Palo Alto/CA), a scripting language for programming graphical user interfaces [9]. The image processing functionality was added using the Tcl/Tk interface of the AVW-2.5 library functions (Biomedical Imaging Resource, Mayo Clinic,

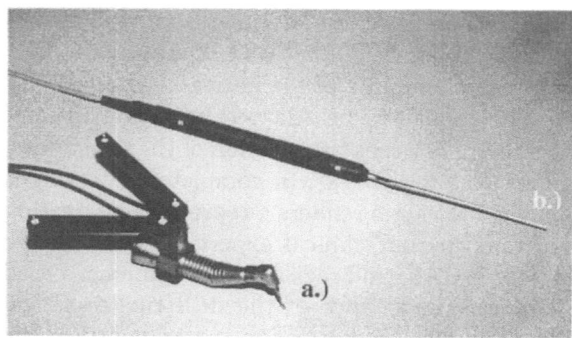

Fig. 1. An implant drill (a) and a 5 degree - of - freedom (dof) probe (b). The position and orientation of the drill bit are measured with the LED assembly mounted to the implant drill. The LED assembly can be rotated relative to the drill handle.

Rochester/MN). A well known software package based on AVW is the Analyze$_{AVW}$ image processing software [12]. A set of routines for communication with the tracking system over the serial port was also developed and can be found under *http://www.bmtp.akh-wien.ac.at/people/birkwo1/home.htm*. Software development was undertaken in ANSI-C using gcc 2.71 (Free Software Foundation, Boston/MA). The system was finally implemented on a Sun Ultra Sparc 10 running Solaris 2.6 (Sun Microsystems, Palo Alto/CA).

2.2   The Optical Tracking System

The optical tracker used was a Flashpoint 5000 system (Image Guided Technologies, Boulder/CO). A set of light-emitting diodes (LED) for position measurement purposes was attached to a frame made of polyamide and epoxy (Figs. 1, 2). The tools have shown good sterilizability by ethylene oxide, formaldehyde or H_2O_2 plasma. Since the probes do not contain additional softening agents and all cavities in the epoxy resin were removed by evacuation during the curing process, no residual accumulation of ethyleneoxide was detected after several sterilization cycles.

2.3   CT Scanning Protocol, Image Postprocessing

We used a clinical Dental CT – scanning protocol (1.5 mm slice thickness, 1 mm table feed, fast incremental scanning, 120 kV, 150 mAs, 512 * 512 matrix, FOV 120 mm) on a Tomoscan SR6000 (Phillips AG, Best, the Netherlands). A Dental CT investigation usually consists of 20 to 40 slices. In order to achive isotropic voxel size, we interpolated the raw scan with our software to cubic voxels using AVW-routines. This resulted in a voxel size of typically 0.25 mm^3.

2.4   Registration Methods

A large number of surface points on the jawbone could be collected by optical or *mechanical methods* through the oral mucosal tissue and would allow for using point-to-surface registration methods. Since collecting the points has been proven

886   W. Birkfellner et al.

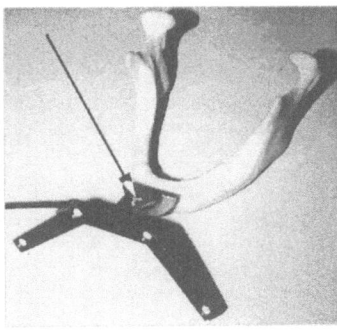

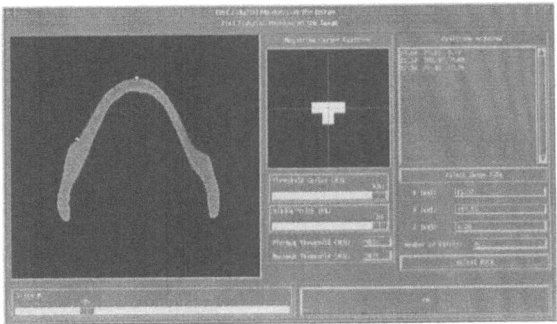

Fig. 2. The reference LED emitter array mounted to a maxilla model. The tool is fixed to the patient by means of a single osteosynthesis screw (inserted through the channel denoted by the arrow) and three sharp pins which penetrate the oral mucosa.

Fig. 3. A screenshot of the dialog for identification of fiducial marker positions. The markers (surgical miniscrews made of titanium) are segmented by simple thresholding. By pointing the cursor to the approximate position of the fiducial on the original CT-scan (left part of the screen), a subvolume is identified. The segmented and magnified view at the cursor position can be seen in the middle of the screenshot. By computing an intensity centroid the exact location of the fiducial is determined.

to be difficult and cumbersome in clinical routine we therefore have tested the performance of two point-to-point registration algorithms [1, 7]. Both techniques utilize implantable fiducial markers and are mathematically equivalent – both solve a general linear least squares problem and yield identical results when using the same input data; the algorithm given in [1] may result in a rigid-body transformation containing a reflection in addition to a rotation. Therefore a larger number of fiducials is necessary. The algorithm in [7] does not show this behavior. To assess whether this difference renders one of the algorithms superior under the special conditions in CAID was an aim of our study. Mathematical algorithms for solving the optimization problem in the registration algorithms (singular value decomposition – SVD, or solution of an eigenvalue problem by Jacobi-transformation) were taken from [11]. Surgical titanium miniscrews used in oral surgery (Leibinger AG, Freiburg, Germany, 2 mm length, 1.8 mm head diameter) were chosen as fiducial markers. Clinical tests had shown that three or four of those miniscrews can be implanted preoperatively under local anesthesia. They show good stability, require little effort by the surgeon and cause only little discomfort to the patient.

Fiducial positions are allocated by identifying a miniscrew on the CT-scan and by segmenting the head of the screw by intensity thresholding using a semi-automatic segmentation technique. The resulting binary image is shown under 5× magnification (Fig. 3). The exact location of the screw head is determined by calculating the intensity centroid within the binary subvolume around the screw. Image processing functionality was again taken from the AVW-library.

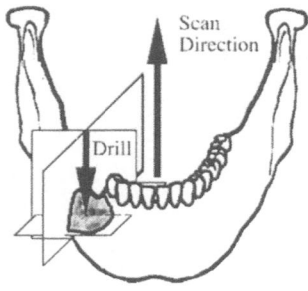

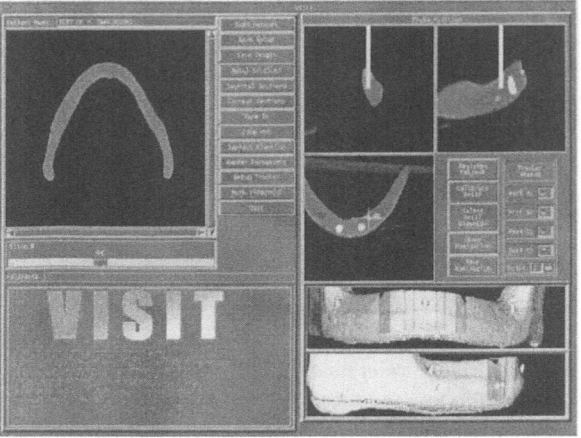

Fig. 4. The reformatted sets of orthogonal slices are determined as a plane perpendicular to the drill bit, a plane normal to a vector which is normal to the drill bit and intersects the central axis of the Dental CT scan, and a plane normal to both of these.

Fig. 5. Visualisation of the current drill position. Like in many other CAS systems, the drill position is visualised by means of three obliquely reformatted views orthogonal to each other (right half of the screenshot). The left half of the window shows the original scan.

Completely automatic detection and segmentation of fiducial positions based on this method is also possible but is not recommended in our application since the performance of the automatic fiducial detection algorithm might be significantly reduced by spray artifacts from metallic materials like dental metallic fillings.

2.5   Visualization Methods

Positioning of the implant drill relative to the jaw was visualized by means of a set of orthogonal slices aligned relative to the implant drill axis. This technique has proven useful in many systems for CAS; the tool coordinate system is chosen according to Fig. 4. One slice is orientated perpendicular to the axis of the drill and another slice is perpendicular to this plane whereby it's normal vector intersects the central axis of the axial CT scan; the third slice is orthogonal to both of these.

2.6   Accuracy Tests

The accuracy of the complete system was tested using five epoxy models of typical situations in implant dentistry. The models were manufactured by casting molds from plastic teaching dummies (Fig. 6). Landmarks for assessing the accuracy of the complete setup (steel spheres, 0.5 mm diameter) were fixed to the surface in addition to the fiducial markers. The landmarks were not used for registration. The total positioning error was asessed as the difference between the positions of the landmarks on the CT-scan and the position of the

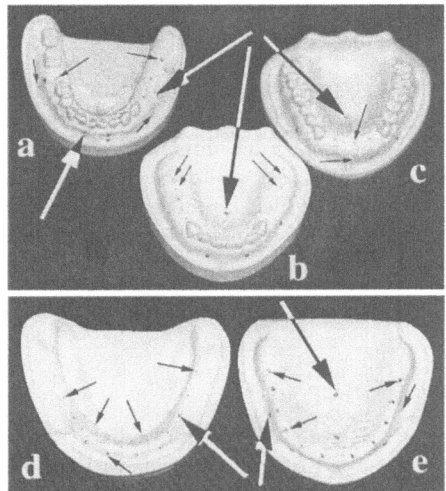

Fig. 6. Partially edentulous models representing typical cases in implant dentistry; a.) represents a mandible with a single gap and a terminal gap, b.) a maxilla model with a terminal gap on both sides, and c.) a maxilla model with a frontal gap. Completely edentulous models with atrophic alveolar ridges were also prepared. d.) is a mandible model, and e.) represents a maxilla. Broad arrows indicate the location of some of the fiducial markers, and small arrows point to some of the landmarks used for assessing the system's accuracy.

landmark after position measurement with the 5 degree-of-freedom (dof) probe transformed back to the CT-volume. The quantities influencing the precision of the navigation system were assessed experimentally as the intrinsic accuracy of the tracking system (or fiducial localization error – FLE), as the error in registration as reported by the cost function of the registration algorithm (fiducial registration error – FRE), and as the error in localization of arbitrary targets (target registration error – TRE). A detailed analysis of these quantites can be found in [4].

3   Results

3.1   Intrinsic Accuracy of the Tracking System — FLE

In a first step, we have estimated the fiducial localization error FLE by taking ten measurements of a fiducial marker on a jaw model while varying systematically the positions of the model and the 5 dof – probe (Fig. 1). The compound error of these point measurements relative to the reference sensor (Fig. 2) for ten different fiducials accounted for 0.69 ± 0.15 mm; details are given in table 1.

3.2   Fiducial Registration Error FRE, Target Registration Error TRE, and the Reliability of Registration Algorithms

The fiducial registration error and the target registration error were also measured by collecting position measurements of the fiducial markers and additional landmarks on the models shown in Fig. 6. The two rigid-body point based algorithms (see section 2.4) were used on identical position data. No difference in the resulting registration error FRE and the localization error TRE (measured by

Measurement #	Fiducial Localization Error - FLE [mm]
1	0.64 ± 0.52
2	0.87 ± 0.36
3	0.63 ± 0.32
4	0.67 ± 0.27
5	0.84 ± 0.29
6	0.91 ± 0.20
7	0.46 ± 0.31
8	0.60 ± 0.29
9	0.74 ± 0.28
10	0.54 ± 0.35
Average	0.69 ± 0.15

Table 1. FLE – The repeatability of fiducial position measurements using the optical tracking system. Each fiducial position was measured ten times while varying the location of the 5-dof measurement probe relative to the model. Positions were measured relative to the reference sensor (Fig. 2).

Table 2. Fiducial registration error FRE, target registration error TRE and the mathematical stability of the SVD-based registration algorithm given in [1] as a function of the number of fiducials used. Values were acquired in the five models shown in Fig. 6 and averaged.

# of Fiducial Markers	Fiducial Registration Error [mm] - FRE -	Target Registration Error [mm] - TRE -	Success Rate of SVD-based Registration Algorithm
3	0.71 ± 0.12	1.23 ± 0.28	40 %
4	0.70 ± 0.12	1.25 ± 0.31	80 %
5	0.76 ± 0.06	1.31 ± 0.28	100 %

comparing the target position transformed to CT-space to the original position in CT space) could be found for these two algorithms. An interesting finding when using three or four fiducials is, however, the fact that the SVD-based algorithm given in [1] occasionally fails. For CAID, the algorithm given in [7] appears to be superior under the aspects of reducing discomfort for the patient during the implantation of the fiducial markers and intraoperative time-requirements during registration; stable values can always be achieved by using only three markers. The usage of up to two additional markers did not improve TRE significantly. On average, FRE was found to be 0.7 mm, whereas TRE typically accounted for 1.3 mm. Results for the five models (Fig. 6) are shown in table 2.

3.3 Software Engineering Aspects of a Modular Software Toolkit for CAS

Within six man-months a prototype of the system was developed. The task of programming a graphical user-interface was significantly simplified by using Tcl/Tk. Since Tcl/Tk, AVW, and our custom developed routines can be used under different operating systems such as Solaris, IRIX, Windows NT and others, this combination appears to be a flexible solution to develop further software applications for CAS.

4 Discussion

Dental CT is becoming a more and more used tool for planning of endosteal implants [5, 15]. Image guidance is a logical adjunct to this method; pathologies of the alveolar ridge due to atrophy or bone augmentation can be easily visualized and might help even experienced oral surgeons to monitor the result to be expected in delicate intraoperative situations. The positive influence on postoperative outcome as well as surgical performance has yet to be assessed.

Despite the small dimension of the oral cavity which implies an inferior signal-to-noise ratio in fiducial localization, our results for TRE in CAID compare well to the accuracy of other CAS applications, and, more important, are close to the resolution of Dental CT (typically 0.25 * 0.25 * 1.00 mm^3) which limits navigation accuracy in general.

Future efforts should focus on reducing the variance of TRE. However, this is achievable by improving the tracker hardware and utilizing dual point-to-point/point-to-surface [8] registration approaches. We consider the usage of surface registration methods to be infeasible in CAID; nevertheless we believe that a point-to-point registration algorithm combined with a surface registration method applied to the small area accessible intraoperatively after surgical preparation of the mucosal flap might improve TRE.

Currently we are in the process of undertaking corpse studies and first clinical trials with our system. Besides refining the planning capabilites of VISIT, the most important visualization problem to be solved might be displaying the drill position in comparison to the planned implant site. The usage of head-mounted augmented reality display technologies for interactive visualisation at the operating field provides a method for achieving this goal. These technologies as well as the implementation of hybrid tracking technologies [3] might also further enhance the clinical impact of this technology.

Besides these technical aspects, the most important point in assessing the clinical relevance of CAID is the comparison of this method to common splint based techniques. From our clinical experience, however, we expect a dramatic improvement in implant placement precision in edentulous patients where templates are bound to fail.

5 Acknowledgment

This study was made possible by the expert advice and the kind help of the following individuals: A. Gamperl (IBMTP, AKH Vienna) and W. Piller (Ludwig-Boltzmann Institute of Nuclear Medicine, Vienna) manufactured parts of the hardware necessary for this study. L. Chamberlain, D. Dick (Image Guided Technologies, Boulder/CO), A. Larson, D. Hanson (Biomedical Imaging Resource, Mayo Clinic, Rochester/MN), and W. Zawodsky (IBMTP, AKH Vienna) helped to solve a number of hard- and software problems. M. Eigenschink (Central Sterilization Unit, AKH Vienna) tested the sterilizability of the probes. This work was supported by the Austrian Science Foundation (FWF) under research grant P12464-MED.

References

1. K. S. Arun, T. S. Huang, S. D. Blostein: "Least-Squares Fitting of two 3-D Point Sets", IEEE Trans Pattern Anal 9(5), 698 - 700, (1987).
2. W. Birkfellner, F. Watzinger, F. Wanschitz et al.: "Systematic distortions in magnetic position digitizers", Med Phys 25(11), 2242 - 2248, (1998).
3. W. Birkfellner, F. Watzinger, F. Wanschitz et al.: "Calibration of Tracking Systems in a Surgical Environment", IEEE Trans Med Imaging 17(5), 737-742, (1998).
4. J. M. Fitzpatrick, J. B. West, C. R. Maurer: "Predicting Error in Rigid-Body Point-Based Registration", IEEE Trans Med Imaging 17(5), 694 - 702, (1998).
5. T. Fortin, J. L. Coudert, G. Champleboux et al.: "Computer - assisted dental implant surgery using computed tomography", J Image Guided Surg 1, 53 - 58, (1995).
6. A. Gahleitner, C. Nasel, S. Schick et al.: "Dental magnetic resonance imaging (dental MRI) as a method for imaging maxillo-mandibular tooth retention structures", RoFo Fortschr Geb Rontgenstr Neuen Bildgeb Verfahr 169(4), 424-428, (1998).
7. B. K. P. Horn: "Closed form solution of absolute orientation using unit quaternions", J Opt Soc Am A 4(4), 629 - 642, (1987).
8. C. R. Maurer, R. J. Maciunas, J. M. Fitzpatrick et al.: "Registration of Head Images to Physical Space Using a Weighted Combination of Points and Surfaces", IEEE Trans Med Imaging 17(5), 753 - 761, (1998).
9. J. K. Ousterhout, "Tcl and the Tk Toolkit", Addison-Wesley, Reading, (1994).
10. O. Ploder, A. Wagner, G. Enislidis et al.: Computer - assisted intraoperative visualization of dental implants. Augmented reality in medicine", Radiologe 35(9), 569 - 572, (1995).
11. W. H. Press, S. A. Teukolsky, W. T. Vetterling, B. P. Flannery: "Numerical Recipes in C - The Art of Scientific Computing, Second Edition", Cambridge University Press, Cambridge, (1992).
12. R. A. Robb: "Three-Dimensional Biomedical Imaging. Principles and Practice", VCH, Weinheim, (1995).
13. P. Solar, S. Grampp, B. Gsellmann et al.: "A computer - aided navigation system for oral implant surgery using 3D -CT reconstruction and real time video - projection", in H. U. Lemke, M. W. Vannier, K. Inamura, A. G. Farman (Eds): Computer Assisted Radiology (CAR 96), Elsevier Science, Amsterdam, 884 - 887, (1996).
14. W. Stein, S. Hassfeld, J. Mühling: "Tracing of Thin Tubular Structures in Computer Tomographic Data", Comput Aided Surg 3(2), 83 - 88, (1998).
15. K. Verstreken, J. Van Cleynenbreugel, K. Martens et al.: "An Image Guided Planning System for Endosseous Oral Implants", IEEE Trans Med Imaging 17(5), 842 - 852, (1998).
16. F. Watzinger, W. Birkfellner, F. Wanschitz et al.: "Computer – aided positioning of dental implants using an optical tracking system - Case report and presentation of a new method", J Craniomaxfac Surg 17(2), 77-81, (1999).

Surface Registration for Use in Interactive Image-Guided Liver Surgery

Alan J Herline[a], Jeannette L Herring[b], James D Stefansic[c], William C Chapman[a], Robert L Galloway[c], Benoit M Dawant[b].

Vanderbilt University, a)Division of Hepatobiliary Surgery and Liver Transplantation, 801 Oxford House, Nashville, TN 37235 and b) Department of Electrical and Computer Engineering and c)Department of Biomedical Engineering.
alan.j.herline@vanderbilt.edu

Abstract: Liver surgery is difficult because of limited external landmarks, significant vascularity and inexact definition of intrahepatic anatomy. Intraoperative ultrasound (IOUS) has been widely used in an attempt to overcome these difficulties, but is limited by its two-dimensional nature, inter-user variability and image obliteration with ablative or resectional techniques. Because the anatomy of the liver and intra-operative removal of hepatic ligaments make intrinsic or extrinsic point-based registration impractical, we have implemented a surface registration technique to localize physical points for liver phantoms and anatomically placed targets within the liver on CT images. Liver phantoms were created from anatomically correct molds with "tumors" imbedded within the substance of the liver. Helical CT scans were performed with 3 mm slices. Using an optically active position sensor, the surface of the liver was digitized according to anatomical segments. A surface registration was performed and RMS errors of the locations of internal tumors are presented as verification. An initial point based marker registration was performed and considered as the standard for error measurement. Errors for surface-registration were 2.9 mm for the entire surface and 2.8 mm for embedded targets. This is an initial study considering the use of surface registration for the purpose of physical to image registration in the area of liver surgery.

1. Introduction

Liver surgeons have relied on preoperative imaging studies to select patients for operative intervention. The "operative planning", however, has been performed in an inexact and general conceptual fashion (i.e., removing the right lobe versus a wedge resection of the right lobe) as opposed to a more precise resection. A recent lead article in the *Annals of Surgery* suggested that preoperative planning with 3-dimensional CT reconstructions and virtual-reality techniques could allow precise preoperative planning and even allow surgeons to "practice" the resection and perhaps minimize operative errors in the actual resection procedure [1, 2]. While this approach could provide CT visualization of planned liver resections, no one has reported a method to execute such an image-guided pre-planned hepatic resection.

One suggested method to provide tomographic information for surgical guidance involves operating room placement of scanners [3].   However, these systems have significant barriers to broad acceptance: 1) These units are very costly on the basis of installation, per procedure costs and intra-operative modification of instruments to avoid magnetic interference. 2) These systems are large and can make standard operations more difficult because of space occupied by imaging equipment. We have initiated studies investigating alternative methods of intra-operative guidance for liver surgery that we believe will provide more tomographic data and be much more cost effective than placing scanners in the OR.

There are a number of initial engineering problems in adapting current guidance systems from neurosurgical procedures for use in hepatic procedures. Given these constraints, obtaining the margin of error demonstrated in neurosurgical systems is probably not feasible and is not needed for hepatic applications. The current gold standard for intra-operative localization is intra-operative ultrasound (IOUS). IOUS has the ability to accurately identify tumors of 5 mm or greater [2]. The liver has a variety of ligamentous attachments to the diaphragm and therefore physical space position is also dependent on the point in the respiratory cycle. The liver deforms and its thin capsule does not add rigidity. Point based registration methods are difficult to implement secondary to the inability to attach markers to the liver clinically. Even intrinsic point based methods become impractical due to the lack of points visible on the pre-operative tomographic images that would then be visible to the surgeon intra-operatively. Initial attempts at this method led to registration errors in the 12 mm range. Given our experience in the area of registration and more recently in the area of surface-based registration, we sought to determine the feasibility of surface registration as a method for physical to image registration for the liver [4,5,6].

2. Methods

2.1 Phantom, Target Creation and Image Acquisition

Phantom livers were constructed from a two component poly (dimethyl) siloxane (rubber silicone). The livers are poured into a plaster mold allowing for the addition of "tumors". The current phantom tumors are cork of various sizes from 4 – 15 mm. In addition to tumors we have placed 4 markers in the liver phantom so that they are evenly spaced and located in various anatomical segments.   The marker system consists of plastic marker posts that are attached to the phantom, imaging markers that generate a high intensity level in CT images, and physical-space markers that contain a hemispherical divot into which the ballpoint tip of a three-dimensional spatial localizer (3DSL) fits precisely [7]. The position of an image marker is defined as its centroid and is determined using the algorithm described in [7]. The liver is scanned using a helical CT scanner, Philips Tomoscan AV scanner with 3mm slices and voxel dimensions of 0.50774 mm/pixel. For these experiments the 6 "tumors" are easily visualized on the images.

2.2 Physical Surface and Point Collection

The physical surface of the liver is digitized using an optically active position sensor and a 3DSL. An optically active position sensor (Optotrak 3020, Northern Digital, Ontario, Canada) is used to detect the IREDs and it can precisely calculate the position of the tip if four of the IREDs are visible. This system is used to locate the position of the markers in physical-space, which correspond to the centroid of the image markers in the CT images. Approximately 900 points are collected from the entire anterior surface of the liver using a probe with a 3mm tip in a manner that could be duplicated in the operating room. Following this and prior to any movement of the liver the surfaces of each of the visible 8 anatomic segments of the liver (figure 1) are collected in consecutive trials of 10-15 seconds and 200-300 points per trial. The final set of data is collected from the edges of each of the 8 visible segments. The image markers placed on the liver phantom   are then removed and replaced with physical

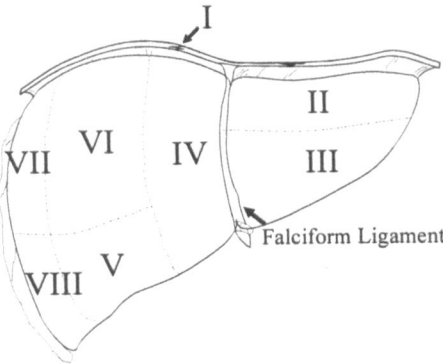

Fig. 1. Liver with the anatomical segments drawn upon the anterior surface. These segments correspond to blood supply for the liver. Segment I is not generally visible and is located on the liver's undersurface.

markers and these points are collected. These points are used for initialization of the surface based registration. The "gold standard" registration is performed using the points as described in [8].

2.3 Image Segmentation and Surface Creation

The phantom liver and the "tumors" are semi-automatically segmented using Midas (in-house image processing software). A triangle set representation of the liver surface is automatically generated using an independently implemented version of the classic marching cubes method developed by Lorensen and Cline [9], and the final representation was generated by simplifying the surface produced by the marching cubes algorithm using the VTK vertex-deletion scheme [10]. The resulting triangle set represents a close approximation to an iso-surface that is characterized by a specific intensity value. This iso-intensity-based approach is well suited to the extraction of the surface of a phantom imaged in isolation, since there are no surrounding tissues to confuse the definition of the surface. The only parameter that the triangulation algorithm requires is an intensity value. The Hounsfield number of the phantom is approximately 400, and the Hounsfield number of the air surrounding the phantom is -1024. There is an offset of 1024 introduced into the intensity values due to the method used to transfer the scans from the CT machine, resulting in average intensity values of about 1400 for the phantom and 0 for the surrounding air. We chose to use an intermediate value of 600 as an input to our intensity-based surface extraction algorithm. A different segmentation method will be required for use with a patient liver.

2.4 Registration

We initially perform a point-based registration using the method described by Maurer [8]. This serves as a "gold standard" for comparison of the surface-based registrations to follow. We perform surface-based registration using an independent implementation [11] of the iterative closest point registration algorithm of Besl and McKay [12]. First, the closest point on one surface is computed for each point in a set of points representing the other surface. In this study, the first surface is a triangle set representation of the liver surface in the CT image, and the point set representation of the second surface is a set of physical space surface points. Second, a transformation is determined by registering these two point sets. This process is iterated until some stopping criterion is satisfied. This method converges to a local minimum of the cost function, which is the root-mean-square (RMS) distance between the corresponding points at the last iteration. Because the physical space surface points we record are the positions of the center of the ballpoint tip of the 3DSL, the recorded surface points are displaced from the actual surface by the radius of the tip. We have not corrected for this and it is a source of error.

Because of the possibility of convergence to a local minimum that is not the correct solution, the algorithm works best when it is initialized with rotations and translations that are close to the exact solution. In this work, the initial registration for the physical points is computed by using the point-based algorithm with the markers and then rotating and translating those points from a corner of the image by progressive amounts for each trial to test the sensitivity of the algorithm to initial conditions.

2.5 Error Calculation

To evaluate the registration error obtained with the surface-based registration method we propose, the following procedure was utilized. First, the four fiducial markers were used to compute a rigid-body transformation between physical and image space using point-based registration of the marker centroids, which were located as described in section 2.2. The image-space coordinates of all the physical points acquired with the 3DSL were then computed using this transformation. For each registration trial performed with the surface-based method being investigated, a physical-to-image transformation matrix was generated and used to compute a second set of image-space coordinates for the physical points. The registration error obtained with the surface-based approach was then computed as the root-mean-square (RMS) difference between the image coordinates obtained with the marker-based registration and the coordinates obtained using our surface-based approach.

A more clinically applicable error is calculated using the position of targets more central within the volume of interest instead of surface points. Our results are examined by looking at the RMS error for both the surface and each of six tumors embedded within the liver phantom for the following cases: 1. surface registration using the total surface, 2. using an individual liver segment's surface 3. using an individual liver segment's surface boundary or edge.

For RMS calculations of target registration errors (TREs) for the six tumors, the CT image points corresponding to each tumor are transformed into physical space using two different transformations. Each tumor is transformed from image space into physical space using the results of the point-based registration. These points establish a "gold standard" position for the tumor. Then, each tumor is transformed from image space into physical space using the results of the surface-based registration which is being tested in these experiments. RMS error is then calculated from these two point sets, and this RMS error is designated the TRE for the tumor.

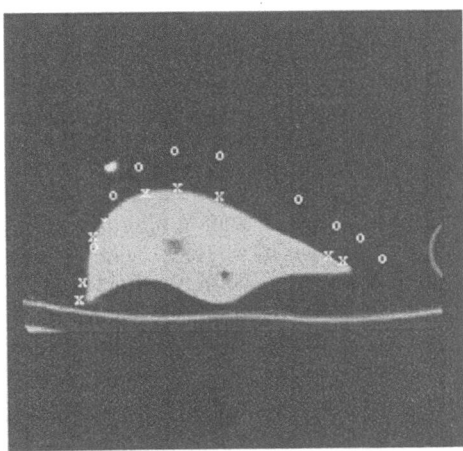

Figure 2. Shown is a CT scan of the phantom liver with o's showing the starting point for the 15 degree rotation and x's showing the results of the surface registration.

3. Results

3.1 Surface Error

Using the markers and posts embedded onto the substance of the liver we obtained a fiducial registration error (FRE) of 0.95 mm. Individual registrations were performed using nine surfaces (eight segments and a total surface) and eight segment boundaries (or edges) for the following three trials: 1. Rotation of 5 degrees and translation of 5 mm 2. Rotation of 10 degrees and translation of 5 mm 3. Rotation of 15 degrees and

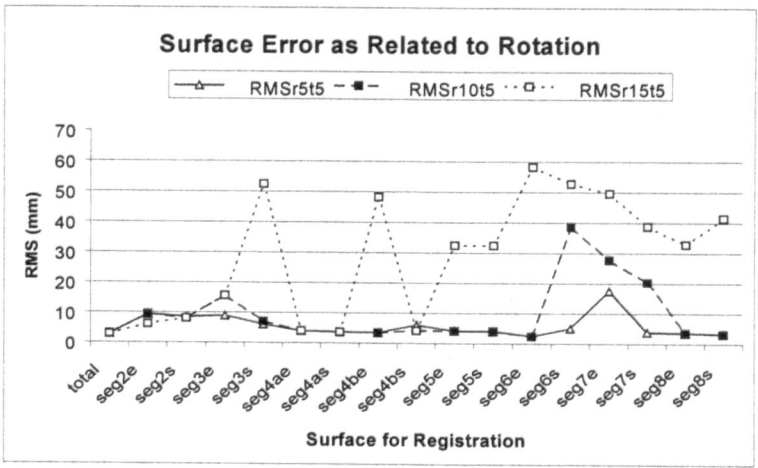

Fig. 2. RMS error for the entire surface using the total surface and various surface segments and their boundaries for registration.

translation of 5 mm. A total of 51 trials were performed to study the RMS error of surface registration with the above points and under the listed starting locations of the physical point set. RMS error is calculated for the entire surface. This is demonstrated on a single slice of the CT scan in figure 1.

The graph for all results is shown in figure 2. The average RMS error using the total surface for registration was 2.99 ± 0.006 mm for the three trials. Using segment VI boundary produced smaller RMS errors (2.6, 2.5 mm) for the trials with 5 degrees and 10 degrees of rotation, respectively. The 15 degree rotation trial produced a 58.4 mm RMS for the segment VI boundary.

3.2 Target Error

Individual registrations were again performed using the nine surfaces and eight segment boundaries as above for the same three rotations and translations of initial points. RMS errors were calculated on six tumors distributed within the phantom in a fashion similar to clinical tumors. RMS errors were calculated for 306 trials differing in tumor localized, surface used for registration and rotation of initial points. The graph for all results is shown in figure 3. The average RMS error for all six tumors using the total surface for registration with all three rotations as initial points was 2.82 mm ± 0.3 mm. The range in error was from 2.45 – 3.35 mm.

4. Discussion

Surface registration has been implemented and used for neurosurgical applications because of the potential for accurate registration in a non-invasive, retrospective manner. While effective from a retrospective standpoint, a good surface fit may not offer a similar level of accuracy for objects beneath the surface. While extrinsic point-based techniques offer robustness appropriate for neurosurgical applications, they are difficult to implement for organs not surrounded by osseous formations and errors are difficult to quantify for intrinsic point-based methods [8]. Our interest has been to develop an image-guided system for hepatic resection and ablation of liver tumors. The liver is a smooth organ with few surface markings. It is not amenable to applied markers or suitable for accurate intrinsic point-based registration. The anatomical location of hepatic tumors is usually determined pre-operatively by tomographic imaging (CT or MR). Ultrasonography can provide intraoperative imaging information regarding tumor location and surrounding vascular anatomy [2], but it requires special expertise to perform and properly interpret. We are investigating the use of endoscopic registration, but feel that surface registration may offer an effective method given the physical constraints of our clinical situation [4].

The errors obtained for tumor localization in the current study are very acceptable for hepatobiliary applications. The small variance between different trials when using a total surface for registration indicates the insensitivity of the algorithm to initial conditions. For transformations calculated only using a segment of the liver's surface we observed the following: 1) as rotations increased error increased dramatically. 2) For those segments with smaller error there was a wider range of error between tumors. Both of these suggest that a single segment's surface may not be adequate for the entire volume of the liver; however, it may not be necessary to obtain a surface from the entire liver to be accurate for a tumor isolated to a single segment.

Our errors can be attributed to several known problems. The centroid of the probe tip is 1.5 mm from the surface of the liver. This can be corrected, but was not in this study. While this correction would increase the accuracy for this study, it may not approach clinical reality as the surface of the liver is deformable even under slight pressure and a consistent surface to 3DSL point distance may not be known. Additionally the presumed physical space locations of the tumors are obtained by the point-based registration using the markers. This is a problem of having centrally located targets whose exact physical locations are not known and error is introduced using this method. We feel tracked ultrasound will be a feasible method to verify the registrations for deeper structures and our group has begun preliminary investigations in this area [13].

5. Conclusions

We are encouraged by our initial work in the use of surfaces from a liver phantom. This work can potentially apply the use of image-guidance for hepatic procedures. There is further design and experiments needed to clarify the amount of surface needed in order to adequately register the liver volumes with physical space and in the area of target design and localization for this application.

6. Acknowledgements

The authors want to acknowledge support from the NSF, BES-9703714 and the NIH NRSA #1 F32 DK 09671-02 SB. They want to thank Cindy Duncan, CRT and Tina Herron, CRT for their invaluable assistance with imaging.

7. References

1. Marescaux, J., *et al.*, *Surgical simulation and virtual reality: the coming revolution.* Ann Surg, 1998. **5**: p. 635-637.
2. Rafaelsen, S.R., *et al.*, *Intraoperative ultrasonography in the detection of hepatic metastases from colorectal cancer.* Dis Colon Rectum, 1995. **38**: p. 355-360.
3. Klotz, H., R. Flury, and P. Erhart, *Magnetic resonance-guided laparoscopic interstitial laser therapy of the liver.* AJS, 1997. **174**: p. 448-451.
4. Herline, A., *et al.*, *Studies in the Feasibility of Interactive Image-Guided Liver Surgery.* Arch. Surg., 1999.
5. Herring, J.L., *et al.*, *Surface-based Registration of CT Images to Physical Space for Image-guided Surgery of the Spine: A Sensitivity Study.* IEEE Trans. Med. Imag., 1998. **17**: p. 743-752.
6. Herring, J.L., *et al. Effect of vertebral surface extraction on registration accuracy: a comparison of registration results for iso-intensity algorithms applied to computed tomography images.* in *SPIE.* 1999. San Diego, CA.
7. Wang, M.Y., *et al.*, *An automatic technique for finding and localizing externally attached markers in CT and MR volume images of the head.* IEEE Trans. Biomed. Eng., 1996. **43**: p. 627-637.
8. Maurer, C.R., *et al.*, *Registration of head volumes using implantable fiducial markers.* IEEE Trans. Med. Imag., 1997. **16**: p. 447-462.
9. Lorensen, W.E. and H.E. Cline, *Marching Cubes: A High Resolution 3D Surface Construction Algorithm.* Computer Graphics, 1987. **21**: p. 163-169.
10. Schroeder, W., M. K., and L. V., *The Visualization Toolkit.* 1998, Upper Saddle River, New Jersey: Prentice Hall PTR.
11. Maurer, J.C.R., *et al.*, *A method for registration of 3-D images using multiple geometrical features.* IEEE Trans. Med. Imag, 1996. **15**: p. 836-849.
12. Besl, P.J. and N.D. McKay, *A method for registration of 3-D shapes.* IEEE Trans. Pattern Anal. and Machine Intell, 1992. **14**: p. 239-256.
13. Beasley R. A., S.J.D., Herline A.J., Guttierez L., Galloway Jr., R. L.. *Registration of ultrasound images.* in *SPIE.* 1999. San Diego, CA.

Model-Updated Image-Guided Neurosurgery Using the Finite Element Method: Incorporation of the Falx Cerebri

Michael I. Miga[1], Keith D. Paulsen[1,2,3], Francis E. Kennedy[1],
Alex Hartov[1], and David W. Roberts[2,3]

[1] Dartmouth College, Thayer School of Engineering, HB8000, Hanover, NH 03755
{michael.miga, keith.paulsen, francis.kennedy, alex.hartov,
david.w.roberts}@dartmouth.edu
http://www.thayer.dartmouth.edu/thayer/
[2] Dartmouth Hitchcock Medical Center, Lebanon, NH 03756
[3] Norris Cotton Cancer Center, Lebanon, NH, 03756

Abstract. Surgeons using neuronavigation have realized the value of image guidance for feature recognition as well as for the precise application of surgical instruments. Recently, there has been a growing concern about the extent of intraoperative misregistration due to tissue deformation. Intraoperative imaging is currently under evaluation but limitations related to cost effectiveness and image clarity have made its wide spread adoption uncertain. As a result, computational model-guided techniques have generated considerable appeal as an alternative approach. In this paper, we report our initial experience with enhancing our brain deformation model by explicitly adding the falx cerebri. The simulations reported show significant differences in subsurface deformation with the falx serving to damp the communication of displacement between hemispheres by as much as 4 *mm*. Additionally, these calculations, based on a human clinical case, demonstrate that while cortical shift predictions correlate well with various forms of the model (70-80% of surface motion recaptured), substantial differences in subsurface deformation occurs suggesting that subsurface validation of model-guided techniques will be important for advancing this concept.

1 Introduction

The realization that intraoperative brain shift can misregister image-guided neuronavigation has generated significant interest in the surgical community. Studies of cortical surface shift during neurosurgery have reported movement on the order of 1 cm with a tendency for displacement to occur in the direction of gravity [1], [2], [3]. Early subsurface shift studies revealed substantial movement on the order of 4-7 *mm* during tumor resection cases [4]. Recently, Maurer et al. reported preliminary results using an interventional MR system to quantify subsurface movement and found significant variability from case to case suggesting that intraoperative motion is somewhat unpredictable based on the type of surgery alone [5]. Interestingly, they found significant shift due to gravity and that deformation across the midline was small indicating that the falx cerebri may play an important role. Clearly, the extent of deformation and mechanical support provided by anatomical anchor points needs to be studied further.

The emerging clinical experience suggests that intraoperative misregistration induced by tissue deformation is a significant problem. To date, solutions have been proposed using intraoperative MR and ultrasonography [6]-[11]. Intraoperative MR has the most appeal given its high resolution and excellent contrast but its expense and cumbersome implementation into the OR have raised some questions about its widespread adoption [6]-[8]. Co-registered ultrasonography overcomes these drawbacks but has poor image clarity which tends to degrade as surgery proceeds [9]-[11]. Alternatively, co-registered ultrasonography may serve an important role in correcting for misregistration when used in conjunction with other methods. The approach we are developing exploits sparsely available intraoperative data, i.e. ultrasonography and cortical surface measurements, in conjunction with a computational model of brain deformation to update preoperative images during surgery thus serving to enhance neuronavigational accuracy as well as realism [12].

To date, explicit modeling of the falx cerebri has been limited largely to the car crash environment [13] which is substantively different than the surgical counterpart, although some initial work has been performed here as well [14]. In this paper, we have taken a surgical case where significant gravity-induced shift was reported and added the anatomical constraint of the falx cerebri to improve the understanding of anatomical anchor points and their influence on subsurface tissue deformation distributions. The model calculations are compared to measurements of the cortical surface taken in the direction of gravity. Additionally, the calculations are compared to their homogeneous counterpart which has been presented elsewhere [15].

2   Methods

The computational geometry is derived from the preoperative MR series of the patient. Using AnalyzeAVW - Version 2.5, the brain and falx cerebri (approximate 2 mm width located between hemispheres) are segmented from the images and a discrete marching cubes algorithm is applied to create a surface boundary description of the extracted volumes [16]. The surface description is then used to generate a tetrahedral mesh [17]. Material heterogeneity is performed by calculating the average voxel intensity in an element and thresholding each tissue type based on the original MR series. Figure 1a is an illustration of the computational geometry with extra refinement about the falx cerebri. The mesh consisted of 25,340 nodes and 139,351 elements. Figure 1b depicts a nodally interpolated representation of the tissue element thresholding on a coronal cross-section in the mesh where the dark surrounding area represents gray matter, the lighter central area represents white matter, and the falx can be seen as the descending division between the hemispheres.

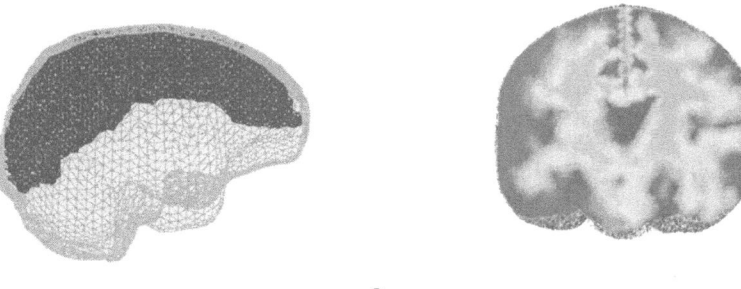

a   b

Fig. 1. Computational representation of the brain: (a) finite element brain mesh with extra refinement about the falx cerebri; (b) element-based thresholding as a means of incorporating heterogeneity.

In previous work, we reported a detailed study measuring the displacement of cortical landmarks in 28 neurosurgical cases using an operating microscope and robotic platform [1]. This same technique was used to track a series of cortical landmarks in the direction of gravity for the clinical case presented in this paper.

3   Computational Model

We have chosen consolidation physics to represent deformation characteristics of the brain [18]. Consolidation describes the continuum as a biphasic medium with a solid matrix saturated with an interstitial fluid. When subjected to load, tissue experiences an instantaneous deformation at the contact area followed by subsequent deformation due to strain-induced hydrodynamic changes. The governing equation describing mechanical equilibrium is,

$$\nabla \cdot G \nabla \mathbf{u} + \frac{G}{1 - 2\nu} \nabla \varepsilon - \alpha \nabla p + (\rho_t - \rho_f)\mathbf{g} = 0. \tag{1}$$

where G is the shear modulus ($G = \frac{E}{2(1+\nu)}$ where E is Young's modulus), ν is Poisson's ratio, α is the ratio of fluid volume extracted to volume change of tissue under compression, ε is the volumetric strain ($\varepsilon = \nabla \cdot \mathbf{u}$), ρ_t, ρ_f are the density of the tissue and surrounding fluid respectively, $\mathbf{g}$ is the gravitational acceleration vector, $\mathbf{u}$ is the displacement vector, and p is the interstitial pressure. Gravitational forces have been simulated as a difference in density between tissue and the surrounding fluid (elements above the resting level of cerebrospinal fluid post-craniotomy/drainage use the density of air for ρ_f).

A continuity equation relating volumetric strain to fluid drainage completes the description,

$$\nabla \cdot k \nabla p - \alpha \frac{\partial \varepsilon}{\partial t} - \frac{1}{S} \frac{\partial p}{\partial t} = 0, \tag{2}$$

where k is the hydraulic conductivity, and $1/S$ is a void compressibility constant. We have adopted the convention assuming full saturation with an incompressible fluid (i.e. $\frac{1}{S} = 0$, $\alpha = 1$). The mathematical framework of coupled equations (1) and (2) has been previously reported in detail [19]. Model validation was performed using an *in vivo* experimental porcine model and demonstrated a 75-85% predictive capability of subsurface deformation [20].

In this paper a series of simulations were performed to understand the impact of the anatomical constraint of the falx cerebri on a real clinical case. The patient was brought to the OR for resection of tumor and surrounding epileptogenic cortex. The patient was supine with head turned 60 degrees to his right and secured in three-point fixation. The falx cerebri extends down between the hemispheres and is securely attached both anteriorly and posteriorly with the inner margin free to deform. In the first simulation considered, there is no special treatment of the falx and the tissue is assumed to be homogeneous. The second simulation (referred to as falx simulation 1) treats the falx as a structure with a stiffness approximately 6 times larger than that of the surrounding parenchymal tissue ($E_{tissue} = 2100\,Pa$, $E_{falx} = 12000\,Pa$) where the nodes along the cortical surface of the falx are fixed. The last simulation (referred to as falx simulation 2) treats the falx as a rigid surface that allows brain tissue to slide (i.e. tangential motion) but not deform (i.e. normal motion) the falx. In all cases the level of cerebrospinal fluid is assumed to be slightly lower than the brain stem elevation when the head is rotated into its surgical orientation.

4   Results

Figure 2 reports an axial cross section in the MR data set and the model-updated image counterparts for the three simulations with the top image showing the undeformed preoperative state and the direction of gravity (white arrow). The difference images highlight the amount of shift by the shading which differs from the background. Although not an exact measure due to out of plane motion, we can observe that falx simulation 1 (pinned falx at the cortical surface) has less motion than the homogeneous model at the interhemispheric fissure which is to be expected. However, simulation 1 does appear to have a small increase in deformation in the right posterior temporal section of the image. Falx simulation 2 also has increased temporal movement and seems to have less shift than falx simulation 1 in the contralateral hemisphere.

Further appreciation of these calculations can be found in Figure 3. Here, the total displacement of the cortical surface is shown on the left and the model cross-section corresponding to the MR slices in Figure 2 is shown on the right where the total displacement is color-coded. As can be anticipated, falx simulations 1 and 2 have less subsurface deformation which is undoubtedly caused by the rigid falx cerebri acting as a central support to the brain tissue. Also, the decrease in contralateral hemispheric motion indicated in Figure 2 is confirmed by the gradient shadings in Figure 3. Another interesting feature is that the area of *maximal deformation has moved* more temporally in both falx simulations which would explain the increased posterior temporal motion findings in Figure 2.

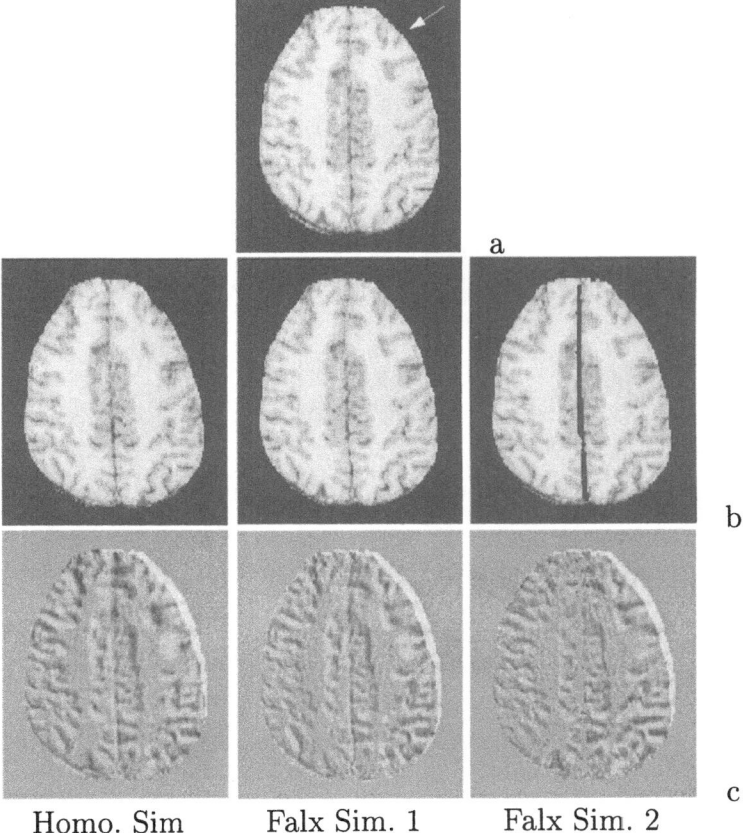

a

b

c

Homo. Sim   Falx Sim. 1   Falx Sim. 2

Fig. 2. Deformed axial MR slice based on model simulations: (a) preoperative slice with gravity designated by white arrow, (b) slice generated from deformed image volume, (c) difference images with shades differing from background indicating shift.

Figure 4 quantifies these changes in displacement between the falx simulation and the homogeneous model. Figure 4b and 4c shows the difference in total displacement along transects through the volume designated in Figure 4a (the largest lateral distance points correspond to the highest gravitational elevation along transect). Predominantly, the homogeneous model experienced more deformation than the falx counterpart (all positive values in Figures 4b and 4c correspond to larger movement by the homogeneous model). Additionally, we can see from Figures 4b and 4c that subsurface displacement can differ between the models by as much as 3 mm and 4 mm, respectively.

Table 1 quantifies the comparison between model calculations and cortical surface measurements with respect to gravity. Also shown is a point by point percent recapture ($\%_{recapture} = 100\% - \frac{|d_m - d_c|d_m}{*}100\%$, where d_m and d_c are measured and calculated displacements, respectively) which estimates the amount

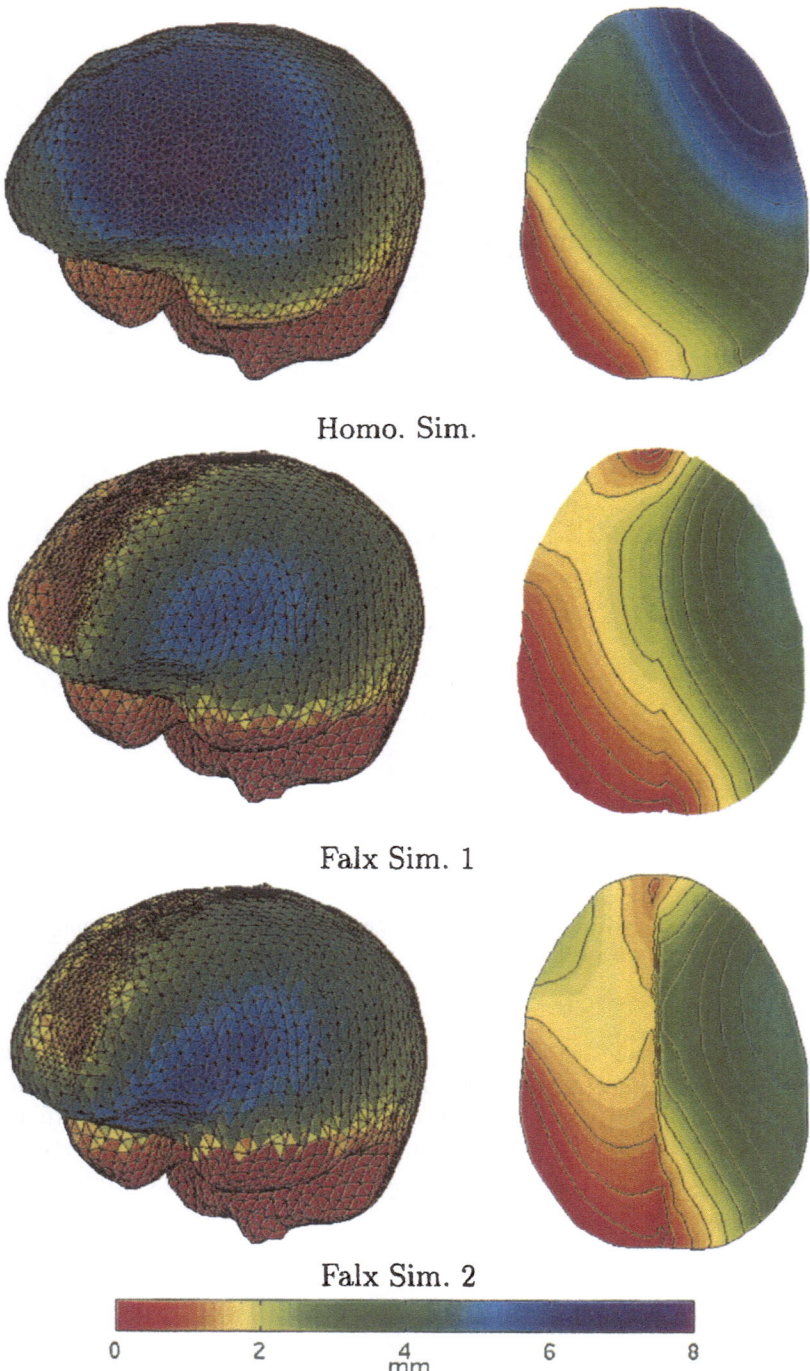

Homo. Sim.

Falx Sim. 1

Falx Sim. 2

Fig. 3. Cortical surface deformation distribution (left) and axial cross section equivalent to MR slice (right) showing total displacement for each simulation.

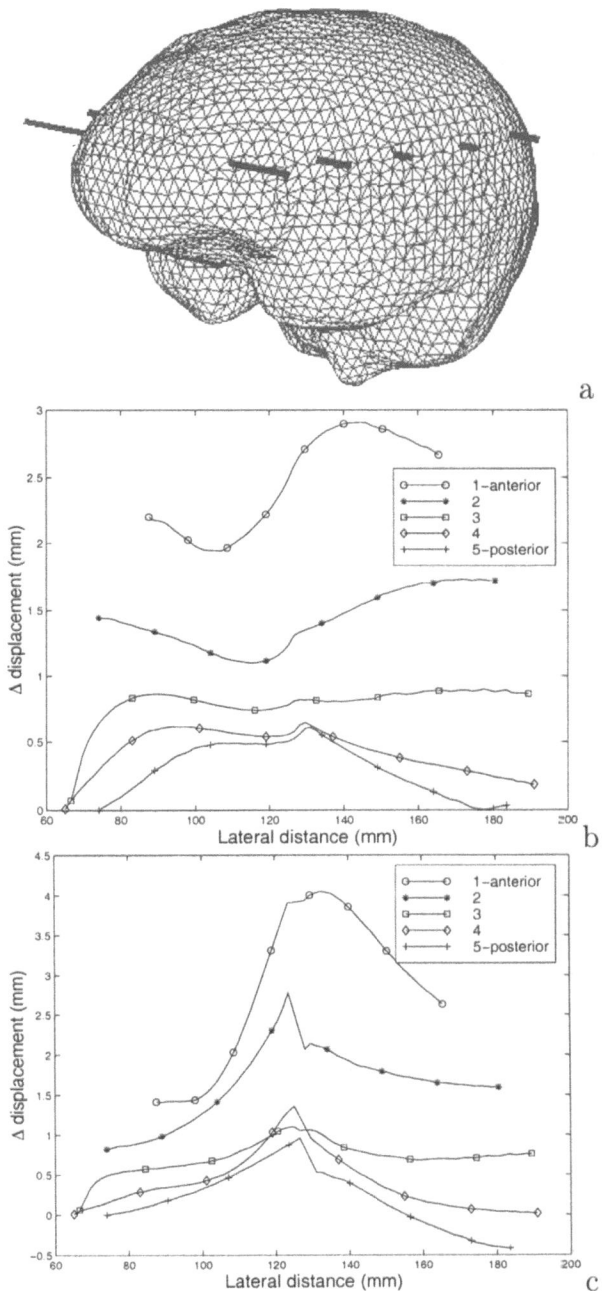

Fig. 4. Total displacement distribution **difference** between homogeneous and falx simulations where the values of total displacement for each simulation is subtracted from the homogeneous counterpart at the same points along each transect: (a) brain mesh volume showing comparison transects; (b) **difference** calculation for falx simulation 1; (c) **difference** calculation for falx simulation 2. The largest lateral distance in (b) and (c) corresponds to highest elevations in the surgically positioned cranium.

Point #	Measured Displ. mm	Homo. Sim Displ. mm ($\%_{recapture}$)	Falx Sim1 Displ. mm ($\%_{recapture}$)	Falx Sim2 Displ. mm ($\%_{recapture}$)
1	6.7	4.7 (70%)	4.3 (64%)	4.9 (73%)
2	4.6	5.2 (87%)	4.6 (100%)	5.2 (87%)
3	4.2	5.6 (67%)	4.9 (83%)	5.6 (67%)
4	3.5	3.5 (100%)	3.4 (97%)	2.9 (83%)

Table 1. Comparison between measured and calculated shift with respect to gravity for all simulations.

of displacement recaptured by the model-guided technique that would have otherwise been added to misregistration error. Here, we see that all calculations qualitatively match the data well, however, falx simulation 1 appears to be the most satisfying in terms of surface data.

5   Discussion

Figure 2 highlights a decrease in contralateral motion illustrated by a decrease in shading differences above the background across the simulations which is confirmed by results observed in Figures 3 and 4. Figure 3 shows significant differences with respect to cortical movement, particularly in the hemisphere of surgical focus with the temporal migration of maximal deformation as well as the sharp change in total deformation in the region of the falx. Further, the gradient images shown in Figure 3 show significant differences in subsurface deformation with the falx serving to damp the communication of displacement between hemispheres. Figures 4b and 4c suggest that the falx cerebri could affect subsurface deformation in the region of surgical focus by as much as 3-4 mm. Table 1 indicates that small differences exist among cortical shift predictions, with all calculations recapturing approximately 70-80% of the gravity-induced motion. Interestingly, falx simulation 2 has less subsurface movement than simultaion 1 when comparing Figure 4b and 4c, yet larger cortical surface movement in Table 1. Recall that simulation 2 has a rigid falx but the tissue is not bound to the falx per se, i.e. gravity can still move the tissue along the falx but because the falx is rigid, contralateral motion will still be inhibited. In falx simulation 1, the falx is part of the continuum and is pinned at the cortical surface (Figure 3, middle left shows a red zero displacement strip extending along the falx) which would undoubtedly dampen surface motion more than in the case of falx simulation 2 which is evident in the Figure 3 axial cross sections where falx simulation 2 has more displacement all along the upper left hemispheric surface.

6   Conclusions

The preliminary investigation reported by Maurer et al. provides impetus for understanding anatomical constraints intracranially and warrants more detailed experimental investigation using interventional imaging systems. The results shown here correlate with Maurer et al.'s initial interventional MR observations which noted that the deformation across the midline seemed to be damped significantly by the falx cerebri. Falx simulation 1 is the most satisfying with respect to cortical displacement measurements (Table 1). As noted in Figures 2-4, simulation 2 did appear to dampen more motion in the contralateral hemisphere resembling the Maurer et al. experience. However, we should note that the stiffness properties used in falx simulation 1 have not been investigated thoroughly and we could anticipate that properties stiffer than those used here may decrease displacement communication between hemispheres even further.

In any case, more detailed investigation needs to be conducted with respect to the stiffness properties as well as the hydrodynamic communication across the falx. Other support structures such as the tentorium cerebelli which supports the occipital lobes of the cerebral cortex as well as the cerebellum also need to be studied. Further, we can anticipate that with more detailed knowledge of anatomical support structures, the accuracy of our model-guided approach to neuronavigation will increase. In addition, the presence of support structures in the brain gives further credence to the possibility of reduced volume calculations which would significantly improve computational speed thus increasing the attractiveness of the model-updating approach.

Acknowledgments: This work was supported by National Institutes of Health grant R01-NS33900 awarded by the National Institute of Neurological Disorders and Stroke. ANALYZE software was provided in collaboration with the Mayo Foundation.

References

1. D. W. Roberts, A. Hartov, F.E. Kennedy, M. I. Miga, K. D. Paulsen, 'Intraoperative brain shift and deformation: a quantitative clinical analysis of cortical displacements in 28 cases', *Neurosurgery*, vol. 43, no. 4, pp. 749-760, 1998.
2. D. L. G. Hill, C. R. Maurer, R. J. Maciunas, J. A. Barwise, J. M. Fitzpatrick, M. Y. Wang, 'Measurement of intraoperative brain surface deformation under a craniotomy', *Neurosurgery*, vol. 43, no. 3, pp. 514-528, 1998.
3. N. L. Dorward, A. Olaf, B. Velani, F. A. Gerritsen, W. F. J. Harkness, N. D. Kitchen, and D. G. T. Thomas, 'Postimaging brain distortion magnitude, correlates, and impact on neuronavigation', *J. Neurosurg.*, vol. 88, pp. 656-662, 1998.
4. H. Dickhaus, K. Ganser, A. Staubert, M. M. Bonsanto, C. R. Wirtz, V. M. Tronnier, and S. Kunze, 'Quantification of brain shift effects by MR-imaging', *Proc. An. Int. Conf. IEEE Eng. Med. Biology Soc.*, pp. 491-494, 1997.
5. C. R. Maurer, D. L. G. Hill, A. J. Martin, H. Liu, M. McCue, D. Rueckert, D. Lloret, W. A. Hall, R. E. Maxwell, D. J. Hawkes, and C. L. Truwit, 'Investigation of intraoperative brain deformation using a 1.5-T interventional MR system:

Preliminary Results', *IEEE Transactions on Medical Imaging*, vol. 17, no. 5, pp. 817-825, 1998.

6. T. M. Moriarty, R. Kikinis, F. A. Jolesz, P. M. Black, and E. Alexander 3rd, 'Magnetic resonance imaging therapy. Intraoperative MR imaging.', *Neurosurg. Clin. N. Am.*, vol. 7, pp. 323-331, 1996.

7. C. R. Wirtz, M. M. Bonsanto, M. Knauth, V. M. Tronnier, F. K. Albert, A. Staubert and S. Kunze, 'Intraoperative magnetic resonance imaging to update interactive navigation in neurosurgery: Method and preliminary experience', *Computer Aided Surgery*, vol. 2, pp. 172-179, 1997.

8. R. Steinmeier, R. Fahlbusch, O. Ganslandt, C. Nimsky, M. Buchfelder, M. Kaus, T. Heigl, G. Lenz, R. Kuth, W. Huk, 'Intraoperative magnetic resonance imaging with the Magnetom open scanner: concepts, neurosurgical indications, and procedures: a preliminary report', *Neurosurgery*, vol. 43, no. 4, pp. 739-748, 1998.

9. J. W. Trobaugh, W. D. Richard, K. R. Smith, and R. D. Bucholz, Frameless stereotactic ultrasonography: Methods and applications. *Computerized Medical Imaging and Graphics*, vol. 18, no. 4, pp. 235-246, 1994.

10. R. M. Comeau, A. Fenster, T. M. Peters, 'Intraoperative US in interactive image-guided neurosurgery', *Radiographics*, vol. 19, no. 4, pp. 1019-1027, 1998.

11. A. Hartov, S. D. Eisner, D. W. Roberts, K. D. Paulsen, L. A. Platenik, M. I. Miga, 'Error analysis for a free-hand three-dimensional ultrasound system for neuronavigation', *Neurosurgical Focus*, vol.6, no. 3, art. 5, 1999.

12. D. W. Roberts, M. I. Miga, A. Hartov, S. Eisner, J. Lemery, F. E. Kennedy, K. D. Paulsen, 'Intraoperatively updated neuroimaging using brain modeling and sparse data', *Neurosurgery*, (submitted), 1999.

13. T. Nishimoto, and S. Murakami, 'Relation between diffuse axonal injury and internal head structures on blunt impact', ASME Journal of Biomechanical Engineering, vol. 120, no. 1, pp. 140-147, 1998.

14. M. Schill, M. Schinkman, H.J. Bender, and R. Manner, 'Biomechanical simulation of the falx cerebri using the finite element method', *Conference Proceedings to the 1996 IEEE Engineering in Medicine and Biology 18th Annual International Conference*, Amsterdam, The Netherlands, pp. 455-456, 1996.

15. M. I. Miga, K. D. Paulsen, F. E. Kennedy, P. J. Hoopes, A. Hartov, and D. W. Roberts, 'Model-updated image guidance: Initial clinical experience with gravity-induced brain deformation', *IEEE Transactions on Medical Imaging*, (accepted), 1999.

16. W. Schroeder, K. Martin, and B. Lorensen, *The Visualization Toolkit: An Object-Oriented Approach to 3D Graphics*, Prentice Hall, New Jersey, 1996.

17. J. M. Sullivan Jr., G. Charron, and K. D. Paulsen, 'A three dimensional mesh generator for arbitrary multiple material domains, *Finite Element Analysis and Design*, vol. 25, pp. 219-241, 1997.

18. M. Biot, 'General theory of three dimensional consolidation', *J. Appl. Phys.*, vol. 12, pp. 155-164, 1941.

19. K. D. Paulsen, M. I. Miga, F. E. Kennedy, P. J. Hoopes, A. Hartov, and D. W. Roberts, 'A computational model for tracking subsurface tissue deformation during stereotactic neurosurgery', *IEEE Transactions on Biomedical Engineering*, vol. 46, no. 2, pp. 213-225, 1999.

20. M. I. Miga, K. D. Paulsen, F. E. Kennedy, P. J. Hoopes, A. Hartov, and D. W. Roberts, 'In vivo quantification of a homogeneous brain deformation model for updating preoperative images during surgery', *IEEE Transactions on Biomedical Engineering*, (in press), 1999.

Assessment of Intraoperative Brain Deformation Using Interventional MR Imaging

Derek L. G. Hill[1], Calvin R. Maurer, Jr.[1,2], Alastair J. Martin[3,4], Saras Sabanathan[1], Walter A. Hall[5], David J. Hawkes[1], Daniel Rueckert[1], and Charles L. Truwit[3]

[1] Division of Radiological Sciences and Medical Engineering, King's College London, 5th floor Thomas Guy House, Guy's Hospital, London SE1 9RT, U.K.
Send correspondence to: Derek.Hill@kcl.ac.uk
[2] Departments of Neurological Surgery and Biomedical Engineering, University of Rochester, 601 Elmwood Avenue, Box 670, Rochester, NY 14642, U.S.A.
[3] Department of Radiology, University of Minnesota, Minneapolis, MN USA.
[4] Philips Medical Systems, Best, The Netherlands.
[5] Department of Neurosurgery, University of Minnesota, Minneapolis, MN, USA.

Abstract. We study brain deformation for a series of 8 resection cases carried out in the interventional MR suite at the University of Minnesota. The pattern of deformation is described qualitatively. We also quantify deformation by identifying anatomical landmarks spread over the brain in pre- and post-resection images, and show these values agree well with the results obtained from an automatic non-rigid registration algorithm. For all but one patient, the deformation was significantly greater ipsilateral to the lesion than contralateral, with the contralateral deformation being of the same order as the precision of the measurements. For the remaining patient, there was bi-lateral deformation of several millimetres. Example deformation fields are shown illustrating the distribution of deformation over the brain. The variability of deformation between subjects was considerable, suggesting the automatic correction of intraoperative deformation without use of interventional images may be difficult to achieve.

1 Introduction

The increasing use of image guided surgery systems for neurosurgery has lead to considerable recent interest in quantifying brain deformation during neurosurgery [1, 3, 4, 8, 7]. Traditional image guided neurosurgery systems determine the rigid body transformation between pre-operative images and an intraoperative coordinate system (eg: defined by an optical localiser). The intraoperative position of tracked pointers, surgical instruments, microscopes or endoscopes can then be related to pre-operative images. These systems can be very accurate, especially if bone-implanted fiducial markers are used [6], provided the rigid body assumption is valid. Any tissue deformation invalidates the rigid body assumption. If the tissue deformation is large compared to the required surgical accuracy, then the overall accuracy of the image guided surgical system will be reduced. Recent studies have shown that the brain surface can deform by 10mm or more underneath a craniotomy even before any resection takes place [4]. In many cases, however, the structures of interest, such as the lesion and adjacent blood

Table 1. Details of eight resection patients studied using interventional MR.

Patient	Age	Gender	lesion position	lesion type
1	53	male	left occipital	lung metastasis
2	5	male	left occipital	astrocytoma with necrosis
3	69	male	left frontal	glioblastoma multiforme
4	3	female	right medial temporal	low grade glioma
5	39	female	right occipital-parietal	meningioma
6	41	female	right frontal	recurrence of oligodendroglioma
7	36	female	superficial left temporal	glioma
8	57	male	left frontal	glioblastoma multiforme

vessels, are well below the surface of the brain, and these may deform substantially less than the brain surface. Since the recent work quantifying brain deformation has concentrated on surface features [3, 4, 8], the deformation of the structures of surgical interest remains unknown.

Interventional imaging combined with suitable image analysis software could potentially provide measurements of brain deformation throughout the head, both near and far from the site of resection. Interventional MR is not currently widely available for this application, but the good soft tissue contrast, high resolution in three dimensions and absence of ionising radiation make it ideally suited to this purpose. In this paper we extend our previous preliminary work [7] by reporting measurements of brain deformation taken on eight patients who underwent neurosurgical resections in the University of Minnesota Interventional MR suite. This paper reports results from twice the number of resection cases we previously reported (eight instead of four), provides more quantitative results, and includes results obtained from 3D deformation maps from all cases.

2   Method

Eight patients undergoing resective surgery at the University of Minnesota were selected for this study. Their lesions and surgical approaches are listed in table 1.

2.1   Image acquisition

In normal use, the interventional MR scanner acquires small numbers of slices in the vicinity of of the resection site with the patient in the operating position immediately prior to craniotomy. Then the patient is re-imaged one or more times during the procedure to check the completeness of the resection. Finally the patient is imaged at the end of the resection. To quantify deformation throughout the brain, we changed the acquisition process to acquire additional sagittal 3D magnetisation prepared rapid gradient echo (MP-RAGE) volume images just before resection, and after resection was complete. These images differ from traditional pre- and post-operative images in that the patient was anaesthetised and lying in the operative position. We refer to them as pre-resection and post-resection images.

Gradient echo images have good resolution, and the 5mT/m readout-gradient used results in relatively little geometric distortion in the read-out direction caused by B0 inhomogeneity [5]. Gradient echo images are, however, sensitive to susceptibility differences in the object being imaged. In particular, there can be signal loss at the boundary between air and soft tissue. Spin echo images do not have this problem. For patients undergoing resections, the brain is exposed to the air and air can enter the head. The magnitude of any brain deformation could, therefore, be exaggerated by signal loss due to susceptibility artefacts. To establish the extend of this problem we also acquired T2 weighted turbo-spin-echo images from some patients.

Images were acquired using a flexible phased array "synergy" coil, which provides good patient access, but produces a less uniform B1 field than a standard bird-cage head coil. As a result, the images acquired in this project have considerable intensity shading.

2.2   Image analysis

We first registered the images to correct for any rigid-body motion between the pre- and post-resection images by maximising the normalised mutual information of the joint probability distribution of the two images [11]. After this rigid alignment difference images were calculated by subtracting the transformed pre-resection images from the post-resection images. Because many of the images had different intensity gains, the difference image inspected was calculated by iteratively determining an intensity scale value that minimises the mean square difference in voxel intensities.

We subsequently applied a non-rigid registration algorithm to correct any remaining non-rigid motion. This non-rigid registration algorithm uses a two-stage transformation model. The first stage captures the global motion of the brain and is modelled by a rigid transformation calculated in the previous step. The second stage captures the local motion of the brain and is modelled by a free-form deformation (FFD) based on B-splines. The non-rigid registration is achieved by maximising the normalised mutual information as a similarity measure between pre- and post-resection images [10]. The algorithm has been previously applied [9] and evaluated for the registration of 3D breast MRI [2].

2.3   Assessment of intraoperative deformation

For each patient, representative 3D points were identified in the frontal, parietal, occipital and temporal lobe of the brain and the lateral ventricles both ipsilateral and contralateral to the lesion. One point was identified in each lobe by a single observer. A point was also marked in the cerebellum. Each point had to be definable in three dimensions, for example a vessel bifurcation, an extrema of curvature of a vessel, or a characteristic 3D feature of a sulcus. The position of the point did, therefore, vary between patients, but for each patient, the same point was identified in both the pre- and post-resection image. The software used to identify points allows the user to measure points on zoomed in images, giving coordinates with sub-voxel precision. The length

Table 2. Qualitative description of deformation from the eight resection cases listed in table 1. For each patient, the table shows whether there was shift in the midline or tentorium (m/t shift), and comments on deformation elsewhere.

Patient	m/t shift?	Comments
1	No	Deformation near lesion. Some subtle change in posterior horns
2	Some	Substantial deformation near lesion, small volume loss in enlarged contra-lateral ventricle, small volume gain in ipsilateral ventricle
3	No	Deformation near lesion; falling of ipsilateral frontal lobe, subtle change in anterior horns
4	No	Deformation at resection site, diffuse ipsilateral gyral deformation, sinking at entry ($\sim$3mm)
5	No	Deformation near lesion. Dark bilateral ventricular rim; little contralateral cortical deformation
6	No	Major resection on one side, bilateral brain deformation $\geq$5mm; Loss of CSF from ventricles and sulci
7	No	Shift under craniotomy $\geq$5mm; little contralateral cortical change; bilateral ventricle volume loss
8	No	Large shift near resection ($\sim$10 mm), substantial bilateral ventricle enlargement

of the vector separating the two points was calculated as a measure of local brain deformation. To assess reproducibility of the measurements, the points were marked six times each by a single observer. There was a gap of several hours between marking the point on the different occasions. The standard deviations of the local deformation measurements was calculated.

In addition to the assessment of intraoperative brain deformation by an observer, the non-rigid registration algorithm was used to calculate a dense deformation field for the entire brain. To avoid influences of deformable or resected tissue on the calculation of the deformation fields, the post-resection images were segmented using Analyze (Mayo Clinic) and the portion of the image volume corresponding to extra-dural material or resected lesion was excluded from the calculation of the similarity measure during the registration process. The node spacing of the algorithm was set at 15mm.

3 Results

3.1 Qualitative description of deformation

In many cases the RF inhomogeneity was quite different in the pre- and post-resection images, and the amount of contrast agent in the scans was different, so there are many intensity changes between the images that do not correspond to tissue deformation. It is, nevertheless, possible to identify tissue deformation independent of the other intensity effects. The observed deformation is described in table 2. Example difference images from patient 6 is shown in figure 1.

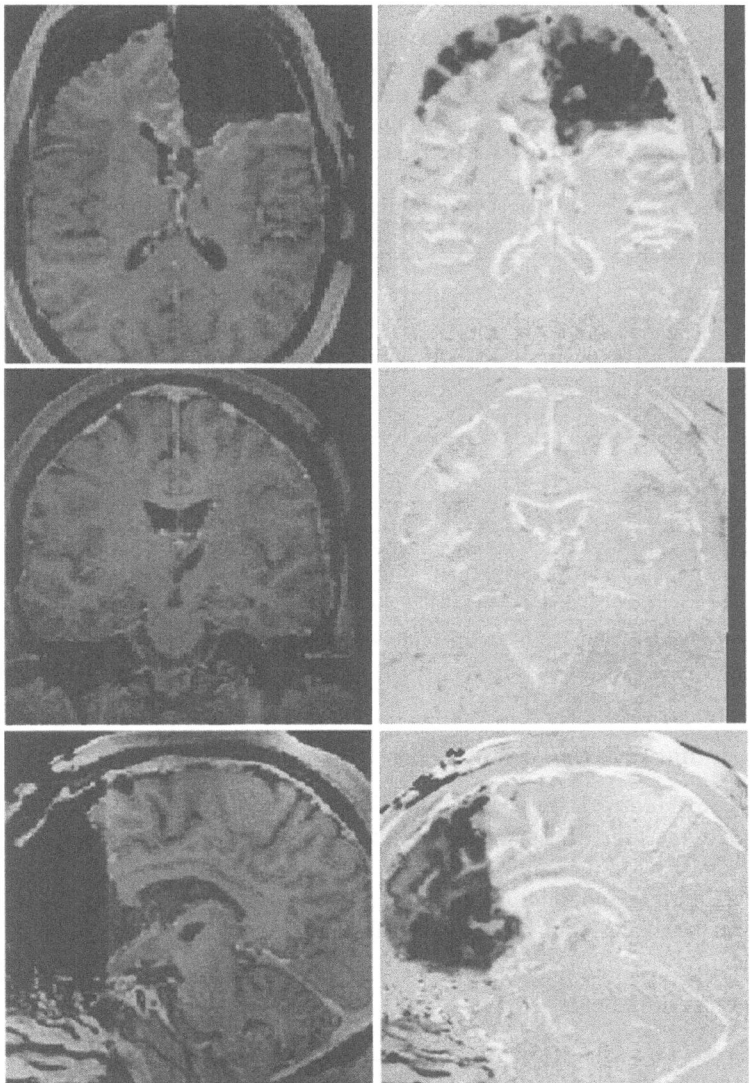

Fig. 1. Example post-resection and difference images from patient 6. The axial, coronal and sagittal images in the left column are re-formatted from the post-resection MP-RAGE volume image. The difference images in the right column are obtained by subtracting the pre-resection image (registered using maximisation of normalised mutual information) from the post-resection image. The dark portions of the frontal lobe indicate resection on the right side and brain deformation alone on the left side side. This was the only patient with substantial bi-lateral deformation. Note also the white line around the lateral ventricles in the difference image: this represents reduction of CSF volume between the pre- and post-resection images.

Table 3. Measurement of deformation (in mm) in different parts of the brain for eight patients. The left side of the table reports distances between 3D anatomical points interactively identified in the post-resection images and registered pre-resection images. Reproducibility studies showed that the standard deviation of these measurements varied between 0.1mm and 0.9mm. The right part of the table shows the deformation at these same positions calculated using the free form deformation algorithm described in the text. Entries marked with a - could not be marked in those datasets (eg: that part of the brain had been resected).

Patient	Interactive measurements								Deformation algorithm values							
	1	2	3	4	5	6	7	8	1	2	3	4	5	6	7	8
	Ipsilateral to lesion															
Frontal lobe	0.5	1.2	2.7	2.6	0.5	-	1.0	1.0	1.0	0.5	1.4	2.4	1.0	-	1.6	0.7
Parietal lobe	1.9	7.7	2.2	0.8	0.7	1.7	-	0.8	1.1	6.0	0.8	0.6	0.2	2.9	-	1.0
Temporal lobe	1.6	-	0.8	-	0.7	0.7	-	1.8	0.6	-	0.3	-	0.3	1.3	-	1.8
Occipital lobe	1.5	-	0.6	1.0	1.6	0.2	0.6	1.7	1.3	-	0.3	1.2	1.9	0.5	1.0	1.0
Lat. ventricle	0.6	0.7	0.9	1.7	0.8	2.1	1.9	3.4	0.4	0.7	0.5	1.0	0.3	0.5	1.9	3.0
	Contralateral to lesion															
Frontal lobe	0.5	1.0	0.5	0.8	0.7	6.0	0.7	0.6	0.6	0.5	0.5	0.5	0.8	6.8	0.5	0.6
Parietal lobe	1.8	0.9	0.5	0.6	0.6	0.7	0.6	1.0	0.6	1.3	0.5	0.5	0.5	0.4	0.3	1.1
Temporal lobe	0.5	0.6	0.4	1.0	0.5	0.5	0.4	0.8	0.2	0.3	1.0	0.3	0.0	0.8	0.3	0.5
Occipital lobe	0.5	2.5	1.0	0.7	0.5	0.5	0.6	0.7	0.3	0.3	0.2	0.3	0.1	0.6	0.4	0.3
Lat. ventricle	0.9	1.2	1.0	1.0	1.3	5.0	1.1	0.6	0.1	0.3	0.3	0.3	0.3	6.0	0.8	0.9
Cerebellum	2.2	0.6	0.5	0.9	0.6	0.9	0.5	0.2	0.3	0.5	0.2	0.2	0.2	1.0	0.3	0.3

3.2 Quantitative assessment of deformation using interactively identified points

The left side of table 3 shows the deformation in different regions of the brain measured by manually marking 3D anatomical points. The standard deviation of the point separations was between 0.1 and 0.9mm. While the reproducibility of marking the points will vary with the point and patient, these measurements suggest that the precision of the deformation values in table 3 is better than 1.0 mm.

3.3 Deformation fields

The non-rigid registration algorithm was run on all eight patients. The algorithm calculates a voxel-by-voxel deformation field. This can be used to transform the pre-resection image into the coordinates of the post-resection image, or it can be used to generate a deformation map, which gives the magnitude and direction of deformation for each voxel. Deformation values calculated by the algorithm for the same points in the brain as used to produce the left side of table 3 are shown in the right side of this same table. 68% of the values from the deformation map are within 0.5mm of the interactively measured values, 90% are within 1.0mm, and 95% are within 1.5mm. This suggests that the results of the automatic non-rigid registration algorithm agree with the interactive measurements to the precision of the interactive measurements. The values where the agreement is less good tend to be points where the interactively measured deformation is higher.

It is clear from both the interactive and automatic measurements that, with the exception of patient 6, deformation ipsilateral to the resection is substantially greater than on the contralateral side. A paired Student t-test was used to test whether these differences are significant. Pooling the results for all eight patients, the null hypothesis that the deformation measurements from both sides of the brain come from the same population is rejected ($P<0.05$ for the interactive measurements; $P<0.01$ for the automatic algorithm).

All the resections were supra-tentorial. It is noticeable that the deformation of the cerebellum was 1mm or less for all cases according to the automatic algorithm, and for all but one case, according to the interactive measurements.

Figure 2 compares difference images obtained by subtracting the transformed pre-resection image from the post-resection image for patient 4. Reformated axial and sagittal slices are shown as these clearly illustrate the deformation below the craniotomy. It is clear from the difference images that transformation using the non-rigid registration algorithm results in better alignment of pre- and post-resection images than using the rigid-body registration algorithm. Figure 3 shows the region around the craniotomy of patient 4 in more detail. The deformation map overlaid on the post-resection image indicates that the deformation corresponding to a falling of the brain away from the craniotomy, in approximately the direction of gravity. This deformation is greatest immediately beneath the craniotomy, and by the time the mid-line is reached, becomes virtually zero. This figure also compares the overlay of the pre-resection image on the post-resection image using the rigid body transformation and deformation field shown. There is much better alignment of both brain surface and ventricles using the deformation algorithm.

4 Discussion

We have assessed intraoperative brain deformation on eight patients who underwent neurosurgical resections in the interventional MR suite at the University of Minnesota. We have described the deformation qualitatively, and quantified the deformation over the brain volume using interactively identified anatomical landmarks. We have also used a non-rigid registration algorithm to automatically calculate a deformation field that gives a deformation magnitude and direction for each voxel in the image. The algorithm used to calculate the deformation field is a modification of an algorithm previously used to non-rigidly register pre- and post-contrast MR mammograms. The algorithm provides deformation values that agree well with interactively measured deformation for all patients. We believe that this non-rigid registration algorithm is useful both for quantifying brain deformation in this on-going study, and is also likely to provide a method for overlaying information from pre-operatively acquired images from MR or other modalities on interventional images. This could, for example, be used to overlay a pre-operative surgical plan, or features of interest onto intraoperatively acquired MR images.

The intraoperative brain deformation for this set of eight patients was quite variable. In some, but not all cases, there was no shift in the midline or tentorium. Similarly, in some, but not all cases, there was very little deformation contralateral to the lesion.

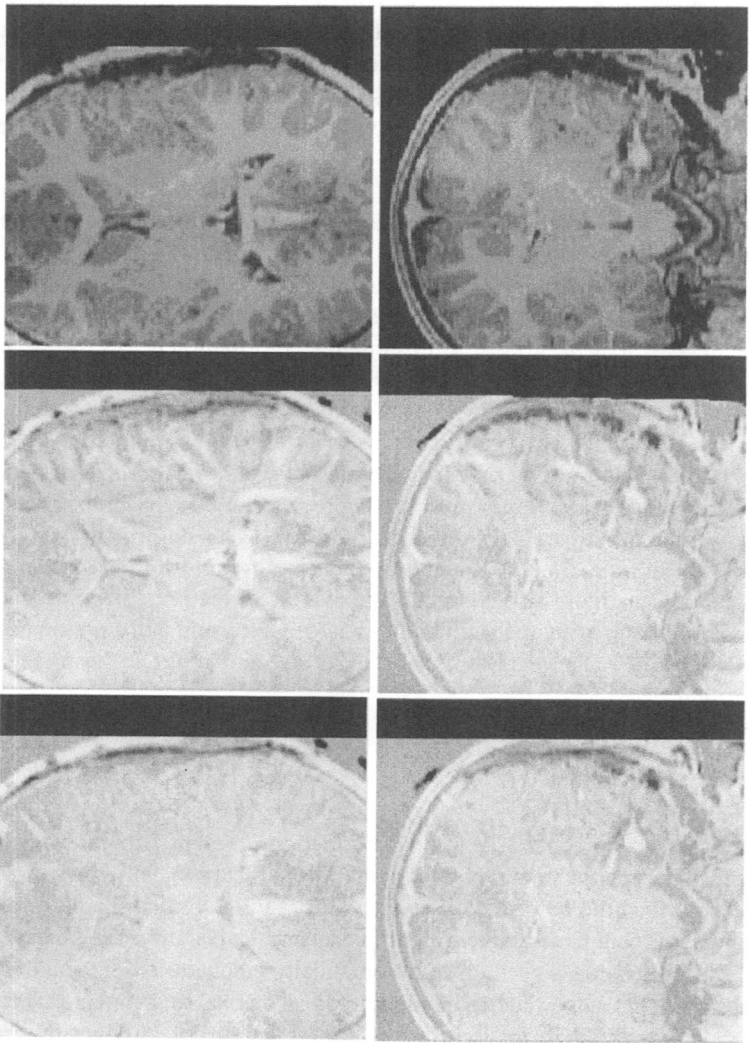

Fig. 2. Example coronal and axial slices from patient 4, showing the transformed pre-resection image subtracted from the post-resection image. The top row shows the post resection images, the middle row the subtraction image produced after rigid body registration, and the bottom row the subtraction image after non-rigid registration. Notice the reduction in residual signal in the subtraction image using free form deformation. The residual difference after free form deformation results from contrast in the post-resection image and differences in RF inhomogeneity, as well as uncorrected tissue deformation. The slices are orientated such that the gravitationally most apendent part of the patient is at the top of the page.

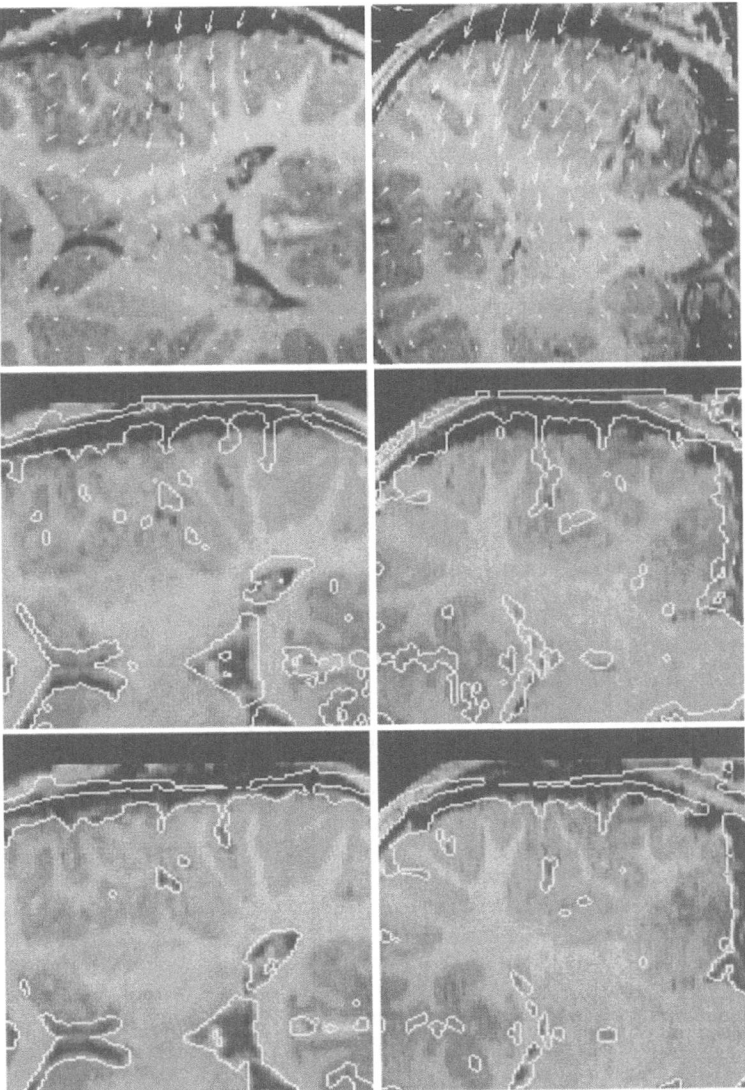

Fig. 3. Brain deformation in the vicinity of the craniotomy for patient 4. All rows show axial and coronal views approximately aligned with the patient's intraoperative position. The top row shows the deformation field overlaid as white arrows on the post-resection image. The length of the vectors have been exagerated for visualization purposes. The middle and bottom row show the boundary of the pre-resection volume overlaid on the post-resection volume using the rigid body (middle) and free-form deformation (bottom) transformation respectively. The free-form deformation algorithm results in better alignment of both the cortical surface and ventricle outlines than the rigid body transformation.

Also, the magnitude of deformation ipsilateral to the resection, but away from the site of surgery was variable. This suggests that the mechanisms of brain deformation are likely to be quite complex. Simple physical models of brain deformation may, therefore, be inadequate for compensating for brain deformation in image guided surgery systems that do not make use of intraoperative imaging.

Acknowledgements

We thank Frans Gerritsen and Joop van Vaals of Philips Medical Systems for assistance and the UK EPSRC (GR/M47294 and GR/L08519) and the EU (EASI project HC1012 under 4th framework programme) for financial support.

References

1. R. D. Bucholz, D. D. Yeh, J. Trobaugh, L. L. McDurmont, C. D. Sturm, C. Baumann, J. M. Henderson, A. Levy, and P. Kessman, "The correction of stereotactic inaccuracy caused by brain shift using an intraoperative ultrasound device", in *CVRMed-MRCAS '97*, J. Troccaz, E. Grimson, and R. Mösges, Eds., pp. 459–466. Springer-Verlag, Berlin, 1997.
2. E. R. E. Denton, L. I. Sonoda, D. Rueckert, S. C. Rankin, C. Hayes, M. Leach, D. L. G. Hill, and D. J. Hawkes, "Comparison and evaluation of rigid and non-rigid registration of breast MR images", *J. Comput. Assist. Tomogr.*, 1999, In press.
3. N. L. Dorward, O. Alberti, B. Velani, F. A. Gerritsen, W. F. J. Harkness, N. D. Kitchen, and D. G. T. Thomas, "Postimaging brain distortion: Magnitude, correlates, and impact on neuronavigation", *J. Neurosurg.*, vol. 88, pp. 656–662, 1998.
4. D. L. G. Hill, C. R. Maurer, Jr., R. J. Maciunas, J. A. Barwise, J. M. Fitzpatrick, and M. Y. Wang, "Measurement of intraoperative brain surface deformation under a craniotomy", *Neurosurgery*, vol. 43, pp. 514–526, 1998.
5. D. L. G. Hill, C. R. Maurer, Jr., C. Studholme, J. M. Fitzpatrick, and D. J. Hawkes, "Correcting scaling errors in tomographic images using a nine degree of freedom registration algorithm", *J. Comput. Assist. Tomogr.*, vol. 22, pp. 317–323, 1998.
6. C. R. Maurer, Jr., J. M. Fitzpatrick, M. Y. Wang, R. L. Galloway, Jr., R. J. Maciunas, and G. S. Allen, "Registration of head volume images using implantable fiducial markers", *IEEE Trans. Med. Imaging*, vol. 16, pp. 447–462, 1997.
7. C. R. Maurer, Jr., D. L. G. Hill, A. J. Martin, H. Liu, M. McCue, D. Rueckert, D. Lloret, W. A. Hall, R. E. Maxwell, D. J. Hawkes, and C. L. Truwit, "Investigation of intraoperative brain deformation using a 1.5 Tesla interventional MR system: Preliminary results", *IEEE Trans. Med. Imaging*, vol. 17, pp. 817–825, 1998.
8. D. W. Roberts, A. Hartov, F. E. Kennedy, M. I. Miga, and K. D. Paulsen, "Intraoperative brain shift and deformation: a quantitative analysis of cortical displacement in 28 cases", *Neurosurgery*, vol. 43, pp. 749–758, 1998.
9. D. Rueckert, C. Hayes, C. Studholme, P. Summers, M. Leach, and D. J. Hawkes, "Non-rigid registration of breast MR images using mutual information", in *First Int. Conf on Medical Image Computing and Computer-Assisted Intervention (MICCAI '98)*, Cambridge, MA, 1998, pp. 1144–1152.
10. D. Rueckert, L. I. Sonoda, C. Hayes, D. L. G. Hill, M. O. Leach, and D. J. Hawkes, "Non-rigid registration using free-form deformations: Application to breast MR images", *IEEE Trans. Med. Imaging*, 1999, In Press.
11. C. Studholme, D. L. G. Hill, and D. J. Hawkes, "An overlap invariant entropy measure of 3D medical image alignment", *Pattern Recognition*, vol. 32, pp. 71–86, 1999.

Ultrasound Probe Tracking for Real-Time Ultrasound/MRI Overlay and Visualization of Brain Shift

David G. Gobbi[1], Roch M. Comeau[2], and Terry M. Peters[1,2]

[1] Imaging Research Laboratories,
John P. Roberts Research Institute, University of Western Ontario,
London ON N6A 5K8, Canada
dgobbi@irus.rri.on.ca, tpeters@irus.rri.on.ca
[2] McConnell Brain Imaging Centre, Montreal Neurological Institute,
Montréal QC H3A 2B4, Canada
roch@nil.mni.mcgill.ca
http://www.bic.mni.mcgill.ca/research/groups/igns/

Abstract. Stereotactic techniques are prevalent in neurosurgery. A fundamental assumption of stereotaxis is that the brain is a rigid body. It has been demonstrated, however, that following a craniotomy the brain tissue will shift by 10 mm on average. We are investigating intra-operative ultrasound, using an optical tracking system to record the position and orientation of the ultrasound probe, as a method of measuring and correcting for brain shift. We have determined that the accuracy to which ultrasound image coordinates can be tracked (including the errors involved in calibration) is better than 0.5 mm within the ultrasound image plane, and better than 2 mm perpendicular to the plane. We apply two visualization methods to compare the ultrasound and the pre-operative MRI: the first is real-time overlay of the ultrasound with the co-planar MR slice, and the second is the real-time texture mapping of the ultrasound video into a 3D view with the MRI. Our technique is demonstrated on a poly vinyl alcohol cryogel phantom.

1 Introduction

1.1 Stereotaxis and Brain Tissue Shift

Pre-operative MR or CT images are used to identify the surgical target and to plan procedures in stereotactic neurosurgery. The images are registered to a surgical coordinate system through a set of fiducial markers visible in the images. The most commonly used fiducials are Z bars attached to the stereotactic frame: a single MR or CT slice through three or more Z bars is sufficient to calculate the coordinate transformation from image coordinates to stereotactic frame coordinates.

Recently, frameless stereotactic systems have been developed which use fiducial markers affixed directly to the skin or the skull. These markers are registered to a 3D tracking system after the patient's head has been immobilized for surgery. The tracking system can then report tool positions in image coordinates.

There is an implicit assumption for both of the above stereotactic methods that the target does not move between the time the pre-operative images are obtained and the time when surgery is performed. This assumption has recently been examined [1][2]. It has been found that for craniotomies, brain tissue will shift by an average of ten millimetres during the operation.

A very general method for dealing with the problem of brain shift is to obtain images during surgery. Imaging modalities that can be used during neurosurgery include interventional MRI and ultrasound.

1.2   Intra-Operative Imaging

For an intra-operative imaging technique to be acceptable, the benefit it provides must outweigh the disruption it causes to routine operating room activity.

Interventional MR units restrict the access the surgeon has to the patient. Much of the standard operating-room equipment is incompatible with strong magnetic fields, including surgical instruments, anaesthesia units and life-support equipment. In addition to the cost of the interventional MR unit itself, the cost of rendering ancilliary equipment MR compatible is high.

Intra-operative ultrasound can be used as an adjunct to existing neurosurgical procedures because it is safe and minimally disruptive. Some advantages of ultrasound are: 1) a conventional ultrasound machine can be used in the operating room, 2) there are no compatibility problems between ultrasound imaging and standard operating room equipment, 3) the ultrasound machine is portable.

The aim of our group and others that work with stereotactic intraoperative ultrasound [3][4][5] is to use ultrasound images to measure brain shift. This is achieved by tracking the position and orientation of the ultrasound probe, such that the ultrasound image is always registered to the stereotactic coordinate system and to the pre-operative images. We sample the probe position/orientation at $20\text{--}60~\text{s}^{-1}$, which makes a real-time MR/ultrasound overlay possible. A still from an overlay done during a surgical procedure at the Montreal Neurological Institute is shown in Figure 1. The ventricles and the falx were used as landmarks to detect brain shift.

Our ultimate goal is to use homologous landmarks in 3D ultrasound and pre-operative 3D data sets to correct the pre-operative images for brain shift via an elastic deformation. We have demonstrated, using a deformable phantom, the 2D deformation of MR images to match ultrasound images [6].

1.3   Tracking Systems and Registration

In order for a tracking system to be useful, two separate calibrations must be performed. The first is required because the coordinate system associated with the surgical tool (e.g. ultrasound image coordinates if the 'tool' is an ultrasound probe) is in general not identical to the coordinate system of the 'tool holder'

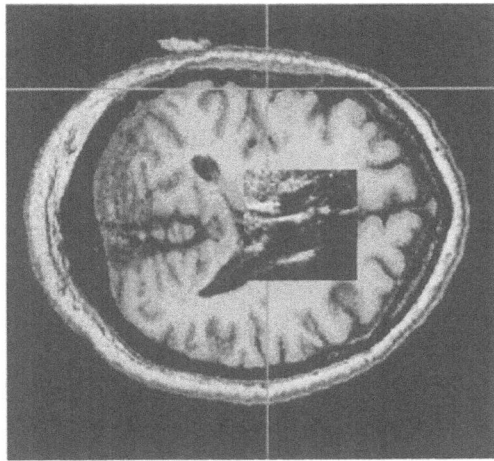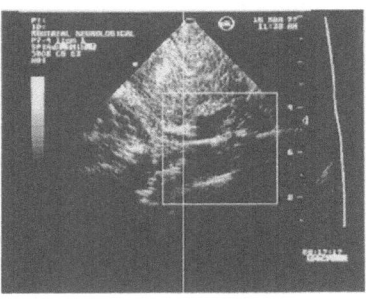

Fig. 1. Left: A still from a MR/ultrasound video overlay which was part of an amygdalohippocampotomy procedure. Right: The ultrasound video still from the overlay, with the overlay ROI outlined.

(the portion of the OTS on which the tracked infared LEDs are mounted). We refer to the transformation between 'tool' and 'tool holder' coordinates as the tool calibration matrix, and denote it $^h_u T$. The procedure we use to find $^h_u T$ for the ultrasound probe is described below.

The second calibration transformation converts tracking-system coordinates (relative to the cameras of the OTS) to a more useful coordinate space (e.g. the pre-operative image space if we are doing an MR/ultrasound overlay). We refer to this transformation as the world calibration matrix, and denote it as $^t_t T$.

These two transformation matrices are combined with the transformation $^t_h T$ returned by the OTS (the transformation between the infrared LEDs and the OTS cameras) to provide the transformation $^p_u T$ between ultrasound image space and pre-operative image space:

$$^p_u T = {}^p_t T \, {}^t_h T \, {}^h_u T \qquad (1)$$

2   Materials and Methods

The primary components of our system are an Aloka SSD-2000 ultrasound scanner with a 5 MHz neuro ultrasound probe (Aloka Co., Ltd, Tokyo 181-8522, Japan), a POLARIS optical tracking system (Northern Digital Inc., Waterloo ON N2V 1C5, Canada, www.ndigital.com), and a 450 MHz Pentium II workstation with video input/output capabilities.

Our image-guided neurosurgery platform, ASP, has been developed using the Visualization Toolkit [8] (VTK). We have added our own classes to VTK to support the POLARIS, video input, and trilinear interpolation of oblique slices from rectilinear image volumes. We chose VTK because it provides a very high-level interface for 3D rendering (making it exceptional for prototyping software), because the source code is available and the addition of custom features is straightforward, and because it is platform-independent across all modern versions of Windows and UNIX.

Our visualization methods were tested on a poly vinyl alchohol cryogel [9] (PVA-C) phantom which we built for that purpose.

2.1   Ultrasound Probe Calibration

It is necessary to determine the calibration transformation which converts ultrasound image coordinates to the tracked infrared LED ('tool holder') coordinates. Our calibration relies on a small phantom, consisting of strings supported by a lucite frame, which is modelled after the Z bars used for frame stereotaxy. The cross section through each Z bar is visible as three bright spots in the image. We manually place a 2.5 mm diameter region-of-interest around each spot, within which the centroid is calculated, to measure the coordinates of the spots.

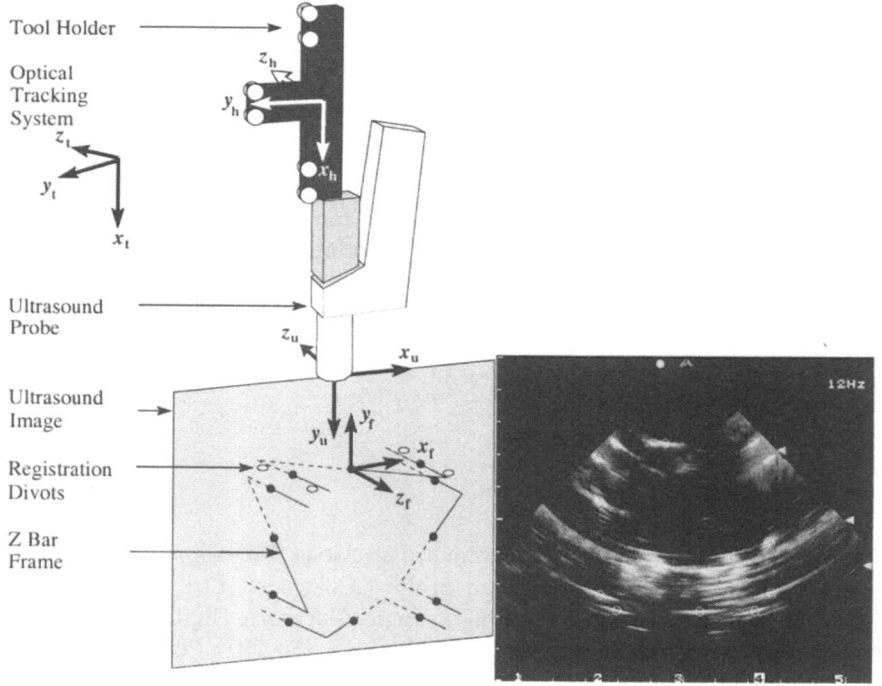

Fig. 2. Ultrasound probe calibration using a Z-bar phantom. One of the annotated images used for a calibration is shown on the right.

Figure 2 displays the coordinate systems involved in the calibration. The calibration matrix to be found is $^{h}_{u}T$, the transformation from ultrasound image coordinates to the tool holder coordinates. The following method is applied:

1. The transformation $^{t}_{f}T$ from frame coordinates to tracking system coodinates is calculated, using four divots at known locations on the frame.
2. For each of the point triplets (Z bar cross-sections) visible in the image, the position $\mathbf{p_f}$ of the central point in frame coordinates is calculated.
3. Each point is converted to probe-holder coordinates using $\mathbf{p_h} = {^{h}_{t}T} \, {^{t}_{f}T} \, \mathbf{p_f}$.
4. For each point $\mathbf{p_h}$ in probe-holder coordinates, there is a homologous point $\mathbf{p_u}$ in ultrasound image coordinates which is the central point of the corresponding Z-bar cross-section triplet. Least-squares minimization is used to calculate the transformation $^{h}_{u}T$ between ultrasound image coodinates and probe holder coordinates.

We have encapsulated the above procedure within a small application which allows the user to grab ultrasound images (the OTS transformation $^{h}_{t}T$ is automatically recorded at the same time), place annotation marks, and apply the above calibration procedure.

2.2   Viewing Options

Our software currently supports 2D and 3D real-time viewing options. In 2D mode, the tracking of the ultrasound probe is used to determine the intersection of the ultrasound image with the pre-operative MR data set. The MR slice which lies at the intersection is interpolated from the MR data set, and is overlaid on top of the live ultrasound video. The overlay is streamed to a video encoder and can be recorded on a VCR. The typical update rate is 4 frames per second. The result is as shown in Figure 1.

For the 3D viewing mode (see Figure 3), the ultrasound video is streamed into ASP, our 3D surgical navigation software, and an alpha (transparency) mask is applied to it. The ultrasound video is then texture-mapped onto a plane within the 3D scene, which is re-rendered with an updated video frame and ultrasound probe position at approximately ten frames per second.

3   Results and Discussion

3.1   POLARIS Accuracy

An accuracy of 0.35 mm RMS is quoted for the POLARIS on its data sheet. Our own measurements of the POLARIS accuracy for our tracked pointer (the tip of which is 180 mm from the origin of the POLARIS tool holder) are given in Table 1. It can be seen that the error in the z coordinate, the depth-of-field coordinate, is greater than that in x or y. As well, the tracking accuracy improves by a small amount when the tool holder is in the same orientation relative to the POLARIS for all measurements.

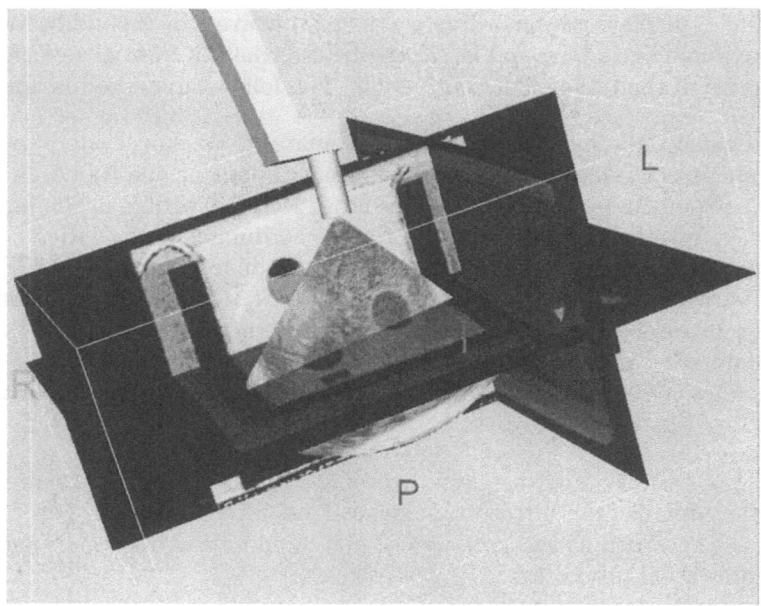

Fig. 3. The ultrasound video is texture-mapped into a 3D view of the MR data.

When several samples are averaged for each registration point, with a small change in the pointer orientation for each sample, the accuracy increases to 0.15 mm. In comparison, fiducials in an MRI with 1 mm^3 voxels can generally be located to within 0.3–1.0 mm.

Table 1. Accuracy of the POLARIS Tracking System

	σ_x [mm]	σ_y [mm]	σ_x [mm]	$\sqrt{\sigma_x^2 + \sigma_y^2 + \sigma_x^2}$ [mm]
similar orientation	0.093	0.114	0.282	0.318
varied orientation	0.157	0.190	0.316	0.401
average 50 samples	0.027	0.079	0.122	0.148

This table is condensed from data included in [6]

3.2 Ultrasound Calibration Accuracy

The accuracy of the ultrasound probe calibration transform ^h_uT was estimated by performing four separate calibrations, using four ultrasound images for each calibration. For all four calibrations the calibration phantom was in the same location, and the phantom was only registered to the OTS once to determine the transformation ^t_fT. Because each of the fiducial divots was registered to within 0.15 mm, the overall error on ^t_fT was on the order of 0.2 mm.

For each of the calibration matrices $^h_uT_i$, a point $\mathbf{p}_u$ in the ultrasound image was converted to tool holder coordinates $\mathbf{p}_{hi} = {}^h_uT_i\,\mathbf{p}_u$. The standard deviation $\sigma_{\mathbf{p}_h}$ of these coordinates is the reproducibility of the calibration. This can be converted into ultrasound image coordinates through the transformation $\sigma_{\mathbf{p}_u} = {}^u_hT\,\sigma_{\mathbf{p}_h}$ where ^u_hT is the inverse of any of the ^h_uT.

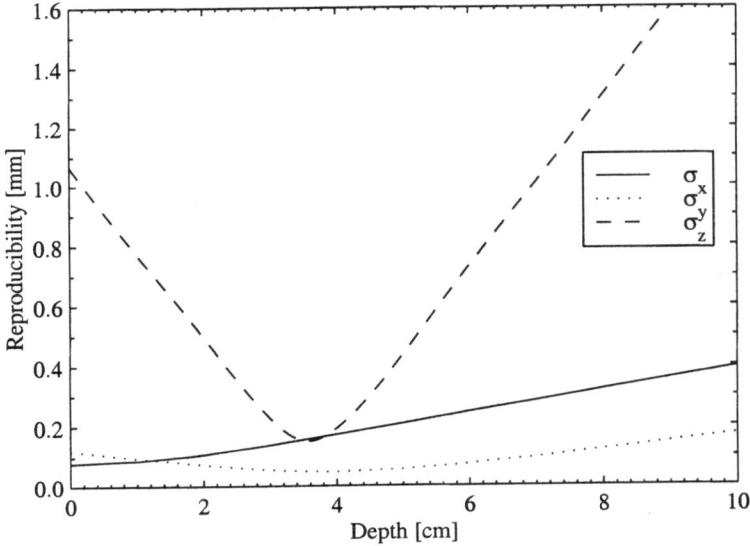

Fig. 4. Reproducibility of the ultrasound probe calibration.

Figure 4 shows the values of $\sigma_{\mathbf{p}_u}$ (broken into x, y, and z components) for points along the y axis (depth axis) of the ultrasound image. The values of σ_x and σ_y are excellent; σ_z is comparable only at 3.5 cm depth (approximately 1 cm below the top Z bar in most of the images used for the calibration).

3.3   Registration Accuracy

The POLARIS tracking accuracy is 0.3–0.4 mm, the accuracy of the registration of the calibration phantom to the OTS is 0.2 mm, and the ultrasound probe calibration reproducibility is better than 0.3 mm in either x or y. The total registration accuracy between ultrasound image coordinates and the OTS coordinates is 0.5 mm or better in x,y and between 0.5 and 2.0 in z. The accuracy in an MR/ultrasound overlay is therefore governed primarily by the error in the registration of the MR, which is usually on the order of 1–2 mm.

4   Conclusion

We have determined that the registration of ultrasound images for use in stereo-tactic neurosurgery can be done to a very high precision, better than 0.5 mm in the x and y directions and around 1 mm in the z direction except at depths greater than 7 cm. This precision is more than sufficient to accurately measure and correct for brain shift. In fact, the accuracy of the measurement of brain shift will be limited by either the accuracy of the registration of the MR images (via conventional stereotactic techniqes) or by the resolution of the MR and ultrasound images.

Acknowledgments

We gratefully acknowledge Kathleen Surry for building our PVA-cryogel phantom and Yves Starreveld for co-developing ASP. Funding for this research is provided by the Medical Research Council of Canada, and scholarship funding for David Gobbi is provided by the Ontario Ministry of Education.

References

1. D. L. G. Hill, C. R. Maurer Jr., R. J. Maciunas, J. A. Barwise, J. M. Fitzpatrick and M.Y. Wang. Measurement of Intraoperative Brain Surface Deformation under a Craniotomy. *Neurosurgery* **43**:514–528, 1998.
2. D. W. Roberts, A. Hartov, F. E. Kennedy, M. I. Miga and K. D. Paulsen. Intraoperative Brain Shift and Deformation: A Quantitative Analysis of Cortical Displacement in 28 Cases. *Neurosurgery* **43**:749–760, 1998.
3. R .D. Bucholz, D. Yeh,, J. Trobaugh, L. L. McDurmont, C. D. Sturm, C. Baumann and M. H. Jaimie. The Correction of Stereotactic Inaccuracy Caused by Brain Shift Using an Intraoperative Ultrasound Device. *CVRMed-MRCAS '97 : First Joint Conference Computer Vision, Virtual Reality and Robotics in Medicine and Medical Robotics and Computer-Assisted Surgery*, Troccaz, J., Grimson, E., Mösges, R., (eds.), Grenoble, France, Springer-Verlag, Berlin, 1997.
4. C. Giorgi and D.S. Casolino. Preliminary Clinical Experience with Intraoperative Stereotactic Ultrasound Imaging. *Stereotactic and Functional Neurosurgery* **68**:54-58, 1997.
5. A. Jödicke, W. Deinsberger, H. Erbe, A. Kriete and D.-K. Böker. Intraoperative Three-Dimensional Ultrasonography: An Approach to Register Brain Shift Using Multidimensional Image Processing. *Minim. Invasive Neurosurg.* **41**:13-19, 1998.
6. R. M. Comeau, D. G. Gobbi, A. Fenster, A. F. Sadikot and T. M. Peters. Detecting and Correcting Brain Tissue Deformation Using Intraoperative Ultrasound Imaging in Interactive Image Guided Neurosurgery. *Canadian Organization of Medical Physicists Conference Proceedings*, 131–133, June 18-20, 1998.
7. R. M. Comeau, A. Fenster and T. M. Peters. Intraoperative US in Interactive Image-Guided Neurosurgery. *Radiographics* **18**:1019-1027, 1998.
8. W. Schroeder, K. W. Martin and W. Lorensen. *The Visualization Toolkit*, 2nd Edition. Prentice Hall, Toronto, 1998.
9. I. Mano, H. Goshima, M. Nambu and I. Masahiro. New Polyvinyl Alcohol Gel Material for MRI Phantoms. *Magnetic Resonance in Medicine* **3**: 921–926, 1986.

A Volumetric Optical Flow Method for Measurement of Brain Deformation from Intraoperative Magnetic Resonance Images

Nobuhiko Hata, Arya Nabavi, Simon Warfield, William Wells, Ron Kikinis, Ferenc A. Jolesz

Image-guided Therapy Program, Department of Radiology

Brigham and Women's Hospital and Harvard Medical School

75 Francis St., Boston, MA 02115, USA
{noby, navabi, warfield, sw, kikinis, jolesz}@bwh.harvard.edu

Abstract. : A method to measure spatial and temporal brain deformation from sequential intraoperative Magnetic Resonance Images (MRI) and its preliminary clinical results are reported. Deformation is estimated with a volumetric optical flow measurement based on local intensity differences. A multi-resolution approach was used to efficiently estimate the deformation. We applied the method to five different cases and the method is highlighted by illustrative features accompanied by five sets of intraoperative MRI scanned before and after dura opening, twice during tumor resection and immediately after dura closure. The maximum cortical surface shift measured was 11 mm and subsurface shift was 4 mm. Volume change was measured by aligning the sequence of intraoperative MR images immediately after the opening of the dura to the images during the tumor resection. The amount of deformation present at each stage of the surgery was visualized. The computed deformation field was most satisfactory when the skin was first segmented and removed from the images prior to the optical flow computation. Magnetic field inhomegeneities as well as administration of contrast agent (Gadolinium-DTPA) were observed to modify the deformation field. The method demonstrated a good capability of intra-operative surface, subsurface and midline shift measurement.

Introduction

The evolution of image-guided neurosurgery raises intraoperative brain shift as a problematic issue, since any spatial discrepancy between coregistered preoperative image and the shifted brain diminishes the accuracy of neuronaviagtion. Kato and Koivukangus [1, 2] pointed out, from their clinical experience with a neuronavigation system, that significant brain shift is observed after cerebrospinal fluid is drained and during tumor resection.

Ideally, more accurate and reliable image-guided-navigation, the preoperative image should be updated and deformed to reflect intraoperative shape change of the brain. This can be accomplished by performing deformable registration of pre- to intra-operative images.

This paper will introduce our approach to assess intra-cranial structural change by optical flow measurement. To gain true intraoperative observation of brain deformations, we performed brain surgeries in an intraoperative Magnetic Resonance Imaging scanner (Signa SP, General Electric Medical Systems, Milwaukee, WI). The scanner has two toroidal magnetic coils and allows access to the surgical field through a 56-cm gap between the magnet coils.

Methods

We developed a method to measure brain deformation from intensity change in sequential MR-images. Deformation is estimated with a volumetric optical flow measurement based on local intensity differences. A multi-resolution approach was used to efficiently estimate the deformation. The method was originally developed for two-dimensional image measurement, and we modified it to process volumetric images.

Optical flow is a method for computing a motion field from images and has been employed mostly in the computer vision and artificial intelligence community since the late 1970's. By definition, optical flow is image velocity approximating image motion from sequential time-ordered images. Optical flow has been applied to motion detection, segmentation and motion-compensated image encoding. Detailed comparison of various optical flow methods appears in Barron and Bauchemin's report [3].

The underlying assumption of optical flow is that image intensity E of a moving point (x,y,z) at a time point t is constant after a short duration of time δt. If a vector (u,v,w) represents a velocity of the point and the intensity of the point doesn't change over the time δt, we can formulate,

$$E(x+u\delta t, y+v\delta t, z+w\delta t, t+\delta t) = E(x,y,z,t) \tag{1}.$$

Assuming that the image intensity varies smoothly with x,y,z and t, we can use a first-order Taylor expansion of the left hand side of (1):

$$E(x,y,z,t) + u\delta t \frac{\partial E}{\partial x} + v\delta t \frac{\partial E}{\partial y} + w\delta t \frac{\partial E}{\partial z} + \delta t \frac{\partial E}{\partial t} \approx E(x,y,z,t) \tag{2}.$$

Dividing by δt, and abbreviating the first-order derivatives by using subscripts, we can obtain

$$E_x u + E_y v + E_z w + E_t = 0 \tag{3}$$

Equation (3) is the optical flow constraint equation to solve for (u,v,w). However, as is in two-dimensional cases, we cannot solve (u,v,w) in the direction of the iso-brightness contours, or along intensity gradient (details in [4] "the aperture problem").

We followed the approach of Horn and Shunck [4] for solving underdetermined optical flow problem.   We construct a total error measure $E(\alpha)$ as the spatial integral of two terms; the first term $E_o = \left(E_x u + E_y v + E_z w + E_t\right)^2$ is the square of the error   from   the   optical   flow   constraint   (3),   and   second   term $E_s = u_x^2 + u_y^2 + u_z^2 + v_x^2 + v_y^2 + v_z^2 + w_x^2 + w_y^2 + w_z^2$ is   a   penalty   that   encourages smoothness:

$$E(\alpha) = \iiint \left(E_o(x,y,z,t) + \alpha^2 E_s(x,y,z,t)\right) dxdydz \qquad (4).$$

α^2 is a relative weight of the two terms and determined by considering the signal-to-noise ration of the second term E_s.

The smoothness constraint E_s was derived from Horn and Shunck's smoothness constraint in the two-dimensional case [4]. The assumption here is that neighboring points on the objects have similar displacements.   We may solve (4) by the calculus of variations [5]. The Euler-Lagrange equations yield:

$$\nabla^2 u = \frac{1}{\alpha^2}(E_x u + E_y v + E_z w + E_t)E_x$$

$$\nabla^2 v = \frac{1}{\alpha^2}(E_x u + E_y v + E_z w + E_t)E_y \qquad (5)$$

$$\nabla^2 w = \frac{1}{\alpha^2}(E_x u + E_y v + E_z w + E_t)E_z$$

where ∇^2 is the Laplacian operator $\nabla^2 = \dfrac{\partial^2}{\partial x^2} + \dfrac{\partial^2}{\partial y^2} + \dfrac{\partial^2}{\partial z^2}$.

We approximate the Laplacians of u, v and w by

$$\nabla^2 u \approx \overline{u}_{i,j,k} - u_{i,j,k} \,, \nabla^2 v \approx \overline{v}_{i,j,k} - v_{i,j,k} \,, \nabla^2 w \approx \overline{w}_{i,j,k} - w_{i,j,k} \qquad (6)$$

where $\overline{u}_{i,j,k}, \overline{v}_{i,j,k}$ and $\overline{w}_{i,j,k}$ denote Gaussian weighted average ($\sigma = 0.75$) of the neighbor points around the point at (i,j,k).

Combining (5) with (6) and isolating u, v and w leads to

$$u = \overline{u} - \frac{E_x(E_x\overline{u} + E_y\overline{v} + E_z\overline{w} + E_t)}{\alpha^2 + E_x^2 + E_y^2 + E_z^2}$$

$$v = \overline{v} - \frac{E_y(E_x\overline{u} + E_y\overline{v} + E_z\overline{w} + E_t)}{\alpha^2 + E_x^2 + E_y^2 + E_z^2} \qquad (7)$$

$$w = \overline{w} - \frac{E_z(E_x\overline{u} + E_y\overline{v} + E_z\overline{w} + E_t)}{\alpha^2 + E_x^2 + E_y^2 + E_z^2}.$$

Equation (7) is a system of linear equations with about 10^8 variables. Direct matrix methods such as Gauss-Jordan are computationally expensive, so we use the iterative Gauss-Seidel method [6].

Using this method, the updated $(u^{n+1}, v^{n+1}, w^{n+1})$ is computed from $(\overline{u}^n, \overline{v}^n, \overline{w}^n)$ using the following iteration:

$$u^{n+1} = \bar{u}^n - \frac{E_x(E_x\bar{u}^n + E_y\bar{v}^n + E_z\bar{w}^n + E_t)}{\alpha^2 + E_x^2 + E_y^2 + E_z^2}$$

$$v^{n+1} = \bar{v}^n - \frac{E_y(E_x\bar{u}^n + E_y\bar{v}^n + E_z\bar{w}^n + E_t)}{\alpha^2 + E_x^2 + E_y^2 + E_z^2} \tag{8}$$

$$w^{n+1} = \bar{w}^n - \frac{E_z(E_x\bar{u}^n + E_y\bar{v}^n + E_z\bar{w}^n + E_t)}{\alpha^2 + E_x^2 + E_y^2 + E_z^2}.$$

E_x, E_y and E_z are approximations to the derivative and computed by averaging finite element differentials in two input images from intraoperative MRI, namely a *reference* image of the brain before deformation and a *target* image after a deformation, and applying Gaussian smoothing ($\sigma = 0.75$). We also approximated partial derivative of intensity over time E_t by subtracting the *reference* the *target* image and applying Gaussian smoothing ($\sigma = 0.75$).

We employed a hierarchical multi-resolution scheme to accommodate different scales of motions with computational efficiency. The multi-resolution speeds up the convergence of the iteration represented by (11). The resolution ratios from the original data are x1/8, x1/4, x1/2 and x1, by downsampling by a factor of two in the slice direction image and smoothing by a Gaussian filter kernel.

After 500 iterations in each resolution, or when convergence is observed, the estimated motion field is passed to the next resolution level using bilinear interpolation, and used as the next initial guess. α^2 was 0.1 in the experiments presented in this paper.

Results

We applied the method to five sets of clinical data both for the evaluation of the method and for quantitative and qualitative evaluation of brain deformation.

In each cases 3D volume SPGR (Spoiled gradient echo recovery) with 60 slices (TR: 28.6ms, TE: 12.8ms, FOV 240x240 mm, matrix 256x128, 1 NEX, 2.5 mm thickness/0 spacing) were obtained before and after dura opening, once or twice during tumor resection, and after dura closure (a total of five series per case). Note that all images are acquired during surgery in the interventional MRI scanner.

Volume change experiment

The first part of the test covered in this section is a volume change test with images from five clinical cases: #1 Lt. frontal mass, 47yo, male; #2 Rt. frontal mass, 49yo, female; #3 posterior fossa mass, 19yo male; #4 Rt. paretal mass, 53yo male; #5 Rt. frontal mass, 36yo, female.

The first part of the test covered in this section is a volume change test. In this test, volume change was measured by comparing the sequence of intraoperative MRI right after the opening of the dura (namely the *reference* data) to the image acquired in the beginning of tumor resection (namely the *target* data). We also measured the volume change after motion correction of *target* image. The motion correction was possible by applying the inverse deformation field (indicating displacement from the *target* data to the *reference* data) to the *target* image. We subtracted aligned *reference* images from *target* images in order to measure mismatched volume based on the intensity difference. From the subtraction images, we counted voxels with over a pre-defined intensity threshold computed from mean image intensity value of graymatter. This mean image intensity was computed from ten rectangular (10x10 pixels) regions randomly but manually selected from the *reference* images.

Average volume change was 10385 mm^3 and motion correction reduced the volume difference to 703mm^3. The result can be also interpreted that the optical flow measurement presented can detect at least 90% of deformation from sequential intraoperative MRI.

Brain deformation analysis

We performed clinical feasibility tests in all of the five cases with qualitative and quantitative analysis of the deformation. Five combinations of image sets are analyzed: (1st) image scanned before dura opening vs. after dura opening, (2nd and 3rd) before dura opening vs. during tumor resection, (4th) before dura opening vs. right after dura closure. This section presents case #4, which has illustrative findings.

Maximum cortical surface shift measured was 11 mm and subsurface shift around ventricle was 4 mm. Volume change was measured by aligning the sequence of intraoperative MRI before opening of the dura to the image acquired immediately after the dura is opened.

Figure 1 shows subtraction images and deformation vector map from case #4. Intraoperatively the cortex showed a consistent sinking, associated with cerebrospinal fluid (CSF) drainage and tumor removal. The elongation of the vectors was judged to depict the clinical finding of a consistent sinking of the cortex. The subsurface movement in the vicinity of the ventricles, away from the region of tumor resection is also detected in the right image.

Figure 2 shows sequential movements of randomly selected points along the gravity direction computed with the method (case #1). Two sites near the cortical surface and ventricle were selected from the image taken before the craniotomy; four points (6 mm apart) in each site were tracked using the volumetric optical flow. In Figure 2, the gravity-directional component of the displacement vectors shows local shifting near the cortex (maximum approximately -8 mm) and ventricle (approximately -2mm). The global shift was observed in the tissue within approximately 10 mm of the surface layer.

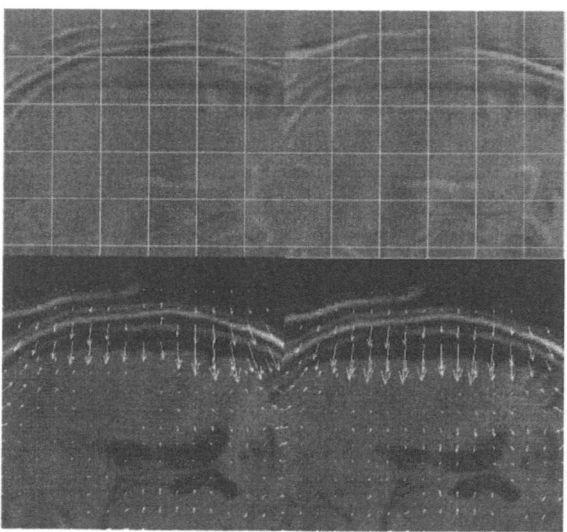

Fig. 1. Subtraction images (top left, after dura opening vs. before dura opening: top right, beginning of tumor resection vs. before dura opening) and deformation vector map (bottom left, after dura opening: bottom right, beginning of tumor resection.) from case #4. The elongation of the vectors depicts the clinical finding of a consistent sinking of the cortex. The subsurface movement in the vicinity of the ventricles, away from the region of tumor resection is also already detected in the right image.

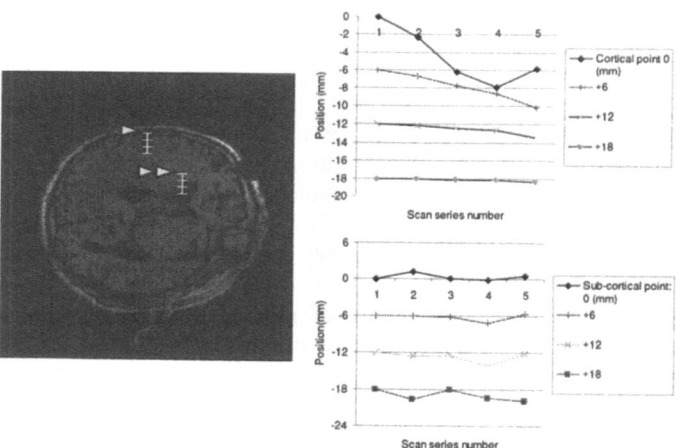

Fig. 2. The brain shift along the gravity direction by tracking four points (each 6 mm apart) at a cortical site (single arrow) and ventricular site (double arrow) with the volumetric optical flow (case #1). The volumetric optical flow of 1st and subsequent series (2nd ~ 5th) yields the displacement of selected points during the surgery.

Discussion

The method proposed in this paper is based on Horn and Shunck's two-dimensional optical flow measurement. We employed a similar smoothness term in the optimization: the sum of squares of partial derivatives of displacements with respect to axis of coordinates. The model applies when we can assume that neighboring displacements are similar, though some studies question this assumption in real camera imagery and proposed other methods with different smoothness constraints. Alternatively, we could employ a smoothness model based on the assumption that the brain deformation field is mostly continuous.

Trobaugh and Bucholz [9] investigated intra-operative brain shift by mounting an ultrasound probe on a tracking sensor and coregistering preoperative MR/CT with intraoperative ultrasound images. The registered ultrasound images were helpful to predict intraoperative brain deformation and update mismatched preoperative images. Another publication [10] discusses three categories of depth movements. Hill [11] and Robert [12] were among the first groups to tackle measurement and quantitative analysis of intraoperative brain surface shift. Hill reported a study measuring the deformation of the dura and brain surfaces between the time of imaging and the time right after dura opening and before resection. In the surgery, the patients were first registered to preoperative images by localizing fiducial markers and performing standard patient-image registration in an image-guided surgery system. Then, they measured the location of multiple points (approx. 60) on the brain surface to compare their position with respect to those in the preoperative images. They reported mean displacements of the brain surface of 5.6-mm before tumor resection. Roberts's study used a ceiling mounted robot microscope system to measure surface displacement during surgery. They determined mean displacement of approximately 10-mm and direction of movement is presumably in the gravity direction.

Freeborough, et. al., [13] measured brain deformation to track Alzheimer's disease by nonlinear registration modified from [14]. Maurer measured the brain shift from pre- and post-operative images scanned in interventional MR setting [15] by a voxel-similarity rigid registration by Studholme et. al. [16]. No qualitative findings about subsurface displacement were in their report except a preliminary result from three-dimensional B-spline-driven deformable registration.

Both the volume change test and clinical test indicated the proposed method is capable of capturing surface and sub-surface shift of the brain. It also enables the deformable registration of pre-deformation image to post-deformation images by applying the computed motion field to the pre-deformation images: such functionality provides the means to warp intra-operative images to match pre-operative images with finer anatomical and physiological imaging capability.

Acknowledgement

NH, RK and WW were in part supported by NSF funding "Engineering Research Center for Computer-Integrated Surgical Systems and Technology" # 9731748. AN was supported by the DFG Grant NA 359/1-1. SW was supported (in part) by grant from National Multiple Sclerosis Society.   WW was supported by Whitaker Foundation.

References

[1]   J. Koivukangas, Y. Louhisalmi, J. Alakuijala, and J. Oikarinen, "Ultrasound-controlled neuronavigator-guided brain surgery," *J Neurosurg*, vol. 79, pp. 36-42, 1993.

[2]   A. Kato, T. Yoshimine, T. Hayakawa, Y. Tomita, T. Ikeda, M. Mitomo, K. Harada, and H. Mogami, "A frameless, armless navigation system for computer-assisted neurosurgery," *J Neurosurg*, vol. 74, pp. 845-9, 1991.

[3]   J. L. Barron, D. J. Fleet, and S. S. Beauchemin, "Performance of optical flow techniques," *Intnational J. Comp. Vision*, vol. 12, pp. 43-77, 1994.

[4]   B. K. P. Horn and B. G. Schunck, "Determining optical flow," *AI*, vol. 17, pp. 185-204, 1986.

[5]   G. M. Ewing, *Calculus of Variations with Applications*. Mineola, NY: Dover Publications, 1985.

[6]   R. Hamming, *Numerical Methods for Scientists and Engineers*, 2nd ed. Mineola, NY: Dover Pubns, 1987.

[7]   P. A. Viola, "Alignment by Maximization of Mutual Information," in *Artificial Intelligence Laboratory*. Cambridge,MA: Massachusetts Institute of Technology, 1995, pp. 155.

[8]   W. M. Wells III, P. Viola, H. Atsumi, S. Nakajima, and R. Kikinis, "Multi-Modal Volume Registration by Maximization of Mutual Information," *Medical Image Analysis*, vol. 1, pp. 35-51, 1996.

[9]   J. W. Trobaugh, W. D. Richard, K. R. Smith, and R. D. Bucholz, "Frameless stereotactic ultrasonography: method and applications," *Comput Med Imaging Graph*, vol. 18, pp. 235-46, 1994.

[10]   R. Bucholtz, D. Y. J. Trobaugh, L. McDurmont, C. Sturm, C. Baumann, J. Henderson, A. Levy, and P. Kessman, "The correction of stereotactic inaccuracy by brain shift using an intraoperative ultrasound device," presented at CVRMed-MRCAS 97, Grenoble, France, 1997.

[11]   D. L. Hill, C. R. Maurer, Jr., R. J. Maciunas, J. A. Barwise, J. M. Fitzpatrick, and M. Y. Wang, "Measurement of intraoperative brain surface deformation under a craniotomy," *Neurosurgery*, vol. 43, pp. 514-26; discussion 527-8, 1998.

[12]   D. W. Roberts, A. Hartov, F. E. Kennedy, M. I. Miga, and K. D. Paulsen, "Intraoperative brain shift and deformation: a quantative analysis of cortical displacement in 28 cases," *Neurosurgery*, vol. 43, pp. 749-760, 1998.

[13]   P. A. Freeborough and N. C. Fox, "Modeling brain deformations in Alzheimer disease by fluid registration of serial 3D MR images," *J Comput Assist Tomogr*, vol. 22, pp. 838-43, 1998.

[14]   G. E. Chiristensen, R. D. Rabbitt, and M. I. Miller, "Deformable templates using large deformation kinematics," *IEEE Trans Image Proc*, vol. 5, pp. 1435-1447, 1996.

[15]   C. R. Maurer, D. L. G. Hill, A. J. Martin, H. Liu, M. McCue, D. Rueckert, D. Lloret, W. A. Hall, R. E. Maxwell, D. J. Hawkes, and C. L. Truwit, "Investigation of intraoperative brain deformation using a 1.5T interventional MR system: preliminary results," *IEEE Trans Med Img*, vol. 17, pp. 817-825, 1998.

[16]   C. Studholme, D. L. G. Hill, and D. J. Hawkes, "Automated 3D registration of truncated MR and CT images of the head," presented at British medicine vision conference, 1995.

Spotlights: A Robust Method for Surface-Based Registration in Orthopedic Surgery

B. Ma   R. E. Ellis   D. J. Fleet

Department of Computing and Information Science
Queen's University at Kingston, Ontario, Canada
Contact: ellis@cs.queensu.ca

Abstract. Fast, simple and effective registration methods are needed in a wide variety of computer-assisted surgical procedures in which readily locatable anatomical landmarks are not available. Surface-based least-squares registration methods can be used, but are susceptible to poor initial pose estimates and to error contamination during intraoperative data collection.

We have developed a fast, statistically robust method for surface-based registration during orthopedic surgery. The method, based on the iterative closest point (ICP) algorithm, fits a set of sparsely measured data points to a planar facet model. A first registration estimate is obtained by having the user contact the anatomy in a set of general anatomical regions (rather than contacting distinctive features). A small number of additional data points are acquired to refine the registration. Starting from the refined estimate, a robust scored perturbation method is used to find a better registration. This is followed by an M-estimate registration that is taken as the final registration. Simulation results show that this method is robust for data sets containing up to 25% gross outliers. The method has been tested *in vitro* on plastic bone models, where it outperformed the least-squares estimate and maintained the required 1mm/2° accuracy. The *in vivo* use of spotlights in computer-enhanced osteotomies of the knee have confirmed the usefulness of the method.

1 Introduction

Registration of a patient to a medical image is often performed by finding a rigid transformation that minimizes the squared residual error between the surgical points and points on a model derived from a 3D medical image. One widely cited surface-based registration method is the iterative-closest-point (ICP) method of Besl and McKay [2]. Two widely acknowledged problems with ICP-like surface registration methods are the need for a good initial estimate and that minimizing the sum-of-squared residual error is optimal only when the measurement errors have Gaussian distributions. If measurements are accidentally taken far from the target anatomy, a least-squares error measure can produce poor results.

Here we present a fast, robust method for surface-based registration that provides reliability and accuracy in the presence of spurious data. The user interface presents the surgeon with a visualization of the target anatomy in which restricted regions, termed *Spotlights*, are individually illuminated; Figure 1 shows an example surface mesh of the proximal tibia and four spotlight regions. Initial contact points, one from each region, are used to compute a registration. Additional points, collected from the exposed anatomy, are then used in a robustly perturbed M-estimation process to refine the final registration estimate. The principal contribution of this work is our consideration of the effects that

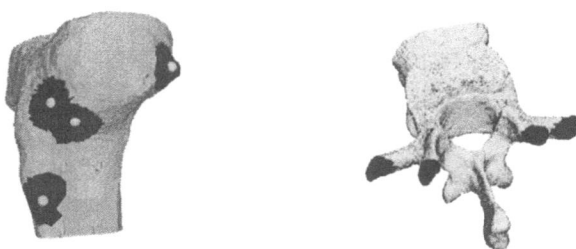

Fig. 1. CT-based surface meshes (not to scale) of a phantom tibia and vertebra, and spotlight regions for registration. The spheres mark the spotlight centers.

local-search methods have on the estimate of the registration. ICP, and previously investigated robust estimators, are susceptible to convergence on a local, non-global minimum. The method presented here is mathematically robust and was designed with the intent of avoiding false local convergence.

2   Robust Surface-Based Registration

Rigid-body surface-based registration is the process of finding a transformation from a set of measured points on the target anatomy to the model surface derived from medical images. Let $P = \{p_i\}$ be a set of n surface-data points measured from the target anatomy by the surgeon, let $X = \{x_i\}$ be the set of all points on the surface model, and let $T(\tau)z = R(\hat{q})z + t$ be a rigid transformation of a point z with pose parameters τ. The registration goal is to find both the rigid-body transformation T and some n-element subset Y of model surface locations X to which the target anatomy locations P project under T. The anatomical points P will not in general project exactly onto Y. A least-squares solution to the surface-based registration can be stated as the minimum, over τ and $Y \subseteq X$, of

$$F_2(\tau, Y) = \sum_{i=1}^{n} \|y_i - T(\tau)p_i\|^2 \tag{1}$$

where $y_i \in Y$. In the general case this is a non-convex minimization problem with multiple local minima.

Statisticians have long been aware of the need for robust methods of parameter estimation [9,14]. Robust methods have been applied widely in the computer vision community for many estimation problems, including pose estimation [6, 10, 11] which is mathematically similar to the registration problem. Grimson *et al.* [5] performed point-to-surface matching by progressively refining the registration using a series of objective functions. Although it was not stated explicitly, their final objective function is the Huber [9] estimate.

Many robust estimation techniques use *M-estimation*, in which the L_2 norm in (1) is replaced with a robust norm to yield an objective function of the form

$$F_M(\tau, Y) = \sum_{i=1}^{n} \rho(\boldsymbol{y}_i - T(\tau)\boldsymbol{p}_i; \sigma) \qquad (2)$$

where $\rho(r; \sigma)$ is the robust norm applied to the residual r, and σ is a scale parameter that depends on the form of the expected error distribution. One robust estimator that has reportedly provided good performance on 3D range data [13] is the Tukey biweight:

$$\rho(z; \sigma) = \begin{cases} \frac{\sigma^2}{2}(1 - (1 - \frac{z^2}{\sigma^2}))^3 & \text{if } z \le |\sigma| \\ \sigma^2/2 & \text{otherwise} \end{cases} \qquad (3)$$

We used ranked scores of perturbations of the least-squares estimator to improve the least-squares surface registration. We then used a robust M-estimator version of ICP to refine the registration further. These estimators form the basis of a fast and accurate method for surface-based registration.

The main stages of our surface-based registration method are

Spotlight: Surface data are gathered intraoperatively. The surgeon contacts points on the exposed anatomical regions that correspond to the spotlights shown on the model.

Centroid: The initial contact points are first matched to the spotlight *centroids* on the model using a simple least-squares minimization method [8].

Patch: The initial contact points are then matched to the spotlight *surface regions* on the model, using a least-squares ICP method.

Refinement: The surgeon then contacts another set of points on the exposed anatomical region. These locations should be chosen to cover the anatomy that will be involved in the image-guided surgery, and should provide sufficient translational and rotational constraints on the registration.

Perturbation: The initial registration is repeatedly perturbed, and residuals are calculated. The perturbation with the largest number of residuals that are all less than a user-supplied threshold is taken as the best registration estimate.

Final: The perturbation registration estimate is refined by use of an ICP algorithm that incorporates the robust Tukey-biweight M-estimator.

Each iteration of the ICP algorithm actually involves two estimation steps: given a registration estimate, one needs to find the set of closest points on the surface to the transformed data points. It is important that this search for the closest points be fast because it is one of the most computationally demanding steps of the algorithm. From these closest points on the surface, one then needs to update the registration estimate.

2.1 Finding Nearest Neighbors on a Surface Model

Given a transformation, at each iteration of the algorithm the ICP method requires solution of the nearest-neighbor problem: For each point p_i and a model X, the point x_i in X that is nearest to p_i under the transformation must be found. If X is a triangulated surface mesh then the facet containing x_i must be found so that x_i can be calculated. Exhaustive search over all facets is impractical for large models.

Although heuristics have been proposed for finding the facet containing the nearest point [1, 12], we can guarantee that a nearest neighbor is always found. For each model facet, we precompute the centroid and the largest centroid-to-vertex distance and record the largest centroid-to-vertex distance found over all facets, R, which is used to build a k-D tree from the facet centroids. To find a nearest neighbor, we first find the nearest centroid and compute its distance r. We then use the region search algorithm of [1] to find all facet centroids within the sphere of radius $R + r$ centered on the data point. Finally, we exhaustively search all returned facets to find the true nearest neighbor.

This algorithm can return a large number of facets, especially when the datum p_i is very far away from the model or if the model contains some unusually large facets. The requirement can be relaxed by limiting the number of returned facets to a fixed number. Compared to exhaustive search, reductions in computation time of more than two orders of magnitude were observed for models that contained tens of thousands of facets.

2.2 Robust Registration Estimation

A robust version of ICP was produced by modifying the process of updating the registration. This requires a solution to the absolute orientation problem, for which Horn's method provides a common least-squares solution.

To obtain an M-estimate of absolute orientation, we use an iteratively reweighted least-squares modification [7,6] of Horn's method [8]. The scale parameter σ in Equation (3), is estimated, following Rousseeuw [14], as a function of the parameters τ by using the median of absolute deviations of the residuals: $r_i(\tau) = y_i - T(\tau)p_i$:

$$\sigma = 1.4826 \underset{i=1..n}{\text{median}} \left(\|r_i(\tau)\| - \underset{j=1..n}{\text{median}}\|r_j(\tau)\| \right) \quad (4)$$

2.3 Refinement of Registration Using Perturbation

Even when started from a reasonable spotlight estimate, traditional ICP and simplistic robust variants suffer from "trapping" by converging to a local non-global minimum of the registration parameters. To alleviate trapping we locally explore the parameter space to find a better estimate, as suggested by Grimson *et al.* [5]. Our implementation explored the effect of rotational parameters on the estimate by assessing sixty-four uniformly distributed axes of rotation. The surgical data were rotated, about their mutual centroid, around each of these axes by ±3 degrees and residual errors were calculated. For each of the 128 rotations, if half of the transformed surgical data had residuals that were less than a provided threshold value (1 mm) then the rotation and maximum residual were noted.

The perturbation that produced the minimum maximum residual for at least half the surgical data was provided as the initial estimate for the final robust iterative calculation of the registration transformation.

3   *In Vitro* Experiments

One application of computer-enhanced orthopedic surgery is to the high tibial osteotomy, for which the surgical exposure is limited to the anterolateral aspect of the proximal tibia. The only distinctive landmarks are the tibial tubercle (which is concealed by the patellar tendon) and the fibular head (which is mobilized from the tibia by osteoclasis). Spotlight registration was examined as an alternative to fiducial registration, which is very accurate but invasive.

As a standard comparison, we also considered the procedure of pedicle-screw insertion into a lumber vertebra, for which the posterior aspect of the ends of the transverse and superior articular processes provide prominent landmarks.

3.1   Materials and Preparation

A plastic tibia and L1-vertebra (Sawbones, Vashon, WA) were instrumented with three titanium-alloy anchor screws of 1.9 mm diameter (Wright Medical Devices) that acted as fiducial markers. The phantoms were imaged by computed tomography, and decimated isosurface models were produced. The tibial mesh contained 34,537 vertices and 68,564 triangular faces, and the vertebral mesh contained 27,096 vertices and 54,904 faces. The fiducial locations in CT coordinates were found using a previously validated center-of-mass calculation [3] and the locations were verified with Roentgen stereogrammetric analysis.

The phantoms were fixed in frames and the fiducial markers were contacted using a six-degree-of-freedom mechanical pointer (FARO Technologies, Lake Mary, FL) to obtain a registration that bore a known error to ground truth [4]. For the tibial phantom, twelve 10 mm×10 mm squares were drawn on the surface in the area of typical surgical exposure and 100 data points were collected for each square, attempting to keep the datum spacing as uniform as possible. For the vertebral phantom, eight 8 mm×8 mm squares were drawn on the surface and data were collected as for the tibial phantom. Four spotlights of radius 10 mm were sampled with 100 data points each from the tibial phantom, and similarly for the vertebral phantom (with spotlights of radius 7.5 mm). Figure 1 shows the 3D tibial model and the spotlight locations.

3.2   Methods

A data set consisted of one point from each spotlight and one refinement point from each square on the surface, yielding a total of sixteen points for the tibial phantom and twelve points for the vertebral phantom. One thousand sets were randomly selected and assessed by six different methods. For all but Method 1, all data in the set were matched to the entire isosurface:

1. Paired-point least-squares registration of initial data to spotlight centers.
2. Scored perturbation registration, starting from the estimate of Method 1.
3. Robust Tukey-estimator registration, starting from the estimate of Method 2.
4. ICP least-squares registration, starting from the estimate of Method 1.
5. Robust Tukey-estimator registration, starting from the estimate of Method 1.
6. Robust Tukey-estimator registration, starting from the estimate of Method 4.

The purpose of Methods 1, 2, and 3 are to provide an overall estimate of robust registration. Method 4 is the traditional ICP registration, to which robust estimates can be compared (it also acts as an initial estimate for a robust estimates). Method 5 is a robust M-estimator started from a naive initial estimate, and Method 6 is a robust M-estimator started from an ICP estimate.

Traditionally the results of a registration with parameters τ are reported in terms of the root-mean-square of the residual errors between the data P and the nearest points $Y \subseteq X$ derived from the model points X. We have previously shown [4] that this fails to describe the errors arising from incorrect estimates of the rotational parameters, so we used an axis-angle decomposition for analysis.

Suppose that the ideal transformation is $T_I(\tau)$. One can form the *residual* transformation between a given $T(\tau)$ and the ideal $T_I(\tau)$ as

$$D(\tau) = T(\tau)T_I(\tau)^{-1}$$

The matrix R_D of the transformation $D(\tau)$ is a rotation about an axis k by an angle θ. This angle is the angular error of the given $T(\tau)$ and is important because the angular error produces an increasingly large positional error of a transformed point as the point is increasingly far from the region from which the registration was derived. By comparison the translational error, which is the translational component of $D(\tau)$, is constant for all points.

To compare the results of surface registrations to the fiducial registration, the surface registration was applied to the measured location of fiducial marker nearest to the spotlight centroid. The distance between the transformed marker and the CT coordinate of the fiducial location was then calculated. The ideal registration transformation is unknown, so $T_I(\tau)$ was taken to be a registration derived from the fiducial markers (which were adjacent to the spotlight regions).

3.3 Results

The experiments produced an ensemble of 1,000 registrations for analysis, which represent a sampling of how the spotlight registration to an anatomical region might perform in practice. For each registration in this ensemble we calculated the angular error as the rotational difference between the sample registration and the fiducial registration. Histograms of the registration results of each method were produced; results for the tibial phantom are shown in Figure 2.

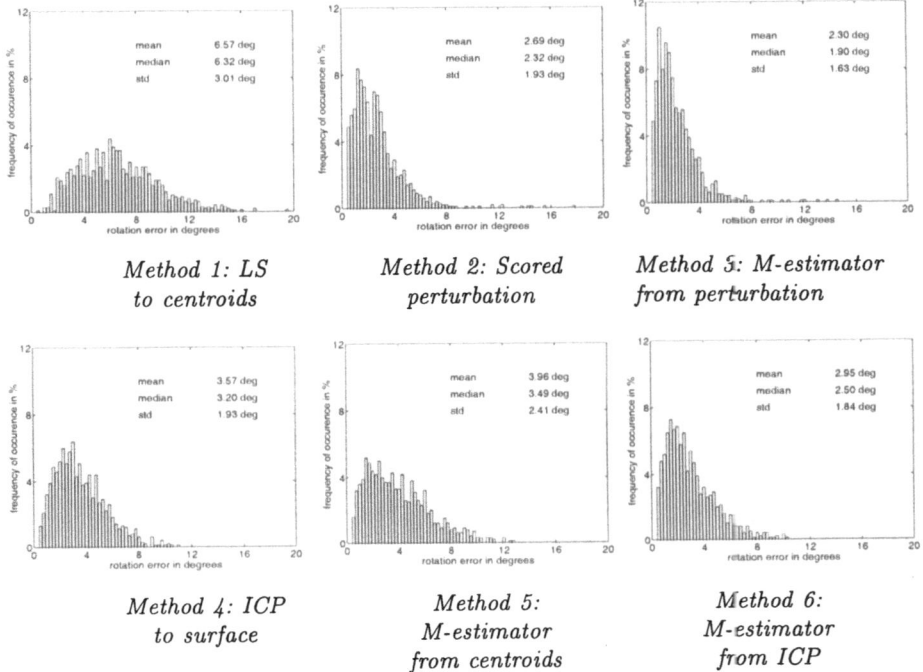

Method 1: LS
to centroids

Method 2: Scored
perturbation

Method 3: M-estimator
from perturbation

Method 4: ICP
to surface

Method 5:
M-estimator
from centroids

Method 6:
M-estimator
from ICP

Fig. 2. Tibial rotational errors from 1000 sets of physical surface data, 16 points per set. Rotational error was calculated as the maximum expected feasible deviation of nearby fiducial points.

4   An *In Vivo* Pilot Clinical Study

Spotlight registration has been conducted on six patients in Kingston General Hospital. Each patient presented with osteoarthritis confined to the medial tibiofemoral compartment and was deemed appropriate for high tibial osteotomy. Five of the six patients were instrumented with the type of fiducial markers used in the *in vitro* study. In each case the process of drilling 4mm Kirschner guide wires for a modified Coventry procedure was performed with the spotlight registration. Registration was validated visually by contacting bony surfaces both within and outside the spotlight regions, and by contacting the fiducial markers when they were present and unmoved by dissection.

The ultimate use of registration is in providing an appropriate treatment, so a standard outcome measure was used. Postoperative A/P radiographs were measured to determine the radiographic angle between the tibial plateau and the tibial shaft. From this angle was subtracted the intended correction angle. The resulting correction errors are tabulated in Table 1.

Table 1. Osteotomy correction errors arising from computer-enhanced surgery with spotlight registration.

Valgus correction error (degrees)	Patient Number					
	1	2	3	4	5	6
	$+1.5°$	$-1.5°$	$-1.5°$	$-1.5°$	$+0.5°$	$-1.0°$

5 Discussion

The *in vitro* results for the tibial phantom demonstrate the utility of robust registration, as well as the sensitivity of robust estimators to the choice of initial estimate. The final M-estimates of the registration had a median rotational error that was about 60% of the conventional ICP estimate. However, if the M-estimator was started from the ICP registrations then the error was a little less than 80% of the ICP estimate, which is significantly different from our method (#3) and from the ICP method (#4). Naive use of the M-estimator, starting it from a closed-form registration to the spotlight centroids, produced registrations for which the median rotational error was almost 10% larger than for ICP.

The *in vitro* results for the vertebral phantom showed that ICP produced accurate registrations, with a median rotational error of slightly more than 2°. With our robust method, starting the M-estimator from ICP produced a stable result for which the median error was about 10% less than that of ICP. This suggests that, for surfaces with numerous distinctive features, traditional least-squares surface registration may be adequate.

The *in vivo* results measure the accuracy of the entire process of computer-enhanced surgery: CT, isosurface extraction, decimation, computer-based planning, registration, the physical processes of resection and reduction, and angular measurement from plain radiographs. The maximum error of 2° in the pilot study compares very favorably with the results by traditional methods.

The main contributions of this work are the development of an intraoperative data-collection scheme that is easy to use, and the implementation of a pair of robust statistical methods for estimating 3D surface registration. The methods have been tested extensively in the laboratory and have been used in early clinical trials. The registration codes run in a few seconds on common UNIX workstations.

Robust statistical methods are important for registration because they provide a sound mathematical basis for attenuating the influence of spurious data. For intraoperative use we suggest that they are superior to manual editing of the data and to *ad hoc* methods of attenuation. However, the implementation of robust methods requires care: robust methods, like nonlinear least-squares methods, can converge to local non-global minima.

Robust surface registration is potentially useful in computer-enhanced surgery. The local nature of the search still leaves the method subject to "trapping", and we recommend that such methods continue to undergo visual verification by the surgeon until validated global registration methods are devised.

Acknowledgments

This research was supported in part by Communications and Information Technology Ontario, the Institute for Robotics and Intelligent Systems, the Natural Sciences and Engineering Research Council, and by an Alfred P. Sloan Research Fellowship to DJF. Interventional procedures were performed in Kingston General Hospital by Dr. Paul Fenton, Dr. Mark Harrison, and Dr John Rudan.

References

1. J. L. Bentley. "Multidimensional binary search trees used for associative searching". *Communications of the ACM*, 18(9):509–517, September 1975.
2. P. J. Besl and N. D. McKay. "A method for registration of 3-d shapes". *IEEE Transactions on Pattern Analysis and Machine Intelligence*, 14(2):239–256, February 1992.
3. R. E. Ellis, S. Toksvig-Larsen, M. Marcacci, D. Caramella, and M. Fadda. "Use of a biocompatible fiducial marker in evaluating the accuracy of ct image registration". *Investigative Radiology*, 31(10):658–667, October 1996.
4. R. E. Ellis, D. J. Fleet, J. T. Bryant, J. Rudan, and P. Fenton. "A method for evaluating ct-based surgical registration". In J. Troccaz, E. Grimson, and R. Mösges, editors, *CVRMed-MRCAS'97*, pages 141–150. Springer-Verlag, March 1997.
5. W. E. L. Grimson, G. J. Ettinger, S. J. White, P. L. Gleason, T. Lozano-Pérez, W. M. W. III, and R. Kikinis. "Evaluating and validating an automated registration system for enhanced reality visiualization in surgery". In N. Ayache, editor, *Computer Vision, Virtual Reality and Robotics in Medicine*, pages 3–12. Springer-Verlag, April 1995.
6. R. M. Haralick, H. Joo, C. Lee, X. Zhuang, V. G. Vaidya, and M. B. Kim. "Pose estimation from corresponding point data". In H. Freeman, editor, *Machine Vision for Inspection and Measurement*. Academic Press, Inc., 1989, pages 1–84.
7. D. C. Hoaglin, F. Mosteller, and J. W. Tukey, editors. *Understanding Robust and Exploratory Data Analysis*. John Wiley & Sons, 1983.
8. B. K. P. Horn. "Closed-form solution of absolute orientation using unit quaternions". *Journal of the Optical Society of America A*, 4(4):629–642, April 1987.
9. P. J. Huber. *Robust Statistics*. John Wiley & Sons, 1981.
10. R. Kumar and A. R. Hanson. "Analysis of different robust methods for pose refinement". In *International Workshop on Robust Computer Vision*, 1990.
11. T. Masuda and N. Yokoya. "A robust method for registration and segmentation of multiple range images". *Computer Vision and Image Understanding*, 61(3):295–307, May 1995.
12. C. R. Maurer, J. M. Fitzpatrick, R. J. Maciunas, and G. S. Allen. "Registration of 3-d images using weighted geometrical features". *IEEE Transactions on Medical Imaging*, 15(6):836–849, December 1996.
13. M. J. Mirza and K. L. Boyer. "Performance evaluation of a class of m-estimators for surface parameter estimation in noisy range data". *IEEE Transactions on Robotics and Automation*, 9(1):75–85, February 1993.
14. P. J. Rousseeuw and A. M. Leroy. *Robust Regression and Outlier Detection*. John Wiley & Sons, 1987.

Automated Registration and Fusion of Functional and Anatomical MRI for Navigated Neurosurgery

T. Rohlfing[1], J. Beier[1], J. B. West[2],
U.-W. Thomale[3], T. Liebig[1], and C. A. Taschner[1]

[1] Department of Radiology, Charité, Campus Virchow-Hospital,
Medical Faculty of Humboldt-University Berlin,
Augustenburger Platz 1, D-13353 Berlin, Germany
{torsten.rohlfing,juergen.beier,thomas.liebig,
christian.taschner}@charite.de
[2] Department of Computer Science, Vanderbilt University,
Nashville, TN, U.S.A.
jayw@vuse.vanderbilt.edu
[3] Department of Neurosurgery, Charité, Campus Virchow-Hospital,
Medical Faculty of Humboldt-University Berlin,
Augustenburger Platz 1, D-13353 Berlin, Germany
uthomale@charite.de

Abstract. A procedure for acquisition, automated registration and fusion of functional and anatomical magnetic resonance images (MRI) is presented and validated. The technique is based upon the acquisition of high-resolution anatomical slices at the same spatial locations as functional images (5 slices). The accuracy of registration of these slices and high-resolution 3D MRI volumes (MP-RAGE imaging) was quantified using adapted data originating from the Vanderbilt retrospective registration project (8 patients). Selecting a subset of slices from that data, the small number of images available from fMRI acquisition was taken into account. Quantitative analysis showed no loss of accuracy caused by the reduced number of slices used for registration. For real patient data, fMRI were fused with MP-RAGE images, thus integrating anatomical images with information about locations of functional areas. Via a case study, the benefits of the described approach for intraoperative navigation using an operating microscope (MKM, Zeiss) are demonstrated.

1 Introduction

Intraoperative navigation in neurosurgery requires knowledge of the exact positions of lesions. In addition, information about the locations of certain functions areas in the operating region helps to protect these risk structures from accidental damage.

Positron emission tomography (PET) and single photon emission tomography (SPECT) deliver suitable information by displaying the spatial distribution of radionuclides inside the patient's body. These nuclides are attached to substances like glucose, and their concentration provides information about local metabolic activity.

An alternative to these techniques is based upon the so-called "BOLD effect" (Blood Oxygenation Level Dependency). MRI gradient echo sequences (e.g. T2*-weighted) are sensitive to blood oxygenation. Exploiting this dependency, functional MRI (fMRI, cf. [1]) is computed from a sequence of plain MRI images. In order to do this, the pixel intensities of the images are correlated with excitations of certain areas of interest.

While PET and SPECT are primarily useful for locating brain lesions, fMRI identifies healthy functional areas of the brain. Using this information, therapy can be planned in such a way as to interfere with these areas as little as possible. For these reasons it is desirable to integrate fMRI rather than PET into the process of planning neurosurgical interventions. Even more benefit is to be expected if fMRI data is also available for navigation during surgery, thus enabling the surgeon to assess the locations of access paths and resections in relation to certain functional regions to be protected [2].

Another advantage of fMRI becomes recognizable as soon as fusion with other modalities is performed, in particular those that display anatomical information. Integrated into the acquisition process, high resolution anatomical slices are collected at the same locations as the fMRI slices.

Voxel-based automatic registration algorithms can then be employed for robust correlation of these slices with another anatomical imaging modality. Such an anatomical-to-anatomical registration is usually easier to achieve than registration of fundamentally different functional and anatomical images.

The present paper first describes the process of data acquisition based upon this principle. Subsequent registration and image fusion of MRI and fMRI are presented next. Registration accuracy is assessed using an adapted set of images originating from the Vanderbilt retrospective registration project [3]. Finally, a patient case is presented, demonstrating the application of the described techniques to intraoperative navigation in neurosurgery.

2   Materials and Methods

2.1   Image Acquisition

MRI data originated from a 1.5T MRI scanner (Gyroscan ACS NT, Philips, Best, The Netherlands). Three different data sets are required:

(*I*) For fMRI computation, 5 slices of T2*-weighted MRI were repeatedly collected using a fast gradient echo sequence. Imaging parameters were: pixel size 1.80 mm×1.80 mm (128×128 pixels), slice thickness 7.0 mm, no gaps. Functional MRI images were computed using evaluation software provided by Philips (Brain Activation Processing Tool, Release 6.1). Functional regions of interest were then identified in fMRI and transferred to one of the original T2*-weighted images (Figure 2).

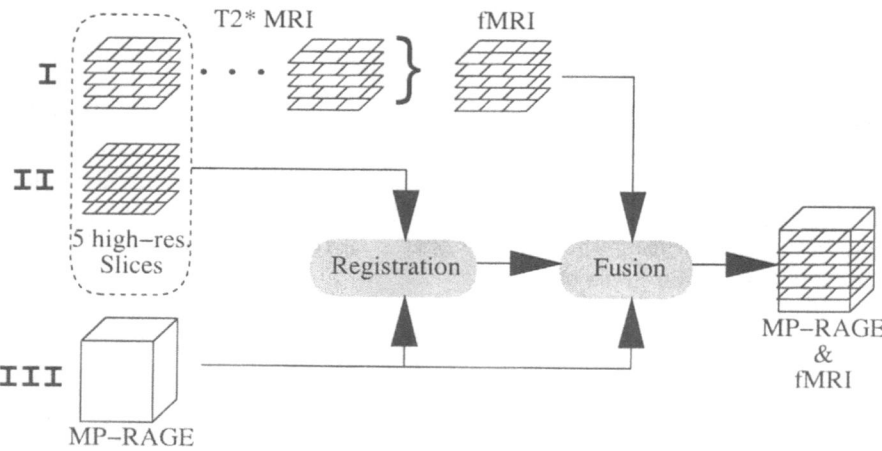

Fig. 1. Flow of image data through the registration and fusion process. A set of 5 T2*-weighted MRI images (*I*) is acquired repeatedly. From this sequence, fMRI images are computed. In addition, 5 high-resolution anatomical images (*II*) are collected at the same locations. These are registered to an MP-RAGE volume (*III*). For fusion with the MP-RAGE data, the resulting transformation can be applied to fMRI as well, because the spatial locations of fMRI slices are identical to those of the T2*-weighted slices as well as the additional anatomical slices.

(*II*) For registration an additional set of 5 anatomical slices was collected. These were measured immediately after the T2*-weighted series and at the very same spatial locations (Figure 2). Parameters for these slices were: pixel size 0.45 mm×0.45 mm (512×512 pixels), slice thickness 7.0 mm, no gaps.

(*III*) For navigation, high-resolution MRI data was collected using an MP-RAGE sequence (called 3D-FFE on Philips scanners). Typical acquisition parameters were: pixel size 0.45 mm×0.45 mm (512×512 pixels), 160 slices, slice thickness 1.0 mm, no gaps.

2.2 Image Processing

As mentioned above, fMRI images were computed from a series of T2*-weighted MRI volumes with a set of equivalent high-resolution slices measured immediately afterwards. For this reason, there is a trivial spatial relationship of functional and anatomical images (Figure 2). This is exploited for registration of fMRI to other anatomical imaging modalities as well. In the present paper for instance, this is a full MP-RAGE volume. Figure 1 illustrates the process.

Registration was performed by optimization of the normalized mutual information similarity measure [4]. The optimum rigid-body transformation was determined by an independent implementation of a multiresolution search algorithm similar to that described in [5]. Afterwards, MP-RAGE and fMRI were fused by an overlay-based technique previously applied to CT and MRI [6, 7].

Patient ID	101	102	104	105	106	107	108	109	
Slices	28-36	28-36	24-32	24-32	32-40	16-24	24-32	24-32	
Offset	81	81	69	69	93	45	69	69	[mm]

Table 1. Selected slices and z-translation offsets for the patients from the Vanderbilt data used for registration accuracy assessment. Every other slice in the range given for each patient was contained in the sparse T2-weighted image (indexing starts with slice #1). To compensate for this modification, the offsets in the second table row were added to the z-translation component of the resulting registration transformations. There original number of slices was 52 for all patients. Patient 103 is not included because no T2-weighted data was available for this patient.

The resulting images showed the ROIs defined in fMRI and the unaltered MP-RAGE data where no ROI was present (Figure 4).

2.3   Validation of Registration Accuracy

Accuracy of image registration was assessed using data originating from the Vanderbilt retrospective registration project [3]. As gold-standard transformations based on bone-implanted fiducial markers [8] are known for that data, the accuracy of the automatic registration algorithm could be quantified. From the data provided by that project, T2-weighted MRI to MP-RAGE registration was chosen to represent the situation of the present study. T2-weighted images were used, because they best matched the properties of the images used for fMRI computation.

From fMRI acquisition as described in section 2.1, only five anatomical MRI slices corresponding to fMRI were available for registration. To reflect this in the registration accuracy assessment, the original T2-weighted volumes of the Vanderbilt data (52 slices) were reduced accordingly. In particular, a subset of only five images with a uniform spacing of 6 mm (twice the original spacing) was selected from the original T2-weighted data. This was done to match the 7 mm spacing of fMRI data as closely as possible without having to apply inter-slice interpolation. Matrix size and pixel calibration of the original images remained unmodified.

In order to focus on regions of diagnostic interest, the range of remaining slices was chosen in such a way as to cover lesions identified independently for each of the patients. Table 1 gives the details about which slices were used from the T2-weighted data of the respective patients. It also contains information about how the resulting transformations had to be processed to be comparable to the available gold-standard registrations.

2.4   Surgical Navigation

After fusion, the resulting images were reformatted to slice images spatially equivalent to the slices of the original MP-RAGE volume. These were written to

Patient ID	101	102	104	105	107	108	109	total	
	mean	2.78	1.81	1.90	2.54	3.43	2.51	2.68	2.59	[mm]
Complete	median	2.81	1.84	1.93	2.55	3.41	2.43	2.74	2.67	[mm]
	max	2.95	1.92	2.55	2.77	4.13	3.33	3.37	4.13	[mm]
	mean	2.39	1.33	1.17	2.38	3.99	2.07	2.08	2.20	[mm]
Sparse	median	2.44	1.29	1.18	2.40	4.05	2.11	2.11	2.16	[mm]
	max	2.98	1.79	1.39	2.51	4.51	2.45	2.46	4.51	[mm]

Table 2. Registration errors compared to the gold-standard for each patient and averaged over all patients (rightmost column). The upper three rows give the results for complete (52 slices, spacing 3mm) data. Below are the results for sparse (5 slices, spacing 6mm) data. Complying with the policy of the original Vanderbilt study, patient 106 was omitted as visual inspection revealed a failed registration.

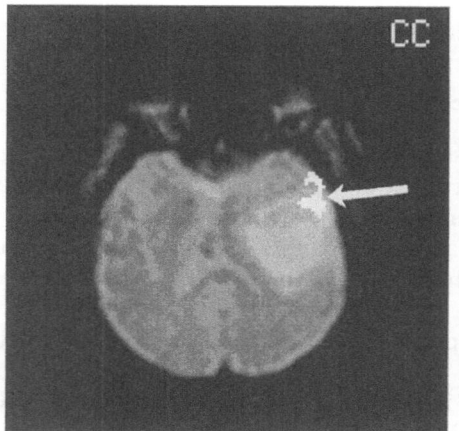 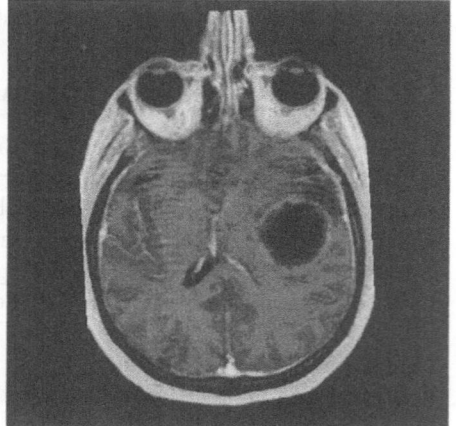

Fig. 2. *Left:* One of the T2*-weighted MRI images with overlaid functional information. The white area (*arrow*) adjacent to the cystic glioma represents Broca's area (motor speech center) identified in fMRI. *Right:* High-resolution anatomical slice measured at the same location.

DICOM files and subsequently communicated to an MKM operating microscope (Zeiss, Oberkochen, Germany) via campus-wide LAN. There, they were used for target definition as well as for intraoperative navigation (Figure 4).

3   Results

Registration Accuracy Assessment. The accuracy assessment results for registration of original and sparse Vanderbilt data are presented in Table 2. T2-weighted to MP-RAGE registration accuracy was not appreciably worse using only 5 slices. In fact, accuracy in terms of median errors was found to be even better in 6/7 cases using sparse data than it was with the complete set of T2 slices considered.

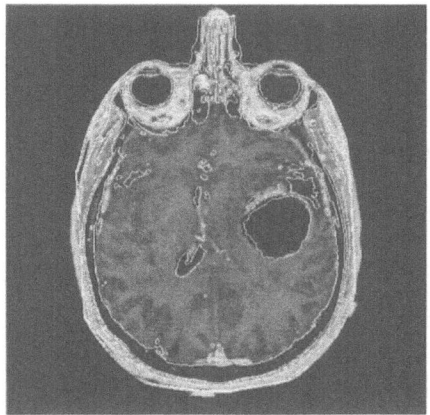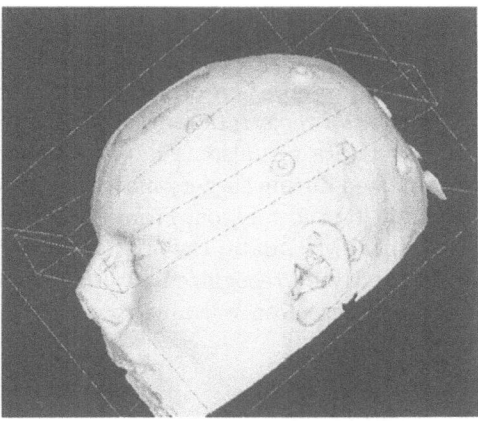

Fig. 3. Multi-modality images demonstrating registration accuracy of MP-RAGE and fMRI. *Left:* MP-RAGE slice overlaid with isolines generated from the accordingly reformatted T2*-weighted image used for fMRI computation. *Right:* spatial relationship of both modalities in 3D space. Bounding boxes represent the extents of MP-RAGE and fMRI volumes. The skin surface was computed by isosurface generation from the MP-RAGE data. On the back of the patient's head, the fiducials used for patient-to-data registration can be seen.

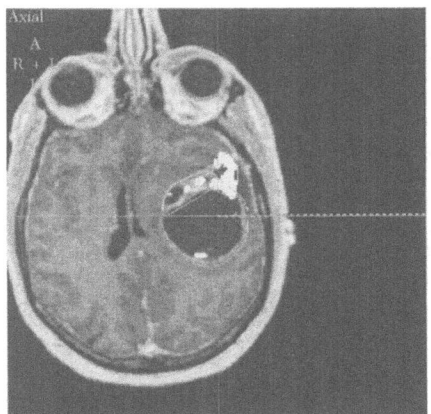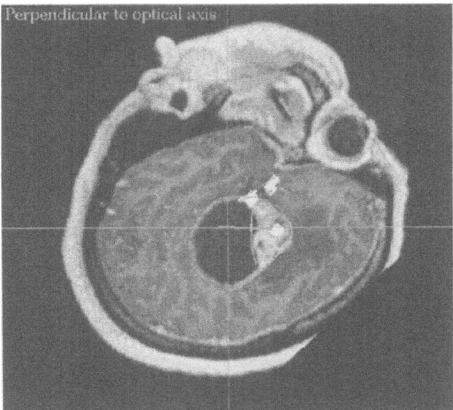

Fig. 4. Fused images corresponding to the operating region. During surgery, the axial image on the left was reformatted along the optical axis (*dashed line*) of the MKM operating microscope. *Right:* Corresponding image reformatted perpendicular to the optical axis is displayed. The cross in the right image represents the exact position the microscope was focused upon when the images were generated. In addition, during surgery planning contours outlining tumor and Broca's area had been defined. These were also overlaid on the microscope view presented to the surgeon for orientation during the intervention.

Case Report. The procedure described above was applied to a patient suffering from a grade II-III (biopsy proved state III) cystic glioma. The anatomical and functional MRI images of this patient are shown in Figure 2. In Figure 3, a combined presentation of MP-RAGE and T2*-weighted MRI provides a visual impression of registration accuracy for this particular patient.

Fused data was also used for navigation during surgery. Figure 4 shows slices reformatted during surgery matching the current location in the operating region looked at by the surgeon. From the ROIs defined in fMRI and overlaid upon the anatomical MRI data, the spatial relationship of tumor, cyst, and Broca's area could clearly be recognized. By this presentation, the neurosurgeon performing the tumor resection was able to minimize damage to the patient's motor speech area.

4   Discussion

A major advantage of fMRI is its inherent support for acquisition of spatially equivalent morphological images. Automated image registration with voxel-based techniques could therefore be performed with high reliability and accuracy.

Using the Vanderbilt data, accuracies found for sparse (5 slices) T2-weighted data were similar to those achieved using the complete set (52 slices) of images. Therefore, the small number of slices available did not impose a severe restriction to accuracy and reliability of the registration (cf. Table 2). The only failed registration (patient 106) could easily be identified by visual inspection. For real patients, this could be compensated for by repeating registration after manual determination of an initial registration estimate.

Two additional facts likely to have caused a decrease in registration accuracy using the Vanderbilt data should also be mentioned. First, in the application described the imaging properties of both data sets (T1-weighted and MP-RAGE MRI) are more similar to each other than the respective Vanderbilt images.

Second, registration accuracy was evaluated for a set of volumes of interest (VOIs) defined in the original images (cf. [3]). A large number of these VOIs, however, was no longer present in the sparse data. Therefore, VOIs neither available for registration, nor contributing to the resulting fusionated images may have caused accuracy to appear worse than it actually was.

5   Conclusions

This paper has demonstrated that the close connection of anatomical and functional MRI imaging can be exploited for easy registration and fusion of both. By comparison to gold-standard transformations in a similar context (Vanderbilt study), registrations using a limited number of slices did not decrease registration accuracy.

Integration of image acquisition, processing, and surgical navigation into a common schedule allowed routine application of the techniques presented. Therefore, usage of functional MRI provides a promising method of gaining insight into relation of anatomical and functional brain structures during navigated neurosurgery.

6 Acknowledgements

This work was funded by Deutsche Forschungsgemeinschaft (DFG), Graduate School 331. For their generous support in doing this research, the authors would like to thank Prof. Dr. Dr. R. Felix, MD (Director of Department of Radiology, Virchow-Hospital), Prof. Dr. W. Lanksch (Director of Department of Neurosurgery, Virchow-Hospital), and Prof. Dr. N. Hosten, MD (Scientific coordinator of Graduate School 331). The images and the standard transformations for registration accuracy assessment were provided as part of the project, "Evaluation of Retrospective Image Registration", National Institutes of Health, Project Number 1 R01 NS33926-02, Principal Investigator, J. Michael Fitzpatrick, Vanderbilt University, Nashville, TN.

References

1. J. Frahm, H. Bruhn, K. D. Merboldt, and W. Hanicke. Dynamic MR imaging of human brain oxygenation during rest and photic stimulation. *J Magn Reson Imaging*, 2(5):501–505, September 1992.
2. U.-W. Thomale, T. Liebig, C. Taschner, T. Rohlfing, J. Beier, A. Rosenthal, et al. Integration of functional MRI data in computer assisted surgery. In H. U. Lemke et al., editors, *Computer Assisted Radiology and Surgery*. Elsevier, June 1999.
3. J. West, J. M. Fitzpatrick, M. Y. Wang, B. M. Dawant, C. R. Maurer Jr, R. M. Kessler, et al. Comparison and Evaluation of Retrospective Intermodality Brain Image Registration Techniques. *J Comput Assist Tomogr*, 21(4):554–566, 1997.
4. C. Studholme, D. L. G. Hill, and D. J. Hawkes. An overlap invariant entropy measure of 3D medical image alignment. *Pattern Recognition*, 32:71–86, 1998.
5. C. Studholme, D. L .G. Hill, and D. J. Hawkes. Automated three-dimensional registration of magnetic resonance and positron emission tomography brain images by multiresolution optimization of voxel similarity measures. *Med Phys*, 24(1):25–35, January 1997.
6. D. L. Hill, D. J. Hawkes, J. E. Crossman, M. J. Gleeson, T. C. Cox, E. E. Bracey, et al. Registration of MR and CT images for skull base surgery using point-like anatomical features. *Br J Radiol*, 64(767):1030–1035, November 1991.
7. N. Hosten, T. Rohlfing, J. Beier, T. Liebig, W. Lanksch, and R. Felix. Registration of CT and MRT images for navigation in image-guided brain surgery. *Radiology*, 209 (P):206, November 1998.
8. C. R. Maurer, Jr, J. M. Fitzpatrick, M. Y. Wang, R. L. Galloway, Jr, R. J. Maciunas, and G. S. Allen. Registration of head volume images using implantable fiducial markers. *IEEE Trans Med Imaging*, 16(4):447–462, August 1997.

AcouStick: A Tracked A-Mode Ultrasonography System for Registration in Image-Guided Surgery

Calvin R. Maurer, Jr.[1,2], Ronald P. Gaston[2], Derek L. G. Hill[2], Michael J. Gleeson[3], M. Graeme Taylor[2], Michael R. Fenlon[4], Philip J. Edwards[2], and David J. Hawkes[2]

[1] Departments of Neurological Surgery and Biomedical Engineering, University of Rochester, 601 Elmwood Avenue, Box 670, Rochester, NY 14642, U.S.A.
Calvin_Maurer@URMC.Rochester.edu
[2] Division of Radiological Sciences and Medical Engineering, King's College London, 5th Floor Thomas Guy House, Guy's Hospital, London SE1 9RT, U.K.
David.Hawkes@KCL.ac.uk
[3] Department of Surgery, King's College London, Guy's Hospital, London, U.K.
[4] Department of Prosthetic Dentistry, King's College London, Guy's Hospital, London, U.K.

Abstract. In this paper, we describe a system for noninvasively determining bone surface points using an optically tracked A-mode ultrasound transducer. We develop and validate a calibration method; acquire cranial surface points for a skull phantom, three volunteers, and one patient; and register these points to surfaces extracted from CT images of the phantom and patient. Our results suggest that the bone surface point localization error of this system is less than 0.5 mm. The target registration error (TRE) of the cranial surface-based registration for the skull phantom was computed by using as a reference gold standard the point-based registration obtained with eight bone-implanted markers. The mean TRE for a 150-surface-point registration is 1.0 mm, and ranges between 1.0 and 1.7 mm for six 25-surface-point registrations. Our preliminary results suggest that accurate, noninvasive, image-to-physical registration of head images may be possible using an A-mode ultrasound-based system.

1 Introduction

Registration of preoperative images with the physical space occupied by the patient during surgery is a fundamental step in image-guided surgery. Image-to-physical space registration is commonly performed using stereotactic frame systems, points, and surfaces. Point-based registration can be accomplished using external anatomic landmarks (e.g., internal and external canthi, nasion, tragus), skin-affixed markers, and bone-implanted markers. Surface-based registration is generally accomplished using the air-skin interface. Registration using the bone surface could remove errors due to deformation of the skin surface between scanning and the operation.

In this paper, we describe a system for noninvasively determining cranial surface points using an optically tracked A-mode ultrasound transducer. These points can be used to perform surface-based image-to-physical registration of three-dimensional (3-D) head images. We develop and validate a calibration method; acquire cranial surface points for a skull phantom, three volunteers, and one patient; and register these points to surfaces extracted from CT images of the phantom and patient.

2   Methods

2.1   System Overview

In pulse echo ultrasound, a short pulse of energy is transmitted into the body. Echoes in the received signal represent sound reflected at interfaces between regions of different acoustic impedance. The intensity reflection coefficient, which is the ratio of the pressure reflected to the pressure incident, is less than 0.1 for most soft tissue interfaces, and is approximately 0.6–0.7 for bone-tissue interfaces [8]. Thus echoes corresponding to bone-tissue interfaces have high signal amplitude and are easily identified. The distance from the transducer to the interface corresponding to an echo is easily calculated as $d = ut/2$, where d is the distance, u is the speed of sound, and t is the time interval between the initial sound pulse and the received echo. Thus our aim is to track the position of an ultrasound transducer and calculate the position of a bone surface point as the position of the transducer face plus the distance to the bone-tissue interface along the ultrasound beam axis.

We use a heavily damped, spherically focused, 10 MHz A-mode ultrasound immersion transducer (part number V312, Panametrics, Waltham, MA). The nominal element size is 6 mm and the focal length in water at 22 °C is approximately 19 mm. The -6 dB beam width at the focal point is 0.4 mm. The -6 dB depth of field is 10 mm.

The transducer is driven with an ultrasonic pulser/receiver (model 5072PR, Panametrics). The damping is set to 50 ohm. The amplifier gain is varied between 0 and 20 dB as necessary to maximize reflected signal amplitude without clipping. The pulse repetition frequency is set to 100 Hz. The pulser/receiver output is connected to a 12-bit, 80 MHz analog-to-digital (A/D) data acquisition board (CompuScope 8012/PCI, Gage, Montreal, Canada) placed in a PC running Windows NT. The A/D board is operated in single-channel capture mode with a sampling rate of 80 MHz. The input voltage range is ±1 V and the input signal is DC coupled. Signal acquisition is controlled by a program written in Microsoft C++ using the win32 API. The A/D board is programmed to collect data continuously and store a fixed number of samples in a circular buffer after a trigger event is detected. The trigger level is set at 500 mV with a positive trigger slope. This provides a reliable and reproducible trigger on the initial signal of the pulser/receiver pulse. We store 8192 samples (102 μs) per pulse. This corresponds to 79 mm if the speed of sound is 1540 m/s.

The ultrasound transducer is optically tracked using an Optotrak 3020 system (Northern Digital, Inc., Waterloo, Ontario, Canada). Twenty infrared light-emitting diodes (IREDs) are mounted on a plastic cylindrical housing attached to a UHF-to-UHF connector (immersion search tube, part number F112, Panametrics) that is screwed into the back of the transducer.

A plastic (polyetherimide, Ultem, General Electric) offset is attached to the transducer. Polyetherimide was used because it can be autoclaved. The tip of the offset is adjustable. It is normally set at about 15 mm from the transducer face so that the transducer focal point is approximately at the cranial surface. The offset is filled with water during data collection and has a hole in the tip for water coupling at the skin surface. The ultrasound transducer, the array of IREDs, and the offset are shown in Fig. 1.

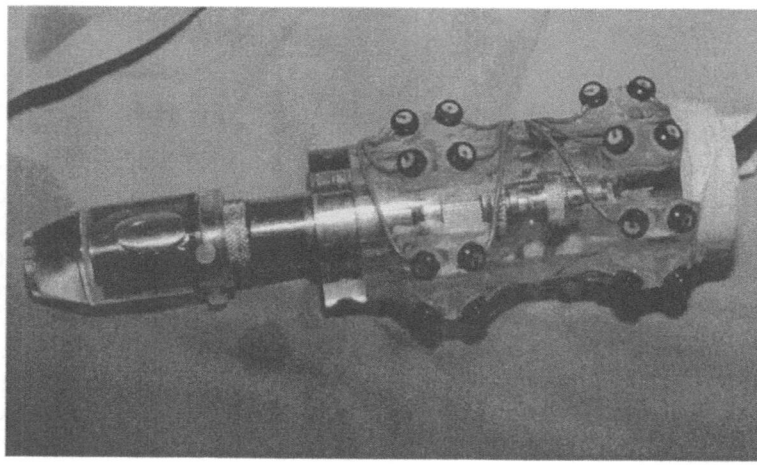

Fig. 1. Photograph showing the A-mode ultrasound transducer, the array of attached IREDs, and the offset.

Echo locations in the received ultrasound signal are determined using the Hilbert transform. The envelope of the received signal is calculated as the magnitude of the analytic signal. The analytic signal of $x(t)$ is the complex signal that has $x(t)$ as its real part and the Hilbert transform of $x(t)$ as its imaginary part. The Hilbert transform is related to the actual data by a $\pi/2$ phase shift. We compute the Hilbert transform in the time domain using a finite-impulse response (moving average) filter of order 60. The filter coefficients were calculated with the Parks-McClellan algorithm using the Matlab (The Mathworks, Inc., Natick, MA) signal processing toolbox function remez. We define the echo locations as the maxima of the echo peaks in the resulting signal envelope. A sample ultrasound signal from a volunteer and the magnitude of the analytic signal are shown in Fig. 2.

2.2 Calibration

The AcouStick is essentially a tracked probe with a variable length tip. Cranial surface positions $\mathbf{p}$ are calculated as $\mathbf{p} = \mathbf{p}_0 + d\mathbf{n}_p$, where $\mathbf{p}_0$ is the position of the transducer, i.e., the 3-D point corresponding to time zero in Fig. 2, $d = ut/2$ is the distance from the transducer to the bone-tissue interface, u is the speed of sound in tissue, t is the time interval between the initial sound pulse and the bone-tissue echo, and $\mathbf{n}_p$ is the unit vector along the direction of the ultrasound beam. Calibration for this system is the process of determining $\mathbf{p}_0$ and $\mathbf{n}_p$.

Our method is a variation of the invariant point method commonly used for calibrating ball-tipped probes. We mount a steel ball on a post attached to a heavy base and place it in a tracked water bath. The diameter of the ball we use is 7 mm. The ultrasound probe is placed in the water and moved until a strong echo reflected from the ball is observed in the ultrasound signal. We calculate the position of the center of the

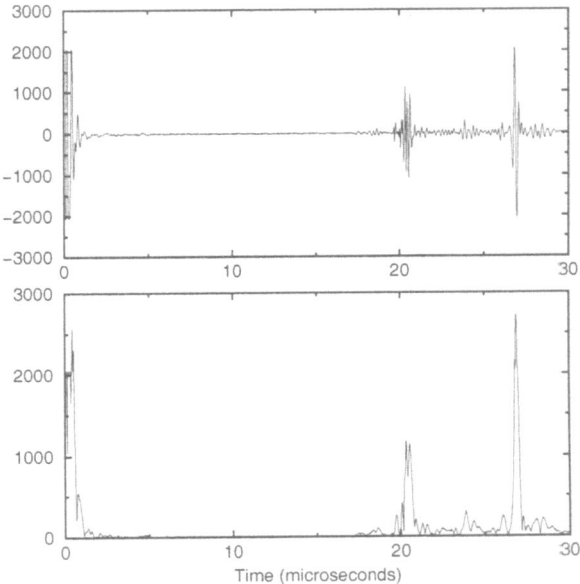

Fig. 2. A sample ultrasound signal from a volunteer (top) and the magnitude of the analytic signal (bottom). The initial sound pulse is at $t = 0$. The first received echo at $t \approx 20 \ \mu s$ corresponds to the water-skin interface. The second echo at $t \approx 27 \ \mu s$ corresponds to the tissue-bone interface. This data is typical of the signals we obtain.

steel ball using $d = ut/2 + r$, where u is the speed of sound in water at the temperature of the bath and r is the radius of the sphere. There are three coordinate systems in this process: the probe coordinate system P, the world coordinate system W defined by the optical position sensor, and the reference coordinate system R defined by an array of IREDs that we place on the water bath. The calculated position of the steel ball in the reference coordinate system, $^R\mathbf{p}_i$, is

$$^R\mathbf{p}_i = {}^R T_{Pi}{}^P\mathbf{p}_i = {}^R T_{Wi}{}^W T_{Pi}(\mathbf{p}_0 + d_i\mathbf{n}_p), \tag{1}$$

where $^R T_{Pi}$ is the rigid-body probe-to-reference transformation, $^P\mathbf{p}_i$ is the position of the steel ball in the probe coordinate system, $^R T_{Wi}$ is the world-to-reference transformation, and $^W T_{Pi}$ is the probe-to-world transformation. The transformations $^R T_{Wi}$ and $^W T_{Pi}$ are provided by the optical tracking system. The subscript i denotes a single measurement. The position of the steel ball in the reference coordinate system, $\mathbf{w}_0$, is fixed, and thus $^R\mathbf{p}_i \approx \mathbf{w}_0$. This relationship is not exact because of measurement error. Thus we iteratively search for the parameters $\mathbf{p}_0$ and $\mathbf{n}_p$ and the most invariant steel ball position $\mathbf{w}_0$ in a least-squares sense, that is, we minimize χ_{cal} defined as

$$\chi_{cal}^2 = \sum_i ||^R\mathbf{p}_i - \mathbf{w}_0||^2. \tag{2}$$

We use a large number of points (approximately 24) collected at different orientations and distances. The probe is hand held and moved until a strong echo is detected. We perform calibration with the offset removed. This allows us to collect points over a wide range of lengths, from approximately $d = 5$ to 60 mm.

2.3   Point Localization Error

To estimate the AcouStick point localization error, we used the AcouStick system to measure the position of 25 5-mm diameter steel balls arranged in a 5×5 grid on a acrylic plate in a water bath. The grid spacing is 10 mm. We performed this measurement in two ways. In the first way, the probe is held with a hand and moved until a strong echo is detected. Each point measurement is obtained from a different orientation. We refer to this approach as the "free hand" method. In the second way, the probe is rigidly held in a clasp that is connected to a micrometer-controlled positioning stage. The probe is translated back and forth in two directions using the micrometer dials until the locally maximum echo amplitude is found as judged by visual examination of the constantly updated analytic signal. We do not use the micrometer readings in any quantitative way. Rather we use the micrometer dials merely to achieve fine translational movement. We refer to this approach as the "fixed orientation" method. Both types of measurements are made over the range of lengths for which the system is intended to be used, that is, from approximately $d = 15$ to 25 mm. We collected two sets of free hand measurements, and two sets of fixed orientation measurements. As the two types of measurements were performed on different occasions, a separate calibration was done for each. Both calibrations were obtained with 24 points. The measured point sets were registered to the known grid positions. The AcouStick localization error was estimated as the residual error after registering these point sets times $\sqrt{N/(N-2)}$, where $N = 25$ [10]. This assumes that the localization error is identical, independent, zero-mean, isotropic, and normally distributed.

2.4   Skull Phantom Experiment

We used the AcouStick system to collect cranial surface points on a plastic skull phantom covered with a layer of gelatin (see left and middle panels of Fig. 3). Eight bone-implanted markers similar to those described in [6] were used for validation. Plastic marker bases were screwed into the top of the skull. A CT image volume of the phantom was acquired using a Philips Tomoscan SR 7000 scanner. The image volume contains 145 axial slices with a slice thickness of 1.0 mm. Just prior to image acquisition, imaging caps containing iodinated contrast were attached to the marker bases. After image acquisition, the phantom was lowered upside down into a latex swimming cap filled with a warm solution of gelatin (150 g/l) that was allowed to set overnight. The thickness of the gelatin varied over the cranial surface from 3 to 16 mm, with a mean thickness of 9 mm. The next day, ten IREDs were glued onto the front of the skull and were used to define the reference coordinate system. Marker bases were identified by manual palpation, small cuts were made in the swimming cap, and physical space caps with a hemispherical divot that corresponds to the centroid of the imaging caps were attached to the bases. Physical space positions of the markers were determined by

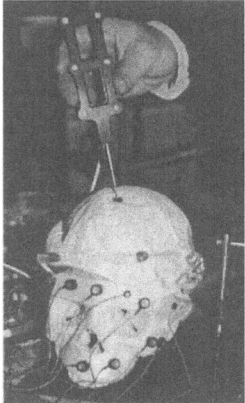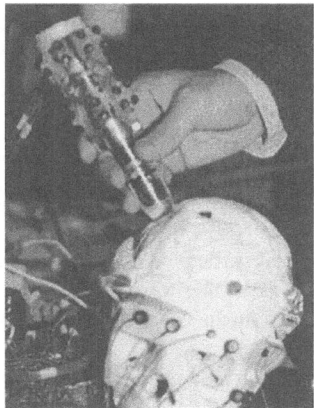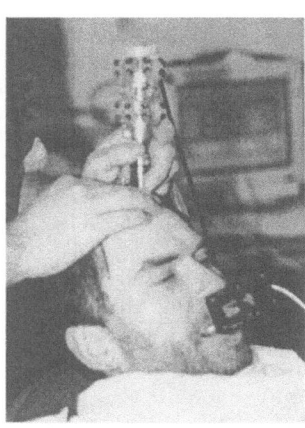

Fig. 3. Localization of markers (left) and collection of cranial surface points (middle) during the skull phantom experiment. Also, localization of skull surface points in one of the volunteer studies (right).

placing an optically tracked ball-tipped probe in the divot of each cap. The AcouStick was calibrated and 150 cranial surface points widely distributed over the head were collected. The speed of sound in the gelatin was determined by measuring the time of flight through a plastic cylinder filled with the same gelatin used to cover the skull. The nominal length of the cylinder was 30 mm. A more accurate length was determined with digital calipers. The speed of sound in water was similarly measured to validate this technique and was found to differ from published values by less than 0.3%.

A triangle set representation of the cranial surface was automatically extracted from the CT image volume [4]. The ultrasonically determined cranial surface points were registered to the image-derived surface model using an independent implementation [5] of the iterative closest point registration algorithm [2]. We calculated the target registration error (TRE) of the surface-based registration by using as a reference gold standard the point-based registration obtained with the eight markers [7]. Specifically, we calculated TRE as the distance between a point in CT mapped from physical space by the reference transformation and its position mapped by the transformation being evaluated. We performed this calculation at the center of every CT voxel inside the head and averaged the resulting values.

2.5 Volunteer and Patient Data

We used the AcouStick system to collect cranial surface points on three volunteers (see right panel of Fig. 3). Each volunteer had a locking acrylic dental stent (LADS). This custom built device attaches to the person's upper teeth. Six IREDs are attached to the LADS and are used to track head movement. The LADS assembly also contains ten fiducial markers similar to those in [6]. This allows the LADS device to also be used for image-to-physical registration if the device can be accurately repositioned. All

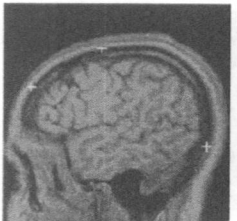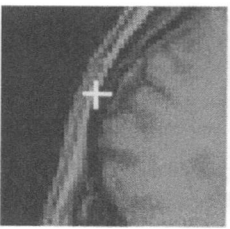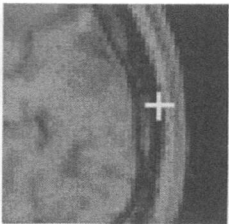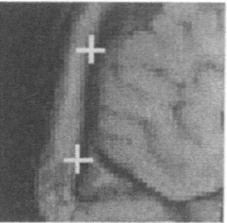

Fig. 4. Ultrasonically determined cranial surface points superimposed as white crosses on four regions from the MR image of a volunteer. The seven surface points shown are representative of those collected, and were transformed to image coordinates using the LADS-based registration.

three volunteers had an MR gradient echo image volume acquired while wearing the LADS. The ultrasonically determined cranial surface points were superimposed on the MR image volume according to the registration transformation provided by the LADS device and then visually examined.

We used the AcouStick system to collect cranial surface points on one patient that underwent surgery for removal of a petrous apex cyst. This patient had a CT image volume acquired as a normal part of his treatment. He was fitted with a LADS device that was used only for tracking of patient movement. The same methods used to extract a cranial surface model and perform surface-based registration for the skull phantom were used for the patient data.

3 Results

Calibrations performed with 24 points typically have a calibration residual error χ_{cal} of about 0.6–0.8 mm. The calibration residual errors of the calibrations used for the free hand and fixed orientation validation measurements are 0.61 and 0.75 mm, respectively. The residual errors after registering the two free hand validation point sets to the known grid positions are 0.48 and 0.53 mm. The residual errors for the fixed orientation validation point sets are 0.13 and 0.16 mm.

The skull phantom cranial surface points determined using the AcouStick were registered to the triangle set representation of the cranial surface that was extracted from the CT image volume. Seven registrations were performed, one using all 150 AcouStick surface points, and six using randomly chosen independent subsets of 25 points each. The surface residual error, i.e., the root-mean-square difference between the surface points and the surface model after registration, is 0.20 mm for the 150-point registration, and ranges between 0.10 and 0.18 mm for the 25-point registrations. The mean TRE over the head volume computed using the eight-marker point-based registration as a reference gold standard is 1.03 mm for the 150-point registration, and ranges between 1.04 and 1.73 mm for the 25-point registrations. The surface points superimposed on CT image slices using any of these surface-based transformations appear visually to lie on the cranial surface.

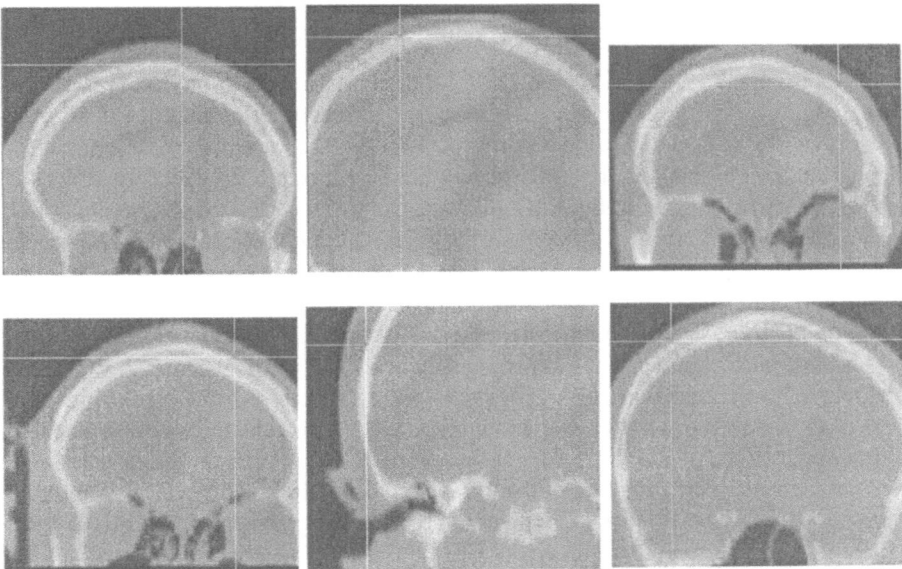

Fig. 5. Sample image slices from the patient CT scan with AcouStick recorded points overlaid as white crosses. The transformation between the AcouStick data and the segmented CT skull surface was determined using surface matching. The slices shown indicate the position of a representative group of six out of 30 points collected from this patient.

The cranial surface points collected from the three volunteers were superimposed on the volunteers' MR image volumes using the LADS-based transformation. For two of these data sets, visual inspection suggests that almost all of the surface points are within one or two voxels of the inner surface of the subcutaneous fat. The voxel dimensions of these images are approximately $1.0 \times 1.0 \times 1.5$ mm. Sample MR slices showing several of these surface points for one of the volunteers are shown in Fig. 4. For the third volunteer, there appears to be a systematic error in the position of the surface points. On one side of the head most of the points lie inside the bone by several millimeters, whereas on the other side of the head the points predominantly lie outside the bone by several millimeters. It is possible that this observation is caused by a systematic calibration or localization error. It is also quite plausible that it results from a LADS relocation error relative to its position during image acquisition.

The 30 cranial surface points collected from the patient using the AcouStick were registered to the triangle set representation of the cranial surface that was extracted from the patient's CT image volume. The surface residual error is 0.17 mm. Sample CT slices showing six of these surface points superimposed using this surface-based registration are shown in Fig. 5.

4   Discussion

We have presented a location device, the AcouStick, for image-to-physical registration in image-guided surgery. The device is based on a tracked A-mode ultrasound transducer. It can be considered to be a point localizer, with a variable length tip, capable of non-invasive penetration of soft tissue and fluids to locate echogenic structures such as bone. Our work builds on the work of Bass, Galloway & Maurer [1], and is related to preliminary work reported by Schmerber et al. [9]. Neither of these earlier papers describe an appropriate calibration technique nor do they contain a detailed validation.

We have described the construction, data analysis, calibration, and initial work on validation of the system. The intrinsic accuracy of the system was measured using an array of steel balls. The free hand measurements, which suggest an accuracy of 0.5 mm, will include latency errors in sensing the probe position and errors due to the finite width of the ultrasound beam (-6 dB beam width is about 0.4 mm at the focal point). The fixed orientation measurements, which suggest an accuracy of 0.15 mm, might underestimate systematic errors in the direction of the ultrasound beam. In practice the system will be used to measure points on surfaces with a radius of curvature much greater than 0.4 mm, but latency errors and systematic errors will be important. Hence we regard 0.15 and 0.5 mm as the lower and upper bounds of the intrinsic accuracy of the system, giving it accuracy comparable to existing contact based pointers.

A phantom test on a skull, with gelatin covering to mimic scalp tissue, showed that the AcouStick could recover image-to-physical registration with a TRE of between 1.0 and 1.7 mm. Location of skull surface points on MR scans of three volunteers wearing a lockable acrylic dental stent (LADS) for registration produced results within 1 or 2 voxels (1 to 2 mm) for two volunteers. For the third volunteer there was a systematic shift of about 3 voxels. Independent experiments [3] yielded a mean TRE for relocation of the LADS for the three volunteers of 0.6, 0.7, and 1.1 mm, respectively. Geometrical distortion, scaling errors, fat shift, etc., could be as high as 2 mm in these MR scans. These experiments therefore indicate an upper limit of the in vivo TRE of about 3 mm and are consistent with a TRE of between 1 and 2 mm. Finally, the data was used to register a CT scan of a volunteer to physical space. This yielded a residual surface registration error of 0.17 mm.

Preliminary results obtained from three volunteers and a patient indicate that the AcouStick has the potential to provide accurate image-to-physical registration of the head without the use of any markers or frames. Calibration currently takes about 20 minutes, and data collection in the operating theater about 15 minutes. The AcouStick may also be usable for non-cranial image-guided surgery applications.

Acknowledgment

C. R. Maurer, Jr. was a Research Fellow at King's College London when this work was performed. He was supported by the EASI project "European Applications for Surgical Interventions" HC1012 of the EU "4th Framework Telematics Applications for Health" program. We are grateful to Philips Medical Systems (Best, The Netherlands) for supporting R. Gaston and for supplying the equipment used in this project. P. J. Edwards

962   C. R. Maurer, Jr., et al.

was supported by the EPSRC GR/L62221. We thank G. Penney for his help and Dr. F. Gerritsen (Philips Medical Systems) for his advice, encouragement, and support.

References

1. WA Bass, RL Galloway Jr, CR Maurer Jr. Surface-based registration of physical space with CT images using A-mode ultrasound localization of the skull. *Medical Imaging 1998: Image Display*, Proc. SPIE 3335: 228–238, 1998.
2. PJ Besl, ND McKay. A method for registration of 3-D shapes. *IEEE Trans. Pattern Anal. Mach. Intell.*, 14: 239–256, 1992.
3. PJ Edwards, AP King, CR Maurer Jr, DA de Cunha, DJ Hawkes, DLG Hill, RP Gaston, MR Fenlon, S Chandra, AJ Strong, CL Chandler, A Richards, MJ Gleeson. A system for microscope-assisted guided interventions (MAGI). *MICCAI '99* (appears elsewhere in these proceedings).
4. A Gueziec, R Hummel. Exploiting triangulated surface extraction using tetrahedral decomposition. *IEEE Trans. Visualization Comput. Graph.*, 1: 328–342, 1995.
5. CR Maurer Jr, GB Aboutanos, BM Dawant, RJ Maciunas, JM Fitzpatrick. Registration of 3-D images using weighted geometrical features. *IEEE Trans. Med. Imaging*, 15: 836–849, 1996.
6. CR Maurer Jr, JM Fitzpatrick, MY Wang, RL Galloway Jr, RJ Maciunas, GS Allen. Registration of head volume images using implantable fiducial markers. *IEEE Trans. Med. Imaging*, 16: 447–462, 1997.
7. CR Maurer Jr, RJ Maciunas, JM Fitzpatrick. Registration of head CT images to physical space using a weighted combination of points and surfaces. *IEEE Trans. Med. Imaging*, 17: 753–761, 1998.
8. W. W. McDicken. *Diagnostic Ultrasonics: Principles and Use of Instruments*. John Wiley & Sons, Inc., New York, 1976.
9. S Schmerber, B Chen, S Lavallee, JP Chirossel, P Cinquin, A Poyet, M Coulomb, E Reyt. Markerless hybrid registration method for computer assisted endoscopic ENT surgery. In: *Computer Assisted Radiology and Surgery 1997*. HU Lemke, MW Vannier, K Inamura, eds. Springer-Verlag, Berlin, 1997, pp. 799–806.
10. R Sibson. Studies in the robustness of multidimensional scaling: Perturbational analysis of classical scaling. *J. R. Statist. Soc. B*, 41: 217–229, 1979.

Synthetic Image Modalities Generated from Matched CT and MRI Data: A New Approach for Using MRI in Brachytherapy[1]

R. Krempien[a], H. A. Grabowski[b], W. Harms[a], F. W. Hensley[a], S. Hassfeld[c], U. Mende[a], M. Treiber[a], M. Wannenmacher[a]

[a] Clinic for Radiology, Department of Clinical Radiology, University of Heidelberg, INF 400, 69120 Heidelberg, Germany
[b] Institute for Process Control and Robotics, Department of Computer Science, University of Karlsruhe, 76128 Karlsruhe, Germany
[c] Clinic for Cranio-Maxillo-Facial Surgery, University of Heidelberg, INF 400, 69120 Heidelberg, Germany

robert_krempien@med.uni-heidelberg.de

Target definition and dosimetric evaluation of brachytherapy procedures is crucial in developing proper technique and has prognostic implications. Accurate definition of tumour volume and organs at risk is essential for treatment planing. CT accurately localise sources, but often poorly delineates tumour volume. Magnetic resonance imaging (MRI) has introduced several imaging benefits such as improved soft tissue definition and unrestricted multiplanar and volumetric imaging. However, MRI has not yet seriously challenged CT for brachytherapy planing in most sites. One main reasons for this is the poor imaging of the applicator dummy markers required for detecting the source dwell positions. Therefore a new system generating synthetic image modalities from matched and fused CT and MRI-data has been developed. The system presented consists of five modules serving for viewing, matching, segmentation, fusion and validation. With the presented new system manual or automatic image registration and fusion of CT and MR-images can be done, enabling the use of the imaging advantages of MRI and CT in brachytherapy planing. Tumour structures or source dwell positions could be measured in any plane in one imaging modality and then copied into the other. With synthetic image-based brachytherapy planing a optimisation of target volume covering and dose distribution to treatment volume and structures at risk could be achieved. These preliminary data show that image registration and fusion is feasible for brachytherapy planing. The procedure integrating synthetic images from CT and MRI into brachytherapy planing has the advantage of precise target volume definition and of better determination of dose within this target taking into account the critical dose at structures at risk. Synthetic images may lead to an improved tumour control and reduced side effects by brachytherapy.

[1] The work is partly being funded by the 'Sonderforschungsbereich Informationstechnik in der Medizin - Rechner- und sensorgestütze Chirurgie' of the Deutsche Forschungsgemeinschaft

1. Introduction

Brachytherapy from the Greek word "brachy - short distance" consists of placing sealed radioactive sources close or in contact with the target tissue. Implantation techniques may be broadly characterised in terms of surgical approach, i.e. interstitial or intracavitary. In modern brachytherapy using afterloading techniques a single stepping radioactive source is introduced into applicators or guides according to a chosen plan with a predetermined geometrical distribution of possible source dwell positions. Individual adjustment of dose distribution in the target volume and structures at risk can be performed by controlling the dwell time used at each dwell position. Before inserting radioactive sources a dummy marking chain representing the source dwell positions is introduced. Methods using radiographs or computed tomography (CT) accurately localise sources [7]. Computerised dosimetry generally has been generated from orthogonal radiographs rendering limited information about spatial relationship between source positions and tumour volume or structures at risk. The CT-based reconstruction allows the individual adjustment and optimisation of the dose distribution to anatomical target volumes [4,16]. But due to the poor soft tissue contrast CT still has limitations in determing target volume and structures at risk [3]. Magnetic resonance imaging (MRI) has introduced several added imaging benefits that may confer an advantage over the use of CT in brachytherapy planing such as improved soft tissue definition and unrestricted multiplanar and volumetric imaging [9]. However, MRI has not yet seriously challenged CT for brachytherapy planing in most sites. The reasons for this include (1) the poor imaging of bone and the lack of electron density information from MRI required for dosimetric calculations; (2) the poor imaging of the applicator dummy required for detecting the source positions due to the lack of source visibility (3) the presence of intrinsic system-related and object-induced MR image distortions [3,9,17].

Synthetic image modalities from matched and fused CT and MRI-data may add the advantages of both imaging modalities [8]. The registration and fusion of medical images, especially the registration of CT and MR images, may be a useful step for brachytherapy planing [12]. The aim of this study was to access the possibilities of synthetic images from registered and fused CT- and MR-Images in brachytherapy planing.

2 Materials and Methods

2.1 Patients and Brachytherapy

In 1998 two Patients (one Patients with cervix carcinoma, one Patients with soft tissue sarcoma) receiving a combined therapy of external beam and brachytherapy have been planned in parallel mode using (1) CT-based brachytherapy planing and (2) brachytherapy planing based on synthetic images of both imaging modalities (CT and

MRI). Target volume, treatment volume, planing volume and the resulting optimised dose distribution was calculated. The dose distribution in structures at risk was also calculated. This was performed by two radiation therapists and one physicist. The brachytherapy planing was performed at the planing system Plato (Nucletron, Netherlands). The patients were either treated with high dose rate (HDR) or pulsed dose rate (PDR) brachytherapy.

2.2 Image acquisition

After positioning of brachytherapy applicators or surgical implantation of brachytherapy guides CT and MRI was performed. Since the examination with a brachytherapy applicator needs a larger variety in patient positioning MRI was performed using a open low field MRI (Picker Outlook 0.23 Tesla). T1-weighted spin-echoes with and without Gadolinium and T2-weighted spin-echoes were used. The geometric distortion of the MRI-facility was investigated by a special phantom using spin-echo sequences. Within 10 cm around the isocentre - the region of interest for brachytherapy-planing- this distortion was below 1 mm [13].

2.3 System overview

For interaction with medical images a system is required which guides the user through several image processing tasks. For that reason a system consisting of five modules was developed. At each time during the image processing task the obtained results can be validated and, if necessary, the task can be repeated.

Viewing: At the beginning of a session, both volumetric data are loaded with the viewer module. This module is designed to exploit as much information as possible from the original slices. In two adjacent windows, the MR and CT images can be visualised in arbitrary planes, the slices can be interpolated, and a histogram-based grey value normalisation can be performed. Other features like picking grey values or cutting regions are available.

Matching: In this module, the images can be registered manually or automatically. The automatic registration takes about one to three minutes for two data sets of about 60 slices. The matched images can be visualised in checkerboard overlay. The automatic registration algorithm is able to register MRI and CT data in over 95 percent of the cases without any interaction. Depending on slice thickness the achieved average accuracy of the calculated transformation was bellow 1 millimetre [11].

Segmentation: In this module, the images can be segmented. Global thresholding and region-growing based seed-point segmentation is available. Up to 15 different structures can be segmented with an index-structure, so that one voxel can belong to two or more structures. Logical operations like (AND, OR, etc.) can be performed with the structures. All segmented structures can be visualised with different volume rendering techniques, like gradient shading, MIP (Maximum Intensity Projection) or

SIP (Summarised Intensity Projection). The module consists of two modes, the *volume mode* and the *slice mode*. In the *volume mode* three dimensional region growing can be used to segment connected structures. Since different structures are sometimes connected via thin regions, the size of the seed point can be chosen. In the *slice mode* fine segmentation can be performed slice by slice. For segmentation, polygon lines are used. The previously registered images are superimposed in one window, while it is possible to blend smoothly between the two images. In the superimposed image, interactive segmentation can be performed slice by slice.

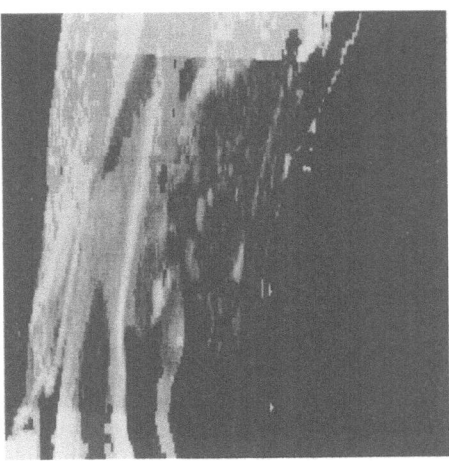

Fig. 1. The MR image and the CT image are fused by the fusion function *addition* (The grey values of both images are added after a certain kind of grey-value adaptation). Since bony structures are represented with high grey values in CT images, while these structures - giving no MRI-signal in T1w- and T2w-images - are represented with low grey values in MR images the result of the addition of both grey values can not exceed a certain threshold. Otherwise a high grey value in CT images corresponds to a high value in MR images which indicates an error in registration at the bony structures. As seen in the above image the bony structures and the skin contour fit well. Reconstruction of the fused images in different planes offer the possibility to validate the matching accuracy. The result of the fusion obtained by multiplication, addition and subtraction can also be used as a new, synthetic modality.

Validation and Fusion: The grey values of the segmented structures can be copied and pasted from one volumetric image into the other (Fig. 4). In order to obtain high accuracy, the segmented regions are re-sampled before insertion. To avoid aliasing effects, the resampling can be performed with different rates. Additionally, the segmented regions can be copied and pasted without copying the grey values, thus enhancing the possibilities of the segmentation task. With the help of that technique, new imaging modalities can be created by a various fusion functions, like addition, subtraction, multiplication of grey values The fusion function can be used for validation (Fig. 1). In the superimposition of the images under different fusion functions, the overall fitness of the obtained matching can be visualised transparently. Also technical validation like the average mean square distance between corresponding landmarks is possible

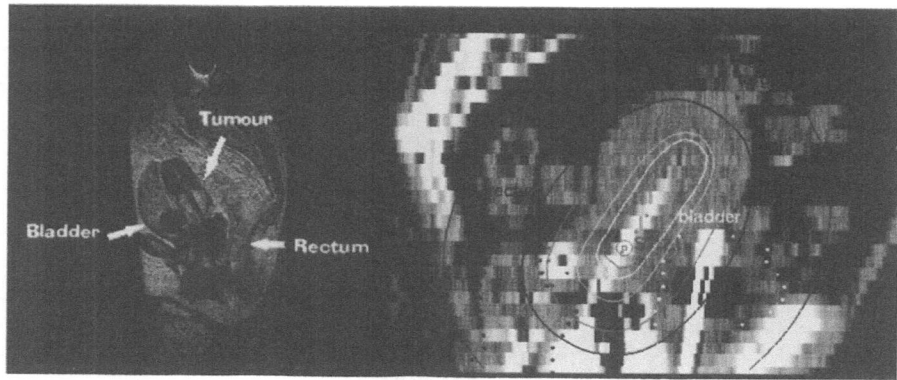

Fig. 2. Cancer of the uterine cervix. **Right:** Sagittal reconstruction of a pelvic CT-scan with brachytherapy applicator in position. In the planing CT the exact tumour localisation and spread and its relationship to the surrounding structures at risk (i.e. rectum, bladder) were very difficult to determine. Thus brachytherapy planing on CT alone may result in miscalculation in target definition and dosimetry within this target. **Left.** In the sagittal pelvic MRI scan the tumour localisation and the relationship to the surrounding tissue is easily visible. The combination of both imaging modalities makes dosimetric optimisation possible with respect to the tumour and the structures at risk.

3 Results

The described system for image registration and fusion can (1) visualise and reconstruct CT and MRI- images in any desired plane (2) manually or automatically register CT- and MRI-images. (3) segment multiple structures using global thresholding and region-growing based seed-point segmentation (4) superimpose the previously registered images and segment manually or automatically structures slice by slice (5) transfer the grey volumes of the segmented structures from one volumetric image into the other and (6) validate the achieved accuracy of the matching and fusion procedure interactively. The automatic registration process takes about one to three minutes for two data sets of about 60 slices. The algorithm is able to register MRI and

CT data in over 95 percent of the cases without any interaction. The average accuracy of the calculated transformation was below 1 millimetre [11].

With the help of the information of both imaging modalities the optimal imaging plane for further brachytherapy planing could be chosen (Fig. 2). After registration structures of interest could be segmented in either one of the imaging modalities. Since MRI has a superior soft tissue contrast possible tumour structures, target structures or organs at risk were segmented in the MRI-data. The applicator dummy markers which were not visible in the MRI could only be segmented in the CT (Fig. 3). The image fusion offered the possibility to merge both information in one image (Fig. 4 left). Since the brachytherapy planing system can only work with Diacom3 data the grey values of the segmented structures from one imaging modality were copied and pasted to the other. These generated synthetic images were retransformed in Diacom3 and imported into the brachytherapy planing system for further planning. The use of the synthetic images leads to a significant adjustment and optimisation of the dose distribution to target volumes and structures at risk.

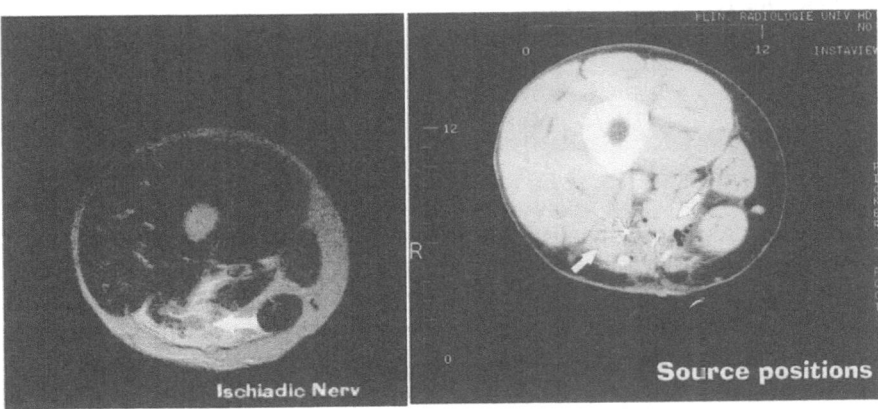

Fig. 3. A patient with liposarcoma in the thigh showed a histological positive tumour margin to the ischiadic nerve. Intraoperativley the decision was made to implant brachytherapy guides for postoperative boost-radiation of the tumour-bed rather than resecting the nerve to preserve the function of the leg. CT (**right**) accurately localises source positions (arrows) but due to the limited soft tissue contrast and the postoperative changes the nerve as the primary target structure was hardly detectable. The MRI (**left**) with its superior soft tissue contrast easily showed the nerve (arrow) but no source positions could be visualised.

For example a patient with liposarcoma in the thigh showed a positive tumour margin to the ischiadic nerve. Since further operating meant to resect the nerve which would have resulted in a paralysed leg the intraoperative decision was made to implant brachytherapy-guides for postoperative boost-radiation of the tumour-bed. The nerve as the primary target structure was hardly detectable in the planning CT alone not only due to the poor soft tissue contrast but due to the postoperative changes. In the MRI the nerve could be easily located and it was possible to segment it precisely (Fig. 3). Since both imaging modalities had been registered it was possible to copy the grey values of the segmented nerve into the planing CT. With the help of these generated synthetic images the nerve and its relationship to the source dwell positions could be determined in one image set (Fig. 4 left). Based on the synthetic images a new dose prescription was applied (Fig. 4 right). The comparison of the CT-based and synthetic image based planing revealed that the nerve as the primary target structure was incompletely covered or heavily overdosed in 30% of the target volume based on CT-planing alone. This could have resulted in early tumour relapse or excessive radiation damage to the nerve. The synthetic image based planing resulted in superior target definition and a determination of dose within this target taking into account the critical doses at structures at risk (Fig. 4). Since there was no predefined correct object to compare against various fusion function like addition, subtraction, multiplication of grey values of the registered images were generated in the validation mode. These fused images were used to validate the matching accuracy comparing different anatomical structures i.e. bone and skin contour. As shown in Figure 1 a good matching result could be achieved.

4 Discussion

Brachytherapy offers two main advantages in radiation therapy [1]: (1) The radioactive source can be applied close to or into the tumour volume, sparing the surrounding tissue which in external beam radiation often limits the dose escalation needed for tumour control. (2) The steep dose gradient (Fig. 2, 4) enables the delivery of radiation doses into the target volume while sparing structures at risk. As shown in Figure 4 a small error in target volume definition can lead to an incorrect enclosure of tumour volume or to a overdose to organs at risk. This may lead to early tumour relapse and severe side effects [14]. Having this in mind the necessity for exact definition of target volume is clearly visible.

Modern brachytherapy using afterloading technique offers the possibility of individual target definition. Since CT is bound to axial scanning and offers limited soft tissue contrast, it is sometimes difficult to determine the exact tumour location and spread [3]. MRI has introduced several added imaging benefits that may confer an advantage over the use of CT in brachytherapy planing. The problem with MRI in brachytherapy-planing is despite the presence of intrinsic system-related and object-induced MR image distortions that MRI cannot visualise the dummy source positions required for detecting the source dwell positions needed for further planing [3,9].

Experiments with contrast agent (i.e. gadolinium) filled applicator guides did not result in satisfactory determination of source positions [6,10]. One method of avoiding the problems associated with MRI is to integrate the superior tumour definition of MRI with the accurate source localisation, the electron density information and the geometric accuracy obtained from CT. This allows for the integration of comprehensive anatomical mapping with functional distribution of the tissues within a single image set [8]. The registration of medical images, especially the registration of CT and MR images, may be a useful step for brachytherapy planing [12]. Manual methods of registering different images sets can be inefficient and error prone. In manual transposition of target information calculated mismatches of up to 8.5 mm between the volumes outlined by CT compared to MRI have been reported [2]. Having in mind the steep dose gradient this certainly is not acceptable. Automated approaches will reduce inter-operator variability and allow more accurate registration between multimodality systems [15]. Problematic for image registration are the image distortions of the MRI.

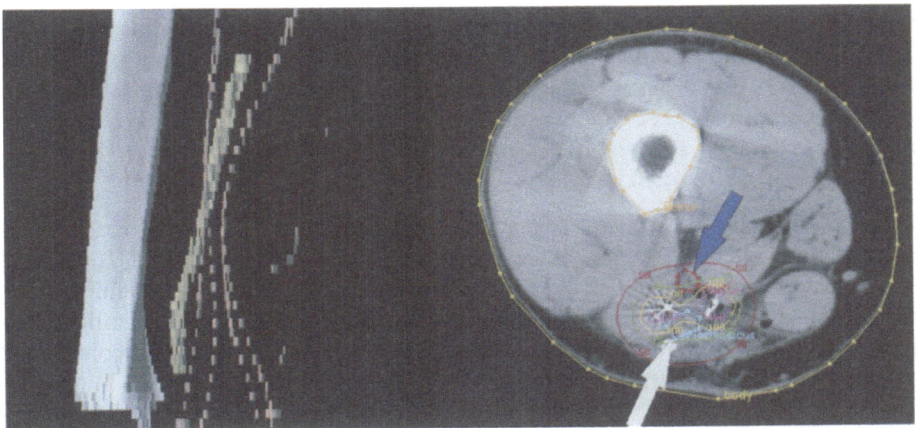

Fig. 4. Left: The ischiadic nerve (yellow structure) is segmented in MRI and the segmented structure can be visualised and positioned in the CT image. The dummy source positions (red) and the femoral bone (blue) are segmented via seed point segmentation in CT. The Position of the nerve can now be visualised in comparison to the source dwell positions. **Right:** The fused synthetic images are added into the Plato brachytherapy planing system. The red circle (blue arrow) was the supposed nerve localisation due to the planing CT, the turquoise circle (white arrow) due to the planing MRI. The 100 cGy isodose/pulse (yellow line) was the enclosing target volume isodose. The use of a CT alone for brachytherapy-planing would have resulted in a heavy overdose of the nerve with a high risk of radiation damage to the nerve in this slice position, in other places a actual miss of the target structure occurred which may have resulted in early tumour relapse.

Since patient positioning and scanning with brachytherapy applicators or guides sometimes is difficult in a high field MRI due to limited space an open low field MRI was used for the planing MRI. The low field MRI shows less patient induced image distortions since they accumulate with higher magnetic field strengths [17]. But the inhomogeneity in the magnetic field due to the open construction resulted in stronger system induced distortions [17]. The measurement of the geometric distortion investigated by a special phantom showed that within 10 cm around the isocentre this distortion was below 1 mm and the phantom investigation offered a possibility to correct these distortions, thus disturbing geometric distortions could be overcome [13]. But distortion of anatomical structures due to patient movements are still problematic. This can result in problems in the automatic registration process, needing manual adjustment. The use of deformable image models using finite element meshes [5] may be a possible solution but needs further investigation.

The presented interactive system allows full automatic registration, based on voxel similarity measurements. After segmentation structures in the matched images can be copied from one image into the other. Tumour structures or source dwell positions can be segmented in one imaging modality and then copied into the other thus enabling the use of the superior soft tissue contrast of the MRI in brachytherapy planing. The planing procedure integrating synthetic images from CT and MRI has the advantage of precise target volume definition and of determination of dose within this target taking into account the critical dose at structures at risk.

5 Conclusion

These preliminary data show that image registration and fusion is feasible for brachytherapy planing. The procedure integrating synthetic images from CT and MRI into brachytherapy planing has the advantage of precise target volume definition and of better determination of dose within this target taking into account the critical dose at structures at risk. Synthetic images may lead to an improved tumour control and reduced side effects by brachytherapy.

References

[1] K.S.C. Choa, C.A. Perez, L.W. Brady *Radiation Oncology: Managment Decisions.* Lippincott - Raven, Philadelphia New York p79-99, 1999

[2] A.W.T. De Valles, M. Abe, R. N: Kjellberg *Transposition of target information from magnetic resonance and computed tomograpy scan images to concentional stereotacic space.* Appl. Neurophysiol. 50:23-32 1987

[3] D.F. Dubois, B.R. Prestidge, L.A. Hotchkiss, W.S. Bice, J.J. Prete *Source localisation following permanent transperineal prostate interstitial brachytherapy using magnetic resonance imaging.* Int. J Radiat. Oncol. Biol. Phys. 39:1037-1041;1997

[4] B. Erickson, K. Albano, M. Gillin *CT-guided interstitial implantations of gynecologic malignancies.* Int. J Radiat. Oncol. Biol. Phys. 36:699-709; 1997

[5] H.A. Grabowski, J. Brief, S. Hassfeld, R. Krempien, J. Raczkowsky, H. Wörn, U. Rembold *Model-based registration of medical images using finite element meshes,* In: H. Lemke, M.W. Vannier, K. Inamura, A.G. Farman (eds.): Proceedings of the 12th International Symposium and Exhibition on Computer Assisted Radiology and Surgery (CAR'98), Tokyo, Elsevier Press, 1998, p. 159-163

[6] W. Harms, R. Krempien, F. Hensley, M. Wannenmacher. Work in progress: Using MRI in brachytherapy planing

972   R. Krempien et al.

[7] F.W. Hensley, W. Harms, R. Krempien, P. Fritz, Ch. Berns, M. Wannenmacher *Analysis of the geometrical accuracy of CT-based interstitial brachytherapy reconstructions.* GEC Estro 1999

[8] K. Kagawa, W.R. Lee, T.E: Schultheiss, M.A. Hunt, A.H. Shaer, G.E. Hanks *Initial clinical assessment of CT-MRI image fusion software in localisation of the prostate for 3D conformal radiation therapy.* Int. J. Radiation Oncology Biol. Phys. 38:319-325

[9] V.S. Khoo, D.P. Dearnaley, D.J. Finnigan, A Padhani, S.T. Tanner, M.O. Leach: Magnetic resonance imaging (MRI): considerations and applications in radiotherapy treatment planing. Radiother. Oncol. 42:1-15; 1997

[10] G. Kovacs, R. Pötter, F.J. Prott, B. Lenzen, T.H. Knocke *The Münster experience with magnetic resonance imaging assisted treatment planing used for high dose rate afterloading therapy of gynaecological and nasopharyngeal cancer.* Advanced Radiation Tumour Response. in: Breit (Ed.): Monitoring and Treatment Planing, Springer Heidelberg 1992: p661-665

[11] P. Pokrandt *Fast Non-Supervised Matching: A Probabilistic Approach,* Proceedings of the 10th International Symposium and Exhibition on Computer Assisted Radiology and Surgery (CAR´96), 1996

[12] J.G. Rosenman, E.P. Miller, G. Tracton, T. Cullip *Image registration: an essential part of radiation therapy treatment planing.* Int. J. Radiation Oncology Biol. Phys. 40:197-205

[13] K. Schubert, F. Wenz, R. Krempien, O. Schramm, G. Sroka-Perez, P. Schraube, M. Wannenmacher *Einsatzmöglichkeiten eines offenen Magnetresonanztomographen in der Therapiesimulation und dreidimensionalen Bestrahlungsplanung.* Strahlentherapie Onkologie 175:225-231, 1999

[14] A. Terahara, T. Nakano, A. Ishikawa, S. Morita, H. Tsujii *Dose-volume histogram analysis of high dose rate intracavitary brachytherapy for uterine cervix cancer.* Int. J. Radiation Oncology Biol. Phys. 35:549-554; 1996

[15] P.A. van den Elsen ;E.J. Pol, M.A. Viergever *Medical image matching - a review with classification.* IEEE Trans. Med. Biomed. Eng. 12:26-39, 1993

[16] K.J. Weeks, G.S. Montana *Three-dimensional applicator system for carcinoma of the uterine cervix.* Int. J Radiat. Oncol. Biol. Phys. 37:455-463; 1997

[17] G Wesby, M.K. Adamis, R.R. Edelmann: *Artifacts in MRI: description, causes and solutions.* In: Edelmann RR, Hesselink JK, Zlatkin MB Eds.: Clinical magnetic resonance imaging. Saunders, Philadelphia, p88-144, 1996

3D Interventional Imaging with 2D X-Ray Detectors

L. Desbat[1], G. Champleboux[1], M. Fleute[1], P.Komarek[1], C. Mennessier[1],
B. Monteil[2], T. Rodet[1], P. Bessou[3], M.Coulomb[4], and G.Ferretti[4]

[1] TIMC-IMAG, IAB, Faculté de Médecine, UJF, 38706 La Tronche France
Laurent.Desbat@imag.fr,
WWW home page: http://www-timc.imag.fr/cami/
[2] TRIXELL, Parc d'Activités Centr'Alp, 38430 Moirans France
[3] Neuroradiology department of the Grenoble University Hospital, 38000 Grenoble
France
[4] Radiology and Medical Imaging department of the Grenoble University Hospital,
38000 Grenoble France

Abstract. Pre-operative images, such as CT or MRI, are often necessary for CAMI. However, they could be replaced by interventional 3D reconstruction from 2D x-ray sensors. 3D reconstruction from classical image amplifiers needs the correction of geometric distortions due to the magnetic fields. We investigate new calibration marker schemes exploiting spectral properties of the x-ray transform. According to Shannon theory, no information is lost with these new schemes, even if the markers can be seen in each image. Numerical experiments from both phantom and real data are provided.

1 Introduction

Computer Assisted Medical Intervention needs numerical information on the patient. This information is treated by computers in order to propose some optimal strategy for the intervention. Then, the surgeon can be assisted during the operation. Medical imaging is an essential source of information available on the patient. Nowadays MRI and CT lead to sufficiently precise information for planning a wide range of interventions. MRI has the essential advantage of being non-invasive. Nevertheless, for complex bone surgery (traumatology, orthopedy), CT and radiologic images remain necessary because of their incomparable quality. However, MRI and CT systems are rather slow and not ergonomic. They are mainly used as pre-operative imaging devices. Moreover, pre-operative images need to be registered with the patient during the intervention. This implies to acquire information on the patient during the intervention for this registration. Intra-operative imaging systems just need to be calibrated. They can be used for the planning but also to guide the surgeon. They offer the possibility to control and optimize dynamically the intervention. They are more flexible. Their use can be optimized for each intervention protocol. Thus, interventional imaging is a natural trend.

Ultrasound and x-ray systems coupled to a localizer are already used during interventions in order to acquire 3D information [3, 12]. For some applications, a limited number of acquisitions is sufficient. Moreover, a prior information can be used to improve the identification of the unknown parameters [8]. In this work we consider 3D reconstruction of attenuation coefficients from image intensifiers. This can produce pre-operative 3D images for planning but also interventionnal 3D images for controling. Since the beginning of 1980s, 3D reconstruction techniques from conical x-ray projections have been greatly improved [7, 11, 5, 14]. Reconstructions of high contrast structures from few projections acquired on image intensifiers have been proposed [15, 4]. Image intensifiers are widespread, relative low cost imaging system already available in most surgical rooms. However, image intensifiers suffer from geometric distortions due to magnetic fields. These distortions must be corrected before the reconstruction. Because the image intensifier distortion depends on the surrounding magnetic field, a dynamic distortion correction needs to be implemented. Indeed, the correction depends on the position and orientation of the image intensifier. Because the modeling of these distortions is very difficult, opaque markers are usually used to estimate the distortion. For a static acquisition, a first image with markers is generally acquired. Then the distortion is estimated. The distortion correction is finally applied to a second image without markers (see [1] for details). This method can hardly be implemented for dynamic acquisition: rapidly removable marker grids are not available and seem difficult to be designed for a rate of more than 10 images per seconds. Moreover, this approach implies a significant increase of x-ray dose on the patient.

In section 2, we first propose a calibration marker geometry that can stay on the image amplifier: it enables a dynamic distorsion correction of 3D tomographic acquisitions with almost no loss of information according to Shannon theory. Spectral properties of the 3D projection data are exploited.

2   3D reconstruction from image intensifiers

For interventional 3D reconstructions from image intensifiers, we need to collect a set of x-ray projections, regularly spaced around the patient. In this paper, we only consider the simplest trajectory of the source and detector around the patient, i.e., one circle. In this work we show that spectral properties of the data can be exploited to design a calibration marker geometry, which is "invisible" in the reconstruction. We first present the idea in 2D tomography. Spectral properties of the 2D Radon transform are shown in section 2.1. A generalization to the 3D x-ray transform is then presented. The main result is that standard sampling schemes (equally spaced projection angles, equally distant sampling of the detector) are redundant. Thus, we can recover the data covered by opaque markers for particular (interlaced) marker distribution schemes. In section 2.2, we present a fast Fourier interpolation formula in 2D. In section 2.3, we present 3D reconstructions from data containing interlaced markers. They are as good as 3D reconstructions from data without marker. This approach is then tested on real data.

2.1 Data spectrum and efficient sampling

Let $g(y)$ be an n-dimensional function to be sampled (for simplicity let $g \in \mathcal{S}(\mathbb{R}^n)$, the Schwartz space of $\mathbb{R}^n$), let $\mathbf{K}$ be the essential support of its Fourier transform $\hat{g}(\xi) = (2\pi)^{-1/2} \int_{\mathbb{R}^n} g(x)e^{-ix\cdot\xi}dx$, more precisely $\int_{\xi \notin \mathbf{K}} |\hat{g}(\xi)|d\xi$ is supposed to be almost zero. The non overlapping Shannon condition associated to a sampling scheme generated by the non singular matrix W, i.e., the sampling set $\{Wl, l \in \mathbb{Z}^n\}$, is that *the sets $\mathbf{K}$ translated on the reciprocal scheme, i.e., $\mathbf{K} + 2\pi W^{-1^t}l, l \in \mathbb{Z}^2$, do not overlap*. If this condition is satisfied, then $g(y), y \in \mathbb{R}^n$ can be estimated from the Fourier interpolation formula:

$$(S_W g)(y) = (2\pi)^{-n/2}|\det W| \sum_{k \in \mathbf{Z}^n} g(Wk)\hat{\chi}_{\mathbf{K}}(Wk - y) \tag{1}$$

with the error estimate

$$\|S_W g - g\|_\infty \le 2(2\pi)^{-n/2} \int_{\xi \notin \mathbf{K}} |\hat{g}(\xi)|d\xi.$$

Thus, geometrical properties of the set $\mathbf{K}$ can be exploited for the choice of W satisfying the non-overlapping Shannon conditions. Efficient sampling is based on the choice of W yielding the most compact non-overlapping conditions. In this case $\det(W^{-1^t})$ is minimal, equivalently $\det(W)$ is maximal, hence the sampling scheme is the sparsest among those satisfying the Shannon conditions. Non-efficient sampling are redundant. This redundancy can be exploited to design opaque marker distribution schemes so that no information is lost on g (only signal to noise is then lost).

In tomography, it is well known that the spectrum of the 2D Radon transform or the 3D x-ray transform has a particular geometry that can be exploited by interlaced sampling schemes [16, 13, 6]. In 2D tomography, we want to sample the Radon transform g of an unknown function f to be reconstructed

$$g(\phi, s) \stackrel{\text{def}}{=} \int_{-\infty}^{\infty} f(s\theta + t\zeta)dt, \tag{2}$$

where $\theta = (\cos\phi, \sin\phi)$ and $\zeta = (-\sin\phi, \cos\phi)$. The Fourier transform of g is defined by

$$\hat{g}_k(\sigma) = \frac{1}{2\pi} \int_0^{2\pi} \hat{g}(\phi, \sigma)e^{-ik\phi}d\phi \text{ with } \hat{g}(\phi, \sigma) = \frac{1}{\sqrt{2\pi}} \int_{-\infty}^{\infty} g(\phi, s)e^{-i\sigma s}ds. \tag{3}$$

It is shown [16, 13] that, if f is essentially b band limited, i.e., if $\int_{|\xi|>b} |\hat{f}(\xi)|d\xi << \int_{\mathbb{R}^2} |\hat{f}(\xi)|d\xi$, the set $\mathbf{K}_2$ is the essential support of $\hat{g}_k(\sigma)$, see figure 1. Thus, the interlaced matrix W_I satisfies the Shannon conditions with twice less points that the standard scheme ($\det W_I = 2 \det W_S$), with

$$W_S = \begin{bmatrix} h_1 & 0 \\ 0 & h_2 \end{bmatrix}, W_I = \begin{bmatrix} 2h_1 & -h_1 \\ 0 & h_2 \end{bmatrix}, \tag{4}$$

where $h_1 = \frac{\pi}{p}, h_2 = 2/q$ and $p \in \mathbb{N}$ is the projection number on $[0, \pi)$ and q is the translation number on a diameter of the reconstruction disk (normalized to the unit disk in this paper). The sampling conditions are fullfilled if p is slightly larger than $\pi q/2 = b$, see [13] and the figure 1.

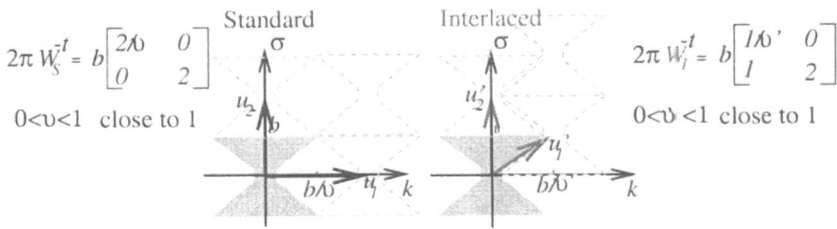

Fig. 1. Sampling condition of the 2D Radon transform in the Fourier space. The set K_2 is shown in gray with translations on the reciprocal scheme generated by the matrix $(W_I^{-1})^t$ (best interlaced scheme, right) and repectively $(W_S^{-1})^t$ (best standard scheme, left). Note that the matrices given in (4) satisfy the sampling conditions if $h_2 = \pi/b$ and $\pi/h_1 = b/\vartheta'$ (in practice $0 < \vartheta' < 1$ close to 1).

In [6], these results have been generalized to 3D tomography. The measured function $f \in C_0^\infty(\Omega)$ is supposed to be essentially b band limited where Ω is the unit cylinder of $\mathbb{R}^3$. The essential support of the Fourier transform $\hat{g}_k(\sigma, \tau)$ of the x-ray transform $g(\phi, s, t)$ is essentially K_3-band limted (see figure 2) where

$$g(\phi, s, t) = \int_{-\infty}^\infty f(s\theta + te_3 + u\zeta)du \text{ and } \hat{g}_k(\sigma, \tau) = (2\pi)^{-1} \int_0^{2\pi} \hat{g}(\phi, \sigma, \tau)e^{-ik\phi}d\phi,$$

with $\zeta \in S^1$ (circle trajectory), i.e., $\phi \in [0, 2\pi]$, $\zeta = (-\sin\phi, \cos\phi, 0)$, $\theta = (\cos\phi, \sin\phi, 0)$, $e_3 = (0, 0, 1)$, $s \in [-1, 1], t \in [-1, 1]$, and where $\hat{g}(\phi, \sigma, \tau)$ is the Fourier transform of g with respect to s and t. This geometry is the classical parallel geometry. It corresponds to a 2D detector turning around the patient with a x-ray source at infinity. Once again, standard sampling grids are redundant and interlaced schemes are twice more efficient. Interlaced hexagonal schemes can be shown to be $4/\sqrt{3}$ more efficient than the best standard grid.

Usual sampling schemes are standard grids. The main idea of this work is to place the calibration markers on a subset of the redundant part of the scheme. Indeed, if an interlaced scheme included in a standard scheme is not affected by the markers, all information in the 3D projection set can be essentially recovered thank to an interpolation formula based on (1). In the next section, we propose a fast interpolation formula for the 2D case. This can be generalized to 3D.

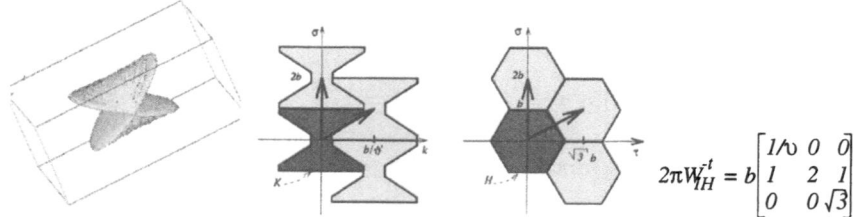

$$2\pi W_{IH}^{-t} = b\begin{bmatrix} 1/\hbar\delta & 0 & 0 \\ 1 & 2 & 1 \\ 0 & 0 & \sqrt{3} \end{bmatrix}$$

Fig. 2. left: 3D visualization of $\mathbf{K}_3$: outside of this isosurface, $|\hat{g}_k(\sigma,\tau)|$ is negligible. Center and right: hexagonal interlaced non-overlapping sets $\mathbf{K}_3 + 2\pi W_{IH}^{-t} l$: $\mathbf{K}_3$ is contained at the intersection of two orthogonal cylinders of respective basis K and the hexagon H.

2.2   Exact Fourier interpolation

Interpolating the lacking data covered by markers allows applying (after interpolation) usual reconstruction methods based on standard schemes. Let us suppose that, in 2D, half of the standard points (in a sub-interlaced geometry see figure 3) are covered by calibration markers and thus are lacking. We want to estimate the complete data $g(W_S l), l \in \mathbb{Z}^2$ from the available sampling points $g(W_I l), l \in \mathbb{Z}^2$. Let us consider the Fourier transform of (1) (with $W = W_I$)

$$\hat{g}_{W_I}(\xi) = (2\pi)^{-1} |\det(W_I)| \sum_{k \in \mathbb{Z}^2} g(W_I k) e^{-i\xi \cdot W_I k} \chi_{\mathbf{K}}(\xi). \qquad (5)$$

From equation (5) $\hat{g}(\xi_l)$ with $\xi_l = 2\pi N^{-1} W_S^{-1} l, l \in \mathbb{Z}^2$ can be computed with DFT, where N is a diagonal matrix $\mathrm{diag}(n_1, n_2)$. Indeed, a simple computation shows that (5) can be re-written

$$\hat{g}_{W_I}(\xi_l) = (2\pi)^{-1} |\det(W_I)| \chi_{\mathbf{K}}(\xi_l) \left\{ \sum_{m \in \mathbb{Z}^2} g\left(W_I \begin{bmatrix} 1 & 1 \\ 0 & 2 \end{bmatrix} m\right) e^{-2i\pi\left(\frac{l_1 m_1}{n_1/2} + \frac{l_2 m_2}{n_2/2}\right)} \right.$$
$$\left. + \sum_{m \in \mathbb{Z}^2} g\left(W_I \begin{bmatrix} 1 & 1 \\ 0 & 2 \end{bmatrix} m + W_I \begin{bmatrix} 0 \\ 1 \end{bmatrix}\right) e^{-2i\pi\left(\frac{l_1 m_1}{n_1/2} + \frac{l_2 m_2}{n_2/2}\right)} e^{-2i\pi\left(\frac{l_2}{n_2/2} - \frac{l_1}{n_1/2}\right)} \right\}.$$
$$(6)$$

In practice, the two previous sums are truncated, considering that the sinogram is periodic. Thus, with $m = (m_1, m_2)$ in (6), m_1 will be restricted to $0, \dots, p$ and m_2 to $0, \dots, q$ (the sinogram is periodic of period 2π in its first variable and must be zero padded in the translation direction from $[-1,1]$ to $[-2,2]$). We will choose $n_1/2 = p$ and $n_2 = q$. Thus, $\hat{g}_{W_I}(\xi_l)$ can be computed from two FFT of dimension $(n_1/2, n_2/2)$, respectively on the points $2W_S \mathbb{Z}^2$ and $2W_S \mathbb{Z}^2 + W_S(-1,1)^t$. Indeed,

$$W_I(m_1 + m_2, 2m_2) = 2W_S(m_1, m_2) \text{ and } W_I(0,1) = W_S(-1,1).$$

The value of $g_{W_I}(W_S k)$ is obtained by inverse FFT on the 2D grid of $\hat{g}_{W_I}(\xi_l)$. In Figure 3 we show a numerical example of this approach based on (6).

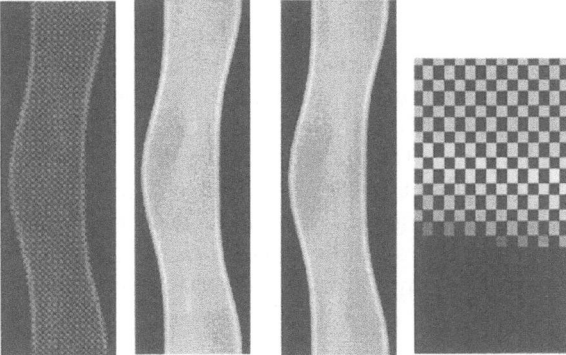

Fig. 3. From left to right: interlaced markers (see the zoom on the right) in a sinogram of $p = 202$ projections on $[0, \pi[$ and $q = 128$ samples ; Fourier interpolation from the available interlaced data ; corresponding complete standard sinogram ; zoom of a part of the sinogram on the left. We see that fast Fourier interpolation yields a good estimation of the complete sinogram, thus of the lacking data.

2.3   3D reconstruction

We can also directly reconstruct the function f from the available data, i.e., not covered by markers. We have seen that they should yield as good reconstruction as from complete data, except from a (small) loss in signal to noise ratio.

We illustrate this approach in figure 4 using algebraic reconstruction techniques. Any kinds of reconstruction methods could be used from interpolated data, but algebraic methods can easily handle irregular geometry and thus avoid the interpolation step. The function f is discretized in a sum of weighted voxel indicators. Then, the following regularized least squares problem is solved with a Conjugate Gradient algorithm:

$$\min_{\mathbf{f}} ||\mathbf{Af} - \mathbf{g}||^2 + \lambda \mathbf{f}^t \Delta \mathbf{f},$$

where $\mathbf{f}$ is the component vector of f according to the voxels, $\mathbf{A}$ is an ART-like matrix ($A_{i,j}$ is the intersection length of the voxel j with the projection line corresponding to the data g_i), $\mathbf{g}$ is the vector of data, Δ is the positive 3D Laplacian and $\lambda (> 0)$ is a regularization parameter automatically chosen by generalized cross validation [9, 10].

The theoretical result on the spectrum of the data is established for parallel geometry, but it can be numerically verified for a conical transform for large radius of the circle path (let say greater than three time the radius of the cylindrical reconstruction region).

3   Discussion

3D x-ray interventional radiology based on image intensifiers implies a dynamic distortion correction. In the case of multiple successive radiology acquired on a circle trajectory, we have shown that the spectral properties of the 3D data can be exploited to design marker schemes. Indeed, from the Shannon sampling theory, the whole information is then still contained in the data not overlapped by the interlaced markers. On the other hand, new generations of digital x-ray detectors [2], such as the PIXIUM 4600 from TRIXELL, do not suffer from distortions: 3D information on the patient (such as 3D reconstruction of bones surface) can be obtained without distortion correction. However, this very promising new technology is just emerging. Dynamic digital detector (¿10 images/s) are not available right now. Years will be needed before digital detectors will replace image intensifiers. That's why distortion correction technology remains of major interest.

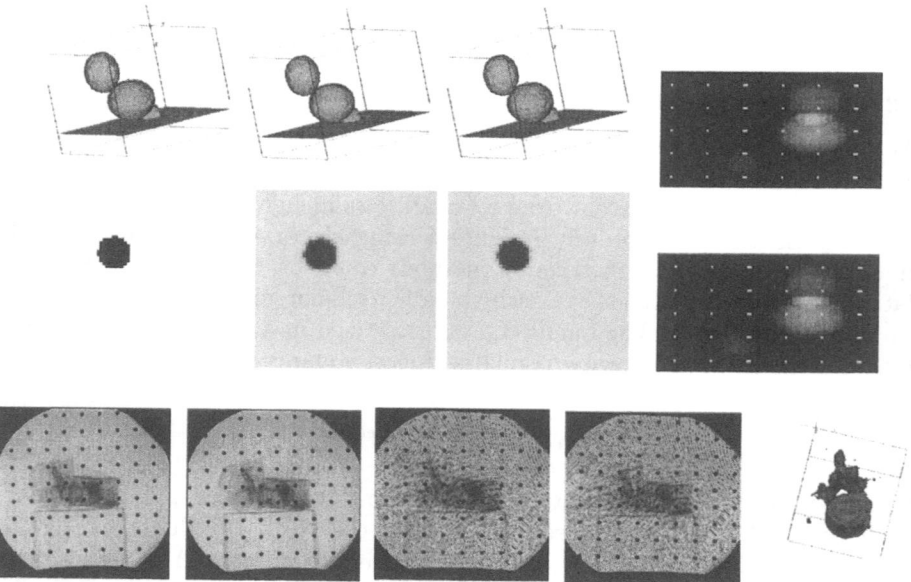

Fig. 4. Top, from left to right: object to be reconstructed; reconstruction from 90 projections with interlaced markers (60 × 50) on [0, π]; reconstruction from 90 projections *without* calibration markers; (right) an even projection with calibration markers. Second line: corresponding cross-section (3 first pictures); (right) an odd projection with translated calibration markers. Third line: even and odd projections of a vertebra; respectively after the distortion correction; 3D reconstruction of a vertebra from 63 projections on [0; 2π] with interlaced calibration markers.

Acknowledgments

This work is supported by a grant of the Région Rhône-Alpes within the project "Santé et HP : de la Vision au Pilotage".

References

1. G. Champleboux, S. Lavallee, P. Sautot, and P. Cinquin. Accurate calibration of cameras and range imaging sensors, the NPBS method. In *IEEE Int. Conf. on Robotics and Automation*, pages 1552–1558, Nice France, May 1992.
2. C. Chaussat, J. Chabbal, T. Ducourant, V. Spinnler, and G. Vieux. New superior detectivity CsI/a-Si 43cm x 43cm x-ray flat panel detector for general radiography provides immediate direct digital output and easy interfacing to digital radiographic systems. In H.U. Lemke, editor, *CAR*, 1998.
3. O. Chavanon, C. Barbe, J. Troccaz, L. Carrat, C. Ribuot, and D. Blin. Computer ASsisted PERicardial punctures : work in progress. *Computer Aided Surgery*, 2(6):356–364, 1997.
4. J.L. Coatrieux and C. Roux. Biomedical imaging: integration of image engineering biology and medicine. In *Contenporary perspectives in three-dimensional biomedical imaging*, chapter 1, pages 3–27. IOS Press, 1997.
5. M. Defrise and R. Clack. Cone-beam reconstruction using shift variant filtering and cone beam backprojection. *IEEE Trans. MI*, 13:186–195, 1994.
6. L. Desbat. Echantillonnage parallèle efficace en tomographie 3D. *C.R. Acad. Sci. Paris, Série I, t. 324*, pages 1193–1199, 1997.
7. I.A. Feldkamp, L.C. Davis, and J.W. Kress. Practical cone-beam algorithm. *J. Opt. Soc. Am. A*, 1(6):612–619, 1984.
8. M. Fleute and S. Lavallee. Nonrigid 3-D/2-D Registration of Images Using Statistical Models. In *MICCAI'99*, 1999. accepted.
9. D.A. Girard. A fast Monte Carlo cross-validation procedure for large least squares problems with noisy data. *Numer. Math.*, 56:1–23, 1989.
10. D.A. Girard. Asymptotic optimality of the fast randomized versions of GCV and C_L in ridge regression and regularisation. *Ann. of Stat.*, 19(4):1950–1963, 1991.
11. P. Grangeat. *Reconstruction d'images tridimensionnelles*. INPG, 1993. Thèse d'habilitation à diriger des recherches.
12. A. Hamadeh, P. Sautot, S. Lavallee, and P. Cinquin. Towards automatic registration between CT and X-ray images : cooperation between 3D/2D registration and 2D edge detection. In *Second Symposium on Medical Robotics and Computer Assisted Surgery Proc. (MRCAS'95)*, pages 39–46, Baltimore, MA, nov. 1995. Wiley.
13. F. Natterer. *The Mathematics of Computerized Tomography*. Wiley, 1986.
14. F. Noo, M. Defrise, and R Clackdoyle. Single-slice rebinning method for helical con-beam CT. *Phys. Med. Biol.*, 44:561–570, 1999.
15. C. Pellot, A. Herment, M. Sigelle, P. Horin, H. Maître, and P. Peronneau. 3D reconstruction of vascular structures from 2 X-ray angiograms using an adapted simulated annealing algorithm. *IEEE trans. Med. Im.*, 13(1):48–60, 1994.
16. P.A. Rattey and A.G. Lindgren. Sampling the 2-D Radon transform. *IEEE Trans. ASSP*, 29:994–1002, 1981.

Reconstruction of 3D Catheter Paths from 2D X-ray Projections

H.-J. Bender[1], R. Männer[2], C. Poliwoda[3], S. Roth[2], and M. Walz[4]

[1] Institut für Anästhesiologie und Operative Intensivmedizin,
Universitätsklinikum Mannheim, Germany
[2] Lehrstuhl für Informatik V, Universität Mannheim, Germany
roth@ti.uni-mannheim.de
[3] Volume Graphics GmbH, Heidelberg, Germany
poliwoda@volumegraphics.com
[4] Institut für Klinische Radiologie, Universitätsklinikum Mannheim, Germany

Abstract. The diagnosis and therapy of intensive care patients requires the usage of several catheters inside the patients chest. The information about the position and path of the catheters inside the patients body is important for the doctor, but is nowadays not part of the clinical routine. One possible source of this information are CT or NMR scans, which lead to an organizational overhead and additional stress for the intensive care patient. To minimize the overhead we implemented an algorithm to extract the 3D path of catheters in the body of the patient from two or more standard X-ray images. The approach is based on only few assumptions, runs completely in three dimensions, and uses the X-ray images only as a guideline for the path reconstruction process. It shows an inherently robust behaviour against misleading structures in the X-ray images, like loops and intersections. The algorithm has been tested with a selection of test images, including images from the clinical routine.

1 Introduction

Intensive care patients often need a multitude of catheters, for example, the central venous catheter for intravenous drips, pulmonary artery catheters to monitor the heart functions, and pleura drainages in case of lung injuries. What all of these examples have in common, is that the exact position of the catheters cannot be verified in the clinical routine. On the other hand the exact position and 3D path of the catheters is important information for the doctor: the risk of lung injuries caused by the catheter, and the success of the pleura drainage depends very much on its position, so knowing the first placement of pleura drainage makes the second placement more apparent. As a second example, the signals of a pulmonary artery catheter which monitors the heart functions, depend very much on its position. The exact position of the catheter tip relative to the heart cannot be controlled without knowing the catheter path and comparing the catheter path with the anatomical situation around the patients heart.

One source of the 3D path information of the catheters are CT or NMR scans. In practice, scanning every patient with catheters to control the position and path of the catheters would introduce a tremendous organizational overhead and additional stress for the intensive care patient. Therefore, CT or NMR scans cannot become part of the standard diagnostic process.

In contrast, 2D X-ray images, even if two or more images from different directions exist, are not the best help to identify the position and path of the catheters in relation to the patients anatomy.

As a result, there are no alternatives to the 3D reconstruction of the catheter position and path to give the doctor additional valuable information about the catheters he has placed. The 3D reconstruction gives the doctor the possibility of viewing the reconstructed catheter path in 3D from all directions, in combination with the X-ray images of the patient.

In this paper we present a method to extract the curve of one or more catheters in 3D space from two or more X-ray images, which is suited in principle for the clinical routine. A special emphasis has been put on the minimization of the number and restrictness of preconditions to allow the algorithm to work with standard X-ray images.

2   Problem Specification and Related Work

Figure 1 shows a typical set of X-ray images from a rotating monoplane X-ray system, which is a standard device to deliver two or more X-ray images of one patient from different directions. Typical catheters can be recognized as tubes with constant thickness and hardly visible edges. In many cases, especially when the catheters are of interest for the doctor, a special strip with high X-ray contrast is added inside the catheters to give a good signal in the X-ray image. The signal of the strip can be used to detect the path of the catheter. The white line, representing the catheter path, is typically not visible in all parts of the image; for example, it can be covered by bone, which absorbs X-ray images as well or better than the catheter material or the contrast strip does.

Because catheters follow anatomical structures and are primarily not intended to be bent, we assume that the 3D catheter path has a restricted curvature. In addition we assume that the geometric parameters of the image producing device are known; especially the projection parameters and the geometric correlation between the single images of the set of X-ray images are important for the catheter path reconstruction process.

As a result we can summarize the following preconditions:

- The catheters itself or a contrast strip appear as one line or two parallel lines with nearly constant thickness or distance in the X-ray images.
- The catheters or the contrast strip are visible in most parts of the X-ray images, and they have detectable edges.

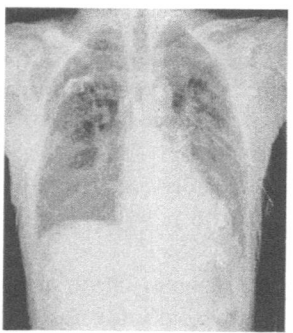
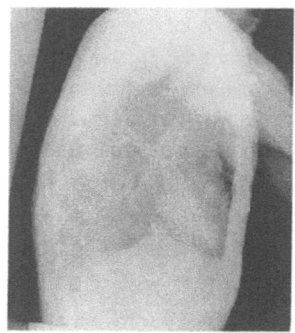

Fig. 1. An example set of X-ray images from a human chest. The pleura drainage at both sides can be recognized, because they contain a strip with good X-ray contrast, visible as thin white lines with constant thickness. The central venous catheter does not contain a contrast enhancing strip and can be seen partly in the upper image, but can only be anticipated in the bottom image.

- The 3D path of the catheters has a restricted curvature. [1]
- The geometric parameters of the X-ray image generating unit are known.

The reconstruction process of 3D paths of catheters out of 2D X-ray images is not a well known topic in literature. Most work related to the position control of catheter inside the human body, describe the reconstruction of the catheter tip only, or describe methods to control the catheters tip with external devices [1][7].

On the other hand, the reconstruction of 3D catheter paths can be compared with technical similar problems like the vessel reconstruction from angiographic images [2][8]. This problem has a similar setup: the goal is to find the 3D path of vessels, which can be seen as a kind of "lines" in the 2D angiographic images. Typical solutions for the vessel reconstruction problem are divided into the distinct steps "preprocessing", "segmentation of the vessels in the 2D images", and "path reconstruction". Because the catheter reconstruction problem does not have to deal with problems of vessel reconstruction like vessel branches and variating diameter of vessels, we decided to combine the "segmentation" of the catheter in the 2D images with the path reconstruction in one iterative algorithm.

3 Catheter Path Reconstruction

3.1 Preprocessing

The algorithm can be divided into two main steps, the preprocessing and the reconstruction loop. The reconstruction process uses the local gradient magni-

---

[1] This need not to be true for the 2D X-ray projections. See Fig. 4 as an example: the *3D helix with low curvature in 3D* has a sinus function with much higher curvature as possible 2D projection.

tude in the X-ray images for the catheter edge detection. The preprocessing step basically has the goal of delivering these gradient magnitude images in a suitable form. To eliminate the usually contained high-frequency noise, first a Gaussian filter is applied to the original images; in addition the images are median filtered, which gives the desired effect that this filter removes noise without destroying the edges of the catheter or its contrast strip. The gradient images are then calculated out of the smoothed images; the absolute value of the gradient is used to produce the gradient magnitude images.

3.2   Catheter Path Reconstruction

The main loop of the catheter path reconstruction process is an iterative process. The main data of the algorithm is a set of points which describe the path of the catheter. The iterative algorithm assumes that a certain amount of points is already available to reconstruct the next point. This is not the case at the beginning of the algorithm; the initial condition of the algorithm is discussed at the end of this section.

The iterative reconstruction process can be divided into the following major steps:

1. Estimation of the catheter direction in 3D and estimation of a new 3D point along the catheter direction.
2. Correction of the 3D point position:
   (a) Projection of the 3D point to the 2D images.
   (b) Detection of the catheter edges in the neighbourhood of the 2D points, giving a corrected catheter centre position in the 2D images.
   (c) Backprojection of the corrected 2D points to form a new 3D point of the catheter path.

The first step is to estimate an actual catheter direction in 3D and a new vertex on the centre of the catheter along its direction. The new vertex is computed in a constant distance to the last known vertex on the catheter centre so that it lies in the actual catheter direction (see Fig. 2). The estimation of the actual catheter direction is done using a main axis transformation of the point cloud containing the last recently generated points of the catheter path.

Since the algorithm works in 3D to use the information of all X-ray images, it is necessary to transform the 3D vertices to the images. This is is done by a homogeneous coordinate transformation using a 4 × 4 matrix for each image [4], which makes it possible to provide the typical conical geometry setup of X-ray image producing devices (see Fig. 2). In addition, the usage of a homogenous coordinate transformation allows it to consider the angle between the X-ray images, as well as other linear coordinate transformations.

After transforming the estimated vertex and the actual direction to the image, the algorithm searches for the edges of the catheter in the local neighbourhood. The search is located on a line, which is orthogonal to the calculated direction and goes through the estimated vertex (see Fig. 3). As the higher

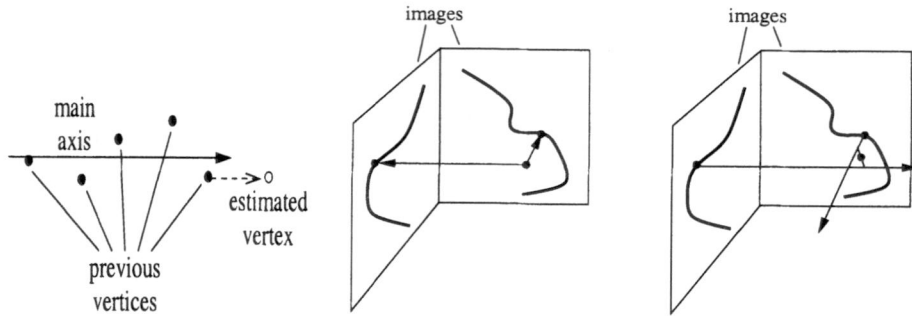

Fig. 2. Left: The first step of each iteration is the estimation of the actual catheter direction and the estimation of a new vertex in 3D. The actual catheter direction is computed using the main axis transformation of the last recently reconstructed catheter path points. Mid: The estimated 3D vertices are projected to the 2D images using a homogeneous coordinate transformation. Right: The backprojection of the corrected 2D vertices to 3D space results in the 3D point with the shortest distance to all projection rays.

greyvalues of the gradient magnitude image correspond to harder edges in the original image, the edges of the catheter are likely to have high greyvalues. To find the catheter edges, the gradient magnitude values along the orthogonal line are evaluated using bilinear interpolation. The interpolated values are weighted with a normal distribution with its expectation value at the estimated position of the edge, which is calculated from the estimated centre and the typical width of the catheter; the standard deviation of the used normal distribution is one of the adjustable parameter of the algorithm. Now the global maximum is searched in the weighted curve. If the maximum value is located in an interval around the expectation value and the value exceeds a lower bound, then the maximum is used as new catheter edge. Otherwise the edge detection process marks the found maximum of the gradient magnitude as invalid. This has the effect that values are ignored which are unlikely to correspond to an edge, because maxima far away from the expected position or soft edges are ignored. If both catheter edges are found by this method, their centre is calculated and saved; if only one edge is found, the most likely centre is calculated from the found edge and the width of the catheter; if no edge is found the original estimated point is taken as probable centre, and no correction of the estimated point in the 2D image occurs.

The catheter centre position correction will be done for each of the images. The corrected 2D positions are used to compute a new three dimensional vertex. A projection ray is casted from each image through the corrected catheter centre position on the images. The vertex having the smallest distance to all of these rays is determined (see Fig. 2). This vertex is taken as the new 3D centre point of the reconstructed catheter.

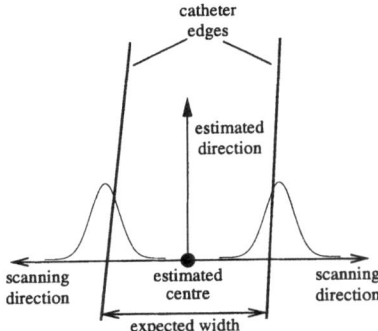

Fig. 3. The estimated catheter centre is corrected by detecting the catheter edges in the 2D images. The edge detection uses a weighted interpolation of the gradient magnitude values, and searches along the "scanning direction", which is orthogonal to the estimated catheter direction.

This whole method is iterated a maximum user definable number of times or until the number of errors exceeds a bound. The error counter is increased when no edge was found on one of the images. Single or only few sequent errors do not have much influence at the reconstruction, because the other images will very likely not show errors at the same time. This approach makes it possible to reconstruct the catheter correctly. This also enables the algorithm to master crossings of the catheter in the projected image.

During the first iterations of the main loop there are not enough preceeding vertices to estimate the actual catheter direction. Therefore, the algorithm uses a starting point and an initial direction, which is used until enough vertices have been calculated. Also the width of the catheter, if not provided externally, has to be determined in the beginning of the reconstruction process. This is done by averaging the distances between the found catheter edges over the first iterations.

4   Results and Discussion

Figure 4 shows a result of the reconstruction process using two test images as input. The algorithm has no problems with the reconstruction of the helix; in particular the circle, as one projection of the helix, will be cycled two times.

As a more realistic example Fig. 5 shows the reconstruction result with X-ray images from the clinical routine. These images show the capability of the algorithm together with its drawbacks. The reconstruction of the pleura drainage tubes is possible because of the good visibility of the strips inside the tubes. The 2D X-ray images contain discontinuities, which have not disturbed the reconstruction process. The central venous catheter is only partially visible in one of the projections and is therefore not reconstructible with the presented algorithm. To allow the reconstruction, the central venous catheter should be marked with the same strips as the pleura drainage contain them.

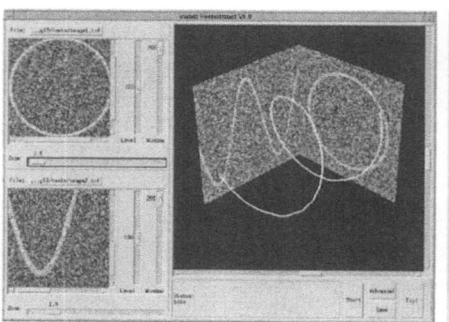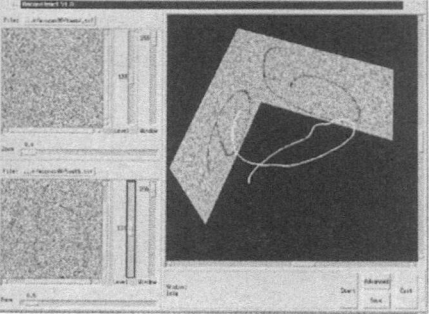

Fig. 4. The left image shows a screenshot of the test application showing two noisy test images for the catheter reconstruction process. The original path (helix) has been reconstructed. The right image shows the reconstruction of two noisy test images with a crossing in one of the images.

We found that the presented algorithm is capable of extracting the 3D path of catheters out of two (or more) X-ray images. But, of course, the algorithm or at least our first implementation is not free of some shortcomings.

First, the algorithm, at least in our implementation, needs a user provided start point and start direction. For the clinical routine, this should be replaced by an automatic process which identifies suitable catheter start points.

In addition, the algorithm has some adjustable parameters which influence the catheter edge detection in the 2D images, and the estimation of a new 3D vertex along the catheter path. The catheter edge detection is controlled by the standard deviation parameter of the Gaussian weighting function, and by the cut-off value which decides if an catheter edge has been found or not. Choosing these parameters badly can reduce the amount and quality of found catheter edge positions, and therefore lead to incorrect reconstruction results. In practice, we found that a certain set of values[2] gives good results, and the parameters are not critical.

The estimation of the new 3D vertex along the catheter path is controlled by the number of known 3D points and the step size. These parameters have much more effect on the quality of the reconstruction process. Since the algorithm extrapolates the linear main axis which approximates a number of vertices, the smoothness of the reconstruction conflicts with the largest possible curvature of the catheter. With increasing number of vertices that are used for extracting the direction, the smoothness improves but the maximum curvature is upper bounded. If the local curvature of the catheter is high, it may happen that the estimated centre vertex is not lying on the catheter anymore. In this case the reconstructed curve will leave the trace of the catheter at this point. A possible

---

[2] The Gaussian weighting function should have a width of approx. 0.5 to 1.0 of the *estimated catheter thickness*. The edge detection cut-off value is set to twice the value of the second maximum of the gradient magnitude image along the scanline.

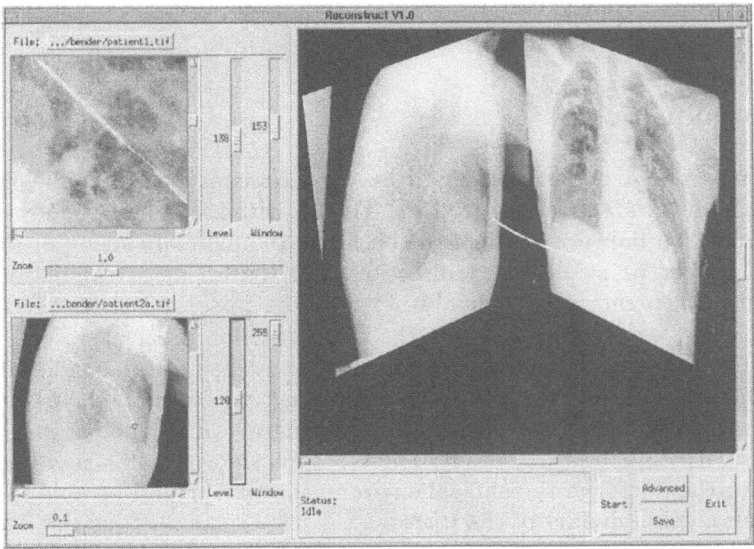

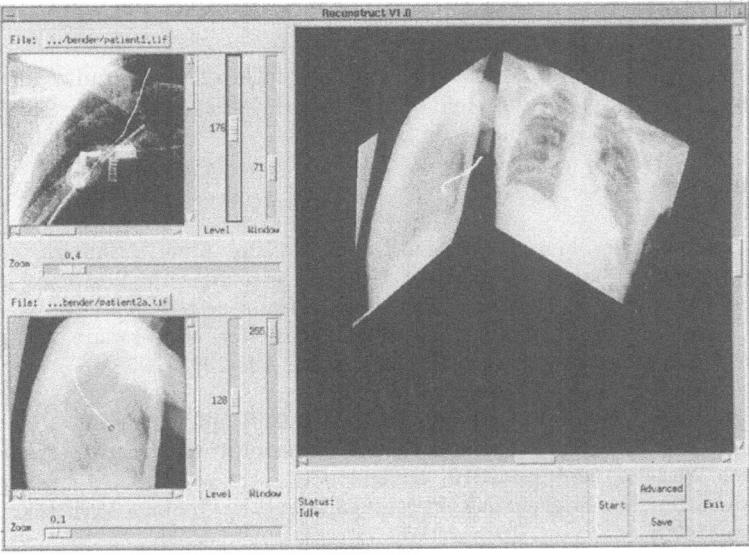

Fig. 5. These two screenshots show reconstruction results with X-ray images from the clinical routine. The upper screenshot shows a situation which has been adapted completely by the algorithm: even the gap in the contrast strip has not disturbed the path reconstruction. The lower screenshot shows the result of the reconstruction of the second pleura drainage of this patient. In this case the gap in the strip could not be crossed because the catheter wire has a non-zero curvature at this place. The linear estimation of new points along the catheter path has the effect that the reconstruction leaves the correct path.

solution to this problem is to use second order extrapolation polynomials, which are an option for further improvement.

5   Conclusion

We have presented an iterative algorithm for the reconstruction of the 3D path of catheters out of 2D X-ray projections. The algorithm contains some weaknesses that should be improved, which are basically the manual setting of the reconstruction start point and start direction, and the linear extrapolation of new catheter path points, which should be enhanced to second order extrapolation to overcome some problems during the reconstruction process.

On the other hand, the algorithm needs a small set of preconditions, which are fulfilled for typical X-ray images containing visible catheter paths, and it needs only standard X-ray images as input data, which can be produced for patients with catheters very easily. Therefore the algorithm can serve as base for a tool for the doctor in the clinical environment, and should be able to improve the accuracy and quality of the therapy.

6   Acknowledgements

The project has been funded by the research fund of the Faculty for Clinical Medicine of the University of Heidelberg with the project number 21/96.

References

1. Hans Starkhammer, Mats Bengtsson, Donald A. Kay, Alan R. Shapiro: Central Venous Catheter Placement Using Electromagnetic Position Sensing: A Clinical Evaluation. http://www.navionbiomedical.com/researc2.htm
2. Hildebrand, A. and Großkopf, S.: 3D Reconstruction of Coronary Arteries from X-Ray Projections. Proceedings of CAR '95, pp. 201-207, 1995
3. Jähne, Bernd: Digitale Bildverarbeitung. Springer-Verlag, Berlin Heidelberg New York (1989), pp. 92ff, 128ff
4. Foley, James D. et al.: Computer Graphics: Principles and Practice (2nd ed.). Addison Wesley (1990), pp. 201ff, 229ff
5. Bronstein, Il'ja N.: Taschenbuch der Mathematik. B. G. Teubner Verlagsgesellschaft, Leipzip (1979)
6. Erbe, W. and Bucheler, E.: Chest radiography for the detection of accidents during intensive care procedures. Prakt Anaesth 1979 Apr; 14(2): pp. 148-53
7. Williams, A.J. and Fraser, R. and Chorley, D.P. and Dent, J.: The Cathlocator: a novel non-radiological method for the localization of enteral tubes. J Gastroenterol Hepatol 1996 May; 11(5): pp. 500ff
8. Klein, J.L. and Hoff, J.G. and Peifer, J.W. and Folks, R. and Cooke, C.D. and King, S.B. 3rd and Garcia, E.: A quantitative evaluation of the three dimensional reconstruction of patients' coronary arteries. Int J Card Imaging 1998 Apr; 14(2): pp. 75-87

Automatic Extraction of Implanted Electrode Grids

Oskar M. Škrinjar[1] and James S. Duncan[1,2]

Departments of Electrical Engineering[1] and Diagnostic Radiology[2],
Yale University, New Haven, CT 06520, USA
oskar.skrinjar@yale.edu,
WWW home page: http://pantheon.yale.edu/~os28/

Abstract. It is common in epilepsy surgery to implant grids and strips
of electrodes between the skull and brain or inside the brain, in order
to localize functional areas. MR scans are currently used for a variety
of image-guided surgical planning tasks, including the localization of the
electrode grids. However, the MR scan taken of a patient with implanted
electrodes is distorted, and it is difficult to visualize and relate the electrode positions to head and brain structures. For this reason we have
developed an automatic algorithm that reliably extracts grids of electrodes from corrupted post-op MR scans. The grid is fitted as a smooth,
curved surface through the estimated electrode positions, properly estimating the orientation of the thin disk-shaped electrodes. The extracted
grid is then displayed in 3D together with the desired brain structures,
coloring the electrodes corresponding to particular functional areas. It
is now much easier to visualize and locate the positions of the important functional areas with respect to other brain structures and plan the
surgery. This method is currently in clinical use within the Department
of Neurosurgery, Yale University and Yale New Haven Hospital.

1 Introduction

During the course of neurosurgery grids and strips of electrodes are often implanted between the brain and skull or inside the brain and are used to map the
brain function. However, in order to effectively use the activation test results,
one needs to be able to relate the electrodes to some of the head and brain structures. This is conventionally done by using the post-op MR scans[1], and looking
for the electrodes in the scan. Clinicians find this approach limiting, however,
since one can look only at individual 2D image slices, and since one typically sees
just a few electrodes in any slice, it is not clear where they are in the grid (e.g.
a grid can have 64 electrodes, arranged in an 8 by 8 matrix), and it is difficult
to relate them to the brain structures. For this reason we have developed a tool
for extracting and visualizing grids of electrodes. The tool extracts the grid as a
whole, not as a set of non-related electrodes, by fitting a smooth, curved surface

---

[1] By post-op MR scan it is meant the MR scan taken after the electrodes have been
implanted

through the estimated centers of the electrodes. A by-product is the ability to reliably estimate the orientation of the electrodes[2]. Knowing the centers and orientations of the electrodes, and the surface of the grid supporting material[3], the whole grid is realistically displayed in 3D, together with brain structures of interest. In addition, the electrodes in the grid corresponding to particular functional areas are colored, further helping establish the correspondence between functional areas and brain structures. By using our tool, it is now much easier to reliably locate the functional areas with respect to the other structures, and plan and guide the surgery.

To the best of our knowledge there are no such methods available in the literature. While our method is automatic, there are two other approaches commonly employed: manual selection of electrodes (see [1]), which it is time consuming, or use of a post-op CT scan for electrode detection. Our first results were reported as an abstract (see [2]), while here we present the full method.

2   Method

The electrodes we use produce sphere-shaped artifacts of about 10 mm in diameter in the MR scan (there is a sphere artifact at the position of each electrode). The artifacts appear to be dark, hide the nearby tissue, and in addition they are often mixed with other head structures that are normally dark (e.g. bone, cerebro-spinal fluid - CSF). Moreover, the wires connected to the electrodes produce artifacts, especially where they are joined together (at the place they leave the skull). Fig. 1 shows typical artifacts in post-op scans.

Because of the artifacts and because of the noise one cannot reliably estimate the positions of the electrodes if they are treated separately, and the orientation of electrodes (the orientation of disks) cannot be estimated at all. The idea here in our work is to treat the grid (e.g. an 8 by 8 grid) as a whole. There are two main reasons to do this. First, this includes prior knowledge (the geometry of the grid is known prior to extraction) and second, the errors in estimating the electrode positions tend to cancel out. Our method is based on a combination of nonlinear and predictive filtering subject to differential geometry constraints. The algorithm fits a smooth, curved surface through the estimated electrode positions, and even if an estimated position is significantly off, the geometric constraints push it very close to its true position. As a by-product, once the surface is fitted, one can find the surface normals at positions of the electrodes and use then to properly orient the electrodes (the disks). The orientation of the electrodes is not as important as their position (the aim is to locate the functional areas), but helps to better visualize the grid by making it more realistic.

The constraint that the grid is deformable but not stretchable is used. If one represents the grid surface as a 2D structure with coordinates $x(s,t)$, $y(s,t)$,

---

[2] Electrodes used at Yale New Haven Hospital are disk-shaped and are 3.8 mm in diameter and about .5 mm in height

[3] The grid supporting material is usually transparent rubber

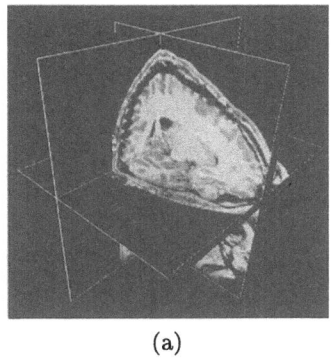
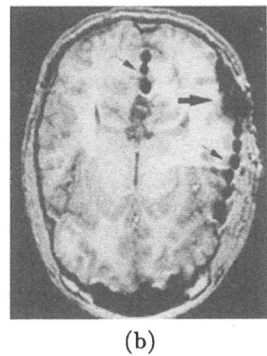

(a)   (b)

Fig. 1. Figure (a) shows three orthogonal sections through a post-op MR scan. One can see the artifacts caused by electrodes of an 8 by 8 grid between the top of the brain and the skull. It is not easy to visualize where those electrodes are in the grid and how they are related to brain structures of interest. Figure (b) shows an axial slice of another patient. The artifacts are usually sphere-shaped (small arrows), but sometimes (big arrow) are so dominant that it is very difficult even for the human eye to locate the electrode positions.

$z(s,t)$, then this constraint reduces to the fact that the integral

$$\int_{s1}^{s2} \sqrt{(\frac{\partial x}{\partial s})^2 + (\frac{\partial y}{\partial s})^2 + (\frac{\partial z}{\partial s})^2} ds \qquad (1)$$

is independent on t, and is invariant under the grid deformation. The same holds if t and s exchange positions.

Due to artifacts and noise it is very difficult in one step to reliably fit a smooth grid of a known geometry that satisfies (1). Rather, the geometry and smoothness constraints are enforced through a few steps, each step introducing some portion of the constraints. The three main steps of the method are: nonlinear filtering, predictive filtering and surface regularization and interpolation.

2.1   Nonlinear filtering

The purpose of this step is to find a set of possible electrode centers. Typically, patients are implanted a few grids and strips of electrodes often totaling to more than a hundred electrodes. Since each electrode causes an artifact that is dark, the first idea was to cross correlate a 3D kernel similar to the sphere-shaped artifact to the 3D post-op dataset. The maxima of the normalized cross-correlation would be possible electrode centers. The problem with this is how to set the kernel. While the center of the kernel has to be a dark sphere, the rest of it has to be "white", or some kind of transition to "white". This pattern depends on the structures surrounding particular electrode, and it is not the same for all electrodes. For this reason, we have moved from linear filtering to nonlinear one, i.e. we do not perform ordinary cross-correlation, but maintain the same basic strategy to look for a sphere-shaped dark region surrounded by lighter tissue. Prior to nonlinear filtering the dataset is smoothed by a 3 by 3 by 3 kernel to reduce the effect of noise. The form of the 3D kernel we use for the nonlinear filtering is shown in Fig. 2(b). Each voxel in the dataset is checked by doing the following steps:

- The kernel is centered at the current voxel.
- If any voxel in the KERNEL CENTER exceeds the THRESHOLD value, the current voxel is discarded and the next one is checked.
- The number of voxel values under the THRESHOLD in the KERNEL SPHERE and over the THRESHOLD out of the KERNEL SPHERE is now counted. The count is called SUM.

The parameters used in the algorithm are summarized and briefly explained in Table 1. All parameters are capitalized. There are two groups of parameters. Grid-related parameters depend solely on the geometry of the grid of electrodes used, and are further described in Fig. 2(a). Artifact-related parameters depend on the effect metal electrodes cause in the imaging system.

Table 1 – Algorithm Parameters			
Type	Parameter	Value	Description
Grid Related Parameters	DISK DIAMETER	3.8 mm	Electrode diameter
	DISK HEIGHT	0.5 mm	Electrode height
	OUTER MARGIN	5.0 mm	Supporting material margin
	DISTANCE	10.0 mm	Inter-electrode distance
Artifact Related Parameters	KERNEL CENTER	7.0 mm	Inner "dark" area
	KERNEL SPHERE	10.5 mm	The whole "artifact"
	MIN DISTANCE	7.0 mm	Minimal electrode distance
	MAX DISTANCE	14.0 mm	Maximal electrode distance
	MIN DIAGONAL	10.0 mm	Minimal square diagonal
	MAX DIAGONAL	17.0 mm	Maximal square diagonal
	THRESHOLD	40	"Dark" is under threshold

Thus, each voxel is either discarded or its position and SUM are recorded. The bigger the sum, more likely the particular voxel is an electrode center. However, there are typically many (thousands) of voxels that were recorded during the nonlinear filtering. At this point the first geometric constraint is introduced. Since electrodes on the grid we use are 10 mm apart (DISTANCE parameter), then any two estimated electrode centers should not be closer than a certain distance (MIN DISTANCE parameter). By imposing this constraint many of the estimated centers are rejected (the estimated centers that are kept are those with higher SUM).

The output of this step is a set of positions that are likely to be close to positions of possible electrode centers. The estimated positions are guaranteed to be at least MIN DISTANCE apart. Typically, a majority of the electrode

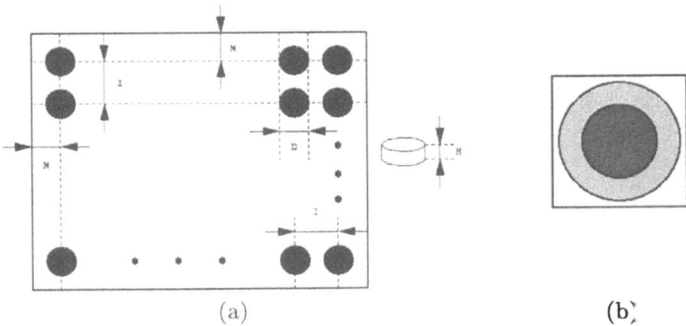

(a)   (b)

Fig. 2. Figure (a) shows the grid related parameters, that define its geometry. The black circles represent the electrodes arranged in a grid, while at right a single electrode is show. M is OUTER MARGIN, D is DISK DIAMETER, H is DISK HEIGHT and I is DISTANCE. Figure (b) shows a section through the 3D kernel. The innermost (the darkest) region is kernel center (its diameter is KERNEL CENTER) and the gray ring together with the kernel center is kernel sphere (its diameter is KERNEL SPHERE).

centers are found, some are missed, and there are some other structures that are wrongly chosen as electrode centers.

2.2   Predictive filtering

The purpose of this step is, using the estimated electrode centers, to label some of them, discard the rest and predict the positions of missing ones. The grid patterns are searched from the largest (typically 8 by 8) to the smallest ones. Each time a pattern is found, the electrodes belonging to that grid are removed from the list of estimated electrode positions, and then next largest grid pattern is looked for. However, since there are typically a few hundred estimated electrode centers, it would be computationally too expensive to check say an 8 by 8 grid pattern against all possible combinations of estimated electrode centers, including cases with missing electrodes. For this reason we first determine what we call "low level topology". We look for all pairs of estimated centers that might be neighboring electrodes on a grid - these pairs are referred to as "links". Any two estimated centers are at least MIN DISTANCE apart (that was enforced in previous step), and two estimated centers make a link if they are at most MAX DISTANCE apart. Next, we look for all sets of four estimated centers that might compose a square on grid, i.e. that make a 2 by 2 "subgrid". A "square" must have sides composed of already determined "links", and its diagonals must be at least MIN DIAGONAL and at most MAX DIAGONAL. An example of estimated centers and "low level topology" is shown in Fig. 3(b).

Now, having the "low level topology" available, it is much easier to search for grid patterns. For each "square" the pattern is searched for by sliding it over that "square". In other words, a pattern is positioned over the current "square", such that the "square" is in position (1,1) in the pattern, this case is checked,

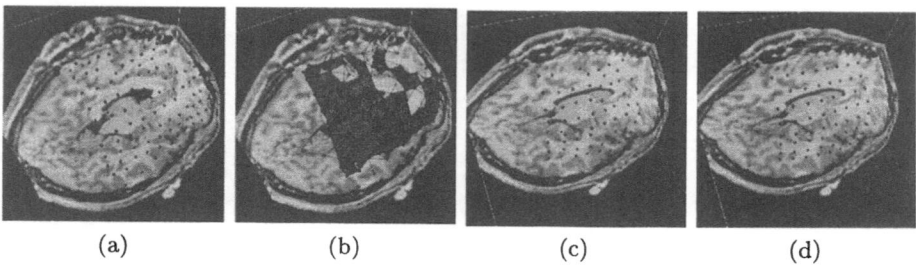

(a)   (b)   (c)   (d)

Fig. 3. Figure (a) shows part of the estimated electrode centers in a post-op MR scan (some of the estimated centers are occluded by the three orthogonal slices through the dataset). One can see a pattern of an 8 by 8 grid, but still the estimated centers are not regularly arranged, some are missing and there are false ones. Figure (b) represents the "low level topology" ("links" and "squares") as defined in the paper. Figure (c) shows the best match for an 8 by 8 grid pattern using the estimated electrode centers and "low level topology", while predicting the missing electrodes. The non-regularity of electrode positions is due to errors in estimated electrode center positions. It is significant in the top row of the grid, since the wires are coming out of the grid at that side causing increased artifacts. Figure (d) shows the electrode positions of the best match after regularization. One can see that the electrode positions form a more regular grid, compared to the one in Figure (c).

then the pattern is moved such that the "square" is in position (1,2) in the pattern, this case is checked, and so on until the "square" visited all positions in the pattern, both for "vertical" and "horizontal" orientation of the pattern (if the pattern has the same number of rows and columns, then "vertical" and "horizontal" orientations are the same, i.e. only one orientation is checked). For a particular case, say when the current "square" is in position (2,4) in the grid pattern, the nodes in the grid pattern neighboring to the square are predicted using the estimated positions of the four vertices of the "square". Predicted node positions that are close to some estimated centers are replaced by them. Further, the new neighboring nodes in the grid pattern are predicted using the the positions of the "square" vertices and already predicted node positions, and so on until the whole pattern is filled. By doing this, the pattern tries to follow the estimated centers, but if some are missing their positions are predicted. Once this process is finished, it is counted how many node positions, links and squares in the pattern match the estimated electrode positions, "links" and "squares" from the "low level topology". This sum is used as a measure to find the best pattern match. Thus, for each "square" the pattern is moved over all positions (and for both orientation), and the best match is determined. An example of the best pattern match is shown in Fig. 3(c).

2.3   Regularization and surface interpolation

The estimated electrode positions and the predicted positions of the missing electrodes have errors. However, those errors tend to cancel when a surface of a know geometry (representing the grid) is fitted through the best pattern match. The reason why the errors tend to cancel is that there is no preferred direction for error in estimated or predicted electrode centers. We suggest the following way to regularize the grid. If r_1, r_2, r_3 and r_4 are positions of four electrodes making a square in the best pattern match (the vertices of the square are connected as follows: 1-2-3-4-1), and

$$x_t = \frac{r_4 - r_1 + r_3 - r_2}{|r_4 - r_1 + r_3 - r_2|}, \; y_t = \frac{r_2 - r_1 + r_3 - r_4}{|r_2 - r_1 + r_3 - r_4|}, \; n = x_t \times y_t, \; a = \frac{x_t + y_t}{|x_t + y_t|}$$
$$d = \frac{a \times n}{|a \times n|}, \qquad \hat{x} = \frac{a + d}{|a + d|}, \qquad \hat{y} = \frac{a - d}{|a - d|}, \quad c = \frac{r_1 + r_2 + r_3 + r_4}{4},$$

then it is not difficult to see that c is the origin, and $\hat{x}$ and $\hat{y}$ are orthogonal unit vectors of a planar coordinate system fitted through the four vertices and centered at the square center. Furthermore, $\hat{x}$ is approximately in direction 2-3 (and 1-4), while $\hat{y}$ is approximately in the direction 1-2 (and 4-3). This is used to improve the vertex positions, knowing the inter-electrode distance (DISTANCE), as follows:

$$\begin{bmatrix} r_1 \\ r_2 \\ r_3 \\ r_4 \end{bmatrix}_{new} = c \begin{bmatrix} 1 \\ 1 \\ 1 \\ 1 \end{bmatrix} + \frac{DISTANCE}{2} \begin{bmatrix} -1 & -1 \\ -1 & 1 \\ 1 & 1 \\ 1 & -1 \end{bmatrix} \begin{bmatrix} \hat{x} \\ \hat{y} \end{bmatrix}.$$

This computation is done for each square in the grid. Since a vertex may be shared by two or four squares, its new position is computed as the average of its new positions in each of the squares it belongs to. Let $\mathcal{R}$ be a vector of all the electrode positions in the grid pattern. Combining previous equations for all the "squares" in the grid pattern, one can relate the electrode positions for two subsequent iterations, as $\mathcal{R}_{k+1} = f(\mathcal{R}_k)$, where k is the iteration index. The entire process is iteratively repeated until the electrodes assume steady state positions, i.e. until $\|\mathcal{R}_{k+1} - \mathcal{R}_k\|_\infty < \epsilon$ [4]. The procedure converges in practice. By doing this, the grid keeps its shape, while enforcing the distances between the electrodes to become closer and closer to the ideal inter-electrode distance. An example of grid regularization is shown in Fig. 3(d).

Regular grids can now easily be interpolated by spline or some other smooth surfaces. However, since the grids are just slightly curved, each square is approximately flat, and practically there is no need to do better than a linear piece-wise interpolation. Due to the aforementioned reasons, this interpolation provides almost a smooth surface and very closely satisfies (1). In addition, the surface can be extrapolated to model the grid-supporting material margins, and the surface normals can be computed to properly orient the disk-shaped electrodes. Two examples are shown in Fig. 4.

---

[4] Infinity norm of a vector is effectively its maximum element

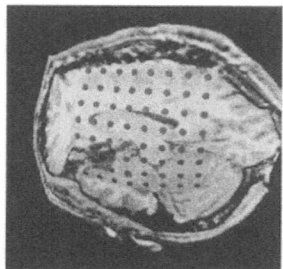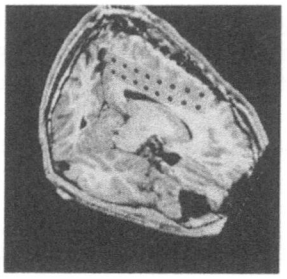

Fig. 4. These two figures show examples of the final electrode grid, represented as a smooth surface with disk-shaped electrodes properly oriented. The electrodes can be colored to denote certain functional areas.

3   Discussion

We tried to describe the algorithm in details, so that anyone interested can reproduce it. We have compared the algorithm output to the manually positioned electrodes, concluding that the error is within 1.5 mm, for most of the electrodes within 1 mm which is sufficient for clinical applications. Our plan for future is to perform extensive validation study of the method, and if necessary to improve it. The whole procedure takes a few minutes on an SGI Octane machine. The method, as currently implemented, works for rectangular grids of electrodes, but can easily be adjusted to work for non-rectangular grids and strips of electrodes as well.

This method is a big step forward in visualization of the electrodes, especially when it is compared to what was used before: either manual clicking on the electrodes, or just mere looking at the slices of post-op MR scans. It is now in clinical use within the Department of Neurosurgery, Yale University.

Acknowledgments

We are thankful to Dr.Dennis Spencer and Kevin McCarthy from the Department of Neurosurgery, Yale University, for useful discussions and for providing us with data.

References

1. A. Chabrerie, F. Ozlen, S. Nakajima, M. Leventon, H. Atsumi, E. Grimson, E. Keeve, S. Helmers, J. Riviello Jr., G. Holmes, F. Duffy, F. Jolesz, R. Kikinis, P. Black: Three-dimensional Reconstruction and Surgical Navigation in Pediatric Epilepsy Surgery. *MICCAI'99, Proceedings*, (1998) 74-83
2. Škrinjar, O., Duncan, J.: Automatic Electrode Grid Extraction from Distorted Post-Op MR Scans. *ISMRM'99, Proceedings* (1999)
3. M. P. do Carmo, Differential Geometry of Curves and Surfaces. Englewood Cliffs, N.J., Prentice-Hall (1976)

The Potential Use of an Autostereoscopic 3D Display in Microsurgery

P. Chios[1] , A C Tan, A D Linney, G H Alusi, A Wright, G.J. Woodgate[2], D. Ezra[2]

Institute of Laryngology & Otology
University College London
330-332 Gray's Inn Road, London WC1X 8EE
http://www.ilo.ucl.ac.uk
[2] Sharp Laboratories Europe Ltd.
Edmund Halley Road, Oxford Science Park
Oxford OX4 4GB
http://www.sle.sharp.co.uk

Abstract. This paper investigates the potential use of a prototype micro-optic twin Liquid Crystal Display (LCD) monitor for stereomicroscopy in microsurgery. The new device displays stereoscopic images via a pair of colour Charge-Coupled Device (CCD) video cameras attached on to a surgical stereo microscope. The paper illustrates the 3D microscope-display system set-up and calibration for stereo viewing. A series of experimental techniques was devised to measure the user-response of the new display system in depth perception of a solid object against the traditional eyepieces of a stereo microscope. As a control, free viewing with the un-aided eyes was also measured. The positional data were collected using a passive mechanical arm. The results showed good correspondence between all three visualisation methods. Error analysis of our numerical findings suggests that the depth accuracy of the new device is well within the precision limits of hand movement for surgical operations. Our study also proves that there are small discrepancies within the sample population of operators using the system. A study based on the psychological and psychophysical factors influencing the system is planned.

1 Introduction

The research group from the Institute of Laryngology and Otology at UCL has been conducting active research in the field of Augmented Reality in Ear, Nose & Throat (ENT) surgery. The aim of the project is to create a tool based on the concept of 'augmented reality' which will allow surgeons to realistically plan, rehearse and execute complex otological and base of the skull surgery. The scientific and technical issues relate to creating dynamic 3D images and involve real time processing, image buffer updating, parallel processing, developing, integrating an accurate tracking technique and creating a suitable human-machine interface for interacting under virtual surgical environment. This paper investigates the display aspect of the project,

---

1 For correspondence, email author at: doros@james.ilo.ucl.ac.uk

for which a binocular stereoscopic surgical microscope is transformed with "electronic eyes" to couple with a "3D TV" for surgery.

1.1   Stereo Vision

Stereo Vision is important for the perception of depth. Each eye uses different images of the same object to form a solid view in the human visual system. The 3D view is achieved by using many of the depth cues such as scenes hidden by opaque objects lying closer to the observer, foreshortening of distant objects by perspectives, shadows cast by oblique illumination, shading of the surface luminance, rotation of the object, and binocular parallax. In stereo microscopy most of these cues disappear and the main one used for perceiving depth is the binocular parallax. This is vital in microsurgery where depth perception is very important.

1.2   Microsurgery

Microsurgery has always been considered as one of the most difficult and delicate types of surgery. This is mainly due to the limited amount of working space and the high density of anatomical structures that exist in the region of interest. The use of binocular operating stereo microscopes is universal, but they limit the surgeon's head movement. This often makes the surgical operation stressful, uncomfortable for the eyes and hence more hazardous for the patient.

The arrangement of devices, tables and stools inside the operating theatre is fairly standard and has not been changed for a long time. Operating ergonomics are essential for any type of operation, and together with health safety protocols, form the design requirements for introducing new devices to the operating theatre.

1.3   Autostereoscopic 3D Displays

The display of stereoscopic images has been the subject of research for many years. Early techniques involved the use of two genlocked, monochrome video cameras which, being attached onto a stereo microscope, could capture the anaglyph created by the microscope's objective lens and intermediate red or green filters. With the use of complementary colour glasses the observer could see an intermediate-magnified stereo image. Recently developed stereoscopic displays differ only a little from the original concepts. Such display systems suffer from uncomfortable eye-wear, reduced image brightness, image flicker and cross-talk levels up to 10% [1].

Autostereoscopic displays that do not require specialised headsets are considered as a more realistic approach to 3D viewing. They offer a greater viewing freedom than the binocular stereo microscope eyepieces and are also useful for multi-view image presentations. However, image quality can be affected by several factors. Cross-talk of the two image channels may occur due to aberrations of the optical system. A limited display bandwidth causes degradation of image quality which results in lower depth perception. Additionally, it restricts the number of views that can be simultaneously displayed. The latter problem can be overcome by using observer tracking displays [2]. The observer's position is normally measured by infrared or video image processing tracking devices.

The current trend in autostereoscopic 3D display development is found in the use of thin film transistor Liquid Crystal Displays. These offer significant advantages such as flatness and thinness, high image resolution, high image contrast and fidelity, good colour quality and low cost. Especially "Twin-LCD' systems are considered of great prospect as they can offer full resolution of the LCD to each to the observer's eye [3].

2   3D Video Microscope

The surgical stereo microscope, one of the main instruments used by the microsurgeons at the time of operation, is usually attached to the end of a side arm of a crane that stands at one side of the operating theatre. The microscope itself is small, light and compact so that it can move freely in all directions.

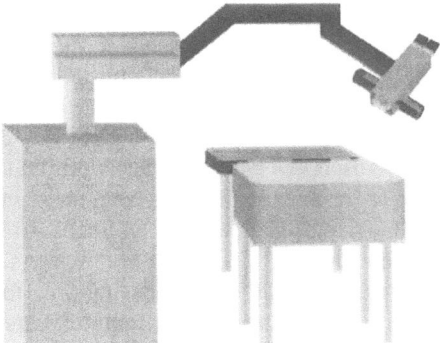

Figure 1: Typical microscope positioning inside the operating theatre

With new demands being introduced to medicine, the microscope structure has changed from its original form. For example, the need for teaching and subsequently for documentation brought forward the idea of splitting the light beam that comes out of the objective lens of the microscope into two identical beams. The first beam then follows its original optical path and enters the eyepiece while the other is directed towards a photographic camera, positioned at the focal plane of the light beam. This photographic camera mounting can be replaced with a video camera-TV adapter arrangement, through which the optical image observed by the microscope can be displayed on a 2D monitor or even recorded on a standard video recorder. In this way, staff inside and outside the operating theatre (*e.g.* consultants, medical students, nurses, etc.) can watch the procedure as if looking through one eye of the stereo microscope.

2.1   CCD Technology

One of the latest advances in the field of video microscopy is based on the recent developments of Charge-Coupled Device (CCD) video cameras. Modern CCD cameras come in a range of sizes designated by the 'inch' notation. The most common ones are the 1/3, 1/2, 2/3 and 1 inch. The field of view of the microscope is determined by the projected image from the eyepiece and is generally larger than the CCD sensor size. For high resolution and colourful visualisation of the images we use the three chips, 1/2 CCD, C-mount Panasonic GP-US522 remote head video camera. The 1/2 inch CCD covers only 20% of the total field of view, but offers a highly magnified video image. The 3 CCD sensors acquire the primary colours (Red, Green, Blue RGB) separately, thus leading to good colour representation.

2.2   Camera mounting

The synthesis of stereoscopic images, captured from a binocular operating stereo microscope can be achieved by placing two video cameras at the distal ends of the beam splitter respectively. The monoscopic images relate to the left and right eye fields of view. When combined and calibrated correctly the two images form a stereoscopic image that can be displayed by an autostereoscopic 3D display monitor. A 10.4-inch prototype Sharp Micro-optic twin-LCD display monitor (courtesy of Sharp Laboratories Europe Ltd) was used to conduct our experimental study. The light beam leaving the microscope's beam splitter is originally focused at infinity. In order to focus the beam to a reasonable distance from the splitter's distal end we use a Zeiss f60 TV adapter. The adapter has manual fine focus, iris selection and a bayonet connection at the camera end.

The precise placement of the CCD active sensing area to focus onto the field of view of each of the microscopic output areas requires careful calibration. A small deviation of 1 mm from the ideal position can result to a distortion of 2 cm between identical monoscopic images even at low magnification factors (*e.g.* x10). Therefore, the correct alignment of the two cameras on the autostereoscopic 3D display requires prior calibration before the cameras are aligned vertically and horizontally using the 3D display itself.

To overcome the above problems we designed and manufactured a prototype coupler that can give a travelling distance for the horizontal x-y plane of ±2.5 mm and on the z direction ±2.5 cm. The x-y translation ensures fine adjustment of the two monoscopic images on the screen, while the z direction movement finds accurately the ideal focusing position of the two cameras before or after the focal point. The coupler has a bayonet base so that it can be coupled to the TV adapter of the microscope. The other end is a C-mount coupling for video camera attachment. It can be locked at any desired position and can afford a maximum camera weight of up to 500 gr. The remote head video camera has negligible weight and does not affect the microscope's overall shape.

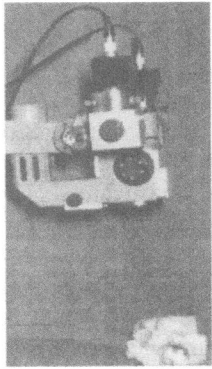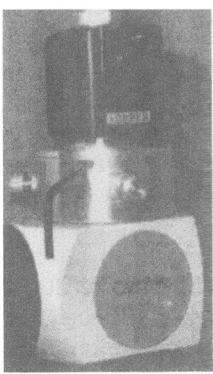

Figure 2: 3D Microscope profile and coupler close-up

3   Prototype Experiment

To test the effectiveness of the prototype Sharp Micro-Optic Twin-LCD monitor as an alternative to the eyepieces of the binocular operating stereo microscope, an observer-response evaluation test was devised. To conduct the experiment, we used a passive robot arm [4] to correctly identify and mark three identifiable points of a miniature model placed under the microscope. We chose 7 test subjects (including the author who is a medical physicist, the rest are all ENT surgeons) to carry out the experiment. The choice of examiners was made on criteria such as ease with microscope use and understanding of the visual information as it appears on the 3D display. A second series of experiments looked into the timed response of the observers on the task of passing a thread through the eye of a needle. In both experiments the microscopic image was viewed through both the 3D-display screen and the eyepieces. All experiments were conducted under a $x16$ magnification factor.

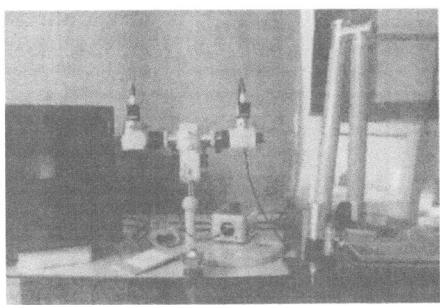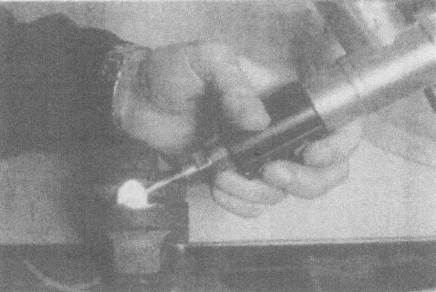

Figure 3: (a) Experimental arrangement of equipment (b) miniature model under the microscope

3.1   Use of 3D mechanical arm for digitising positions

The passive robot arm used in our experiment is a multiple axis-articulated arm with a spherical working volume of 2.4 metres. It has a 0.25 inch ball probe attached to its working end and a 1-inch reference sphere placed at its base. The mechanical arm is counterbalanced and temperature compensated, with six or seven degrees of freedom. It has optical encoders, placed at each of six joints, which combine to provide complete point position $(x\text{-}y\text{-}z)$ and orientation $(i\text{-}j\text{-}k)$. Three-dimensional digitised measurements are taken between the distance of the ball probe and the origin at the reference sphere. It operates using a standard PC and can be used as a stand-alone 3D-measurement system. The 3D mechanical arm has an accuracy of ±0.075 mm and has a calibration procedure to maintain correct operation.

3.2   Calibrating The System

Calibration of the 3D microscope-display-arm system is carried out manually and in sequence of steps before the start of the experiment.

Initially, the focusing level of each camera is individually adjusted by placing an edge-enhanced object under the microscope. At each step, the cameras are alternatively selected to adjust to the same focus level. Therefore, both cameras have the same zooming and focusing levels.

The next calibration step involves the alignment of the two monoscopic images on the autostereoscopic 3D display. This is done with the use of a cross-hair grid that is situated at the focal plane of the microscope's objective lens. The grid has a diameter of 30 mm. This ensures that the region illuminated by the microscope's light source is covered when an objective lens of 250 mm focal length is used. Next, the left and right displayed images are centred by superimposing the grid. A coarse alignment is accomplished at low magnification factors $(x6)$ using $x\text{-}y$ translation of the camera coupler and then fine alignment is achieved at higher magnification factors $(x16, x25$ and $x40)$. Correct alignment of the two monoscopic images is achieved only when they overlay each other in the final display. When alignment is complete, the two couplers are locked at this fixed position.

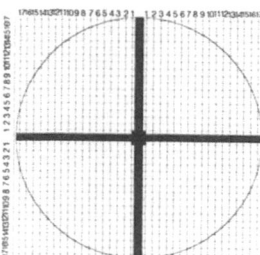

Figure 4: Calibration grid (numbers denote mm distance from the grid's origin)

Finally, the passive robot arm is calibrated. This is done by measuring 27 points on the circumference of the 1-inch sphere with the arm's probe. The x-y-z co-ordinates of the probe location are displayed on the PC screen [5].

3.3   The experimental protocol

Each operator starts the experiment by trying to identify 3 marked points on the object under the microscope via the autostereoscopic 3D display. He then attempts to bring the arm's probe in the focusing region of the microscope. The probe is not expected to make contact with the designated points on the object. This ensures that the positioning of the probe is driven by visual feedback and not by a motor reflex due to touching. To correctly register a 'hit', the x-y-z position is recorded by pressing a button on the probe's handle. In addition, each time the operator registers a point he then must remove the probe from the microscope's viewing region before carrying on with the next one. This prevents the user from getting to same position via 'memory effect'. This procedure is repeated 5 times for each of the designated points. The whole exercise is then repeated again using the microscope eyepieces only. Finally, without the aid of any magnification device, the exercise is done by means of free viewing of the object. The latter gives the operator more depth cues to work with.

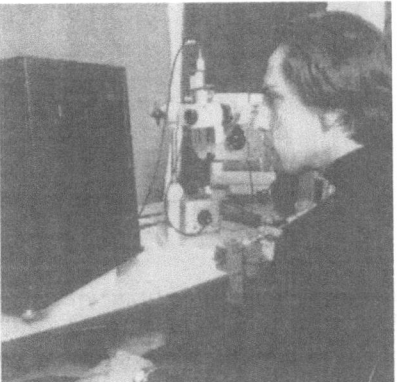
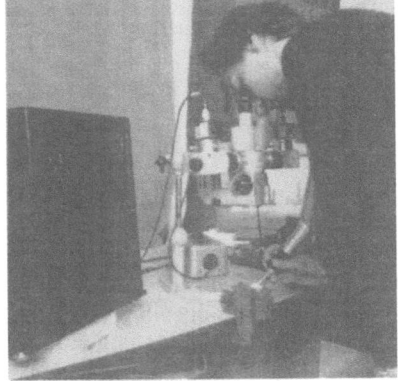

Figure 5: Operator performing the experiment using
(a) the Sharp autostereoscopic 3D display and (b) the microscope eyepieces

The second series of experiments evaluates the time response of each operator when asked to carry out the simple task of passing a thread through the eye of a needle while looking through the eyepieces. This is a representing experiment that takes place at the early stages of microsurgical training. The same experiment is repeated with the examiner looking through the autostereoscopic 3D display and finally, a standard 2D display (*i.e.* monoscopic display by switching off one of the image channels).

4   Results

4.1   3D Autostereoscopic Display vs Binoculars

The results showed that there is a correlation between the display and the eyepieces for one of the operators in the *x*, *y* and *z* directions for the second target point on the model. Other graphs for the remaining operators, which are not shown here, exhibit very similar patterns.

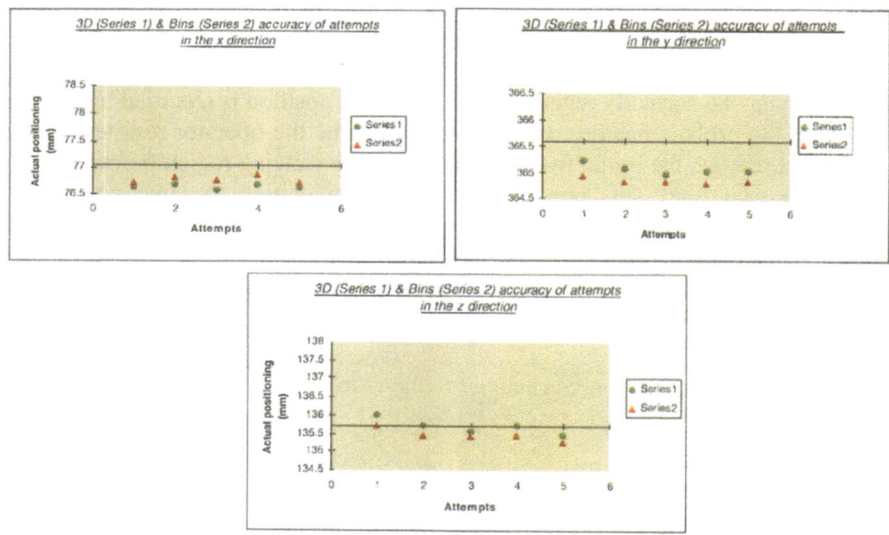

Figure 6

The experiment uses the free viewing value as the gold value from which the other two measuring techniques are compared. In the chart for x direction above, 77.041 mm is the gold value while Series 1 represents the deviation using the autostereoscopic display and Series 2 represents the deviation under the binocular eyepieces of the microscope. This 'gold value' is used as a reference value throughout the experiment. Likewise, similar gold values are used for the charts in the y and z directions.

The above graphs show little differences between the 3D display and eyepieces measurements for the individual's attempts in 'hitting' the target point. The following figure shows the overall correlation between each pair of results for all operators. This suggests that there is a matching trend in visual perception of the Sharp autostereoscopic 3D display to that achieved by the stereo microscope eyepieces.

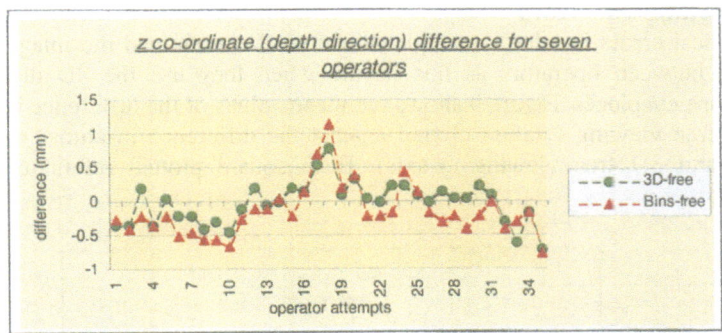

Figure 7: Correlation pattern between the autostereoscopic 3D display and the eyepieces of the microscope.

The overall x, y and z difference for all operators hitting the second marked point is -0.091 mm, 0.064 mm and 0.121 mm respectively. This implies good accuracy and precision in readings.

The time-response measurements show clearly the importance of depth information when the operator works in three-dimensional space. Additionally, we notice that the viewers response when using the autostereoscopic 3D display is very similar to when they use the microscope eyepieces.

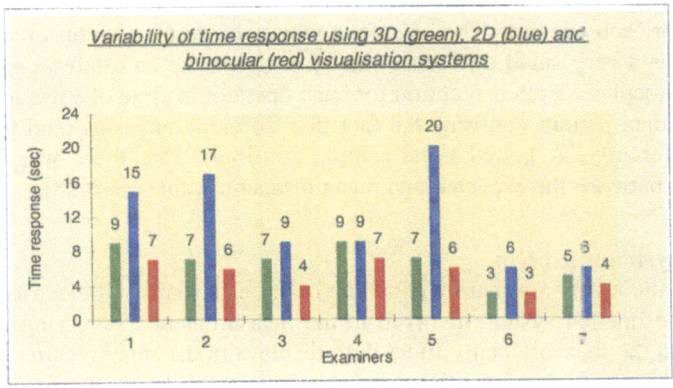

Figure 8: Graphical representation of results from the time study

4.2   Error Analysis

In order to validate the accuracy and precision of the Sharp autostereoscopic 3D display we conducted an error analysis. We divided possible sources of error into two categories, statistical and systematic.

4.2.1   Statistical errors

Statistical errors are due to sample selection. We examined the image perception variance between operators as this occurs when they use the 3D display or the microscope eyepieces. Figure 9 shows the mean values of the difference in binoculars and 3D free viewing (y-axis) plotted against the difference in autostereoscopic 3D display and 3D free viewing (x-axis). Each square plotted refers to a different observer.

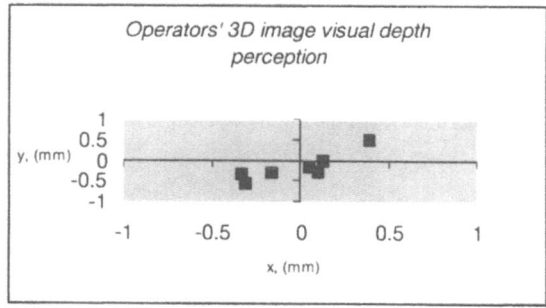

Figure 9

The figure clearly illustrates the way all operators view depth information from both visualisation media. Note that position mean differences are very small with all values lying very close to zero, thus implying only small discrepancies between both the Sharp 3D autostereoscopic display, the binocular stereo microscope with free viewing for each operator. The line along which the points are clustered demonstrates that there is a very small difference indeed between the autostereoscopic 3D display and the binoculars depth perception for each operator in spite of variations in operator bias. The data pattern confirms the fact that different surgeons tend to interpret the image differently. A paired t-test sample confirmed that there was no significant difference between the expected and mean measured values ($t{\approx}0.83$).

4.2.2   Systematic error

Systematic errors are mainly concerned with electronic and electrical deficiencies of the experimental system involved in the measurements. Justifying that the optics involved in the measurements affect both displays in the same fashion we considered errors in the accuracy of the 3D mechanical arm and the depth resolution from the pixel arrangement of the Sharp 3D display.

The active window of our prototype Micro-optic twin-LCD monitor was placed at a distance of 270 mm from the back LCD panel. Every operator was positioned at 270 mm from the window plane. At this position the specific prototype offers optimum three-dimensional visual information. The average interpupillary distance of the operators was 60 mm. Mathematical calculations of the Euclidean problem suggest that there is a 0.16 mm window in the depth axis in which the viewer can see the 3D image. This error is comparable to the 0.121 mm error in the operator-response graph of depth perception.

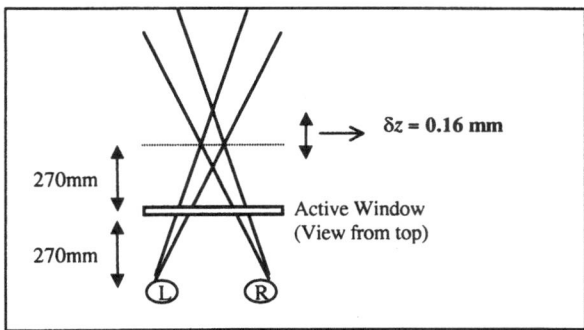

Figure 10: Depth variations in pixel arrangement of display

5   Discussion

The results showed that there's a correlation between the viewing properties of the Sharp Micro-optic twin-LCD autostereoscopic display and the eyepieces of the surgical microscope. Great emphasis is given in the perception of depth as this is very important to the acting ENT surgeon while he/she performs a surgical operation. Equally, the results establish the accuracy and precision in viewing three-dimensional objects using the new 'heads up' display.

The initial response of the clinical subjects who tried the experiment was positive to the use of this new viewing device. The device was found to be easily adaptable, accommodating to the eyes and offers natural viewing conditions. Similar results are also noted by other research groups as in laparoscopic [6] and endoscopic [7] surgery. It is envisaged that autostereoscopic 3D displays offer opportunities for lengthy surgeries. The additional benefit of the 'electronic eye' is that the image can also be routed to other display monitors located outside the operating theatre. This would introduce educational benefits for training purposes.

6   Conclusion/Future Experiment

At the present time, the use of stereoscopic displays has become a necessity in the practice of microsurgery. In ENT surgery, the use of stereo microscopes is unavoidable but uncomfortable for the surgeon. The system we have configured allows a 'heads up' 3D display where stereoscopic images can be seen in the same way as when viewed through the eyepieces of the microscope.

The experimental data indicate that the accuracy of the system is almost identical to that of the eyepieces. Depth recognition measurements of a microscopic model result to deviations of less than 1 mm, the average surgeon's hand movement precision. Also, the time study verified that human observers can accommodate the 3D image from the monitor freely and comfortably. Furthermore, studies for lower magnification levels (x10) showed similar result with slightly higher discrepancies between the two three-dimensional visualisation media. Finally, we feel that the Sharp autostereoscopic 3D display can be easily used in the implementation of augmented reality computer-assisted surgery.

Our experiment was laboratory-based and tried by seven clinical users. However, we noticed a few variations in the perception of the 3D image between different observers. This implies the possible intervention of psychological factors. Previous studies have shown direct association between surface curvature, and image spatial separation [8]. We will examine how this theory has interfered with our prototype monitor. We are in the process of running clinical trials using the 3D display.

The results of the experiment encourage the use of the Sharp Micro-optic twin-LCD monitor for stereo viewing of microsurgical procedures. The system is still only a prototype and work in theatre ergonomics will be needed for the optimum design of the 3D microscope-display system.

Acknowledgements

Our group would like to thank the Defeating Deafness charity organisation for their financial support of the project. We would also like to thank Sharp Europe Laboratories Ltd. for their constant support, help and assistance with the 3D viewing prototype.

References

[1] P.J. Bos, Liquid-crystal shutter systems for time multi-plexed stereoscopic displays, D.F. McAllister (Ed.), Stereo Computer Graphics and Other true 3D Technologies, Princetown University Press, Princetown, pp. 90-118, (1993)

[2] Graham J. Woodgate et al, Autostereoscopic 3D display systems with observer tracking, Signal Processing: Image Communication 14, pp. 131-145, (1998)

[3] D. Ezra et al, New autostereoscopic display system, Proc. SPIE 2409, pp. 31-40 February 1995,

[4] FaroArm Silver 8, Faro Technologies Inc., Florida, USA

[5] Caliper 3D for Windows manual, Faro Technologies Inc., Florida, USA, (1997)

[6] N.A. Dodgson et al, Autostereoscopic 3D Display in Laparoscopic Surgery, Proc of CAR'95, H U Lemke et al (Ed.), Springer-Verlag Berlin, pp. 1139-1144, (1995)

[7] J. Woodham, Amin Javer, "Heads-Up-FESS"- working from the TV monitor, FESS Special Feature, ENT News, vol. 7, no. 5, pp. 19-20, November/December 1998

[8] W. Curran, A. Johnston, Three-dimensional Curvature Contrast-Geometric or Brightness Illusion?, Vision Res., vol. 36, no. 22, pp. 3641-3653, (1996)

A Progressive Cut Refinement Scheme for Revision Total Hip Replacement Surgery Using C-arm Fluoroscopy

Jianhua Yao[1], Russell H. Taylor[1], Randal P. Goldberg[1], Rajesh Kumar[1], Andrew Bzostek[1], Robert Van Vorhis[2], Peter Kazanzides[2], Andre Gueziec[3], J. Funda[3]

1 Computer Science Department, The Johns Hopkins University, Baltimore, MD, USA
2 Integrated Surgical Systems, Davis, CA, USA
3 IBM T.J. Watson Research Center, Yorktown Heights, NY, USA

Abstract. We describe a new method to cut a precise, high quality cavity in Revision Total Hip Replacement surgery (RTHR) using a set of intra-operative C-arm fluoroscopic images. With respect to previous approaches, our method provides the following new features: (1) a novel checkerboard plate was designed to correct the geometric distortion within fluoroscopic images. Unlike previous distortion correction devices, the plate doesn't completely obscure any part of the image, and the distortion correction algorithm works well even when there are some overlaid objects in field of view; (2) a novel corkscrew fiducial object attached to the robot end-effector was designed, and a 6D pose estimation algorithm based on the 2D projection of the corkscrew is developed and used in robot-imager registration and imager co-registration; (3) we propose a progressive cut refinement scheme and an iterative cut location algorithm which utilizes image subtraction and 2D anatomy contour matching techniques. Several cutting experiments and some simulated experiments have been conducted to assess our techniques. The results indicate that our scheme is a promising method for RTHR application.

1. Introduction and Previous Works

Our research is part of a joint project with Integrated Surgical System (ISS), at Davis, CA., to develop a computer integrated system to assist surgeons in revision total hip replacement surgery (RTHR). RTHR is performed after a patient had PTHR (Primary Total Hip Replacement Surgery) and the implant fails for some reason. RTHR is a much more difficult operation, because less bone tissue remains and a precise, high quality canal is required [1].

In PTHR and RTHR, a surgical robot is needed to mill a precise cavity for the femoral implant. The robot trajectory is planned preoperatively based on a CT scan of the femur and the CAD model of the implant. Then the robot trajectory is executed after the intra-operative registration between the robot and the femur [1, 2]. Accurate robot-to-patient and robot-to-image registrations are essential to RTHR surgery. Registration techniques have included: implanted fiducials as in ROBODOC® [3], 3D-3D anatomy based registration [4], and 2D-3D anatomy based registration [4-6]. Among these, 2D-3D anatomy based registration is the most favorable one because it is less invasive, but it also presents significant technical challenges.

Our developments of a computer integrated RTHR system started about four years ago. Taylor, Joskowicz *et al.* [1, 2] proposed the initial system. Some of their ideas have been investigated in the current research. Gueziec *et al.* [5, 7] explored the feasibility of anatomy based registration using fluoroscopy. The goal of our research is to direct the robot to cut a precise cavity using intra-operative portable C-arm fluoroscopy as guidance. We propose a series of new methods and system to solve this problem. Section 2 addresses the overview of the system first. Then a new method for fluoroscopic image spatial distortion correction is described in section 3. In section 4 we present a novel pose estimation device that can be attached to the robot end-effector and provide a method to compute the transformation between robot and imager geometry and as well as perform co-registration between different imager geometry. In section 5, the experimental protocol is introduced. A progressive cut refinement scheme is elaborated in section 6. Finally we discuss several experiments we have done so far and our future plan.

2. System Overview

Our current work is applicable for execution of pre-surgical plans based either on preoperative CT images or on multiple intra-operative 2D X-ray images. The flow chart in Figure 1(left) illustrates the former option. First the cut cavity is planned based on the preoperative CT volume. During preoperative setup, a corkscrew-shaped fiducial object is mounted on the robot's cutter and a calibration procedure is performed to determine the corkscrew-to-robot transformation (section 4). In the intra-operative stage, the femur is placed in a fixation device that holds it in a fixed but unknown position relative to the robot. Multiple C-arm images are grabbed. The registrations among robot, patient and imager are conducted using our pose estimation algorithm and the anatomy or fiducial based registration method (section 4, 5). Then a small progressive cut is executed by the guidance of the images. After the cut, another set of images is taken in similar C-arm poses as those used for initial registration. The real cut cavity is detected using a digital subtraction technique and is compared to the expected cavity (section 6). Then the registration between the robot and patient is updated based on the discrepancy between the real cavity and the expected cavity. The procedure is iterated until we get the final cut.

A typical flow for intraoperative X-ray based plans is shown in Figure 1(right). Such a case can arise in RTHR if CT reconstruction artifacts are so severe that CT-based planning is impractical or if unexpected circumstances during surgery make re-planning necessary. In this case, the femur is placed into a fixation device that holds it stationary with respect to the robot and multiple C-arm X-ray images are taken as before. A cut cavity shape is determined and its desired pose is determined interactively using an "image spreadsheet" [1, 2] in which the projected contours of the cavity are superimposed on the X-ray images. Iterative cutting proceeds as before.

We have prototyped our method and experimentally demonstrated it on dental acrylic phantoms and simulated images. Figure 2 is a typical experimental setup. The de-warping plate is placed over the C-arm detector. The corkscrew for pose estimation is attached to a ROBODOC® cutter. A dental acrylic phantom held by a box holder is used for these cutting experiments to evaluate our method.

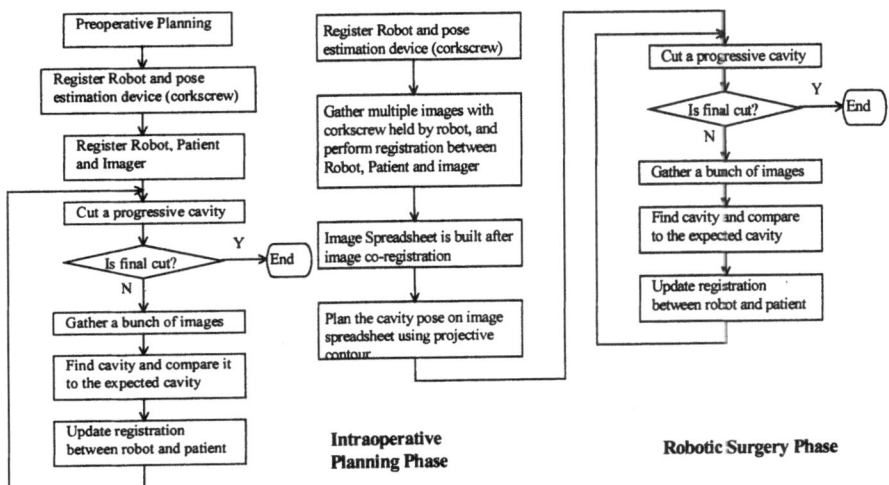

Figure 1. (left) Procedure flow for CT-based plans;
(right) Procedure flow for multiple x-ray based plans.

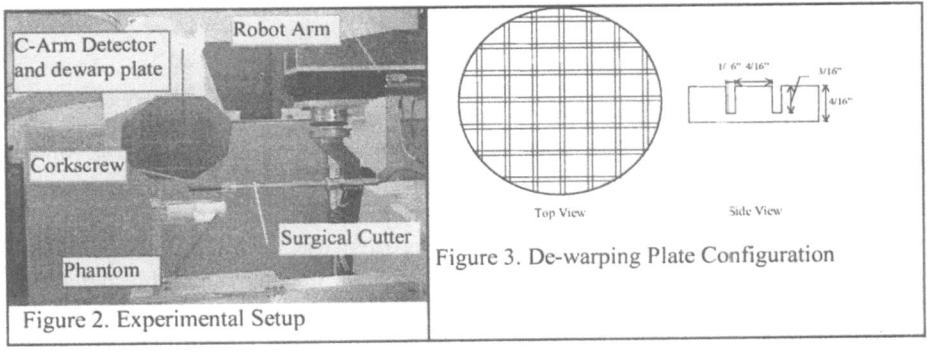

Figure 2. Experimental Setup

Figure 3. De-warping Plate Configuration

3. Intrinsic Image Calibration

Intrinsic imaging parameters correspond to image warping, focal length, pixel scaling, and image center, and can be computed by analyzing an image of a calibration object. Schreiner's method [8] was used to compute the C-arm focal length, the pixel scaling and the image center. We assume that these parameters do not change under different C-arm poses. Using fluoroscopic X-ray imaging for quantitative measurement requires precise calibration of the imager to remove the spatial distortions caused by the intensifier. Boone [9] provided the theory and analysis of the nature of the distortion and proposed some techniques to correct it. Schreiner [8] implemented Boone's method by placing a grid of radiopaque beads over the C-arm detector.

In our distortion correction approach, a 1/4 inch thick semi-radiolucent aluminum plate is placed over the detector of the fluoroscopic C-arm (Figure 2). Horizontal and vertical grooves with 3/16 inches deep and 1/16 inch wide are machined in the plate in a square pattern on 1/4 inch intervals (Figure 3). These grooves show up as pale lines on the x-ray images, and provide enough contrast to be found in the log image by delicate image processing methods. Other objects are still clearly visible with the checkered pattern as background. It has some advantages for cases such as ours, where the C-arm may be placed in multiple unpredictable poses during the procedure, thus making a separate preoperative distortion correction calibration impractical. In particular, the checkerboard geometry does not completely obscure any part of the image, allowing it to remain in place during the procedure although there is some sacrifice of contrast.

We have investigated various ways to use this checkerboard plate to compensate for fluoroscopic image distortion. Methods examined include Piecewise Polynomial Mapping Algorithm, Thin Plate Spline Morphometric Algorithm [10], and Two-Pass Scanline Algorithm [11]. Our current preferred choice is a variant of Two-Pass Scan-

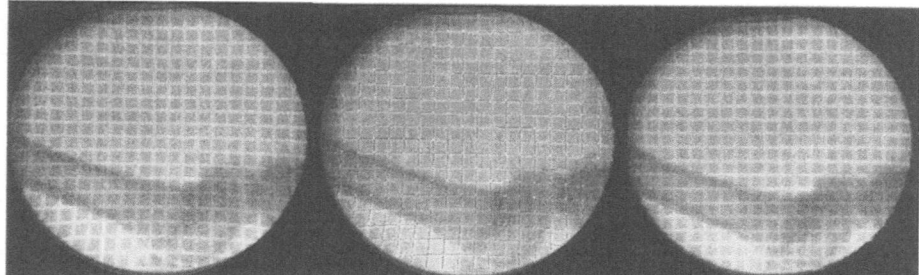

Figure 4: Image de-warping Results. (Left) Fluoroscopic x-ray image of a smoked ham. The white lines correspond to grooves cut into an aluminum de-warping calibration plate. (Middle) The same image after the grooves have been located. (Right) De-warped image.

line Algorithm. Sample images can be found in Figure 4.

The accuracy of the distortion correction process was verified by following experiments: First one image with the checkerboard plate was taken and the spatial distortion of the image was corrected, and the lookup table was saved. Then a bead pattern was attached over the plate, and another image was taken. The bead pattern image was then de-warped using the saved lookup table. The beads were detected in the image and distances between pairs of beads computed. Comparison of the computed distance and the actual distance between beads in the bead pattern gives an assessment of the accuracy of the de-warping algorithm. The mean error was 0.12 mm on the central area and 0.25mm on the marginal area while the beads were 20mm apart. (Pixel size is approximately 0.32mm). This shows that our distortion correction methods provide reasonably accurate results.

4 C-arm Pose Estimation and Extrinsic Calibration

For extrinsic calibration, the task is to compute the transformation between the C-arm coordinate system and other intra-operative coordinate systems such as the patient's anatomy, the robot, and the surgical tool.

Our current research provides image-based methods for the co-registration of the portable C-arm without extrinsic tracking device. Our strategy relies on identifying features within a single X-ray image of a known 3D arrangement of fiducials and computing the appropriate transformation. These considerations have led us to explore a calibration fiducial geometry consisting of a 5/4-turn "corkscrew" spiral and four circular rings surrounding a central shaft, as shown in Figure 5. The initial embodiment is designed to be held in the JHU/IBM LARS™ robot and the ROBODOC® orthopedic cutter. It is fabricated from autoclavable polyamide with a steel central shaft and copper wire filled grooves machined into the outside of the polyamide rod.

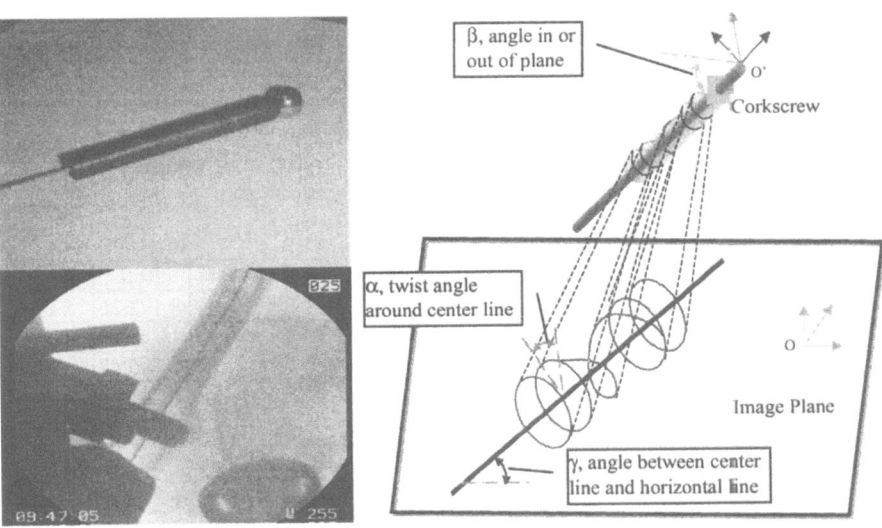

Figure 5. Corkscrew fiducial object. (left top) Corkscrew fiducial object. (left bottom) Introaoperative x-ray image of corkscrew object. (right) Projection of corkscrew

The fiducial geometry of the corkscrew has the property that its 6D pose can be computed from a single projected 2D image. Calculation of these parameters is accomplished by applying delicate image segmentation algorithms and a series of Hough transforms to the subject image, calculating a subset of the parameters using different parts of the fiducial geometry as following (Figure 5): The centerline of the shaft provides one rotation and one translation parameter, both in the plane of the image, restricting the centerline of the fiducial to lie on a plane in 3D space. The ellipses projected by the four rings give the other two translations as well as a rotation into or out of that plane. The first translation is determined by the position of the pattern of ellipses along the centerline. And the distance between the ellipses determines the fiducial's distance from the image plane (one translation in 3D). The phase angle of the projection of the helix directly determines the twist rotational angle. The shape of the projected helix also determines whether the corkscrew rotates into or out of the image plane, i.e. the sign of angle β. After finding and computing the geometry parameters of the corkscrew projection on the 2D image, the transformation between the image coordinate system (O) and the corkscrew coordinate system (O') can be constructed. The algorithm is pretty robust due to the use of the Hough transform and the geometric constraints between different parts. The corkscrew can be used for pose estimation of C-arm geometry and co-registration between two C-arm poses. By attaching this corkscrew to the robot's end effector and conducting a pre-operative corkscrew-robot registration, the registration between the robot and the imager can be computed.

We conducted the following experiments to assess the accuracy of our method. The corkscrew was mounted on the LARS^{TM} robot's end-effector. One image of the corkscrew was taken first. Keeping the C-arm pose unaltered, the robot joint was then translated or rotated. Then another image was taken after the movement. The corkscrew movement (i.e. the movement of the robot end-effector) between the two images was computed based on the pose estimation algorithm. Then the computed movement was compared to the real movement of the robot. Table 1 and Table 2 show the results. The results indicate that the rotation accuracy is around 1°-2°. The error of the roll angle is large because the secondary radius of the ring can not be computed accurately especially when the angle is small. The results also show that the average translation error is under 0.5 mm along the direction parallel to the image plane (Axis x, y), and can be larger than 1.0mm along the focal length direction (Axis z).

Trial	Robot Rotation Angle(°)			Computed Rotation Angle(°)			Error (°)		
	Twist	Roll	Pitch	Twist	Roll	Pitch	Twist	Roll	Pitch
1	30	15	15	30.28	17.26	14.82	0.28	2.26	0.18
2	60	30	30	59.53	31.76	29.34	0.47	1.76	0.66
3	90	45	45	88.95	44.17	47.07	1.05	0.83	2.07
						Average Error	0.60°	1.62°	0.97°
						Standard Deviation	0.33°	0.59°	0.80°

Table 1. Rotation Error Assessment in Corkscrew Pose Estimation Method

Trial	Robot Translate (mm)			Computed Translate (mm)			Error (mm)		
	X	Y	Z	X	Y	Z	X	Y	Z
1	5	5	5	5.04	5.13	5.61	0.04	0.13	0.61
2	10	10	10	9.73	10.39	11.25	0.27	0.39	1.25
3	15	15	15	14.2	14.35	13.62	0.8	0.65	1.38
						Average Error	0.37	0.39	1.08
						Deviation	0.32	0.21	0.34

Table 2. Translation Error Assessment in Corkscrew Pose Estimation Method

5. Cutting Experiment

We have conducted some cutting experiments using the orthopedic cutter and dental acrylic phantoms. Extensive tests were carried out on plastic bones and foam test blocks in order to verify basic system accuracy and to gain confidence in overall system behavior. The following is a general procedure for a cutting experiment.

Step 1: The corkscrew is attached to the cutter mounted on the end-effector. A separate procedure is performed to calibrate the robot and the corkscrew, i.e. $F_{robot\text{-}corkscrew}$.

Step 2: Several images of the corkscrew and the phantom are taken. Then the registration, $F_{corkscrew\text{-}imager}$, between the corkscrew and the imager is computed using the corkscrew pose estimation algorithm in Section 3. The registration $F_{femur\text{-}imager}$ between the femur and the imager is obtained using the femur anatomy or fiducial beads (at present fiducial beads are used). Finally the registration between femur and robot is written as

$$F_{robot-femur} = F_{robot-corkscrew} \cdot F_{corkscrew-imager} \cdot F_{imager-femur}$$

<u>Step 3</u>: The cutter is moved to the starting position, and a predefined shape is cut.

The cavity position was estimated by measuring wall thickness using calipers to get the assessment of the errors. With the angular separation of about 50 degree between two C-arm views, we observe a cavity placement error of about 0.5mm in one direction in the cutting plane but as large as 1.5 mm in the other direction. A number of factors may count for this result: the limited angular separation between views, the particular method used to cut the test cavity, the calibration error in setup. In any case, these results led us to explore a progressive cutting scheme described in Section 6.

6. Iterative cut cavity location algorithm

We are investigating a progressive cutting scheme to improve the placement accuracy: First a small cavity is cut. Then an iterative cut cavity location algorithm is applied to compute the discrepancy between the real cut pocket and the cut model, then the registration between the robot and femur anatomy is adjusted accordingly. On the next cut, a larger pocket is cut and the process is repeated until the final desired shape is cut. The idea of progressive cutting is straightforward. The problem is how to measure the error after each cut using the fluoroscopic C-arm. We developed an iterative cut cavity location algorithm to solve this problem.

The idea of the iterative cut cavity location algorithm is outlined: The cut cavity model and its transformation relative to the femur is planned in the pre-operative stage. After each cut, several images of the cut cavity and corkscrew from different view angles are taken. The C-arm geometry of each image is constructed using the corkscrew pose estimation algorithm. On each image, an image subtraction technique (section 6.3) is employed to generate the 2D contour of the cut cavity, denoted as C_c. The projective apparent contour C_m (section 6.1) of the cut cavity model is built. A 2D contour registration algorithm (section 6.2) is applied to get the 2D transformation between C_c and C_m. Then the 2D transformation between contours is back-projected to a 3D transformation. Finally the transformation between the real cut cavity and the cut model is updated (Section 6.4). The above procedure is iterated on all images. Then the transformation is used to update the registration between the robot and the femur.

6.1 Projective Apparent Contour of 3D model

An algorithm to generate the 2D projective apparent contour of a 3D surface model was developed. A 3D surface model is a list of 3D triangular facets. Given the view geometry, the projective apparent contour is the projection of a set of edges on the surface, such that the facet on one side of the edge is visible while the facet on the other side is invisible.

6.2 2D contour registration algorithm

There are two stages in the computation of the 2D transformation between two contours. During the first stage the initial 2D transformation is computed using first and second order moments of the contour. Second stage is an Iterative Closet Point algorithm. It involves using Least-Square-Error method to recursively update the transformation. It usually takes two or three iterations to converge in the second stage.

6.3 Digital Subtraction

On the image of the cut cavity, the edge of the cavity can be very blurred, it is impractical and inaccurate to rely on an edge detector or image gradient to detect the contour of the cavity. We turned to digital subtraction technique for solutions [12]. One image is taken before the cutting and the C-arm pose is marked. After the cut is done, the C-arm is moved back to the marked position and another image is taken. The digital subtraction of these two images can provide meaningful information. Under ideal conditions, this subtraction image can detect subtle changes. If the two C-arm poses are different, structured noise exists. Fortunately in our case the C-arm pose is marked, so the difference between two imager poses should be small. Furthermore the outer contour of the femur hardly changes before and after the cut, the 2D contour transformation algorithm in section 6.2 can be employed on them to compute the 2D transformation between two images. Then one image is rotated, translated and scaled to make the two images have maximal mutual information. After that the two images can be subtracted without too much structured noise. We tested this idea on some simulated images generated from a CT set. (Figure 6).

6.4 Computational Analysis

The objective of this algorithm is to compute $?F$, i.e. the transformation between the real cavity and the cavity model.

The cavity model frame relative to the C-arm coordinate system can be written as $F_{v-m} = F_v^{-1} F_m$, where F_v is the C-arm coordinate frame and F_m is the cut cavity model coordinate frame. Based on F_{v-m}, the model projective contour C_m is generated, then the 2D contour transformation algorithm is employed to get the 2D translation $(?x, ?y)$, 2D rotation angle $??$ and rotation center (x_0, y_0).

Distance from the cavity model to the C-arm source along the focal length direction can be written as $d = \left(F_m.P - F_v.P\right) \circ F_v.R.Rz$, where $F_v.R.Rz$ is the viewing direction, and $\circ$ is the dot product between two vectors.

The 3D transformation between the real cavity and the cavity model $\Delta F_c = T_2^{-1} R_1 T_2 T_1$, and $T_1 = Translate(\Delta x \cdot s_x \cdot d / f, \Delta y \cdot s_y \cdot d / f, 0)$, $R_1 = Rotation\ (\Delta\theta, Z - Axis)$, $T_2 = Translate(x_0 \cdot s_x \cdot d / f, y_0 \cdot s_y \cdot d / f, 0)$, and f is the focal length of the C-arm and (s_x, s_y) is the pixel size of the 2D image.

So the cumulative transformation $?F_w$ can be denoted as $\Delta F_w.P = F_v.R \cdot \Delta F_c.P$ and $\Delta F_w.R = F_v.R \cdot \Delta F_c.R$. Then the Cavity Model frame and the cumulative transformation can be updated by: $F_m = \Delta F_w \cdot F_m$ and $\Delta F = \Delta F_w \cdot \Delta F$

The above computing procedure is iterated on all images. Finally the transformation between the real cavity and the cavity model is got.

6.5 Results

We have tested our ideas on some simulated images. An algorithm was developed to generate the simulated fluoroscopic image from a CT data volume based on the attenuation rule. The simulated image is very realistic except that there is no spatial distortion. The process of cutting a pre-defined cavity from the CT volume can also be simulated by subtracting the cavity volume from the CT volume. Figure 6 is a set of simulation images generated from a CT set of a patient femur.

Table 3 provides some numerical assessment of our method. During this experiment, a cut cavity (in the shape of an implant) is first preplanned relative to the femur. Then the cut cavity is perturbed with various transformations, and a simulated cutting of the perturbed cavity is executed on the femur. Then the Iterative Cavity Location algorithm is employed to recover the perturbation transformation. Figure 6 illustrates the images simulated in trial 4 of table 3.

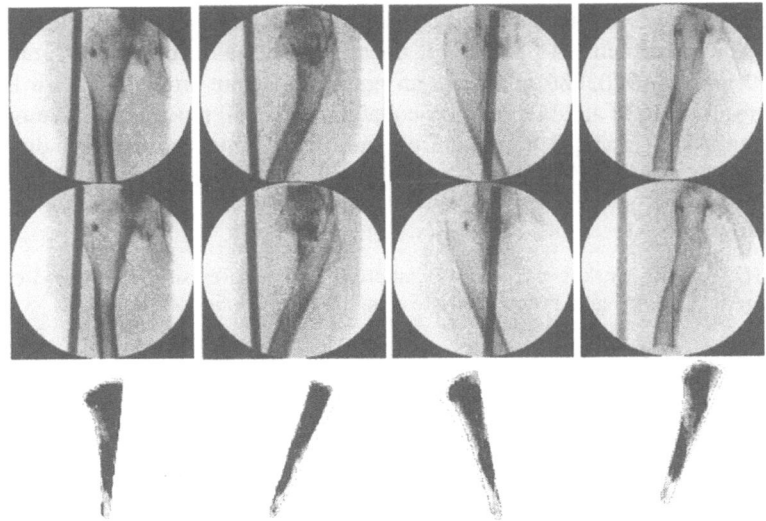

Figure 6 Images Used on Iterative Cavity Location Algorithm. Row 1 are images before the cutting; row 2 are those after cutting; and row 3 are their subtraction after removing the noises and enhancing the contrast, and superimposed by the contours of real cavity (red lines) and projective model contours (green line).

Trial	Expected Transformation						Computed Transformation						Trans Error (mm)	Rotation Error (°)
	X	Y	Z	Roll	Pitch	Yaw	X	Y	Z	Roll	Pitch	Yaw		
1	2.00	1.00	0.00	0.00	0.00	0.00	1.93	1.05	0.01	0.00	0.00	0.00	0.09	0.00
2	-2.00	1.50	1.00	0.00	0.00	0.00	-2.09	1.42	0.94	0.03	0.00	-0.01	0.13	0.03
3	0.00	0.00	0.00	-3.00	3.00	3.00	0.11	-0.05	0.07	-2.18	3.49	1.67	0.14	1.64
4	1.00	-2.00	-3.00	3.00	2.00	2.00	0.56	-2.21	-3.30	2.47	2.37	0.43	0.57	1.70
												Average	0.23	0.84
												Std Dev	0.23	0.96

Table 3 Results of Recursive Cavity Location Algorithm

7. Discussions and Future Plans

The system and method described in this paper demonstrates the feasibility of cutting a precise pocket using the C-arm fluoroscopy. We have been able to demonstrate an-order-of magnitude improvement in the precision by the progressive refinement scheme in revision total hip replacement (RTHR) surgery. Based on the preliminary results, our research shows that a fluoroscopy based registration method and progressive cutting scheme is a promising alternative for RTHR as well as other orthopedic surgery procedures.

A number of areas must be further investigated, including the anatomy based registration methods. We plan to further assess the accuracy of the corkscrew pose estimation algorithm under different circumstance. We also plan to integrate an independent validation system to assess the accuracy of our system.

8. Acknowledgements

This work was partially funded by NIST Advanced Technology Program Cooperative Agreement No. 94-01-0228. It benefited from NSF equipment grants CDA-9529509 and EIA9703080 and from an equipment grant from Intel. We thank our colleagues from IBM and ISS for their collaboration in all phases of this research. Leo Joskowicz, Alan Kalvin, Bill Williamson, and Brent Mittelstadt perhaps deserve special thanks, as does Rod Turner, MD from New England Baptist Hospital.

References

[1] R. H. Taylor, L. Joskowicz, et al, "Computer-Integrated Revision Total Hip Replacement Surgery: Concept and Preliminary Results," Medical Image Analysis, vol. 3, pp. 1-18, 1999.

[2] L. Joskowicz, R. H. Taylor, et al, "Computer Integrated Revision Total Hip Replacement Surgery: Preliminary Report", pp. 193-202, presented at MRCAS, 1995.

[3] R. H. Taylor, B. D. Miittelstadt, et al, "An Image-Directed Robotics System For Precise Orthopaedic Surgery," in Computer-Integrated Surgery, Technology and Clinical Applications, R. H. Taylor, Ed., 1995, pp. 379-396.

[4] S. Lavallee, et al, "Anatomy-Based Registration of Three Dimensional Medical Images, Range Images, X-Ray Projections, and Three Dimensional Models Using Octree-Splines," in Computer-Integrated Surgery, R. H. Taylor, et al, Eds., 1995, pp. 115-144.

[5] A. Gueziec, P. Kazanzides, et al, "Anatomy Based Registration of CT-scan and Intraoperative X-ray Images for Guiding a Surgical Robot," IEEE Transactions on Medical Imaging, special issue on IMAGE GUIDANCE OF THERAPY, 1998.

[6] A. Hamadeh, P. Sautot, et al, "Towards automatic registration between CT and X-ray images: cooperation between 3D/2D registration and 2D edge detection," presented at Second Annual International Symposium on MRCAS, Baltimore, MD USA, 1995.

[7] A. P. Gueziec and J. Funda, "Evaluating the Registration of 3D Points to 3D Lines with Application to the Pose Estimation in a Projective Image," IBM RC 20560, 1996.

[8] S. Schreiner, et al, "A system for percutaneous delivery of treatment with a fluoroscopically-guided robot," presented at Joint Conf. of Computer Vision, Virtual Reality, and Robotics in Medicine and Medical Robotics and Computer Surgery, Grenoble, France, 1997.

[9] J. M. Boone, J. A. Seibert, et al, "Analysis and correction of imperfections in the image intensified-TV-digitizer imaging chain," Medical Physics, vol. 18, pp. 236-242, 1991.

[10] F. L. Bookstein, Morphometric tools for landmark data, Geometry and biology: Cambridge University Press, 1991.

[11] G. Wolberg, Digital Image Warping: IEEE Computer Society Press Monograph, 1990.

[12] G. Levy, "Robotic Control for Digital Subtraction Radiography," in Electrical Engineering. Rutgers, the State University of New York, 1994, pp. 145.

MR Compatibility of Mechatronic Devices: Design Criteria

Kiyoyuki Chinzei[1], Ron Kikinis[2], and Ferenc A. Jolesz[2]

[1] Mechanical Engineering Laboratory, AIST, MITI
1-2 Namiki, Tsukuba, 305-8564 Japan
chin@mel.go.jp
[2] Department of Radiology, Brigham and Women's Hospital
Francis St. 75, Boston, MA 02115, USA
{kikinis, jolesz}@bwh.harvard.edu

Abstract. Criteria to design MR (Magnetic Resonance) compatible mechatronic devices, e.g., surgical robots, are discussed. Some of critical interactions between MRI and mechatronic devices are discussed. Experimental results of the effects from several passive and active mechanical elements are demonstrated.

Some passive elements, e.g., ball screw and linear guide have point contacts therefore, they are required to be made of hard smooth surfaces. Both beryllium-copper and a new stainless steel were examined. Effects from ultrasonic motor were also examined. They didn't show any image shift. Significant degradation of signal noise ratio was not observed, too. Based on these results, we developed a five d.o.f. MR compatible surgical manipulator.

1 Introduction

MR compatibility has been a tough hurdle for device developers, in particular, for mechatronic developers who want to design robot. It is believed that the common standard mechanical parts cannot be used in MR environment because they usually contain ferromagnetic components. However, open configuration scanners have opened a door to the intraoperative use of MRI, where actuated parts have been used in some of the surgical equipment, e.g., respirator, etc [1].

Shellock intensively studied this subject and issued a guidebook of the compatibility to many medical devices [2]. Schenck defined magnetic MR compatibility and classified numerous materials [3]. GE Medical System disclosed its guideline in the homepage to design MR compatible devices for its intraoperative scanner [4]. It provides quite comprehensive and descriptive information about how developers should test the compatibility of their products.

Hynynen has developed MR guided focused ultrasound system [5]. It was actuated by ultrasonic (piezoelectric) motors. Masamune developed an MR compatible surgical manipulator, which also employed ultrasonic motors [6]. One of the authors has developed a few mechanical instruments which were intended to be used in MR environment.

This paper will illustrate the criteria to design mechatronic devices to be MR compatible, assuming their use with open configuration scanners. This paper first reviews the MR compatibility, then summarizes any possible interaction between the mechatronic devices and the MR imaging. The effects caused by several metal samples and mechanical parts in the intraoperative MR scanner are demonstrated.

2   MR Compatibility

The most descriptive and practical definition of MR compatibility is found in [4]. It describes the experimental protocols to evaluate compatibility, which is introduced in this paper [4].

First [4] defines *MR environment* as, the area of influence, in particular, inside the 5 Gauss line. 'Influence' can be more than magnetic, as discussed in Section 3. Then [4] states that a foreign device is *MR safe* when it does not add risk to human or any equipment by placing it in the MR environment, however, it may effect imaging quality.

Finally, [4] defines *MR compatibility* of a foreign device as;

- it is MR safe,
- its use in the MR environment does not affect imaging quality,
- it operates as designed in the MR environment.

In addition, [4] defines location and timing *zones*, where MR compatibility with respect to each zone should be stated. The zones are defined as followings:

Zone 1 device may remain in the image's region of interest and in contact with the patient during the surgical procedure and imaging.

Zone 2 device may remain in the imaging volume and in contact with the patient during the surgical procedure and imaging, but the device is not in the region of interest.

Zone 3 device is used within the imaging volume, but removed during imaging or when not in use.

Zone 4 device can be used in the magnet room during the surgical procedure if it is kept a distance of more than 1 m from the magnet center or outside the 200 Gauss line. [1]

3   Interaction between MRI and Mechatronic Devices

3.1   Definition of Mechatronic Device

In this paper, we refer to *mechatronic devices*, e.g., robot, as the composite of the *mechanical* and *control (electric)* parts. The mechanical part is composed from four elements: *structural element, passive and active mechanical devices,* and *sensors*. The control part can be outside the MR environment, therefore this paper is concerned with the behavior of the mechanical parts.

---

[1] The distance should be appropriately interpreted depending on the scanner.

3.2 Possible Interaction

Here are various phenomena that can happen when a mechatronic device is placed adjacent to MRI scanner and is driven it during imaging.

Effect 1: Magnetic field affects mechanical devices. The strong static magnetic field can affect ferrous parts in the passive and active devices. This may result unexpected behaviors. For example, standard springs often do not function as expected inside zone 3.

Effect 2: RF pulse affects sensors. High-impedance sensors can induce the RF (radio frequency) pulse depending on the distance from and directivity of the RF coil. It is not easy to eliminate such induced signals. However, optics based sensors, e.g., optical encoders, can be free from this, if photo sensors and its amplifier are placed carefully.

Effect 3: Foreign objects affect magnetic field. The effect of ferromagnetic objects to the homogeneity of the magnetic field is obvious. In fact, even paramagnetic object can have an effect if it was conductive due to the eddy current in zones 1 to 2.
Most of standard mechatronic devices are magnetically very incompatible.

Effect 4: Foreign objects affect RF probe. The RF probe is a receiver antenna and is tuned to the resonance frequency. Foreign objects that are dielectric or conductive, and are adjacent to the probe, typically in zones 1 to 2, can affect the property of the antenna.

Effect 5: Wiring introduces noises. MR magnet room is an RF shield room. It cuts off electric noise from the outside and vice versa.
The wire to the device can act as an antenna radiating electric noise from the outside, regardless of the distance from the scanner. It significantly affects the image quality, in particular, its signal to noise ratio.

Effect 6: Foreign resonant objects affect gain controller. The gain controller of the signal receiver can be mistuned in the presence of a large source of resonance signal in zone 1 when the imaging object has weak signal. This can occur when the imaging object is small in volume and a hydraulic or water driven actuator is in zone 1.

4 Design Criteria

4.1 Device Design

Structural Element. Many non-ferrous metals, ceramics, plastics, and composite materials are non-magnetic. Due to cost, strength and easiness of manufacturing, non-ferrous metals are the second best.

Austenitic stainless steels (300 series) are neither ferromagnetic, nor paramagnetic. Their magnetic susceptibility range from 10^{-1} to 10^{-3}. Titanium and Aluminum are well known as MR compatible, but they are not ideally paramagnetic, hence they require some compromise if they were to be used in zones 1 to 2. Other materials are often too soft except ceramics, which are too hard and brittle.

Passive Mechanical Devices. Gears, wire drive, cam, bearings, ball screw, linear guide, etc. are in this group. A variety of plastic parts are available. They are fine if rigidity is not required. Ceramic devices are expensive, brittle, and can be heavy. However, they are very hard and rigid. Ceramic bearings are widely available.

When frictionless is important, some devices, e.g., bearings, ball screws, etc., need the point contacts to transfer the load, hence they should have precise dimension and should be smooth as well as hard. Therefore, plastic parts are not suitable for this kind.

We examined ball screws made by paramagnetic metals, as will be described later.

Active Mechanical Devices. Actuators, clutches, and brakes fall into this category. Majority of these are electromagnetic device and practically impossible to use inside zone 3.

Ultrasonic (piezoelectric) motor can be the substitute for electromagnetic motor [7, 8]. Commercial non-magnetic products are available, however, they are electrically driven hence caution against any EMI (electromagnetic interference: discussed later) is required. Fluidic actuators, e.g., hydraulic or pneumatic actuators, can be also magnet free in principal. Transmission mechanisms, such as drive shafts, gears, and wires, allow the actuator to be placed away from MR scanner therefore compatibility criteria can be relaxed.

As far as actuators are concerned, there are other alternatives, however, it has been difficult to find good alternatives to electromagnetic clutches and brakes.

Sensors. Most of modern sensors are electric, which can emit noise to the imaging, and can receive signals from the RF pulse. The former can be improved by applying the general techniques against EMI, unless it is used in zones 1 to 2. Since the noise is a series of sharp pulses, standard EMI techniques, such as rejecting the common mode noise, are not effective, therefore it is a better practice to decouple the sensor and its wire from the RF coil.

As a solution the measured media should be placed far from the magnet. A case study was an optical encoder. Its photodiodes were located outside the magnet room and fiber optics were used to guide the signals to the optic sensors. This technique was shown to be effective.

4.2   Electromagnetic Interference (EMI)

EMI can occur even if the electric device is placed in zone 4. To minimize EMI, the following techniques must be considered:

- Wires and circuit should be properly shielded,
- Cables of appropriate size and impedance should be used,
- Twisted pair cables are recommended,
- Shield should be properly grounded. Large ground loop should be avoided,

- Switching regulator and DC-DC converter, etc., should be avoided,
- Opto-isolation should be considered if necessary,
- Inline noise filters are often effective, etc.

5   Alternative Devices and Simple Experiments

Some alternative materials and devices were examined using the intraoperative MR scanner Signa/SP (GE Medical Systems, Milwaukee, WI, 0.5 tesla/60 cm, active shielding).

5.1   Hard Paramagnetic Metal Chips in Zone 1

The passive mechanical devices require precise dimensions, smooth and hard surface materials. As a substitute to steels, the following materials were tested: three austenitic stainless steels (type 304, 316, YHD50), and a beryllium-copper (BeA-25-HT; abbreviated as Be-Cu). YHD50 is a non-standardized new stainless steel (Hitachi Metals Ltd., Tokyo, Japan). Table 1 lists surface hardness and magnetic susceptibility of typical metals.

Table 1. Hardness and magnetic susceptibility of typical metals

	Hardness (HB)	χ ($\times 10^{-6}$)
Be-Cu	300-380	4
YHD50	420	1900
Type 440C stainless steel	580	10^9
Type 316 stainless steel	<187	9000
Al	<150	20.7 [3]
Ti	>100	182 [3]

(Values from unpublished measurements by NSK Ltd. (Tokyo, Japan) otherwise indicated.)

Method. Five sample chips (stainless steels type 304, type 316, YHD50, YHD50 with surface hardening treatment, and Be-Cu) were prepared (Fig. 1). These had the identical cylindrical shapes of 20 mm in height and 20 mm in diameter. Each sample was put in $NiCl_2$ solution so that its axis was aligned to the magnetic axis. We acquired a 2D scan that axially intersected the sample. Sequence was GRE, TE/TR: 30/150 msec, FOV: 260×260 mm, slice thickness: 4 mm, bandwidth: 15.6 kHz, flip angle: 30 degrees.

Result. Every metallic object produced a void (dark) shadow that had no resonance signal. The object also distorted the magnetic field around it. The larger the void was the larger distortion.

Beryllium-copper showed the smallest void. YHD50 was the second best followed by the stainless steel type 316, type 304 which was the worst (Fig. 2).

YHD50 after surface treatment showed larger void, which meant degradation of paramagnetism. It is known that austenitic stainless steel is so delicate that it can cause phase transfer to ferromagnetic by the cold working, e.g., bending [9]. MR compatibility should be assessed using the final products. Figure 3 shows the assessment of the final products of ball screws made of beryllium-copper and YHD50.

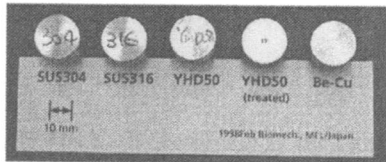

Fig. 1. Sample chips. From left, stainless steel type 304, type 316, YHD50, surface treated YHD50, and Be-Cu.

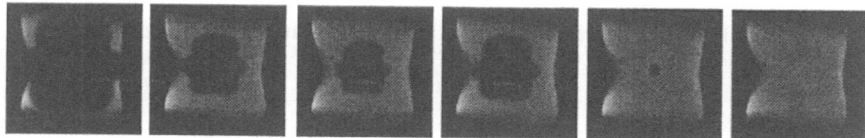

Fig. 2. Effect by metallic samples. From left, stainless steel type 304, type 316, YHD50, surface treated YHD50, Be-Cu, and the control, respectively. Void is caused by the distortion of the magnetic field.

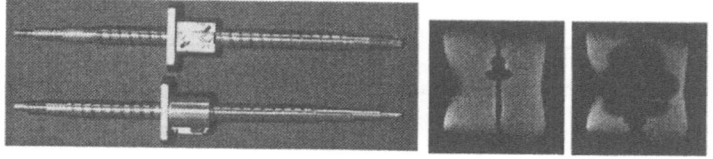

Fig. 3. Be-Cu (upper), YHD50 (lower) ball screws, and the effect by Be-Cu (center), YHD50 (right) ball screws.

5.2   Ball Screws in Zones 2-3

Two ball screws were examined; one made of YHD50 and another was made of beryllium-copper.

Method. We put each ball screw in the scanner and observed the effect which appeared in the image by changing the distance between the screw and the center of imaging volume. The distances were selected at 240, 330 and 520 mm. The ball screw was aligned parallel to the magnetic axis, or perpendicular to it. The control image was taken without the screw.

The imaging object was a spherical phantom of $CuSO_4$ solution. The imaging sequence was SE, TE/TR: 17/400 msec, bandwidth: 15.6 kHz, FOV: 240×240 mm, Slice thickness: 5 mm. As the phantom was kept immobilized, the images should stay identical.

Result. The obtained images looked identical. Thus, we list here the subtraction of the control image (Fig. 4).

To evaluate noise, Signal to noise ratio (SNR) was calculated:

$$SNR = Pcenter/SDcorner .\qquad(1)$$

Where *Pcenter* is the mean value of 40×40 pixels area at the center of the image, *SDcorner* is the standard deviation of 40×40 pixels area at the lower right corner [4]. Table 2 lists the SNR values. The high SNR values correspond to high image quality. Note that, image shift and significant loss of SNR were not observed.

Table 2. Signal to noise ratio (SNR) of images with ball screws.

(distance from isocenter)	240	330	520 (mm)
Be-Cu ball screw (parallel)	55.6	65.5	59.4
Be-Cu ball screw (perpendicular)	–	58.4	56.9
YHD50 ball screw (parallel)	57.5	56.6	62.9
YHD50 ball screw (perpendicular)	–	60.7	61.9
Control (no ball screw)		59.1	

5.3   Actuator: Ultrasonic Motor (USM) in Zones 2-3

Method. An ultrasonic motor was placed in the scanner and the effect in imaging was observed. The motor was USM-60N1 (Shinsei Kogyo Corp., Tokyo, Japan; Fig. 5). The method described in Section 5.2 was repeated. The motor was driven at 75% of its maximum speed, or unplugged from its amplifier.

Result. Figure 6 shows the subtraction of the control, and Table 3 lists the SNR values.

Results show that there was neither image shift nor significant degradation of SNR values regardless of the motor being driven.

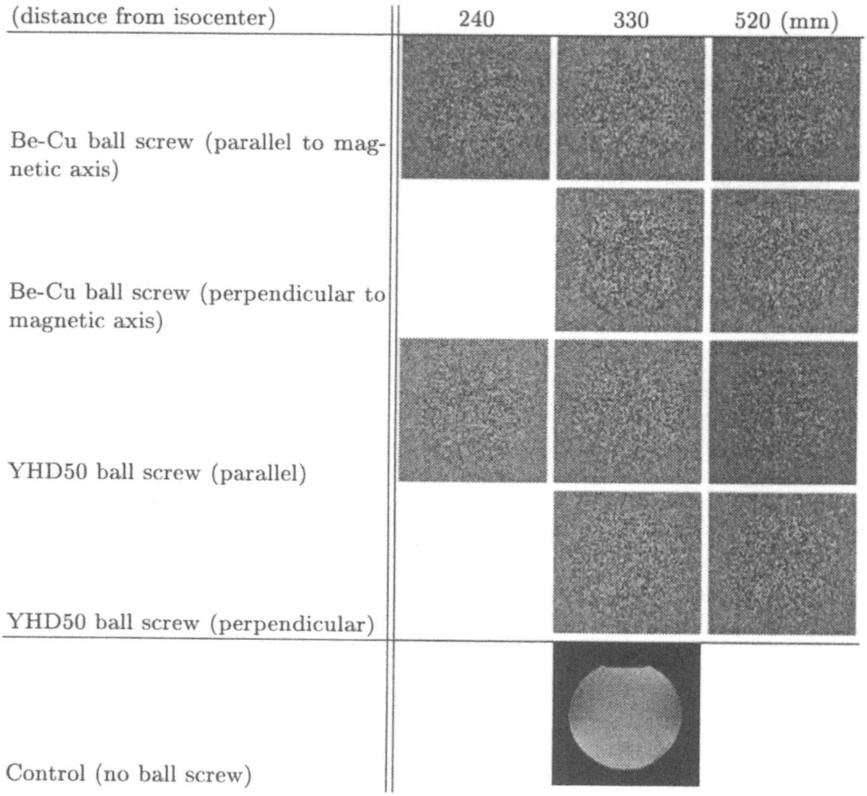

(distance from isocenter)	240	330	520 (mm)
Be-Cu ball screw (parallel to magnetic axis)			
Be-Cu ball screw (perpendicular to magnetic axis)			
YHD50 ball screw (parallel)			
YHD50 ball screw (perpendicular)			
Control (no ball screw)			

Fig. 4. Image shift by ball screws. Subtracted images are listed and no shift is found. (The ball screw could not be located perpendicular at 240 mm from the isocenter.)

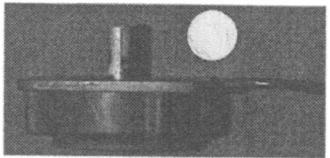

Fig. 5. Ultrasonic motor

Table 3. Signal to noise ratio (SNR) of images with ultrasonic motor driving during imaging.

(distance from isocenter)	240	330	520 (mm)
Motor ON 75 % of max speed	54.4	64.0	55.5
Motor OFF, unplugged from amplifier	58.4	55.8	59.2
Control (no object)		59.1	

(distance from isocenter)	240	330	520 (mm)
Motor ON 75 % of max speed			
Motor OFF, amplifier unplugged			
Control (no object)			

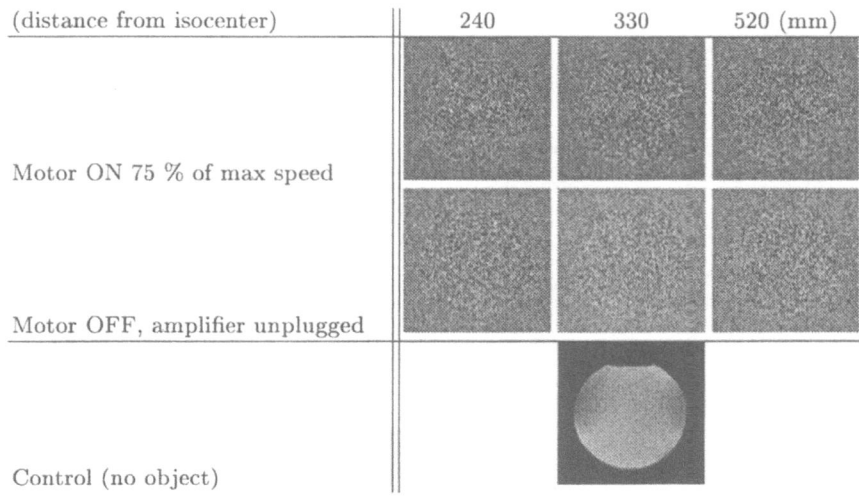

Fig. 6. Image shift by driving ultrasonic motor during imaging. Subtracted images are listed and no shift is found.

6   Discussion

Possibility of MR compatible precise mechanisms. Though these results are not meant to guarantee the acceptance of volumes or shapes of the foreign objects, they cast a spotlight to the possibility of MR compatible precision mechanisms. The results obtained from the study of the ball screw is encouraging to develop similar devices, such as linear guide.

Application: An MR compatible manipulator. The results have mainly been applied in the 5-axes surgical manipulator (Fig. 7). It is optimally designed for the intraoperative scanner and scheduled to be at the test stage shortly. It will be part of an image guided surgical assist system, which will integrate pre-operative planning and intra-operative MRI.

It was designed to guide surgical tools, such as biopsy needle, or pointing devices according to the preoperative planning. The manipulator consists of the main mechanical body and the tool holder hang from the former. The main body is placed above surgeon's head so that it does not block the surgeon accessing the patient. The tool holder contains neither delicate mechanical parts nor sensors, and is exchangeable and sterilizable.

It is a Cartesian type robot consisting of an X-Y-Z table with an additional horizontal X-Y table. Each table has a rigid arm and the ends of these arms, the tool holder, link together by two pivoted joints. Every table unit is composed from a ball screw and a pair of linear guides that are made of YHD50 or beryllium-copper. The actuators are the ultrasonic motors. All the sensors are optical and their circuits are placed outside the magnet room. Fiber optics are used for signal transmit.

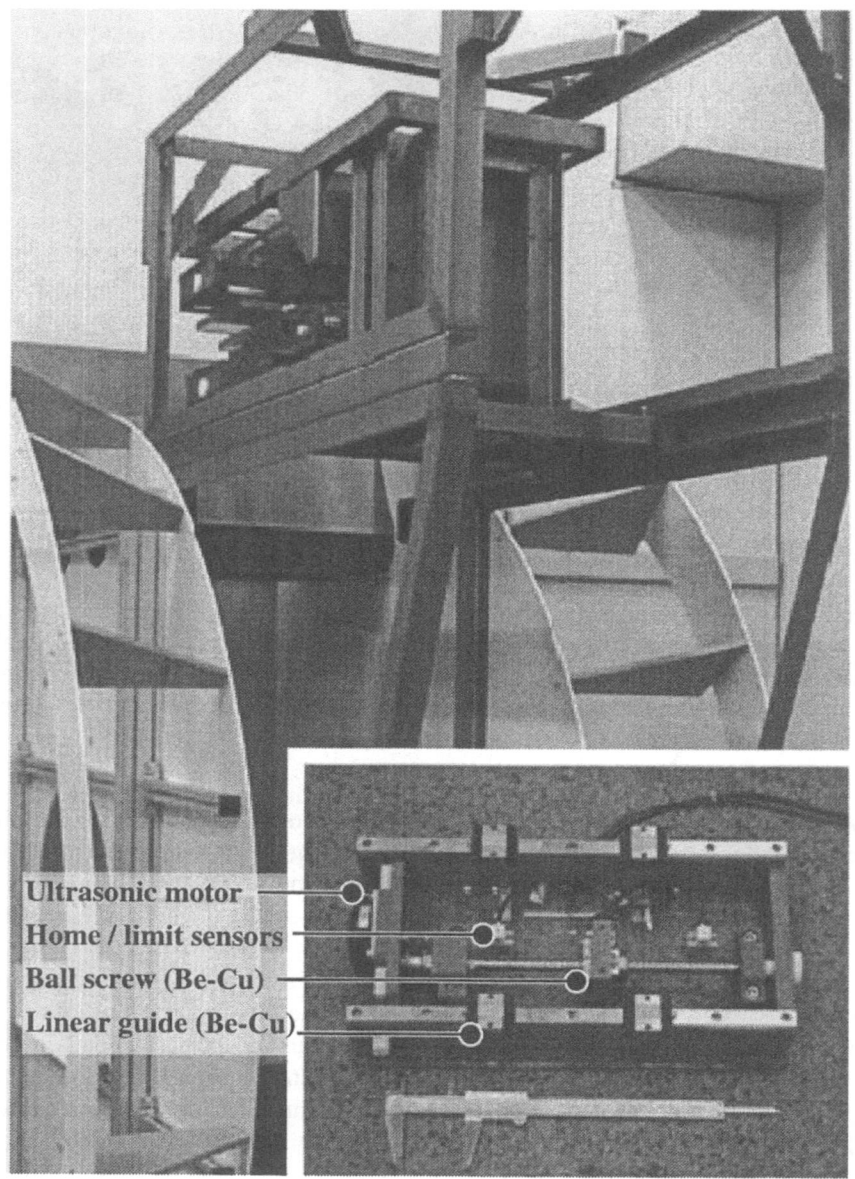

Fig. 7. Five d.o.f. MR compatible manipulator for the intraoperative MR scanner (main), and a linear motion table unit (bottom), made from MR compatible devices described in this paper.

7   Conclusion

The definition of MR compatibility was reviewed and the criteria to design mechatronic devices to be MR compatible were discussed.

Low susceptibility / high hardness stainless steel YHD50 and beryllium-copper (Be-Cu) as well as other standard stainless steels (type 304 and type 316) were examined in zone 1 of an intraoperative MR scanner. Be-Cu was proven to be best performance to other materials, followed by YHD50. Ball screws made of these metals and an ultrasonic motor placed separately in zones 2-3 didn't show significant loss of SNR nor any image shift.

Though the result didn't guarantee the acceptable amount or shape of these objects, it encourages the possibility of the use of MR compatible components. Based on these results, an MR compatible surgical manipulator was approved for development.

Acknowledgements

The main part of this work has been funded by AIST, MITI, Japan. The application system described in Section 6 is bilaterally funded, in the US side by NSF ERL "Computer Integrated Surgical Systems and Technology" #9731748.

References

1. Jolesz, F.A., Morrison, P.R., Koran, S.J., et.al.: Compatible instrumentation for intraoperative MRI: expanding resources. *JMRI*, 8(1) (1998) 8–11
2. Shellock, F.G.: Pocket Guide to MR Procedures and Metallic Objects: Update 1998. Lippincott-Raven publishers, Philadelphia (1998)
3. Schenck, J.F.: The role of magnetic susceptibility in magnetic resonance imaging: Magnetic field compatibility of the first and second kinds. *Med. Phys.*, 23(6) (1996) 815–850
4. GE Medical Systems (ed): MR Safety and MR Compatibility: Test Guidelines for Signa SP^{TM}. Version 1.0, http://www.ge.com/medical/mr/iomri/safety.htm October (1997)
5. Hynynen, K., Darkazanli, A., Unger, E., Schenck, J.F.: MRI-guided noninvasive ultrasound surgery. *Med. Phys.*, 20 (1992) 107–116
6. Masamune, K., Kobayashi, E., Masutani, Y., et.al.: Development of an MRI compatible Needle Insertion Manipulator for Stereotactic Neurosurgery. *J Image Guided Surgery*, 1 (1995) 242–248
7. Sashida, T., Kenjo, T.: Introduction to Ultrasonic Motor (Chouonpa Motor Nyuumon; written in Japanese). Sogo Denshi Shuppan, Tokyo, (1991)
8. Crivii, M., Jufer, M.: Piezoelectric ultrasonic motor - design and comparison. *In proc Annu Symp Incremental Motion Control Syst Devices*, 23 (1994) 35–40
9. Bendel, L.P., Shellock, F.G., Steckel, M.: The effect of mechanical deformation on magnetic properties and MRI artifacts of type 304 and type 316L stainless steel. *JMRI*, 7(6) (1997) 1170–1173

A Steady-Hand Robotic System for Microsurgical Augmentation

Russell Taylor[1], Patrick Jensen[3], Louis Whitcomb[2], Aaron Barnes[2], Rajesh Kumar[1], Dan Stoianovici[4], Puneet Gupta[3], ZhengXian Wang[1], Eugene deJuan[3], Louis Kavoussi[4*]

The Johns Hopkins University
Baltimore, Maryland, USA

[1]Department of Computer Science, Whiting School of Engineering
[1]Department of Mechanical Engineering, Whiting School of Engineering
[3]Wilmer Eye Institute, Johns Hopkins Medical Institutions
[4]James Buchanan Brady Urological Institute, Johns Hopkins Medical Institutions

Abstract: This paper reports the development of a robotic system designed to extend a human's ability to perform small-scale (sub-millimeter) manipulation tasks requiring human judgement, sensory integration and hand-eye coordination. Our novel approach, which we call "steady hand" micromanipulation, is for tools to be held simultaneously both by the operator's hand and a specially designed actively controlled robot arm. The robot's controller senses forces exerted by the operator on the tool and by the tool on the environment, and uses this information in various control modes to provide smooth, tremor-free precise positional control and force scaling. Our goal is to develop a manipulation system with the precision and sensitivity of a machine, but with the manipulative transparency and immediacy of hand-held tools for tasks characterized by compliant or semi-rigid contacts with the environment.

1. Introduction

This paper describes the first steps in an ongoing development of a robotic assistant for microsurgery and other precise manipulation tasks. It reports a new robotic system developed to extend a human's ability to perform small-scale (sub-millimeter) manipulation tasks requiring human judgement, sensory integration and hand-eye coordination. Our approach, which we call "steady hand" micro-manipulation is for tools to be held simultaneously both by the operator's hand and a specially designed robot arm (figure 1). The robot's controller senses forces exerted by the operator on the tool and by the tool on the environment, and uses this information in various control modes to provide smooth, tremor-free precise positional control and force scaling. The result will be a manipulation system with the precision and sensitivity of a machine, but with the manipulative transparency and immediacy of hand-held tools for tasks characterized by compliant or semi-rigid contacts with the environment.

Humans possess superb manual dexterity, visual perception, and other sensory-motor capabilities. We manipulate best at a "human scale" dictated by our physical

We gratefully acknowledge the support of the National Science Foundation under grant #IIS9801684, the Engineering Research Center grant #EEC9731478, and in cooperation with the Whitaker Foundation on grant #ST32HL07712. General lab infrastructure was partially supported by NSF equipment grants CDA-9529509 and EIA9703080 and by an equipment grant from Intel. This work was also funded in part by Johns Hopkins internal funds.

size and manipulation capabilities and roughly corresponding to the tasks routinely performed by our cave man ancestors. Tasks that require very precise, controlled motions are difficult or impossible for most people. Further, humans work best in tasks that require relative positioning or alignment based on visual or tactile feedback. We do not come equipped with an innate ability to position or fabricate objects accurately relative to arbitrary measuring standards or to perform tasks based on non-human sensory feedback. For these tasks, we rely on machines. A good machine tool, for example, can routinely measure and fabricate parts to a precision of ≈ 2.5 μm (≈ 0.001 inch). Fine-scale tasks such as microsurgery require both precise manipulation and human judgement. Other tasks may require combining precise manipulation with sources of information (assembly specifications, non-visible-light images, etc.) that are not naturally available to a human. We thus have a choice: either automate the human judgement aspects of the task (difficult at best and often impossible) so that a machine can automatically perform the task or else find a way to use a machine to augment human manipulation capabilities while still exploiting the human's natural strengths.

Most prior robotic micro-manipulation systems have emphasized traditional master-slave and telerobotic manipulation. Our approach might offer several advantages compared to these systems in the context of micromanipulation. These include: 1) simplicity; 2) potentially cheaper implementations; 3) a more direct coupling to the human's natural kinesthetic senses; 4) straightforward integration into existing application environment; and 5) greater "immediacy" for the human operator. The principal drawbacks are the loss of the ability to "scale" positional motions and the loss of the ability to manipulate objects remotely. These are certainly important abilities, but we believe there are many tasks in which they are not crucial and for which a simpler alternative is more attractive. These advantages are especially attractive in applications like microsurgery, where surgeon acceptance is crucial and where approaches that do not require a complete re-engineering of the surgical workstation are much easier to introduce into practice.

2. Robotically Assisted Micro-Manipulation

Mechanical systems have been developed which extend the capability of human operators using telerobotic principles [1] including virtual training [2], manipulation of objects in hazardous environments [3], remote surgery [4, 5], and microsurgery [2, 6-10]. In general, telerobotic devices rely on an operator commanding the motion of a robot using a secondary input device. The operator may reside in close proximity to the robot, observing its motions through a microscope as in microsurgery or may be many miles away as in space exploration. In both cases, the operator is an integral part of the system and has direct control over how the manipulator moves. An ideal teleoperated system would be transparent to the operator and give the impression of direct control. The input device manipulated by the operator may be either passive, such as a trackball, joystick or stylus, or made up of active devices such as motors. An active input device allows forces imposed on the robot to be measured, scaled and mimicked at the input device to be subsequently felt by the operator.

Several systems have been developed for teleoperated microsurgery using a passive input device for operator control. Guerrouad and Vidal [11] describe a system designed for ocular vitrectomy in which a mechanical manipulator was constructed of curved tracks to maintain a fixed center of rotation. A similar micromanipulator [12] was used for acquiring physiological measurements in the eye using an electrode. While rigid mechanical constraints were suitable for the particular applications in which they were used, the design is not flexible enough for general purpose microsurgery and the tracks take up a great deal of space around the head. An ophthalmic surgery manipulator built by Jensen et al. [8] was designed for retinal vascular microsurgery and was capable of positioning instruments at the surface of the retina with sub-micron precision. While a useful experimental device, this system did not have sufficient range of motion to be useful for general-purpose microsurgery. Also, the lack of force sensing prevented the investigation of force/haptic interfaces in the performance of microsurgical tasks.

Many microsurgical devices [2, 6, 7, 9, 10] are based on force-reflecting master-slave configurations. This paradigm allows an operator to grasp the master manipulator and apply forces. Forces measured on the master are scaled and reproduced at the slave and, if unobstructed, will cause the slave to move accordingly. Likewise, forces encountered by the slave are scaled and reflected back to the master. This configuration gallows position commands from the master to result in a reduced motion of the slave and for forces encountered by the slave to be amplified at the master. While a force-reflecting master-slave microsurgical system provides the surgeon with increased precision and enhanced proprioception, there are some drawbacks to such a design. The primary disadvantage is with complexity and cost since two mechanical systems, one for the master and one for the slave, are required. Another problem with telesurgery in general is that the surgeon is not allowed to directly manipulate the instrument used for the microsurgical procedure. While physical separation is necessary for systems designed to perform remote surgery, it is not required during microsurgical procedures. In fact, surgeons are more likely to accept assistive devices if they are still allowed to directly manipulate the instruments.

2.1 Shared Autonomy and Cooperative Control

There is a large body of literature concerning provably stable control techniques for robots. Standard paradigms include 1) pre-programmed trajectory control of position [13, 14] and force [15, 16]; 2) fully autonomous robots (e.g. [17-19]); and 3) master-slave teleoperators (e.g., [20-22]). In our case, we are interested in developing provably stable controls for cases where both the robot and the human manipulate a single tool in contact with a compliant environment. The work most relevant to this includes that of Kazarooni [23-25] who developed exoskeletons to amplify the strength of a human operator.

Kazarooni et al. [23-25] report a linear systems analysis of the stability and robustness of cooperative human-robot manipulator control systems in which the manipulator scales-up the human operator's force input by a factor of ≈ 10. The authors report a stability analysis of this closed-loop system (comprising a dynamical model of both the robot arm and the human arm) is complicated by the fact that precise mathematical plant models do not exist for either the hydraulically actuated robot and the operator's human arm. In consequence, in [23-25] the authors perform a robustness analysis to develop stable robot force-control laws that accommodate wide variation in both human and robot arm dynamics. In contrast, we propose to address the control problem of cooperative human-robot manipulator systems in which the manipulator scales-down the human operator's force input by a factor of ≈0.1. To achieve this scaling-down of human input we anticipate comparable (or greater) difficulties to arise from unknown human arm dynamics, we can construct the system using electrical motors (rather than hydraulic motors) for which accurate dynamical models are available. A number of authors (e.g., [22, 26]) have investigated "shared autonomy" and for cooperative control of teleoperators, typically with space or other "remote" applications where time delays can affect task performance. There has also been some work (e.g., [27]) on control of robots working cooperatively with humans to carry loads and do other gross motor tasks relevant for construction and similar applications. Within the area of surgery, we have long used "hands on" guiding of robots for positioning within the operating room (e.g., in the "Robodoc" [28-30] hip replacement surgery system and in the JHU/IBM LARS system [31-38] for endoscopic surgery). Davies et. al.[39-41], have combined hands-on guiding with position limits and have demonstrated 3 DOF machining of shapes in the end of a human tibia.

At JHU, we have been using the LARS robot [31] to perform a variety of "steady hand" tasks combining hand guiding, active control, and safety constraints in neuroendoscopy and other areas. In one experiment using the LARS robot-assisted evacuation of simulated hematomas was found to take longer (6.0 min vs 4.6 min) than freehand evacuation but was found to remove much less unintended material (1.5% vs 15%) [36]. We have also made some preliminary experiments using the LARS for micro-manipulation [42], although the compliance of the LARS upper linkage severely limits the benefit gained.

3. A Robotic System for Steady-Hand Micro-Manipulation

3.1 Design Goals

Table 1 summarizes the performance design goals for our system. Cooperative micro-manipulation requires capabilities not commonly found in conventional robots or teleoperator systems. Typically, these tasks will be performed by a human operator looking through a microscope while grasping a "handle" on the instrument or tool being used to perform the task. In the tasks that we are considering, we believe that motion "scaling" (in the sense that a 1 cm human hand motion might cause a 100 μm instrument motion) is much less important than smooth motion naturally aligned with the human's own kinesthetic senses. Pulling on the tool's handle should produce intuitively natural translation and orientation motions.

We are interested in manipulation tasks requiring very precise positional control, with controlled end-effector motion resolution on the order of 3-10 μm, when rotational motion is decoupled at the tool tip and 5-25 μm tip resolution when motion is decoupled about a fulcrum point 2 cm from the tool tip (i.e., when a point 2 cm from the tool tip remains fixed in space). Our strong preference is for relatively low power actuators with high-reduction, non-backdrivable joints. Such systems are relatively easy to monitor, stop, and stay put once stopped. For a clinical system, we also require some form of redundant position sensing. Although the current

Base (XYZ) assembly	(Off-the-shelf)
Work volume	100 mm × 100 mm × 100 mm
Top Speed	40 mm/sec
Positioning resolution	≈2.5 μm (0.5 μm encoder res.)
RCM orientation assembly	**(Custom)**
Link length	100 mm
Range of motion	Continuous 360°
Top speed	180°/sec
Angular resolution	≈0.05 ° (0.01° encoder res.)
End-of-arm/guiding assembly	**(Custom)**
Range of motion	±2cm; 360° continuous
Positioning resolution	0.5 μm; 0.1° (tentative)
Top speed	40 mm/sec; 180°/sec

Table 1. Steady-Hand Robot Design Goals

implementation (intended for pre-clinical research) does not have this feature, future implementations will have this feature.

We are primarily interested in manipulation tasks with a reasonable degree of contact compliance between the tool and the environment being manipulated. In the case of microsurgery, this compliance is provided by the tissue being manipulated. Our goal is moderate bandwidth (3-5 Hz) control and scaling of interaction forces, with tool tip forces ranging from ≈0.001 N to ≈0.01 N, depending on specific application, and human interaction forces ranging from ≈0.03N to ≈3 N. We also wish to provide higher bandwidth sensing and haptic feedback of force discontinuities, and to explore the usefulness of such feedback in micro-manipulation tasks. One option under consideration is the addition of vibrotactile displays [43]

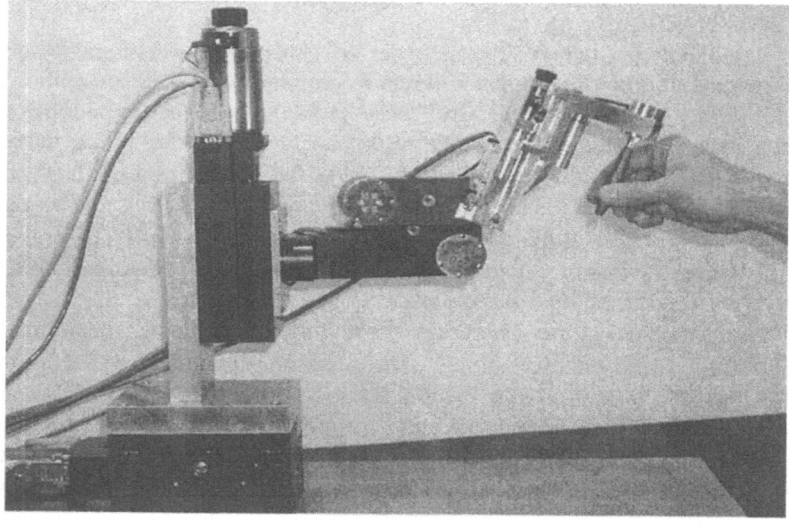

Figure 1. Current version of the steady hand manipulator

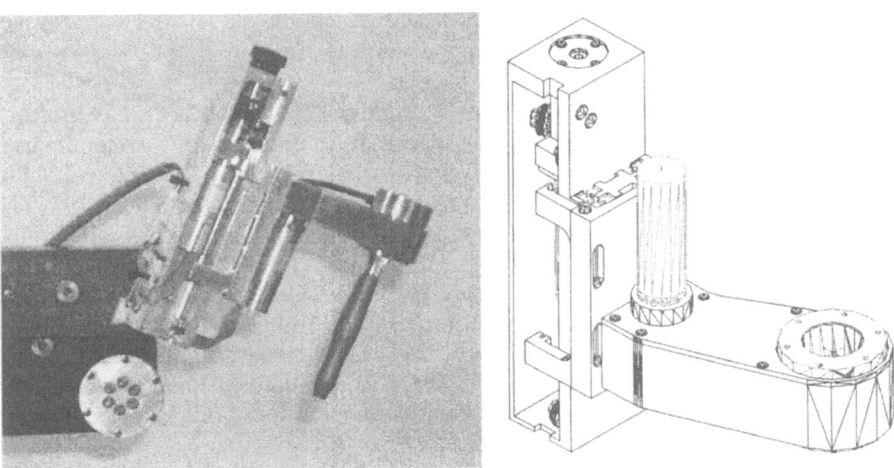

Figure 2. Photograph (left) and drawing (right) of insertion and rotation stages

3.2 System Design and Implementation

3.2.1 Manipulator and mechanical components

We have emphasized modularity in development of our steady hand system. The manipulator itself (Figure 1) kinematically decouples surgical instrument translational and rotational motions and consists of four modular components. The *XYZ translation assembly* is constructed with off-the-shelf motorized micrometer stages from New England Affiliated Technologies of Lawrence, MA.. Each axis has 100 mm of travel, can travel at speeds >40 mm/sec and has a positioning resolution of <2.5 μm (0.5 μm encoder resolution).

The *remote center-of-motion (RCM) orientation assembly* provides two rotations about a "fulcrum" or remote motion center point located in free space approximately 100 mm from the robot. The current compact design [44, 45] weighs 1.6 Kg and may be folded into a 171 × 69 × 52 mm cube. The RCM design is very well adapted to microsurgical augmentation, since it permits us optimize actuators to combine relatively rapid reorientations about a fixed point with very precise and relatively slow translational motions. Its kinematic properties make it appropriate for a number of endoscopic and percutaneous applications, and it has been used clinically at JHU for placing needles into the filling system of the kidney under fluoroscopic guidance [46, 47].

The *instument insertion stage* provides linear displacement along the tool axis passing through the remote motion center. The axis utilizes a two-stage telescoping crossed-roller slide mechanism driven via a cable by an encoded DC servo motor. The insertion stage can travel at speeds of ≈30 mm/sec and has a positioning resolution of ≈5-10 μm (1.5 μm encoder resolution). The rotation end-effector provides rotation about the tool axis and the mounting surface for the force sensor with guiding handle. The *instrument rotation stage* is driven by a timing belt attached to a encoded DC servo motor. It provides a 360° continuous range of motion and is expected to travel at speeds of ≈120°-180°/sec with a positioning resolution of ≈0.05°-0.10° (0.01°encoder resolution).

The current *force sensing handle* uses a commercially available 6DOF force sensor (Model: NANO-17 SI 12/0.12, ATI Industrial Automation, NC) to capture user forces. The force sensor is read using a 12-bit ISA bus F/T controller card with up to 7800Hz sampling rates, and has 0.025N resolution in Z and 0.0625N in XY. The force sensor is mounted on the instrument rotation stage with its z-axis parallel to the instrument insertion stage of the robot.

A variety of surgical instruments such as picks, forceps, needle holders and scissors are required during microsurgical procedures. To utilize the benefits offered by the cooperative control algorithms of steady hand augmentation, these microsurgical tools must be equipped with sensitive, multidimensional force sensors. Our initial approach uses silicon strain gauges configured into bridges located within the surgical tool handle.

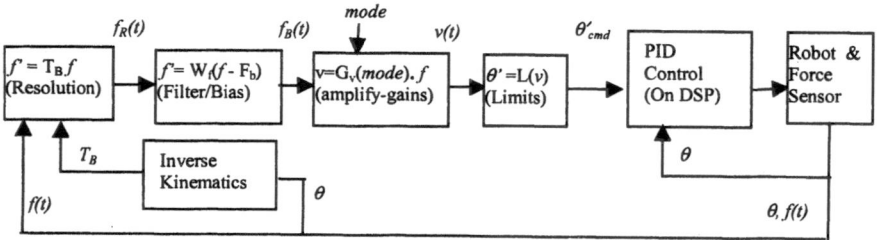

Figure 3. Controller block diagram. The notation is as follows. *f(t)*: sampled forces *(f_x, f_y, f_z)*; *f_R(t)*: forces resolved in the robot base frame, *f_B(t)*: filtered and biased forces; *F_b* :bias force forces *(f_bx, f_by, f_bz)*, in the robot base frame; T_B : transformation from force sensor frame to robot base frame; *mode*: Base X,Y joints and insertion joint (mode 1), or RCM rotation joints and insertion joint (mode 2); G_v(*mode*): joint velocity proportional gains, based on user selected *mode*; *v(t)*: joint velocities for selected joints; *θ*: joint position feedback from encoders; *θ'_cmd*:commanded joint velocities.

3.2.2 Control System

The robot hardware control runs on a Pentium-II 450MHz PC with the Windows NT operating system. An 8-axis DSP series controller card (PCX/DSP, Motion Engineering Inc, CA) is used to control the robot. The card provides servo control using a 40MHZ Analog Devices ADSP-2105 processor. It also has support for user digital and analog input, output lines. The PC also houses the ISA force sensor controller.

Although we anticipate that the control algorithms will eventually be quite sophisticated, the current method (illustrated in Figure 3) is very simple. User forces are sensed from the force sensor attached axially to the handle held by the user. The z axis of the force sensor is aligned with the axis of insertion of the robot and the other two axis are aligned when the instrument rotation stage is at zero. The force sensor is calibrated by computing a bias force with no external forces on the sensor. This bias force is stored in the robot base coordinate frame. During compliant motion, the system samples the current forces, and resolves them to the robot base frame. These resolved forces are offset by the bias and noise filtered using a simple filter (W_f). This biased signal is then amplified by gains G_v .The velocities computed are limited by user specified limits. The commanded velocity is then supplied to the PID controller on the DSP.

4. Current Status and future evolution

Mechanical integration of the steady hand manipulation system is complete Experiments designed to evaluate the augmentation value of steady-hand manipulation are currently being performed. Initial indications are that the basic design assumptions of a stiff robot with force control are valid for surgical manipulations at a micro-scale. In one experimental study comparing unassisted human versus steady hand performance in inserting a 10-0 surgical needle into holes of diameter ranging from 150 μm to 250 μm, the steady hand system improved success rates from 43% unassisted to 79% for 150 μm holes and from 49% unassisted to 78% for 250 μm holes [48].

Our immediate goal is a rigorous evaluation of the completed system as a microsurgery augmentation aid, using test environments developed by our colleagues at JHU's Wilmer Eye Institute and CMU [49-52]. We will compare the system in-vitro and in cadaveric models both against unassisted humans and against alternative methods for reducing physiological tremor (e.g., [50, 53]). Subsequently, we hope to begin evaluation of a clinical system. Initial targeted applications will include epiretinal surgery and retinal vein cannulation under direct surgeon control.

A second stage will combine the steady hand system with various real time imaging modalities (video from optical microscopes & endoscopes (e.g., [54], optical coherence tomography, etc.) in order to produce an enhanced mosaic image of the patient's eye. This information will be made available to the surgeon, for example, by image injection into the surgical microscope or by a suitable video display.

This "information enhanced" surgery system will gradually evolve into a more capable surgical assistant. Initial tasks will be rather simple. We anticipate the development of graceful ways to hand off control between the surgeon and the robot for the performance of specific surgical macros. For example, the surgeon may guide an injection instrument to the vicinity of a blocked vein, but rely on a specialized function incorporating visual servoing and force sensing to perform cannulation and injection of clot-dissolving drugs. Other examples include such "third hand" tasks as pointing a micro-endoscope at designated anatomical features or following the surgeon's instrument movements, force-controlled retraction, or the like. As this repertoire of functions increases, the system will become an increasingly effective partner in surgical treatment.

5. Summary

Our approach extends earlier work on cooperative manipulation to microsurgery and focuses on performance augmentation utilizing both force and position control. Our goal is to develop a manipulation system with the precision and sensitivity of a machine, but with the manipulative transparency and immediacy of hand-held tools for tasks characterized by compliant or semi-rigid contacts with the environment. The design is highly modular and represents one step in the evolution of a family of robotic surgical devices. Although our first focus is retinal microsurgery, we believe that our approach is more general. Other applications will include neuroendoscopy, ENT, and microvascular surgery.

References

1. Sheridan, T.B., *Teleoperation, telerobotics and telepresence: a progress report.* Control Engineering Practice, 1995. 3(2): p. 205-214.
2. Hunter, I.W., *et al., Ophthalmic microsurgical robot and associated virtual environment.* Computers in Biology and Medicine, 1995. 25(2): p. 173-182.
3. Mindell, D.A., *et al. JasonTalk: A standard ROV vehicle control system.* in *IEEE/MTS OCEANS'93.* 1993.
4. Satava, r., *Robotics, telepresence, and virtual reality: A critical analysis fo the future of surgery.* Minimally Invasive Therapy, 1992. 1: p. 357-363.
5. Green, P., *et al., Telepresence: Advanced Teleoperator Technology ofr Minimally Invasive Surgery (abstract).* Surgical Endoscopy, 1992. 6(91).
6. Charles, S., *Dexterity enhancement for surgery.* Proc First Int'l Symp Medical Robotics and Computer Assisted Surgery, 1994. 2: p. 145-160.
7. Misuishi, M., *et al. Dexterity enhancement for a tele-micro-surgery system with multiple macro-micro co-located operation point manipulators and understanding of the operator's intention.* in *First joint conference computer vision, virtual realtiy and robotics in medicine and medical robotics and computer-assisted surgery.* 1997. Grenoble, France: Springer.
8. Jensen, P.S., *et al., Toward robot assisted vascular microsurgery in the retina.* Graefes Arch Clin Exp Ophthalmol, 1997. 235(11): p. 696-701.
9. Salcudean, S.E., S. Ku, and G. Bell. *Performance measurement in scaled teleoperation for microsurgery.* in *First joint conference computer vision, virtual realtiy and robotics in medicine and medical robotics and computer-assisted surgery.* 1997. Grenoble, France: Springer.
10. Schenker, P.S., H.O. Das, and R. Timothy. *Development of a new high-dexterity manipulator for robot-assisted microsurgery.* in *Proceedings of SPIE - The International Society for Optical Engineering: Telemanipulator and Telepresence Technologies.* 1995. Boston, MA.
11. Guerrouad, A. and P. Vidal, *S.M.O.S.: Stereotaxical Microtelemanipulator for Ocular Surgery.* Proc. of the Annual Int'l Conf. of the IEEE Engineering in Medicine and Biology Society, 1989: p. 11:879-880.
12. Pournaras, C.J., *et al., New ocular micromanipulator for measurements of retinal and vitreous physiologic parameters in the mammalian eye.* Exp Eye Res, 1991. 52: p. 723-727.
13. Dinsmoor, C. and P. Hagermann. *Fanuc robotics system r-j controller.* in *Proceedings of International Robots and Vision Automation Conference.* 1993. Detroit Michigan USA.
14. Sakakibara, S. *A two-armed intelligent robot assembles mini robots automatically.* in *Proceedings of the 1996 IEEE IECON. 22nd International Conference on Industrial Electronics, Control and Instrumentation.* 1996. Taipei Taiwan.

15. Whitcomb, L.L., A. Rizzi, and D.E. Koditschek, *Comparative experiments with a new adaptive controller for robot arms.* IEEE Transactions on Robotics and Automation, 1993. **9**(1): p. 59-70.

16. Whitcomb, L., L.,, et al., *Adaptive model based hybrid control of geometrically constrained robot arms.* IEEE Transactions on Robotics and Automation, 1997. **13**(1): p. 105-116.

17. Suzuki, H. and S. Arimoto, *Visual control of autonomous mobile robot based on self-organizing model for pattern learning.* Journal of Robotic Systems, 1988. **5**(5): p. 453-470.

18. Krotkov, E. and R. Simmons. *Performance of a six-legged planetary rover: power, positioning and autonomous walking.* in *Proc IEEE Int Cong Proc Robt Aut.* 1992. Nice, France.

19. Yoerger, D.R., A.M. Bradley, and B.B. Walden, *Autonomous benthic explorer deep ocean scientific auv for seafloor exploration: Untethered on station one year without support ship.* Sea Technology, 1992: p. 50-54.

20. Xu, Y. and T. Kanade, *Space robotics: Dynamics and control.* 1993, Boston, MA USA: Kluwer.

21. Morikawa, H. and N. Takanashi. *Ground experiment system for space robots based on predictive bilateral control.* in *IEEE Conf on Robotics and Automation.* 1996. Minneapolis, MN USA: IEEE Press.

22. Guo, C., T.J. Tarn, and A. Bejczy. *Fusion of human and machine intelligence for telerobotic systems.* in *IEEE Int Joint Conf on Robotics and Automation.* 1995. Nagoya, JP: IEEE Press.

23. Kazerooni, H. *Human/robot interaction via the transfer of power and information signals -- part i: Dynamics and control analysis.* in *Proc IEEE Int Conf on Robotics and Automation.* 1989.

24. Kazerooni, H. *Human/robot interaction via the transfer of power and information signals -- part ii: Dynamics and control analysis.* in *Proc IEEE Int Conf on Robotics and Automation.* 1989.

25. Kazerooni, H. and G. Jenhwa, *Human extenders.* Transaction of the ASME: Journal of Dynamic Systems, Measurement and Control, 1993. **115**(2B): p. 218-90, June.

26. Cho, Y., T. Kotoku, and K. Tanie. *Discrete-event-planning and control of telerobotic part mating process with communication delay in geomtric uncertainty.* in *IEEE Conf on Intelligent Robots & Systems.* 1995. Pittsburgh, PA USA: IEEE Press.

27. Yamamoto, Y., H. Eda, and X. Yun. *Coordinated task execution of a human and a mobile manipulator.* in *IEEE Int Conf on Robotics and Automation.* 1996. Minneapolis, MN USA: IEEE Press.

28. Bargar, W., et al. *Robodoc Multi-Center Trial: An Interim Report.* in *Proc. 2nd Int. Symp. on Medical Robotics and Computer Assisted Surgery.* 1995. Baltimore, Md.: MRCAS '95 Symposium, C/O Center for Orthop Res, Shadyside Hospital, Pittsburgh, Pa.

29. Taylor, R.H., et al., *An Image-directed Robotic System for Precise Orthopaedic Surgery.* IEEE Transactions on Robotics and Automation, 1994. **10**(3): p. 261-275.

30. Mittelstadt, B.D., et al. *The Evolution of a Surgical Robot from Prototype to Human Clinical Trial.* in *Proc. Medical Robotics and Computer Assisted Surgery.* 1994. Pittsburgh.

31. Funda, J., et al. *Image Guided Command and Control of a Surgical Robot.* in *Proc. Medicine Meets Virtual Reality II.* 1994. San Diego.

32. Eldridge, B., et al., *A Remote Center of Motion Robotic Arm for Computer Assisted Surgery.* Robotica, 1996. **14**(1 (Jan-Feb)): p. 103-109.

33. Funda, J., et al. *Optimal Motion Control for Teleoperated Surgical Robots.* in *1993 SPIE Intl. Symp. on Optical Tools for Manuf. & adv. Autom.* 1993. Boston.

34. Funda, J., et al. *An experimental user interface for an interactive surgical robot.* in *1st International Symposium on Medical Robotics and Computer Assisted Surgery.* 1994. Pittsburgh.

35. Funda, J., *et al. Comparison of two mainpulator designs for laparoscopic surgery.* in *1994 SPIE Int's Symposium on Optical Tools for Manufacturing and Advanced Automation.* 1994. Boston: October.

36. Goradia, T.M., R.H. Taylor, and L.M. Auer. *Robot-assisted minimally invasive neurosurgical procedures: first experimental experience.* in *Proc. First Joint Conference of CVRMed and MRCAS.* 1997. Grenoble, France: Springer.

37. Taylor, R.H., *et al.*, *A Telerobotic Assistant for Laparoscopic Surgery*, in *IEEE EMBS Magazine Special Issue on Robotics in Surgery.* 1995. p. 279-291.

38. Taylor, R.H., *et al.*, *A Telerobotic Assistant for Laparoscopic Surgery*, in *Computer-Integrated Surgery*, R. Taylor, *et al.*, Editors. 1996, MIT Press. p. 581-592.

39. Harris, S.J., *et al. Experiences with robotic systems for knee surgery.* in *Proc. First Joint Conference of CVRMed and MRCAS.* 1997. Grenoble, France: Springer.

40. Ho, S.C., R.D. Hibberd, and B.L. Davies, *Robot Assisted Knee Surgery.* IEEE EMBS Magazine Sp. Issue on Robotics in Surgery, 1995(April-May): p. 292-300.

41. Troccaz, J., M. Peshkin, and B.L. Davies. *The use of localizers, robots, and synergistic devices in CAS.* in *Proc. First Joint Conference of CVRMed and MRCAS.* 1997. Grenoble, France: Springer.

42. Kumar, R., *et al.*, *Robot-assisted microneurosurgical procedures, comparative dexterity experiments*, in *Society for Minimally Invasive Therapy 9th Annual Meeting, Abstract book Vol 6, supplement 1.* 1997: Tokyo, Jaban.

43. Kontarinis, D.A. and R.D. Howe, *Tactile Display of Vibratory Information in Teleoperation and Virtual Environments.* Presence, 1995. **4**(4): p. 387-402.

44. Stoianovici, D., Cadeddu, J., A., Whitcomb, L., L., Taylor, R., H., Kavoussi, L., R.,. *A Robotic System for Precise Percutaneous Needle Insertion,.* in *Thirteenth Annual Meeting of the Society for Urology and Engineering.* 1988. San Diego.

45. Stoianovici, D., *et al. A Modular Surgical Robotic System for Image-Guided Percutaneous Procedures.* in *Medical Image Computing and Computer-Assisted Interventions (MICCAI-98).* 1998. Cambridge, Mass: Springer.

46. Cadeddu, J.A., *et al.*, *A Robotic System for Percutaneous Renal Access Incorporating a Remote Center of Motion Design.* Journal of Endourology, 1998. **12**: p. S237.

47. Bishoff, J.T., *et al.*, *RCM-PAKY: Clinical Application of a New Robotic System for Precise Needle Placement.* Journal of Endourology, 1998. **12**: p. S82.

48. Kumar, R., *et al. Performance of Robotic Augmentation in Microsurgery-Scale Motions.* in *2nd Int. Symposium on Medical Image Computing and Computer-Assisted Surgery.* 1999. Cambridge, England.

49. Humayun, M.U., *et al.*, *Quantitative measurement of the effects of caffiene and propranolol on surgeon hand tremor.* Arch. Opthomol., 1997. **115**: p. 371-374.

50. Riviere, C.N. and N.V. Thakor, *Modeling and canceling tremor in human-machine interfaces.* IEEE Eng. in Med. & Biol. Magazine, 1996(May/June): p. 29-36.

51. Riviere, C.N. and P.K. Khosla. *Microscale measurement of surgical instrument motion.* in *2nd Intl. Conf on Medical Image Computing and Computer-Assisted Interventions (MICCAI 99).* 1999. Cambridge, England.

52. Riviere, C.N. and P.K. Khosla. *Intraoperative tremor monitoring for vitreoretinal microsurgery.* in *2nd Intl. Conf on Medical Image Computing and Computer-Assisted Interventions (MICCAI 99).* 1999. Cambridge, England.

53. Riviere, C.N. and P.K. Khosla. *Augmenting the human-machine interface: improving manual accuracy.* in *Proceedings of the IEEE International Conference on Robotics and Automation.* 1997. Albuquerque.

54. Jensen, P.S. and J. de Juan, E., *In-vivo microscopy using gradient index of refraction (GRIN) lens endoscopy.* Journal of Biomedical Optics, 1999((in review)).

Optimising Operation Process for Computer Integrated Prostatectomy

Q. Mei*, S.J. Harris*, R.D. Hibberd*, JEA Wickham†, B.L.Davies*

* Mechatronics in Medicine Laboratory, Imperial College, London SW7 2BX, England
† Department of Surgery, Guys Hospital, London SE1, England

Abstract. A method to optimise the whole process of operation/vaporising the prostate tissue using a prostatectomy robot to relieve urethra blockage is presented. The cavity that closely satisfies the surgeon defined model can be created by robot in half of the time that done manually. The desired vaporising region can even be reshaped during the operation, resulting in new optimised vaporising sequence that excludes the region already operated. The method also excluds vulnerable regions from operation for safety. All models maintained benefit for pre/intra/post-operation evaluation. The method exhibits a promising future for the application of robotic prostatectomy and robotic surgery on soft tissue in general.

1. Introduction

The **PROBOT** (PROSTATE-CTOMY **ROBOT**), a computer integrated prostatectomy system, has been developed in the **MIM** Lab, Imperial College to aid in the resection of prostate tissue. [**Fig. 1**]. Aspects of the design that have been considered are the graphical user interface, safety of the hardware and software, the use of real-time ultrasound imaging, 3D modelling, sterilisation of the system etc [**1-3, 9**]. The PROBOT has already been tried on 18 patients with

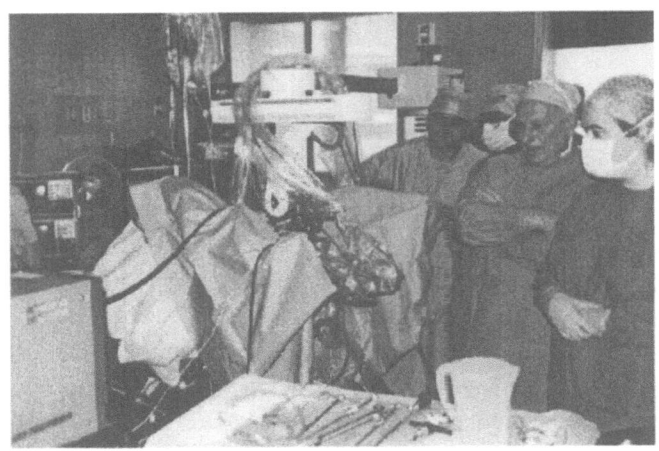

Fig. 1- the PROBOT is in operation
(The surgeon is monitoring the screen)

satisfactory result except that the overall operation time is approximately 1.5 times slower than its manual counterpart [9].

This paper mainly focuses on the optimisation of the vaporising process. Improved with new optimising software of the operation/vaporising process, the PROBOT can be expected to finish the operation within half of the time that done manually.

Prostate enlargement is a common disease among men over certain age and quite often this results in a blockage of urethra for which an operation called **TURP** (TransUrethral Resection of Prostate) is required to create a cavity inside the prostate and restore the normal passage of urine. A typical manual operation of such takes about 40 minutes or less to finish and takes away about 10 grams of prostate tissue [8].

By nature, the prostate can be regarded as a soft object that is fixed in position inside the men's body. The region around the urethra between penis and prostate is very flexible which allows the vaporising instruments to move transurethrally in different angles. When being operated upon, the inside of the prostate may deform locally, but the prostate as a whole generally maintains both its position and shape. A rigid model can thus be generated and processed based on transurethral ultrasound image slices, which makes the robotised operation feasible.

An essential part of the **PROBOT** is a specially designed motorised frame that is capable of creating a cone shaped cavity at desired positions [**Fig. 2**]. Mounted on the frame with an ultrasound probe, automatic ultrasound imaging can be carried out. Otherwise mounted with vaporising instrument, cystoscope and video camera, the system can perform prostatectomy operation, or non-bleeding vaporising procedure with clear on-line video monitoring.

The strategy for optimising the operation/vaporising process is based on matching the surgeon defined regions on recorded US images with corresponding pre-arranged, maximum mechanically feasible, overlapping cones, to generate the vaporising sequence with least number of vaporising actions (or vaps).

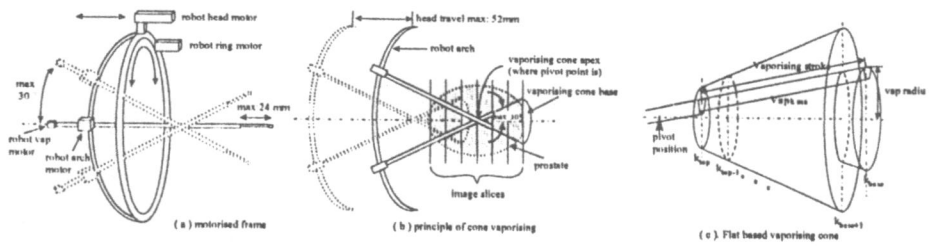

Fig. 2 - Model of the motorised frame and principle of (extended) cone-shape vaporising

2. Registration

Registration is normally concerned with relating the reference systems associated with different modalities to the rigid or elastic geometric transforms [4-6]. However, the registration of **PROBOT** is very straightforward. At the beginning of the surgery, the bladder neck and verumontanum (a clearly visible landmark that should never be resected) are first registered to the **PROBOT** via direct viewing from the cystoscope. Then, automatic transurethral ultrasound imaging is performed between the two end positions of the prostate. US (ultrasound) image slices, perpendicular to the urethra or central axis, are recorded at 5 mm intervals in the computer by means of a frame grabber integrated into the system. Subsequently, any geometric element on these image slices is directly transferred into the co-ordinate system of the motorised frame. The physical distortion from the 'soft' feature of prostate tissue caused by the imaging process has a negligible effect, as this distortion will be the same for the vaporising instrument because they share the same working mechanism.

3. Surgeon defined model

Having acquired computer based US images, the surgeon can now mark on each what region or area should be removed. A 3D **surgeon defined model** is thus obtained:

$$\textbf{Model}_{def} = \{ \textbf{Area}_{def\,i} \} \text{ and } \textbf{Area}_{def\,i} = \{ \textbf{dist}_{def\,ij} \} \quad |(i = 0,1, \cdots, I; j = 0,1, \cdots, 359)$$

Where **Area**$_{def\,i}$ is a **surgeon defined area** on ith image slice; {**dist**$_{def\,ij}$ } is the boundary for **Area**$_{def\,i}$ and **dist**$_{def\,ij}$ is the distance from the centre (urethra) to the boundary, at individual radial angle **j** on ith image; **I** is the largest index number of an image.

The anterior surfaces of prostate are covered by abundant loose fat that includes the preprostatic *venous plexus* [7], which is a vulnerable region susceptible to heavy bleeding during prostatectomy operation. As shown in **Fig. 3**, this region is located in the upper 120° part of the prostate, and slightly away from the urethra or where the

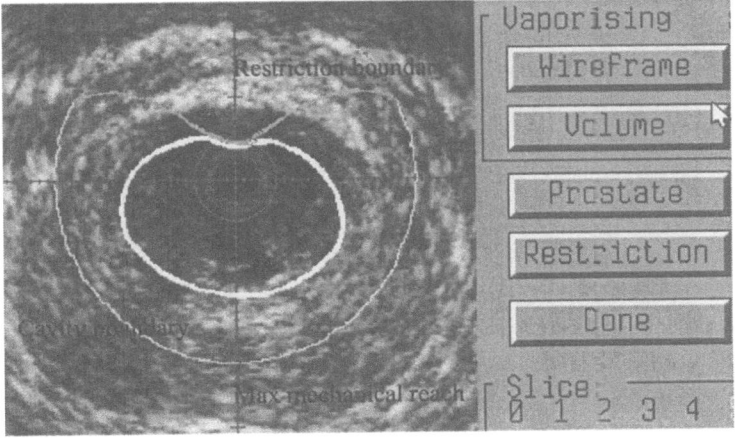

Fig. 3- Restriction boundary for safe cavity model definition

sheath of the motorised frame is anchored. A *restriction boundary* is given there, so that this vulnerable region will be excluded from the operation. The *restriction boundary* can be pre-set or edited to satisfaction for each slice. Together with the boundary of maximum mechanical reach on other parts, a region is formed where surgeon can define the boundary of cavity model.

4. Mechanically feasible model

One way to create the cavity of **surgeon defined model** is to cover it with a number of *maximum* "mechanically feasible" overlapping cones. By careful planning, the relationship between the distance of the verumontanum and bladder_neck, and the least number of cones, is worked out as that shown in **Table 1**. These cones are positioned from the verumontanum towards the bladder_neck at 5 mm intervals. The opening radius of the cone at the verumontanum is controlled by *press_depth* (a parameter from the user interface) for the purpose of reducing the risk of hitting the verumontanum. An example is shown in **Fig. 4.**

Table 1 - Relationship between the distance between bladder neck   and verumontanum and total number of cones

Dist (veru - bladder)	<=25 mm	<=33 mm	<=38 mm	<=43 mm	<=48 mm	<=52 mm
Number of slices	<= 6	= 6/7	= 7/8	= 8/9	= 9/10	= 10/11
Number of cones	1	2	3	4	5	6

(The distance between verumontanum slice and its neighbouring slice can be 1/2/3/4/5 mm; otherwise always 5mm)

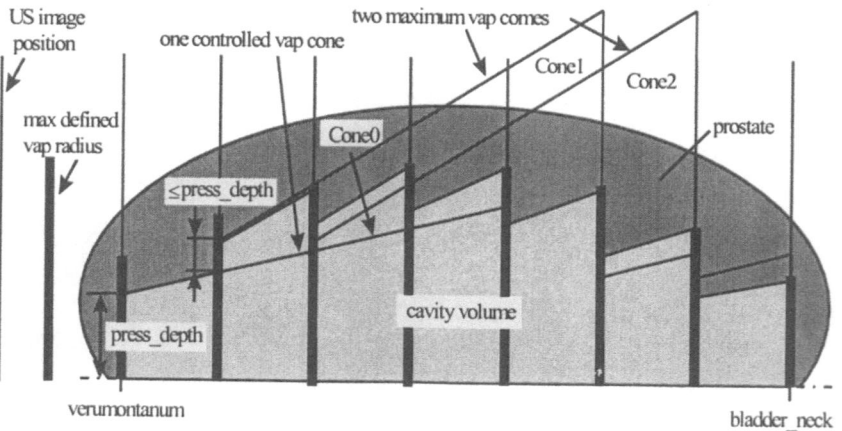

Fig. 4 - Section diagram of using pre-arranged cones to maximumly cover the desired vaporising volume

Given a surgical case, the corresponding **mechanically feasible vaporising model** can be obtained:

$$\mathbf{Model_{fea}} = \bigcup_{k=0}^{k=K} \mathbf{Cone}_{\text{fea } k}$$

$$\mathbf{Cone_{fea\ k}} = \{\ \mathbf{vap_{k\ mn}}\ \}\quad |\ (\ m = 1, 2,\ \cdots, M_k;\ \ n = 0, 1,\ \cdots, N_{mk}\ )$$

Where **K** is the largest possible index number of a cone. Each cone consists of a series of **vaporising** actions which starts from the inside to outside, and first in a clockwise then anti-clockwise way (to avoid entangling wires). M_k is the number of vaporised rings of cone k; N_{mk} is the largest number of a **vap** for ring **m** of cone **k**. Both M_k and N_{mk} are controlled by *vap_depth*, which controls how deep each vap will vaporise the tissue, and *vap_width*, which controls the distance between each neighbouring vaps. These also come from the user interface.

The above model can also be expressed as

$$\mathbf{Model_{fea}} = \{\ \mathbf{Area}_{\text{fea } i}\ \}\qquad |\ (\ i = 0, 1,\ \cdots, I\ )$$

Where **Area** $_{\text{fea } i}$ is the intersection of pre-arranged vaporising cones and slice **i**, or:

$$\mathbf{Area}_{\text{fea } i} = \bigcup \mathbf{area}_{i\ k\ mn}\quad |\ (\ k = 0, 1,\ \cdots,\ K;\ m = 1, 2,\ \cdots,\ M_k\ ;\ n = 0, 1,\ \cdots,\ N_{mk}\ )$$

Where $\mathbf{area}_{i\ k\ mn}$ is the intersection of $\mathbf{vap}_{k\ mn}$ and slice i.

5.   The final vaporising model

Obviously, part of the pre-arranged **mechanically feasible model** may operate outside the ***surgeon defined model***. Appropriate adjustments should be made so that there should be no vaps to operate outside the **Model_{def}**.

In other words, the final vaporising model should be, ideally, the intersection of the **surgeon defined model** and the **mechanically feasible model**, which can be expressed as follows:

$$\mathbf{Model_{final}} = \{\ \mathbf{Area'_i}\ \}\qquad |\ (\ i = 0, 1,\ \cdots, I\ )$$

$$\mathbf{Area'_i} = \bigcup \mathbf{area'}_{i\ k\ mn}$$

Where $\mathbf{area'}_{i\ k\ mn} = \mathbf{vap}_{k\ mn} \bigcap \mathbf{Area}_{def\ i}$ $|(\ k=0,1,\cdots,K; m=1,2,\cdots,M_k; n = 0, 1,\cdots,N_{mk}\ )$

or $\mathbf{Model_{final}} = \{\ \mathbf{vap'_{k\ mn}}\ \}$

where each $\mathbf{vap'}_{k\ mn}$ operates within **Model_{def}**.

6.   Optimising the generation of vaporising sequence

The aim of optimising the vaporising sequence is to generate from **Model**$_{final}$, a vaporising sequence that will be finished in the shortest time. From the design of **PROBOT**'s motorised frame, the control parameters for lth vaporising action (**vap**$_l$) are:

1. The distance to the pivot from the last position on the central axis to control the head travel motor(h_l)
2. The eccentric angle of the vap off the central axis to control the arch motor (a_l)
3. The angle of the vap off $0°$ home position on slice to control the ring motor (r_l)
4. The vaporising stroke to control the vap motor (d_l)

Let the vaporising sequence be: [vap$_l$ (h_l , a_l , r_l , d_l)], $1 \leq l \leq L$ (L is the total number of vaps) and h_0 , a_0, r_0, d_0 be the origin of all motors. The total time **T** spent on executing this vaporising sequence can be calculated by the sum of the time for each vaps (t_l):

$$T = \sum t_l \qquad\qquad 1 \leq l \leq L$$

t_l can be calculated by the sum of the t_{hl} , t_{al} , t_{rl}, and t_{dl} , where t_{hl} is the time spent for the head travel to move the sheath to the given pivot position h_l from h_{l-1} ; t_{al}: arch rotation from a_{l-1} to a_l ; t_{rl}: ring rotation from r_{l-1} to r_l; and t_{dl}: vaporising motor for a stroke(forward and backward). The time spent on communication can be neglected. So we have:

$$t_l = t_{hl} + t_{al} + t_{rl} + t_{dl}$$

The optimisation objective is to minimise **T**. This could be decomposed into the following five sub-objectives: i.e., to minimise L; minimise t_{hl}, t_{al}, t_{rl}; and t_{dl} .

Since these five parameters are not independent of each other, a reasonable principle is to give higher priority to the more time consuming parameters. Based on experience with PROBOT, priority has been set in the following sequence:

1. Minimise **L**
2. Minimise t_{hl}, , t_{al} , t_{rl}
3. Minimise t_{dl}
4. Minimise t_{hl}, , t_{al} , t_{rl}

To minimise **L** (the total number of vaps), it is necessary to maximise the amount for each vap or to use a full stroke where possible. It is also necessary to avoid repetitive vaps, which means it has to be remembered where all the previous vaps have reached, so that the subsequent vaps can be generated more effectively.

When vaporising a positioned single cone, t_{hl} will be zero, t_{al} and t_{rl} will be a small constant (decided by *vap_depth* and *vap_width*). t_{dl} is decided by the vaporising stroke.

Based on the analysis above, an optimisation algorithm called **max-stroke vaporising by cones** has been developed. It always finds, among the cones left, the one that has the maximum stroke.

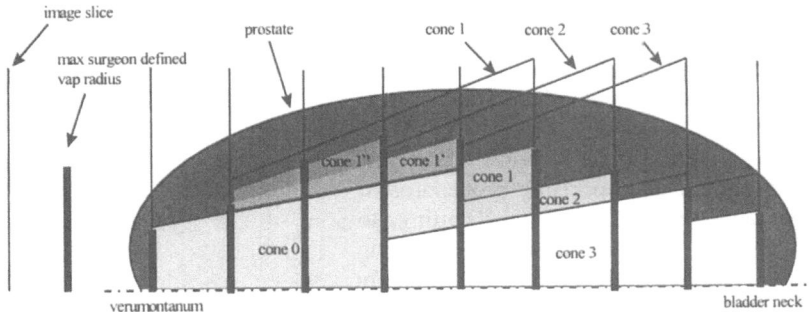

Fig. 5- Principle of max-stoke vaporising by cones

The principle of the algorithm is shown in **Fig. 5** and the 3D shape of the cavity is shown in **Fig. 6.** Without optimisation, to finish the cavity of $model_{def}$, the total time spent will be the summation of time spent on 4 individual cones (cone 0 to 3), or, the time is proportional to the *summation* of the section areas of 4 individual cones. With optimising, the total time is only proportional to the *union* of these 4 section areas.

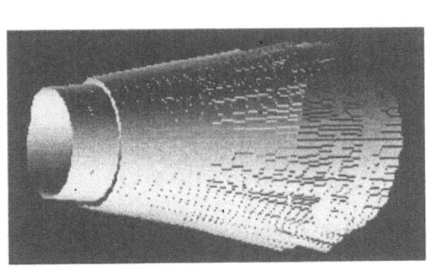

Fig. 6 - An Example of 3D shape of the cavity created by **PROBOT**

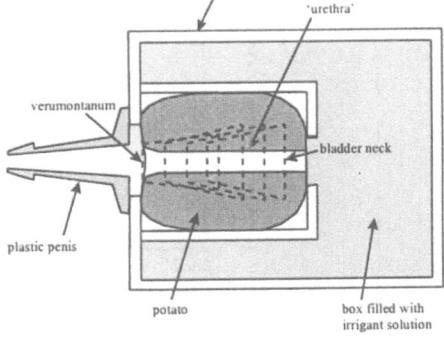

Fig. 7- Potato test settings

Moreover, a new mechanism of **two way vaporising** (both forward and backward vaporising) is introduced, by which a further 1/3 of operation time can be saved comparing to **one way vaporising** (backward only).

7. Results of experiments

The system with optimisation has gone through 25 potato tests [9], a traditional practice before live patient trial [**Fig. 7**]. Repeatability is within 1.5 mm on the maximum diameter of the cavity and 5 mm of cone spacing is good [**Fig. 9**].

It can be seen, from **Table 2**, the difference between the maximum diameter defined and maximum diameter obtained is within 0.75 mm with standard deviation being within 0.51mm.

Table 3 and **Fig. 8** show the time (minutes) spent on vaporising procedures. It can be seen that with two way cutting, to create a cavity of 10 cc/gram, the vaporising procedure can be finished in approximately 20 minutes, which is the half of the time that done manually. For the largest prostate (about 50 mm long with 11 slices) that **PROBOT** is able to operate, the two way vaporising procedure can be finished in less than half an hour.

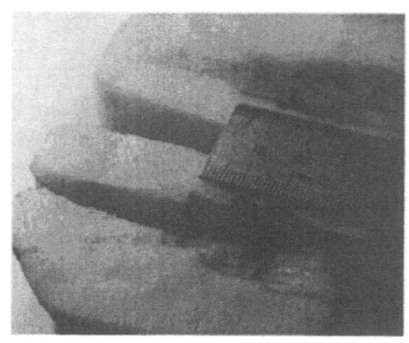

Fig. 9 - An example of the section shape of the potato after the "operation"

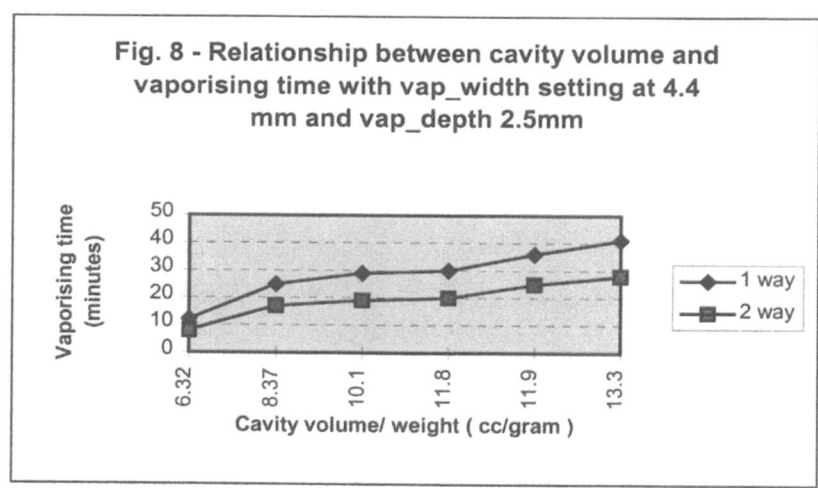

Fig. 8 - Relationship between cavity volume and vaporising time with vap_width setting at 4.4 mm and vap_depth 2.5mm

Table 2 - Experiment data 1

length	num	Max	max vap	D mean &
mm	Cases	Def D	standard	deviation
25	3	23mm	22.75	-
30	2	21mm	20.25	0.35
35	11	24mm	23.67	0.51
40	2	22mm	21.25	0.35
45	5	22mm	21.4	0.42
50	2	22mm	21.25	0.35

Vap_width: 4mm; vap_depth 1.7mm

Table 3 - Experiment data 2

Test	slices	press	vaps	volume	1 way (min)	2way (min)
1	6	3.5	49	6.32	12	8
2	7	3.5	105	8.37	25	17
3	8	3	122	10.06	29	19
4	9	2.5	128	11.78	30	20
5	10	2	154	11.87	36	25
6	11	2	173	13.33	41	28

Vap width: 4.4 mm; vap depth: 2.5mm which are acceptable by urologists.

8. Regenerating the optimised vaporising sequence

While vaporising is in process, it is likely to occur that the surgeon defined cavity model needs to be reshaped because of, say, hitting blood vessels or being too close to the capsule of the prostate. Then the software needs to re-generate the optimised vaporising sequence that should efficiently exclude the region that has already been vaporised rather than start vaporising from the scratch.

The surgeon re-defined model can be expressed again as:

$$\text{Model}_{\text{re-def}} = \{ \text{Area}_{\text{re-def } i} \} \quad | \, (\, i = 0, 1, \cdots, I \,)$$

$$\text{Area}_{\text{re-def } i} = \{ \text{dist}_{\text{re-def } ij} \} \quad | \, (\, j = 0, 1, \cdots, 359 \,)$$

The model for the cavity region that has already been created can also be expressed as:

$$\text{Model}_{\text{vaped}} = \{ \text{Area}_{\text{vaped } i} \} \quad | \, (\, i = 0, 1, \cdots, I \,)$$

$$\text{Area}_{\text{vaped } i} = \{ \text{dist}_{\text{vaped } ij} \} \quad | \, (\, j = 0, 1, \cdots, 359 \,)$$

So the required vaporising model can be expressed as:

$$\text{Model}_{\text{def}} = \{ \text{Area}_{\text{def } i} \} = \{ \text{Area}_{\text{re-def } i} - \text{Area}_{\text{vaped } i} \} \quad | \, (\, i = 0, 1, \cdots, I \,)$$

$$\text{or } \text{Area}_{\text{def } i} = \{ \text{dist}_{\text{re-def } ij} - \text{dist}_{\text{vaped } ij} \} \quad | \, (\, j = 0, 1, \cdots, 359 \,)$$

The generation of optimised vaporising sequence for this model is the same as that described in section 6.

9. Conclusions

This paper describes different stages involved in optimising the operation/vaporising process in a computer integrated prostatectomy system. The pre-arranged maximum *mechanically feasible overlapping cones* ensure that the surgeon defined model is completely covered so that any unnecessary under-vaporising can be avoided. Generating the optimised vaporising sequence with *max-stroke vaporising by cones* ensures the sequence will be generated in the least number of vaporising actions. With two way vaporising, this sequence can be finished in half of the time that done manually. Re-generating the optimised vaporising sequence, to exclude the region already vaporised, makes the system more practical. Vulnerable regions are excluded from the operation. This adds to the system safety functionality. As the whole vaporising sequence is generated before the start of actual vaporising, the graphical simulation of the vaporising process can be fully realised [3, 9]. While the vaporising procedure being finished automatically, surgeon can sit aside and just monitor, releasing him from otherwise a very demanding task [Fig. 1].

In short, after the above optimisation method is implemented, the prostatectomy operation carried out by **PROBOT** can be finished faster, safer, nicer and with better pre/intra/post-operation evaluations.

10. References

1. Davies, B. L., Hibberd, R.D., Ng, W.S., Timoney, A., Wickham, J.E.A.,   **"Mechanical Constraints - The Answer to Safe Robotic Surgery?"** J.de Innovation et Technoogie en Biologie et Medecine, France, Vol. 13 No. 4. pp425-436, Sept. 1992.

2. Harris, S.J., Mei, Q., Arambula-Cosio, F., Hibberd, R.D., Nathan, MS, Wickham, JEA, Davies, B.L., **"A Robotic Procedure for Transurethral Resection of the Prostate"**. Second Annual International Symposium on Medical Robotics and Computer Assisted Surgery, John Wiley & Sons, Inc., Baltimore, USA, November 1995. pp264-271.

3. Mei, Q., Harris, S.J., Arambula-Cosio, F., Hibberd, R.D., Nathan, MS, Wickham, JEA, Davies, B.L., **"PROBOT - A Computer Integrated Prostatectomy Robot System"**, Procedings of Fourth International Conference on Visualization in Biomedical Computing, Hamburg, Germany. Sept. 22-25, 1996

4. LAVALLÉE, S, et al., **Image-Guided Operating Robot: A Clinical Application in Stereotactic Neurosurgery,** p343-352, COMPUTER INTEGRATED SURGERY Technology and Clinical Applications, The MIT Press, 1996.

5. Kall, B. A. **Computer-Assisted Surgical Planning and Robotics in Stereotactic Neurosurgery,** p353-362, COMPUTER INTEGRATED SURGERY Technology and Clinical Applications, The MIT Press, 1996.

6. Taylor, R. H., et al., **An Image-Directed Robotic System for Precise Orthopaedic Surgery,** p379-398, COMPUTER INTEGRATED SURGERY Technology and Clinical Applications, The MIT Press, 1996.

7. Fornage, Bruno D. **Ultrasound of the prostate**, Chichester : Wiley Press, 1988.

8. Nathan, M.S., Wickham, J.E.A., **"TVP: a cheaper and effective alternative to TURP"**, Minimum Invasive Therapy & Allied Technology, 1996, :5: pp292 - 296.#

9. Mei, Q., **"PROBOT - A Computer Integrated Prostatectomy System"**, PhD thesis, Imperial College, May 1998.

A Passive Positioning and Supporting Device for Surgical Robots and Instrumentation

A. Grey Lerner, M.S.[2], Dan Stoianovici, Ph.D.[1,2], Louis L. Whitcomb, Ph.D.[2], and Louis R. Kavoussi, M.D.[1]

[1] James Buchanan Brady Urological Institute, Johns Hopkins Medical Institutions, Johns Hopkins University, Baltimore, Maryland, USA
[2] Department of Mechanical Engineering, Whiting School of Engineering Johns Hopkins University, Baltimore, Maryland, USA

Abstract. The recent development of compact surgical robots and instrumentation raise the need of a suitable mechanism for positioning and support in the proximity of the operative field. The accuracy of the surgical instrument and surgical procedure heavily relies on the ability of the supporting device to provide a sturdy base under the payload and dynamics of the instrument.

We present a compact and sturdy passive mechanical arm equipped with a central braking system that can be easily manipulated to desired locations and firmly locked in place. The arm presents serial link architecture comprising two links and three joints: spherical-rotational-spherical. To ease the maneuverability of the arm, one degree of freedom of the spherical joint at the base has been blocked, yielding six overall degrees of freedom.

The novelty of the arm relies in the special design of the braking mechanism that simultaneously locks all the joints using one single electric motor. The arm design is simple yet safe. One of its safety features is the power-fail-safe design rendered by the normally locked braking mechanism unlocked by a low-voltage electrical actuator.

The arm is designed for stand-alone use in the operating room as an independent module, representing the latest member of a growing family of surgical robotic modules under development at our institution.

1 Introduction

A significant research effort is presently dedicated to the development of purpose-built surgical robotic systems. As compared to industrial types, these robots present distinctive features such as safety, sterility, and compactness making them appropriate for surgical environments. The reduced size, compact geometry, and lightweight of the mechanical structure are important robotic requirements necessary for satisfying ergonomic requirements in the operating room [2], [4]. Moreover, for image guided procedures the robot design must allow access within the limited working space of existing medical imagers [5], [6].

A shortcoming of the compact design is the reduced working envelope of the robot [7]. Although sufficiently large for performing the surgical procedure at hand, the working envelope is too narrow for providing global positioning over the patient from a base to the operated organ. A positioning and supporting device is thus required in order to initially locate the robot at the operative site and to sustain it during the procedure. The accuracy of the robot/instrument and the clinical outcome of the procedure heavily rely on the ability of the supporting arm to provide a fix reference base for the operation under the payload and dynamics of the robot/instrument. Thus such arms are required to be lightweight, compact, sturdy, and easy to position.

Several arms have been developed for supporting instrumentation on the operating table. They range from simple passive knob-locked clamps for organ retraction and instrument holding to active robotic holders providing actuated orientation of laparoscopic instruments (AESOP - Automated Endoscope and System for Optimal Positioning, Computer Motion, Inc., Goleta, CA). Several of these are equipped with joint position sensors [5]. The locking mechanisms employed are either individual for each joint or central, providing simultaneous locking of all joints. The common actuation used for the locking mechanism is manual [1] yet pneumatic (Leonard Arm, Leonard Medical, Inc., Huntingdon Valley, PA) and piezoelectric actuation [2] have been proposed. Several devices are either in the experimental stages of development while other are already commercially available, approved by regulatory committees, and clinically used (AESOP, Leonard). Generally, the existing systems well perform the particular task that they have been designed for. Nevertheless, in demanding applications such as the support of compact surgical robots and precision instrumentation, these arms present the common shortcoming of insufficient stiffness and payload capability.

This paper reports the design and performance evaluation of an arm capable to provide a steadier support of larger payloads, the Grey Arm. The compact and ergonomic characteristics of previous designs have been maintained while improving overall safety and maneuverability. The design is protected by a provisional patent of invention [3].

2   Methods

The main design requirements for the Grey Arm were specified according to the shortcomings of existing designs: increased stiffness and payload capability. For ergonomic and ease of use reasons, the arm was required to provide free, frictionless motion of the end-effector in the unlocked state. The locking mechanism requirement was to simultaneously engage all joints from one simple command. For the safety of operation in the event of power failure, the locking mechanism was required to present a normally locked configuration. Detailed specifications are given in Table 1. The SRS (spherical - revolute - spherical) kinematic architecture of the arm has been imposed as a design requirement due to the positive experience of previous SRS arms for providing a large working envelope in a compact design. In addition, initial specifications required the arm to be passive in order to achieve simplicity and cost efficiency. Electrical actuation of the

Table 1. Design specifications

CONSIDERATION	SPECIFICATION
Weight	$\leq$ 10 Kg for comfortable single person operation
Degrees of freedom	$\geq$ 6 preferable 6
Workspace	Spherical with 0.35 m radius
End-effector	Easy attachment
Architecture	Spherical - Revolute - Spherical joints (SRS)
Payload	$\geq$ 10 Kg
Actuation	Passive
Brakes	Simultaneous for all joints,
	normally locked, electrical actuation preferred
Locking time	$\leq$ 250 ms
Power	Electrical $\leq$ 24V
Rigidity	$\geq$ 10 Hz natural frequency
Stiffness	$\geq$ 0.4 N/μm ($\sim$250μm deflection for 10 Kg load at end effector)
Materials	Non-corrosive

braking mechanism was preferred for its reliable, noiseless, and clean operation. Safety required a low voltage electrical supply.

Figure 1 presents a schematic of the Grey Arm. The arm comprises a proximal link (1) and a distal link (2) connecting three joints (3,4,5). The middle joint (4) is revolute while the base joint (4) and the distal joint (5) are spherical.

The base of the arm is mounted via a tapered shaft (6) to a custom clamp (not represented) that mounts on a fixed support such as the rail of the operating room table. The surgical instrument or robotic system is connected as an end-effector at the distal joint (5) through a custom-made adapter (8). Both the base clamp and the end-effector adapter are simple and easy to manufacture. They can be machined depending on the desired base and end-effector of the given application.

2.1 Degrees of freedom

The arm may be configured so that when unlocked it exhibits either seven or six overall degrees of freedom (dof). This wrench-adjustable configuration may be easily set depending on the application at hand and the preference of the surgeon.

The freedom of the arm results from the type and number of its joints. As previously described, the Grey Arm presents a spherical-cylindrical-spherical joint architecture altogether yielding seven (3+1+3) degrees of freedom. In this situation the arm presents one redundant degree of freedom creating ambiguity in the orientation of the arm for a given end-effector location. This is, with more than six dof the linkage position is not unique. For the surgeon positioning the arm this translates into the requirement of holding not just the end-effector but also

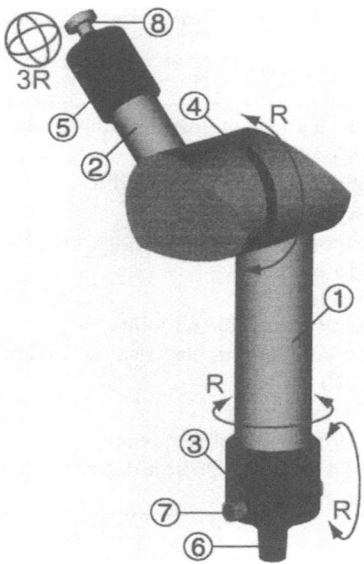

Fig. 1. Grey Arm: Architecture and degrees of freedom

the arm, which sometimes may be impractical. However, the 7-dof configuration of the arm is necessary in case that specific orientations of the arm are desired.

Constraining the spherical (ball) joint at the base to only two rotational dof leads to less ambiguity in the positioning task. Ball joints are compact, simple, and free to rotate in three dimensions. By contrast, common 2-dof rotary joints, which are implemented by serially linking a pair of revolute joints, lead to a bulkier more complex assembly. A novel design was used to implement a ball joint with only two rotational dof (Figure 2).

The 2-dof ball joint employs a spherical ball (1) with an equatorial groove of semi-circular cross section (2) and a pair of spring loaded ball plungers (3) mounted into the socket of the joint (4). The plungers face opposite sides of the sphere (1) such that their spring loaded balls (5) ride smoothly in the mating equatorial groove (2). In this arrangement, one rotational dof is constrained while rotations R_α and R_β are free. This constrain is active as long as the moment applied in the constrained direction is low. After a certain limit, which is determined by the plunger spring, the balls (5) leave the equatorial groove (2) and the blocked dof is released. This threshold is set so that under normal operation the joint is constrained, while under intentional action of the surgeon the constrain is bypassed allowing the arm to change orientation. In case that this operation mode is impractical for a certain clinical procedure the plungers (3) may be unloaded or completely removed thus rendering a regular 3-dof spherical joint.

This scheme allows the construction of a 2(3)-dof rotary joint while maintaining the compactness and simplicity of the classic spherical joint. In addition,

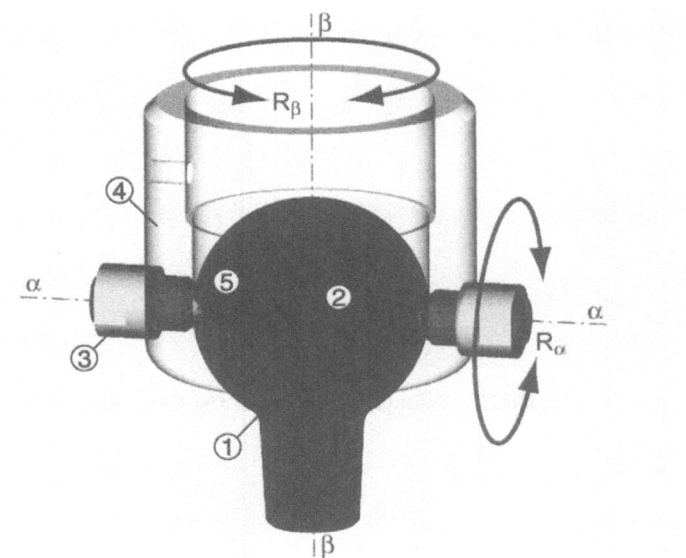

Fig. 2. The two degrees of freedom ball joint at the base of the Grey Arm

the ball-based scheme allows the addition of a simple locking mechanism of the joint, as presented next.

2.2   Central Active Locking Mechanism

All joints of the arm are locked from one single electrical motor through a special mechanism that generates and transmits the locking force independent of the orientation of the arm. Figure 3 presents a planar axial cross section through the arm when the joints are oriented such that their axes are contained into the plane of the section. The links represented by the hallow tubes (4) and (17) are rigidly fixed into the ball sockets (3) respectively (19) and into the hubs of the middle joint (13) respectively (16). The electrical motor (6) used for the prototype is a 21.2W power 12V nominal voltage motor with a 159:1 planetary gear head (MicroMo Electronics: 3042W012CR+30/1 159:1). The motor is mounted into the housing (5) that is constrained to rotate into the link (4). The motor engages a planar cam mechanism represented by the thrust bearing (7), the cam (8), the pair of spherical balls (9), the balls race (10), and the cam follower (11). Figure 4 presents an isometric view of the cam (8), balls (9), and follower (11) represented transparent. Part numbers coincide with those in Figure 3. For clarity, in this representation the race of the ball race (10) has been hidden.

   The cam (8) presents a pair of helical grooves of semi-circular cross section (22), end to end spanning 1.5 mm in height over 130° each. The depth of the helical groove is a quadratic function of the helical angle, such that the mechanism provides large displacement at the beginning and large force at the end

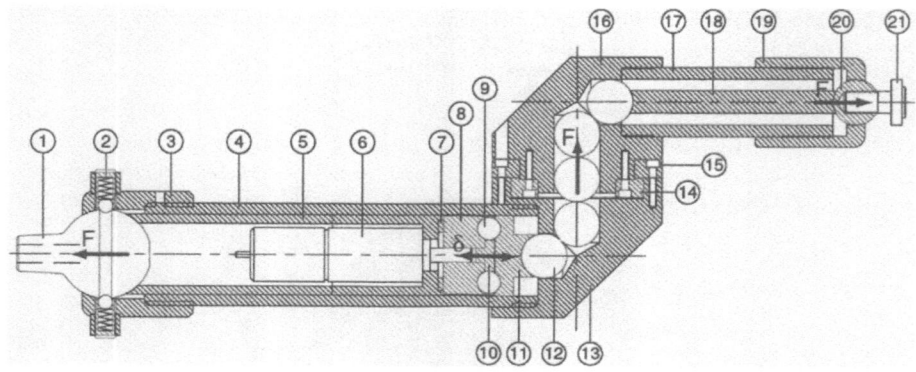

Fig. 3. Axial cross section of the Grey Arm

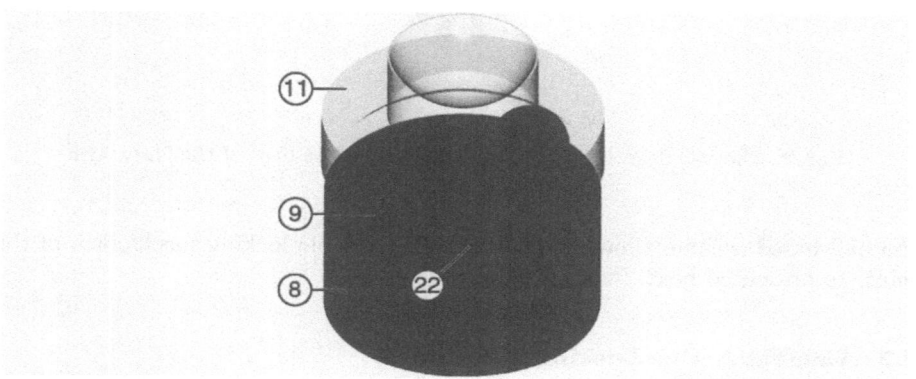

Fig. 4. The planar cam mechanism with load-carrying ball bearings

of the locking stroke. The race of balls (10) presents a small ball plunger (not represented) oriented radial which is in permanent contact with the inner part of the link (4). This is necessary in order to insure the engagement of the balls (9) between the cam (8) and the follower (11) independent of the arm's orientation.

The cam mechanism generates an axial displacement δ (Figure 3). A transmission mechanism comprising a series of spherical balls (12) and the spacer rod (18) propagates the displacement from the proximal joint (1) through the middle joint (14,15) to the distal joint (20). The chain of internal components is constrained within the outer components of the arm. Braking occurs when the length of the transmission chain (1,5,8,9,11,18,20), which is controlled by the electrical motor (δ), exceeds the length of the conformed space (3,4,13,16,17,19). This is guaranteed by the setting the cam displacement to be greater than the free travel in the transmission. An initial adjustment is used to fine tune the outer chain length by tightening the socket (19) on the distal link (17) such that in the unlocked state there is no braking force generated into the joins.

The cam displacement δ generates compressive forces throughout the entire internal path balanced by tensile forces in all outer components. This yields equal braking forces F in all joints regardless of the relative orientation of the distal and proximal links. A reversed arrangement for the middle joint comprising the braking disks (14,15) was necessary in order to achieve braking the under tensile forces. The disks (14,15) are pushed together when the normal force F attempts to spread the central joint, thus causing friction forces that block the joint.

2.3 The electronic circuitry

The Grey Arm is a modular component in that it functions independently only requiring a low voltage DC power supply. All components, including the electronic circuitry for motor control and the command buttons, are integrated into the arm. A power connector is mounted into the proximal sphere (1). The power is transmitted through a rotary connector to the electronic board located inside the proximal link between the ball (1) and the motor (6).

The command is based on two momentary buttons mounted on opposite sides of the proximal link. The arm unlocks when the buttons are simultaneously pressed. The arm locks as soon as at least one button is released. While the buttons are pressed the motor spins continuously in the unlocking direction. When a button is released the motor reverses for a short period that is timed to provide full locking of the arm. A current amplifier is used to limit the motor current. No encoders are required for operation.

3 Results

Two prototypes of the Grey Arm have been developed. The second generation improved upon esthetics and modularity. Figure 5 presents a photograph of the second prototype Grey Arm (1) supporting the driver (2) PAKY [6] of the trocar needle (3) under an x-ray fluoroscope (4) (C-Arm). The arm (1) is mounted by means of a clamp (5) on a rigid custom side rail (6) of the operating room table. The operation of the Grey Arm is simple and intuitive. The arm is normally locked and two buttons (7) must be pressed before the arm will unlock. While holding both buttons closed, the arm's 6/7-dof are fully available for completing the positioning task. Upon release of either button, the arm locks rigidly in place (approx. 200 ms locking time), fixing the position and orientation of the end-effector mounted at the distal joint.

Tests have been performed to assess performance and reliability. Experiments reviled that the Grey Arm prototype is concurrent with the design specifications (Table 2).

High stiffness of the arm was imperative due to the nature of the task. Figure 6 presents the results of stiffness measurement experiments performed on the Grey Arm. The graph of the displacement versus load at the end-effector reveals sub-millimeter deflections realized at the end of the arm under full load.

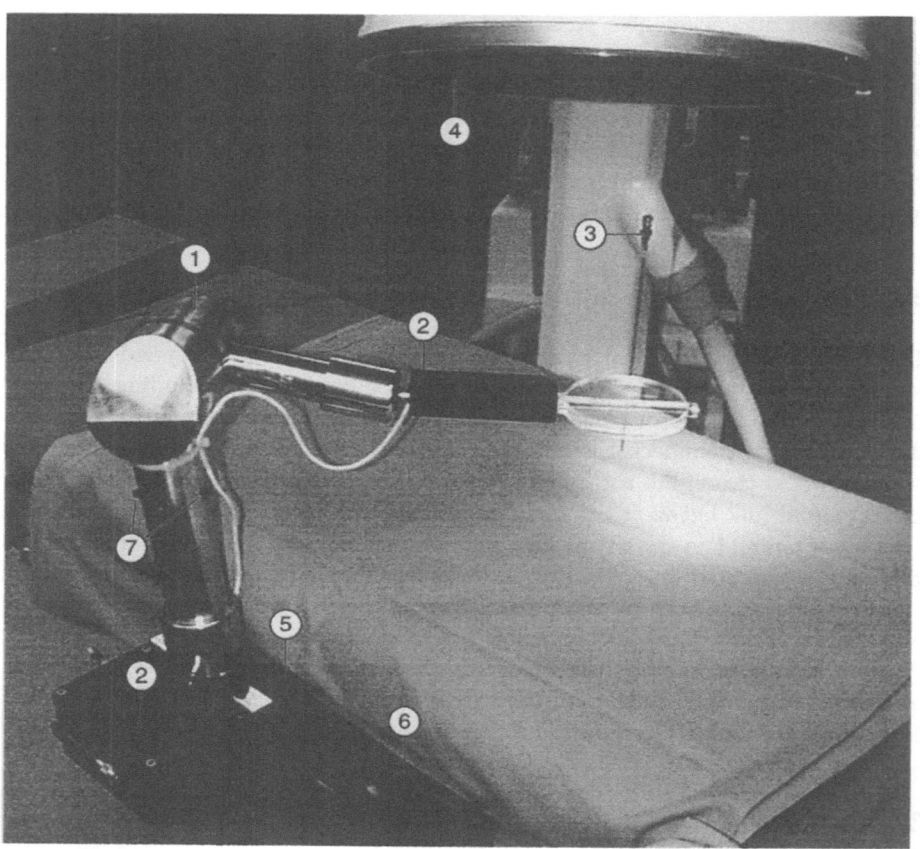

Fig. 5. The Grey Arm supporting the PAKY needle driver

Additional tests have been performed to assess the arm's rigidity by performing measurements of the natural frequency of the arm. An accelerometer interfaced with a digital spectrum analyzer was used to determine the natural vibration modes on the Grey Arm. The arm was found to be very rigid with a natural frequency of approximately 45 Hz.

The Grey arm significantly increased upon the payload capability, rigidity, and safety of previous designs. For example, the piezoelectric arms developed at the Aachen University of Technology, Germany [2] exhibit 35N - 50N payload capability and 100 ms lock time using 200V - 1000V electrical power. Our design revealed a four times increase of payload (200N), uses a safe voltage supply of 24V DC, while slightly increasing the braking time to 200 ms.

During testing, the Grey Arm did not malfunction and proved to be reliable. The Grey Arm presents several features that insure safe operation. The arm is normally locked, hence power failures do not lead to arm unlocking. In addition, dual buttons insure that unlocking does not occur inadvertently. The arm oper-

Table 2. Achieved and specified design considerations

CONSIDERATION	SPECIFICATION	PROTOTYPE
Weight	$\leq$ 10 Kg	6.65 Kg
Degrees of freedom	$\geq$ 6 preferable 6	6 or 7
Workspace	Spherical with 0.35 m radius	0.4 m
End-effector	Easy attachment	M12 x 1.5 thread
Architecture	Spherical - Revolute - Spherical joints (SRS)	SRS
Payload	$\geq$ 10 Kg	19 Kg
Actuation	Passive	Yes
Brakes	Simultaneous, normally locked, electrical	Yes
Locking time	$\leq$ 250 ms	200 ms
Power	Electrical $\leq$ 24V	24V
Rigidity	$\geq$ 10 Hz natural frequency	45 Hz
Stiffness	$\geq$ 0.4 N/μm	0.7 N/μm
	($\sim$250μm @ 10 Kg)	(137μm)
Materials	Non-corrosive	Aluminum, stainless steel, teflon

ates on a low power supply, which is safe for the patient as well as the medical personnel. While firmly fixed in the locked position, the arm could forcibly be moved should a situation necessitate such action.

Clinical experiments with the Grey Arm supporting the RCM-PAKY system [7] will soon commence. The system will be initially used for performing image guided percutaneous renal access in the operating room using a portable x-ray imager.

4   Conclusion

A fully functional Grey Arm prototype has been designed and manufactured. Testing of the device shows that it meets or exceeds all given design specifications. Clinical trials will begin in the near future.

The design includes two new features: the architecture of the central locking mechanism and the design of the 2-dof spherical joint. With these features, the compact-ergonomic characteristic of previous designs has been maintained while improving overall safety, reliability, maneuverability, rigidity, and payload capability. The arm is intuitive and simple to use.

The arm shares the attributes of compactness and modularity of the robotic systems / surgical instruments for which will provide support on the operating table. This stand-alone device requires no additional components and operates on a DC power supply.

This type of device may prove to be highly useful for holding, supporting, and stabilizing a great variety of robotic and conventional surgical devices. We are hoping to begin clinical use of this device in the near future.

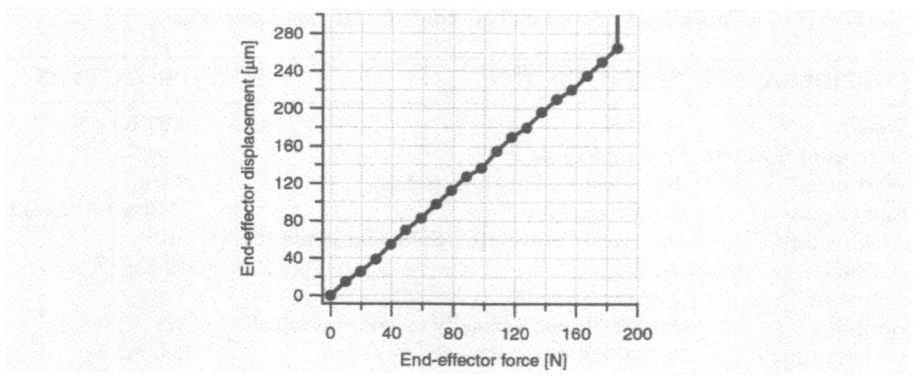

Fig. 6. Stiffness diagram for the Grey Arm

Acknowledgements

We thank Mr. Leonard Bonell of Leonard Medical Inc., Huntingdon Valley, PA for partially supporting the research involved in the development of the prototype. This research was also supported in part by the National Science Foundation under grants BES-9625143 and EEC-9731748.

References

1. J. A. Cadeddu, D. Stoianovici, L. R. Kavoussi. Robotics in urologic surgery. *Urology*, 49(4):501–507, 1997.
2. S. Erbse, K. Radermacher, M. Anton, G. Rau, W. Boeckmann, G. Jakse, H. W. Staudte. Development of an Automatic Surgical Holding System Based on Ergonomic Analysis. *1997 CVRMed - MrCas, Lecture Notes in Computer Science*, Springer-Verlag, 1205:737–746, 1997.
3. G. A. Lerner, D. Stoianovici, L. L. Whitcomb, L. R. Kavoussi. A Passive Positioning Device for Surgical Robots and Instrumentation. *Provisional patent of invention*, DM-3489, 1998.
4. P. Potamianos, B. L. Davies, R. D. Hibberd. Intra-operative imaging guidance for keyhole surgery methodology and calibration. *Proc. First Int. Symposium on Medical Robotics and Computer Assisted Surgery*, Pittsburgh, PA., 98–104, 1994.
5. P. Potamianos, B. L. Davies, R. D. Hibberd. Intra-operative registration for percutaneous surgery. *Proc. Second Int. Symposium on Medical Robotics and Computer Assisted Surgery*, Baltimore, MD., 156–164, 1995.
6. D. Stoianovici, J. A. Cadeddu, R. D. Demaree, H. A. Basile, R. H. Taylor, L. L. Whitcomb, W. N. Sharpe Jr., L. R. Kavoussi. An Efficient Needle Injection Technique and Radiological Guidance Method for Percutaneous Procedures. *1997 CVRMed - MrCas, Lecture Notes in Computer Science*, Springer-Verlag, 1205:295–298, 1997.
7. D. Stoianovici, L. L. Whitcomb, J. H. Anderson, R. H. Taylor, L. R. Kavoussi. A Modular Surgical Robotic System for Image Guided Percutaneous Procedures. *1998 MICCAI, Lecture Notes in Computer Science*, Springer-Verlag, 1496:404–410, 1998.

Robot-Assisted Diagnostic Ultrasound – Design and Feasibility Experiments

S.E. Salcudean, G. Bell, S. Bachmann, W.H. Zhu,
P. Abolmaesumi, and P.D. Lawrence

University of British Columbia
Department of Electrical and Computer Engineering
Vancouver, B.C., Canada, V6T 1Z4
tims@ece.ubc.ca
WWW home page: http://www.ece.ubc.ca/~tims

Abstract. Motivated by the need for providing a better user interface for ultrasound technicians, a teleoperation approach to diagnostic ultrasound examinations is proposed in this paper. In this approach, the ultrasound probe is positioned by a robot, with the operator, the robot controller, and an ultrasound image processor having shared control over its motion.

An inherently safe, light, backdrivable, counterbalanced robot has been designed for carotid artery examinations. Its design, as well as experiments demonstrating effective free-motion and force control, are presented. The feasibility of using visual servoing for motion in the plane of the ultrasound probe has also been addressed. Using a modified image correlation algorithm, tracking of the carotid artery for periods of time in excess of ten seconds has been demonstrated.

1 Introduction

Medical ultrasound exams often require that ultrasound technicians hold the transducers in awkward positions for prolonged periods of time, sometimes exerting large forces. Not surprisingly, a number of studies indicate that they suffer from an unusually high incidence of musculoskeletal disorders (e.g. [1]).

Motivated initially by the need to alleviate these problems and present a more ergonomic interface to the ultrasound technician, the authors have embarked upon the development of a teleoperation system for medical ultrasound. The system consists of a master hand controller, a slave manipulator carrying the ultrasound probe, and a computer control system that allows the operator to remotely position the ultrasound transducer relative to the patient's body. The problem considered first as a test-bed for robot-assisted ultrasound was that of carotid artery examination. This examination is carried out to detect occlusive disease in the left and right common carotid arteries - a major cause of strokes.

A robot-assisted ultrasound examination system would provide other, not only ergonomic, benefits. For instance, since the location of the ultrasound transducer can be determined via the forward kinematics of the slave manipulator, three-dimensional ultrasound images can be reconstructed from a series of two-dimensional image slices [4]. Remote probe positioning could also be used in teleradiology. Although a number of methods for transmitting ultrasound images have been proposed in the literature [3], none allow the radiologist to view *and manipulate* the ultrasound transducer at the remote site. The ability to position the ultrasound transducer in response to acquired ultrasound images would also be of benefit to image guided interventions (e.g., percutaneous pericardial puncture) and registration with past examination records or images obtained with other imaging methods (e.g., MRI).

This paper presents significant steps towards a robot-assisted ultrasound examination system. Based on ultrasound transducer position and force measurements taken during carotid artery examinations, a novel fully counterbalanced robot suitable for placing the ultrasound transducer in contact with a patient was designed and is presented in Section 2. The motion of the robot arm and the hand controller of the proposed ultrasound are based on measured positions and forces, acquired ultrasound images, and/or taught position and force trajectories. Several modes of control are discussed in Section 3, including the control of the transducer using ultrasound image tracking, for which the image Jacobian is derived. The feasibility of feature tracking in ultrasound images is discussed in Section 4, where it is shown that a modified correlation method can be used to track the carotid artery over periods of time as long as ten seconds. This will enable users of the system to apply image servoing techniques such as those described in [2], and can be used to follow along an anatomical feature such as a carotid artery, or to keep a feature, such as the tip of a needle, within the image plane.

2   Ultrasound Robot Design

2.1   Measured Motion/Force Requirements

The range of ultrasound probe motions and forces was measured during carotid artery examinations. These involve duplex imaging of the distal end of the common carotid artery and the proximal ends of the internal and external carotid arteries, both longitudinally and transversely, from the clavicle to the mandible on both the left and right sides of the neck.

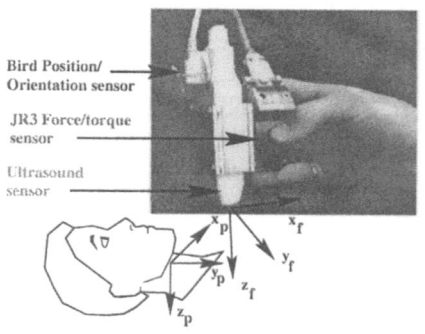

Fig. 1. Apparatus for force-torque-pose experiment

A 5MHz ultrasound transducer used in the examination was fitted with a JR^3 force/torque sensor and the magnetic field sensor of an ATC The Bird^{TM} electromagnetic position and orientation sensor, *as shown in Fig. 1.* The Bird's magnetic field generator was placed near the patient's neck. The ultrasound technician then carried out a carotid artery examination on the patient, holding the force/torque sensor instead of the ultrasound transducer (Fig. 1).

Metallic objects in the proximity of magnetic sensors are known to cause significant measurement errors. These were quantified for our experimental setup by placing the instrumented ultrasound transducers in a number of known locations and reading the sensor measurements. An average error of less than 1% was found in orientation, and less than 30% for translation. The measured motion range and the maximum forces encountered are tabulated in Tables 1 and 2. The uncertainty in translational motion range is not of significant concern, as the translational workspace of the robot must be significantly larger than measured in order to comfortably place the ultrasound probe against the patient. The orientation range can be approximated by the right elliptical cone

$$(\tan 15°)^2 x_p^2 + (\tan 35°) y_p^2 = z_p^2, \quad z_p \leq 0, \quad (1)$$

shown, with the measured orientation data, in Fig. 2. Note that the transducer must be able to rotate by $\pm45°$ about its longitudinal axis everywhere within this right elliptical cone in order to scan transversely and longitudinally.

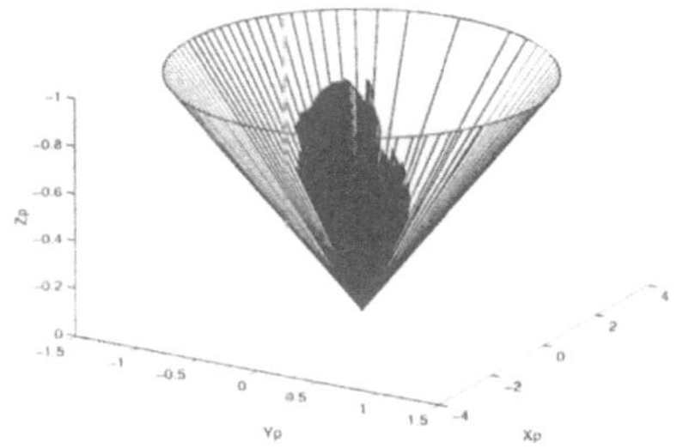

During these experiments, the maximum velocities recorded, of the order of 0.2 m/s and 260°/s, occurred during a switch to a different scanning area or during probe re-orientation. The average velocities were very small, of the order of 5 mm/s and 3°/s.

Fig. 2. Orientation range

Translation Range		Angular Range	
Axis	Translation	Axis	Rotation
x_p	130 mm	x_p	35,-50 deg
y_p	150 mm	y_p	-75,75 deg
z_p	100 mm	z_f	-45, +45

Table 1. Probe Motion Estimate

Force Range		Torque Range	
Axis	Force	Axis	Torque
x_f	3.8 N	x_f	0.4 Nm
y_f	4.2 N	y_f	0.7 Nm
z_f	6.4 N	z_f	0.1 Nm

Table 2. Probe Force Estimate

2.2 Robot design

A robot used for ultrasound probe positioning must be safe under any circumstance, including power failure, and should move fast enough to allow the ultrasound examination to take place at a pace close to that achieved by the unassisted sonographer. Therefore, the robot should be light and of limited force ability to allow relatively rapid probe motion in a safe manner. The robot joints should be backdriveable so that the arm could be pushed out of the way if necessary and controlled effectively in force mode. In addition, the robot should cover the required range of motions and forces described above. Because of the large orientation workspace required, the orientation and translation of the probe tip should be approximately decoupled. Otherwise, the entire robot arm has to be moved in order to accommodate probe orientation changes.

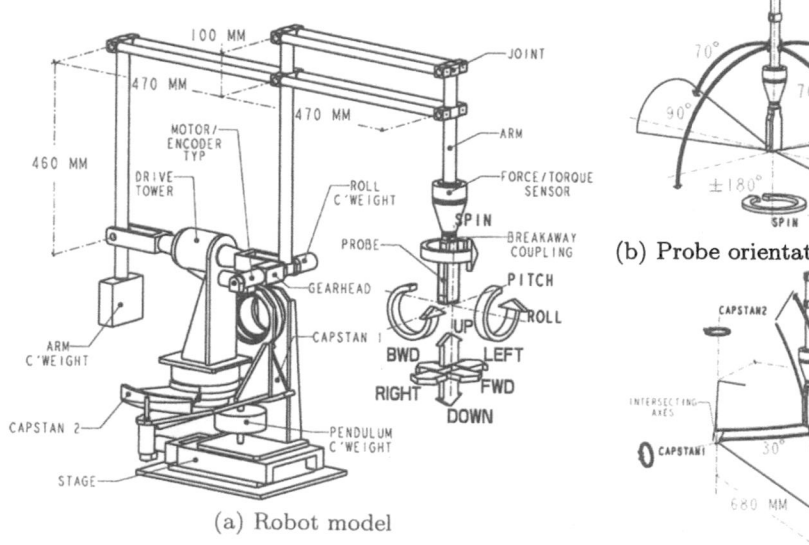

(a) Robot model

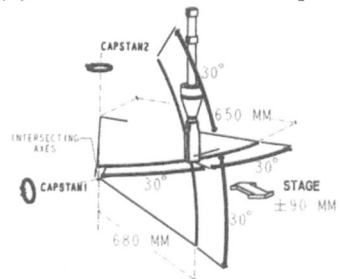

(b) Probe orientation workspace

(c) Probe tip position workspace

Fig. 3. Ultrasound robot design and workspace

This implies that the arm force capability has to be increased beyond a safe level, or that the arm has to be slowed down beyond an acceptable performance level. A number of design options, such as the use of a spherical wrist, were eliminated by testing whether the range of orientations in the elliptical cone (1) could be attained without interference and with reasonable link lengths. The only remote-center wrist structure that was found to satisfy the orientation range requirement was a rotating parallelogram linkage as used in the LARS robot [5]. The parallelogram linkage used in our design is different because of the need to counterbalance the arm.

The solid model of the robot is shown in Fig. 3, and a photograph is shown in Fig. 4. The robot is placed at the head of the bed, with the labeled LEFT, FWD and DOWN directions coinciding with the x_p, y_p, and z_p axes of Fig. 1, respectively.

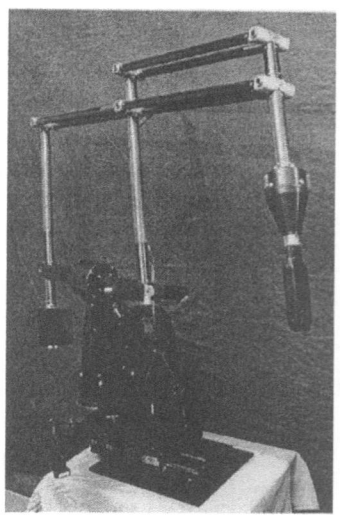

Fig. 4. Photograph of the ultrasound robot

The probe is mounted on a breakaway magnetic coupling and its spin motor is housed in a cone that attaches to a JR^3 force/torque sensor supported by a light and stiff parallelogram linkage. Constructed with carbon-fiber tubes and magnesium joints, this linkage weighs less than 2.4kg including the ultrasound probe and its spin motor. A rigid drive tower with an offset motor rolls the parallelogram linkage. Two revolute intersecting axes actuated by capstan drives move the probe up-down and left-right, and are mounted on a low friction (<0.007 N-m) linear stage that moves the probe along the neck of the patient. Each capstan is mounted on a single crossed-roller bearing, and each uses 1 mm diameter coated, annealed, steel cable, pre-loaded with a tensioning device.

Revolute axes were chosen over translational stages in order to maximize the workspace and minimize the inertia seen at the probe. Note that the parallelogram wrist is rolled to one side or the other during most of the carotid artery examination, and therefore most of the probe normal force

Axis	Trans. ratio	Motor	Force/Torque @ Current
Roll	93.6:1	Maxon 90	12.28 N m @ 2.5A
Pitch	50:1	Maxon 90	6.56 N m @ 2.5A
Capstans	40:1	Maxon 90	10.50 N m @ 5A
Spin	1:1	Maxon 20	0.18 N m @ 5A
Stage	0.49 $\frac{rad}{mm}$	Maxon 90	15 N* @ 2.5A
Probe Force			10-15 N**

* software limited   ** configuration dependent

Table 3. Actuation system characteristics

is controlled by capstan 2, which moves the least mass and therefore allows for higher bandwidth force-control.

Three adjustable counterweights were used to fully balance the robot. The roll and arm counterweights place the center of mass of the parallelogram linkage at a fixed point on the linkage roll axis, independently of the ultrasound transducer orientation. Because of mechanical interference (e.g. between the arm counterweight and the capstan), the roll axis had to be placed above capstan 1, creating an unstable inverted pendulum with the center of mass above the capstan 1 axis. This center of mass of this pendulum was moved below the capstan 1 axis by a pendulum counterweight.

As seen in Fig. 3 (b),(c), the ultrasound transducer workspace significantly exceeds the specified requirements.

3   Teleoperation and Shared Control

A signal flow diagram and the present hardware implementation for the teleoperation system are illustrated in Fig. 5.

During the ultrasound examination, the operator controls the ultrasound machine as usual, but moves a hand-controller or joystick instead of the ultrasound probe. Some of control modes that have been tested or are envisaged are:
Master-slave mode without force feedback, with the ultrasound transducer velocity and force tracking a joystick displacement as described in the next subsection. A SpaceMouse/Logitech Magellan [6] was used as a joystick. Experimental results are described in Section 4.
Master-slave mode with force feedback, as described in [8], using the handcontroller described in [7]. Feasibility experiments have been carried out [8].
Shared operator/robot controller mode, in which the two modes specified

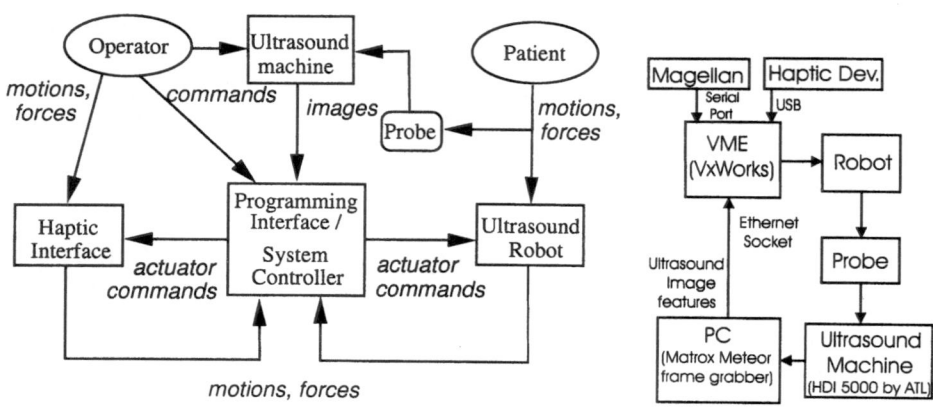

Fig. 5. Signal flow and present hardware implementation for the teleoperation system

above might be used along some of the degrees of freedom, but not others. For example, the probe force along its beam center axis z_f could be controlled or kept within safe pre-specified values by the robot controller.

Shared operator/robot controller/image processor control, in which visual servoing can be used to control up to three degrees of freedom - the translation and rotation of the ultrasound transducer in the plane of the ultrasound beam, while the operator and robot controller control the other degrees of freedom. The image Jacobian obtained below demonstrates that indeed the three degrees of freedom in the ultrasound image plane are controllable, while the ability to track features in ultrasound images over tens of seconds with a modified image correlation technique has also been demonstrated and is summarized in Section 4.

3.1 Force/velocity control

Because the robot is counterbalanced and velocities are small, the robot dynamics simplify to

$$M(\theta) \cdot \ddot{\theta} = \tau - J^T \cdot F \tag{2}$$

where $\theta \in R^6$ denotes the robot joint variables, $M(\theta) \in R^{6 \times 6}$ is the joint space mass matrix, $\tau \in R^6$ denotes the control torques, $J \in R^{6 \times 6}$ is the Jacobian matrix, and $F \in R^6$ is the force/moment exerted on the patient.

The control approach is illustrated in Fig. 6. Its objective is to let a linear combination of the ultrasound probe velocity and scaled force track the joystick command (displacement), i.e.

$$\dot{X} + K_f \cdot F = \text{Command}, \tag{3}$$

where $\dot{X} \in R^6$ denotes the linear/angular velocity of the end-effector and K_f is a *force scaling matrix*. When in free motion where $F = 0$, the ultrasound transducer Cartesian velocity tracks the command; while in contact motion where

$\dot{X}$ is very small, the contact force is controlled by the command proportionally. There is no explicit switching between the contact and free motion states.

The   joint   space   control   law   in   Fig.   6   is   designed   as

$$\tau = M(\theta) \cdot \left[\ddot{\theta}_d + \lambda \cdot \dot{e} \right]$$
$$+ K_s \cdot S + K_I \cdot S^* \qquad (4)$$
$$\ddot{\theta}_d = C \cdot (\dot{\theta}_d^* - \dot{\theta}_d) \qquad (5)$$
$$S = \dot{e} + \lambda \cdot (e + \zeta) \qquad (6)$$
$$\dot{S}_i^* = \begin{cases} S_i & \underline{S}_i^* \leq S_i^* \leq \overline{S}_i^* \\ 0 & \text{otherwise} \end{cases} \qquad (7)$$
$$\zeta_i = \begin{cases} \delta_i - e_i, & e_i + \xi_i > \delta_i \\ -\delta_i - e_i, & e_i + \xi_i < -\delta_i(8) \\ \zeta_i & \text{otherwise} \end{cases}$$

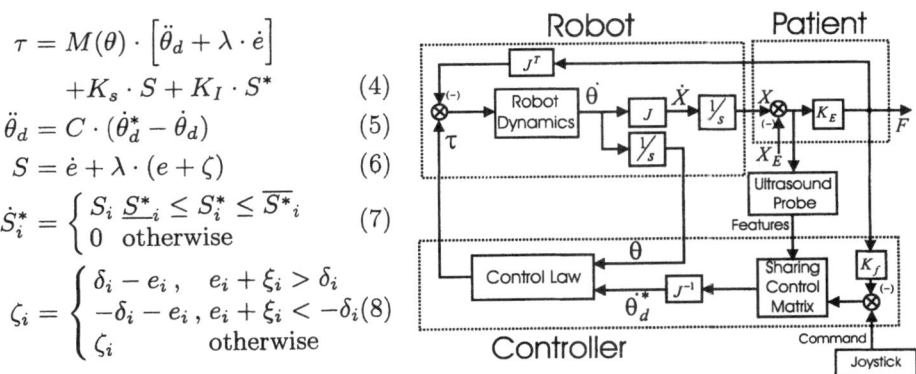

Fig. 6. Velocity/force control

where $e = \theta_d - \theta$, the subscript i denotes the ith entry of a vector, $\lambda > 0$ is a control parameter determining the compliance of the robot arm, δ is a vector of small positive threshold elements, and K_s and K_I are two positive-definite gain matrices. C is a filter parameter, and S^* is an integral term with lower and upper bounds $\underline{S}^*$ and $\overline{S}^*$, respectively.

The control law (4) implements a joint-space PID controller with saturated integral terms and mass and acceleration feedforward, modified by a "reset" function ζ defined in (8) that never allows position errors to be large. Under normal operation, absolute joint position errors will be limited by δ_i, i.e. $\mid (e + \zeta)_i \mid \leq \delta_i$. Should the patient or the ultrasound technician attempt to push the robot out of the way, ζ becomes active in such a way that the absolute position errors are still bounded by δ. Should the robot return to normal operation, it will stay close to where it was released, with an error determined by the size of δ. Note that the reset function does not require force sensor input. The natural low stiffness of the arm allows it to be moved away by pushing on any part of the arm linkage. The proportional and integral control terms are not allowed to increase, and therefore wind-up effects (the robot swinging when the patient's push subsides) do not exist.

The contact force F is handled in two ways. First, it is treated as a disturbance in the robot dynamics and is compensated by S^*. Second, F is measured by the force sensor and is used to achieve the control objective (3).

3.2   Visual Servoing and Feature Tracking

Visual servo-control [2] could be used to control motion in the plane of the ultrasound beam. Its feasibility can be determined by examining the ultrasound image Jacobian J_v, which relates differential changes in image features to differential changes in the configuration of the robot [2]. Let p_i be a feature point in the plane of the ultrasound beam with coordinates $[^f x_i, \ ^f y_i, \ ^f z_i]^T$ in the probe-attached frame. Assuming an orthographic projection model with scale a for the ultrasound image and that p_i remains in the image plane, the coordinates of p_i in the two-dimensional ultrasound image become $[0, u_i, v_i]^T = [0, a^f y_i, a^f z_i]^T$. It can be shown that

$$\begin{bmatrix} \dot{u}_i \\ \dot{v}_i \end{bmatrix} = \begin{bmatrix} 0 & -a & 0 & v_i & 0 & 0 \\ 0 & 0 & -a & -u_i & 0 & 0 \end{bmatrix} {}^f\dot{X} = J_{v_i} {}^f\dot{X} \qquad (9)$$

where ${}^f\dot{X}$ are the translational and angular end-effector velocities in end-effector coordinates. If several points are considered in the image, similar pairs of rows will be added to (9). The rank of the resulting Jacobian is at most three. Two or more feature points non-colinear with the origin will generate a Jacobian of rank three. Thus, as expected, with non-trivial ultrasound images, it is possible to control the motion of the ultrasound transducer in its image plane.

4   Experimental Results

4.1   Teleoperation Control

The control approach proposed in Section 3.1 was implemented with the hardware described in Fig. 5, with the mass matrix identified at the nominal configuration of the robot (shown in Figure 3) by applying small joint torques. Figs. 7 to 9 demonstrate the effectiveness of the control law while the operator controls the robot in vertical motion. Scaling parameters were set such that the maximum 1.5 mm joystick motion corresponds to a transducer velocity of 0.18 m/s and a force of 36 N. Actual forces are limited to 20 N by the robot capability and to 10 N by software and hardware.

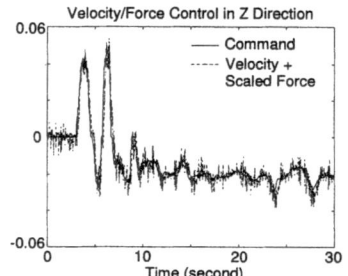

Fig. 7. Tracking of velocity plus scaled force vs command in the z_p direction

Free motion with velocity tracking is displayed until approximately $t = 10s$, when the probe contacts a person's forearm until $t = 30s$.

Fig. 7 illustrates the excellent tracking between the command and the linear combination of velocity and scaled force. Fig. 8 shows excellent velocity tracking in free motion, but not in contact motion. Fig. 9 demonstrates excellent tracking of scaled force in contact motion. It is clear that the both position and forces are followed precisely with appropriate switching between free motion and contact.

Some of the safety features built into the controller and robot design were also successfully tested. The robot could be easily moved away with a single hand, and would remain put in the position in which it was left by the operator. Turning the motor current drivers off left the robot in equilibrium.

4.2   Feature Tracking in Ultrasound Images

Motion tracking of a region of interest in B-mode ultrasound images was demonstrated before (see, e.g., [9]), but with different goals. Of particular interest to the

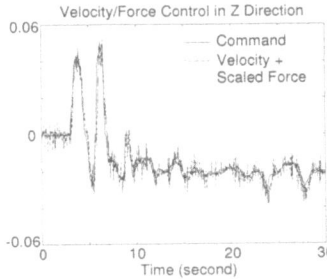

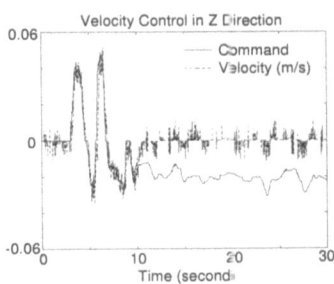

Fig. 8. Velocity tracking   **Fig. 9.** Force tracking

problem of visual servoing and shared control is the ability to track images over a long period of time. A normalized cross-correlation technique was modified for this purpose and is presented here.

Video-images from an ultrasound examination were obtained. Typical transverse scans clearly showing the carotid artery are shown in Fig. 10. The video images were digitized and processed using a 233 MHz Pentium II PC with a Matrox Meteor frame-grabber.

In a normalized cross-correlation technique, a sub-block of the image (in this case, a 128 × 128 pixel area containing the carotid artery) acquired at time t_i is shifted in its vicinity looking for a best correlated match with a fixed sub-block of the same size in a prior frame t_k. If k is fixed, the best correlation is sought relative to a fixed or reference image. Applying the cross-correlation method in this way leads to little drift, but high sensitivity to image deformation. If $i - k$ is fixed, the best correlation is sought relative to an image acquired a fixed time offset relative to the current frame. Applying the cross-correlation method in this way leads to little sensitivity to image deformation, but to significant drift, as the shift estimate is being integrated. A mixed approach was implemented that seeks the best correlation relative to multiple frames at times $t_k, t_{k-2}, t_{k-4}, \cdots, t_{k-2^n}$, where n is fixed.

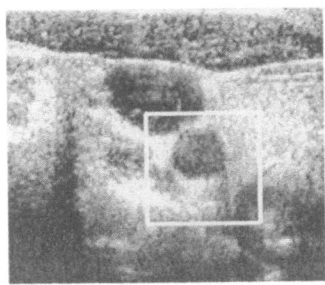

(a) Initial image.

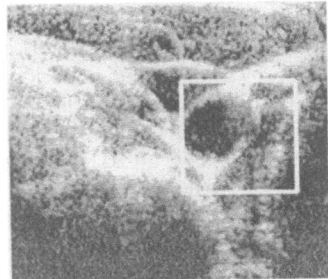

(b) Final image.

Fig. 10. Images of the carotid artery taken ten seconds apart.

Assuming only translational displacements, image sub-blocks of 128 × 128 of the carotid artery could be tracked at 30 frames/second most often in the range of 5 to 10 seconds, and for as long as 30 seconds.

5   Conclusions

A robot-assisted system for performing ultrasound examinations was proposed in this paper with the goal of providing a more ergonomic interface for sonographers. A prototype problem, that of carotid artery examination, was considered. A novel safe robot with a large workspace was designed and built and its control in velocity/force mode was demonstrated. The feasibility of tracking ultrasound image blocks over significant time intervals was also demonstrated. In the immediate future, the system will be used to explore the use of operator-computer shared control of the ultrasound probe and ultrasound image servoing. It is hoped that other applications of the system, including the ability to acquire 3-D images and to perform precise registration, will also be developed.

6   Acknowledgments

Discussions with Prof. David Lowe and Dr. Paul Trepanier, help with imaging from Henry Wong, machining and robot construction by David Fletcher and Peter Vautour are gratefully acknowledged. This work is supported by the Canadian IRIS Network of Centres of Excellence project SAL.

References

1. H. E. Vanderpool, E. A. Friis, B. S. Smith, and K. L. Harms, "Prevalence of carpal tunnel syndrome and other work-related musculoskeletal problems in cardiac sonographers," *Journal of Occupational Medicine*, vol. 35, pp. 604–610, June 1993.
2. P. I. Corke, *Visual Control of Robots: High Performance Visual Servoing*, John Wiley & Sons Inc., 1996.
3. J. W. Sublett, B. J. Dempsey, and A. C. Weaver. Design and implementation of a digital teleultrasound system for real-time remote diagnosis. In Proceedings of the 1995 Sympo-sium on Computer-Based Medical Systems, pages 292-298, 1995.
4. J. F. Brinkley, W. E. Moritz, and D. W. Baker. Ultrasonic three-dimensioanl imaging and volume from a series of arbitrary sector scans. Ultrasound in Medicine and Biology, 4:317-327, 1978.
5. R. H. Taylor, J. Funda, B. Eldridge, S. Gomory, K. Gruben, D. LaRose, M. Talamini, L. Kavoussi, and J. Anderson. A telerobotic assistant for laparoscopic surgery. IEEE Engineering in Medicine and Biology Magazine, 14(3):279-288, May/June 1995.
6. Hirzinger, G., Dietrich, J., Gombert, B., Heindl, J., Landzettel, K., Schott, J., "The sensory and telerobotic aspects of the space robot experiment ROTEX," in *Int. Symp. on Artificial Intel., Rob. and Aut. in Space*, (Toulouse, France), Sept. 30-Oct. 2, 1992.
7. S.E. Salcudean and N.R. Parker, "6-DOF Desk-Top Voice-Coil Joystick", *Symp. Haptic Interfaces for Virtual Env. and Teleop. Syst., Intl. Mech. Eng. Congr. Exp.*, DSC-Vol. 61, pp. 131–138, Dallas, Texas, Nov. 16-21, 1997.
8. W.H. Zhu and S.E. Salcudean, "Teleoperation with Adaptive Motion/Force Control", 1999 *IEEE Intl. Conf. Rob. Aut.*, pp. 231–237, Detroit, USA, May 1999.
9. E.J. Chen, I.A. Hein, J.B. Fowles, R.S. Adler, P.L. Carson, and W.D. O'Brien Jr., "A Comparison of the Motion Tracking of 2-D Ultrasonic B-Mode Tissue Images with a Calibrated Phantom", 1991 IEEE Ultrasonic Symposium, pp. 1211-1213.

Accuracy and Repeatability of Joint Centre Location in Computer-Assisted Knee Surgery

Kevin B. Inkpen & Antony J. Hodgson

Department of Mechanical Engineering
University of British Columbia, Vancouver, BC, Canada

Abstract. **To properly align knee prostheses, we must accurately define the mechanical axis which joins the hip and ankle centres. Current computer-assisted techniques rely on markers pinned not only to the distal femur and proximal tibia, but also to the pelvis and calcaneus, thereby increasing pain and the risk of infection. To eliminate these pins remote from the knee, we are designing non-invasive "trackers" that are strapped to the patient's pelvis and foot and are insensitive to skin motion. We mounted our prototype trackers on a fresh cadaver alongside conventional bone pin markers in the pelvis and calcaneus, and located the hip and ankle centres 30 times. We then dissected out and digitized the femoral head. Results from the hip tracker were excellent, the mean centre being within 0.2 mm (ML) and 1.3 mm (AP) of the physical centre of the femoral head (all results at 95% confidence limit). Compared to the digitized centre, the hip tracker introduces mechanical axis error of less than 0.07° (frontal plane) and 0.25° (sagittal plane) 95% of the time, while the pelvic bone pin introduces 0.03° (frontal) and 0.14° (sagittal) error. Results were not as good at the ankle: although there was no significant difference in mean ankle centre location between the foot tracker and the calcaneus bone pin (P = 0.09 in ML, P = 0.08 in AP), both means differed from the anatomical ankle centre (digitized midpoint between malleoli) by 5-7 mm, a mechanical axis difference of ~0.5°. Compared to the digitized mechanical axis, overall axis definition will be within 1.2° (frontal) and 0.9° (sagittal) using bone pins and 1.3° (frontal) and 2.0° (sagittal) using non-invasive trackers 95% of the time. For both methods, almost all error arises from bias and lack of precision at the ankle. We conclude that bone pins at the hip are unnecessary for sub-degree accuracy, but that better methods of locating the ankle centre should be investigated.**

1 Introduction

We are developing computer assisted total knee replacement (TKR) tooling that eliminates intramedullary rods and improves alignment accuracy without introducing additional imaging requirements (such as preoperative CT scans) or invasive procedures (such as bone pins remote to the operating site). Current non-computer assisted techniques have overall limb alignment standard deviations (SD) of 2.5° to 3.0° ([1],[2],[3]). Since alignment errors of as little as 3° have been shown to cause poor outcomes [4] and normal asymptomatic knees are typically within 1° of neutral alignment [5], our goal is to achieve a SD of 1°; this improvement will be large enough to potentially improve outcomes and will enable us to assess the effect of alignment on implant longevity. Prosthesis alignment begins with an accurate definition of the mechanical axis (the line between the hip and ankle centres) since this axis is the datum to which bone cuts and the resulting alignment are referenced. Additional errors are introduced when positioning the knee centre and joint line relative to the mechanical axis and when making the bone cuts, so we must be able to define the mechanical axis to a SD well within 1° in order to reach our overall alignment accuracy goal.

The computer assisted TKR technique developed by Leitner [6] defines the mechanical axis intraoperatively using a 3D optoelectronic localizer. They find the hip centre by tracking a point at the distal femur in a reference frame rigidly pinned to the pelvis as they move the femur through its range of motion. Similarly, they find the ankle centre by tracking a marker pinned to the talus or calcaneus in a coordinate frame rigidly pinned to the tibia. In contrast to conventional TKR, this technique requires two incisions and bone pin holes remote from the operating site which increases the patient's pain and risk of infection. In an effort to eliminate bone pins remote from the operating site, we have designed and tested devices that are strapped to the patient intraoperatively and used to track the motion of the pelvis and the foot without requiring incisions or immobilization. In this paper we compare the accuracy and repeatability of mechanical axis definition using our prototype non-invasive hip and foot trackers to results using bone pins, and we compare both methods to the mechanical axis defined by digitizing the femoral head and ankle centre.

2 Methods

2.1 Hip and Foot Tracker Design

In order to minimize artifacts due to relative motion caused by skin sliding over bone, we designed our hip and foot trackers to constrain all six degrees of freedom by applying six reaction forces only normal to the bone (see Figure 1; note that proximal-distal components of forces are not shown). The trackers are fully adjustable to accommodate different patients and seating forces are applied by straps. Each tracker has an optical marker array rigidly attached.

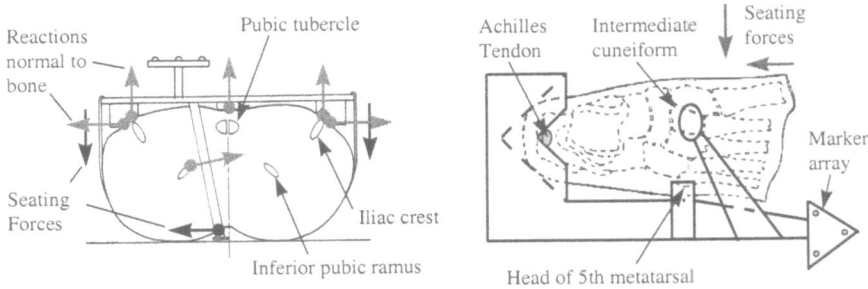

(a) Transverse section (looking proximally) through pelvis   (b) View looking distally on right foot.

Fig. 1. Hip tracker (a) and foot tracker (b) schemes

2.2   Setup and Procedure

We adjusted the hip and foot trackers and strapped them to a fresh cadaver (female, 89 y.o., 1.45 m tall, 760 mm hip-ankle). We drove bone pins (4 mm dia) into the ilium, distal femur, proximal tibia, and calcaneus on the right side, and rigidly attached one array of three infrared emitting diodes (IREDs) to each bone pin.

We used a Flashpoint 5000 localizer (Image Guided Technologies, Boulder, CO, USA), which has a typical accuracy of ~0.5 mm [7] to track the markers. We found that its noise level (SD of reported IRED position under static conditions) was ~0.12 mm at the typical poses in our study. For digitizing, we used the 135 mm two-emitter point probe supplied with the localizer. Each coordinate frame is defined by an array of 3 IREDs arranged in an equilateral triangle, 120 mm on a side for the pelvis and hip tracker and 60 mm on a side at the femur, tibia, calcaneus, and foot tracker. We recorded the transforms between all the coordinate frames in anatomic position, with a flat surface pressed against the soles of the feet to approximate the ground plane. We then digitized the distal tips of the malleoli and defined the midpoint between them as the anatomic ankle centre.

To find the hip centre, we recorded 50 points from a single IRED on the distal femur array as the femur was moved slowly through the maximum range of motion possible, creating a 'cloud' of data points in the pelvic bone pin coordinate frame. At each of the 50 sampling points, we also recorded the pose of the hip tracker marker array. We found the hip centre in pelvic bone pin coordinates by fitting a sphere (by least squares) to the data and also found the corresponding centre in hip tracker coordinates by expressing each data point in hip tracker coordinates using the homogeneous transform recorded at that point, fitting a sphere, and transforming the resulting centre back to pelvic pin coordinates using the anatomic position transform. We repeated this procedure 30 times, producing 30 pairs of hip centres. Similarly, we calculated 30 ankle centres in the tibial coordinates by tracking one IRED each on the foot tracker and calcaneus pin arrays. All resulting centres are in tibial coordinates and can be compared directly. We also recorded the poses of the foot tracker and calcaneus arrays at each sampling point so that we could detect their relative motions.

2.3   Data Analysis

All centres are expressed in coordinates aligned with the body axes (ML = medial/lateral, AP = anterior/posterior, PD = proximal/distal). We consider the digitized results to be the control and compare them to each of the two treatments (trackers and bone pins) separately to find maximum expected errors. To compare the bone pins to the trackers, we analyze the differences between them in each direction under the null hypothesis that the mean difference is zero. All groups of 30 centres and differences were normally distributed (checked using normal scores plots), so we used standard t-tests. Based on the variance of the differences in each direction, we can detect differences between the bone pins and the trackers of 0.25 mm (ML) and 0.76 mm (AP) at the hip and 4.7 mm (ML) and 5.2 mm (AP) at the ankle 95% of the time (95% power).

The angular error in defining the mechanical axis is proportional to the joint centre location errors and inversely proportional to the mechanical axis length. To be conservative, we have used the mechanical axis length (750 mm) for a 5th percentile female (mean of Japanese and Swedish populations; ~1.5 m tall) for computing all angular errors.

To portray the motion of the trackers relative to the bone pin frames, we compute changes in the vector between the nominal joint centre and the origin of the tracker coordinate frame as the limb is moved; we plot these changes on a 5° grid representing the limb motions (e.g., flexion & abduction); each motion vector represents the average motion in the surrounding 5°x5° neighbourhood and the magnitude will depend on the location of the tracker coordinate frame.

3   Results

Figures 2 & 3 show average range of motion across the 30 trials, digitized joint centres, and the resulting groups of centres from both the trackers and the bone pins. Frontal plane motion of the hip tracker is shown in Fig. 4. Motion plots of the hip tracker in the sagittal plane and the foot tracker are not shown due to space limitations. Relative to the ilium pin coordinate frame, the mean magnitude of movement of the hip tracker coordinate origin was 3.2 mm (range 2.0 mm to 3.8 mm). Relative to the calcaneus pin coordinate frame, the mean magnitude of movement of the foot tracker coordinate origin was 22 mm (range 14 mm to 26 mm).

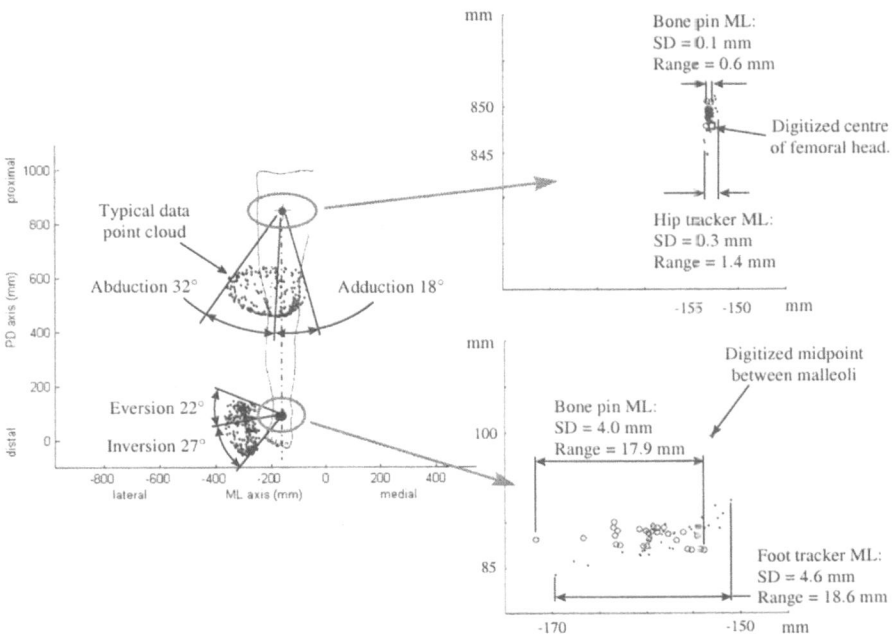

Fig. 2. Frontal plane view, mean centres and ranges of motion, 30 trials

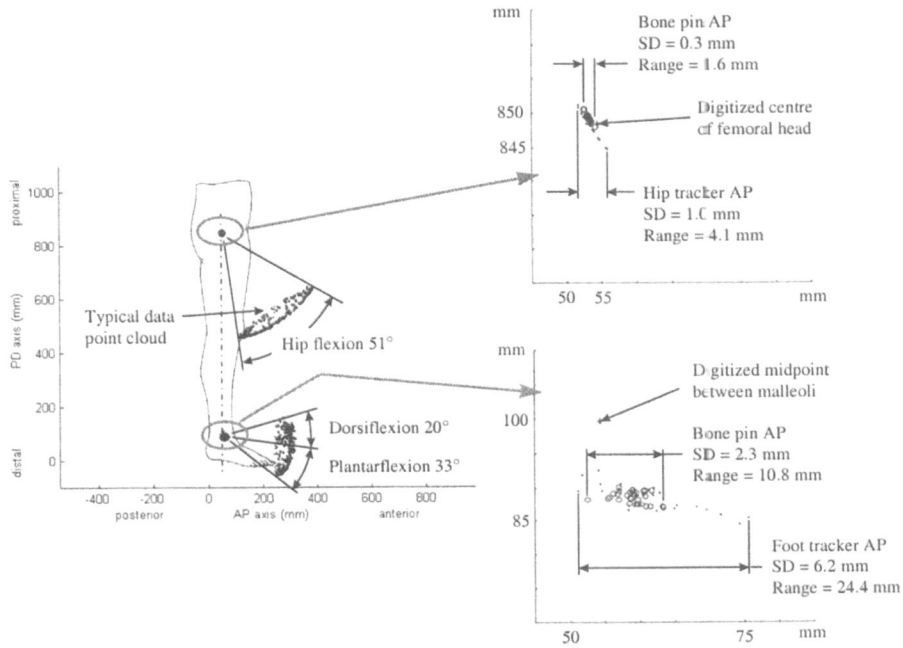

Fig. 3. Sagittal plane view, mean centres and ranges of motion, 30 trials.

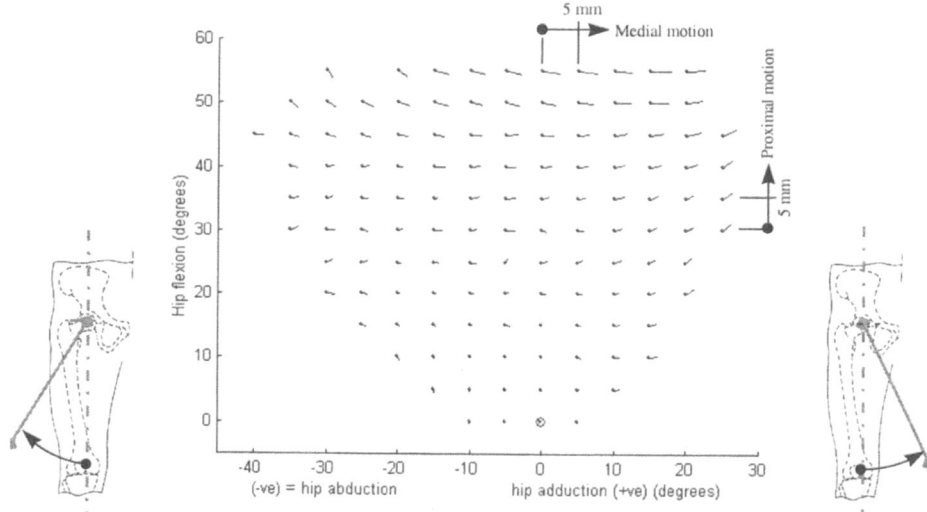

Fig. 4. Motion of hip tracker in frontal plane vs. femur position, mean of 30 trials

4.0 Discussion

The mean hip centre found using the hip tracker is 0.09 mm medial (95% CI -0.03 to 0.21, P = 0.14), 0.94 mm posterior (95% CI 0.58 to 1.3, P < 0.001), and 0.11 mm distal (95% CI -0.43 to 0.66, P = 0.67) to the digitized femoral head centre. Mechanical axis definition using the pelvic bone pin will be within 0.03° (frontal plane) and 0.14° (sagittal plane) of the digitized result 95% of the time (at 95% confidence).   Although the hip tracker results are ~3x more variable, the corresponding mechanical axis errors are still very low at less than 0.07° (frontal) and 0.25° (sagittal) 95% of the time. Compared to the pelvic bone pin, the mean hip centre found with the hip tracker was 0.23 mm medial (95% CI 0.10 to 0.35, P< 0.001) and 0.17 mm anterior (95% CI -0.21 to 0.55, P = 0.37). In PD, which has little effect on the mechanical axis definition, the tracker mean was 1.1 mm distal (95% CI 0.51 to 1.7, P < 0.001). The motion of the hip tracker relative to the ilium is comparable to motion found by Lea [8] for a pelvis immobilizer. The directions of motion are as expected, with a medial shift particularly in flexion and adduction due to the thigh contacting the rod passing through the crotch. Results using the hip tracker may be worse for obese patients, and some bruising may occur at the iliac crests; we are therefore continuing to test and refine our hip tracker.

At the ankle, both the foot tracker and bone pin methods are highly variable and produce mean centres distinctly different from the digitized ankle centre (midpoint between the distal tips of the malleoli). The calcaneus bone pin mean is 6.7 mm lateral, 4.7 mm anterior, and 11 mm distal to the digitized point, resulting in a mean 0.51° abduction and 0.36° flexion difference in mechanical axis definition. The foot tracker mean is 4.6 mm lateral, 7.0 mm anterior, and 11 mm distal to the digitized point, resulting in 0.35° abduction and 0.54° flexion. Mechanical axis definition using the calcaneus bone pin will be within 1.26° (frontal plane) and 0.80° (sagittal plane) of the digitized result 95% of the time (at 95% confidence). The corresponding errors using the foot tracker are within 1.23° (frontal) and 1.72° (sagittal). Note that compared to the bone pin, the mean ankle centre found with the foot tracker was not significantly different at 2.0 mm medial (95% CI. -0.31 to 4.39, P = 0.09), 2.4 mm anterior (95% CI -0.29 to 4.98, P = 0.08), and 0.13 mm distal (95% CI -0.74 to 0.47, P = 0.65). The foot tracker was significantly less precise in the AP (P < 0.001) and PD (P < 0.001) directions but ML precision was not significantly different (P = 0.21).

We would expect some difference between digitized and motion tracking results at the ankle because they are really two different measurements: The digitized ankle centre roughly corresponds with the centre of rotation of the talus alone [9], making the mechanical axis pass roughly through the centre of area of the talo-crural joint, while the calcaneus bone pin and the foot tracker motions include the effects of the subtalar joint, with its externally rotated and inverted axis of rotation. Therefore, by using calcaneus motion tracking and sphere fitting at the ankle, we are modelling a biaxial joint complex as a spherical joint. In pilot studies, we have found tracking a bone pin in the talus to be the most imprecise method, particularly in the frontal plane (as expected due to limited inversion/eversion). Considering that virtually all existing studies and techniques of lower limb alignment refer to the midpoint between the malleoli, we consider the digitized ankle centre to be the current 'gold standard'. The current results suggest that either an explicitly biaxial representation of the ankle joint complex or a robust method of digitizing the ankle centre should be investigated as an alternative to fitting a sphere to tracked motions of a bone pin or a foot tracker.

As found in [10], we expect the main source of alignment error in a passive guidance system to be the implementation. Bone cutting errors of up to 1° are expected with current techniques [11], and error will also be introduced in finding the appropriate references at the knee [12]. Mechanical axis definition error arises from the sum of the variances and biases at the hip and ankle, so we can see from the current study that the ankle centre definition contributes almost all of the error. As implementation errors will add to registration error, the current results show that even if bone pins are used at the ankle, it will be difficult to achieve sub-degree accuracy in final limb alignment.

5.0 Conclusions

We conclude that for sub-degree alignment accuracy in computer assisted knee surgery, bone pins at the hip can be eliminated, but at the ankle a robust method of digitizing the joint centre should be developed as an alternative to motion tracking methods.

Acknowledgements

Thanks to Dr. Robert W. McGraw, UBC/Vancouver General Hospital Dept. of Orthopaedics, Dr. Thomas Oxland, UBC Division of Orthopaedic Research, and Dr. Vlad Stanescu, UBC Dept. of Anatomy for their assistance.

References

1. Elloy MA, Manning MP, Johnson R: Accuracy of Intramedullary Alignment in Total Knee Replacement. Journal of Biomedical Engineering, 14 (5), 1992, pp. 363-370
2. Ishii Y, Ohmori G, Bechtold JE, Gustilo RB: Extramedullary vs. Intramedullary Alignment Guides in Total Knee Arthroplasty. Clinical Orthopaedics (318), 1995, pp. 167-175
3. Jessup DE, Worland RL, Clelland C, Arredondo J: Restoration of Limb Alignment in Total Knee Arthroplasty: Evaluation and Methods. J. Southern Orthopaedic Assoc. 6 (1), 1997, pp. 37-47
4. Jeffery RS, Morris RW, Denham RA: Coronal Alignment After Total Knee Replacement. J. of Bone and Joint Surgery (British Ed.) 73-B, 1991, pp. 709-714
5. Nguyen C, Bryant JT, Cooke TDV, Chow D: Alignment and Geometry of the Normal Knee in Stance. J. of Bone and Joint Surgery (British Ed.) 71-B(3) 1989, pp. 346
6. Leitner F, Picard F, Minfelde R, Schulz H-J, Cinquin P, Saragaglia D: Computer Assisted Knee Surgical Total Replacement. In: Troccaz, J., Grimson, E., Mosges, R. (eds): CVRMed-MRCAS '97. Lecture Notes in Computer Science Vol. 1205, Springer-Verlag 1997, pp. 627-638.
7. Chassat F, Lavallee S: Experimental Protocol of Accuracy Evaluation of 6-D Localizers for Computer-Integrated Surgery: Application to Four Optical Localizers. In: Wells, W; Colchester, A; Delp, S. (eds): Medical Imaging and Computer Assisted Intervention (MICCAI'98). Lecture Notes in Computer Science Vol. 1496, Springer-Verlag 1998, pp. 421-430.
8. Lea JT, Mills A, Watkins D, Peshkin M, Kienzle T, Stulberg SD: Registration and Immobilization for Robot-Assisted Orthopaedic Surgery. In: DiGioia, Kanade, Taylor, eds: First International Symposium on Medical Robotics and Computer Assisted Surgery (MRCAS) 1994. Shadyside Hospital, Pittsburgh, PA, USA, pp 63-68.
9. Lundberg A, Svensson OK, Nemeth G, Selvik G: The Axis of Rotation of the Ankle Joint. J. of Bone and Joint Surgery (British Ed.) 71-B, 1989, pp. 94-99
10. Moody JE, DiGioia AM, Jaramaz B, Blackwell M, Colgan B, Nikou C: Gauging Clinical Practice: Surgical Navigation for Total Hip Replacement. In: Wells, W; Colchester, A; Delp, S. (eds): Medical Imaging and Computer Assisted Intervention (MICCAI'98). Lecture Notes in Computer Science Vol. 1496, Springer-Verlag 1998, pp. 421-430.
11. Otani T, Whiteside LA, White SE: Cutting Errors in Preparation of Femoral Components in Total Knee Arthroplasty. Journal of Arthroplasty, Vol 8, No 5, Oct. 1993 pp. 503-510.
12. Inkpen KB, Emrich RJ, Hodgson AJ: Probe Design to Robustly Locate Anatomical Features. In: Wells, W; Colchester, A; Delp, S. (eds): Medical Imaging and Computer Assisted Intervention (MICCAI'98). Lecture Notes in Computer Science Vol. 1496, Springer-Verlag1998,pp.335-342.

Microscale Tracking of Surgical Instrument Motion

Cameron N. Riviere and Pradeep K. Khosla

Center for Medical Robotics and Computer Assisted Surgery, The Robotics Institute
Carnegie Mellon University, Pittsburgh, PA
{camr,pkk}@ri.cmu.edu   www.mrcas.ri.cmu.edu

Abstract. An apparatus for accurate three-dimensional tracking of the tip of a microsurgical instrument has been developed for laboratory use. The system is useful for evaluation of microsurgical instrument designs and devices for accuracy enhancement (both robotic devices and active hand-held instruments), as well as for assessment and training of microsurgeons. It can also be used as a high-precision input interface to microsurgical simulators. The system involves illumination of the workspace and optical sensing of the position of a small reflective ball at the instrument tip, and therefore requires no wiring connection to the instrument being tracked. Sensing is performed by two position-sensitive photodiodes, placed orthogonally. The rms noise per coordinate is presently 7 microns. Preliminary results are presented. The photodiodes exhibit some degree of nonlinearity, which can be calibrated. The goal is to achieve an rms noise level of 1 micron. This is expected to be attainable via a synchronous detection scheme which has not yet been implemented.

1 Introduction

The need for high accuracy is intrinsic to microsurgery [1]. Vitreoretinal microsurgeons, unassisted by accuracy enhancement devices, are capable of accuracy to well below 100 μm for brief periods of time [2]. Vitreoretinal microsurgery is among the most demanding of specialties in terms of positioning accuracy; there appears to be some consensus within the field on the goal of 10 μm accuracy [3]. Thorough evaluation of microsurgical accuracy enhancement devices (whether robotic manipulators [4–7] or active hand-held instruments [8]), as well as more traditional passive instruments, therefore requires sensing of instrument tip position in three dimensions, and with accuracy to less than 10 μm. A sensing apparatus meeting these requirements would also be useful for assessment and training of surgeons, as well as comprehensive characterization of erroneous manual motion at the microscale (including non-tremorous components [2]), and could be used as a high-precision input interface for microsurgical simulators.

Ease of manipulation and avoidance of fatigue are important in microsurgery, and as a result, hand-held instruments are of course designed to be lightweight. In order to keep the sensing apparatus from altering the dynamics of the motion to be tracked, it is desirable to avoid configurations that require physical contact between sensor and instrument, or that require significant added mass to be attached to the instrument.

Numerous commercial systems are commonly used in tracking surgical instruments [9], including Optotrak systems (Northern Digital, Waterloo, Can.) [10], the miniBird (Ascension Technology Corp., Burlington, Vt.) [11], and Fastrak (Polhemus, Colchester, Vt.) [12]. These systems, as available off the shelf, offer high accuracy, but not high enough for the present application, and all require that a sensor module be attached to the instrument, usually resulting in a significant change in its mass. Another system, recently developed specifically for evaluating vitreoretinal surgical instruments and surgeons, is the Johns Hopkins MADSAM system [13], which utilizes Hall effect sensing. It provides accuracy to a few microns, and requires attaching only a magnet of 0.23 g mass to the instrument tip. The drawback of MADSAM is that it only tracks in one dimension. One technology that offers a promising alternative is the position-sensitive detector, or lateral-effect photodiode. A two-dimensional position-sensitive detector is an analog sensor that puts out currents related to the x and y position of a light spot on its active surface. Position-sensitive detectors are frequently used in remote position sensing applications [14, 15]. They require no contact with the sensed object, and feature high position resolution and fast response [14], although they also often have significant thermal drift. Direct illumination from lasers or light-emitting diodes (LEDs) is typically used for sensing, but a reflective approach is also possible. The Apparatus to Sense Accuracy of Position (ASAP) has been developed for laboratory use, to meet the need for non-contact three-dimensional tracking of the tip of a microsurgical instrument, without adding significant mass to the instrument, for applications in surgical performance evaluation, analysis, training, and simulation, and for testing of engineered devices for accuracy enhancement.

2   Methods

ASAP is a system for measurement of surgical instrument tip position in three dimensions. A hexagonal array of seven Hewlett-Packard HLMP-DG08 red (626 nm) high-power light-emitting diodes (LEDs) illuminates the workspace. The LEDs are pulsed at 1 kHz with 50% duty cycle. A white aluminum oxide ball 1.6 mm in diameter is affixed to the tip of a typical hand-held vitreoretinal microsurgical instrument. The instrument itself, and all other surfaces within view, are painted flat black. Reflected light from the ball is received by two photodiode sensors facing in orthogonal directions, each one oriented at 45 with respect to the LED array, providing sensing in three dimensions, with redundant measurement along the vertical axis. Each sensor is fitted with a red optical bandpass filter and a lens (Nikkor 50 mm 1:2). This reflective approach obviates electrical connection to the instrument tip. Each sensor is mounted on a linear motion stage, and positioned roughly 10 cm from the back of the lens, putting it about 20 cm from the workspace.

The photodiode sensors used in the system are pincushion-type position-sensitive detectors (PSDs) (S2044, Hamamatsu Corp., Bridgewater, N. J., USA). This type of sensor is a planar photodiode with an electrode at each of its four corners. Each electrode is connected to ground via a load resistor. A common fifth pin of the detector may be grounded, or biased by several volts. Incident light represents a photocurrent that then flows to ground via the load resistor, generating an analog signal. PSDs are characterized by high position resolution and fast response compared with other detectors such as charge-coupled devices. PSDs are quite susceptible to thermal drift; in order to avoid the effects of this, ASAP uses AC excitation of, and coupling to, the PSDs.

In the ASAP system, a 5.11 kΩ load is used for each signal, in parallel with a capacitance of 0.0068 µF. The voltage across the load is input to an instrumentation amplifier. The instrumentation amplifier output passes through a passive high-pass filter with 330 Hz cutoff. This signal is full-wave rectified and amplified, and then low-pass filtered with a 20 Hz second-order cutoff. This cutoff frequency is selected to minimize noise while allowing capture of the full bandwidth of hand motion, including the nominally 8-12 Hz physiological tremor band. The total gain of the circuit is 90 dB.

A special-purpose analog-to-digital converter card for PSDs (DAS-PSP, Magen Scientific Corp., New York, N. Y., USA) is used to acquire the signals and calculate the position of the light spot on each photodiode [16]. The system samples data at 2 kHz, downsampling to 100 Hz.

Looking into the front of the PSD, moving counterclockwise from the lower left, let $u_1, v_1, u_2,$ and v_2, respectively, be the signals from the four electrodes. For the pincushion-type PSD, the coordinates (x and z for the first PSD) of the light spot on the photodiode surface are calculated as follows [17]:

$$x = L \left(\frac{(u_2 + v_1) - (u_1 + v_2)}{u_1 + u_2 + v_1 + v_2} \right) \tag{1}$$

$$z = L \left(\frac{(u_2 + v_2) - (u_1 + v_1)}{u_1 + u_2 + v_1 + v_2} \right). \tag{2}$$

The second PSD likewise yields coordinates y and z, respectively. The system is shown in Figure 1. Figure 2 displays ASAP with a mannequin face that has been prepared for realistic simulation of vitreoretinal microsurgery, including a sclerotomy to accommodate the surgical instrument.

3   Results

The root-mean-square noise in each of the three coordinate measurements is 7 µm. The position resolution of the system resulting from the discretization is approximately 0.2 µm. The linearity of the system is largely determined by the linearity of the PSDs. Hamamatsu reports typical nonlinearity of ±40 µm within a 0.9 mm radius of the center, and ±70 µm within a 4 mm × 4 mm square,

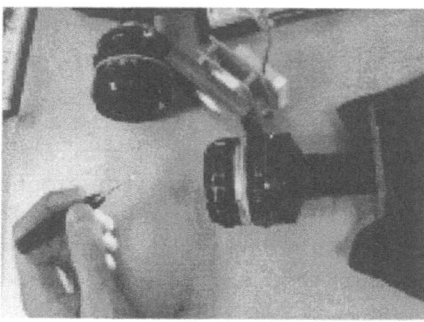

Fig. 1. The ASAP 3-D position measurement system for microsurgical evaluation. The LED array, lenses, and black instrument with white reflective ball are all visible.

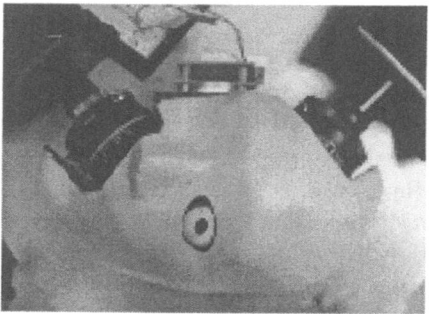

Fig. 2. The vitreoretinal microsurgery testbed constructed using ASAP for sensing within the simulated eye.

excluding the previous circular region. The workspace is a roughly cubical region with a volume of approximately 90 mm^3.

Sample results from the ASAP system are displayed in Figures 3 through 5. Figure 3 presents a tracing of an orthogonal frame made with the instrument mounted on a manually operated 3-D linear stage. Nonlinear calibration has not yet been performed, and the nonlinearity in the system may be seen, e.g., in the departure of the frame's z-axis from the vertical. The figure also makes the repeatability of the system evident, as each of the three line segments in the figure is traced twice (one in each direction). Figure 4 represents a freehand attempt at a similar figure. Figure 5 presents a sample of data recorded while a subject holding the instrument attempted to keep it motionless, along with a recording of the system noise for comparison.

4   Discussion

To our knowledge, the data presented here represent the first recordings ever made of microsurgical instrument motion in three dimensions with this degree

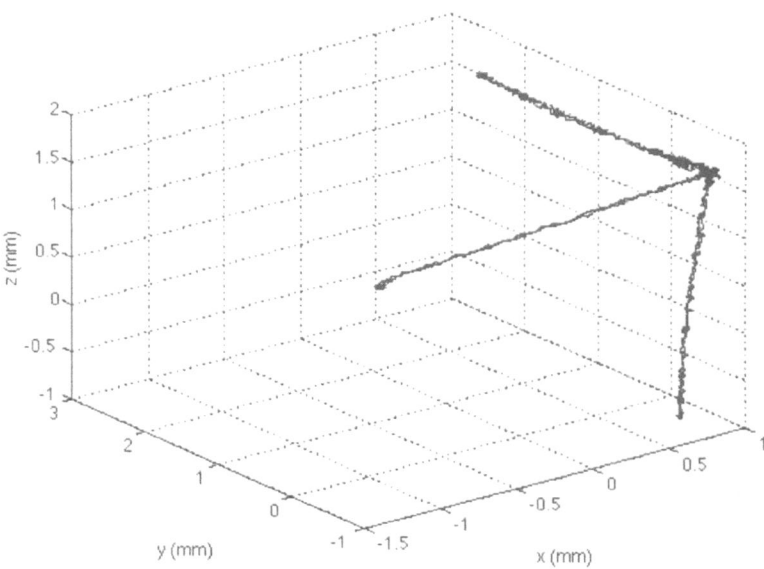

Fig. 3. Tracing of an orthogonal frame with surgical instrument mounted on a manual 3-D linear stage. In the course of the motion, each segment was traced twice (once in each direction).

of accuracy (7 μm rms noise). The goal of the project is accuracy to 1 μm. This goal is expected to be attainable through the use of synchronous detection [15], which is the next step in the development of ASAP, and nonlinear calibration. The characteristic PSD nonlinearity evident in the system can be calibrated out, as the detectors are repeatable to submicron levels [14]. This work is in progress. As noted earlier, drift is already suppressed via AC excitation and coupling. The position detection error in ASAP, after nonlinear calibration, then consists largely of the noise.

Upon attaining the goal of 1 μm accuracy, the system will be used in experimentation to obtain full 3-D quantification of instrument tip motion by vitreoretinal microsurgeons. These studies will lead to better understanding and modeling of involuntary and inadvertent components of the motion, especially non-tremorous components, which are little understood. This information is expected to enable the development of better algorithms and techniques for suppressing or compensating positioning error during microsurgery. In the future, ASAP will be applied also for evaluation of active devices for microsurgical accuracy enhancement, as well as new ergonomic designs for passive instruments.

The ASAP system described here can be duplicated at relatively low cost— less than US$2000, excluding the cost of an IBM-compatible personal computer to operate the system. The system is intended for use in the laboratory, not in the operating room, where optical tracking of the instrument tip is problematic.

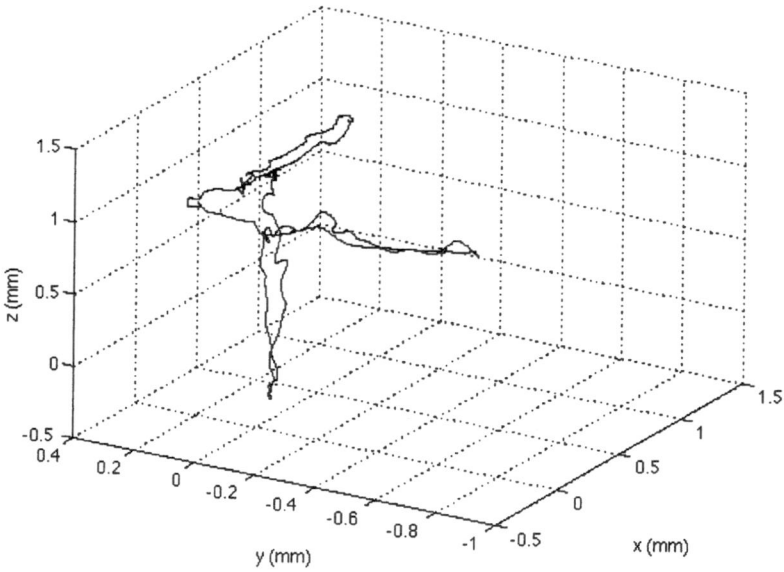

Fig. 4. Freehand tracing of an orthogonal frame. In the course of the motion, each segment was traced twice (once in each direction).

A separate effort in our laboratory involves inertial tracking of intraoperative instrument motion [18].

Plans for future work include not only further improving the accuracy, but also enlarging the workspace to approximately 1 cm³. Reducing the size of the marker ball would increase the workspace somewhat, but would also decrease the signal-to-noise ratio, as its decreased surface area would decrease the incident light to the sensors. Another possibility, conversion to a different PSD with larger active area, is presently being planned. The new PSDs will be from the DL series of UDT Sensors, Inc. (Hawthorne, Ca.), which offers superior linearity [14]. Readjustment of the optics may also be necessary.

5   Conclusion

A laboratory system for three-dimensional non-contact tracking of microsurgical instrument tip position has been developed. Optical tracking of a small reflective ball at the instrument tip is accomplished using two position-sensitive detectors. The system is presently accurate to approximately 7 μm. Development is ongoing toward the goal of 1 μm accuracy. Preliminary results have been presented.

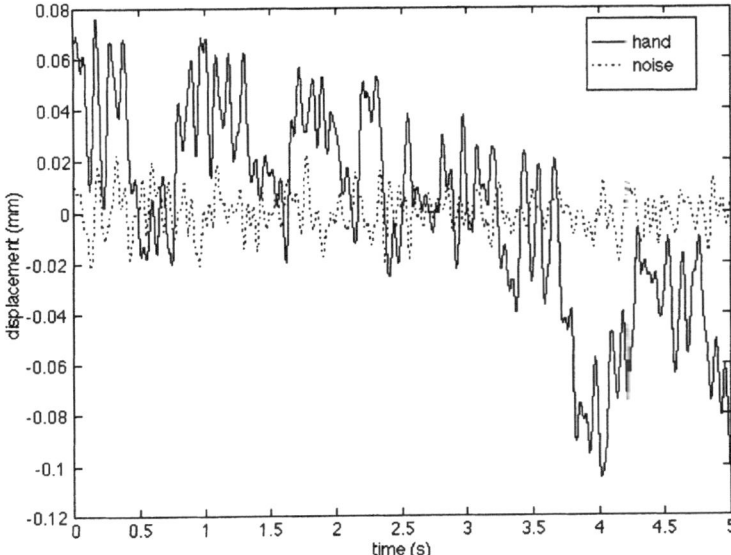

Fig. 5. Sample of data recorded while subject attempted to hold instrument motionless. The solid line depicts the motion in x, a horizontal coordinate. Both physiological tremor and lower-frequency aperiodic erroneous motion are visible. The dotted line presents, for comparison, a sample of the system noise in x taken from a separate recording made moments earlier.

6   Acknowledgments

Funding is provided by the Johnson & Johnson Focused Giving Program. The authors are grateful to Mr. C. Wen for software programming, Drs. M. Siegel and V. Brajovic for advice, Dr. R. Hollis for the use of equipment, and Mr. Jerry Lim for construction of the mannequin.

References

1. Patkin, M.: Ergonomics applied to the practice of microsurgery. *Austr. N. Z. J. Surg.* 47 (1977) 320-239.
2. Riviere, C. N., Rader, R. S., Khosla, P. K.: Characteristics of hand motion of eye surgeons. Proc. 19th Annu. Conf. IEEE Eng. Med. Biol. Soc., Chicago (1997).
3. Charles, S.: Dexterity enhancement for surgery. In: Taylor, R. H., Lavallée, S., Burdea, G. C., Mösges, R. (eds.): *Computer Integrated Surgery: Technology and Clinical Applications.* MIT Press, Cambridge (1996) 467-471.
4. Hunter, I. W., Doukoglou, T. D., Lafontaine, S. R., Charette, P. G., Jones, L. A., Sagar, M. A., Mallinson, G. D., Hunter, P. J.: A teleoperated microsurgical robot and associated virtual environment for eye surgery. *Presence* 2 (1993) 265-280.
5. Schenker, P. S., Barlow, E. C., Boswell, C. D., Das, H., Lee, S., Ohm, T. R., Paljug, E. D., Rodriguez, G., Charles, S. T.: Development of a telemanipulator

for dexterity enhanced microsurgery. Proc. 2nd Intl. Symp. Med. Robot. Comput. Assist. Surg. Wiley, New York (1995) 81-88.

6. Salcudean, S. E., Ku, S., Bell, G.: Performance measurement in scaled teleoperation for microsurgery. In: Troccaz, J., Grimson, E., Mösges, R. (eds.): CVRMed-MRCAS'97. Lecture Notes in Computer Science, Vol. 1205. Springer-Verlag, Berlin Heidelberg New York (1997) 789-798.

7. Mitsuishi, M., Watanabe, H., Nakanishi, H., Kubota, H.: Dexterity enhancement for a tele-micro-surgery system with multiple macro-micro co-located operation point manipulators and understanding of the operator's intention. In: Troccaz, J., Grimson, E., Mösges, R. (eds.): CVRMed-MRCAS'97. Lecture Notes in Computer Science, Vol. 1205. Springer-Verlag, Berlin Heidelberg New York (1997) 821-830.

8. Riviere, C. N., Rader, R. S., Thakor, N. V.: Adaptive canceling of physiological tremor for improved precision in microsurgery. *IEEE Trans. Biomed. Eng.* 45 (1998) 839-846.

9. Simon, D. A. Intra-operative position sensing and tracking devices. In: Troccaz, J., Grimson, E., Mösges, R. (eds.): CVRMed-MRCAS'97. Lecture Notes in Computer Science, Vol. 1205. Springer-Verlag, Berlin Heidelberg New York (1997) 62-64.

10. Simon, D. A., Jaramaz, B., Blackwell, M., Morgan, F., DiGioia, A. M., Kischell, E., Colgan, B., Kanade, T.: Development and validation of a navigational guidance system for acetabular implant placement. In: Troccaz, J., Grimson, E., Mösges, R. (eds.): CVRMed-MRCAS'97. Lecture Notes in Computer Science, Vol. 1205. Springer-Verlag, Berlin Heidelberg New York (1997) 583-592.

11. Tseng, C.-S., Chung, C.-W., Chen, H.-H., Wang, S.-S., Tseng, H.-M.: Development of a robotic navigation system for neurosurgery. In: Westwood, J. D., Hoffman, H. E., Robb, R. A., Stredney, D. (eds.): Medicine Meets Virtual Reality. Studies in Health Technology and Informatics, Vol. 62. IOS Press, Amsterdam (1999) 358-359.

12. Sherman, K. P., Ward, J. W., Wills, D. P. M., Mohsen, A. M. M. A.: A portable virtual environment knee arthroscopy training system with objective scoring. In: Westwood, J. D., Hoffman, H. E., Robb, R. A., Stredney, D. (eds.): Medicine Meets Virtual Reality. Studies in Health Technology and Informatics, Vol. 62. IOS Press, Amsterdam (1999) 335-336.

13. Rader, R. S., Walsh, A. C., Awh, C. C., de Juan, E., Jr.: Manual stability analysis of vitreoretinal microsurgery tasks. *Ergonomics*, in review.

14. Schaefer, P., Williams, R. D., Davis, G. K., Ross, R. A.: Accuracy of position detection using a position-sensitive detector. *IEEE Trans. Instrum. Meas.* 47 (1998) 914-919.

15. Ma, J.: Precision optical coordination sensor for cooperative 2-dof robots. M.S. report, Carnegie Mellon University (1998).

16. Daghighian, H. M.: Optical position sensing with duolateral photoeffect diodes. *Sensors* (Nov. 1994) 35-40.

17. Large-Area Position-Sensitive Detectors datasheet. Hamamatsu Corp., Bridgewater, N. J., USA (1988).

18. Gomez-Blanco, M. A., Riviere, C. N., Khosla, P. K.: Intraoperative tremor monitoring for vitreoretinal microsurgery. Submitted to Medicine Meets Virtual Reality 8 (2000).

On the Feasibility of a Moving Support for Surgery on the Beating Heart

A. L. Trejos[1†], S. E. Salcudean[1‡], F. Sassani[1†], and S. Lichtenstein[2]

[1] Department of Mechanical Engineering [†]/ Department of Electrical Engineering [‡],
University of British Columbia, Vancouver, BC, Canada, V6T 1Z4. tims@ece.ubc.ca
[2] Department of Cardiovascular Surgery, St. Paul's Hospital 1081 Burrard,
Vancouver, BC, V6Z 1Y6

Abstract. In this paper the use of a heart-tracking hand support is proposed to allow coronary artery bypass grafting surgery to take place on the beating heart. Requiring only a three-degree-of-freedom motion platform that tracks a point on the surgical site, this method eliminates the tissue damage associated with the use of physical heart stabilizers and provides a much cheaper alternative to six-degree-of-freedom master-slave systems.

To demonstrate the feasibility of such an approach, a motion platform with a motion range and frequency typical of coronary motion was designed and built. A task typical of suture placement was executed on this platform by twenty six subjects, while (i) the platform was stationary, (ii) the platform was in motion with the subjects' hands attached to it, and (iii) the platform was in motion but the subjects' hands were not attached to it. This system simulates the use of a motion tracking platform with perfect tracking performance. Mono and stereo vision systems were also mounted to the platform to provide subjects with a visually stable view. Accuracy and task completion time were measured.

Relative to the stationary platform case, only a 10% loss of accuracy and 40% increase in completion time were noted when the platform was in motion but the subjects' hands were attached to it. When the hands were not attached, a significantly higher 50% loss of accuracy and 100% increase in task completion time were noted. Task completion time was improved when a visually stable view was also provided, but accuracy results were inconclusive due to problems with the vision systems used.

1 Introduction

Coronary artery bypass grafting (CABG) surgery requires complex grafts on the surface of the heart. While a bloodless anastomotic field can be easily achieved by a temporary coronary occlusion [2], achieving the motionless surgical field required for such delicate work is much more challenging and requires cardiopulmonary bypass with the use of a heart and lung machine. While performing the circulation and filtration of blood that allow the heart to be stopped, such a machine has many damaging effects on the patient's blood, and leads to high surgery costs and long recovery times [1].

Previous studies have been made to allow CABG surgery to be performed on the beating heart. The proposed methods work by stabilizing the surgical area on the surface of the heart, either by pressure on the tissue [3,4] or by attaching an apparatus using suction [5,6]. The use of stabilizers that work by pressure have

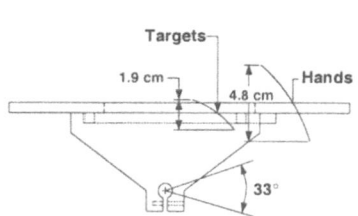

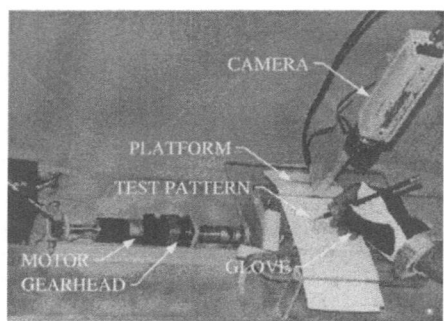

Fig. 1. Platform Motion   **Fig. 2.** Moving Platform

the disadvantage of allowing grafts to be performed only on the top surface of the heart. Stabilizers that work using suction have the disadvantage of damaging the heart tissue, even when used for short periods of time [7].

In principle, the master-slave robotic systems that have been developed to perform minimally invasive heart surgery [9, 10] could be modified to allow tracking of the heart motion by the endoscope and surgical instruments carried by the slave robot. The slave robot motion relative to the surgical site would follow the motion of the master robot, giving the user of the master robot the impression of working on a stationary surgical field. However, such a system would be extremely complicated, and likely would require at least six-degree-of-freedom systems for each of the master and the slave robots.

In this paper, the use of a motion platform that moves the hands of the surgeon in synchrony with the heart motion is proposed for CABG surgery. Such a motion platform would track the position of or the forces on a selected anastomosis site by using optical or mechanical sensors and a feedback control system, and would work in practice if (i) near-zero relative motion could be achieved between the moving platform and the surgical site, and (ii) surgeons could perform delicate tasks such as anastomosis on a moving surgical site as long as their hands are moved with the site.

The objective of this paper is to prove the latter point. Perfect tracking is simulated by having the operator perform a task on the same platform to which the hands are attached. The paper also aims to determine the need for a vision system that provides a stable view of the hands, tools and workspace.

If a system as proposed above did work in practice, it would have the following advantages:

- cardiopulmonary bypass and its damaging effects would be eliminated,
- damaging effects on heart tissue due to stabilization forces would be drastically reduced or eliminated,
- the surgeon's dexterity would be largerly preserved because the tools are manipulated directly without the loss of dexterity imposed by teleoperation,
- low cost relative to teleoperation systems, as only a 3-DOF platform is required, as opposed to 6-DOF master and slave robots for each instrument.

A moving hand support that moves in synchrony with the heart was independently proposed recently in [8], where it was suggested that the heart motion be paced by the platform motion controller. Pacing the heart motion instead of following it can lead to large tracking errors and has clear clinical disadvantages.

Equipment	Brand \Model	Characteristics
Motor	Maxon \RE035-071-34EAB200A	90 Watt DC, Stall Torque 1.1 Nm
Gearhead	Sterling Inst. \ S9117A-PG010	Planetary, Ratio 10:1, single stage
Camera	Philips \VC72505T	Color CCD
Cameras	Pulnix \TM-545	Monocrome CCD, 510 x 492 pixels
Stereo Goggles	Keiser Electro-optics \ VIM 500	Color, 180000 pixels, 4:3 ratio

Table 1. Equipment details

2   Experimental setup

2.1   Moving Platform

To test the ability of a human to perform a task on a moving target while the hands are being moved with it, an experimental platform was built. The motion of the platform roughly imitates the heart motion through an oscillatory rotation around a shaft. Figure 1 shows the vertical displacement in centimeters of the hand and the targets caused by a 33° rotation of the shaft.

The hand of the subject can be attached to the platform by means of a glove fixed to it, so that it tracks the platform. To provide a guide for the task to be performed, a piece of paper having a suture target pattern (see section 2.2) can be inserted and fixed at a desired position. This simulates perfect tracking of the surgical site by the hand, since both the hand and the target are fixed to the moving platform. It is possible to attach one or two cameras to the platform so that the workspace can be seen either on a TV screen (1 camera, mono vision) or on a pair of goggles (2 cameras, stereo vision).

Figure 2 shows a photograph of the platform with one camera mounted on it. Table 1 shows the details of the equipment used in the system.

Figure 3 shows a diagram of the functional components of the system. The desired platform angle was generated by a PC as a pulse width modulated (PWM) signal. This was converted to a reference voltage for a standard PID motor controller loop.

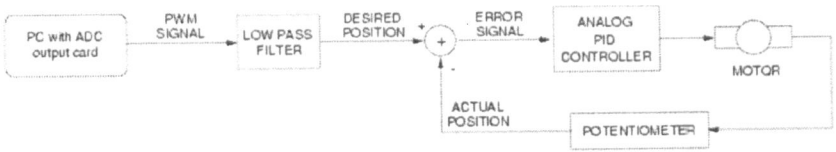

Fig. 3. Functional Components of the System

The original waveform used by the program was determined by measuring the motion of the medial coronary artery of a pig's heart which was then scaled to a human heart [6]. Figure 4 shows a typical plot of the actual motion of the targets as a function of time.

2.2   Task and Test design

The task performed simulates a simple suturing process. It consists of marking with a pen one single dot inside each of the circles of a pattern as seen in Figure

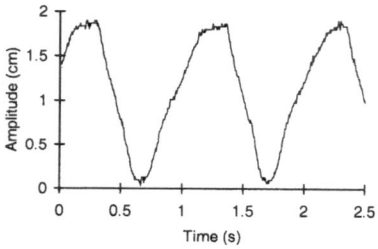

Fig. 4. Typical motion plot

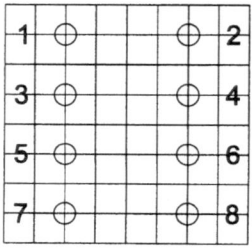

Fig. 5. Test pattern

5, in the order shown by the numbers. The diameters of the circles, the grid spacing and the respective target size assigned for the four different sizes used are shown in Table 2.

Target Size	Diameter (mm)	Grid Spacing (mm)
1	3.43	4.76
2	2.29	3.18
3	1.73	2.38
4	1.14	1.59

Table 2. Test pattern dimensions

A total of seven different tests were performed, as follows:

1. Stationary platform and direct visualization of the workspace. This situation simulates suturing on an arrested heart.
2. Stationary platform and visualization of the workspace on a TV screen. This test was added as a reference to Test 6 below.
3. Stationary platform and visualization of the workspace through stereo goggles. This test was added as a reference to Test 7 below.
4. Platform in motion and no attachment of the hand. This test simulates suturing on the beating heart without any stabilization help.
5. Platform in motion, hand attached to it and direct visualization of the workspace. This test simulates suturing on the surface of the beating heart with the hands being moved to track the surgical site.
6. Platform in motion, hand attached to it and visualization of the workspace on a TV screen. These are the same conditions as in Test 5, with the subjects seeing a stationary two-dimensional image of the surgical site.
7. Platform in motion, hand attached to it and visualization of the workspace through stereo goggles. To provide depth perception, two cameras and a pair of stereo goggles were used to produce a three-dimensional image.

The hand that was attached to the platform during tests 5 to 7 depended on whether the subject was left or right handed.

2.3 Testing

Twenty six subjects were tested, comprised of three cardiac surgeons, one professor and twenty two graduate students. The age of the subjects ranged from

Score	Characterisitcs of the mark
6	A neat dot inside the target
5	A smear inside the target or one neat dot in contact with the circle
4	A smear in contact with the circle
3	A neat dot outside the circle but inside the four quadrants surrounding the target
2	A smear outside the circle but inside the four quadrants surrounding the target
1	A smear or a dot that is outside the four surrounding quadrants

Moving Platform Testing

Subject's Information
Name:
Age:
Sex:
Occupation:

Subject's Evaluation on Moving Platform
After performing each task, score each according to the following scale:
4-Very High 3-High 2-Average 1-Low 0-None

Please feel free to add comments and suggestions. The numbers from one to seven correspond to each of the tests made, which are:
1. Steady platform and direct vision.
2. Steady platform and use of the image from the camera (mono vision).
3. Steady platform and use of the image from the camera (stereo vision).
4. Moving platform and no attachment of the hand.
5. Moving platform, hand attached and direct vision.
6. Moving platform, hand attached and steady image (mono vision).
7. Moving platform, hand attached and steady image (stereo vision).

Discomfort   1 — 2 — 3 — 4 — 5 — 6 — 7 —
Fatigue   1 — 2 — 3 — 4 — 5 — 6 — 7 —
Concentration   1 — 2 — 3 — 4 — 5 — 6 — 7 —
Difficulty   1 — 2 — 3 — 4 — 5 — 6 — 7 —

Comments and suggestions:

Fig. 6. Questionnaire

Table 3. Accuracy scoring scale

22 to 49 years of age. Seven were older than 30 years of age and nineteen were younger. Seven subjects were female and nineteen were male. Two of the subjects were left handed.

Although surgeons perform training exercises similar to the task performed, none of the other subjects had any experience in performing such tasks. For this reason they were allowed to practice as much as they felt was necessary. Each subject was told to perform the task as accurately and quickly as possible, giving greater importance to the accuracy than to the speed. Each of the subjects performed the seven tests in a random order.

After each test, subjects were asked to fill out the subjective questionnaire shown in Fig. 6.

Three of the subjects were asked to perform the test set an additional two times with the goal of determining whether there was a learning process involved when performing the task.

2.4 Quantification of Performance

The two factors measured to judge performance were task completion time and the accuracy and neatness of the mark made with the pen. To measure accuracy the scoring scale shown in Table 3 was used. If two marks were made, the one further away from the target was considered for scoring purposes.

3 Experimental Results

Table 4 shows the measured values for task completion time and accuracy for Test 1. These values are averaged over the 26 subjects. The standard deviations are indicated.

Target Size	Accuracy Score	Completion Time (s)
1	46.6 ± 2.4	6.52 ± 2.6
2	47.2 ± 1.3	6.04 ± 2.0
3	47.3 ± 1.4	6.08 ± 2.1
4	45.5 ± 2.5	6.31 ± 2.2

4	Very High
3	High
2	Average
1	Low
0	None

Table 4. Average results for test 1   **Table 5.** Scoring scale

For each subject, all measured values were normalized with respect to the test where the platform was stable and the same vision system was used. The graphs show the average results obtained by the twenty six subjects. The error bars show the standard deviation of the measurements from the average.

3.1   Results obtained from tests with direct vision

Figures 7 and 8 show the decrease in accuracy and increase in the task completion time, respectively, that result from a moving platform compared to a stationary platform for the four different target sizes (see Table 2). The results show that without the hand support, the accuracy decreases by more than 50% when performing the task on the smallest pattern size. When the hand is attached to the platform this reduction is less than 11%, even for the smallest targets.

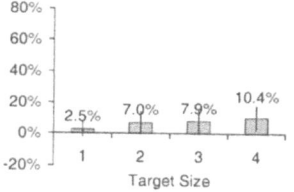
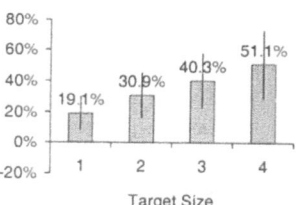

(a) Hand attached   (b) Hand not attached

Fig. 7. Decrease in accuracy

When the hand is attached and the platform is in motion, the average task completion time is increased by around 40% with respect to when the platform is stationary, independent of the target size. This shows a considerable improvement over unattached hand, where the increase in task completion time is doubled.

3.2   Results from the use of different vision systems

Further analysis was made to determine the advantages or disadvantages of using different vision systems to provide a steady image of the workspace. The results are compared to the test with direct vision in Figures 9 and 10.

These graphs show that the accuracy is reduced by approximately 15% for the smallest target using mono vision and 18% using stereo vision. These values

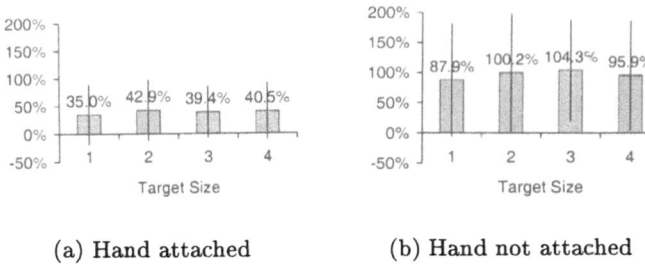

(a) Hand attached   (b) Hand not attached

Fig. 8. Increase in task completion time

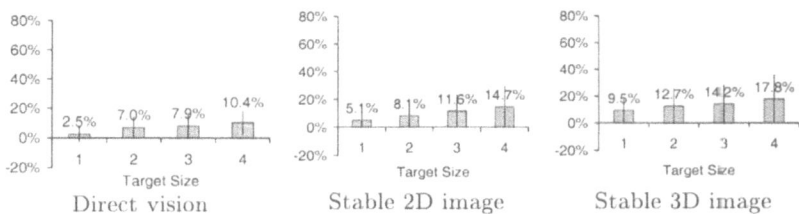

Direct vision   Stable 2D image   Stable 3D image

Fig. 9. Decrease in accuracy when using different vision systems

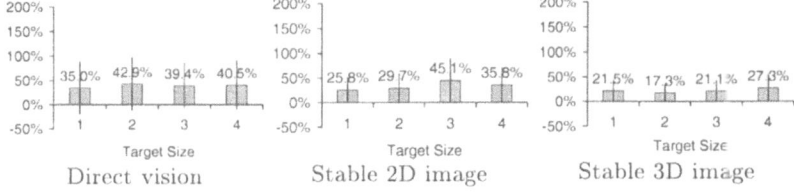

Direct vision   Stable 2D image   Stable 3D image

Fig. 10. Increase in completion time when using different vision systems

are both greater than for direct vision. On the other hand, the stereo vision system produces the least increase in task completion time - less than 30% for all the target sizes.

3.3   Questionnaire Results

The graphs in Figure 11 show the results of the subjective evaluation made by each test subject. The scale used by the subjects for scoring purposes is shown in Table 5. The test number shown corresponds to the list given in Section 2.2.

As can be seen from the graphs, subjects found the test with no hand support and the platform in motion (Test 4) to be the most uncomfortable, fatiguing and difficult one, as well as the one that required the most concentration. When the

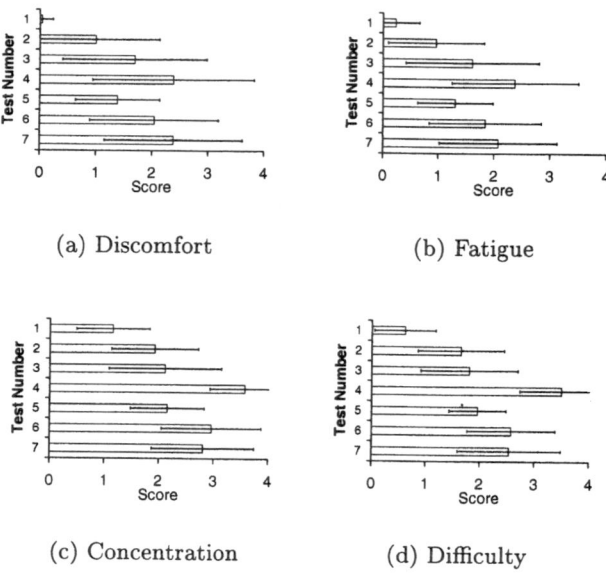

(a) Discomfort   (b) Fatigue

(c) Concentration   (d) Difficulty

Fig. 11. Questionnaire results

platform was stationary, the test with direct vision (Test 1) was perceived to be the easiest and simplest to perform. Looking at the image on the TV screen (Test 2) in 2D or with the goggles (Test 3) in 3D caused the task to be more difficult and to require higher concentration. In addition, the use of the goggles produced the greatest discomfort and fatigue.

These results are consistent with the results obtained when the platform was in motion (Tests 5, 6 and 7), although there is a general increase in all the factors due to the motion.

3.4   Results of the Learning Process

The results obtained when three of the subjects repeated the test two more times show that there is no general tendency for an increase in accuracy or decrease in task completion time for the second or third performances. In some cases there is improvement, but not in all the tests.

4   Discussion

The direct vision results demonstrate that when the hand moves in synchrony with the task space, there is a significant improvement in the accuracy achieved. Using a vision system to provide a steady image of the workspace and the hand did not further improve the accuracy of results; however, there are several factors that have to be taken into account when analyzing these results. The TV screen used in the 2D system is located in front of the subject, causing the workspace to be seen as a vertical surface instead of a horizontal one. In addition, there is lack of depth perception. When using the stereo goggles, although the 3D image provided depth perception, problems arose due to the low resolution of the image (17 pixels across smallest target) and the fact that the image was located at the edge of the depth of field of the camera.

Due to the nature of the surgical task, magnification of the workspace is a necessity. Without the use of a vision system, capable of following the motion of the heart, the surgical area would likely pass out of the field of view of the magnification apparatus. It is believed that if a clear and magnified stereo image is provided, the results obtained could be as good or better than those obtained when looking at the surgical area directly.

When analyzing the results obtained for task completion time, it was noticed that there was a high degree of variability among the subjects, as seen from the large standard deviations shown in the graphs. This variability was noticeable in all of the tests, including those performed when the platform was stationary (Table 4). The main cause of this variability is the random order in which the tests were performed — it was common for subjects to decrease completion time from the first tests to the last. This makes it difficult to obtain conclusive results from the graphs; however, the analysis was made based on the general tendency, showed by the average value obtained from all the subjects.

There was an increase in the task completion time when performing the task with the platform in motion regardless of the vision system used. This increase in time is considered to be much less than that required for the use of the heart and lung machine (approximately 80 minutes); therefore, the approach is still viable.

The increase in task completion time when using the stereo vision system was slightly less than when using the 2D system or direct vision. By offering a stable, 3D image of the workspace, the motion of the platform did not degrade performance as much as with the other vision systems. This agrees with the results of the questionnaire which indicate that the 3D image reduced the concentration requirements and perceived difficulty of the task.

The results from the questionnaire also indicate that there is a need to improve the design of the apparatus. The levels of discomfort, fatigue, concentration and difficulty experienced by the subjects when the platform was in motion can be reduced by a better design of the support and the vision system.

It is worth noting that there is no significant performance improvement to be realized by repeating the tests several times. This is demonstrated by the tests used to evaluate the learning process. Also, the ability to perform the tests was not influenced by surgical skill, as the performance of the three surgeons was very similar to the other, unskilled subjects.

5   Conclusions and Future Work

A new method based on a moving hand and/or tool support that tracks the motion of the heart has been proposed for performing coronary artery bypass grafting surgery on the beating heart. This method involves small or zero forces on cardiac tissue and could provide a low cost alternative to master-slave systems in offering a less invasive surgery, with reduced recovery time and secondary effects.

Twenty six subjects evaluated the feasibility of this approach by executing a task on a moving platform while their hands were attached to it. The situation simulated the use of a motion platform that tracks the surgical site perfectly. The experimental results show that it is possible to perform accurate tasks while the hands are being moved in synchrony with the workspace.

The results obtained when using the moving hand support are clearly improved as compared to those when it was not used. The average accuracy of the tasks was nearly unaffected (more than 90%). Average task completion time was increased by approximately 40%. Although our data show no improvement realized by providing a stationary image, the results could change significantly for the better if a high resolution stereo vision system were used.

The need for a magnified image justifies the need for a vision system that follows the motion of the workspace. The vision system used should provide a stable stereo image with very good resolution and clarity.

Potential improvements to the apparatus include an ergonomically designed support that guides and supports the hand comfortably. Adjustments to allow the tool that is being used to also be attached and moved in synchrony with the heart would be beneficial. The main future work will involve evaluating methods to track the heart motion in real time and designing a mechanism that produces the required platform motion.

Acknowledgments

This study has been supported by the Canadian IRIS/PRECARN Network of Centres of Excellence, Project SAL. Special thanks to Terence Gilhuly for his helpful work and ideas.

References

1. J.W. Kirklin and B.G. Barratt Boyes, *Cardiac Surgery: Morphology Diagnostic Criteria, Natural History, Techniques, Results and Indications*. New York, USA: Churchill-Livingstone Press, 1993.
2. Robert W. Emery, ed., *Techniques for Minimally Invasive Direct Coronary Artery Bypass (MIDCAB) Surgery*. Philadelphia, PA: Hanley and Belfus, Inc., 1997.
3. Piet W. Boonstra, "Local immobilization of the left Anterior Descending Artery for Minimally invasive Coronary Bypass Grafting," *Annals of Thoracic Surgery*, Vol. 63, pp. S76-8, 1997.
4. Guidant CVS Group, "Cardiovascular Products," 1998. http://www.guidant.com/cvs /product/vasoview.html
5. Cornelius Borst, "Coronary Artery Bypass Grafting without Cardiopulmonary Bypass and without interruption of Native Coronary Flow using a novel Anastomosis Site Restraining Device ("Octopus")," *Journal of American College of Cardiology*, vol. 27, no.6, pp. 1356-64, May, 1996.
6. Terence Gilhuly, "Optical and Physical Heart Stabilization for Cardiac Surgery," April, 1998. Master's Thesis, Department of Electrical Engineering, University of British Columbia
7. David C. Youmans, Ethicon Endosurgery. Personal Communication.
8. Paul W. Mayer, "Relative motion canceling platform for surgery," Feb. 15, 1999. U.S. Patent No. 5871017.
9. Computer Motion "Robotic Surgical System Enabling Minimally Invasive Microsurgery," 1998. http://www.computermotion.com/old/zeus.htm.
10. Tala Skari "The Cutting Edge: Heart surgery enters the age of robotics," *Life*, Special Issue, pp. 14–23, Fall, 1998.

A Testbed System for Robotically Assisted Percutaneous Pattern Therapy

Andrew Bzostek[1], Aaron C. Barnes[2], Rajesh Kumar[1], James H. Anderson[3], Russell H. Taylor[1]

[1] Department of Computer Science, The Johns Hopkins University
[2] Department of Mechanical Engineering, The Johns Hopkins University
[3] Department of Radiology, The Johns Hopkins University

Abstract. This paper presents a second generation prototype image-guided robotic system for percutaneous delivery of surgical devices and therapeutic agents, with potential applications in the treatment of liver cancer and other malignancies. The system is intended to deliver these devices and therapies more consistently and accurately than a physician can achieve freehand. This capability will permit the treatment of smaller lesions, will enable the physician to better achieve optimized patterns of therapy distribution, and will allow for more rapid re-targeting for multiple lesions. The system will allow treatment of patients for whom surgery is contraindicated and could potentially replace major surgery, reducing patient morbidity and mortality, as well as the cost of treatment. The new prototype system uses new, modular hardware and software components, which improve its accuracy, usability, and flexibility as compared to the first generation prototype. Techniques for image processing, both in 2D and 3D images, planning, and fiducial registration have also been developed. *In vitro*, the system achieves submillimetric accuracy in the placement of simulated treatment devices from a preoperative plan generated from 3D imagery. Some initial *in vivo* considerations have also been addressed, and work is ongoing in this area.

1 Introduction

Providing therapy in a minimally invasive manner can afford significant improvement to traditional surgery for a variety of procedures, and in many cases such techniques are already accepted as the preferred form of treatment.

With an estimated 500,000 to 1 million new hepatocellular carcinoma (HCC) cases annually, liver cancer is, globally, one of the most common malignancies [1]. Though approximately 16 thousand new cases of liver and biliary passage cancer are diagnosed each year in the US [2], with increasing hepatitis incidence in this country, the incidence of HCC is expected to increase significantly.

Developing minimally invasive treatments for liver malignancies has attracted significant interest. Such treatments seek both to reduce the invasiveness associated with lesion resection, and to provide treatment in cases for which surgical resection is not indicated. Surgical resection is associated with some patient morbidity and mortality, but it remains the standard for treatment of both primary and metastatic hepatic tumors.

However, even for patients for whom disease is confined to the liver, surgery is often not an option, because of an inoperable lesion location, associated co-morbid conditions, or the lack of sufficient hepatic parenchyma reserve to tolerate a major resection.

Percutaneous treatment modalities offer local control and potential prolongation in survival for patients with liver tumors, while reducing the risk associated with standard liver resection [3]. Methods under investigation include ethanol injections [4], cryotherapy [5], radiofrequency ablation [6,7], interstitial radiation [8], and laser hyperthermia [9]. Using real-time ultrasound or fluoroscopy for guidance, these therapies are typically delivered freehand. It is often difficult to approach small lesions (< 2 cm), specific tumor regions are difficult to target, and larger lesions often require multiple applications to a given tumor. The clinical value of these therapeutic approaches could be significantly improved with the ability to deliver these therapies more precisely in a planned pattern.

We are currently developing a system that will assist in the percutaneous placement of treatment patterns [10],[11],[12],[13],[14]. The system utilizes preoperative 3D imaging (CT or MRI) for planning and uses intraoperative, real-time fluoroscopy to guide a robotic system to align and deliver therapy to target locations. The ability to consistently place a therapy pattern with high accuracy will not only improve currently available treatments, but will also foster the development of new therapies which rely on it.

This paper presents this system and preclinical validation results. The rest of the introduction will discuss previous work and our target clinical procedure. In Section 2, we will present the hardware and software components of the new prototype system. Section 3 presents the results from a series of validation experiments, including an in vitro, end-to-end assessment. The paper will conclude with a discussion of the implications of these results as well as our path for future work.

1.1   Previous Work

There has been some previous work dedicated to image-guided needle placement in soft tissue. Some of these systems rely on the fixed relationship between the treatment delivery system and the image, e.g. [15], and some, e.g. [16],[17] use only a passive positioning aid. One previous system, the Picker PinPoint does address problem of pattern placement, but this system uses a passive manipulator fixed in a known way to a single, proprietary imaging system. We believe that use of an active positioning device imparts significant benefits, including higher accuracy, repeatability and speed of alignment, that justify a more complex system. Additionally, not having to rely upon *a priori* knowledge of imager to positioning device fixation makes the system significantly more flexible, both in terms of reachable anatomical targets, and the choice of guidance imaging modality.

1.2   The Target Procedure

We are investigating a broad range of percutaneous scenarios, but in order to focus our discussion, have defined a reference procedure, which has been described more fully in [11]. For the discussion here, suffice it to say that fiducials, hand implanted prior to 3D planning imagery, serve as guides for target registration under intraoperative, biplanar fluoroscopy. Also, for each planned treatment insertion, reregistration, alignment, needle insertion, treatment deposition, and needle removal must be completed within a single breath-hold (~20 sec)

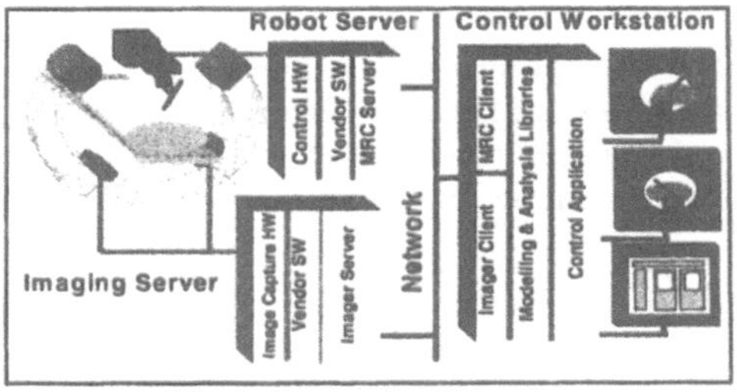

2 Methods

Fig. 1. System Architecture

2.1 Hardware

As discussed in previous papers [10],[11], previous tests were conducted using a LARS surgical robot developed at IBM research and a treatment insertion device.

The current prototype system uses an XYZ translation platform and a simulated treatment injector from the Hopkins Modular Robotic Family. The current robot is positioned via a cart-mounted U-frame and 3 passive, lockable degrees of freedom. This configuration allows it to reach into the field of view (FOV) of the intraoperative imaging system without impeding patient positioning, restricting its work volume or interfering with the collected images.

We have constructed a second-generation injector for our automatic injection system described in [11]. This injector is designed to overcome the first-generation injector's shortcomings, including a relatively violent release mechanism and asymmetric intravenous point needle, both of which contributed to significant simulated therapy seed shift upon release. The improved injector utilizes a computer controlled release mechanism. This release mechanism allows adjustment for varying therapy size and verification of therapy release. The simulated therapy consists of a 0.5" length of 13-gauge stainless steel hypodermic tubing. held via a diamond tipped trocar matched to the inner diameter of the tubing. The therapy rod is released from the injector by withdrawing the trocar from within the tubing.

Intraoperative computational capabilities are provided by a group of workstations connected by a local area network. Currently, only two workstations are used, one of which provides robot control and the other which both captures images and provides a user interface and application level control.

2.2 Software

The new prototype robotic system is controlled through the Modular Robot Control (MRC) Library developed at JHU, which provides Cartesian level control. Image capture and processing are done via a image control library written on top of Matrox Imaging's MIL library

The basic imager calibration and robot registration techniques used have been presented elsewhere [11]. In previous experiments, a mean image-guided placement accuracy of 0.43 mm [14] and intra-operative plan-based pattern placement with an accuracy of 0.52 mm [11]. In order to allow the system to accurately create, register, and execute planned patterns created from preoperative 3D imaging, several new algorithms have been developed.

Bead Image Processing. Fundamental to the accuracy of the system is its ability to find the centers of spherical fiducial markers, both in tomographic and projective imaging. In order to maximize the system's accuracy, we have developed two novel techniques which improve the accuracy of these measurements.

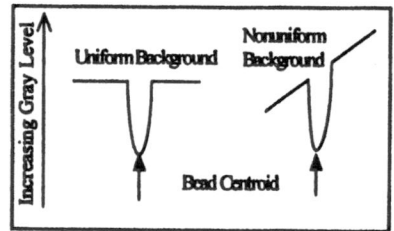

Projective Fluoroscopic Imagery. The most basic technique for finding the projection of the center of a bead in a fluoroscopic images is weighted centroid determination. Two problems arise, though, when the bead of interest is projected over a region of non-uniform density. First, it can be quite difficult to identify seeds automatically, second (see **Figure 2**) such a region will skew the determination of the center downward along the gray level gradient. For small, dense spheres, this is only a small problem, however, when using the larger, less radioopaque markers, the calculated centers are often skewed by several pixels. In order to remove this affect, we have developed a novel technique, which processes a single image to remove most of the background influence.

Given a log image of a fiducial, our technique uses pixels in an annular neighborhood at a distance r from the pixel of interest to calculate the direction of the gradient, then corrects the pixel's value by subtracting the average value of pixels at distance r in the direction perpendicular to the calculated gradient. The technique can be applied efficiently, for small r, over entire images, and can thus be used prior to any bead localization. The first step is to calculate the estimated gradient vector $\mathbf{V}$:

$$\mathbf{V} = \sum_{d \in S}\left[\left[I(t+d) - I(t-d)\right]\frac{\mathbf{d}}{|\mathbf{d}|} \right]$$

where t is the target pixel, $\mathbf{d}$ is a displacement selected from the set S of all integral vectors in the annular neighborhood and $I(\mathbf{p})$ is the image intensity at position $\mathbf{p}$. Once $\mathbf{V}$ is calculated, calculating $I'(t)$, the corrected intensity, is simply:

$$I'(t) = I(t) - \frac{I\left(t - r\hat{\mathbf{v}}_\perp\right) + I\left(t + r\hat{\mathbf{v}}_\perp\right)}{2}$$

where r is the average annular radius, $\hat{\mathbf{v}}_\perp$ is the unit vector in the direction perpendicular to $\mathbf{V}$, and I of a non-integral position is the linear interpolation from the position's four integral neighbors.

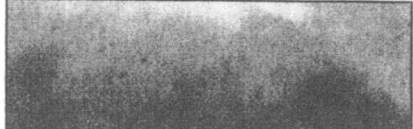

Fig. 3. Beads implanted in a porcine liver. The right image shows the results of applying the linear gradient correction with a radius of 3 pixels followed by a 3x3 gaussian smoothing operation to the left image, a raw fluoroscopic image after a log correction to linearize its density response.

This correction is calculated identically for all pixels within the region of interest, thus r is set to twice the radius of the beads we are interested in finding. This technique not only allows for the accurate calculation of projected bead centers [see section 3 for results], but is also quite useful for separating out beads in a complex image (see fig. 3).

Volumetric Images. Our system also relies upon the accurate localization of the fiducial beads in the 3D preoperative planning image. This is particularly important in the interslice direction (Z), where the resolution can be as small as 1/10 that in the two intraslice directions When faced with similar problems, Hanson, et al [18] and Lewis et al[19,20] chose to use fiducials which are large and implanted in bone, while Ellis et al[21] utilizes details of the slice geometry in CT scanners to localize small, very dense tantalum spheres, which, while nicely visible on fluoroscopic imagery, cause artifacts in CT.

Currently, we are working with 1/8" Aluminum Oxide fiducials. The material was chosen, both for its biocompatibility and its balance of contrast in fluoroscopy and lack of artifacts in CT. Unfortunately, many clinical CT scans have an interslice distance of 3mm, just smaller than the bead diameter. This leads to a inaccuracies when using the standard weighted centroid calculation for determining the bead center in the Z direction. To solve this problem, we have derived a method which uses the known geometry of the fiducial to allow us to much more accurately find its center in this direction.

Given a sphere of radius r centered at the origin, the area A of a slice at signed distance $| d | <= r$ from the center is given by: $A = \pi s^2 = \pi(r^2 - d^2)$, (figure 4) where s is the radius of the circular slice. Such a slice divides the sphere into two regions. Without loss of generality, we can assume that the normal to the slice is along the z direction and that it is displaced in the positive z direction. Thus the volume of smaller of the two regions is:

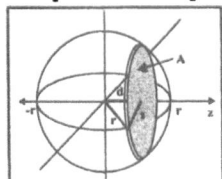

Fig 4. Slicing a sphere

$$V_1 = \int_d^r A(z)\,dz$$

$$= \frac{2}{3}\pi r^3 - \pi d \left[r^2 - d^2 / 3 \right]$$

and the volume of the larger region is $V_2 = \frac{2}{3}\pi r^3 + \pi d \left[r^2 - d^2 / 3 \right]$. The sum and difference are:

$$V_{SUM} = \frac{4}{3}\pi r^3$$

$$V_{DIFF} = 2\pi d \left[r^2 - d^2 / 3 \right]$$

For a sphere with uniform density δ, these can be converted to masses simply by multiplying each by this δ. This factor, though, can be removed by taking the ratio of the two values:

$$R_V = \frac{V_{DIFF}}{V_{SUM}} = \frac{3}{2}\left[\frac{d}{r} - \frac{1}{3}\frac{d^3}{r^3} \right]$$

Given a known radius and a measurement of the mass on each side of the cut, we would like to solve for the offset of this cut. Solving for a cubic equation in d, we get:

$$d^3 - 3r^2 d + 2r^3 R_V = 0$$

where r is known and R_v is measured. Since the zeros of the derivative with respect to d, $3d^2 - 3r^2$, occur when $|d| = r$, and we've assumed that $|d| <= r$, we only need to solve for the central root, which will be real. In fact, since this region of the equation is monotonic, we can use a binary search to find an arbitrarily accurate estimate for d in time proportional to the log of the inverse of the size of the desired maximum error.

In a tomographic image set where the slice spacing is equal to the slice thickness, we can take the two sliced volumes as the portions of the sphere on either side of a voxel (slice in the Z direction) boundary, and d is the boundary's distance to the sphere's center. In order to find a value proportional to the total mass on each side, the partial mass of sphere within each voxel is esimated using an approximate density value for the background, which can be estimated for the neighborhood of the sphere. Once d is calculated, the sphere's center position in the direction perpendicular to the cut is simply the cut's position plus d. This technique shows promise for the precise, slice spacing-independent calculation of the fiducials' centers. (see section 3.4 for results)

Planning. We have developed a system for planning the arbitrary path brachytherpies that our prototype can implement. This system uses user input to select an approach direction, then projects the problem into 2D, where it is solved using a modified gradient descent method. The target points are then projected back into lines, whose depth and length are calculated to cover the target. While this is only an initial prototype planner and still requires significant verification, it provides a useful platform for testing the rest of the system.

Pattern Registration. Given 3D positions for fiducials in two spaces, we now need to: 1. find the correct pairing of these positions, and 2, find the best fit transformation between them. Unfortunately, the intraoperative set may either be incomplete-- containing points not matched in the preoperative one, or may have deformed. In order to make the specified problem solvable, we will assume that there is a known upper bound on the displacement the non-rigid deformation causes from the best fit rigidly transformed location, and that the fiducials are at least twice this far apart. These assumptions are not unreasonable, given the spacing of the fiducials (~1-2 cm) as compared to the level of non-rigid motion we've observed in fiducials within the same lobe of a porcine liver (up to ~3mm).

Our algorithm iteratively solves for both the matching and transformation, first matching an arbitrary triple of points, then iteratively pairing the remaining best fit pairs and updating the transformation. If the matching is unsatisfactory, then a different initial set of three beads from set 1 are chosen and the procedure repeated. If m, the number unmatched beads in set 1 is less than 1/3 the number of beads in the set, this will take at most m attempts. Each application of this algorithm takes, worst case, time proportional to n^5, though in practice it is generally much smaller because there tend to be very few candidate matches for the 2nd and 3rd points in the initial pairing, given a match for the 1st.

Once the matching and best-fit transformation has been established, small perturbations in the intraoperative fiducial positions are easily handled. This process has been automated and takes less than a second on inexpensive computational hardware.

Phantom Construction. We constructed *in vitro* phantoms for each of our experiments. These phantoms consisted approximately cylindrical plastic containers, approximately 4 inches in diameter, and approximately 4 inches tall. These containers were filled with agarose gel at 1.3% concentration. Tumor phantoms were created by creating a smaller cylinder of 1.3% agarose with a suspended Barium solution. Fiducials were 1/8" radius Aluminum Oxide spheres.

3   Experimental Results

Table 1. Results from *in-vivo* bead motion study

Comparison	Condition	N (beads)	Avg Error (mm)	Max Error (mm)
Within Sessions	Different Poses	336	0.75	1.59
	Same Pose	100	0.40	0.87
Between Sessions	Different Poses	40	1.11	2.12
	Same Pose	7	1.15	2.18

3.1   Bead Stability/ Deformation

Bead stability and non-rigid deformation are a concern, so we have conducted studies to gain a better appreciation of the motion which *in vivo* implanted beads will undergo. Two in-vivo experiments were conducted in which a set of beads were implanted manually and imaged in several poses, in two sessions separated by several days. The results in table 1 represent residual errors in bead location prediction after using a thin-plate spline based on a sub-set of the fiducials to correct for their deformation. Table 1 summarizes the results from the first study.

The second study yielded some interesting, if less quantitative results. For this study, a small set of beads were implanted within a lobe different from the primary insertion site, and within the primary lobe, some fiducials were implanted more superficially than others. Insufficient beads were available to do a good TPS correction, but within a group of fiducials implanted within the interior of the primary lobe, deformative motion was small (approx. 1mm without correction). Beads implanted more superficially showed more significant deformation (approx. 3 mm max without correction), and beads implanted in different lobes showed quite significant deformation (5-10 mm max).

3.2   Bead Localization in Fluoroscopic Images

While our background subtraction has significantly improved the general automaticity of our application (and thus time to realign), we also wanted to quantify the improvement in bead center finding achieved by the algorithm. To do so, we imaged a phantom with 7 fiducials implanted. Their centers were determined using the 3D weighted-centroid method, from a 3mmx3mm CT scan, then from a pair of fluoroscopic images using weighted centroid, both before and after background correction w/ an $r=7$. The sub-pixel centroids differed by an average of 1.58 pixels (~.3mm), though it should be noted that without background correction, care had to be taken to select seed points which actually corresponded to the centers of beads, while after background correction, these seeds could be determined semi-automatically. The 3D point sets were then registered to the set calculated from CT. The set without background correction showed a residual error of 1.68 mm, while the set after correction showed a residual error of 1.2 mm, demonstrating that most of the error represented by the difference in the image positioning occurred in the centers found prior to the background correction

3.3   CT Plan Placement

In order to quantify the end-to-end accuracy of our system, in vitro, we conducted a study in which a tumor phantom was suspended in undoped agarose gel. 7 fiducials were implanted by hand surrounding the tumor model A 3mmx3mm CT scan was collected, and a plan was created based on this scan. At that time, the fiducials were localized using only the standard weighted centroid method. The plan called for 9 rods to be inserted. After random

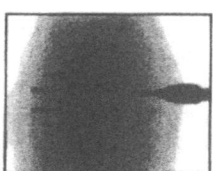

Fig. 6. Fluoroscopic image of implantation

initialization, the plan converged in 32 iterations to an approximately circular pattern, with one treatment placed at the center of the tumor. The experiment then moved to a biplanar fluoroscopic suite. After calibrating the imagers (avg residual error in fiducials = 0.49 & 0.37 pixels) and registering the robot (placement error (n=8) (mm): mean = 0.314, max = 0.489, std dev = 0.194), the phantom was placed in the working volume and imaged. The fiducials were isolated and a registration performed. [mean error = 1.35 mm]. Using the robot, the simulated treatment rods were inserted. Between each insertion, the phantom was moved away from its starting position, replaced approximately, and the fiducial positions relocalized automatically [mean residual = 1.28 mm, time < 1sec]. After all of the rods were implanted, fluoroscopic images were taken to measure the position of the implanted rods. The fiducial locations in this image were registered to the CT-based positions (mean residual = 1.20 mm), and this transformation applied to the bottom positions of the treatment rods. After removing known systematic displacements, their positions showed an average error of 0.765 mm, max of 1.38 mm, and a standard deviation of 0.339 mm.

3.4   CT Bead Localization

To verify the accuracy of our 3D bead center calculation, a phantom containing 8 fiducials was created. Two 3mm x 3mm CT scans of the phantom were collected, with the phantom rotated by approximately 90 degrees between scans. In each of the scans, the position of each of the fiducials was calculated using both a weighted centroid and our sliced-sphere technique. We then registered the point sets created by the different techniques within and between images (see table 2)

Table 2. RMS Error (mm) when registering fiducials. Comparison between techniques and images (WC = Weighted Centroid, SS = Sliced-Sphere)

		Volume 1		Volume 2	
		WC	SS	WC	SS
Volume 1	WC	--	0.547	0.731	0.601
	SS	0.547	--	0.600	0.271
Volume 2	WC	0.731	0.600	--	0.560
	SS	0.601	0.270	0.560	--

Our sliced-sphere technique shows almost a 3-fold improvement in RMS error when compared to the weighted centroid technique (.27mm vs ..73.mm) Even more importantly, it shows significantly less directional bias than those from the weighted centroid method, by comparing errors in the relative Z directions when registering point sets from both different images and different techniques (.55 mm vs .22mm).

4   Discussion

Though some work remains in validating the improved accuracy cf the sliced-sphere fiducial localization technique, the system has demonstrated more than adequate baseline performance *in vitro* Many obstacles remain in the creation of a clinically viable system, including work on the injector end effector, planning system, and overall system robustness. From an engineering standpoint, however, the primary challenge that remains is to translate good *in vitro* performance into an *in vivo* setting. The primary obstacle to this goal is the deformation of the soft tissue targets. This deformation occurs both because of natural motion of the organ, and, intraoperatively, due to the insertion of the implantation needle. We have demonstrated that even a naïve non-rigid deformation model can account relatively well for the first source. Deformation due to needle insertion is a much greater challenge. We are currently pursuing work to use force measurements in conjunction with our imaging capabilities to characterize and hopefully, minimize and correct for, this kind of non-rigid motion.

5   Conclusions

In this paper, we have presented a prototype system for the precise and accurate percutaneous placement of patterns of therapy, with application to the treatment liver cancer as well as other malignancies. It uses an automated alignment and injection system which allows for the consistent, rapid alignment which is highly advantageous in this environment. We have presented image processing and fiducial registration techniques which have allowed us to build such a system. In particular, we have demonstrated a novel analytic geometry-based fiducial localization technique which offers almost a 3-fold improvement in RMS residual error when compared to the current standard. Most significantly, we have demonstrated a high level of end-to-end system accuracy in non-deforming in-vitro models, with a mean placement error of 0.75 mm.

6   Acknowledgements

The authors would like to acknowledge the work of Steve Schreiner in the development of the first generation prototype system. The research reported in this paper was supported in part by NSF/Whitaker Foundation for Cost Reducing Health Care Technology Grant #5T32HL07712, in part by NSF Grant #EEC9731478, in part by NSF equipment grant #CDA-9529509 and in part by Johns Hopkins University internal funds.

References

1. J. R. Wands and H. E. Blum, "Primary Hepatocellular Carcinoma," *The New England Journal of Medicine,* vol. 325, pp. 729-731, 1991.

2. C. C. Boring, et al., Cancer Statistics, 1994," *Cancer Journal for Clinicians*, vol. 44, pp. 7-26,1994.

3. P. D. Schneider and J. P. McGahan, "Percutaneous Approaches to Liver Neoplasms," in *Minimally Invasive Surgery*, J. G. Hunter and I. Sackier, Eds. New York: McGraw Hill, 1993, pp. 255-263.

4. T. Levraghi, A Salmi, and L Bolondi, 'Small hepatocellular carcinoma: percutaneous alcohol injection - results in 23 patients," *Radiology*, vol. 168, pp. 1313-1317,1988.

5. T. S. Ravikumar, "The Role of cryotherapy in the management of patients with liver tumors", *Adv Surg* 30:281-291, 1996.

6. A. E. Siperstein, S. J. Rogers, P. D. Hansen, A. Gitomirsky, "Laparoscopic thermal ablation of hepatic neuroendocrine tumor metastases," *Surgery* 122:6, 1146-1155, Dec 1997.

7. J. McGahan, P. Browning, and J. Brock, 'Hepatic ablation using radiofrequency electrocautery," *Investigational Radiology*, vol. 25, pp. 267-270,1990.

8. R. Holt, R. Naunta, and T. Lee, "Intraoperative interstitial radiation therapy for hepatic metastases from colorectal carcinomas," *Amer. J. of surgery*, vol. 54, pp. 231-233,1988.

9. J. Hahl, R. Haapiainen, and J. Ovaska, "Laser-induced hyperthermia in the treatment of liver tumors," *Lasers Surg Med*, vol. 10, pp. 319-321, 1990.

10. J. H. Anderson, et al., "Image-Guided Percutaneous Robotic Assisted Therapy,' presented at Annual Fall Meeting of the Biomedical Engineering Society, The Pennsylvania State University, 1996.

11. S. Schreiner, J. H. Anderson, R. H. Taylor, J. Funda, A. Bzostek, A. C. Barnes, "A System for Percutaneous Delivery of Treatment with a Fluoroscopically Guided Robot," *Proceedings of the First Joint Conference of CVRMed-MRCAS*, pp 747-756, Grenoble, France, 1997.

12. S. Schreiner, J. Funda, A. C. Barnes, and J. H. Anderson , "Accuracy Assessment of a Clinical Biplane Fluoroscope for Three-Dimensional Measurements and Targeting," presented at SPIE Conference on Medical Imaging, Newport Beach, CA, 1997.

13. A. Bzostek, S. Schreiner, A. C. Barnes, J. A. Cadeddu, W. W. Roberts, J. H. Anderson, R. H. Taylor, L. Kavoussi, "An Automated System for Precise Percutaneous Access of the Renal Collecting System", *Proceeding of The First Joint Conference of CVRMed-MRC.AS*, Grenoble, France, 1997.

14. S. Schreiner, et al., "Accuracy Assessment of a clinical biplane fluoroscope for three-dimensional measurements and targeting," presented at SPIE Conference on Medical Imaging, Newport Beach, CA, 1997.

15. F. Burbank, S. H. Parker, "Stereotactic Core Breast Biopsy," *Surgical Technology International II*, pp. 179-186, 1993.

16. P. Potamianos, B. L. Davies, and R. D. Hibberd, "Manipulator Assisted Renal Treatment," *Proc. ARA/IFR Int. Conf. Robots for Competitive Industries*, Brisbane, Australia, pp. 214-227, 1993.

17. P. Potamianos, B.L Davies, and R.D. Hibbard, "Intra-operative Registration for Percutaneous Surgery," Proceedings of the 2nd Annual Symposium on MRCAS, Baltimore, MD, pp. 156 - 164, 1995.

18. W. H. Hanson, H. A. Paul, B. Williamson, and B.D. Mittelstadt, "Orthodoc: A computer system for presurgical planning." *Proceedings of the 12th IEEE Medicine and Biology Conference*, 12: pp 1931-1932, Philadelphia, 1990.

19. J. T. Lewis, R. L. Lewis Jr., S. Schreiner, "An ultrasonic approach to localization of fidcial markers for interactive, image-guided neurosurgery part I: principles," *IEEE Transoactions on Biomedical Engineering*. v. 45 n. 5, pp 620-630, May 1998.

20. S. Schreiner, R. L. Galloway Jr., J. T. Lewis, : "An ultrasonic approach to localization of fidcial markers for interactive, image-guided neurosurgery part II: implementation and automation," *IEEE Transoactions on Biomedical Engineering*. v. 45 n. 5, pp 631-641, May 1998.

21. R. E. Ellis, S. Toksvig-Larsen, M. Marcacci, "Use of a Biocompatible fiducial marker in evaluating the accuracy of computer tomography image registration," *Investigative Radiology*, v. 31, n. 10, pp 658-667, Oct 1996.

Performance of Robotic Augmentation in Microsurgery-Scale Motions

Rajesh Kumar[1], Tushar M. Goradia[3], Aaron C. Barnes[2], Patrick Jensen[5], Louis L. Whitcomb[2], Dan Stoianovici[2,4], Ludwig M. Auer[6], Russell H. Taylor[1]

[1]Department of Computer Science
[2]Department of Mechanical Engineering
[3]Department of Neurosurgery
[4]Department of Urology
[5]Microsurgery Advance Design Laboratory
Johns Hopkins University, Baltimore, Maryland, USA,
[6]Institute of Applied Sciences in Medicine (ISM-Austria)

Abstract. This paper is part of the development process of a microsurgical "cooperating" assistant. To evaluate its applicability to augment fine surgical motions, we test precision and operator perception in simple microsurgical scale pick and place motions. Such motions are common in microsurgical procedures(e.g. micro-vascular anastomosis). The experiments test the users' ability to position a common surgical tool to 250, 200 and 150 micrometer accuracy. These experiments were performed using two test platforms. The new "steady hand" robot designed for microsurgery and the LARS robot (a laparoscopic camera holding robot) adapted for this purpose. Comparative results for several parameters including time, success rate, error rate, number of attempts are included. Comparison of performance of the two robots for these tasks is also included. The results support our claim that the new "steady hand" robot augments human performance for microsurgery-scale motion

1   Introduction

For the purpose of microsurgical applications, cooperative control systems promise significant advantages. A "steady hand" robot (e.g. [1]) can provide guidance, and enforce safety constraints. It can also use compliance models taking into account procedure-specific issues such as tissue properties and thereby provide tactile sensing for the human surgeon. A cooperative control system has the advantage of integrating safety and information integration into the procedure without taking away control from the human surgeon. This allows the surgeon's superior intelligence and experience to be used with greater precision and safety than before.

A first step towards cooperating could be tremor reduction with a stiff robot. If such a system only is used to position surgical tools at the surgical site, the performance of the system would depend upon the performance of the robot and ease of use We discuss use of tremor reduction to increase accuracy of pick-and-place motions at the limits of human motor motion. These motions are required e.g. for micro-vascular surgery when small blood vessels are anastomosed. The task of anastomosis often involves the use of a very fine suture which is attached to a correspondingly small needle. The needle guides the suture material in and out of the vessel wall as the ends of the blood vessels are physically conjoined. Binocular magnification provides clear detail of the vessels and sutures but has little effect on the natural tremor of the surgeon. When the size of these tasks approaches the limit of human dexterity(10s of micrometers), tremor-reducing devices may provide benefit.

1.1 Previous Work

Lengthy procedures that require fine resolution motions are good candidates for robotic assistance ([2],[3],[4]). Other minimally invasive tasks ([5],[6]) limit visual and proprioceptive feedback. Automation has already been applied in several procedures ([7],[8]) in neurosurgery. Other microsurgical fields have also seen increasing use of computer and imaging technology. Troccaz ([9]) designed a system that used a passive robotic arm to provide guidance with dynamic constraints. ACROBOT (Davies, [10]), Cobots (Peshkin, [11]) are other examples of synergistic systems. Active tremor cancellation ([12]), an alternative to passive compensation is also being investigated. Analysis and representation of tactile properties of tissues ([13]) and development of better tactile guidance systems are also current topics of research ([14]). Use of force and tactile feedback for guidance in simulators ([15]) and real robotic systems ([16],[17],[18]) has also been published previously. Master-slave systems have been previously designed for use in microsurgical procedures ([19],[20]) and evaluated ([21],[22]). Human performance issues in these surgical procedures have also been studied ([23],[24]). Most performance evaluation studies of microsurgical tasks use time of completion as a major indicator ([25],[26],[27]). Simulators have also been used to compare/assess surgical skill ([28]). Since complex microsurgical tasks are difficult to quantify automated performance comparisons in the past have used visual inspection by the experimenter (e.g. [22]) or an observer. Authors have also previously looked at comparative performance issues ([29]).

2 Methods and Materials

2.1 Hardware

We use the new "steady hand" robot ([1]) as the first platform for these experiments. Designed for microsurgical applications this is a 7-degree-of-freedom manipulator. It has 3 XYZ translation stages at the base for coarse positioning, two rotational degrees of freedom at the shoulder (the RCM linkage, [30],[31]), an instrument insertion and an instrument rotation stage. The instrument rotation stage was not used for this experiment. A force sensor (ATI Industrial Automation Inc.) is built in the end-effector. This force-sensor can be used to make the robot move in compliance to forces applied at the end-effector. This robot has a remote center of motion. It has an overall positional accuracy of 10s of microns. It is a stiff and slow robot.

The second platform for these experiments was a LARS robot([32]). Designed for camera holding applications in laparoscopic surgery, LARS is a 7 degree-of-freedom manipulator. It has three translation stages at the base, two rotational degrees of freedom at the shoulder, an instrument insertion stage and an instrument rotation stage. LARS also has a force sensor built in the end-effector. LARS also has a remote center of motion. The robot has a stage resolution of 50 microns, and overall positional accuracy close to 100 microns. LARS is a slow robot and its upper linkages have only limited stiffness.

2.2 Software

The new "steady hand" robot uses a PC based controller system consisting of a DSP card for servo control and WIN32 operating system for application development. The modular robot control(MRC) library developed at JHU provides Cartesian level control. The application for these experiments was written using the library. LARS is controlled by a dedicated PC controller, and a more powerful remote PC computer networked to this controller provides the user and application interface.

We compare the accuracy and reliability of performing a highly precise task (repeated placement of microsurgical needle into various sizes of holes (250um, 200um, 150um) under magnified vision at 40-fold magnification). The experiment is performed by six users with and without the aid the robot as well as by the robots alone. The goal is to analyze long-term performance under the human stress-situation of working at the border of motor-space-resolution against time, while avoiding mistakes. Parameters are time to completion and number of errors per unit of time, or number of completed tasks in a given time vs. number of mistakes.

The experiment was performed using common microsurgical tools and a datum surface. The surgical tool was a commonly used 10-0 microsurgical needle held with the help of a needle holder. The datum surface consists of a sandwich of two metallic sheets separated by an insulating surface. This sandwich contains patterns of holes of the same size placed 8 and 2 mm apart in interleaved fashion. These were duplicated for the three different sizes of the holes (250, 200 and 150 microns). The lower sheet is the success surface, and the upper the error surface. Both surfaces are connected to I/O lines of the robot, and so is the microsurgical needle. Any closure of circuit generates a success or error event. An accounting algorithm keeps track of successes and errors. The thickness of the upper (error plate) is 100 microns, and the insulating surface is 50 microns thick. This makes the holes 150 microns deep. Up to 40 fold magnification microscope was used as a visual aid for the experiment. Three different versions of the pick-and-place experiments were performed. These versions were

1.   Unassisted Series - the surgeon used only the conventional techniques to perform the pick-and-place operations
2.   Hand Held Series - the needle holder was attached rigidly to the force sensor at the end-effector of the robot. The robot complied to user applied forces
3.   Autonomous Series - the robot is registered to the plates and performs the task autonomously.

Autonomously, the robot was registered to eight corner holes of the pattern and interpolated the location of the rest. The users performed each of the first two modes of the experiment for a fixed interval of time. The robot was programmed to attempt pick-and-place operations for the same interval of time. Data collection was automatic as the accounting algorithm monitored the digital inputs of robot to which the error and data surfaces were connected.

3   Results

Six different users performed the experiments for each robot. The hand-held manipulator version of the experiment resulted in better average success percentage than the conventional procedure performed by unaided user for the LARS robot. The LARS robot performed consistently with the same accuracy and better than all the three other modes for 200 and 150 microns autonomously. For the new "steady hand" robot, the robot outperformed all other modes and made very few mistakes. Users found both robots easy and convenient to use.

Size of Holes	Unassisted	LARS Robot		Steady Hand Robot	
		Hand-held	Autonomous	Hand-held	Autonomous
250um	48.8%	56.0%	53.0%	77.8%	98.4%
200um	46.3%	50.8%	50.0%	76.7%	97.7%
150um	43.0%	46.0%	48.0%	79.0%	96.5%

Table 1. Comparison of performance in the three modes. The success rate (in %) for microsurgical pick and place operations is given above. The new steady hand robot significantly improves the success rate for both assisted and autonomous modes.

Table 1 compares the success rates of the three modes of the experiment. The average success percentages were 48.8, 46.3, and 43 percent for the three hole sizes in the unassisted series (single factor ANOVA, $p<0.0001$). The hand-held-manipulator series for LARS resulted in 56, 50.8, and 46 percent successes (Single factor ANOVA, $p<0.02$) and reduced the errors significantly (paired t-test, $p<0.01$). Size of holes did not significantly influence the result. The new "steady hand" robot, the hand-held-manipulator series resulted in 77.8, 77.6, and 79.0 percent successes and size of holes did not significantly influence the performance.

Size of Holes	Unassisted	LARS Robot		Steady Hand Robot	
		Hand-held	Autonomous	Hand-held	Autonomous
250um	120.5	65.0	58.0	29.6	5.0
200um	110.0	76.8	62.0	27.0	7.0
150um	107.0	66.8	65.0	25.0	11.0

Table 2. Average Number of Erroneous attempts for the experiment. The new steady hand robot significantly decreases errors for all pick and place motions.

Table 2 lists the number of erroneous attempts. For LARS robot, the total number of attempts as well as the average success percentages decreased with decreasing hole size, except autonomously where the LARS robot performed the same number of attempts with decreasing number of successes. This could be attributed to increase in the difficulty of the task with decreasing hole diameter.

For the new "steady hand" robot, the number of attempts, and success percentage remained approximately constant. This is because of superior accuracy of the robot, so the decreasing size of holes did not pose a significant problem. The new "steady hand" robot-human system therefore has a better accuracy than measured using untrained, unskilled users in this experiment. Further tests will need to be conducted with smaller motions and skilled, trained users to better estimate the accuracy of the system.

Size of Holes	Unassisted	LARS Robot		Steady Hand Robot	
		Hand-held	Autonomous	Hand-held	Autonomous
250um	236.5	148.5	125.0	129.0	315.0
200um	206.1	149.6	125.0	107.0	311.0
150um	189.3	144.1	125.0	107.3	320.0

Table 3. Total Number of attempts for the experiment. These are average number of trials completed over 10 minutes.

Table 3 compares the total number of attempts for various modes of the experiment and table 4 shows average times between attempts. The larger time required for the new "steady hand" robot is expected in part due to the simple force proportional velocity control used. However, given the superior success rates, in this case slow motion is justified.

Size of Holes	Unassisted	LARS Robot		Steady Hand Robot	
		Hand-held	Autonomous	Hand-held	Autonomous
250um	2.7	4.1	4.8	4.6	1.9
200um	2.9	4.0	4.8	5.6	1.9
150um	3.3	4.2	4.8	5.6	1.9

Table 4. Average time between attempts (in seconds). The increase in time with new steady hand robot as a hand held manipulator may be due to the lack of training and the simple force proportional velocity control used.

For autonomous series, LARS could not be programmed to go any faster and still achieve good results because of its limited accuracy. The new "steady hand" robot is faster than all other modes of the experiment. The mistakes made by the robot autonomously are due to the simple control (PD control for positioning), and manufacturing tolerances in the datum grid.

4.   Discussion and Conclusions

Present experience shows that the robotic system is less prone to mistaken movement patterns and can perform the given task repeatedly with the same performance. The results thus suggest that the robot can extend human capabilities by assisting with microsurgical tasks at a greater spatial resolution than humanly possible. As a consequence, the robot may improve the safety of delicate microsurgical procedures at very high magnification, where human motor-skill is artificial and overall space-orientation is also lost. In addition, given the well-known phenomenon of human tiring and loss of attention with increasing time, robotic assistance may benefit lengthy microsurgical procedures.

LARS has a relatively high stage resolution of 50 microns and positional accuracy close to 100 microns: two-thirds the size of smallest holes. Also, it has limited stiffness in its arm linkages. The new "steady hand" robot significantly increases the pick and place accuracy without significantly affecting the operator perception(from reported ease of use). Training is also likely to be a factor (as previous studies have also reported, e.g. [22]), the users were mostly computer science graduate students with no robotic or microsurgical training. Their unfamiliarity with motions at this scale suggests that performance would improve with skilled and trained users.

Several other factors such as mistakes made in positioning the needle, spacing between sutures, etc are important quantifiers of surgical skill. These factors are difficult to evaluate without an automated testing platform. Further experiments in evaluating these and other parameters are planned.

5.   Summary

Several groups, including Davies ([10]), Troccaz ([9]), Peshkin ([11]), and ours have been exploring cooperative manipulation approaches to surgery. There have also been a number of telesurgical systems proposed for microsurgery (e.g. [19],[20],[21]). This paper reports the first experiments we are aware of to quantitatively assess the performance enhancement of microsurgical manipulation using the cooperative approach.

6.   Acknowledgements

The authors gratefully acknowledge the support of the National Science Foundation under grant #IIS9801684, the Engineering Research Center grant #EEC9731478. Some of this work was also supported in part by NSF Grant #5T32HL07712 from the NSF Whitaker Foundation Program for Cost Reduction in Health Care, and by The Johns Hopkins University internal funds. The LARS robots were produced by IBM research and donated to The Johns Hopkins University as part of a generous equipment grant. We also acknowledge the support of the users for these experiments.

References

1   Taylor R.H, Barnes A, Kumar R, Gupta P, Jensen P, Whitcomb L.L, de Juan E., Stoianovici D., Kavoussi L, A Steady-Hand Robotic System for Microsurgical Augmentation, accepted for publication in MICCAI'99.

2   Charles S T, Schenker P S et al., Development of a Telemanipulator for dexterity enhanced Microsurgery, MRCAS'95, Baltimore, USA, pp81-88

3   Charles Steve, Dexterity Enhancements for Surgery in Computer Integrated Surgery, MIT press. pp467-471.

4   Kelly Patrick J, Computer-Assisted Neurosurgery in Computer Integrated Surgery, MIT press, pp301-306.

5   Auer L M, Deinsberger W, NiederKorn K, et al., Endoscopic versus medical treatment of spontaneous intracerebral hemorrhage, Journal of Neurosurgery, 1989, 70:pp 530-535.

6   Auer, L.M., Robots for Neurosurgery?, Minimally Invasive Techniques for Neurosurgery: Current Status and Future Perspectives,.eds. Bauer, B.L., Hellwig, D., Springer Verlag, 1998, pp. 243-249.

7   Glauser D, Fankhauser H, Epitaux M, Hefti J L, Jaccotte A , neurosurgical robot minerva – final results and current developments, MRCAS'95, Baltimore, USA, pp24-30.

8   Ryan M J, Erickson R K, Levin D N, Pelizzari C A, MacDonald R L, Dohrmann G J, Frameless stereotaxy with real-time tracking of patient head movement and retrospective patient image registration, MRCAS'95, Baltimore, USA, pp1-7.

9   Delnondedieu Y, Troccaz J, PADyC: a passive arm with dynamic constraints. A prototype with two degrees of freedom, MRCAS'95, Baltimore, USA, pp173-180.

10   Davies B.L. , Fan K.L., Hibberd R.D., Jakopec M., Harris S.J., ACROBOT – Using Robots and Surgeons Synergistically in Knee Surgery, 8th International Conference on Advanced Robotics, CA, USA,1997

11   Colgate J.E., Wannasuphoprasit W., Peshkin M.A., Cobots: Robots for Collaboration with Human Operators, Proceedings of the International Mechanical Engineering Congress and Exhibition, Atlanta, GA, 1996, DSC-Vol. 58, pp. 433-39.

12   Riviere C N, Rader R S, Thakor N V, Adaptive real-time canceling of physiological tremor for microsurgery, MRCAS'95, Baltimore, USA,pp89-96.

13   Basdogan C, Ho C-H, Srinivasan M A, Small S D, Dawson S L, Force Interactions in Laparoscopic Simulations: Haptic Rendering of Soft Tissues, MMVR'98, San Diego, US, pp.385-391.

14   Kontarinis D A, Howe R D, Tactile display of vibratory information in teleoperation and virtual environments, Presence, 1995, 4(4):pp. 387-402.

15   Yagel R, Stredney D, et al, Multisensory Platform for Surgical Simulation, IEEE virtual Reality Annual International Symposium, Santa Clara, US, 1996, pp. 72-78.

16   Taylor R H, Funda J, LaRose D, Treat M, A telerobotic system for augmentation of endoscopic surgery, IEEE Engineering in medicine and biology society, 1992, pp. 1054-1056.

17   Lavallee J, Troccaz S, Gaborit L, Cinquin P, Benabid A L, Hoffman D, Image guided robot: a clinical application in stereotactic neurosurgery. IEEE Int. conf. on Robotics and Automation, Nice, France, 1992, pp. 618-625.

18   Troccaz J, Peshkin M, Davies B L, The use of localizers, robots and synergistic devices in CAS, CVRMed-MRCAS'97, Grenoble, France, pp. 727-736, 1997.

19   Mitsuishi M, Watanbe H, Nakanishi H, Kubota H, Izuka Y, Dexterity enhancement for a tele-micro-surgery System with Multiple Macro-micro Co-located Operation Point Manipulators and Understanding of the Operator's Intention, CVRMed-MRCAS'97, Grenoble, France, pp. 821-830, 1997.

20   Mitsuishi M., Iizuka Y. Remote Operation of a Micro-Surgical System, Proceedings of IEEE International Conference on Robotics and Automation(ICRA'98), Leuven, Belgium 1998

21   Krapohl B. D., Zins J .E., Siemionow M., Computer Assisted Microsurgery: Introduction of a new robotic arm, 4th International Symposium on Computer Assisted Orthopedic Surgery, Davos, Switzerland,March 1999.

22   Salcudean S.E., Ku S., Bell G., Performance Measurement in Scaled Teleoperation for Microsurgery, Proceedings of CVRMed-MRCAS'97, Springer-Verlag Lecture Notes in Computer Science, March 1997, Vol. 1205, pp.789-798.

23   Sheridan Thomas B, Human factors in Tele-inspection and Tele-surgery:Cooperative manipulation under Asynchronous Video and Control Feedback, Proceedings of MICCAI'98, Springer-Verlag Lecture Notes in Computer Science, October 1998, Vol. 1496, pp368-376.

24   Vasilakos K., Glass L., Beuter A., Interaction of tremor and magnification in motor performance task with visual feedback, Journal of Motor Behavior, June 1998, Vol.30(2),pp 158-168.

25   Starkes, Janet L., Payk Irene, Hodges Nicola J., Developing a standardized test for the assessment of suturing skill in novice microsurgeons, Microsurgery, 1998, Vol 18, pp.19-22.

26   Tendick F., Bhoyrul S., Way L. Comparison of Laparoscopic Imaging Systems and Conditions Using a Knot Tying Task, Journal of Image Guided Surgery, vol. 2, no. 1, 1996.

27   Kavoussi L.R, Moore R. G., Adams J. B., Partin A. W., Comparison of robotic versus human laparoscopic camera control, Proceedings of MRCAS'95,Baltimore, USA, 1995, pp284-287.

28   O'Toole R., et al, Assessing Skill and Learning in Surgeons and Medical Students Using a Force Feedback Surgical Simulator, Proceedings of MICCAI'98, Springer-Verlag Lecture Notes in Computer Science, October 1998, Vol. 1496, pp.899-909.

29   Kumar R, Goradia T M, Taylor R H, Auer L M, Robot-Assisted Minimally-Invasive Neurosurgical Procedures: Dexterity Experiments, SIMT'97, Kyoto, Japan.

30   Stoianovici D., et al, An Efficient Needle Injection Technique and Radiological Guidance Method for Percutaneous Procedures, CVRMed-MRCAS'97, Grenoble, France March 1997.

31   Stoianovici, D., Whitcomb, L.L., Anderson J.H., Taylor R.H., Kavoussi L.R., A Modular Surgical Robotic System for Image Guided Percutaneous Procedures, Proceedings of MICCAI'98, Lecture Notes in Computer Science, Springer-Verlag, ,1998 Vol. 1496, pp.404-410.

32   Taylor, R.H., et al., A Telerobotic Assistant for Laparoscopic Surgery, in Computer-Integrated Surgery, eds R. Taylor, et al., , MIT Press. 1996, pp581-592.

Intra-operative Application of a Robotic Knee Surgery System

S.J.Harris[1], M.Jakopec[1], J.Cobb[2], B.L.Davies[1]

[1] Imperial College of Science, Technology and Medicine, Exhibition Road, London,
SW7 2AX, UK
[2] The Middlesex Hospital, Mortimer Street, London, W1N 8AA, UK
Email address: s.j.harris@ic.ac.uk
WWW home page: http://www.me.ic.ac.uk/case/mim/

Abstract. A robotic system is described with associated components for registration and fixation capable of performing total knee replacement (TKR) surgery. The robot uses an active constraint concept allowing it to work with the surgeon, allowing him to cut flat planes required for a standard TKR prosthesis in the tibia and femur. The human-computer interface for this co-operative scheme is described. Experiments are described that test the robot's basic accuracy. Trials with plastic bone phantoms have been used to calibrate the system, after which tests on cadaveric legs have shown a good fit between the bone and prosthesis.

1 Introduction

Total knee replacement has become a common procedure, in particular to restore functionality and reduce the pain caused by sports injury and by degenerative diseases of the bones in the elderly. Typical prosthetic knees consist of a tibial insert, a femoral insert and a patella component. To implant a prosthesis successfully it is necessary to remove sections of bone from the tibia and femur, forming precisely shaped ends to the bones that match the prosthesis components so they can be accurately mated. Typically a single flat plane is cut across the tibia, while five planes are required in the femur. In addition to obtaining the correct shape of cut for each bone, it is also necessary to ensure correct alignment between the cuts in the two bones to provide the patient with the correct post-operative gait. Failure to provide a good match between prosthesis and bone will result in a poor prosthesis fit, which can cause pain for the patient, excessive wear on the prosthesis and the need for revision surgery. The use of cement to fill the gaps left by a poor fit can result in poor bone alignment. Poor alignment can result in an incorrect gait for the patient and excessive wear on the prosthesis.

The surgical procedure for prosthesis implantation involves the sequential use of a large number of jigs and fixtures for alignment along with oscillating saws and drills for removing bone. The sequential nature of the jigs can result in the accumulation of errors in the cuts made, while it is possible for the blade of the oscillating saw to flex, resulting in curved rather than flat planes.

It was decided that a robot would be capable of cutting the planes with good geometrical precision, allowing a good fit between prosthesis and bone, as has been shown with the *Robodoc* system for hip joints [1]. A special purpose robot was chosen, with forces and displacements just adequate for the task, to best ensure safety at reasonable cost. However, the bones of the knee vary considerably in their hardnesses, varying from very hard surfaces on the femoral condyles, in the case of arthritic joints, to very soft tissue in the medullary canal. It was thought that to allow an autonomous robot (such as *Robodoc*) to remove this variety of bone would require extensive sensing abilities to allow it to alter the cutter speed and force to suit. Providing such senses would increase the complexity of the system and greatly increase its cost. As one of the objectives of the system was to produce a cost effective system, a concept was developed whereby the robot provided the geometrical accuracy for the cuts, while the surgeon provided the intelligence and sensing ability to judge the optimum cutting speed and cutting pattern. The surgeon controls the robot using a force sensitive joystick mounted on the end-effector as close to the milling bit as possible, allowing him/her to feel the forces between bit and bone. The robot responds to the surgeon's forces on the joystick, either moving the cutter with him, allowing regions to be cut, or resisting his motion, preventing him from cutting too much bone, or from damaging surrounding soft tissue. This concept of *active constraint* [2] provides a synergy between the surgeon and robot (called the *Acrobot*), allowing each to use their skills optimally. The robot essentially provides a 'virtual jig' within which the surgeon can move, allowing him to remain in total control of the cutting process. The photograph of Fig. 1 shows this interaction in progress. The robot is a four-axis device, with three axes (pitch, yaw and in/out action) directly under the surgeon's control. The computer controls the fourth axis to select the optimum position for performing a side-milling action to obtain the prosthesis mating planes. The robot itself has a limited reach but with high local precision, and cannot reach all the cutting planes directly, so a gross positioning system (provided by Armstrong Healthcare Ltd.) is used to hold the robot and rotate it to allow access to these surfaces. The overall configuration of the robot within the gross positioner is shown in Fig. 2.

2   Pre-operative Planning

A planning system has been developed to allow CT images of the bones to be viewed in various orientations [3]. From these images bone axes can be determined and the prosthesis components correctly aligned with them. Once the prosthesis model is in the correct position over the bone model, the planning system analyses the cutting planes required to fit the prosthesis and generates outlines of the bone that these cutting planes pass through. These outlines, along with the equations for each of the cutting planes will form the constraint boundaries for the robot. The outlines are computed to extend to the limits of the bone as projected onto each of the cutting planes, ensuring that the robot is only capable of cutting bone, and preventing it from moving into, and damaging, soft tissue.

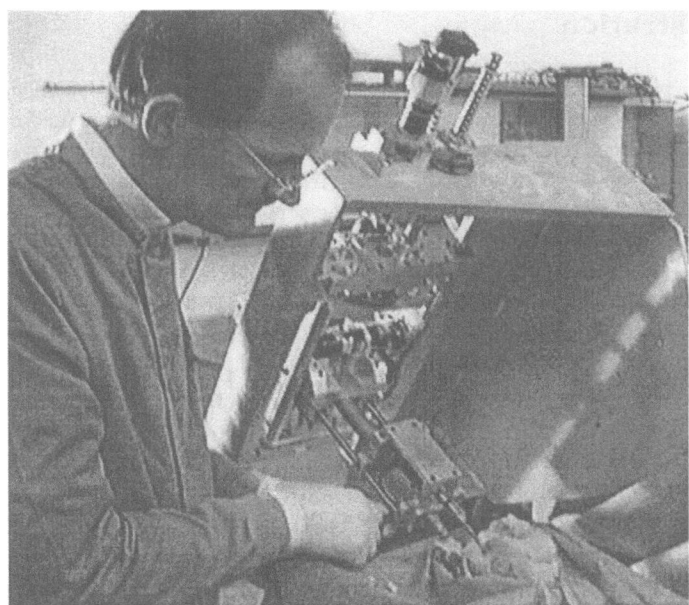

Fig. 1. The robot and surgeon interaction - note the surgeon drives the robot using the handle on the end-effector

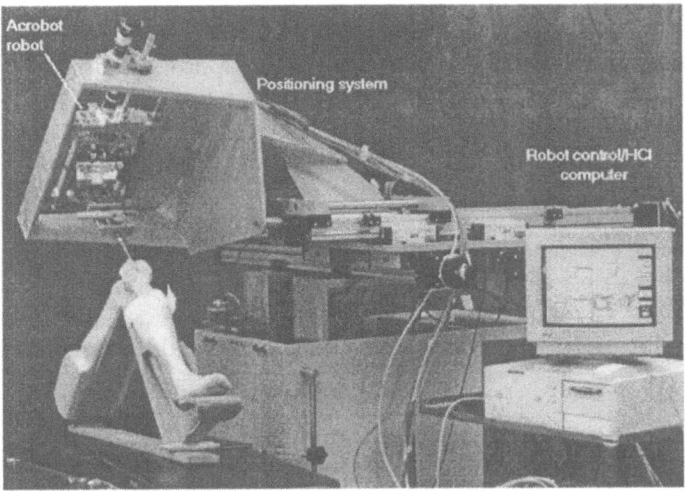

Fig. 2. The overall system showing *Acrobot*, positioning system and control computer

3 Registration

In addition to planning the cuts, the pre-operative planning system performs the first stage of the registration procedure. This procedure maps the bone and the cutting geometry from the CT based co-ordinate system (used pre-operatively) to the physical co-ordinate system used (intra-operatively) by the robot. Registration is performed using fiducial marker screws. For cadaver and plastic bone studies, 2.7 mm x 10 mm titanium cortex screws were used. These cause relatively little distortion in CT images. Their positions and orientations are extracted automatically by the pre-operative planning system. Position and orientation information is passed to the robotic system along with the cutting geometry when the surgeon has completed the planning stage.

Registration with the physical bone is performed by docking a registration tool, attached to the end-effector of the robot, into the heads of each of the fiducial marker screws. Four screws are placed in the femur (two, either side of the condyles) and four in the tibia (three around the edge, just below the tibial plateau) and one a little lower anteriorally. The screw positions are a compromise between the best spread of positions for maximum accuracy and positions that are possible, given the anatomy and geometry of the knee. To locate in each of the screw-heads a ball-ended probe is used. As the geometry of the robot does not allow a single probe to be docked in all the screw-heads, the registration tool comprises a 'tree' of five ball-probes positioned in orthogonal directions - Fig. 3. The planning computer uses the orientation and position of a screw relative to the bone to determine the best of the five probes to access a particular screw. The probe is locked to the end-effector using a rotational quick-release clamp, based on the cam locking mechanism of a typical endoscope. Using a ball-end to the probe ensures that once firmly docked into place, the centre of the ball will remain at a constant location irrespective of the approach angle of the probe.

Each bone is registered individually, as their relative orientations will differ from those in the CT scans. Once the locations of the screws have been recorded for a bone, a transformation matrix is generated to convert from CT based co-ordinates to robot based co-ordinates. The process used to generate this matrix is a least-squares error minimisation technique [4]. In addition to providing the transformation, the algorithm used generates a root mean square error, giving an indication of the match between the CT and physically measured co-ordinates. This is presented to the surgeon since a large error may indicate that one or more screws has not been accurately located, and should be re-registered.

4 The Human-Computer Interface (HCI)

Communication between the surgeon and the robot is via two paths. To indicate required cutting direction and speed, the surgeon applies forces and displacements directly on the robot's end-effector, making the robot itself an inherent part of the HCI. The robot's ability to adjust its stiffness, allowing the surgeon to feel changes in its behaviour as he approaches constraint boundaries provides

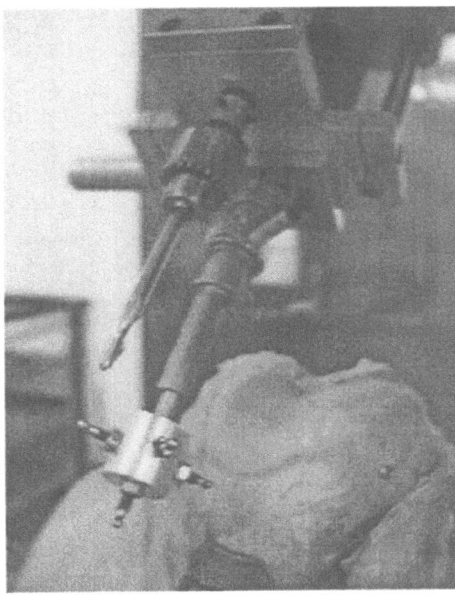

Fig. 3. The registration device showing the 'tree' of ball-ended probes

a natural two way interaction between surgeon and robot. In addition to this
physical interface, the surgeon can visualise the position of the robot's cutter
relative to the cutting surfaces, and can gauge his progress using a video display.
He also has control of the overall functioning of the system using an on-screen
control panel. Controls enable him to select between registration and cutting
modes, and to select the appropriate cutting plane. Fig. 4 shows a typical screen
display. Three views of the prosthesis planes and cutter are available, shown
in differing orientations. The fourth view shows the surgeon's progress on the
current plane with cutting depth above the current plane colour coded. For a
perfectly flat plane, this display should be a uniform colour). Changes in colour
on this display indicate differences in cutting depths in 0.1 mm increments. Cutting 1 mm too deep (which requires a considerable excess force from the surgeon)
results in the over-cut region being shown in red on the screen.

The display panels are re-sizeable, allowing the surgeon to concentrate on a
particular view. Normally, the surgeon will focus on the 'cutting progress' panel.

The HCI been designed to be consistent across all functions, with the display
above maintained throughout, with additional dialogue boxes provided as necessary - for example during registration to indicate that the surgeon has docked
the tool into the head of a fiducial screw and is ready to mark its position.

In use with surgeons, the HCI has proven easy to learn and intuitive to use,
even by novices to the system. The use of the robot as a dynamic, programmable
jig provides the user with the flexibility to control the order of cutting and an

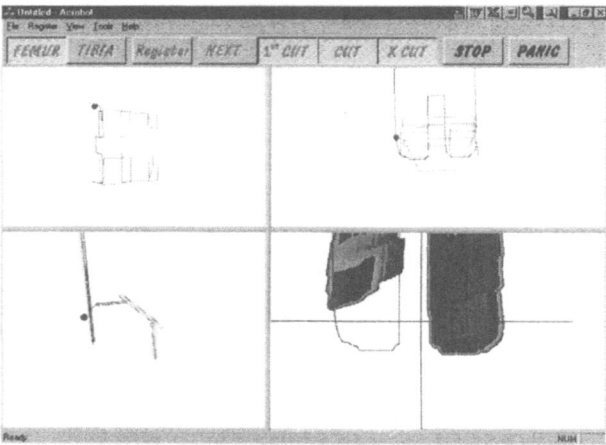

Fig. 4. The HCI showing three views of the cutter position and cutting depth

aspect of direct control lacking in either autonomous or tele-operated systems. However, treating the robot as a jig does require one novel aspect of training for the surgeon. Normally, orthopaedic work requires high forces from the surgeon to cut through bone with an oscillating saw, and to rest it firmly against the jigs used in manual surgery. The assistance provided by the robot allows the surgeon to use much less force, requiring him to reduce his applied forces.

5   Fixation of the Leg

Because the bones are registered before cutting, as it was decided that continuous dynamic tracking during surgery would not be a cost-effective solution, it is imperative that the bones remain firmly fixed in place during the procedure.

A metal framework has been developed (Fig. 5) that supports the leg with the knee bent more acutely than 90° allowing good access to the tibial plateau and the posterior femoral planes. A support holds the foot, which should be rigidly held in a cast to prevent distal movement of the leg. A clamp around the tibia provides proximal support for this bone, ensuring a stable working environment. Similarly, a clamp provides stability for the distal femur, while the thigh is strapped to its support to prevent proximal leg movement. The support is clamped to the operating table, and the table clamped to the passive positioning system. This prevents relative motion between the leg and robot.

6   System Tests and Results

Basic tests have shown that the robot controller could produce flat plains, as required for the prosthesis, and had good positional accuracy [3]. Subsequent tests have been performed on plastic bone phantoms and cadaveric legs.

6.1   Plastic Phantom Tests

Three "Sawbones" plastic bones had fiducial markers inserted into them and were CT scanned with a resolution of 0.39 mm/pixel and a 1 mm slice spacing. Pre-operative plans were made using these CT images, and constraint outlines produced from the CTs and a computer model of a medium sized prosthesis. These outlines were passed to the robot control system and legs cut.

The initial plastic bone trial resulted in a poor cut with the near-parallel anterior and posterior cutting planes required for the femoral component being spaced 37 mm apart instead of the required 43.6 mm. Registration however proved a close match between bone and CT. It was discovered that the poor fit was as a result of bending of the robot's in/out axis and some distortion to the passive frame caused by the surgeon's cutting forces on the plane. This resulted in a mis-match between the physical position of the robot and its perception of the cutter position. Bending errors were not apparent during registration because this was a low-force procedure that did not distort the system.

Subsequently, an additional strengthening shaft was added to the robot's in-out axis to give a more rigid structure. An extra supporting brace was also added to the passive positioner to prevent distortion of this component. Having updated the robot a second trial, performed in a similar manner, resulted in an improved fit for the femoral component, with the distance between anterior and posterior planes increased to 41 mm. The error of 2.6 mm still evident was the result of a small amount of bending and backlash in the system when under force from the surgeon. Calibration experiments were performed to determine compensation required for this error. The third trial was performed and the anterior-posterior plane spacing after cutting was measured to be 43.8 mm, i.e., 0.2 mm greater than the ideal, but well within the tolerances expected by the surgeons, and within the design tolerances of the prosthesis itself.

6.2   Cadaver Trials

Having obtained good results with the plastic bone tests, two cadaveric legs (one left and one right) had fiducial markers inserted into the femur and tibia, and were scanned using the same CT resolution as for the plastic bones. Scans were made approximately 3 days after insertion of the screws. The scans were processed using the pre-operative planning system. Cutting outlines and plane positions were produced and fiducial marker positions determined. These were passed to the robot control system. The prosthesis position was selected by the surgeon and adjusted to minimise the possibility of femoral notching.

The right leg was cut first, five days after screw insertion. Registration of the tibial fiducial markers was performed. A low (0.2 mm RMS) error between physical and scanned screw positions was obtained indicating a good match between the pre-operative screw positions from the CT and the physical positions. The tibial plateau was then cut, using a side-mill action. Shallow marker holes were also cut by the robot into the tibial plateau to allow the standard manual tibial punch to be located relative to the planned orientation. It was decided that the punch should be used to provide the hole and slots for the tibial component fixing shaft and fins (rather than drilling out bone with the robot) as the punch compacts the bone mass preserving, rather than removing it.

Registration of the femoral fiducial markers was then performed, and a low RMS error (0.2 mm) was again noted indicating a good geometrical match between the CT and physical screws. Initially, the anterior femur was cut followed by the posterior femur, using a side-milling action. The robot was rotated using the gross positioner and the anterior and posterior sloping faces were cut, again using a side milling action. Finally, the distal femur face was cut using an end-mill action. The robot was then rotated using the gross positioner and the tibial fiducial markers were registered.

The femoral trial piece was fitted, and the femoral component shaft fixing hole made in the medullary canal. The trial piece was removed and the tibia punched. Finally, the prosthesis components were implanted without cement and found to be a good fit, with little gap between the bone and the prosthesis surface. As was planned, no femoral notching was observable, with the top of the anterior femoral component lying on the anterior femoral surface.

The left leg was cut after a further two weeks. Registration of the tibia was performed, and it was discovered that the RMS error was greater than previously (0.8 mm) and it was noted that there was some movement in the screws as the tool was docked with them, indicating some loosening of the screws within the caderveric specimen. Since tightening them would have adjusted their position relative to the CT data in another undefined manner they were left unaltered and the registration accepted. The tibial plateau was then cut as for the right leg. The femur was then registered, with an RMS error of 0.5 mm, and cut as for the right leg, and prosthesis components implanted without cement.

The pre-operative plan was designed to avoid femoral notching, and the femoral component was found, after cutting, to lie on the anterior femoral surface, as shown in Fig. 5. The leg was tested in extension and flexion and the two prosthesis components were found to mate, giving a good range of motion.

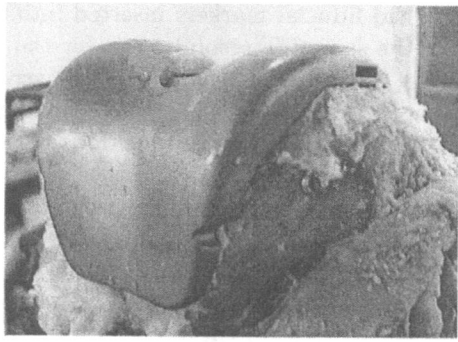

Fig. 5. Cadaveric leg with prosthesis trial piece in position showing high quality of fit.

7   Conclusions

We have successfully demonstrated robotic knee surgery on plastic phantoms and human bones. The system integrates pre-operative imaging and modelling, a force controlled robot and gross positioning system to produce cuts in bones well matched to the prosthesis. The milling cutter used to remove bone was capable of producing smooth, flat surfaces, allowing good contact between bone and prosthesis surfaces enabling cementless procedures to be performed. The fixation system ensures that the bone remains rigidly in place, allowing for registration at the beginning of the cutting procedure, without the need for continuous registration methods. The fiducial screw markers and clamping system have shown themselves to be an accurate registration method, providing a good match between the pre-operative planning and intra-operative stages of the process. However, the insertion of screws into the patient's leg prior to CT-scanning and surgery is not an ideal approach, and future studies will investigate the use of anatomical feature matching. The pre-operative and intra-operative systems together allow the surgeon to position the prosthesis correctly, avoiding problems such as femoral notching, while the provision of a simple HCI allow him to use the system with minimal training. The active-constraint concept that enables the surgeon to work with the robot leaves him in control of the system at all times, increasing his confidence in the end-result, while allowing him to use his intelligence to determine cutting speeds and forces.

The post-operative range of motion in the leg and good mating between the prosthesis components and bone show that the surgery were successfully planned pre-operatively. Intra-operatively the robot successfully reproduced these plans to produce an excellent fit between bone and prosthesis, and well aligned prosthesis components.

8   Acknowledgements

We would like to acknowledge the financial assistance of the UK Department of Health and the 'LINK' Medical Implants Fund in support of this project.

References

1. Bauer, A., Börner M., Lahmer A., *"Robodoc - Animal Experiment and Clinical Evaluation"*, Proc. of CVRMed-MRCAS'97, pp561-564
2. Harris, S.J., Lin, W.J.,Fan, K.L., Hibberd, R.D., Cobb, J., Davies, B.L., *"Experiences with Robotic Systems for Knee Surgery"*, International Symposium on Medical Robotics and Computer Assisted Surgery. Proc. of CVRMed-MRCAS'97, Lecture Notes in Computer Science, 1205, pp 757-766, Springer Verlag Press, March 97
3. Harris, S.J., Jakopec M., Cobb, J., Hibberd, R., Davies B.L., *"Interactive pre-operative selection of cutting constraints, and interactive force controlled knee surgery by a surgical robot"*, Proc. of MICCAI'98, pp 996-1006
4. Besl P.J., McKay, N.D., *"A Method for Registration of 3-D Shapes"*, IEEE Trans. On Pattern Analysis and Machine Intelligence, Vol 14 No 2., Feb 1992, pp 239-256

Image-Based Control of Interactive Robotics Systems

Andreas Hein and Tim C. Lueth

Surgical Robotics Lab (SRL), Clinic for Maxillofacial Surgery, Charité Virchow-Hospital,
D-13353 Berlin, Germany
{a.hein, t.lueth}@ieee.org
http://www.charite.de/rv/mkg/srl/index.html

Abstract. In this paper a robotics system is described which supports the surgeon during drilling and shaping operations. The special feature of this system is the fusion of control commands by the surgeon and control commands derived directly in real-time from the image data of the patient. This interactive control of a robotics system leads to a cooperation between the surgeon and the robotics system. Because the robotics system can directly access to the image data within every control cycle it provides a higher accuracy and an enhanced safety of drilling operations. A tool for the quantitative analysis of the image data, the interactive control system of the robotics system and the first application in Anaplastology is presented.

1   Introduction

Surgery is a relatively new and a rapidly growing field of application for robotics technology. Robots can be used to enhance the accuracy and the dexterity of a surgeon, can decrease the tremble of the human hand and can amplify or reduce the movements and/or forces applied by the surgeon. Especially in fields of surgery where the human hand is the limiting factor for further optimization of the surgical techniques –like in neurosurgery, orthopedic and maxillofacial surgery– robotics technology can be applied.

The drilling or shaping of bone structures is of great importance for surgery. In contrary to soft tissue a static model of bone structures derived from CT images can be used. Currently, these operations are carried out by the surgeons free hand during an intervention. In the near of sensitive regions the manual handling can lead to complications due to inaccuracies or shattering of the drill or shaper.

Especially in maxillofacial surgery the accuracy of an intervention is of paramount importance due to the high social and aesthetic impact of the face. Therefore, the positioning and moving of drills or shapers with a high accuracy is desirable. Additional difficulties in maxillofacial surgery are the restricted access to the bone structures through small incisions, the swelling of tissue during the intervention, and the small distance to vital organs or structures.

This paper presents the image-based control of the first interactive robotics system developed for the application in maxillofacial surgery at the Surgical Robotics Lab

(SRL) at the Virchow hospital (Fig. 1). The concept of the semi-active robot controlling will be refined and the interactive use of the robot based on different information entities will be explored.

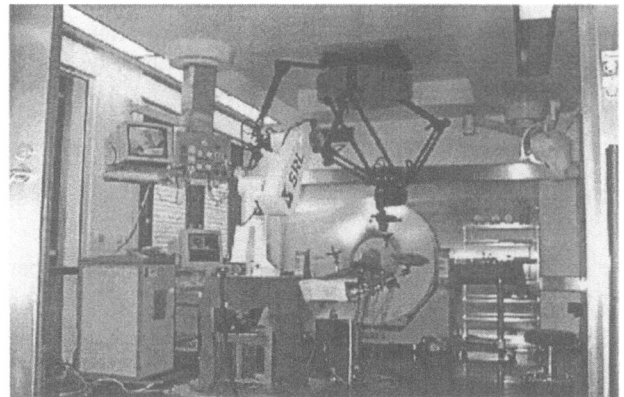

Fig. 1: Experimental OR at the Virchow hospital

2 State of the art

During the last 10 years, robotics techniques have been introduced to operating theaters for only a few surgical applications. The first systems were used in neurosurgery for the guidance of surgical instruments like biopsy needles, catheters, or microscopes [1][2][3][4]. After an initial registration of the patient (determination of the transformation matrix between the image data of the patient, the patient at the intraoperativ position and the robot base frame [5]) the manipulators are used to approach points planned in the preoperative image data. During the treatment the manipulators are either switched off or the brakes are locked.

Active robotics systems are used in orthopedic surgery and for laparoscopic applications. The Robodoc system has been developed for the milling of holes exactly fitting for a hip prosthesis [6]. This system works fully automatic during the operation. That means, the robot executes exactly the preoperative planned movements and can react to environmental changes only with an interruption of the program.

The only interactively controllable robotics system for invasive application has been designed for knee surgery [7]. This experimental 2-link arm is force controlled and can be guided by the surgeon manually to the cutting position at the knee bone. The workspace of the cutter is restricted by decreasing controller gains in the near of the boundaries.

The most successful commercial robotics system is the AESOP system by Computer Motion. This camera holding and positioning system has been designed for laparoscopic surgery and has been used in over 30,000 cases [8]. These systems can be interactively used during the operation like the microscope holding systems SurgiScope by Elekta and the MKM by Zeiss.

In addition to the author's system [12], in maxillofacial surgery only two systems are under development. The system described in [9] consists of a passive manipulator used for positioning instruments. The disadvantage of passive systems is the time consuming positioning procedure and the impossibility to move along desired trajectories with force constrains. The other system [10] is an experimental automatic system that is not designed for interactions with the surgeon. Such systems seem not to be suitable for real applications in maxillofacial surgery.

3 Description of the treatment

To approach the complex field of this surgery and to collect first experiences in drilling and shaping operations the placement of implants for the fixation of an extraoral ear epithesis has been selected as the first application of the robotics system at the SRL.
The medical indication for ear epithesis is given in the case of the resection of the ear due to a tumor resection or the destruction of the ear due to an accident. If a reconstruction fails, an artificial ear can either be modeled using the mirror-image of the CT images of the other side's ear or by a manual procedure using impressions. Fig. 2 shows a scheme for the determination of the optimal implant positions around the center of the ear. The implant manufacturer suggests that the implants should be placed on a circle with a diameter of about 2 cm around the ear channel within the marked areas.

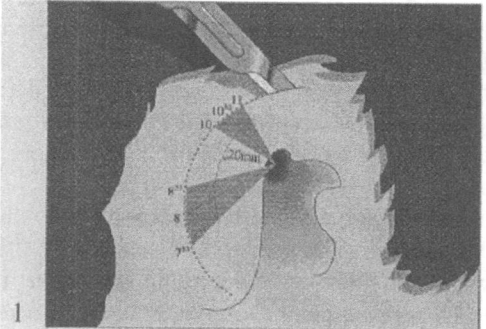 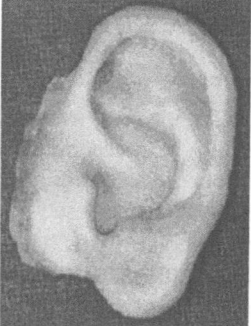

Fig. 2: Planning of the implants' position and placing of the implants [11] (left) and an artificial ear (right)

Using a robotics system for the drilling of the holes and the placement of the implants decreases the number of needed implants to two instead of three. This is caused by the higher stability of the implants. The stability is increased due to a better analysis of the bone structure and due to the exact placement of the implants at the pre-planned positions. Especially, the avoidance of hitting mastoid cells (air-filled cavities in the near of the central ear) increases the stability and decreases the risk of infections. To fix the artificial ear a superconstruction has to be mounted at the implants. An artificial ear –as shown on the right side of Fig. 2– will be clipped onto the superconstruction. The construction consists of distance pieces and a bridge between the distant pieces. The preoperatively known positions of the implant and the supercconstruction allow the fabrication of the ear epithesis before the treatment and supply the patient with the ear right after the healing phase. Currently, the patient must wait months for the epithesis because the implant positions are determined after the interventions by impressions.

4 Architecture of the robot controller

The SurgiScope by Elekta is used as the basis for the development of the robotics system for maxillofacial surgery. This system is originally aimed at the carriage of a microscope for neurosurgery. For invasive applications the controller software and the tools have been changed [12]. The robotics system consists of a parallel manipulator, an infrared navigation system, a control cabinet with the computer for the navigation system and the control computer of the manipulator, and the drilling machine. The drilling machine consists of a drilling station and the hand piece that is mounted to the manipulator.

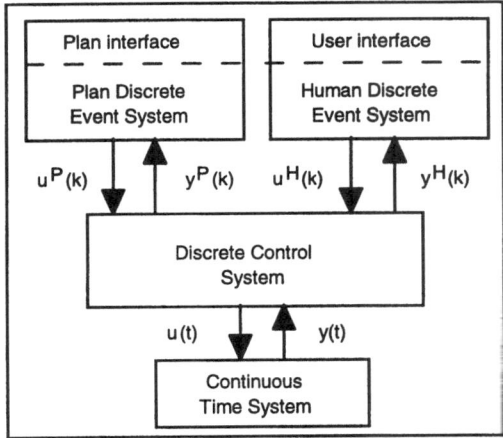

Fig. 3: Architecture of the interactive robot controller [13]

The hand piece of the drilling machine is an unmodified standard surgical hand piece that is mounted to the manipulator by a special construction. Its motor is connected to a station that controls the speed and the force of the drilling machine.

From the perspective of a robot control system which has two distinct information sources this system can be divided into a Human Discrete Event System (HDES) with the user interface, a Plan Discrete Event System (PDES) with the plan interface, a Discrete Control System (DCS), and a Continuous Time System (CTS). Fig. 3 shows an overview of the system.

The PDES is a finite state machine, which encodes the general command sequence for a type of intervention. Additionally, it contains specific patient data as target positions $^I t$ and registration points $^I p$ in respect to the image data coordinate system, and paths between working points outside the patient model. Depending on the current state s^P of the PDCS an elementary operation $o(k)$ in the DCS will be activated by the command

$$u^P(k) = (o(k),{}^I t,{}^I p, path) \tag{3}$$

Each elementary operation terminates by setting one condition out of the vector $y^P(k)$ true and then the PDCS switches to the next state, which corresponds to the true condition. Depending on the active elementary operation $o(k)$ and the current position and velocity of the TCP in respect to the image data coordinate system

$$y^H(k) = (o(k),{}^I p_{TCP},{}^I \dot{p}_{TCP}) \tag{4}$$

the HDES generates a command

$$u^H(k) = ({}^I \dot{p}_{TCP}) \tag{5}$$

that will be delivered to the DCS.

In addition to $y^H(k)$, the HDCS gets a force/torque vector through the user interface, which consists of a force-torque sensor. It should be noticed that the HDES can not distinguish exactly between a user's intervention and an interaction of the manipulator with the environment.

In the DCS the manipulator (CTS) will be controlled by a position, velocity and/or force scheme. The position of the manipulator is given by the vector $y(t)$ that consists of the six encoder values of the joints. The output of the DCS is the vector $u(t)$ that consists of the six values for the DAC for each joint motor.

5 Image-based control

None of the currently known robotics systems are directly using the medical image data like CT or MRI. Most of the systems derive trajectories or target points from the image data during a preoperative planning process. Therefore, an intraoperativ change of treatment parameters is not possible. In case of small changes or misinterpretation of the image data by the surgeon the robot supported treatment has to be interrupted. This may be acceptable as far as a change to conventional treatment methods is possible, but new treatment methods introduced by the advantages of robotics systems eventually do not allow a change.

To avoid these difficulties the described concept of the robot application for maxillo-facial surgery provides the real-time access to image data from a predefined region of interest. That means on one hand the surgeon has the full image information plus pre-operative defined abstractions during the whole intervention (paths, targets, etc.). On the other hand the robot controller uses the image data as normal sensor data.

In the application of the robotics system for the placement of the implants the image data are used to give the surgeon a direct feedback where the optimal drilling positions can be found. A slice through the images is computed which starts at the current tool position in the images and has the orientation of the working direction of the drilling machine. Using an approximated interval of hounsfield units for the bone the thickness of the skull bone can be determined.

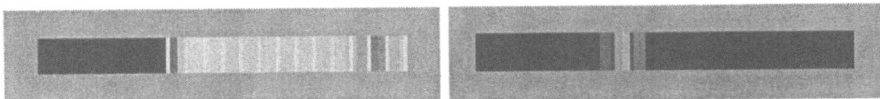

Fig. 4: Slices through the CT images in the working direction of the drill. The thickness of the bone is determined in this section using a fixed threshold. The vertical lines indicate the thickness of the first bone segment. The distance between the lines is 1mm. The segment starts at the drill position (*left side of each segment*) and is 2cm long. In the *left segment* enough bone is below the drill. In the *right segment* the bone is to thin.

A virtual wall is erected in front of bony structures if the bone structure is thinner than the currently used depth of the drill (3 or 4mm). Therefore the robot's movements are stopped if the TCP approaches the bone. In this way the surgeon can „feel" where the placement of the implants is possible through a haptic interface.

In this case the Human Discrete Event System (HDES) computes the velocity of the system based on the desired velocity, the distance to the surface of the skull bone $dist(^I p_{TCP})$, and its computed thickness $thick(^I p_{TCP})$:

$$u^H(k) = (^I \dot{p}_{TCP}) = O(F_u, dist(^I p_{TCP}), thick(^I p_{TCP})) \tag{6}$$

The desired velocity is computed by the force input of the surgeon F_u. This force control scheme has been described in [13]. A main influence on the successful application of the image-based control of a robotics system is the accuracy of the spatial mapping of the real patient to the coordinate system of the robot. The accuracy depends on two transformations:

$$^{pat}T \xrightarrow{\;f\;} {}^{ct}T \xrightarrow{\;g\;} {}^{rob}T \tag{7}$$

f transforms the real patient into an image coordinate system. The transformation contains quantification errors and errors due to the movement of the patient. For CTs the error depends on the slice distance and the window size of the image. An usual voxel size is $2.0 \times 0.5 \times 0.5 mm^3$. g is the transformation between the image coordinate system and the base coordinate system of the manipulator. This transformation is computed after the registration. Inherent errors in g arise from non-rigid fixation of the patient, movements of soft tissue, the type of markers, and measurement errors. The amount of errors in g varies between a few tenths and a few millimeters. The image data part of the robot controller display is shown in Fig. 5. The maximum size of the region of interest is about 150 pixel×150 pixel×30 slices. Using such a RoI size the image data will be updated with a frequency of 10Hz, which is the frequency of the navigation system.

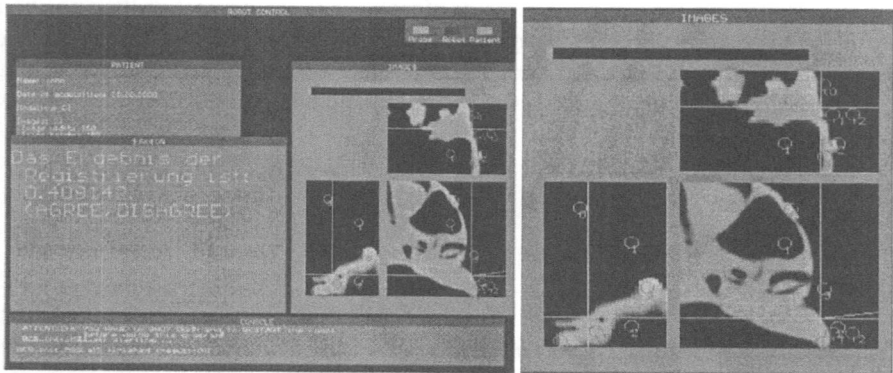

Fig. 5: Screen of the robot controller (left) and a detail of the real-time displaying window with CT data from a plastic scull (right). From the original CT image (in the right window) coronal and sagittal slices (left and above the original slice) and a slice in the working direction (left top) is calculated and the current tool position is superimposed.

6 Conclusions

In the paper new concepts for an interactively usable robotics system have been described. Advantages of this concept are the better acceptance by the surgeons, the improved safety of the procedure, and the easy adaptation of the treatment to the actual requirements.

The usability of the interactive tool control has been approved be surgeons in experimental operations at phantoms. The control has been accepted and the first experiments have shown the overall system's suitability for the implant fixation. Up to now, experiments have been carried out with stereolithographic models of a head, where a superconstruction with a preoperative known size has been mounted at the implants. The measured thickness of the bone in CT images depends to a great extend on the chosen window of houndsfield values. Depending on the window the measured bone thickness differs in a great extend. Further research work has to be done to determine an optimal window for measuring the bone thickness and inaccuracies caused by individual differences of the bone structure have to be determined.

Acknowledgment

This research work has been performed at the Department for Maxillofacial Surgery, Prof. Dr. Dr. Juergen Bier, within the Surgical Robotics Lab, Prof. Dr. Tim C. Lueth,

Medical Faculty Charité, Humboldt-University Berlin. The work has been supported by the Deutsche Forschungsgemeinschaft with the Graduiertenkolleg Temperaturab-hängige Effekte (granted to Prof. Dr. Dr. h.c. R. Felix, Prof. Dr. N Hosten) and by the Real-Time Control Group, Prof. Dr.-Ing. Guenter Hommel, of the Technical University Berlin. Parts of the research have been supported financially by the Deutsche Krebshilfe (granted to Prof. Dr. Dr. J. Bier, PD Dr. P. Wust) and the Berliner Sparkas-senstiftung Medizin (granted to Prof. Dr. T. Lueth, Dr. Dr. Ernst Heissler, Prof. Dr. Dr. Berthold Hell). Special thanks to the companies Elekta, Metalor and Philips for their support of the project. We would like also to thank Thomas Hölper, Edgar Schüle, Dr. h.c. Hervé Druais, Dr.-Ing. Armin Freybott, and W. Scholz. Their personal engagement was the basis for this challenging research.

References

1. Kwoh, Y. S. *et al.*: A robot with improved absolute positioning accuracy for CT guided stereotactic surgery. Trans. on Biomedical Engineering, Vol. 35, No. 2 (1988) 153-161
2. Lavallée, S.: A new system for computer assisted neurosurgery. Proc. 11th IEEE Engineer-ing in Medicin and Biology Conf., Seatle, November, (1989) 926-927
3. Glauser, D. *et al.*: Conception of a robot dedicated to neurosurgical operations. Proc. 5th Int. Conf. on Advanced Robotics, Pisa, (1991) 888-892
4. Watanabe, E. *et al.*: Open surgery assisted by neuronavigator, a stereotactic articulated sen-sitive arm. Neurosurgery, Vol. 28, No. 6 (1991) 792-800
5. Lavallee, S.: Registration for Computer-Integrated Surgery: Methodology, State of the Art. In Taylor, R. H., S. Lavallee, G. C. Burdea, R. Mösges (eds.), Computer-Integrated Surgery, Technology and clinical Applications, MIT Press, (1996) 77-98
6. Taylor, R. H. *et al.*: An Image-Directed Robotic System for Precise Orthopaedic Surgery. IEEE Trans. on Robotics and Automation, Vol.10, No.3 (1994) 261-275
7. Ho, S. C. *et al.*: Force control for robotic surgery. ICAR IEEE Int'l. Conf. on Advanced Robotics, (1995) 21-31
8. Jacobs L. K., V. Shayani, J. M. Sackier: Determination of the learning curve of the AESOP robot. Surg Endosc, Jan; 11(1) (1997) 54-55
9. Cutting, C., Bookstein, F., Taylor, R.: Applications of simulation, morphometrics and ro-botics in craniofacial surgery. In Taylor, R. H., S. Lavallee, G. C. Burdea, R. Mösges (eds.), Computer-integrated surgery: technology and clinical applications, MIT Press, (1996) 641-662
10.Bohner, P. *et al.*: Operation planning in cranio-maxillo-facial surgery. Medicine Meets Virtual Reality 4 (MMVR4'96), San Diego, California, (1996)
11.Brånemark System® product information for fixure placement - surgical procedure - cranio-facial rehabilitation
12.Lueth, T.C. *et al.*: A Surgical Robot System for Maxillofacial Surgery. IEEE Int. Conf. on Industrial Electronics, Control, and Instrumentation (IECON), Aacher, Germany, Aug. 31-Sep. 4, (1998) 2470-2475
13.Hein, A. and T.C. Lueth: Robot Control in Maxillofacial Surgery. Sixth International Sym-posium on Experimental Robotics, Sydney, Australia , March 26-28, (1999) in print

Extracting Features from Tactile Maps

Parris S. Wellman[1], Robert D. Howe[1]

[1]Division of Engineering and Applied Science, Harvard University, Cambridge, MA 02138
parris@hrl.harvard.edu,howe@deas.harvard.edu

Abstract. Tactile imaging is a newly developed mechanical sensing technology for documenting the properties of hard lumps contained in soft tissue. An examiner strokes a scan head across tissue that contains a mass and images of the distributed contact pressure between the head and the tissue are recorded. We have developed models that predict these pressure distributions from geometric and material properties. We then use inversion algorithms developed from these models to extract lump size and shape. In a limited clinical trial on 24 surgical patients, lump size was estimated with less than 17% mean absolute error when compared with ex-vivo size measurements. This is more than twice as accurate as either clinical breast examination or ultrasound examination of the same lumps. This result demonstrates that tactile imaging has the potential to improve the accuracy of clinical breast examination.

1 Introduction

The sense of touch is an invaluable and widely applied clinical tool, particularly for the detection and diagnosis of breast cancer, where a palpable lump is the most common symptom of the disease [1]. Palpation often plays a primary role in monitoring benign breast lumps for change as they are often not visible on mammograms or in ultrasound images because of breast density or scarring. In these cases, CBE is the most effective tool for monitoring a breast for changes in time. The problem with this method is that it is difficult to accurately verbalize and record tactile sensations, prompting one physician to remark "I can only deplore tumor size expressed in terms of fruits, nuts, or vegetables, but ... medical students ... continue to prefer these agricultural analogies" [2]. Even assessing the size of a lump can be problematic, as one study reports that nearly 100% change in the size of a lump is required for it to considered a noticeable clinical change [3]. A method for accurately recording tactile sensations from physical exams would make CBE more objective, and could greatly improve the ability to detect changes.

Many new breast examination technologies have been proposed but the typical intended application has most often been screening, where the primary challenge is the detection of the presence of a lump in the breast [4,5,6,7]. In contrast, the monitoring application we describe assumes that the lump has been detected, and the challenge is to accurately document parameters such as lump size, shape, and hardness. Sarvazyan [8] has proposed a method that uses distributed pressure measurement to estimate the properties of breast and prostate lumps. He uses an iterative solution of a finite element model in order to estimate the properties of these lumps but has only demonstrated it in the prostate. Several new imaging modalities also show promise for characterizing breast lumps, including magnetic resonance and ultrasound elastography [9,10]. However, these techniques require elaborate and relatively expensive imaging systems and skilled technicians.

This paper reports the development of a system that uses simple algorithms for extracting breast lump features from measurements of contact pressure. The clinician strokes a "scan head" containing an array of pressure sensors over the breast. Signal processing algorithms assemble a "tactile map" of the breast and estimate lump parameters such as size and shape. The goal is to provide objective and repeatable documentation of palpation information in a form that is easily understood by the clinician and even the patient. These images may be incorporated into the patient record as a means of tracking lump changes across time. The technique is designed to be inexpensive, noninvasive, quick, and easy to use. It will enable follow-up examinations to be conducted frequently with minimal risk and inconvenience.

In subsequent sections we discuss mathematical forward models that relate geometric and material properties of the breast to pressure distributions measured on the surface of the scan head. We use these forward models to develop inversion algorithms that can be used to extract the size of palpable lumps. Finally we discuss the system performance in a limited clinical trial of 24 breast surgery patients.

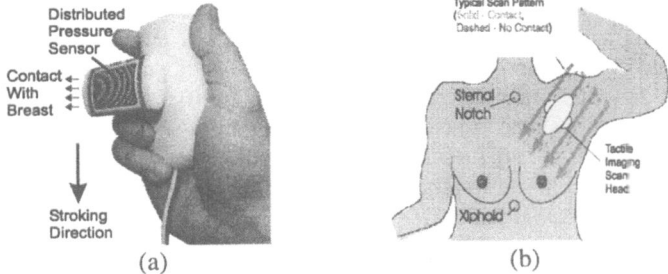

(a)   (b)

Fig. 1. – (a) The scan head of the tactile imaging system. The indentor portion of the scan head is an array of piezoresistive pressure sensors (16 rows by 26 columns, 1.5mm spacing). A magnetic position tracker is located in the head. (b) The patient is placed supine with the ipsilateral arm over the head to stabilize the breast and minimize tissue thickness. The clinician begins the examination by indicating the location of the readily palpable sternal notch and xiphoid to facilitate comparison of follow-up examinations. The clinician then presses the indentor into the breast near the mass, and strokes the sensor repeatedly over the area of the mass and its immediate surroundings. The skin surface is lubricated to minimize friction.

1.1 System Description

Figure 1(a) shows the tactile imaging system "scan head" that the physician strokes over the breast. The array of piezoresistive pressure sensors mounted on its surface have a range of 0-34kPa and are calibrated before each use using a pressure bladder. A magnetic tracker in the handle senses the relative position and rotation of each pressure image. A computer samples the tracker and pressure sensor array every 5 milliseconds. The tactile mapping algorithm assembles these individual pressure frames, or *tactile images*, to form a composite *tactile map* of the mass.

2 Methods

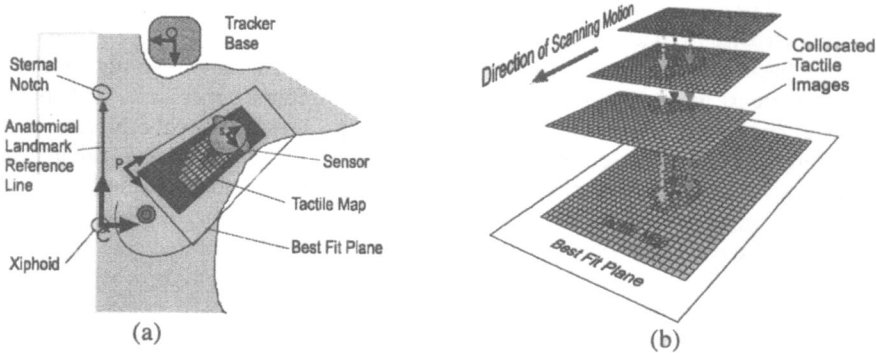

(a)   (b)

Fig. 2 –(a) A tactile map is registered to the patient using coordinate frame C, determined by the sternal notch and xiphoid. Frame S is the location of the scan head during each image, frame P is the best-fit plane frame and Frame O is the base frame for the position tracker. (b) A tactile map is created by collocating each image, projecting and averaging the values onto the plane that best fits the sensor motion in the neighborhood of the mass.

The shape of the indentor was designed to provide a nearly uniform pressure distribution when pressed into homogeneous tissue [11], to minimize the dynamic range required for the pressure sensors and to simplify the signal processing. Analysis shows that this shape is nearly a section of a circular cylinder, but the exact shape depends on the tissue stiffness and the indentation pressure applied by the user [12]. Indentor size was chosen to require a comfortable range of applied force. Finite element analysis showed that for normal breast tissue (15-25 kPa modulus), [13] and anticipated user-applied pressures (5-14 kPa), the pressure variation across the indentor is within 7.5% of mean.

Clinician stroking technique and patient placement must be controlled in order to obtain repeatable results; typical technique is shown in Figure 1(b). An audible tone assists the clinician in maintaining the desired average pressure range while the breast is lubricated to reduce friction. The clinician continues stroking until the tactile map, created in real time on the monitor, reflects the palpable extent of the mass. The tactile map combines the pressure images in a form that is readily interpreted. It also averages multiple images to reduce noise from the transducer, technique variations and small mass motions. Just before making a tactile map, the examiner indicates the sternal notch and the xiphoid using the scan head as shown in Figure 2(a). This provides an alignment reference for future examinations of the patient. Producing a tactile map from the scans made by the examiner can be summarized in three steps

i.   Determine the best-fit plane on which to project the data from the motions of the examiner in the neighborhood of the lump.

ii.   Eliminate pressure frames outside the pressure range of interest and normalize the remainder using the average of the frame to account for the remaining variation in pressure level.

iii. Collocate and average the frames on the best-fit plane to form the composite *tactile map* as shown in Figure 2(b).

Once the maps are constructed, we need to use inversion algorithms to extract lump features. To develop these algorithms we first develop forward models that predict the pressure distribution given the geometric and material properties. We use these models to develop inversion algorithms.

2.1 Forward Models

The most common form of cancer is infiltrating ductal carcinoma [14] which forms in the lactiferous ducts and then spreads through the tissue layers. In our observation these lumps, as well as other non-cancerous masses, become palpable when they project into the fat layer overlying the glandular tissue. We consider the breast to be a three-layer model: a layer of fat, a layer of normal glandular tissue and the rigid chest wall, as shown in Figure 3(a) with a single palpable mass that forms at the boundary of the glandular tissue and fat. We also assume that the tissue is elastic and isotropic, and like other biological tissue is nearly incompressible [15]. Other researchers have solved various aspects of this problem [16,17,18,19] but no analytic solution exists for the full case presented here. We use a finite element model with geometry in Figure 3(a) to determine the relationship of these properties to the output pressure distribution. Because the indentor is much longer than it is wide, see Figure 1(a), we solve the problem with a two-dimensional plane strain model. This model is sufficient because we are only looking for trends to develop inversion algorithms.

We assume that the indentor and chest wall are rigid, the normal glandular tissue is ten times as stiff as the surrounding fat, and the fat has an elastic modulus of 5 kPa, based on our measurements of the elastic properties of breast tissues [20]. Most palpable masses exhibit a nonlinear relationship between stress and strain so we will examine the effect of this change in modulus by varying the ratio of the tumor stiffness to the surrounding tissue stiffness. The indentor is pressed into the tissue under constant force as it slides across the surface.

It is also desirable to have an analytical expression that predicts the pressure at any point on the surface of the indentor as a function of its location, the geometric and material properties. We represent the indentor face pressure distribution for each location of the indentor along the surface of the tissue as the weighted sum of two pressure distributions. The first, P_1, is the pressure distribution across the face of the indentor that would be produced if there were no lump present. The second, P_2, is the difference between the pressure distribution far from the lump, P_1 and P_0, which is the pressure distribution on the face of the indentor when it is centered on the lump. Figure 3(b) shows these distributions, where $P_2 = P_0 - \alpha P_1$ and $\alpha = 0.5$ is an arbitrary parameter chosen to be sure that $P_2 > 0$.

In Figure 4(a) we see that there is some variation in the shape of the pressure distribution far from the lump that depends upon the thickness of the tissue. We use a model which is motivated by Hertz' classic solution [21]

$$P_1(s,t) = \begin{cases} P_0(t) \cdot \left(1 - \left(\dfrac{s}{a(t)} \right)^2 \right)^{\frac{1}{2}} & -w \leq s \leq w \\ 0 & \textit{otherwise} \end{cases} \tag{1}$$

where $2w$ is the width of the head (2.4 cm), $P_o(t)$ and $a(t)$ were determined by fitting the curves in Figure 4(a) with Equation 1. The curves in Figure 4(b) can be fit with a Gaussian distribution that is a function of location along the surface of the tissue, x, lump diameter, d, stiffness ratio of tumor to surrounding fat E_2/E_1, and depth ratio from the surface of the tissue to the center of the lump, h/d, as,

$$P_2(x,d,E_2/E_1,h/d) = g(d,E_2/E_1,h/d) \cdot e^{-\left(\frac{x^2}{2\sigma(d,E_2/E_1,h/d)^2}\right)} \tag{2}$$

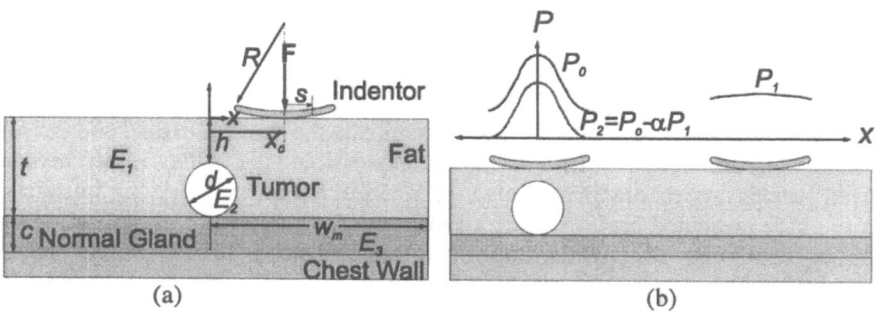

(a)   (b)

Fig. 3 – (a) The geometry of the plane strain model which has been idealized to contain only a single focal mass and three layers of tissue. (b) The pressure distributions modeled in the empirical fit.

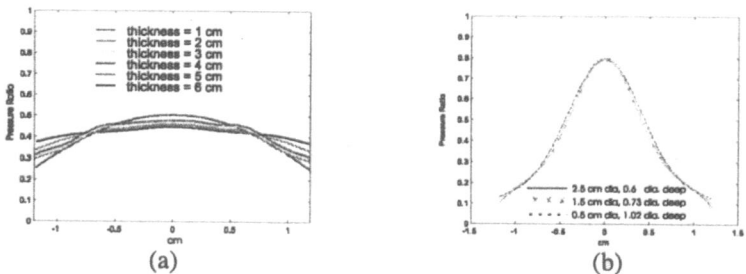

(a)   (b)

Fig. 4 – (a) Pressure frames, from finite element models, FEM, for size different tissue thickness, P_1, on the face of the indentor with the center of the indentor far from the lump. (b) Pressure frames (FEM), P_0, with the indentor centered on the lump for 3 different cases.

We must also develop a two dimensional analog to the tactile map. A tactile map is nothing but the spatial average of all pressure values for a given set of pressure frames. We can also view this average as the average of all pressure curves formed by an individual element on the face of the indentor as it slides across the surface. We change variables to $s=x-x_c$ and write each of these curves as

$$P_{surface}(x,s,d,E_2/E_1,h/d) = P_2(x,d,E_2/E_1,h/d) \cdot \left(\frac{P_1(s,t)}{\max(P_1(s,t))}\right)^2 + \kappa(x_c,d) \cdot P_1(s,t) \tag{3}$$

where the P_1^2 term a good fit to the finite element model data as the indentor slides off of the lump, $x - x_c$ is restricted to the head width , and

$$\kappa(x_c, d) = \begin{cases} 0.5 \cdot \left(1 + \dfrac{8}{3d}|x_c|\right) & 0 \le |x_c| \le \dfrac{8}{3}d \\ 1 & otherwise \end{cases} \tag{4}$$

The equation for the map is just the average of all of the curves. We evaluate this expression to reveal that the map is Gaussian, with the same standard deviation as equation 2 and different amplitude.

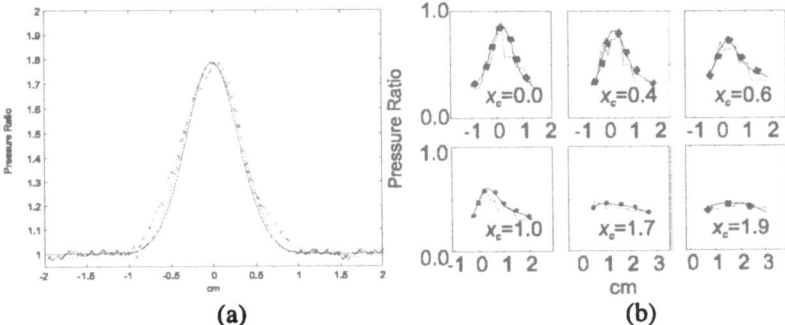

(a)   (b)

Fig. 5 – (a) Comparison for same geometry of the centerline of the tactile map and the two dimensional maps from finite element and empirical models (x – centerline of map, solid line – FEA model, dotted line – empirical model). There is less than a 2.6% mean squared difference between the three curves. (b) Individual pressure frames for a silicone rubber breast model with a 1.25 cm diameter, 0.825 diameter deep rigid spherical inclusion (dotted = empirical model, solid = FEA model, thick solid = actual data).

2.2 Forward Model Validation

In order to verify that the finite element and empirical models give equivalent results, a set of trials on four different silicone rubber breast models (d=1.25cm, h/d=0.825; d=1.55cm, h/d=1.0; d=1.55cm, h/d=1.4; and d=1.875cm, h/d=1.2) were conducted. The pressure frames and tactile maps were compared along the centerline of the indentor to the model derived results. Figure 5(a) shows an illustrative result. The average mean square difference between the model frames and the real data frames is less than 15%, primarily because of the noise in the real data.

To be sure that the empirical model accurately reflects the finite element results, they were compared on a frame by frame level. Figure 5(b) shows a representative set of frame by frame pressure curves for four lumps. The tests spanned a range of lump sizes from 0.5 cm to 2.5 cm in diameter, and depth ratios h/d from 0.6 to 1.8 diameters. Table 1 summarizes the mean squared error figures for ten cases. The average mean squared difference for these frames is less than 4.2%, while the average for all frames in a map it is 4.3%. The finite element and empirical models were also compared on the map level, and Table 2 summarizes the results.

Table 1 – Mean squared difference, MSD, between the empirical model and the finite element models for the indentor frames centered on the lump. Average MSD = 4.3%.

h/d	d=0.5cm	d=1.0	d=1.5	d=2.0	d=2.5
0.6	4.1%	4.3%	4.1%	4.1%	4.2%
1.8	4.1%	4.2%	4.2%	4.0%	4.1%

Table 2 – Mean squared difference between the empirical model and the finite element models for the composite maps. Average MSD = 2.5%.

h/d	d=0.5	d=1.0	d=1.5	d=2.0	d=2.5
0.6	2.4%	2.7%	2.5%	2.3%	2.2%
1.8	2.3%	2.5%	2.4%	2.5%	2.6%

2.3 Inverse Models

Because the rubber model data and the finite element and empirical models showed good agreement in the test cases, we ran a larger set of models to determine the trends that would be present in the tactile maps. These tests spanned all possible combinations of mass diameters 0.5, 1.0, 1.5, 2.0 and 2.5 cm, mass depths of 0.6, 0.8, 1.0, 1.2, 1.5 and 2.0 diameters, and mass stiffness to fat stiffness ratios of 2,5,8,10 and 100 times. These maps are Gaussian and can be fit with

$$P_{map}(x) = a \cdot e^{-\left(x^2/2\sigma\right)} + 1. \tag{5}$$

There are some combinations of lump size and depth that lead to identical output pressure distributions, for a given stiffness ratio. More cases overlap if the lump stiffness is varied. However, Figure 6 makes it clear that the stiffness of the lump makes very little difference to the width of the pressure distribution for lumps greater than eight times as stiff as the fat. Fortunately, our measurements of the elastic properties of breast lumps show that they are at least eight times as stiff as the fat tissue [22]. We ignore the distribution width variations because of stiffness and assume that all lumps are hard ($E_2/E_1 = 100$).

The models reveal that the width of the distribution increases with lump depth and also show that the percent change in width of the pressure distribution (referenced to 1 diameter deep) can be fit with the allotropic relationship, $\Delta\sigma = ea^f$ where e and f are real numbers, and is shown in Figure 7(a). Figure 7(b) reveals that σ is linearly related to the lump diameter at one diameter depth. Therefore

$$d = m \cdot (\sigma/\Delta\sigma) + b. \tag{6}$$

In order to extend this inversion algorithm to the full tactile map, we observe that the three dimensional maps created with the real system also appear to be Gaussian and we minimize the squared error between the map and

$$P_{map}(x, y) = a \cdot e^{-\left(\frac{x^2}{2\sigma_x^2} + \frac{y^2}{2\sigma_y^2}\right)} + 1. \tag{7}$$

We use Equation 6 to determine the two diameters, d_x and d_y of the lump from the fit.

3 Clinical Testing

To test the hypothesis that tactile imaging is more accurate than clinical breast examination (CBE) or ultrasound at assessing size, a limited trial involving surgery patients was performed. We compared size estimates from the various methods with accurate size measurements of the masses after excision. After informed consent was obtained, subjects received mammograms, ultrasound examinations and CBEs following the usual course of treatment. One of the two surgeons in the study made three to five tactile maps of each mass prior to surgery using different stroking techniques. Maximum and minimum sizes were estimated in each of the maps as described above. The maximum size from CBE and ultrasound were recorded. After excision, the mass was bisected parallel to the plane of the tactile map and the palpable extents were measured using a caliper. One African-American and twenty-three Caucasian women participated in the study; ages ranged from 39 to 84 years old. Patients presented a total of 19 infiltrating ductal cancers, 2 fibroadenomas, 1 lobular carcinoma, 1 Phyllodes tumor, 1 papilloma and 1 patient with fibrotic adipose tissue.

Figure 8(a) shows an illustrative tactile map of an infiltrating ductal carcinoma and Figure 8(b) shows a photograph after surgical excision and bisection. Figure 9 presents a comparison of the maximum size estimates from ultrasound, CBE and tactile imaging, respectively, to the ex vivo size measurements made in the clinic. The average standard deviation of size estimated from multiple maps for a single mass is 15% (2.6 mm). The percent mean absolute error (MAE) between ultrasound and ex vivo measurements is 34%, for CBE it is 47% and for tactile imaging it is 17%, which makes tactile imaging more than twice as accurate as either clinical breast examination or ultrasound using this inversion algorithm. The slope of the best fit line with zero intercept for maximum size estimates from tactile imaging as compared to ex vivo size measurements is 1.04 ($r^2 = 0.64$), while for CBE it is 1.26 ($r^2 = 0.39$) and for ultrasound it is 0.90 ($r^2 = 0.14$). We have not presented size information from the mammograms, since only the presence or absence of a mass was typically reported. Of the 25 masses, 24 were visible in mammograms, one was not palpable and one was not visible on ultrasound.

4 Conclusions and Future Work

The inversion algorithms presented here performed well in clinical tests made on real breast lumps, and provided accuracy that was at least twice as accurate as either clinical breast examination or ultrasound breast examination. This validates that the model is useful to obtain results in the real clinical situation, and confirms that we have taken an appropriate approach. There are many improvements that could be made to the model, including elliptical rather than spherical lump geometry, mobile rather than well fixed lumps and non-linear tissue stiffness. Non-linear stiffness is important because it has been shown that tissue stiffness, and the change in tissue stiffness with strain are related to histological diagnosis [23,24]. These enhanced models could make it possible to develop feature extraction algorithms that enhance the utility of tactile imaging by taking it from a documentary to a diagnostic role.

5   Acknowledgements

We gratefully acknowledge the support of the Whitaker Foundation and Assurance Medical. We thank the entire team at Assurance Medical who made this project possible. We would also like to thank Drs. Edward Dalton, Kenneth Kern, Matthew Freedman, David Krag and Prof. Eric Grimson for many fruitful discussions.

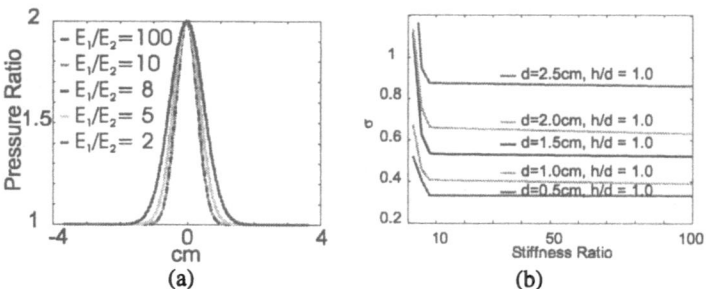

Fig. 6 – (a) Two-dimensional (FEA derived) tactile maps for a 0.5cm diameter lump, 1.0 diameter deep. (b) The width changes by less than 5% after the stiffness ratio exceeds 8.

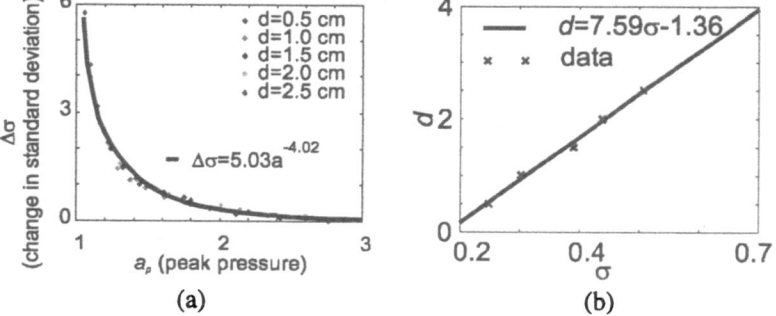

Fig. 7 – (a) The change in width of the pressure distribution, referenced to 1 diameter in depth, is related to the peak of the pressure distribution by an allotropic relationship. (b) At 1 diameter in depth, the fit parameter σ is linearly related to the diameter of the lump, d.

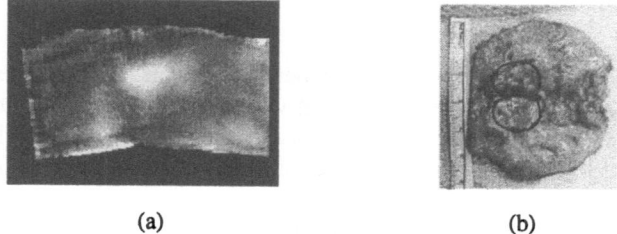

(a)   (b)

Fig. 8 – (a) Tactile map of an infiltrating ductal carcinoma. White = highest pressure. The lump is in the center of the map and the sternum is along the lower edge of the map. (b) Photograph of the same mass after surgical excision and bisection parallel to the imaging plane (the black ellipses are the approximate edge of the bisected halves of the tumor). The tactile map size is 15.7 mm by 13 mm while its ex vivo palpable size is 16 mm by 12 mm

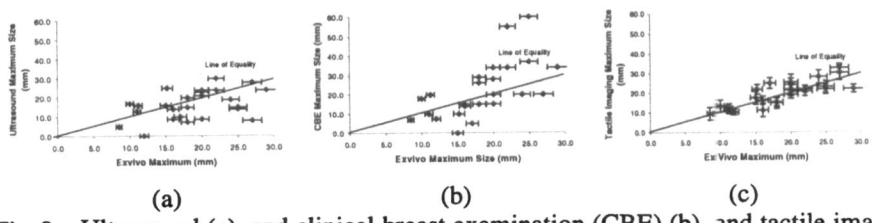

Fig. 9 – Ultrasound (a), and clinical breast examination (CBE) (b), and tactile imaging (c) for 24 subjects (25 masses). Error bars are +/- 5% deviation of the ex vivo size measurements (multiple measurements made by multiple examiners) and +/- one standard deviation of the images made of each mass. One ultrasound or CBE examination was performed; no error bars are shown. One mass was not palpable (zero diameter in CBE) and one was not visible on the ultrasound (zero diameter).

References

1. Dixon JM and Mansel RE. Symptoms Assessment and Guidelines for Referral. BMJ. 309;722-726, 1994 Sep. 17.
2. Haagensen CD. Diseases of the Breast, 3rd Edition. p521-527 Philadelphia, Saunders 1986.
3. Lavin PT. Flowerdew G. Studies in variation associated with the measurement of solid tumors. Cancer. 46(5):1286-90, 1980 Sep 1.
4. Dario P, Bergamasco M and Sabatini A. Sensing body structures by an advanced robot system. Proceedings of the 1988 IEEE ICRA. vol.3 (1988) 1758-63.
5. Frei EH, Sollish BD, Yerushalmi S, U.S. Patent # 4,250,894, (1981)
6. Gentle, C.R. Mammobarography: a possible method of mass breast screening. *J. Biomed. Eng.*, Vol. 10. April 1988.
7. Koganezawa K, Takanishi A, Sugano S eds. Development of Waseda Robot: The Study of Biomechanisms and Kato Laboratory (3rd Edition). Waseda University. 1991.
8. Sarvazyan AP. Knowledge-Based Mechanical Imaging. Proceedings of the 10th IEEE Symposium on Computer-Based Medical Systems. p120-125, 1997.
9. Cespedes I, Ophir J, Ponnekanti H and Maklad N. Elastography: elasticity imaging using ultrasound with application to muscle and breast in vivo. Ultrasonic Imaging. (1993) 15(2):73-88.
10. Manduca A, Muthupillai R, Rossman PJ, Greenleaf JF, Ehman RL. Visualization of tissue elasticity by magnetic resonance elastography. Proceedings of Fourth International Conference on Visualization in Biomedical Computing (VBC'96). p.xii+610, 63-8 22-25 Sept. 1996
11. Konofagou E, Dutta P, Ophir J, Cespedes I. Reduction of stress nonuniformities by apodization of compressor displacement in elastography. Ultrasound in Medicine & Biology. 22(9):1229-36, 1996.
12,21. Johnson, KL. Contact Mechanics. Cambridge University Press. 1987.
13,23. Krouskop TA, Wheeler TM, Kallel F, Garra BS, Hall T, The Elastic Moduli of Breast Prostate Tissues Under Compression, *Ultrasonic Imaging*. 20:151-159, (1998).
14. Harris JR, Lippman ME, Morrow M and Hellman S. Diseases of the Breast. Lippincott-Raven. 1996.
15. Fung YC. Biomechanics: Mechanical Properties of Living Tissues 2nd Edition. Springer Verlag, NY. 1993.
16. Goodier, J.N. Concentration of stress around spherical and cylindrical inclusions and flaws. *Phil. Mag.*, 7(22):678. 1936.
17. Eshelby, J.D. The determination of the elastic field of an ellipsoidal inclusion and related problems. *Proc. R. Soc. Lond.*, A 241:376-396.
18. Yu, H. Y. and Sanday, S.C. Elastic field in joined semi-infinite solids with an inclusion. *Proc. R. Soc. Lond.* A 434:521-530. 1991.
19. Fearing, R. S. and Hollerbach, J. M. Basic solid mechanics for tactile sensing. *International Journal of Robotics Research*, 4(3):40-54, Fall 1985.
20,22,24. Wellman, PS and Howe, RD. The Mechanical Properties of Breast Tissues In Compression. Harvard BioRobotics Laboratory Technical Report #99003. 1999.

Finite Element Model
of a Fetal Skull
Subjected to Labour Forces

R. J. Lapeer and R. W. Prager

Department of Engineering, Cambridge University, Cambridge, UK

Abstract. The objective of this research is to study the deformation of a human fetal skull when subjected to labour forces. The shape of the fetal skull is recovered from a laser-scanned replica model. A combined technique of thin-plate spline surface fitting and an advancing front triangulation method provide a valid mesh model for finite element analysis. The skull is assumed to be a shell object and contains about 64,000 shell elements. The area around the parietal bones is subjected to a pressure load, exerted by the uterine cervix during the first stage of labour. The analysis investigates the influence of four parameters in the model. The resulting deformations agree with previous findings in terms of shape of deformation but are smaller in terms of degree of deformation. This may imply that moulding of the fetal skull during the birth process cannot be solely modelled by the short-time effect of a static load but effects such as hyper-elastic behaviour of the sutures, visco-elastic behaviour of the cranial bones and sliding contact between the head and surrounding tissues should be considered.

1 Introduction

In obstetrics, mechanical concepts are undeniably of major importance. Despite being applied for more than a century, for example the use of mechanical tools such as the forceps and more recently the vacuum extractor for operative delivery, these concepts are usually based on *mechanisms* of labour rather than *mechanics* of labour [1]. Mechanisms of labour are primarily concerned with fetal *movements* of which the majority occur in the second stage of labour. Mechanics of labour is however a much wider concept, involving both the first and second stage of labour and focusing on theoretical mechanical concepts rather than practical issues which are aimed at the delivery of the baby.
From as early as 1861, Kristeller ([1]) attempted to measure the forces during labour by inserting balloons into the uterus via the vagina. Many investigations to measure the forces, and more specific the amniotic pressure and the pressure between the fetal head and the cervix during the first stage, have followed since. The most recent results, amongst many, are from Lindgren [2], Rempen [3] and Antonucci [4].
Bell [1] gave an excellent overview in the early 70's on the mechanical issues of

human parturition. His work is an invaluable contribution since it covers possibly all the work done until 1972.

In the early 90's, the *computerised birth simulation* became a fashionable topic. Wischnik et al. [5] simulated birth by reconstructing the geometry of the birth canal and the fetal head by means of MRI images and the Marching Cubes algorithm [6]. Similar work was done by Geiger [7] and later on by Liu et al. [8]. The idea behind a birth simulation is to allow an obstetrician to assess the probability of a successful vaginal delivery a sufficient time before the actual event. The simulation could for example indicate possible complications such as *cephalo-pelvic disproportion*. This would allow the obstetrician to plan an *elective Caesarian section* rather than risking an *emergency Caesarian section* at the time of delivery. One important issue which was not covered in depth in the work of Wischnik, Geiger and Liu is the moulding of the fetal skull during delivery.

McPherson and Kriewall performed invaluable research in 1980 regarding the biomechanics of fetal head moulding. They evaluated the elasticity modulus of fetal cranial bone from seven stillborn babies [9] and analysed the behaviour of the parietal bones when subjected to the amniotic pressure, AP, and the head-to-cervix pressure, HCP, using a finite element model [10].

A realistic model of the biomechanical behaviour of the fetal skull when subjected to labour forces would allow to significantly improve the reliability and accuracy of a computerised simulation of birth and would also contribute to the investigation of *post-natal pathological conditions* caused by *excessive head moulding*.

The objective of this research is to improve this model by extending the analysis on the parietal bones as performed by McPherson and Kriewall to the fetal skull in its entirety. This requires a more accurate shape model and a more detailed analysis of deformation because of increased complexity.

2   Shape recovery and mesh generation

2.1   Data acquisition

Considering the fact that the cranial bones of the fetal skull are very thin compared to their surface dimensions [9], a shell-based model is justified[1]. Thus, the reconstruction of the outer surface would be sufficient to build a finite element mesh model composed of shell elements.

A surface model of a fetal skull was derived from laser-scanning a life-size model of a real fetal skull, designed and manufactured by ESP Ltd.

The purpose-built laser scanner from the Dept. of Medical Physics at UCL was developed for the simulation of maxillo-facial surgery [12]. A team of laser light is fanned out into a line and projected onto the object surface. When the line is viewed obliquely by a CCD camera it is curved, reflecting the shape of the surface at the intersection with the laser beam. The scanned object is placed on

---

[1] This abstraction has even been used to model adult skulls as reported by Hosey [11].

a turntable hence a matrix of data points around the surface is obtained. The collected data usually consists of between 20,000 and 60,0000 3D coordinates of points lying on the anatomical surface. Individual points can be recorded with a precision better than 0.5 mm. The triangulation of the data points is straight-forward because they form an ordered grid of points. One shortcoming of the laser-scanning system is the inability to scan the top and bottom part of the object. This requires the acquisition of several datasets to obtain data across the entire object. Furthermore, the acquisition suffers from bad connections (tri-angles with high aspect ratio) because data points are missing in concavities, noise due to interfering objects such as the supporting table, incorrect surface patterns because of vibrations and an unclosed gap between the first and last ar-ray of scanned points. In total, four datasets were acquired. To arrive at a single, complete and valid shape/mesh model the following operations were necessary:

1. Noise removal for each selected dataset: a customised software tool, the in-teractive mesh-modelling toolkit (*immtk*) allows easy removal of noise.
2. Registration of the selected datasets: based on the conventional approach of landmark matching followed by least-squares parameter estimation of an affine transformation.
3. Selection of valid parts of each selected dataset, resulting in a set of regis-tered, unconnected patches (Figure 1a).
4. Connection of the loose parts and interpolation of sections of missing data, to obtain a valid and complete mesh model. The methodology is outlined in the next section.

2.2 Surface interpolation, mesh generation and mesh optimisation

Thin-plate spline surface interpolation The thin-plate spline model is ideal for surface interpolation, when a significant part of the surface data is missing or invalid, because it minimises bending energy. An explicit thin-plate spline surface with radial basis function [13] is defined as :

$$z = f(x,y) = -U(r) = -r^2 \log(r^2) \tag{1}$$

where the coefficient of the radial basis function

$$r = \sqrt{(x^2 + y^2)} \tag{2}$$

The thin-plate spline surface parameters can be obtained from a set of valid data points on an unconnected or falsely connected patch, selected by the user.

Surface patch triangulation The first algorithm involves triangles *growing* from the centre of the surface towards the outer boundary Γ. The *invariant* of the algorithm ensures that generated triangles do not penetrate the boundary. When the *post-condition* is reached, i.e. no triangles can be further expanded,

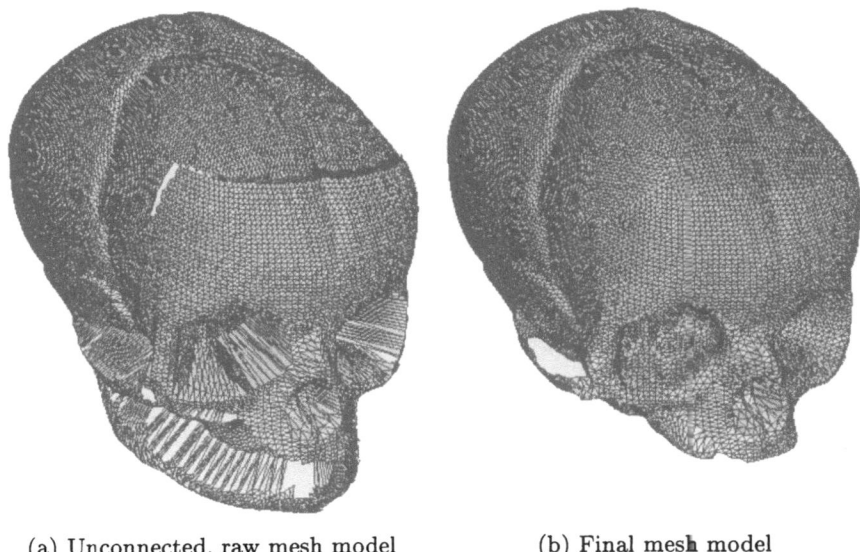

(a) Unconnected, raw mesh model   (b) Final mesh model

Fig. 1. Skull models before and after surface interpolation and remeshing.

an internal boundary is created from the interior triangles. A second algorithm, which we call the *welding* algorithm, connects the interior boundary to the original boundary Γ. The welding algorithm is based on the *advancing front principle*. The advancing front principle was originally developed by Lo [14] and has since widely been used in algorithms for finite element mesh generation and adaptation.

Mesh optimisation and refinement In finite element analysis (FEA), it is important that the elements in the mesh have a good aspect ratio to minimise numerical errors during the calculation of the stiffness matrix and the element normals.

The aspect ratio, ar, of a triangle can be defined as the ratio of the longest edge and the perpendicular distance from this edge to the opposite triangle vertex. The best aspect ratio is exhibited by the equilateral triangle: $ar = 1.1547$. Two simple approaches to optimise the aspect ratio of the mesh are the adjustment of a vertex towards the centre of its surrounding polygon on the surface, also known as Laplacian smoothing, and edge swapping. NAFEMS [15] advises: $ar \leq 4$.

Another important concept in FEA is the number of elements in the mesh model. This parameter is crucial to the accuracy of the solution of the analysis, as the latter converges to the exact solution of the problem, as the number of elements is increased [16]. Cubic spline interpolation of the boundary edges allows the creation of new vertices at arbitrary distances on the boundary. The algorithm described in the previous section can thus generate meshes of arbitrary refinement.

Results Figure 2 shows meshes of a parietal bone [17]: The original mesh (a), the optimised mesh using Laplacian smoothing and edge swapping (b) and a newly created mesh with refinement (c).

Figure 1b shows the connected and optimised mesh of the fetal skull.

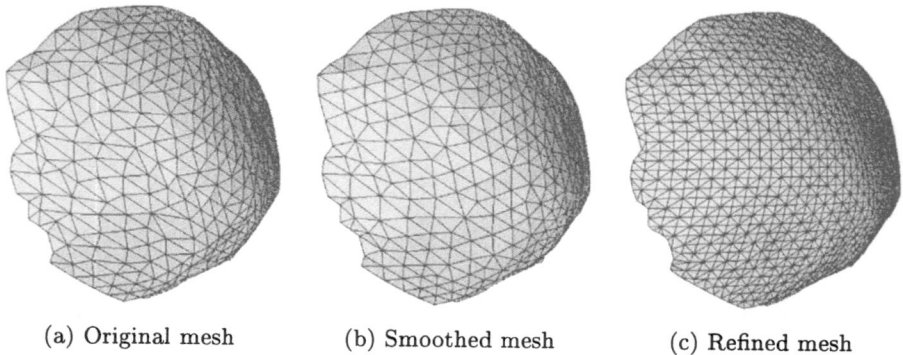

(a) Original mesh   (b) Smoothed mesh   (c) Refined mesh

Fig. 2. Mesh models of a parietal bone.

3   Finite element analysis of the fetal skull

3.1   General concepts

The accurate description of a physical problem using a finite element model is sensitive to an array of possible errors [18]:

- Modelling error: Whatever the analysis method, we do not analyse the actual physical problem but the mathematical model of it. To arrive at such a model, we make assumptions which do not always reflect the exact behaviour of the problem.
- Numerical error: The numerical output has been rounded and truncated during the course of the analysis. Numerical errors are usually small but some modelling practises can significantly increase them.
- Discretisation error: The physical structure which we analyse and the mathematical model have infinitely many degrees of freedom (d.o.f.) whilst the finite element model has a finite number of d.o.f. This implies that the discretisation error will tend to zero as the number of elements increases but will never become zero.

3.2   Experiment: initial setup

The ABAQUS/Standard software was used to perform the analysis.

Geometry:

- The fetal skull model contains 63,413 elements which is sufficient to describe the geometry of the skull in detail (average triangle dimensions < 1 mm.) and the field variable under investigation, i.e. deformation.
- The mandible is left out since it is not a fixed part of the cranium and is unlikely to contribute to the moulding process.
- The thickness of the shells of the cranial vault is initially set to 0.75 mm., an average value of the thickness of parietal and frontal bones as reported in [10].
- The thickness of the maxilla, palate and skull base is set to 2 mm. - an estimate based on the thickness of the palate of the fetal skull model.
- The thickness of the fontanelles is initially set to 0.75 mm. - the same value as for the cranial bones.

Direction of the axes: See Figures 4 and 5a.

Elements: Constant strain elements (ABAQUS S3R) for both the fontanelle/suture structures and the bones of the fetal skull. The S3R shell element in ABAQUS provides accurate results in most loading situations and is valid for thin- and thick-shell problems. However, due to its constant bending and membrane strain approximations, high mesh refinement is required to capture pure bending deformations or solutions to problems of high strain gradients.
The bones of the cranial vault, i.e. parietal and frontal bones, temporal bones and occipital bone, are modelled with thin-shell elements. Figure 3 shows a view of the skull base which is composed of thick-shell elements to emulate its stiffer behaviour.

Material properties: Based on findings reported by McPherson and Kriewall [9].

- Fetal cranial bone (at term)[2]: orthotropic, plane stress,
  $E_1 = 3.86e3$ MPa, $E_2 = 0.965e3$ MPa, $G_{12} = 1.582e3$ MPa,
  $G_{13} = G_{23} = 1.582e3$ MPa, $\nu = 0.08$
- Fontanelles and sutures: isotropy assumed, $E = 31.5$ MPa, $\nu = 0.45$, values of the properties of the dura mater as reported by McElhaney [19].

Boundary conditions: Three nodes at the base of the skull, located at the left and right tympanic ring and the middle of the palate respectively are fully built-in to avoid rigid body displacement. Three extra nodes on the maxilla to avoid rotation about the x-axis.

---

[2] E_i is Young's modulus in the ith local direction,
 G_{ij} is the shear modulus in the plane with normal in the ith local direction and force in the jth direction, ν is Poisson's ratio.

Loads: The loading of the skull is modelled at the first stage of labour where the head is in contact with the cervix. The pressures are average values based on values reported in [2–4]:

- amniotic pressure, *AP*: 50 mmHg. - above the suboccipito-bregmatic plane,
- head-to-cervix pressure, *HCP*: 250 mmHg. - below the suboccipito-bregmatic plane.

Figure 4 shows the pressure distribution: the light-coloured area above the *SOB* plane (positive z-direction) is subjected to amniotic pressure. The dark-coloured band just below the *SOB* plane (negative z-direction) is the head-to-cervix pressure. The light-coloured area beyond the high pressure region is not subjected to any loading.

Analysis: Static analysis assuming non-linear geometry.

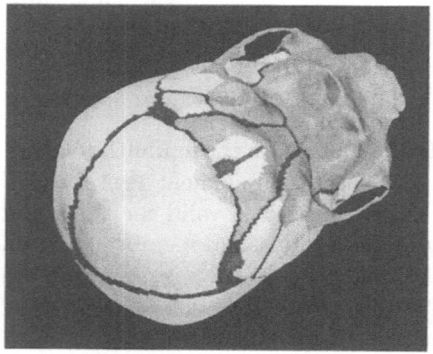 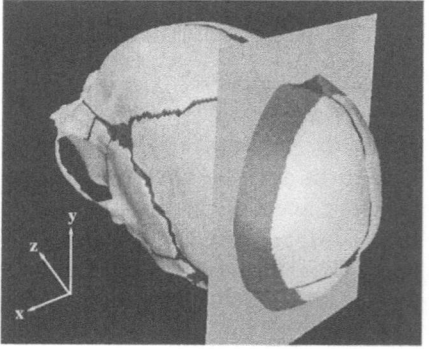

Fig. 3. Fetal skull base: The dark-grey region is composed of thick-shell elements.

Fig. 4. Pressure distributions - *AP*: above the *SOB* plane; *HCP*: dark-coloured band below the *SOB* plane.

3.3   Objectives

In this preliminary experiment we aim to assess the deformation of the bones of the cranial vault. McPherson and Kriewall [10] analysed the deformation of the parietal bones when subjected to the amniotic pressure and cervical pressure during the first stage of labour.

The current analysis extends the investigation to the behaviour of the entire skull and assesses the sensitivity of the results towards changes of the thickness of the bones and sutures, the elasticity and shear moduli and the pressure. Table 1 reports the parameter settings for each analysis. The first analysis is based on the average values as reported earlier. In subsequent analyses, the values of the elasticity and shear moduli, shell thickness and maximum pressure are set to such boundary values, within their valid range, as to increase the moulding effect. Evaluations are based on measurements of the bi-parietal diameter, BPD, the sub-occipito bregmatic diameter, $SOBD$, the orbito-vertical diameter, $OrVD$ and the maxillo-vertical diameter, $MaVD$, before and after moulding (See Figure 5).

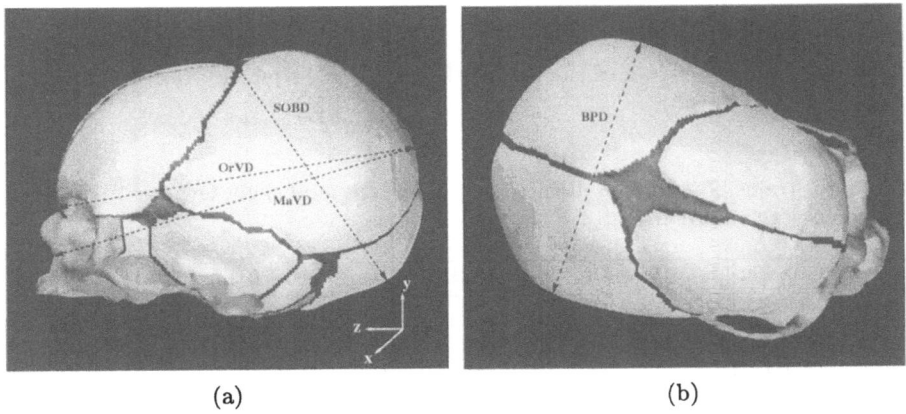

(a)   (b)

Fig. 5. Diameters for evaluation of fetal skull moulding.

Table 1. Analysis parameters.

Analysis	E_1 (MPa)	E_2 (MPa)	G_{12} (MPa)	G_{13} (MPa)	thickness bone (mm)	thickness sut/font (mm)	HCP (MPa)
1	3.860E3	0.965E3	1.582E3	1.582E3	0.750	0.750	-33.33E-3
2	2.830E3	0.570E3	1.160E3	1.160E3			
3	3.860E3	0.965E3	1.582E3	1.582E3		0.375	
4					0.600	0.600	
5					0.750	0.750	-53.28E-3

3.4 Results

Table 2 reports:

- The values of the BPD, $SOBD$, $OrVD$ and $MaVD$ as reported by Sorbe and Dahlgren [20]: they performed a clinical trial on 319 deliveries, without complications, measuring the diameters shortly after birth and three days

later. If we consider restitution of the skull as the inverse process of moulding then the diameters measured after three days correspond to the original
dimensions whilst those measured shortly after birth correspond to the dimensions after moulding. In Table 2, row 0 reports the *original* diameters;
row 1 reports the elongation(+) or compression(-) after moulding[3].
- The values of the *BPD*, *SOBD*, *OrVD* and *MaVD* as a result of our
  analysis. Row 0 reports the original diameters[4]. Subsequent rows report the
  strain after moulding for each analysis as reported in Table 1.
- All reported values are in mm.

Figure 6 shows the shape of the skull before and after deformation (deformation
magnification = 10.0).

Table 2. Strains of four main diameters (mm.) of the fetal skull. Own results, L-P, are
compared with results from S-D [20].

Diameter	S-D(0)	S-D(1)	L-P(0)	L-P(1)	L-P(2)	L-P(3)	L-P(4)	L-P(5)
BPD	105.00	0.00	89.75	-0.07	-0.05	-0.21	-0.11	-0.03
SOBD	117.10	-1.70	88.71	-0.36	-0.42	-1.07	-0.68	-0.63
OrVD	126.90	+2.20	119.35	+0.10	+0.13	+0.25	+0.20	+0.17
MaVD	140.50	+1.90	129.28	+0.13	+0.15	+0.30	+0.24	+0.20

4   Discussion

Before we compare the results of our simulation with the measurements from
Sorbe and Dahlgren, we first discuss the effects of the change of parameters
amongst the different analyses[5], as shown in the lower section of Table 2:

- In analysis 3, the fontanelle/suture thickness was set to a lower bound based
  on values as reported in [21]. It appears to have the most significant effect
  to the stiffness of the skull. This observation is to some degree supported by
  the results from analysis 4.
- Changing the stiffness parameters of the cranial bones to a lower bound
  (analysis 2) does not seem to have a major effect. The explanation lies in
  the inherent stiffness of a shell-shaped object.
- Finally, the increase of the head-to-cervix pressure to a value of 400 mmHg.
  (analysis 5) has a significant effect on all diameters except on the *BPD*. A

---

[3] In the further course of this text we will refer to elongation/compression as *strain*.
This variable is however not the same as the strain, ϵ, which is commonly used in
stress analysis and is dimensionless.

[4] The diameters as measured by Sorbe and Dahlgren are larger because of the skin!

[5] Remember: Analysis 1 involves the initial settings.

possible explanation, similar to the previous one, is based on the stiffness of a shell: the BPD is measured near to, or possibly exactly on, the parietal tuberosities. The latter display the highest curvature of the parietal bone, hence increasing the pressure will have less effect than for example decreasing the bone thickness (analysis 4).

The resulting strains are direction-wise (i.e. elongation vs compression) in complete agreement with the measurements from Sorbe and Dahlgren [20] for the $SOBD$, $MaVD$ and $OrVD$: the $SOBD$ decreases during moulding whilst the $MaVD$ and $OrVD$ decrease. The magnitudes are however significantly smaller for the $MaVD$, $OrVD$ and $SOBD$, the latter to a lesser extent for the configuration of analysis 3. Possible explanations are:

- Effects such as hyper-elastic behaviour of the fontanelles/sutures [21] and visco-elastic behaviour of the skull bones [22] have not been considered. These effects would increase the strains significantly under the same material properties and loading conditions.
- The variable thickness of the skull as reported in [9, 10], varying from higher values at the ossification centres of the bone to lower values at the periphery, will decrease the overall stiffness.
- The measurements reported by Sorbe and Dahlgren [20] are not entirely accurate:
  - Measurements as reported in Table 2 were performed by a photographic method. The advantage of this procedure, as opposed to the use of obstetric callipers, is the elimination of the effect of the skin, the latter resulting in a significant underestimate of the true value. The drawback however is the inability to correctly position the skull, hence parallax errors on the measurements result.
  - The inter-observer variance (from ten different observers on a single child) was 2.7 mm. for the $SOBD$, 2.1 mm. for the BPD, 2.8 mm. for the $OrVD$ and 2.3 mm. for the $MaVD$.

Sorbe and Dahlgren did not find significant changes for the BPD. Our results show a small decrease of the BPD, significant though because of the non-stochastic nature of our 'measurements'.

Figure 6 shows the lifting of the parietal bones when subjected to the cervix pressure. This phenomenon is commonly known by obstetricians and paediatricians and has also been reported in [10] and [23]. However, the figure shows that the frontal bones lift as well. Since they are mainly subjected to the amniotic pressure, some of the effect might come from the parietal bones.

5   Conclusion

An accurate model on the behaviour of the fetal skull during and shortly after delivery is of major importance to the obstetric and paediatric community. We presented a preliminary analysis on this behaviour by assessing the deformation

of a fetal skull when subjected to pressures during the first stage of labour.
The shape of the skull was acquired from laser-scanned data. The acquisition
of a CT dataset, though difficult to obtain for a healthy newborn, could be an
improvement in terms of more accurate modelling of the internal structures of
the skull[6].

The combined surface interpolation/mesh generation method allows us to create
a valid, compatible and optimised mesh-model. This method works well for level
surfaces but further improvement towards a fully 3D implementation should be
considered to avoid 'patching' of general 3D surfaces such as the skull.

The results of the FEA do correspond with measurements as reported in [20] in
terms of *shape of deformation*, however, the *degree of deformation* is significantly
lower. Possible explanations to the *over-stiffness* of our model were mentioned
in the previous section.

The model as presented in this study, despite being significantly more accurate
than the previous model of McPherson and Kriewall [9], can still be considerably
improved by:

- consideration of the skin: the elastic properties of the skin would reduce the
  effect of the pressures on the cranium,
- consideration of the incompressibility of the brain: the model should include
  a parameter to allow for deformation without change of volume,
- the effect of the entire dura mater rather than fontanelles and sutures only,
- geometric modelling of the inner structures of the skull from data obtained
  from a CT dataset of a fetal or newborn head,
- more reliable values of material constants and dimensions,
- more accurate measurements of pressure distributions as exerted on the fetal
  skull, during the first and second stage of labour,
- the consideration of the second stage of labour, when the fetal head is in
  contact with the soft tissues of the birth canal and the bony pelvis,
- to model the problem using *sliding contact* analysis rather than *static* analysis.

Fetal head moulding is a phenomenon with both positive and negative aspects.
The positive aspect manifests itself during the birth process where the moulding
of the skull allows the fetus to pass through the birth canal even when the
dimensions of the latter are restricted. On the contrary, excessive head moulding
can result into pathological conditions, shortly after birth or even a long term
thereafter. A realistic model of the biomechanical behaviour of the fetal skull
when subjected to labour forces would significantly improve the *sensitivity* and
specificity of a *computerised simulation of birth*, used as a tool for timely decision
on mode of delivery. It would also contribute to the investigation of *post-natal
pathological conditions* caused by *excessive head moulding*.

The model as presented in this paper is therefore a big step forwards into a
better understanding of the *mechanics of fetal head moulding* and its potential
applications.

---

[6] Care should be taken however since the resolution of conventional CT images is of
the order of magnitude of the thickness of the cranial bone.

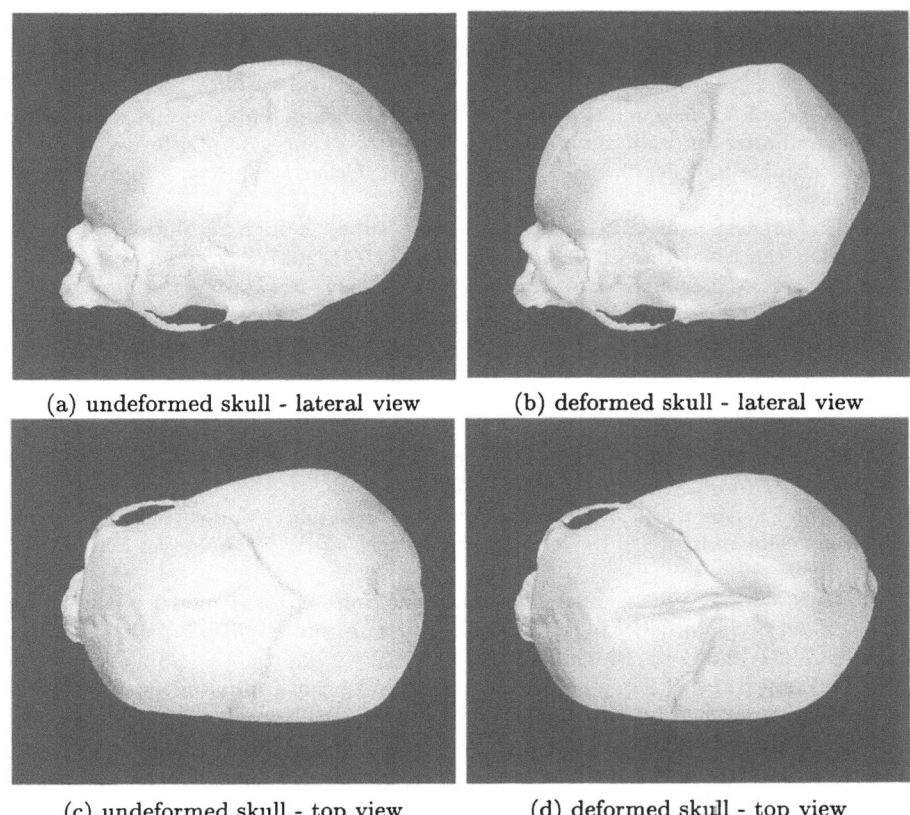

(a) undeformed skull - lateral view   (b) deformed skull - lateral view

(c) undeformed skull - top view   (d) deformed skull - top view

Fig. 6. Fetal skull before and after moulding (deformation magnification = 10).

Acknowledgements

We wish to thank Dr. Robin Richards from the Dept. of Medical Physics at UCL for his help (and patience) to obtain the laser-scan data of the fetal skull model.

References

1. F. Bell. *The bio-mechanics of human parturition: A fundamental approach to the mechanics of the first stage of labour.* PhD thesis, University of Strathclyde - Glasgow, 1972.
2. L. Lindgren and C.N. Smyth. Measurement and interpretation of the pressures upon the cervix during normal and abnormal labour. *J. Obstet Gynaec. Brit. Cwlth*, 68:901–915, 1961.
3. A. Rempen and M. Kraus. Pressures on the fetal head during labour. *J. Perinat. Med*, (19):199–206, 1991.

4. M.C. Antonucci et al. Simultaneous monitoring of the head-to-cervix, intrauterine pressure and cervical dilatation during labour. *Med.Eng.Physics*, 19(4):317–326, 1997.

5. A. Wischnik et al. Zur prävention des menschlichen geburtstraumas i.mitteilung: Die computergestützte simulation des geburtsvorganges mit hilfe der kernspintomographie und der finiten-element-analyse. *Geburtshilfe und Frauenheilkunde*, 53:35–41, 1993.

6. W.E. Lorensen and H.E. Cline. Marching cubes, a high resolution 3d surface construction algorithm. *Computer Graphics*, 21(4), 1987.

7. B. Geiger. *Three-dimensional modeling of human organs and its application to diagnosis and surgical planning*. PhD thesis, Ecole des Mines de Paris, April 1993.

8. Y. Liu, M. Scudder, and M.L. Gimovsky. Cad modeling of the birth process part ii. In H. Sieburg, S. Weghorst, and K. Morgan, editors, *Health Care in the Information Age*, pages 652–666. IOS Press and Ohmsha, 1996.

9. G.K. McPherson and T.J. Kriewall. The elastic modulus of fetal cranial bone: A first step towards an understanding of the biomechanics of fetal head moulding. *Journal of Biomechanics*, (13):9–16, 1980.

10. G.K. McPherson and T.J. Kriewall. Fetal head molding : An investigation utilizing a finite element model of the fetal parietal bone. *Journal of Biomechanics*, (13):17–26, 1980.

11. R.R. Hosey and Y.K. Liu. A homeomorphic finite element model of the human head and neck. In R.H. Gallagher et al., editor, *Finite Elements in Biomechanics*. John Wiley and Sons, Binghamton USA, 1982.

12. A.D. Linney et al. Three-dimensional visualization of computerized tomography and laser scan data for the simulation of maxillo-facial surgery. *Medical Informatics*, 14(2):109–121, 1989.

13. F.L. Bookstein. *Morphometric tools for landmark data*. Cambridge University Press, New-York, 1991.

14. S.H. Lo. A new mesh generation scheme for arbitrary planar domains. *Int.J.Num.Meth.Eng*, 21:1403–1426, 1985.

15. NAFEMS. *A Finite Element Primer*. National Agency for Finite Element Methods and Standards, Glasgow, Schotland, 1987.

16. K-J. Bathe. *Finite Element Procedures*. Prentice-Hall, Englewood Cliffs, New-Jersey, 1996.

17. R.J. Lapeer and R.W. Prager. 3d shape recovery of a newborn skull using thin-plate splines. *Computerized Medical Imaging and Graphics*. In Press.

18. R.D. Cook. *Finite Element Modeling for Stress Analysis*. John Wiley, USA, 1995.

19. J.H. McElhaney et al. Mechanical properties of cranial bone. *Journal of Biomechanics*, 3:495–511, 1970.

20. B. Sorbe and S. Dahlgren. Some important factors in the molding of the fetal head during vaginal delivery - a photographic study. *Int.J.Gynaecol.Obstet.*, (21):205–212, 1983.

21. D.L. Bylski, T.J. Kriewall, et al. Mechanical behaviour of the fetal dura mater under large deformation biaxial tension. *J.Biomechanics*, 19(1):19–26, 1996.

22. Y.C. Fung. *Biomechanics*. Springer-Verlag, USA, 1993.

23. P. Govaert. *Cranial Haemorrhage in the Term Newborn Infant*. Mac Keith Press - Cambridge University Press, London, 1993.

Modeling the Dynamics of a Human Liver for a Minimally Invasive Surgery Simulator

F. Boux de Casson and C. Laugier

INRIA Rhône-Alpes / GRAVIR
38330 Monbonnot Saint Martin, France
{Francois.Boux-de-Casson, Christian.Laugier}@inrialpes.fr
http://www.inrialpes.fr/sharp

Abstract. *Minimally invasive surgery techniques will probably be widely used in the near future for a large number of surgical procedures. However, these procedures are difficult to learn and high-fidelity computer simulation will be of great help to acquire these skills. In this paper, we describe how we have modeled a human liver for the purpose of developing an interactive dynamic simulator. This model makes use of a combination of 2D and 3D spring-dampers meshes to represent the heterogeneous mechanical characteristics of the liver. The related models and algorithms have been designed in order to obtain real-time responses to the operator actions, done using a virtual tool . . .*

1 Introduction

1.1 Motivations and Addressed Problems

Minimally invasive surgery techniques, i.e. surgery performed with instruments inserted through small incisions rather than by making a large incision to expose operation site, will probably been widely used in the near future for a large number of surgical procedures. The main advantage of this new technique is the reduced trauma to healthy tissue which is the leading cause of post-operative pain and long hospital stay of the patient. Consequently, minimally invasive surgery leads to significantly reduce the hospital stay and rest periods (and therefore the procedure's cost), at the expense of more difficult techniques performed by the surgeon. Such techniques require a long training period for the practitioner, involving appropriate computer graphics and Robotics tools. Thanks to the recent advances in computer graphics and processor technologies, it is now possible for researchers to begin exploring the issues involved in creating high-fidelity computer simulations of medical procedures. Such simulations require not only accurate geometric models of anatomical structures, but also realistic dynamic physical models for various tissues.

The purpose of this paper is to address this issue under a particular instance of the problem : how to model a human liver for obtaining a realistic real-time dynamic simulation of the liver behavior. The main characteristics of the problem that have to be considered for that purpose are that :

- The practitioner has to interact with the virtual liver using various interfaces (including a haptic interface). Consequently, the simulation process must satisfy real-time constraints. Moreover this simulation process must include appropriate procedures for detecting collisions and processing physical interactions;
- The simulated objects have complex geometric shapes, are volumetric and often non homogeneous. Both 2D and 3D models have to be used to obtain correct behaviors, and to make it possible to simulate the effects of physical interactions (collisions, cutting ...);
- The involved bodies seldom present a heterogeneous dynamic behavior, and tissues having various mechanical properties are in interaction (e.g. bones, muscles and blood).

In this paper, we propose a dynamic model of the liver which takes care into account the three previous characteristics. This model makes use of a combination of 2D and 3D spring-damper meshes to represent the heterogeneous mechanical characteristics of the liver. It allows to simulate in real-time the deformations of a liver subjected to interactions with a virtual tool. Such simulation includes body deformations, collision detection and physical interaction processing (e.g. sliding on the surface of the virtual liver using a virtual tool). This work has been performed within the framework of the French AISIM project aimed at developing techniques for computer assisted surgery.

1.2   Related Work

One of the main difficulty when developing a simulator for surgical operation, relies in the fact that the system allows interaction with a human operator in real-time, at least visually. The first simulators used 2D models (like in [3]), but such approach do not allow the simulation of complex physical interactions, like cutting operations, because all simulated bodies are hollow. The model proposed by Sagar et al.[12] allows a more realistic tissue simulation but it is exclusively dedicated to the simulation of interventions on the eye.

D. Terzopoulos and K. Waters [13] make use of a heterogeneous multi-layer spring-damper mesh to model a human face and to produce realistic facial animations. A bi-phasic elasticity is used to represent the nonlinear characteristics of the skin. But no geometrical collision detection and physical collision computation are implemented, which do not allow to interact with the model. Furthermore, because the model isn't volumetric, it's not relevant in our case.

M. Bro-Nielsen and S. Cotin [2] propose a volumetric model based on finite element method. This model makes it possible to simulate in haptic real-time volumetric objects composed of 500 nodes (inside and on the surface). But only an *homogeneous* elastic behavior is simulated. Moreover it is not possible to slide *on the surface of the model* with a virtual tool, but only to apply forces on the nodes of the external mesh.

2   Modeling the Liver

2.1   Main Physical Characteristics of a Human Liver

The liver is an organ located under the diaphragm, on the right, and weighs approximately 2.3 kg. Its mainly used to filter blood and to ensure a constant concentration of glucose.

From the mechanical point of view, the liver is a very malleable body (its exact shape strongly depends on the bodies which are in contact with it). It is composed of two major parts :

1. an internal friable material, the "Parenchyma", which includes a complex vascular network (see fig.1);
2. an elastic skin called "Capsule of Glisson".

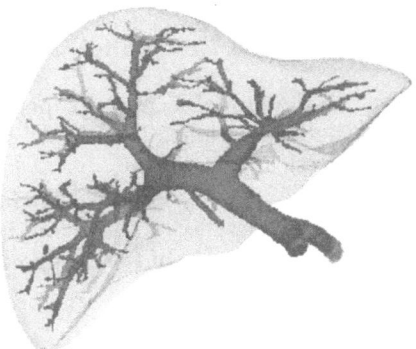

Fig. 1. A human liver, along with its intern vascular network.

Intuitively, one could coarsely represent the liver by a sponge filled with an incompressible liquid and covered by an elastic skin. Since the liver is primarily composed of blood (an incompressible fluid) one can reasonably suppose that its volume remains constant[1].

2.2   Outline of the Model

The experimental knowledge acquired by peoples working in the framework of the French AISIM project (including a surgeon), along with the study of some surgical interventions videos, have shown that the Parenchyma is a volumetric deformable body made of a material so friable that it can be cut or destroyed without using a sharp tool : the simple fact of compressing appropriately the Parenchyma is sufficient to "break it up" (and thus cutting operations can be done in this way, see fig.2).

Other previous experimental studies has also shown that the Capsule of Glisson is mainly an elastic skin (i.e. a 2D elastic surface), which may easily be broken by the interaction with an external rigid tool [4].

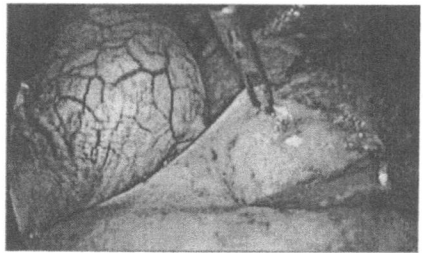

Fig. 2. Laparoscopic operation : Parynchyma and Glisson Capsule.

Consequently a heterogeneous model is required for modeling the behavior of the liver. In the sequel, we show how we have modeled the liver using two main components : a 2D component for modeling the Capsule of Glisson and a 3D component for modeling the Parenchyma. Each of this models include a geometrical and a physical component.

2.3   Geometrical Component of the Model

The geometric component of the model is used for performing the display operations and for detecting the interactions. This model is also used as a spatial frame for constructing the physical component.

We have chosen to make use of 2D mesh of triangles (see fig.3), for representing the Capsule of Glisson, and a tetrahedric mesh for the Parenchyma (i.e. the interior of the liver). The triangular facets of the skin correspond to the external faces of the tetrahedra of the internal 3D mesh.

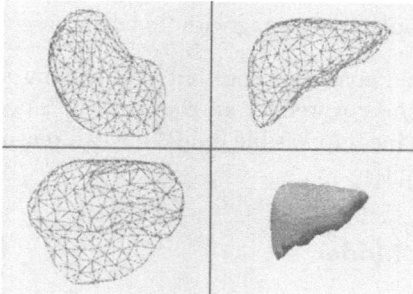

Fig. 3. A 2D mesh, representing the Capsule of Glisson of the liver (the associated 3D mesh representing the Parenchyma is not shown in the drawings).

2.4   Physical Component of the Model

The physical component of the model is used to compute the deformations of the liver resulting from the application of a set of external forces. These forces are either applied by the operator using the virtual tool (for instance controlled using a haptic interface), or generated by the physical interactions with other virtual objects of the scene.

The physical component is constructed from the 2D and 3D meshes (geometrical component of the model), by associating point masses to the nodes of the previous meshes and by adding spring-damper connectors between appropriate local subsets of point masses (see below). Two types of connectors are used for constructing this network : the "Linear Springs" and the "Torsion Springs" (see fig. 4).

The linear springs (denoted LS) are viscous-elastic components, whose main property is to give a viscous-elastic response to tensile forces. They are modelised by the following linear equation :

$$\boldsymbol{F}_a = (-\lambda \Delta d - \mu \dot{d}) \boldsymbol{k}_a \tag{1}$$

where Δd is the relative variation of the distance between the two connected point masses, and $\dot{d}$ is the relative speed of the previous two point masses.

The torsion springs (denoted TS) are used to define angular viscous-elastic constraints between three connected point masses. Such connectors are used to maintain some curvature properties of the surface (represented by a 2D mesh) by giving a viscous-elastic response to torsion forces. They are modelised by the following equation :

$$\boldsymbol{F}_b = (-\lambda \Delta \theta - \mu \dot{\theta}) \boldsymbol{k}_b \tag{2}$$

where $\Delta \theta$ is the relative variation of the angle described by the three connected point masses and $\dot{\theta}$ is the relative angular speed of the two point masses (see fig. 4).

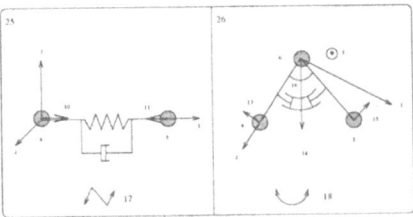

Fig. 4. The two different kinds of connectors

In order to model the heterogeneousness of the liver, the connectors of the 2D mesh and of the 3D mesh are parameterized in such a way that they exhibit different mechanical characteristics :

- The Capsule of Glisson is modelised using almost quasi-elastic linear and torsion connectors (i.e. the viscous components are negligible). This approach allows us to obtain the elastic behavior previously mentioned (§2.1), and to bring back the Capsule of Glisson to its initial shape when no force is applied on it.

– The Parenchyma is modelised by a network of point masses and linear spring-damper connectors located respectively on the nodes and the edges of the 3D geometrical mesh. This network is constructed using quasi-viscous linear connectors (i.e. the elastic component is negligible). This approach allows us to obtain a plastic behavior (the internal material can easily be deformed, but it cannot go back alone to its initial shape).

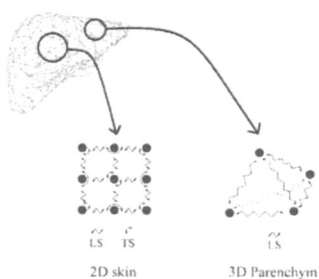

Fig. 5. The hybrid mesh approach. A 2D and a 3D spring-damper meshes are used to model respectively the Capsule of Glisson and the Parenchyma.

The combination of the two previous models (the elastic skin and the viscous volumetric internal material) gives us the required global behavior for the virtual liver (the behavior of a "sponge full of liquid covered by an elastic skin").

3   Outline of the Underlying Simulator System

The dynamic simulation of the liver has been achieved using the AlaDyn3D system developed by the SHARP research team.

This system allows the construction of complex physical scenes involving various interacting objects with different physical properties (deformable, rigid, friction, etc.) [9].

Object modeling The geometrical properties of an object are represented by a set of points and polygons which describe the surface of the object, and its interior. From this data the inertial matrix of rigid objects can be constructed through classical rigid body mechanics. For deformable objects the inertial properties of an object are implicitly defined by the distribution of the mass on its surface. These masses are interconnected by spring-damper connectors along the edges of the polygons, describing the constraint between pairs of masses.

Processing physical interactions Further, to detect the interaction between objects in a scene, a collision detection algorithm must be used. It is well known that collision detection is a computationally expensive task and a potential bottleneck in every application that aims to achieve real-time performance, such as in this case. For this reason it is essential to optimize the routines to their maximal extent. Gilbert et al.[7] have developed an algorithm which calculates, in linear time $O(n)$, the positive distance between the two convex bodies, and gives an approximation of the negative distance when 'small' inter-penetrations occur. Joukhadar et al.[10] extended this algorithm in order to obtain, in linear time, the points of contact on two deformable concave objects, as well as the direction of the contact and the volume of inter-penetration.

Once a collision has been detected an appropriate response must be computed. There exist several collision response models but for deformable objects the penalty method seems to be the most appropriate (N.B. impulse based methods make the assumption that a collision happens in a infinitely small interval of time, this clearly not being the case when dealing with deformable objects; see [5] for more details). Using this approach the force applied at a given point of an object where a collision has taken place is given by

$$F_c = \begin{cases} (-\lambda v - \mu \dot{v} v)k & \text{if } v < 0 \\ 0 & \text{otherwise} \end{cases} \tag{3}$$

where λ is the rigidity factor of the collision, μ is a damping factor (which represents the dissipation of energy), v the volume of inter-penetration, and k the contact direction.

Dynamic Equations Integration The integration method used in this simulator is the well-known explicit Newton-Euler. Using this method, point i of an object has the following update formulae.

$$v_i^{t+\Delta t} = v_i^t + \Delta t a_i^t$$
$$x_i^{t+\Delta t} = x_i^t + \Delta t v_i^t \tag{4}$$

where Δt is the time step used and x_i, v_i and a_i are respectively the position, the speed and the acceleration of the point. This integration method, known for it small time step problem when dealing with rigid objects, is good enough for our application, because we are dealing with soft object.

Finally, an important stage is the parameters identification. Indeed the elasticity and viscosity of each spring of the mass-spring model must be defined, in order to match with the real behavior of the simulated objects. A genetic algorithm, described in [8], allows us to do this for each object, with respect to real data.

4   Implementation and Experimental Results

The machine used for these tests was a biPentiumII 300 (one of the two processors was in fact used for OpenGL software display). The AlaDyn3D system has been used and we have implemented in C++.

About the Real Time Constraint The implementation constraint imposed by the real-time requirement depend on the type of media which is used to communicate with the system. Indeed, the frequency which is needed for a visual output is really smaller that the one which is required to process a haptic output. For instance, S.J. Lederman et al.[11] recommend frequencies of about 300 Hz for a good perception of the forces and about 1000 Hz to feel the textures.

For graphic interfaces a rate of 25 images is usually used.

Quantitative Results We have used as input a 2D mesh of the liver imported from the project "Visible Man". This 2D mesh has been pre-processed in order to reduce the number of facets, to smooth it, and to obtain the internal tetrahedric mesh (which has been calculated using the GHS3D[6] software of INRIA).

Then we have used this 2D and 3D meshes to generate the spring-dampers network (see §2.4). For the purpose of the dynamic simulation, the model of the liver has been placed in an empty space, without gravity, but with a slight environmental viscosity. A virtual tool, simulated by a rigid object controlled in position by the operator, makes it possible to apply forces to the model of the liver, and to follow compliantly the external boundaries of the virtual liver.

Table 1 shows the numbers of states of the system calculated per second of simulation according to the mesh used.

facets	tetrahedrons	states calculated per second
1224	6291	0.3
500	1974	12
320	1576	20

Table 1. Experimental results obtained for three layers of representation of the liver

We thus obtain a "comfortable" visual real-time performance for the coarsest grid and a "satisfactory" real-time performance for the intermediate mesh. For the finest mesh, the simulator was not fast enough to provide real-time simulations.

In the experiments, the simulations of the liver responses to various actions of the operator has shown qualitatively realistic behaviors : the liver was locally deformed under the effects of the forces applied using the rigid virtual tool and it went back to its initial shape as soon as no forces is applied to it. It was also possible to smoothly slide along its external surface, using the virtual tool.

Furthermore, if the operator, after having strongly pressed the liver, withdraws the tool, the liver didn't return fully to its initial shape (since it was submitted to a plastic deformation, see fig.6). This is due to the strong viscosity of the connectors of the Parynchyma, and simulates the malleable characteristic of the liver. Nevertheless, a real liver should finally come back slowly to its initial shape, that is not modelised in our case.

Although the constant volume constraint is not implemented in our simulator, we have observed that the volume of our liver model doesn't change more than 5%, according the operator applies small forces.

This model presents *qualitatively* a mechanical behavior which is closed to that of a real liver. It remains to find the exact numerical values of the parameters of elasticity and viscosity of the Parenchyma and the Capsule of Glisson. However, no force/displacement physical data is available yet, because of the difficulty in making the measurements *in vivo* (the liver being made up mainly of blood, its dynamic behavior is very different when not irrigated, because blood coagulates quickly). Such data should be available within the scope of the AISIM project, in a few months.

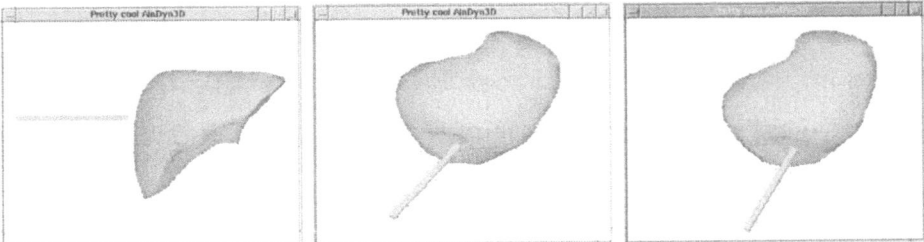

Fig. 6. An example of simulation. On the left is the initial configuration, on the middle and right is the system during manipulation

5   Conclusion and Perspectives

We have presented a heterogeneous volumetric model of the liver based on a mass-spring model. In conformity with the reality, our model presents two different dynamic behaviors for the Parenchyma and the Capsule of Glisson. The optimized collisions detection algorithm of AlaDyn3D makes possible to interact on the model in visual real-time using a virtual tool controlled in position.

But it's important to remember that the elasticity and viscosity parameters of our model were chosen intuitively, to obtain a good *qualitative* behavior at a good simulation frequency, so we strongly need real strain/displacement data to adjust our model.

The current work focuses on the three following points:

- The implementation of an algorithm allowing us to *interactively* modify the topology of the liver, and thus to carry out cutting operations;
- The identification and modification of the parameters of some connectors of the internal 3D mesh, in order to obtain a viscous-elastic behavior for modelising the internal vascular network of the liver (see fig.1);
- The optimization of the model in order to obtain a haptic real-time interface, thanks to the use of a dynamic refinement algorithm of the spring-damper mesh or an other numeric scheme for the integration of dynamic equations.

Acknowledgments

We thank the Epidaure team of the INRIA for the figure 1, as well as the Web site http://www.LAPAROSCOPY.COM/ for the illustration 2. Various people of the team working on AlaDyn3D also helped us: Ammar Joukhadar, Anton Deguet and Diego d' Aulignac.

References

1. O. Antonelli. Modélisation d'un foie humain. Master's thesis, Diplome d'ingénieur en Mathématiques Appliquées et Calcul Scientifique, 1998.
2. M. Bro-Nielsen and S. Cotin. Real-time volumetric deformable models for surgery simulation using finite elements and condensation. In *Proceedings of Eurographics*, volume 15, pages 57–66, 1996.
3. S.A. Cover, N.F. Ezquerra, J.F. O'Brien, R. Rowe, T. Gadacz, and E. Palm. Interactively deformable models for surgery simulation. In *Proceedings of ICRA*, pages 68–75, 1993.
4. P.J. Davies. Mathematical modelling for keyhole surgery simulation : spleen capsule as an elastic membrane. In *Journal of theoretical medecine*, 1998.
5. A. Deguet, A. Joukhadar, and C. Laugier. Models and algorithms for the collision of rigid and deformable bodies. In P. K. Agarwal, L. E. Kavraki, and M. T. Mason, editors, *Robotics: the algorithmic perspective*, pages 327–338. A K Peters, 1998. Proc. of the Workshop on the Algorithmic Foundations of Robotics. Houston, TX (US). March 1998.
6. P.L. George and H. Borouchaki. *Delaunay Triangulation and Meshing - Applications to Finite Elements*. Éditions Hermès, 1998.
7. E. G. Gilbert, D. W. Johnson, and S. S. Keerthi. A fast procedure for computing the distance between objects in three-dimentional space. In *Proc. of the IEEE Int. Conf. on Robotics and Automation*, 1988.
8. A. Joukhadar, F. Garat, and C. Laugier. Parameter identification for dynamic simulation. In *Proc. of the IEEE Int. Conf. on Robotics and Automation*, volume 3, pages 1928–1933, Albuquerque, NM (US), April 1997.
9. A. Joukhadar and C. Laugier. Dynamic simulation: Model, basic algorithms, and optimization. In *Proc. of the Workshop on the Algorithmic Foundations of Robotics*, Toulouse (FR), July 1996.
10. A. Joukhadar, A. Wabbi, and C. Laugier. Fast contact localisation between deformable polyhedra in motion. In *Proc. of the IEEE Computer Animation Conf.*, pages 126–135, Geneva (CH), June 1996.
11. S.J. Lederman and D.T. Pawluk. Lessons for the study of biological touch for robot tactil sensing. In *Advanced tactil sensing for robotics*, 1900.
12. M.A. Sagar, D. Bullivant, G.D. Mallinson, P.J. Hunter, and I. Hunter. A virtual environment and model of the eye for surgical simulation. Proc. SIGGRAPH '94 (Los Angeles, CA), pages 205–212. ACM SIGGRAPH, 1994.
13. D. Terzopoulos and K. Waters. Physically-based facial modelling, analysis, and animation. In *The journal of visualization and computer animation*, 1990.

EyeSi – A Simulator for Intra-ocular Surgery

Markus A. Schill[1], Clemens Wagner[1], Marc Hennen[1], Hans-Joachim Bender[2], and Reinhard Männer[1]

[1] Lehrstuhl für Informatik V, Universität Mannheim, B6,26, D-68131 Mannheim, Germany, http://www-mp.informatik.uni-mannheim.de
[2] Institut für Anästhesiologie und Operative Intensivmedizin, Fakultät für klinische Medizin Mannheim der Universität Heidelberg, D-68135 Mannheim, Germany
markus.schill@ti.uni-mannheim.de

Abstract. We present a computer-based medical workstation for the simulation of a vitrectomy that allows training and rehearsal of eye surgeons. The surgeon manipulates two original instruments inside a cardanically suspended mechanical model of the eye. The instrument positions are tracked by CCD cameras and monitored by a PC which then renders the scenery using a computer graphical model of the eye and the instruments. Stereoscopic images are presented to the user through two small LCD displays that are mounted to the system and emulate the stereo microscope used in real operations. The simulator offers the training of intra-ocular navigation as well as first approaches to interaction with pathological tissues using mass-spring and 3D-ChainMail models. All operations (tracking, rendering, collision detection, tissue manipulation) are computed in real-time on a PC.

Introduction

Operating inside the eye is one of the most demanding tasks in microsurgery: the involved structures are extremely sensitive, the field of view is limited and the operation is performed under a microscope, making hand-eye coordination very difficult. In general, two instruments are inserted into the eye. One is a lamp that lights the operation area. The other one is an operative instrument, used to interact with the pathological tissue. There are several operative devices which mainly differ in the way they interact with the tissue. They range from simple picks and cutters to highly sophisticated instruments like the vitrector. In the following we will focus on the vitrector which performs both sucking and cutting. With the vitrector, the vitreous humor, a gelatineous substance filling the eye, is removed and the eye is refilled with a clear liquid. This process is called vitrectomy and is performed in almost all intra-ocular surgeries to either remove an opaque vitreous humor or to obtain free access to the background of the eye.

Figure 1 illustrates a vitrectomy. Typical pathologies which make intra-ocular surgery necessary include the mentioned opaque vitreous humor, diabetic retinopathy and detached retinas. In case of diabetic retinopathy the surgeon

has to peel off pathological membranes covering the retina. In this case the vitrector can also be used to remove these membranes. From the simulation point
of view the vitrector is one of the most demanding operative instruments.

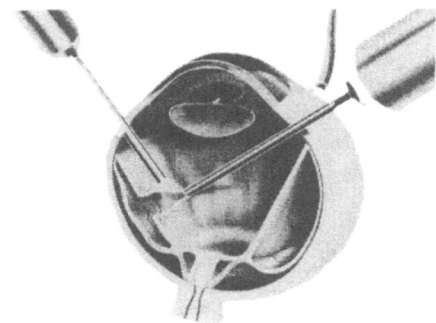

Fig. 1. Illustration of a vitrectomy. The vitrector is inserted from the right, the lamp
from the left side. Picture taken from Freyler: Augenheilkunde (1985)

Interacting with pathological tissues in the eye is very difficult. But even
the pure navigation of the operative instruments inside the eye is a delicate
task. Collisions with the highly damageable retina can be fatal and have to
be avoided in any case. The stereo microscope, used in eye surgery, provides
three dimensional view, which is a first means of orientation inside the eye. To
estimate the distance between a surgical instrument and the retina, the surgeon
additionally uses the strong shadow the instrument casts onto the retina with
the lamp.

Currently surgeons acquire practical knowledge in intra-ocular surgery entirely by assisting an experienced surgeon. This takes usually two years and
bears risks for the patients and the surgeons. The risky, long, and expensive
training could be very much improved by using a simulation system that provides the surgeon with a realistic operation environment.

Previous Work on Eye Surgery Simulation

There are several projects which have dealt with eye surgery simulations in the
past ([6], [4], [1]). [4] and [6] focus on the simulation of cataract surgery. They
either use Finite Element simulations to calculate tissue reaction or previously
measured interaction forces. The first could not be accomplished with interactive
rates whereas the latter is limited to pre-defined interaction points. In addition
[5] describes a current project at the University of Illinois which also aims at
the development of a vitrectomy simulator. The project emerged from [1], the
development of an anatomical eye atlas. Based on this atlas, the simulation

provides detailed graphics which also include periphery of the eye like eye muscles and parts of the face. In contrast to [6] and [4], [5] uses mass spring models to achieve interactive simulation rates. All mentioned projects use OpenGL surface graphics and expensive graphics workstations for rendering.

From our point of view, the Illinois simulator, as presented in [5], lacks an adequate mechanical setup. An eye model is absolutely necessary to provide realistic instrument handling and a simulation of the eye's movement during surgery. Also, including a high precision tracking of instruments- and eye motion is a prerequisite for a correct simulation: the scale of real motion and simulated feed back must be the same.

The *EyeSi* Simulator for Intra-ocular Surgery

Within the EyeSi project a computer-based training workstation for eye surgeons is developed. A prototype allowing the training of membrane peeling is already operational. To reach a high degree of immersion all important aspects of the surgery have been modeled, including the mechanical setup of the surgeon's complete operation environment.

The *EyeSi* Simulator consists of a model of the operation table, a mechanical eye in which original instruments can be inserted, an optical tracking system for two instruments and the eye motion, an off-the-shelf PC which generates the real-time computer graphics, and stereo glasses that replace the operation microscope.

Mechanical Setup

A mechanical eye with gimbal suspension was designed and placed on a model of the operation table. Like the real eye in its orbital cavity the mechanical eye provides three rotational degrees of freedom. Springs with appropriate spring constants were used on all three rotational axes to model the back driving forces of the eye muscles. The eye model has two small holes at the positions where the instruments are to be inserted. Real operative instruments are used in the simulation. Figure 2 shows a picture of the eye model with the two instruments inserted.

To model the stereo microscope a pair of active high resolution LCD stereo glasses are used. The arm holding the glasses has two joints and allows the user to individually adjust their position similar to the real microscope. Figure 3 gives an overview of the complete mechanical setup.

Optical Tracking

During an eye surgery the two instruments are fixed at the insertion points. The tip of each instrument has 3 translational degrees of freedom. In addition the instruments can be rotated. The eye can be tilt in three axes, adding another

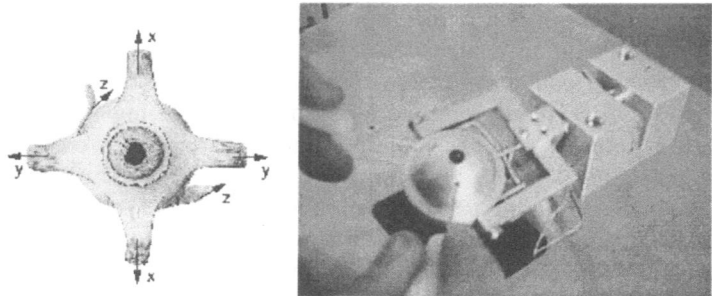

Fig. 2. The real eye in its orbital cavity has three rotational degrees of freedom (left). In the mechanical model, this behavior is modeled by a gimbal suspension and springs which pull teh eye back into its rest position. (right) eye model with two instruments inserted.

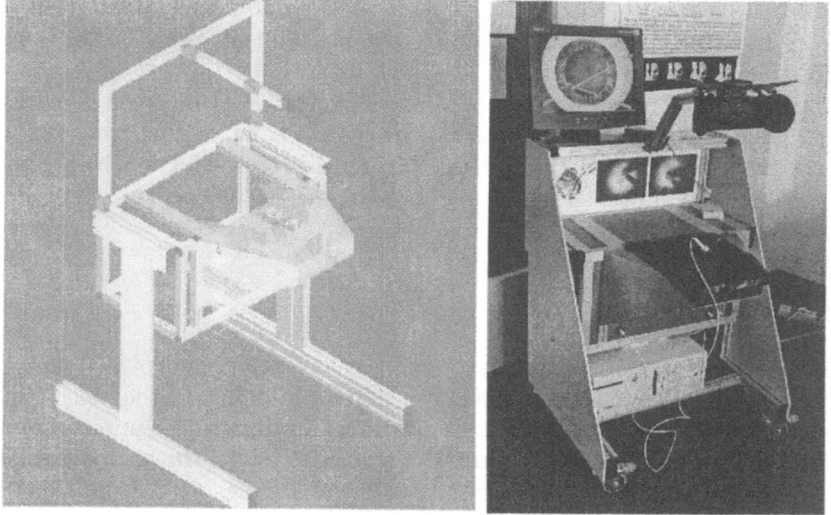

Fig. 3. CAD model of the mechanical setup (left). The current simulator prototype (right).

3 degrees of freedom to the system. All these movements must be identified in real-time. We use an optical tracking system for this task.

Optical tracking systems provide high accuracy and work contact free. Unfortunately we did not find a commercial solution that meets our requirements of narrow setup space (the tracking system has to fit into the body of the simulator) and high accuracy in the small volume of interest, essentially the eye volume (approx. $3 \times 3 \times 3 \ cm^3$). Together with the Fachhochschule Mannheim — Hochschule für Technik und Gestaltung, a solution based on three CCD cameras was developed. Each one is equipped with a digital signal processor (DSP) which can be used to analyze recorded images. The cameras are mounted under the operation table looking from below into the eye model. All instruments and the equator of the eye are marked with small light sources. The DSP in each camera is used to find the projections of the light spots on the CCD sensor and to determine the center of mass of each light spot. These values are then transfered to the PC. As the cameras see the scenery under different angles the stereoscopic back projection can be used with two of the camera images to calculate the positions of the light sources in space. The third camera is automatically activated when an occlusion occurs on one camera. The position of the instruments and the orientation of the eye are then updated accordingly in the computer graphical model.

The equator of the eye model is marked with two light emitting diodes (LEDs) which is sufficient to track its three rotational degrees of freedom. Mounting LEDs to the operative instruments was not feasible because of their small size and possible destruction by mechanical contact during simulation. Instead we abraded the tips of two of the original lamps to uncover the optical fiber inside. The other end of the fiber was connected to a LED. Since the instruments showed sufficient irradiation from their tips and produce good signals on the CCD sensors we used lamps to model all other instruments in the simulator.

Our tracking algorithm currently delivers 4 LED positions at 17 Hz. It returns the position of one light spot within 14 ms. We achieve an inplane accuracy of < 0.1 mm ($\approx \frac{30mm}{512Pixel}$). The depth accuracy (z-resolution) is about a factor four worse (≈ 0.3 mm). The spatial resolution of the current tracking system is sufficiently high for the simulated type of retinal surgery. It lies in the same range as the tremour that is observable in a setup like the one used in this kind of surgery. Unfortunately the time resolution of the current tracking system is not high enough for a tremour analysis. (Nyquist´s theorem: max. 8.5 Hz tremour frequency is detectable with the 17 Hz sampling rate of the tracking system.)

Visualization

The computer graphical model is based on anatomical data from literature. It is currently rendered using OpenGL surface graphics. The textures used for the iris and the retina are digitized photographies from real eyes. The graphical model includes light effects and shadows. The lamp produces a spot light and the instrument casts a strong shadow on the retina. As mentioned above this shadow is one important means of navigation for the surgeon. The other one is the 3D-view through the stereo microscop. The stereo buffer of OpenGL is used to produce stereo images. Stereo glasses with two high resolution mini LCDs present the calculated pictures to the user. Each LCD has a resolution of 800×600 and supports truecolor (16.7 million colors).

We achieve interactive framerates on a Pentium 400 MHz PC and a graphics adapter with hardware OpenGL support. Rendering the computer graphical model is currently the most time consuming step in the simulation. However, the rendering speed could easily be enhanced by using a graphics adapter with higher triangle throughput.

We are currently upgrading the simulator to include volume visualization. The transparent vitreous humor will be visualized using the volume visualization software developed at the Lehrstuhl für Informatik V, Universität Mannheim [7], [3], and provided by Volume Graphics GmbH[1].

Up to now simple geometric intersection calculations are used to detect collisions between instruments and eyeball. Due to the spherical shape of the eye ball this can be accomplished very fast. As soon as collisions with more complex shapes have to be considered, e.g. pathological tissues in the eye, collision detection becomes more expensive. In order to accelerate collision detection in these cases we are currently evaluating a new hardware supported approach.

Biomechanics

Based on 3D-ChainMail [2] an Enhanced ChainMail algorithm for the simulation of inhomogeous materials was developed [8]. This algorithm was successfully tested and will be used in the simulator for the modeling of the vitreous humor. It is currently ported to the *EyeSi* development platform. The Enhanced ChainMail algorithm has advantages over mass-spring regarding numerical stability. This is particularly true for 3D modeling.

However, since there was an immediate need for membrane simulation, a mass spring model was implemented. It produces good results within the known limitations of mass spring models (see below). The model consists of a triangulated mesh of mass points and springs. The governing equation is

$$F_i = \left(\sum_j^N \frac{x_j - x_i}{\|x_j - x_i\|} (C_{i,j} \|x_j - x_i\| - R_{i,j}) \right) - D_i \dot{x}_i \qquad (1)$$

where F_i is the force on mass i, $C_{i,j}$ is the spring constant of the spring between i and j, $R_{i,j}$ is the length of this spring and D_i the damping of spring i.

The biomechanical properties of the model were derived phenomenologically in an iterative process together with an experienced surgeon. With this approach convincing behaviour of soft membranes was achieved. Figure 4 shows an example of membrane peeling off the retina. A membrane tissue with approximately 1,500 mass nodes can be solved within < 10 ms and runs in the inner simulation loop.

The drawbacks of conventional mass spring systems were experienced when simulating stiffer structures. The system then showed a tendency to numerical instability. Moreover, also in cases were soft membranes were simulated, well conditioned boundary constraints had to be chosen: to avoid a collapse of the triangulated mesh the tissue had to be fixed allong its rim.

---

[1] http://www.volumegraphics.com

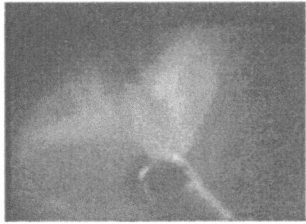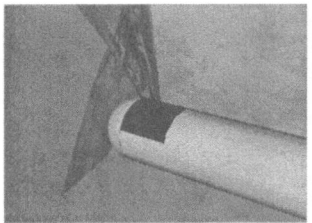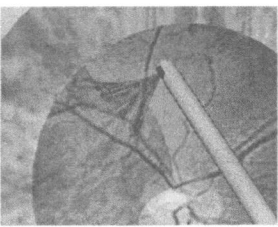

Fig. 4. Video capture (left) and simualtion snapshots (center and right) showing membrane peeling.

Results

We present a simulator for the training of intra-ocular surgery which incorporates all essential details from the real operation senario. Currently it is possible to exercise the manipulation of instrument inside the narrow space of the eye. Biomechanical models allow interaction with pathological tissues. The actual prototype contains the training of membrane peeling off the retina.

Figure 5 gives a comparison between simulation and real operation. The top row shows screen shots from the simulator, the bottom row video captures from a real surgery. The images illustrate that the simulation is very close to reality: light effects, shadow, eye's background and instruments are modeled conform to the real surgery.

Great importance is also attached to the handling of instruments during the simulation. The mechanical eye (see Figure 2) provides a tactile feedback which is very close to what a surgeon experiences when operating a real eye.

The plattform currently used is off-the-shelf-pc hardware. Depending on the actual simulation task we achieve frame rates between 12Hz and 25Hz. The first rate is for a simulation with membrane in stereo mode where all frames need to be rendered twice, the latter for mono mode. The frame rate breakdown when switching from mono to stereo mode illustrates the bottleneck in OpenGL performance of the current hardware.

If necessary, performance can easily be improved by upgrading the engaged hardware. In particular, future biomechanical modeling might require the change to a multiprocessor system.

We have not yet accomplished clinical evaluation studies, but the prototype will be tested in the Klinikum Mannheim as soon as possible. Nevertheless we received very positive feedback from the eye surgeons who have tried the simulator so far.

Discussion

First estimations claim that by the use of the *EyeSi* simulator the current period of education (two years) can be cut down by at least three months.

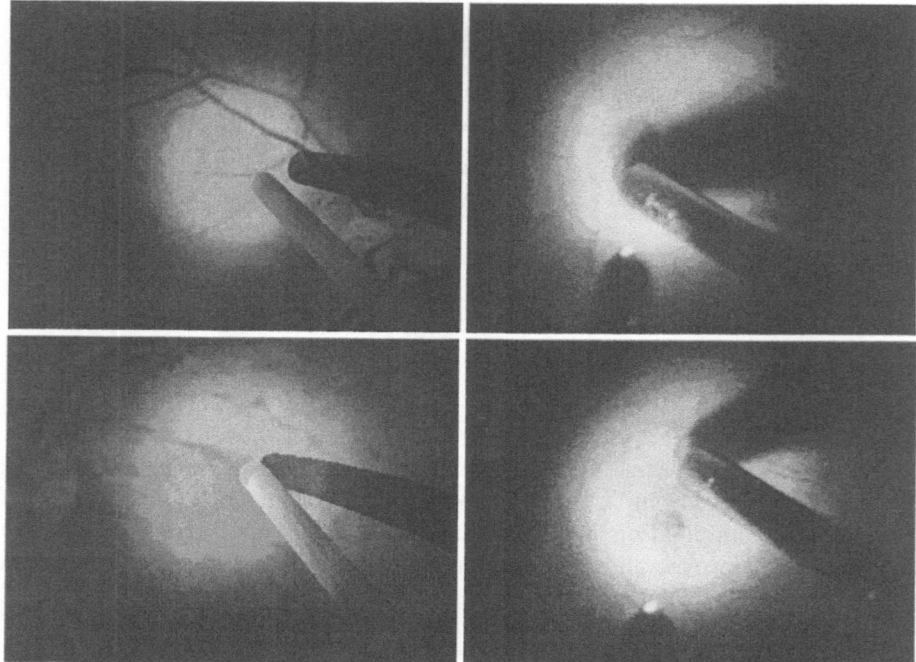

Fig. 5. Comparison: Screenshots from the simulation on the left, video captures from a real surgery on the right.

In addition to training the simulator can also be used for the development of new operative instruments and techniques. New instruments can rapidly be prototyped in a simulation. New operation techniques can be developed, tested, demonstrated and taught to colleagues.

Currently an enhanced tracking system is under development which provides about one order of magnitude higher resolution in time and space. This will be obtained by changing the camera type from area to line camera. Volume modeling for biomechanics with the Enhanced ChainMail Algorithm and the usage of volume visualization is work in progress. Up to now the rotation of the operative instruments is not tracked. This will be fixed in the near future.

Future developments will include a training curriculum for surgeons in education. The program will provide a performance analysis informing the trainee about his training success in terms of accuracy and time needed to complete the task.

Acknowledgement

The authors would like thank Dr. Fridolin Scheuerle and Gerhart Hospach from EM Gerätebau, Mannheim, for generously supporting the *EyeSi* project.

Dr. Michael Knorz greatly improved the simulator with his contributions from the eye surgeon's point of view.

Bausch & Lomb Surgical GmbH, Germany supplied the instruments used in the simulator.

Thanks also to SONY Deutschland GmbH for providing the stereo glasses LDI 100.

References

1. Biomedical Visualization Laboratory at University of Illinois. Model of the Eye. http://www.bvl.uic.edu/bvl/eye/.
2. S. Gibson. 3D ChainMail: A Fast Algorithm for Deforming Volumetric Objects. In *1997 Symposium on Interactive 3D Graphics*, pages 149 – 154, Providence, RI, USA, April 1997.
3. A. Gröpl, T. Günther, J. Hesser, J. Kröll, R. Männer, C. Poliwoda, and C. Reinhart. Interactive Operation Planning and Control with VIRIM. In *Proc. Medicine Meets Virtual Reality 4*, pages 121–133, San Diego, CA, January 1996.
4. Gordon D. Mallinson Mark A. Sagar, David Bullivant and Peter J. Hunter. A Virtual Environment and Model of the Eye for Surgical Simulation. In *SIGGRAPH '94, Anual Conference Series*, pages 205–212, July 1994.
5. Paul F. Neumann, Lewis L. Sadler, and Jon Gieser M.D. Virtual Reality Vitrectomy Simulator. In Alan Colchester William M. Wells and Scott Delp, editors, *Medical Image Computing and Computer- Assisted Intervention - MICCAI '98*, pages 910 – 917, Cambribge, MA, USA, October 1998. Springer.
6. Medical College of Georgia & IMTC at GeorgiaTech. Simulation of a Catheract Surgery. http://www.oip.gatech.edu/MMTLPROJ/eye.html.
7. Markus Schill, Christof Reinhart, Thomas Günther, Christoph Poliwoda, Jürgen Hesser, Martin Schinkmann, H.-J. Bender, and R. Männer. Biomechanical Simulation of Brain Tissue and Realtime Volume Visualisation. Integrating Biomechanical Simulations into the VIRIM System. In *Proceedings of the international Symposium on Computer and Communication Systems for Imageguided Diagnosis and Therapy, Computer Assisted Radiology*, pages 283 – 288, Berlin, Germany, June 1997.
8. Markus A. Schill, Sarah F.F. Gibson, H.-J. Bender, and R. Männer. Biomechanical Simulation of the Vitreous Humor in the Eye Using an Enhanced ChainMail Algorithm. In Alan Colchester William M. Wells and Scott Delp, editors, *Proc.Medical Image Computing and Computer-Assisted Intervention - MICCAI '98*, pages 679 – 687, Cambridge, MA, USA, October 1998. Springer.

The Mesh-matching Algorithm : A New Automatic 3D Mesh Generator for Finite Element Analysis

Béatrice Couteau[1], Yohan Payan[2], Stéphane Lavallée[3], and Marie-Christine Hobatho[1]

[1] Laboratoire de biomécanique. INSERM U305
Centre Hospitalier Hôtel Dieu Toulouse - France
[2] Laboratoire TIMC/IMAG – UMR CNRS 5525 – Faculté de Médecine
Domaine de la Merci, La Tronche - France - Yohan.Payan@imag.fr
[3] PRAXIM Le Grand Sablon, La Tronche - France

Abstract. This paper deals with Finite Element (FE) modeling of human body structures. More specifically, it focuses on the FE mesh generation process, which is a long and tedious task in the case of irregular and non-homogeneous structures. Whereas for regular and symmetrical bodies, some automatic mesh generators have been developed, no robust system is provided for living structures, which are, by definition, non-homogeneous, irregular and patient-specific. This paper proposes a new algorithm, called the mesh-matching (M-M) algorithm, that automatically generates patient-specific 3D meshes for FE models of structures with complex geometry. It assumes that the shape which is studied is sufficiently close to a known standard model for which a mesh has been already generated by an expert. The algorithm proposes then to use a registration method, in order to infer the standard finite element mesh to the data. The M-M algorithm is tested on five human femurs.

INTRODUCTION

The rapid development of medical imaging technology has first provided the accurate visualization of the internal anatomical structures. Secondly, it has been extended to the planning and simulation of medical procedures as the navigation and immersion to 3D anatomical data-sets. Then, physical and physiological mathematical models of human organs based on medical imaging techniques were developed. The Finite Element (FE) Method is one of these modelling technique. It is a numerical analysis which provides an approximate solution to a wide variety of engineering problems, like continuum mechanics problems for example ([16]). The FE method is first based on the "meshing process" consisting in the division of the body into small volumes (called the "elements"), which are connected by "nodes". Consequently, the discretization of the problem is made by computing the mechanical equations for each node.

In the orthopaedic domain, the clinical relevant of the Finite Element Method is the understanding of the mechanical behavior of bone structures. It may be used to analyze the influence of either a pathology or a prosthesis design on the stress field. This method has great potential for pre-clinical testing of new design implants or for simulating pre-operative implantations. But the difficulty of this method lies in the irregularities of the geometrical and mechanical properties of the bone structures. Due to those irregularities, 3D meshing is a difficult process which requires a huge amount of manual labor. For this reason, many two dimensional bone models have been developed in the orthopaedic research field, thus offering the possibility of high 2D mesh refinement, with a limited manual intervention ([2], [3], [15], [21]). In practice, bone 3D FE analysis have to respect some compromises in terms of homogeneity ([19], [13]), symmetry ([8]) or mesh refinement ([19], [20]). Moreover, 3D models, based on average bone geometry, have also been developed ([12], [22]), loosing thus any patient-oriented specificity. An automatic method generating patient-specific 3D meshes, for FE models with irregularities, appears thus as a non trivial problem and has already been studied among the literature ([10], [9]). For animation purposes (facial animation for example), several algorithms have been proposed to automatically create 3-D meshes. In the context of soft tissue modeling for surgery simulation, Cotin et al. ([4]) have used simplex-meshes representations ([6]) to mesh volumetric models. But those mesh-generation methods are not always available in standard commercial FE software as they don't include the geometrical rules of the elements. In this paper, a new method is proposed to automatically generate a 3D FE mesh of any patient anatomical structures from already defined meshes based on atlas structures. This method is called the mesh-matching (M-M) algorithm and automatically provides the 3D meshing of human structures. The method has been tested on five different human femurs In section 1, the automatic mesh- generating method will be introduced. Section 2 will describe the procedure tested on five femurs. Finally, results will be discussed with some perspectives to quantitatively validate the method.

1   THE MESH-MATCHING (M-M) METHOD

Building finite element models for complex shapes is often a tedious task that requires user interaction. Our mesh-matching (M-M) algorithm assumes that the shape which is studied is sufficiently close to a known model for which a mesh has been already generated (the "standard" femur in this paper). The algorithm proposes to use a registration method to infer the finite element mesh to the data. Elastic registration is an important element of 3-D medical image analysis. In our case, the main objective of elastic registration is to deform an atlas to correspond with patient images. In a more general sense, elastic registration is the process by which an object is deformed to match another object (see [11] for more details about registration techniques). The elastic registration algorithm is defined by the estimation of a volumetric transform $\mathbf{T}$ between two coordinate systems R_A and R_B. A point with coordinates (x_a, y_a, z_a) in R_A has coordinates (x_b, y_b, z_b) = $\mathbf{T}(x_a, y_a, z_a)$ in R_B. Obtaining such a transform is the main issue and many technical solutions exist. However, the approach always consists in minimizing the disparity between a set of features F_A extracted in R_A and a set of features F_B extracted in R_B. Once such a transform has been estimated, it can be used to transform a reference object O_A of R_A into a new object O_B in the coordinate system R_B : this process is usually defined as inference. The elastic registration method we have retained for our M-M algorithm was introduced by Szeliski and Lavallée ([17]), and was characterized by three main features (see [18] for more details) :

- Representation of the elastic transform **T**, with the introduction of the notion of hierarchical adaptive oct-tree splines.
- Disparity function between model and data, with the minimization of a distance between two sets of surface points.
- Optimization procedure, with the use of a combination of Levenberg-Marquardt and Conjugate Gradient techniques in a hierarchical space.

Representation of the elastic transform **T** : Szeliski and Lavallée ([18]) searched a transform **T** which is the combination of a rigid-body transform RT, a global warping W and a local displacement function S built on a hierarchical and adaptive grid of displacements basis (*oct-tree splines*) :

$$\mathbf{T_p} = RT \circ W \circ S \tag{1}$$

where **p** is a vector gathering the 6 parameters that define RT, the 12 to 30 parameters that define W and the thousands of local displacement vectors that define S.

Disparity function between model and data : Let $\mathcal{M} = \{M_i, i = 1...N_1\}$ and $\mathcal{P} = \{P_i, i = 1...N_1\}$ be the sets of model and patient features, obtained by segmentation algorithms (e.g. a Canny-Deriche filtering on 3-D images). The elastic registration algorithm minimizes a least-squares criterion $E(\mathbf{p})$, as :

$$E(\mathbf{p}) = \sum_{i=1}^{N1} \frac{1}{\sigma_i^2}[dist(\mathcal{P}, \mathbf{T_p}(M_i))]^2 + \mathcal{R}(\mathbf{p}), \tag{2}$$

where $\mathcal{R}$ defines a regularization term which is applied to S in order to obtain a smooth displacement function. It is, in this implementation, a weighted sum of zero order and first order regularization terms (see [18] for the exact expressions); σ_i^2 is the variance of the noise of the measurement i ([1]); $dist$ is the distance between the set $\mathcal{P}$ and a point M_i' (transformed by **T**). Usually the features are simply 3-D surface points of the object surface in both the Atlas and Patient spaces. But it is also possible to use 3-D points with image gradients. In that case, the distance $dist$ is a 6-D distance function, as proposed by Feldmar and Ayache ([7]) :

$$dist(\mathcal{P}, M_i') = \min_{P_j \in \mathcal{P}} d_{6D}(P_j, M_i') \tag{3}$$

with

$$d_{6D}^2(P_j, M_i') =$$
$$(x_{P_j} - x_{M_i'})^2 \quad +(y_{P_j} - y_{M_i'})^2 \quad +(z_{P_j} - z_{M_i'})^2 +$$
$$\alpha(Gx_{P_j} - Gx_{M_i'})^2 +\alpha(Gy_{P_j} - Gy_{M_i'})^2 +\alpha(Gz_{P_j} - Gz_{M_i'})^2$$

where α is a weighting factor and P_j and M_i' vectors defined with 3D positions of coordinate and gradient points :
$$P_j = (x_{P_j}, y_{P_j}, z_{P_j}, Gx_{P_j}, Gy_{P_j}, Gz_{P_j}) \text{ and}$$
$$M_i' = (x_{M_i'}, y_{M_i'}, z_{M_i'}, Gx_{M_i'}, Gy_{M_i'}, Gz_{M_i'}).$$

Optimization procedure : The optimization of $E(\mathbf{p})$ is performed using the Levenberg-Marquardt algorithm ([14]) and a modified conjugate gradient algorithm in the hierarchical representation of $\mathbf{T}$, in order to smooth the solution and to speed up the minimization. First of all, initial registration is performed by aligning one particular point known in both data sets while rotation is simply provided by the patient coordinate systems defined in the headers of images. Therefore, rigid-body transform parameters are estimated. Then, the global warping parameters are added, the local displacement vectors for a coarse level of the octree-spline are used, and finally, the octree-spline is refined until a given resolution level is reached (see [18] for more details) .

2   THE FINITE ELEMENT MODELING OF BONE STRUCTURES USING THE M-M METHOD

FEMUR ACQUISITION Transverse CT images (Siemens, DRH2) were performed on 6 cadaveric femurs (2 females and 4 males). One millimeter thick slices were performed at 3mm interval for the epiphyses and at 20mm interval for the diaphyseal region. Each image was subjected to an edge detection to separate bone contour lines. The output file of the image processing was a neutral file (in an IGES format) containing the external contours of the cortical bone (connected by bi-parametric surfaces). The 3D surfaces of the bones were then read via the Patran Software V7.5 (MSC Nastran, Los Angeles, CA, USA).

The 3D reconstruction of one of the femur (the "standard" or "reference" femur) was manually meshed by an expert, with hexaedric (8 nodes) and wedge (6 nodes) finite elements. The FE model (figure 1.a) was composed of 3572 elements and has been experimentally validated by means of a vibrational technique and an extensometric measurement ([5]). The 3D surfaces of the other five femurs were automatically meshed with 2D elements (quads and triangles) in order to obtain the external nodes of the bone structure. Figure 1.b gives an example of this automatic meshing for one patient femur.

To allow a complete analysis of the stress field in this patient's femur, a manual volumetric meshing should be performed, which would again require a large amount of labour. Conversely, the M-M algorithm proposes to exploit the work already done on the standard femur, by inferring its 3D mesh to the nodes from the patient's femur.

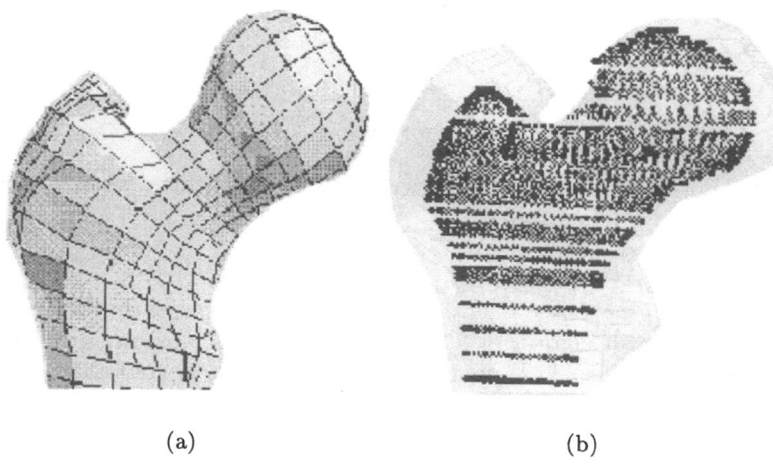

(a)   (b)

Fig. 1. 3D finite element mesh of the standard femur (a) and its superimposition with the patient's femur 3D surfacic nodes. (b)

APPLICATION OF THE M-M METHOD The 3D model of the standard human femur (figure 1.a) takes into account bone irregularities. From this 3D FE model, the points located at the surface of the bone are extracted. The matching algorithm is then required to match this standard femur surface with data collected on a new patient femur surface. Figure 2.a plots the standard femur surface (blue points) superimposed with surface points (contour lines in purple) from one of the patients femurs. The matching algorithm computes, for each patient femur, the global volumetric transformation **T**. Figure 2.b plots the results of one given patient, with the matching of the blue points on the femur surface.

Once surface points have been segmented on the Atlas and on the patient images, the elastic volumetric registration takes less than 30 seconds on a DEC Alpha 5000 workstation.

The last process of our M-M method is the computation of the final 3D FE meshing, of each femur. To do this, the global transformation T is applied to the standard 3D FE model to generate, by inference, the patient 3D meshing of the patient's femur (this step requires less than 10 seconds). Figure 3 illustrates the mesh generation of one patient based on the standard femur mesh transformation.

3   RESULTS AND DISCUSSION

One of the main difficulty encountered during the mesh generation process applied to complex structures lies in the shape rules of the elements which have to

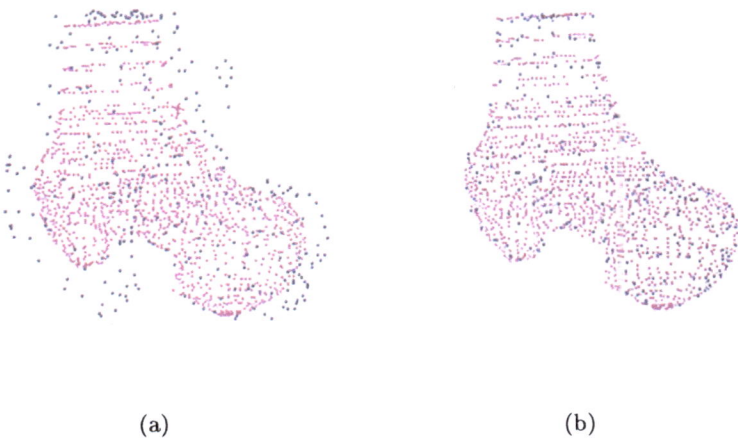

(a)   (b)

Fig. 2. Illustration of the matching of one patient's femur. (a) : Superimposition of patient's femur contour lines (purple) with points collected at the surface of the standard femur (blue). (b) : Results of the matching algorithm

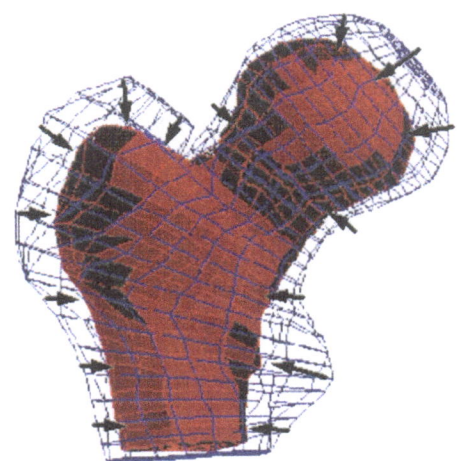

Fig. 3. Inference of the M-M algorithm : generated 3D mesh of the FE patient's femur (red), superimposed with the standard 3D mesh (blue wireframe). Black arrows illustrate the inference of the surfaces.

respect a range of geometrical distortions. For example, FE skew angles, aspect ratio, warp angles, collapses, or twist angles have to respect some specific constraints in order to achieve a complete and correct FE analysis. The application of the M-M method on the femurs from the five patients demonstrates four successfull transformations and one failure transformation. Transformations have been tested by applying a mechanical compressive load onto the FE models of the femurs from patients. A successfull analysis means that the mesh transformation does not involve errors relative to the geometry of the elements. Conversely, a failure analysis is due to elements with a non-reasonable geometrical distortion. In our unique failed transformation, the mesh shows geometric shape failure in 13 elements, which would thus require the manipulation of an expert on those elements. Although the remaining work for the expert is simplified in comparison with building the mesh from scratch, the method is not entirely automatic for that case. It is interesting to focus here on those 13 elements which are all located at the lower part of the model. The difference between this femur and the others consists in its vertical length (15mm longer than the other ones). It would thus be interesting to quantitatively evaluate this phenomena.

CONCLUSION

The M-M method aims at generating automatically 3D meshes for FE analysis of human body structures. It was tested on five femurs, showing an attractive success rate. This method enables to build a FE mesh in less than 1 minute (compatible with a standard FE software). One femur among five presented geometric shape failure in 13 elements which were located at a specific part of the model. In this perspective, in order to avoid manual operation, it would become interesting to develop an algorithm that would locally modify the failed elements of the final 3D mesh. This point, associated with a more quantitative number of tests, will define the main future developments of this complete automatic mesh generator.

ACKNOWLEDGEMENTS

Richard Szeliski and Eric Bittar are acknowledged for their contributions on the elastic registration algorithm used in this paper.

References

1. P.J. Besl and N.D. McKay. A new method for registration of 3-d shapes. *IEEE Transactions on Pattern Analysis and Machine Intelligence*, 14(2):239–256, 1992.
2. T.D. Brown, M.E. Way, F.H. Fu, and A.B. Ferguson. *Finite Elements in Biomechanics*. Gallagher R.H. et al. eds, New York: John Wiley, 1982.
3. D.R. Carter, R. Vasu, and W.H. Harris. Stress changes in the femoral head due to porous ingrowth surface replacement arthroplasty. *Journal of Biomechanics*, 17:737–747, 1984.

4. S. Cotin, H. Delinguette, and N. Ayache. *Real Time Volumetric Deformable Models for Surgery Simulation.* Vizualisation in Biomedical Computing, K. Hohne and R. Kikinis eds., Springer, 1990.

5. B. Couteau, M.C. Hobatho, R. Darmana, J.C. Brignola, and J.Y. Arlaud. Finite element modelling of the vibrational behaviour of the human femur using ct-based individualized geometrical and material properties. *Journal of Biomechanics*, 31:383–386, 1998.

6. H. Delinguette. *Simplex meshes: a general representation for 3d shape reconstruction.* Proceedings of Int. Conf. on Computer Vision and Pattern Recognition (CVPR'94), Seattle, USA., 1994.

7. J. Feldmar and N. Ayache. Rigid, affine and locally affine registration of free-form surfaces. *Int. J. of Computer Vision*, 18(2):99–119, 1996.

8. R. Huiskes and J.V. Heck. Stresses in the femoral head-neck region after surface replacement. a three-dimensional finite element analysis. *Trans. Orthop. Res. Soc.*, 6:174, 1981.

9. J.H. Keyak, M.G. Fourkas, J.M. Meagher, and H.B. Skinner. Validation of an automated method of three-dimensional finite element modelling of bone. *J. Biomed. Eng.*, 15:505–509, 1993.

10. J.H. Keyak, J.M. Meagher, H.B. Skinner, and C.D. Mote. Automated three-dimensional finite element modelling of bone: a new method. *J. Biomed. Eng.*, 12:389–397, 1990.

11. S. Lavallée. *Registration for Computer-Integrated Surgery: Methodology, State of the Art.* Computer Integrated Surgery, R. Taylor, S. Lavallée, G. Burdea and R. Mosges eds., Cambridge, MA: MIT Press, 1996.

12. J.C. Lotz, W.C. Hayes, and T.N. Gerhart. The structural contribution of cortical and trabecular bone in the femoral neck. *Trans. Orthop. Res. Soc.*, 13:232, 1988.

13. H. Oonishi, H. Isha, and T. Hasegawa. Mechanical analysis of the human pelvis and its application to the artificial hip joint - by means of the three dimensional finite element method. *Journal of Biomechanics*, 16:427–444, 1983.

14. W.H. Press, B.P. Flannery, S.A. Teukolsky, and W.T. Vetterling. *Numerical Recipes in C: The Art of Scientific Computing.* Cambridge University Press, Cambridge, England, 1992.

15. E.F. Rybicki, F.A. Simonen, and E.B. Weis. On the mathematical analysis of stress in the human femur. *Journal of Biomechanics*, 5:203–215, 1972.

16. H.R. Schwartz. *Finite Element Methods.* London: Academic Press, 1984.

17. R. Szeliski and S. Lavallée. Matching 3-d anatomical surfaces with non-rigid deformations using octree-splines. *Geometric Methods in Computer Vision II, SPIE*, San Diego., 2031:306–315, 1993.

18. R. Szeliski and S. Lavallée. Matching 3-d anatomical surfaces with non-rigid deformations using octree-splines. *Int. J. of Computer Vision*, 18(2):171–186, 1996.

19. S. Valliappan, N.L Svensson, and R.D. Wood. Three dimensional stress analysis of the human femur. *Comput. Biol. Med.*, 7:253–264, 1977.

20. H.H. Vichnin and S.C. Batterman. Effects of cortical bone anisotropy on prothesis stem stresses. *Trans. Orthop. Res. Soc.*, 7:277, 1982.

21. H. Weinans, R. Huiskes, and H. Grootenboer. The mechanical effects of fibrous tissue interposition at the cement-bone interface in tha. *Trans. Orthop. Res. Soc.*, 13:502, 1988.

22. A.M. Weinstein, J.B. Koeneman, and T.M. Hansen. Finite element analysis of a composite material hip stem. *Proc. 13th Ann. Meet. Soc. Biomat.*, page 264, New-York, June 1987.

Optimization Approaches for Soft–Tissue Prediction in Craniofacial Surgery Simulation

Matthias Teschner, Sabine Girod, and Bernd Girod

University of Erlangen-Nuremberg
Telecommunications Laboratory
Cauerstr. 7, D-91058 Erlangen, Germany
Phone: +49-9131-8528904, Fax: +49-9131-8528849
teschner@nt.e-technik.uni-erlangen.de
http://www-nt.e-technik.uni-erlangen.de/~teschner/

Abstract. A system for interactive, 3–D, craniofacial surgery simulation is presented. It is used for the 3–D simulation of osteotomies of the facial and skull bones and for the prediction of soft–tissue changes caused by bone movement. The result of the simulation process is a 3–D, photorealistic model of the patient's postoperative appearance that can be viewed from any position.

The system is based on the individual preoperative bone structure of a patient's skull derived from a computer tomography scan and on the patient's photorealistic, preoperative appearance obtained by a laser scanner. The elasto–mechanical properties of the multi–layer soft–tissue are represented by springs. The model incorporates additional features such as skin turgor, gravity, and sliding bone contact.

The prediction of soft–tissue deformation due to simulated bone movement is computed using an optimization approach. Several optimization methods have been tested and compared with regard to robustness of the simulation result and to computational costs.

While the osteotomy simulation can be performed interactively, the computation of the corresponding soft–tissue changes usually takes less than 10 seconds even in sophisticated cases. Tests have been performed on a SGI O2 R10000, 175MHz. The system is able to simulate bimaxillary osteotomies, physiological jaw movement and has been used in the planning process in case of a craniosynostosis.

1 Introduction

The success of complex craniofacial surgical procedures is critically dependent on careful planning. The planning process is aimed at the restoration of functionality and at the improvement of the patient's aesthetics. There are two principal methods of planning surgeries based on models. One method is to build physical models that are generated from CT scans, e. g., stereolithography. These realistic models improve osteotomy planning and allow accurate manufacturing of transplants. Moreover, these models can be used for educational purposes and demonstrations. While physical models provide information on the bone structure, they do not contain knowledge of the soft–tissue, which is of importance to assess the patient's aestethics. The second method of planning craniofacial surgical procedures is to utilize medical imaging for generating computer models [1], [2], [3], [4], [5], [6], [7]. Computer models are more flexible than physical models and are able to provide more information by integrating several modalities. A multimodal computer model of the bone structure and soft–tissue can be used for simulating osteotomies as well as for assessing the patient's appearance. Various simulations can be performed with less additional effort compared to physical models. This is especially helpful in cases where various surgical options are possible.

In our laboratory, we have investigated methods for cranicfacial surgery simulation based on 3–D computer models since 1993 [8], [9]. In this paper, a refined system is presented, that uses an optimization approach for fast soft–tissue simulation. The paper is organized as follows. In the next section the generation of the 3–D computer models of the bone structure and the face surface is described. In Section 3 the structure and parametrization of the soft–tissue model is described. In Section 4 optimization methods are compared that are used to estimate the soft–tissue deformation due to bone realignment. Simulation results are presented in Section 5.

2   Data Acquisition

Triangle meshes that describe the surface of the face and the bone structure of the head are the basic elements of the simulation process. These meshes are built using two different sensory modalities. A CT scan provides the anatomically correct representation of the bone structure and a laser scanner records a photorealistic, 3–D model of the patient's face. The triangle mesh that represents the surface of the bone structure is generated by segmenting bone from the CT scan and applying the Marching–Cubes–algorithm [10] to the result. An implementation of these methods is adopted from [6]. The triangle mesh that represents the face surface is computed from the depth and color map of the laser scan.

Both modalities are registered by exploiting corresponding cephalometric landmarks of the laser scan and the skin surface taken from the CT scan [6].

3   Soft–Tissue Model

Given the triangle meshes that represent the skull and the face, the soft–tissue model is generated. In recent years, several soft–tissue models based on springs or finite elements have been developed [3], [5], [6], [11], [12], [13]. As computational costs for finite–element methods are high and these methods seem to be less suitable for interactive applications, in our work, a mesh of springs is utilized. The springs are categorized according to their location and function (Fig. 1):

- *Layer springs* represent soft–tissue layers. In order to model differentiated elasto–mechanical properties of soft–tissue layers, each layer is represented by a particular class of springs. The number and the thickness of soft–tissue layers are variable. Simulations have been performed with one, three, and five layers.
- *Bone springs* represent connections between bone and soft–tissue. Only some regions of the soft–tissue are connected to the underlying bone structure. To mimic sliding contact, these connections are modeled using springs.
- *Boundary springs* prevent the soft–tissue model from undergoing global transformation. Due to the fact that the face model does not include the complete head surface but only the facial region, these springs anchor the face and the underlying soft–tissue in space.

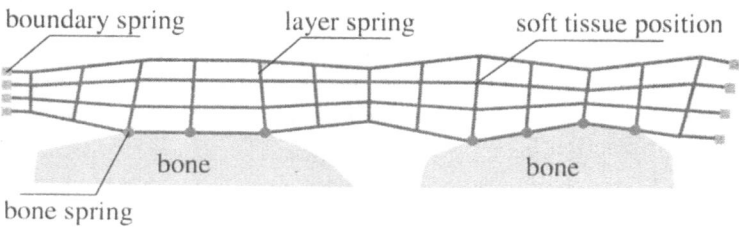

Fig. 1. Soft tissue model.

A spring is characterized by a spring constant k, which describes its stiffness, and by a length l. Every spring class is parametrized with a particular spring constant to model the elasto–mechanical properties of the corresponding soft–tissue layer. Bone springs and boundary springs are parametrized with a comparatively large spring constant. The length of bone springs and boundary springs is zero. The springs that represent the skin surface are given a certain strain. This strain corresponds to the skin turgor. Setting the natural length of all surface springs to $c_{turgor} \cdot l$, with $0 < c_{turgor} < 1$, introduces a certain strain. The difference of l and $c_{turgor} \cdot l$ corresponds to the desired skin turgor.

A *soft–tissue position* is characterized by a location $P \in \mathbb{R}^3$ and a mass m in order to enable simulation of gravity. Every soft–tissue layer is parametrized by an overall mass, which is distributed according to the topology of the representing soft–tissue positions.

Due to the masses and the strain of the surface there are forces at each soft–tissue position. In order to prevent the model from changing without performing any bone realignment and obtaining a stable equilibrium of the mesh, the sum of these forces has to be zero. This is achieved by determining appropriate strains for all springs, given the strain of the skin surface.

4   Soft–Tissue Deformation

The described soft–tissue model is used to estimate soft–tissue deformation due
to simulated bone realignment. Basically, the soft–tissue deformation is computed by applying an optimization method that minimizes the energy of the
spring mesh. In the initial state of the simulation process the energy is zero. The
energy is increased by performing bone transformation. An optimization process
deforms the spring mesh in order to minimize the energy. The energy function

$$f(P_0, P_1, \ldots, P_{N-1}) = \lambda \sum_i k_i (l_{0i} - l_i)^2 + (1 - \lambda) \sum_j (v_{0j} - v_j)^2 \qquad (1)$$

depends on $3 \cdot N$ independent variables determining N soft–tissue positions
$P_i \in \mathbb{R}^3$. It mainly captures differences between initial spring lengths l_{0i} and
current spring lengths l_i and differences between initial volumes v_{0i} and current
volumes v_i. The values k_i are spring constants, and λ $(0 < \lambda < 1)$ weights the
influence of both terms of the function. The values v_i and v_{0i} are volumes of
basic elements of the soft–tissue. The volume consists of prisms.
    The initial state of the mesh is characterized by $l_i = l_{0i}$ for every spring.
Bone movement leads to $l_i \neq l_{0i}$ and $(l_{0i} - l_i)^2 > 0$ for certain bone springs and
to $f(P_0, P_1, \ldots, P_{N-1}) > 0$. Now, new soft–tissue positions P^* are computed by
minimizing f. These values P^* describe the deformed soft–tissue:

$$P_0^*, P_1^*, \ldots, P_{N-1}^* = \arg\min f(P_0, P_1, \ldots, P_{N-1}). \qquad (2)$$

During the minimization process there are no additional restrictions applied
to the soft–tissue positions P apart from the energy function. All soft–tissue
positions are considered in the minimization process, regardless of the simulated
bone realignment.
    Four optimization methods have been compared with regard to computa-
tional costs and robustness of the result (Tab. 1). All optimization methods are
iterative processes. They terminate if the difference of two P^* or the difference
of two evaluations of f in successive steps is tolerably small. This tolerance can
be chosen. On one hand, it influences the accuracy of the minimum, on the
other hand it has an effect on the computation time. The slightly different minima found by the optimization algorithms (Tab. 1) are due to this tolerance.
Some methods require the calculation of partial derivatives. The methods differ
in the amount of allocated memory. The order of additional memory that is
needed by an optimization method is important due to the fact that its amount
is dependent on the number of soft–tissue positions. If the model consists of 3000
positions, then the energy function (1) has 9000 parameters and an optimization
method that requires memory in order of N^2 would need a multiple of $81\,MByte$
memory instead of a multiple of $9kByte$ for an algorithm with order of N. All
optimization methods are described in [14].
    Tests have shown that the conjugate gradient method provides reliable re-
sults and is very efficient with regard to memory and computational complexity.

Optimization method	Order of additional memory	Requires partial derivatives	Time $[s]$	min f
Conjugate gradient, parabolic interpolation	N	yes	0.60	4.33
Conjugate gradient, derivative based	N	yes	2.21	4.33
Direction set (Powell)	N^2	no	81.43	4.33
Variable metric (quasi–Newton)	N^2	yes	2.91	4.30

Table 1. Comparison of optimization methods using a synthetic data set, the energy function (1), and performing an exemplary bone movement. 138 soft–tissue positions P_i, 986 springs, 144 volumes (SGI O2, R10000, $175MHz$). N is the number of parameters of the energy function.

Parabolic interpolation is used for 1–D sub–minimization due to the quadratic form of f. Although partial derivatives of the energy function are calculated by this optimization method, its computational expense is comparatively low because of the similarity of the energy function and its partial derivatives. The partial derivatives are responsible for fast convergence of the optimization process and fast convergence reduces the number of function evaluations.

In addition to computational costs another important criterion of an minimization algorithm is the quality of the minimum found. It cannot be guaranteed that the minimum P^* is the global minimum, and it is difficult to prove that fact in a space with $> 10^3$ dimensions. A method to check the robustness of the minimum P^* is to perform a certain bone movement in different ways and to compare the results. If only a small movement is performed, the distance of the initial soft–tissue positions P and P^* is small, f is comparatively small, and the global minimum is likely to be found. For example, translating a bone by 0.1mm ten times or translating a bone by 1mm once should lead to the same P^*. Several tests using the multidimensional conjugate gradient method have been performed and all minima have been reliable.

5   Results

Table 2 and Fig. 2–4 show examples of simulations performed. The soft–tissue prediction is tested with two individual patient data sets. Several simulations of bone movement have been applied to each model. The last column of Tab. 2 shows the maximum time needed by the optimization process. All tests have been performed on a standard workstation SGI O2, R10000, 175MHz. Fig. 5 shows parts of the simulated planning process in case of a craniosynostosis. In this case, only cutting of the bone structure and its realignment has been simulated.

6   Conclusion

In this paper, a new, efficient and robust approach to soft–tissue prediction has been presented. It is based on an optimization method and has been tested with

Fig.	Number of soft–tissue positions	Number of springs	Number of volumes	Max. simulation time [s]
2, 3	754	6067	874	1.1
4	2092	16547	2820	3.3

Table 2. Model parameters and simulation speed.

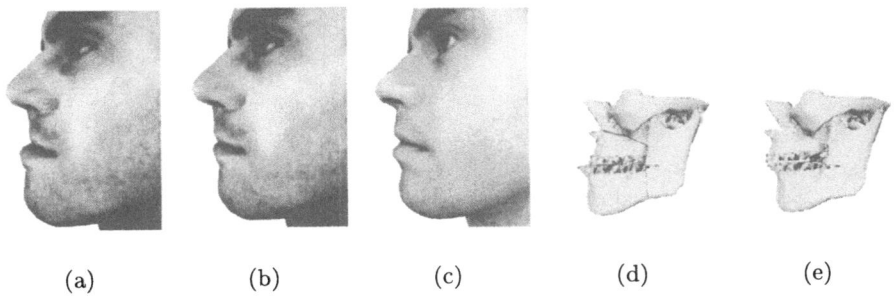

(a)   (b)   (c)   (d)   (e)

Fig. 2. Craniofacial surgery simulation for patient 1. a) Preoperative appearance. b) Simulated postoperative appearance. c) Postoperative appearance. d) Preoperative bone structure. e) Simulated postoperative bone structure. The upper jaw is repositioned 4mm forward and 2mm upward anteriorly and 4mm posteriorly. The lower jaw is moved backwards 5mm.

several individual patient data sets. The soft–tissue prediction is integrated in a system for craniofacial surgery simulation. It simulates bimaxillary osteotomies and physiological jaw movement and predicts the soft–tissue changes caused by bone realignment. Ongoing work focuses on the integration of interactive collision detection and collision response algorithms into the system to enable a realistic simulation of bone movement and transplants. As well as estimating the patient's static postoperative appearance and simulating physiological bone movement, the visualization of the patient's post–operative facial expressions is very useful. Therefore, it is planned to add muscles to the existing soft–tissue model. Further, it is intended to register very accurate measurements of the jaws with the CT scan, in order to consider the occlusion of the jaws in the planning process.

7   Acknowledgement

This work is supported by the Deutsche Forschungsgemeinschaft DFG (SFB 603, Project C4). Patient data have been provided by the Maxillofacial Surgery Department of the University of Cologne, by the Maxillofacial Surgery Department of the University of Erlangen–Nuremberg, and by the Childrens' Hospital of the University of Erlangen–Nuremberg.

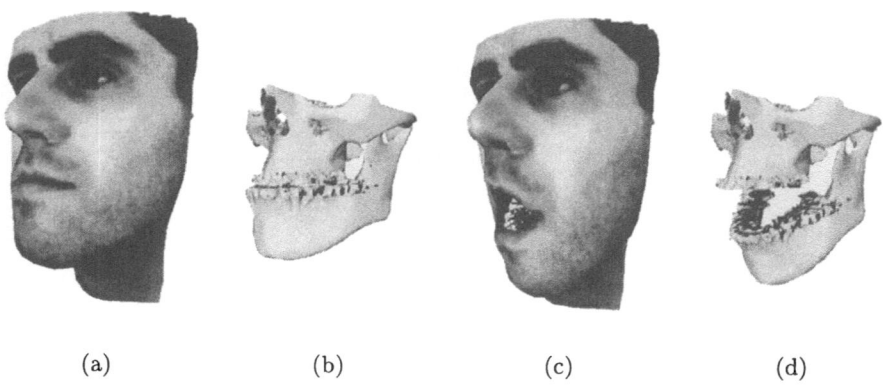

(a)   (b)   (c)   (d)

Fig. 3. Simulated physiological lower jaw movement for patient 1.

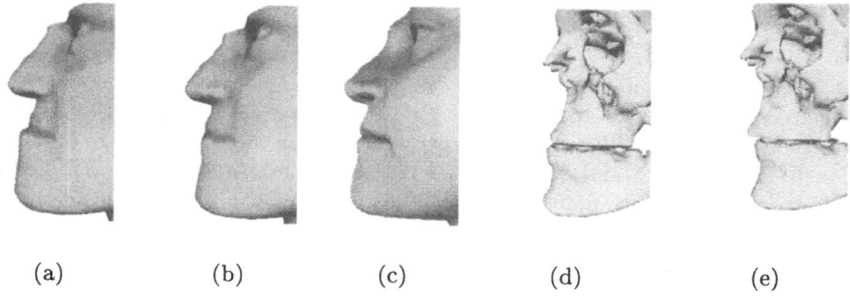

(a)   (b)   (c)   (d)   (e)

Fig. 4. Craniofacial surgery simulation for patient 2. a) Preoperative appearance. b) Simulated postoperative appearance. c) Postoperative appearance. d) Preoperative bone structure. e) Simulated postoperative bone structure.

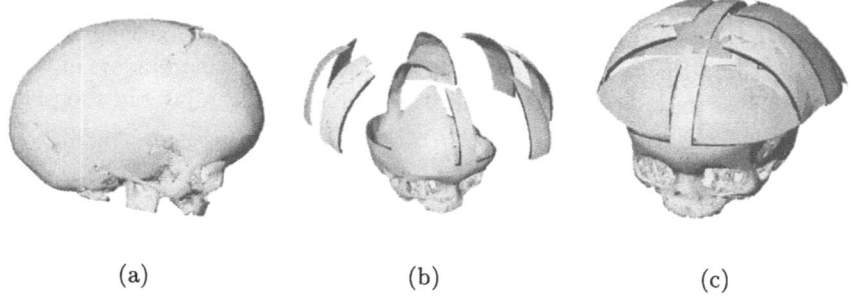

(a)   (b)   (c)

Fig. 5. Planning process in case of a craniosynostosis. a) Reconstructed preoperative skull. b) Segmentation of the Cranial Vault. c) Reconstruction of the Cranial Vault.

References

1. R. H. Taylor, S. Lavellee, G. C. Burdea, R. Mösges. *"Computer Integrated Surgery – Technology and Clinical Applications"*. MIT Press, Cambridge, Massachusetts, USA, 1996.
2. R. Kikinis, H. Cline, D. Altobelli, M. Halle, W. Lorensen, F. Jolesz. "Interactive Visualization and Manipulation of 3D Reconstructions for the Planning of Surgical Procedures". In *Proceedings of Visualization in Biomedical Computing VBC '92*, pages 559–563, 1992.
3. H. Delingette, G. Subsol, S. Cotin, J. Pignon. "A Craniofacial Surgery Testbed". *Technical Report 2119, Institut National de Recherche en Informatique et Automatique, (France)*, 1994.
4. R. A. Robb, B. M. Cameron. "Virtual Reality Assisted Surgery Program". *Medicine Meets Virtual Reality III: Interactive Technology & the New Paradigm for Healthcare*, January 1995.
5. M. Bro-Nielsen. "Finite Element Modeling in Surgery Simulation". *Proceedings of the IEEE: Special Issue on Virtual & Augmented Reality in Medicine*, 86(3):524–530, March 1998.
6. E. Keeve, S. Girod, R. Kikinis, B. Girod. "Deformable Modeling of Facial Tissue for Craniofacial Surgery Simulation". *Computer Aided Surgery*, 3(5), 1998.
7. P. Bohner, P. Pokrandt, S. Haßfeld. "Simultaneous Planning and Execution in Cranio-Maxillo-Facial Surgery". In *Medicine Meets Virtual Reality 4 (MMVR4)*, 1996.
8. S. Girod, E. Keeve, B. Girod. "Soft Tissue Prediction in Orthognatic Surgery by 3D CT and 3D Laser Scanning". *Journal of Oral and Maxillofacial Surgery Suppl.*, 51:167, 1993.
9. E. Keeve, S. Girod, P. Pfeifle, B. Girod. "Anatomy–Based Facial Tissue Modeling Using the Finite Element Method". In *Proc. IEEE Visualization*, 1996.
10. W. E. Lorensen, H. E. Cline. "Marching Cubes: A High Resolution 3D Surface Construction Algorithm". *SIGGRAPH '87, ACM Computer Graphics*, 21(4):163–169, 1987.
11. W. Maurel, Y. Wu, N. Magnenat Thalmann, D. Thalmann. *"Biomechanical Models for Soft Tissue Simulation"*. Springer, Berlin, Germany, 1998.
12. H. Delingette. "Toward Realistic Soft-Tissue Modeling in Medical Simulation". *Proceedings of the IEEE: Special Issue on Virtual & Augmented Reality in Medicine*, 86(3):524–530, March 1998.
13. R. M. Koch, M. H. Gross, D. F. Bueren, G. Frankhauser, Y. Parish, F. R. Carls. "Simulating Facial Surgery Using Finite Element Models". *SIGGRAPH '96, ACM Computer Graphics*, 30, August 1996.
14. W. Press, S. Teulolsky, W. Vetterling, B. P. Flannery. *"Numerical Recipes in C"*. Cambridge University Press, Cambridge, Massachusetts, USA. 2nd edition, 1992.

Modeling the Dynamics of the Human Thigh for a Realistic Echographic Simulator with Force Feedback

D. d'Aulignac[1], M. C. Cavusoglu[2], and C. Laugier[1]

[1] GRAVIR Laboratory
INRIA Rhône Alpes
38330 Montbonnot Saint-Martin, France
{Diego.D_Aulignac, Christian.Laugier}@inrialpes.fr
[2] Robotics and Intelligent Machines Laboratory
University of California, Berkeley
Berkeley, CA 94720
mcenk@eecs.berkeley.edu

Abstract. This paper proposes a mass-spring model of the dynamics of a human thigh based on real data acquired. Using a force sensor mounted on a robot arm the deformation of the thigh with respect to an external force is measured. The stress-strain curves we obtained exhibit a strong non-linearity due to the incompressibility of the human tissue. Hence, we propose a two-layer model of the thigh using both linear and non-linear visco-elastic springs to simulate the observed behaviour. The parameters of the springs are estimated using a least-squares minimisation method. Finally, we discuss the feasibility of our model as part of a fully functional simulator coupled with a haptic interface to train practitioners for echographic exams.

1 Introduction

Echography, in general terms, exploits the information which an acoustic signal provides when it is reflected off a structure to determine the position and shape of the latter. The frequency of these acoustic signals lie within the range of 1MHz and 12 MHz, thus higher then the sounds which are perceptible by humans. Therefore, they are also referred to as *ultrasounds*.

Even though they had already been discovered by P. Curie in 1880, they would have to wait until the 1970's to find an application in the field of medicine. Since, they have been widely used as an inexpensive and non-traumatic means of diagnosis. A common exam is the echography of the thigh to detect a thrombosis in the vein. A healthy vein will compress under the influence of an external force while a vein affected by thrombosis will only partially or even not at all compress, depending on the stage in the evolution of the illness. Depending on the pressure the practitioner applies with the echographic probe on the thigh, he will get an image from which the current state of the vein can be deduced, and hence a possible thrombosis diagnosed.

However, the learning process of this procedure is somehow long and only after approximately 1000 echographic exams an acceptable competence in acquired. The first 500 exams will have to be carried out under the supervision of an experienced practitioner. Virtual environments present an alternative to the conventional medical training scheme. It is possible to create an interactive 3D simulation environment, where the doctors can manipulate or cut dynamically and geometrically correct models of organs and tissues with an haptic interface. The idea is similar to using flight simulators to train pilots. Virtual environments give an environment where there is no risk to a patient, and therefore less stressful. They are interactive and three dimensional contrary to books. Virtual environments also give a unique advantage, as it is possible to generate arbitrary anatomies and pathologies, so that the doctors can be trained for cases that are not frequently encountered.

The goal of this work is to lay the groundwork for the development of an echographic simulator with force feedback. In the final system, the trainee will be looking at artificially generated echographic images, and interacting with a computer simulated dynamical thigh model through a haptic interface. Constructing realistic but computationally efficient models is the main challenge in developing a virtual reality training simulator. In this application it is necessary to have models for deformable tissue being manipulated by the doctor as well as models to construct artificial echographic images.

In this paper, a dynamic model of the human thigh based on experimentally determined deformation characteristics will be presented, followed by a discussion of the results and future directions.

2   Previous Work

Henry [4] examined how a set of echographic images could be used to construct a more general model that would take into account the orientation and pressure exerted with the probe on the thigh. The approach is based on an interpolation method; from a real set of echographic images taken, it will build an echographic image for *any* position and orientation of the probe (see Figure 1 and 2)[1]. Further it is possible to deform the interpolated image obtained with respect to the pressure that is applied to the probe. The criteria on which this deformation depends includes important factors such as the arterial and venous pressure. By modifying these criteria we can simulate a set of pathologies on which medical students could be trained for the identification of the latter.

However, for a meaningful echographic simulation it is of paramount importance to consider the forces involved in such a procedure since they will dictate the deformation of the tissue, and therefore, the subsequent image that is acquired. Laffont [7] was the first to study the implications of the dynamics of such a system which are essential in the development of a realistic simulator coupled to a haptic interface. He based his model on a system of inter-connected springs.

---

[1] Figures kindly provided by the TIMC-GMCAO project

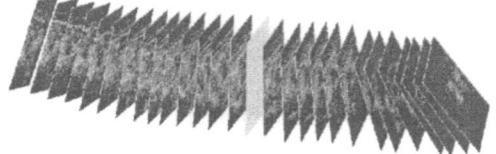

Fig. 1. Creating an image from a set of real echographic images. The highlighted image was obtained by interpolation.

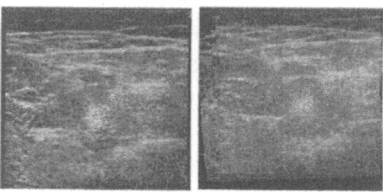

Fig. 2. On the left we can see the real image, and on the right the image obtained by interpolation.

Such a type of approach has already been successfully applied to areas such as facial animation [8] and have the decisive advantage of being easy-to-implement and faster than finite-element simulation, even though lately considerable speed-ups have been achieved in this domain through the use of pre-calculated matrices. This has resulted in, for example, the real-time simulation with force-feedback of the human liver [2] based on the *Visible Human* dataset. However, the model used is inconvenient in the sense that the assumption is made that the tissue is hyper-elastic and linear in its deformation. This is clearly not the case. As bio-mechanical experiments confirm the stress-strain curve of human tissue is non-linear. [8] tackles this problem by using a three-layer model which takes into account the properties of the epidermis, the fatty sub-cutaneous tissue, the muscle, and the bone. The great difficulty for such a system lies in the identification of the parameters of the individual springs that will give the same results to an external force being applied as the measurements in the real world.

3   Modeling of the Thigh

We have constructed a dynamic model of the human thigh based on experimental measurements of its elasticity.

3.1   Experimental Setup and Data Acquisition

In order to model an object such that its behaviour corresponds to reality, measurements must be taken on the real object. In this case we are interested in the deformation of the thigh with respect to an external force which is applied. Intuitively we can affirm that the deformation of the thigh is not the same depending on the shape of the object used to provoke this deformation, or more precisely, the contact surface of that object. Since our aim is to build a generic simulation which will allow a physically correct behaviour which is almost independent of the object we choose to deform the thigh with, two different objects have been used to measure the behaviour of the thigh in terms of penetration distance with respect to the external force being applied.

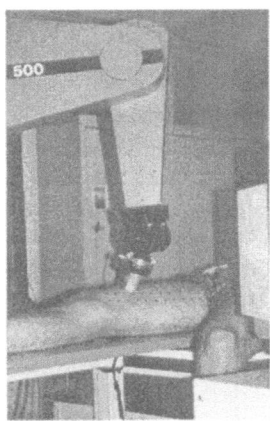 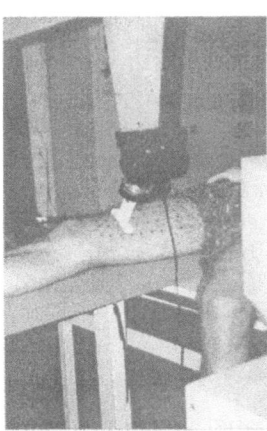

Fig. 3. The two probes used for measuring the behaviour of the thigh.

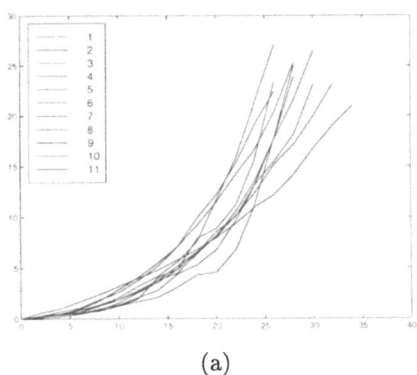 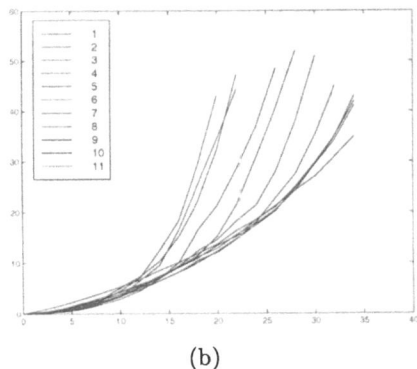

(a)   (b)

Fig. 4. Plot of the reaction force in function of the penetration distance at 11 different points on the thigh using a probe with a punctual contact (on the left) and the pseudo-echographic probe with a larger contact surface (on the right).

The first of these has a tip of pyramidal shape to provoke a punctual force response, while the second one has the same contact surface area as a typical echographic probe. These pseudo-probes are then mounted on a force sensor which in turn is mounted on a PUMA articulated arm. The probe is then positioned perpendicularly to the surface of the thigh at each of 64 points where measurements will be taken. These points are regularly distributed over the area where the echography is performed when trying to detect a thrombosis in the vein. The robotic arm then advances $2mm$ using the reference of the end effector, i.e. the probe pushes along the axis which is normal to the surface of the thigh at the given point. The force is recorded and the procedure is repeated up to an upper force limit.

Figure 4a shows the non-linear relationship between the penetration distance and the reaction force at 11 different points along the thigh. The difference in the curves can be accounted for due to the fact that the thigh is not homogeneous (e.g. in some regions fatty tissue might be pre-dominant, while in others there may be very little separating the epidermis from the bone).

Figure 4b plots the values of the forces for the same points as above but using the second probe with a larger contact surface. As one might expect this results in a larger force for the same penetration distance since the external force applied is distributed over a much larger area.

The assumption is that from these two distinct sets of data it will be possible to make a model which will respond correctly to not only to the two probes used for measurement purposes, but also other probes of a different shape.

3.2   Model construction

Based on the experimental data and the computational requirements, a two layer lumped element model is chosen. The two layer model is composed of a surface mesh of masses, linear springs and dampers, and a set of nonlinear springs orthogonal to the surface to model volumetric effects by giving normal support to the surface mesh (See Figure 5). Two layer models were also used by several authors in the literature, for example in [8]. The deformation-force relation of the nonlinear springs are of the form

$$f(x) = \frac{x}{ax + b} \qquad (1)$$

The nonlinear spring response is chosen to model the incompressibility of the thigh after a certain deformation. In the model, the values of the surface elements are chosen uniform whereas the parameters of the nonlinear spring vary around the mesh to model heterogeneous nature of the thigh mentioned above, while keeping the number of unknown parameters small.

Parameter Estimation Estimation of the model parameters from experimental measurements is a critical part of the modeling. We have used a two step optimisation approach based on nonlinear least squares estimation. In the two step approach, the experimental data is first fit to a simple model without the surface elements, and the results of this fit is used as the initial conditions for the estimation of the parameters of the complete model. This approach is chosen to avoid problems with local minima.

One thing to note here is that the parameter estimation is based on a simplified interaction model between the tissue and indentor, making the assumption

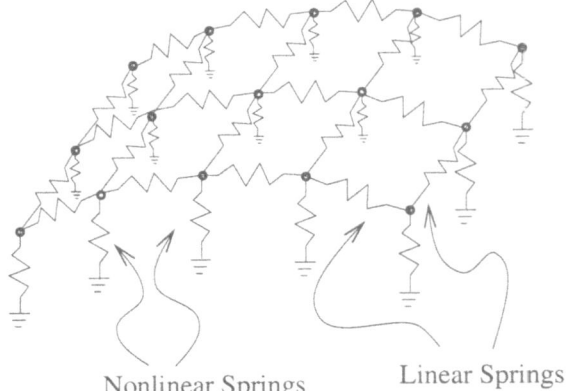

Nonlinear Springs   Linear Springs

Fig. 5. Two layer model of the thigh.

that the probe will principally act on one spring, since the contact area is small. In this simplified interaction model, the nodes that are not in contact with the probe are kept stationary. This simplifies the force calculation as only a small number of springs are deformed for any given dataset.

The mean absolute error between the measured values and the values estimated by the model is 1.05 Newtons, with standard deviation 1.84 Newtons, over the whole dataset. This is equivalent to an approximate error of 5 percent. The distribution of the error can be seen in Figure 6, showing how many of the values estimated by the model exhibit a given error with respect to the real measurements.

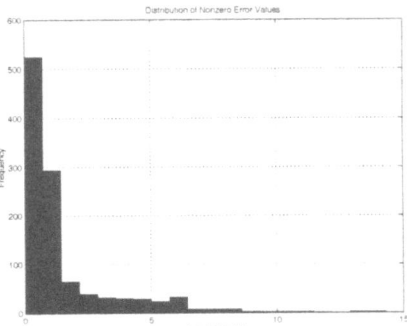

Fig. 6. Frequency distribution of the error between the measured values and the values estimated by the model.

4   Results

Figure 7 shows the model as it has been built in our simulation system [5]. A force is being applied on the thigh using a probe which provokes a deformation which is in accordance with the measurements taken. For collision detection between the objects the algorithm outlined in [6] is used, while the response to a collision is determined by the approach described in [3].

For the integration of the dynamic, differential equations we use *implicit integration* as discussed in [1] and using a conjugate gradient solver [9]. This approach compares favourably to the well-known explicit methods in cases where springs are stiff, allowing to take bigger timesteps, and therefore, gain in overall execution time.

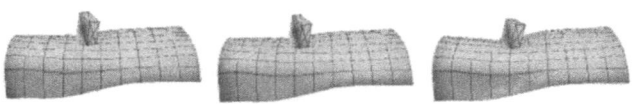

Fig. 7. Model viewed on the simulation system's graphical interface.

The computational speed on a Silicon Graphics R10000 machine is in the order of 100 frames per second of animation, which lets us envisage our simulation system as part of a working echographic simulator which operates in real-time.

5   Discussion

We are at the stage where we can simulate accurately the deformation of the thigh under a static load for a variety of objects used to provoke this deformation. However, what is missing are measurements about the damping and friction coefficients. The first is important in the sense that it defines how fast the tissue will react to a change in external force being applied to it, and the latter due to the fact that the practitioner *slides* the probe down the inner side of the thigh to capture the echographic images. This friction coefficient is influenced by the gel that is typically applied on the thigh to avoid the presence of air between the probe and the tissue, which in turn might influence the quality of the echographic images that are acquired.

We believe that these coefficients may either be adjusted manually using the feedback provided by an experienced practitioner or that additional measurements may be necessary. Once these last problems resolved the primary goal will be to integrate the resulting model with the echographic image creator presented in Section 2 and a force feedback device of type PHANToM built by SensAble Technologies.

6   Conclusions

In this paper we have presented and constructed a model of a human thigh from measurements taken in the real world. We emphasise the point that the human thigh is not linear in its elasticity and introduce the use of non-linear springs for this application and propose a possible solution for the identification of the parameters of the springs. Further, from experimental results of the simulation using the proposed model we believe in the feasibility of our approach as a part of a real-time system which will allow realistic force feedback and the automatic generation of echographic images which takes into account the current deformation.

Acknowledgements We would like to thank Etienne Dombre and François Pierrot at the LIRMM laboratory (Montpellier, France) for their kind assistance while taking the measurements at their lab. Also thanks to the GMCAO project at the TIMC lab in Grenoble, and in particular to Jocelyne Troccaz for her help. This work was partially supported by an INRIA grant within the framework of the AISIM initiative and the France-Berkeley Fund.

Related web sites For more information on the project visit our project homepage: http://www.inrialpes.fr/sharp/modelisation/index-en.html

References

1. D. Baraff and A. Witkin. Large steps in cloth simulation. In *Computer Graphics (Proc. SIGGRAPH)*, pages 43–54, 1998.
2. M. Bro-Nielsen and S. Cotin. Real-time volumetric deformable models for surgery simulation using finite elements and condensation. In *Proceedings of Eurographics*, volume 15, pages 57–66, 1996.
3. A. Deguet, A. Joukhadar, and C. Laugier. Models and algorithms for the collision of rigid and deformable bodies. In P. K. Agarwal, L. E. Kavraki, and M. T. Mason, editors, *Robotics: the algorithmic perspective*, pages 327–338. A K Peters, 1998. Proc. of the Workshop on the Algorithmic Foundations of Robotics. Houston, TX (US). March 1998.
4. D. Henry. *Outils pour la modélisation de structure et la simulation d'examens échographiques.* PhD thesis, Université Joseph Fourier, Grenoble (FR), 1997. (in french).
5. A. Joukhadar and C. Laugier. Dynamic simulation: Model, basic algorithms, and optimization. In *Proc. of the Workshop on the Algorithmic Foundations of Robotics*, Toulouse (FR), July 1996.
6. A. Joukhadar, A. Wabbi, and C. Laugier. Fast contact localisation between deformable polyhedra in motion. In *Proc. of the IEEE Computer Animation Conf.*, pages 126–135, Geneva (CH), June 1996.
7. P. Laffont. Simulation dynamique pour le diagnostic de thromboses veineuses. Mémoire de Diplôme d'Etudes Approfondies, Université de Savoie, Chambéry (FR), 1997.
8. Y. Lee, D. Terzopoulos, and K. Waters. Realistic facial modeling for animation. In *Computer Graphics* Proceedings, Annual Conference Series, Proc. SIGGRAPH '95 (Los Angeles, CA), pages 55–62. ACM SIGGRAPH, August 1995.
9. W. H. Press, B. P. Flannery, S. A. Teukolsky, and W. T. Vetterling. *Numerical Recipes in C.* Cambridge Univ. Press, 2 edition, 1992.

Visualization for Planning and Simulation of Minimally Invasive Neurosurgical Procedures

L.M. Auer[1], A. Radetzky[2], C. Wimmer[1], G. Kleinszig[1], F. Schroecker[2], D.P. Auer[4], H.Delingette[5], B.Davies[3], D.P. Pretschner[2]

[1] Institute of Applied Sciences in Medicine, ISM, Salzburg, Austria
[2] Institute for Medical Informatics, Technical University of Braunschweig, Germany
[3] Imperial College, London, GB
[4] Max Planck Institute for Psychiatry, Munich, AG-NMR, Germany
[5] INRIA, Sophia Antipolis, France

Abstract. A unit for training and simulation as well as for planning of minimally invasive operations of the brain is presented, called ROBO-SIM, for virtual patient positioning, planning of the surgical approach to a target in the depth, for anatomical orientation in the operating field and for manipulations of the virtual tissue. Methods are described for the visualization of the outer body surface (head), the virtual operating field in the depth of the brain, virtual surgical instruments and deformations (displacement, fragmentation) of the virtual tissue by simulated surgical manipulations. Mainly volume-rendered data from 3D-MRI are used. Surface views of the whole dataset are used for virtual patient positioning. For virtual endoscopic visualization of the small operating field within cavities of the brain (ventricles, cysts), a volume rendering application of "Volumizer" has been developed, called "Flight-Volumizer". Elastodynamic tissue deformation is achieved by a viscoelastic model on the surface of the cavities, which is simulated by neuro-fuzzy systems.

1. Introduction

With the advent of computer-assisted methods in surgery, image-guided planning has become an increasingly accepted procedure in neurosurgery under the term of "neuronavigation". As robotic manipulators are being considered to augment precision of microsurgical steps [1-3], complex preoperative planning and simulation is mandatory and will represent an important part of the total duration of a robot-assisted operative procedure. Therefore, the development of surgical simulators, comparable to flight simulators, has been initiated in a number of institutions. However, creation of the illusion of reality, which is most important for simulation and training of surgical manipulations, such as the real-time visualization of movements during manipulations, or the transfer of tactile sensations to the surgeon, or the visualization of the effect of robotic activities, have remained a formidable challenge for high-end graphical computing and other disciplines.

With the concept presented in this paper, the authors propose the use of a combination of volume- and surface-rendered data for visualization tools in a simulator for minimally invasive procedures. 3D-MRI datasets of the brains from actual patients are used to create views from the outer surface of the head (fig. 1) as well as from inner surfaces such as the ventricular system or cystic brain lesions by aid of virtual endoscopy (fig.4) [4-6].

2.   Methods and Present State of Development

The integral setup called ROBO-SIM is designed for manipulator-assisted virtual procedures through a trepanation in the skull of 1-2cm diameter and a miniaturized approach of few millimeters diameter to target areas in the depth of the brain and its ventricular system. The present version of the system consists of a set of real instruments including a real neuro-endoscope mounted onto a passive manipulator arm with encoders and brakes (Impulse Engine, Immersion Corp., San Jose, USA) for the implementation of force-feedback and other constraints. In a more elaborate version as a planning station of the operating system ROBOSCOPE (project of the EU-Telematics programme), the system will include a robot arm, NEUROBOT, which is used by the surgeon as an active manipulator with inbuilt robotic capabilities such as active constraints, backtracking and a steady-distance tool. The surgeon who is planning and performing a virtual surgical procedure is thus working with the real instruments to be used for actual surgery, while looking onto a virtual scenario of the operating field, created by aid of a 3D-MRI-dataset of an actual patient.

For simulations, 3D-MRI-datasets from a 1,5T Signa echo-speed whole body scanner (GE Medical Systems, Milwaukee, USA) are used. The hardware platform for the development and use of the system is an Onyx2 Infinite Reality (Silicon Graphics, Mountain View, USA) as well as SGI O2-workstations and conventional PCs. The Onyx2 is equipped with two R10000 processors (195 Mhz), 640 MB main memory and 64 MB texture memory. The graphics subsystem of the Onyx2 is a Infinite Reality2 graphics board with two channels, 4 graphics engines and one Raster Manager. The Onyx2 is only needed for the real-time visualization and manipulation of the 3D-MRI-dataset.

Figure 1 shows the graphical user interface and the functionality of ROBO-SIM. On the upper left corner, the virtual 3D viewer is demonstrated, where a view onto the patient´s head is shown (Volume Rendering). The wheels and buttons at the sides of the viewer provide control functions, i.e. to rotate and trans-late the virtual camera. The three MR images at the bottom of the user interface show the orthogonal cross-sections of the patients MR 3D-dataset. These images are peri-odically updated with the position of the virtual camera. A red marker in these images indicates the current camera position. The orientation of the virtual camera is represented by a red arrow, and a yellow arrow indicates the up-direction. A manipulator box gives the possibility to change the position and orientation of the camera. The figure shows the axial cross-section with the manipulator to update the camera parameters. With the *view selector* button it is possible to switch to the transendoscopic view and to switch the ventricular surface model on or off. The position and orientation of the virtual endoscope, and in the "Endo" mode also the virtual camera is controlled by the Impulse Engine. The position of the camera in this mode is also displayed in the crossections and updated periodically. Different kinds of virtual instruments can be selected with the *Toolselector*-Menu. With the *Toolmovement*- Slider it is possible to control the instruments' length along the endoscope axis. The *Window/Level*-Sliders are used to adjust the threshold level for the 3D view. With the *Inputfile*-Textfield, different patient datasets can be loaded. If there is an existing surface model in addition to the volume data, it is possible to display this model in the reconstructed 3D-volume as indicated above.

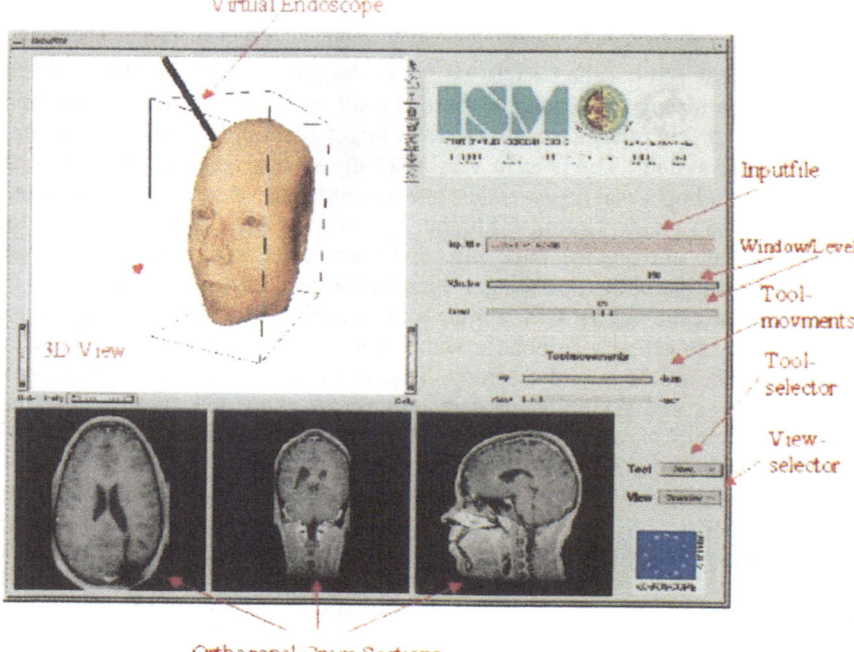

Fig. 1. The user interface of the simulator ROBO-SIM shows a view of the surface of the 3-D-MRI-dataset as well as 3 planes of tomograms.

2.1. Method of Virtual Endoscopy for Visualization of the Virtual Operating Field

Before the development of software for virtual endocopy, various existing systems have been evaluated for their applicability in the frame of ROBO-SIM; detailed descriptions of this work are given elsewhere [7]. As a consequence of these analyses, a new software for virtual endoscopy was developed, called *"Flight Volumizer"*, which uses the Advanced Programming Interface (API) OpenGL "Volumizer" [8] from Silicon Graphics as a basis. "Volumizer" is a volume rendering technique, a so-called *PARC* Algorithm (Polygon Aided Ray Casting), which uses tetrahedrons as volumetric primitives. This algorithm is highly accelerated for the efficient *Infinite Reality Graphics* hardware of the SGI Onyx2.

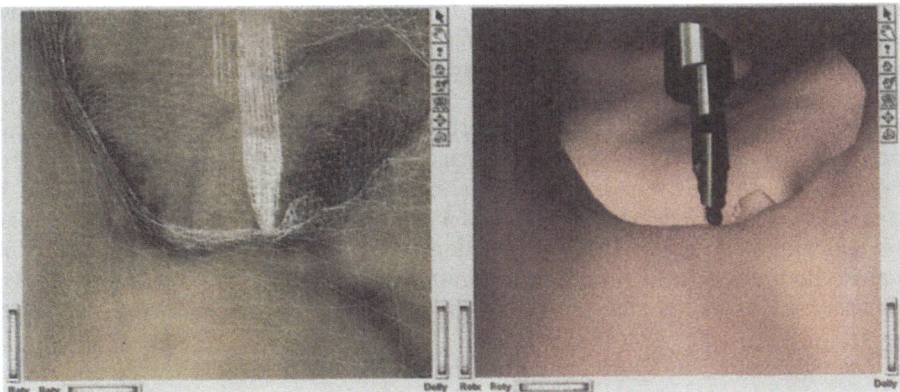

Fig. 2. Virtual endoscopic views of the lateral ventricle (left: surface-rendered image, right: view with Flight-Volumizer) with a virtual instrument applied transendoscopically. The right picture shows the overlay of the mesh underlying the surface rendering and the 3D dataset visualized with Volumizer. Each triangle on the surface is one face of a volumetric primitive at the same time.

Another advantage of "Volumizer" is the separation of the 3D dataset in *Geometry* (a set of volumetric primitives) and *Appearance* (voxel volume). Thus, Volumizer allows deformations and fragmentations by transforming the geometry without alterations of the voxel volume. Fragmentations are achieved by clipping the appearance on the geometry.

Besides, most of the voxel volume is not visible in virtual endoscopy because the usual view is transendoscopic. Therefore, only a small part of the 3D dataset has to be visualized, which is called the 'field of view'. The field of view is defined by the visibility limit of the virtual camera mounted onto the endoscope. In most cases this would be a cone or, for visualization on a monitor, a pyramid (the 'view-frustum'). The tip of the view-frustum is located in the camera, and its basis is perpendicular to the camera's objective. Only the volumetric primitives inside the view frustum are in the field of view, and only these tetrahedrons have to be shown. Thus, by disabling all other tetrahedrons, it is possible to increase the rendering speed considerably.

Furthermore, virtual deformations only have

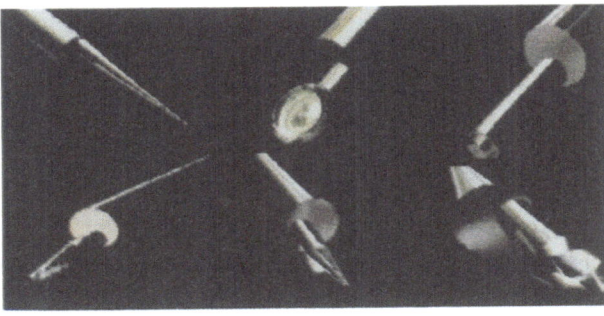

Fig. 3. Set of virtual instruments, which are introduced through the endoscope (scissors, biopsy forceps, grasping forceps, curette, needle, suction tube).

to be applied to the tetrahedrons inside the view frustum and thus simplifying the required algorithms (see section 2.4.2). The software is developed using C++ and the object oriented 3D-toolkit Open Inventor [11], where Volumizer's functionality is fully integrated.

Besides visualization of ventricular surfaces of the volume-rendered dataset, a surface rendered model of the ventricular surface, coregistered with the volume-rendered dataset, may be used for visualization; alternatively, a combination of both can be used. The surface models were generated as a preprocessing step by aid of a semiautomatic segmentation tool [9]. The resulting surface model was integrated in the virtual environment (OpenInventor SceneGraph) in addition to the volume dataset. The transparency of certain intensities can be set with the *Window/Level*-sliders (see fig.1).

The view shown in figure 2 is intentionally different from a transendoscopic view in order to provide a better overview of the situation from a technical standpoint. Primarily, however, visualization of the operating field for virtual surgery would be transendoscopic. Therefore, the number of volumetric primitives inside the view-frustum would be much less, because the endoscope is directly facing the ventricle's surface. Using a transendoscopic view, interactive frame rates of approximately 10 frames per second are possible with a volume-rendered dataset. The virtual instruments available for selection by the surgeon are shown on fig.3.

2.2. Visualization of Virtual Patient Positioning and Approach Planning

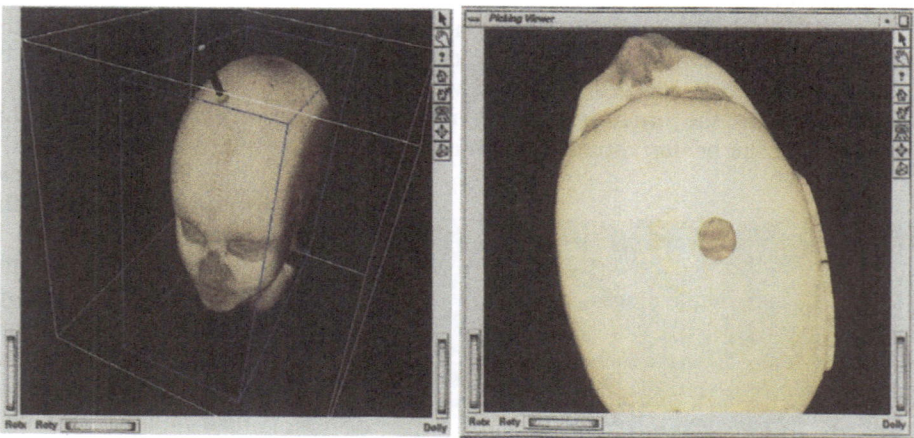

Fig. 4. Following positioning of the virtual patient, a port of entry into the skull (trepanation) is selected by aid of the "virtual craniotomy" tool, which allows to view the cerebral cortex for decisionmaking.

For virtual positioning of the patient's head, it is possible to translate and rotate the dataset with respect to the virtual endoscope using a manipulator box, which surrounds the entire head and can be freely translated and rotated. For the simulation of a trepanation, the virtual burrhole is placed and adjusted to the underlying anatomy of the brain surface (fig.4). This virtual burrhole is defined by a cylinder with a height of 8 mm along the negative gradient of the surface. The volume around the cylinder is filled with a geometry of tetrahedrons, which replaces the standard geometry consisting of a tetrahedrated cube containing the whole dataset. As a result, the entire head exept the skullbone with a selected radius at the desired position is visualized (fig.4).

As a next step in the virtual planning procedure, the target point for arrival of the instrument in the depth of the operating field may be selected by respective placement of the tip of the virtual instrument. The viewing direction inside the dataset can be freely chosen to allow e.g. virtual transendoscopic visualization or a view onto the tip of the instrument in relation to the surrounding anatomical structures (fig.5).

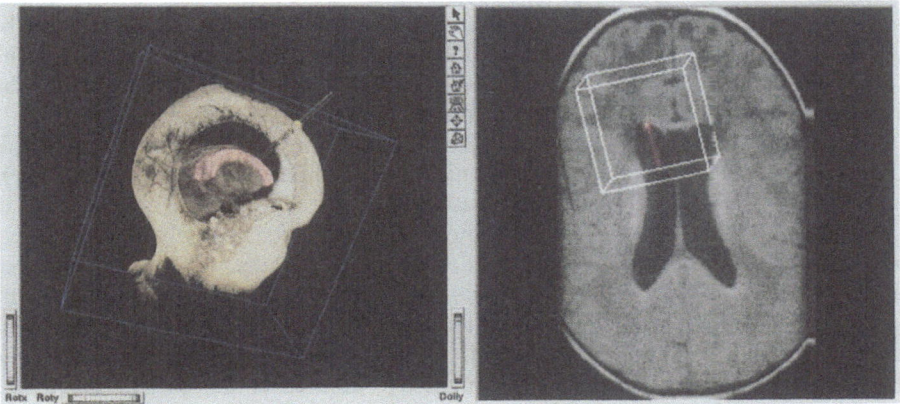

Fig. 5. Planning of the target point is possible by placing the tip of the instrument such as the virtual endoscope (left) or by selecting a point in the tomograms, using the respective selector box (right). The figure on the left is an overlay of a semi-translucent volume-image and the patient's surface-rendered ventricular system.

2.4. Elastodynamic Tissue Deformation

To simulate deformable tissues, a dynamic component is required. Every tissue has an assigned mass, elasticity and viscosity. The appearance or behavior of any deformation depends on these parameters to a great part[1]. To describe these physical conditions, a viscoelastic model can be used [16].

One of the first applications of viscoelastic models for the simulation of elastic deformable models was developed by Terzopoulos et al. [14]. Some improved techniques were presented, for example, in [15-18]. One of the main problems of these approaches is the difficulty to derive the parameters of the physical model – thus leading to an insufficient biological realism [17] – and the high computational demands during simulation. Furthermore, some of these approaches can not be used if

---

[1] Further parameters (depending on the used model structure) are, for example, friction and fragility. These parameters are not considered in the following, but they can be defined by the presented approach, too.

cuts have to be performed. To resolve these problems, a neural network architecture [19] was developed, which is able to simulate viscoelastic models [21]. In this way it is possible to learn the parameters of the physical model and to speed up the simulation by use of problem specific propagation[2] procedures. Furthermore, a fuzzy system was implemented to initialize the network parameters if some prior knowledge about the model, like stiffness, elasticity or shiftability, is available [12, 21].

Viscoelastic Models. In viscoelastic models [16] the whole mass of the elastic objects (e.g. virtual organs) is divided up between the mass points of the model, which are represented as nodes in a mesh. Every node of the mesh can be connected elastically or viscously to its neighbors. The connections are represented as viscoelastic elements. By use of this model, deformations, transections, coagulations etc. can be performed virtually. This is done by applying external forces to the nodes of the mesh, which are affected by collisions with virtual instruments. Also, the displacement of a node can be given and the resulting forces can be calculated.

Viscoelastic models of deformable objects can be simulated 'as a whole', which is comparable to the computation of conventional differential equation systems. This is called total deformation [20] and can be used especially if the objects are not fixed or connected with other objects. However, the total deformation can only be used in real time with small objects consisting of only a few hundred nodes, whereas the complex surface of the ventricle shown in fig. 2 has about 20000 nodes. However, for a realistic impression only deformations within the view-frustum have to be simulated. This can be done with local deformation [20]. A local deformation is the same as a total deformation except that the local deformation is limited to the part of the tissue, which is directly influenced by the contact with an instrument. Using traditional deformation models, this leads to insufficient realism because local deformation is a heavy simplification of the real dynamic system. Another approach uses neuro-fuzzy systems [22] for the simulation of viscoelastic models [21]. With neuro-fuzzy systems, the deformation behavior can be learned or given by simple linguistic terms regardless of the simplification done by local deformation. Not the exact physical model but the visual realism is imitated. For surgical simulation, it is sufficient if a virtual deformation appears real to an expert surgeon.

A comprehensive introduction of the simulation with neuro-fuzzy systems is given in [13, 21].

Virtual Deformations and Fragmentations. In general, virtual deformations of 3D datasets can be simulated by transforming the volumetric primitives of Volumizer's geometry. However, the geometry has to be connected with a viscoelastic model in such a way as to fill the whole visible dataset without intersections of volumetric primitives. One approach is to create viscoelastic models, which are inspired by crystal structures. In [10] an algorithm is presented, which can be used to fill a diamond crystal structure with volumetric primitives. Diamond crystals, represented as viscoelastic models, have the opportunity that large volumes can be filled with

---

[2] Propagation is the computation process of neural networks. In this case it is similar to algorithms for solving systems of differential equations [13].

comparatively few springs and nodes. By connecting the viscoelastic model with the volumetric primitives, deformations of 3D datasets can be simulated simply by deforming the viscoelastic model.

However, simulating deformations of the whole volume is not necessary if an additional surface model exists. For example, the segmented surface of the ventricle shown in fig. 2 can be used to create a geometry of tetrahedrons starting from the ventricle's surface in direction of the brain surface and the skull. Each triangle of the surface defines the base of a prism, which can be described by three tetrahedrons. The surface itself is defined by a viscoelastic model, whose visualization is optional. In case of a collision with a virtual instrument, the surface is deformed using local deformation (see fig. 6). This causes a transformation of the prisms and thus a deformation of the 3D dataset. The generation of the prisms is very fast so that they can be created within the view-frustum during visualization. Thus, only the visible part of the volume has to be shown and deformed.

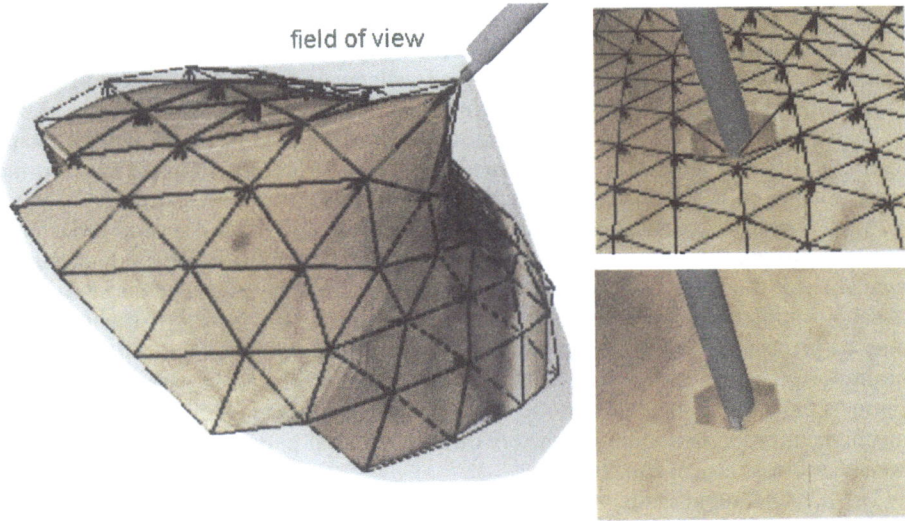

Fig. 6. Virtual deformations and fragmentations of a MR-dataset by use of an endoscope. Only the tetrahedrons inside the view-frustum are shown (left). On the right side a fragmentation is done by clipping on Volumizer's geometry.

Another advantage of this approach is the possibility for an easy implementation of fragmentations, e.g. virtual removal of tissue by aid of a biopsy forceps. By changing the mapping between the geometry and the appearance (cp. section 2.2) the voxel volume is clipped instead of deformed (see fig. 6). At the first contact with the forceps, the volume is deformed until the forceps is closed. Then, the deformation of the volume at the collision points remains permanent, which can be done by relaxing the involved springs. The next step is to change the mapping of geometry and appearance to clip the volume at this location. The fragmented volume remains in the dataset, but it is excluded from rendering by the clipping function of Volumizer.

3. Discussion

Simulation of microsurgical manipulations and their visualization has become technically possible on a widely acceptable financial level of graphic computing. In several more years, hardware costs for the same computing power will be substantially reduced, or significantly more possibilities will be available for the same amount of money.

Several important factors of surgical simulation can already be dealt with by newest technical development such as visualization of the virtual operating field of an actual patient's anatomy and of elastodynamic tissue properties, propagation of some force feedback to the surgeon, manipulation with real instruments while seeing virtual instruments in the virtual operating field similar to the aspect in real surgery.

The simulation of bleeding, considered as an important factor for simulation of surgery in other body regions, is a minor factor in minimally invasive neurosurgery for the following reason: one of the basic strategies of surgical manipulations through minimally invasive approaches is preventive hemostasis by coagulation; this means that tissue is coagulated before it is removed, whenever a disturbing extent of hemorrhage can not be excluded with very high probability.

Typical colors of classical landmarks for endoscopic neurosurgery will be visualized by aid of a deformable surface model of these structures supplied with surface structure and color from a typical example of real endoscopic microsurgery.

More detailed force feedbacks and tactile sensations will not create a major progress for minimally invasive neurosurgery, because very little tactile information is available for the surgeon in real surgery, caused by friction-resistance during transendoscopic application of microinstruments. Individual mechanical tissue properties may be preselected with the present state of development; additional information will be imported by aid of a model database for a number of pathologies. However, the same as the individual color of patient's tissues as mentioned below, simulation of the mechanical properties of single voxels of an individual patient's tissue will remain a considerable technical challenge.

However, a number of other important factors still represent a major technical problem and thus a formidable challenge: one is the basic color of an individual patient's brain tissue, and more so, the individual color of pathology such as an individual tumor. Here, the solution might be to create a database of typical examples from real surgery, at least from the surface texture of a pathological tissue (individual colors of volumes of interest as such as the interior of tumor will remain very complicated).

Yet another factor which plays an important role in creating the illusion of a real situation during virtual surgery is the behavior of intracranial tissue compartments as a consequence of changes in intracranial pressure as well as of intracranial volume compartments: Changes in pressure of the irrigation fluid causes characteristic floating movements of the septum pellucidum and other thinwalled structures. Moreover, removal of larger amounts of intracranial volume such as cerebralspinal fluid or cyst fluid or tumor cause a readaptation of the remaining tissue compartments according to physical conditions in the closed system of a cranial cavity. Thus, physiological parameters such as the intracranial pressure – volume relationship will remain a challenge for the creation of a perfectly simulated surgical scenario, realistic enough to allow the use of such device for comprehensive training of real surgery.

In summary, promising progress has been made in the creation of virtual worlds for a simulator of minimally invasive neurosurgery, however, several problems such as individual physiological factors will remain a formidable technical challenge.

References

1. Benabid-AL; Cinquin-P; Lavalle-S; Le-Bas-JF; Demongeot-J; De-Rougemont-J. Computer-driven robot for stereotactic surgery connected to CT scan and magnetic resonance imaging. Technological design and preliminary results. APPL-NEUROPHYSIOL. 50/1-6 (153-154) 1987

2. Davies, B.L., Ng, W.S., Hibberd, R.D., "Prostatic Resection; an example of safe robotic surgery." Robotica, Cambridge University Press, Vol 11, pp561-566, 1993.

3. Goradia, T.M., R Taylor, Auer LM. Robot-Assisted Minimally Invasive Neurosurgical Procedures: First Experimental Experience. Lecture Notes in Computer Science 1205, Springer 1997, pp319-22

4. Auer LM, Auer D.P., JF Knoplioch. Virtual Endoscopy for Planning and Simulation of Minimally Invasive Neurosurgery. Lecture Notes in Computer Science 1205, Springer-Verlag 1997, pp 315-18

5. Auer D.P., Auer LM. Virtual Endoscopy. A new Tool for Teaching and Training in Neuroimaging. Int.J. of Neuroradiol. 4, 1998, 3-14.

6. Auer, L.M., Auer, D.P. Virtual Endoscopy for Planning and Simulation of Minimally Invasive Neurosurgery. Neurosurgery 43, 1998, 529-548.

7. Kleinszig, G., Auer, D.P., Auer, L.M., Virtuelle Neuro-Endoskopie. Proc. OGBMT, Vienna 1998.

8. Grzeszczuk R, Henn C, Yagel R. Advanced Geometric Techniques for Ray Casting Volumes. In: Course Notes, 4, SIGGRAPH'98, 1998.

9. Delingette, H., General Object Reconstruction based on Simplex Meshes, INRIA Techn. Report No 3111, Feb. 1997

10. Radetzky, A., Wimmer, C., Kleinszig G., Brukner, M., Auer, L.M., Pretschner, D.P. Interactive Deformable Volume Graphics in Surgical Simulation. In: International Workshop on Volume Graphics, 1999.

11. Wernecke J. The Inventor Mentor. New York: Addison-Wesley, 1994.

12. Radetzky A, Nürnberger A, Pretschner DP. Elastodynamic Shape Modeler: A Tool to Define the Deformation Behavior of Virtual Tissues. In: RadioGraphics, 2000; 20(3) (to appear)

13. Nürnberger A, Radetzky A, Kruse R. A Problem Specific Recurrent Neural Network for the Description and Simulation of Dynamic Spring Models. Proc of the Int Joint Conference on Neural Networks, 1998; 468-473.

14. Terzopoulos D, Platt J, Barr A, Fleischer, K. Elastically deformable models, In: Computer Graphics, 1987; 21(4): 205-214.

15. Terzopoulos D, Fleischer K. Deformable Models, The Visual Computer, 1988; 4:306-331.

16. Terzopoulos D, Fleischer K. Modeling inelastic deformation: Viscoelasticity, plasticity, fracture. In: Computer Graphics, 1988; 22(4):269-278.

17. Cotin C, Delingette H, Ayache N. Efficient Linear Elastic Models of Soft Tissues for real-time surgery simulation, INRIA report no. 3510, INRIA Sophia Antipolis, 1998.

18. Cotin C, Delingette H, Ayache N. Real-time elastic deformations of soft tissues for surgery simulation, INRIA report no. 3511, INRIA Sophia Antipolis, 1998.

19. Rojas R. Neural Networks - A Systematic Introduction, Berlin: Springer, 1996.

20. Radetzky A, Nürnberger A, Teistler M, Pretschner DP. Elastodynamic shape modeling in virtual medicine. In: Proc. of Int Conference on Shape Modeling and Applications, IEEE Computer society, 1999; 172-178.

21. Radetzky A, Nürnberger A, Pretschner DP. Simulation of elastic tissues in virtual medicine using neuro-fuzzy systems, Kim, Y.; Mun, S.K. (ed), In: Medical Imaging 1998: Image Display. Proc. of SPIE Vol. 3335, 1998; 399-409.

22. Nauck D, Klawonn F, Kruse R. Foundations of Neuro-Fuzzy Systems, New York: John Wiley & Sons Inc., 1997.

Acknowlegements

This project is supported by the Austrian Ministery of Research (grant to ISM) and by the European Commission, programme telematics (nr. 4.018, Coordinator Dr.V.Paul, IBMT, Fraunhofer Institut für Biomed. Technik, AG Medizin-Telematik, St.Ingbert, D).

The consortium includes, besides the institutions of the authors and IBMT, Katholiek Univ. Leuven, Belgium, Silicon Graphics Inc., Cortaillod, Switzerland, Fokker-Controls, Amsterdam, The Netherlands, Kretz-Technik, Zipf, Austria, and a consortium of clinical validation centers from the departments of Neurosurgery of the Universities of Greifswald, Germany, Ghent, Belgium, Copenhagen, Denmark, Creteil/Paris, France, Nijmegen, The Netherlands).

A Simulation Environment for Maxillofacial Surgery Including Soft Tissue Implications

Filip Schutyser[1], Johan Van Cleynenbreugel[1],
Joseph Schoenaers[2], Guy Marchal[1], and Paul Suetens[1]

[1] Laboratory for Medical Image Computing (ESAT and Radiology) K.U.Leuven,
[2] Departement of Stomatology and Maxillofacial Surgery,
University Hospitals of Leuven, Herestraat 49, B-3000 Leuven, Belgium
Filip.Schutyser@uz.kuleuven.ac.be

Abstract. This paper describes work in progress in the area of planning and prediction of maxillofacial surgery. We focus on true 3D problems which cannot be addressed by conventional 2D cephalometric radiographs. Examples are bilateral repositioning of the zygoma's or treating facial asymmetries. The environment being developed arose from the need of patients for prediction of their expected post-op outlook and from the need of surgeons for better support to reach the desired result. Our simulation environment adheres to a scene-based approach in which CT image-derived visualizations and additional 3D photographs (showing the face surface and its natural complexion) are co-presented and manipulated. Tools for non-planar osteotomy are included. Repositioning of bone fragments is made possible. Furthermore, a voxel displacement formalism is presented to account for soft tissue implications. Combining these simulation tools, a qualitative prediction of the facial outlook is obtained. Results are shown for a case of hypoplastic zygoma repositioning.

Keywords Image guided therapy, maxillofacial surgery simulation, osteotomy, soft tissue modelling

1 Introduction

The human face plays a key role in interpersonal relationships. Indeed, facial outlook is of utmost importance in recognizing and remembering another person. Consequently, people are very sensitive to changes in this outlook. In the case of facial malformations (caused by e.g. car-accidents, tumors, congenital dysmorphologies, ...) this concern is even more severe as maxillofacial surgery is often required. The important question "What will I look like after surgery ?" is not always easy to answer, however.

To predict expected surgical results, an image based simulation system can be considered. However the success of such an approach depends on how it deals with requirements specific to maxillofacial prediction:

- Natural facial perception is 3D. Standard cephalometric images usually show lateral projections only, which is certainly not the facial impression obtained by looking at one-selve's in a mirror.
- The repositioning of bone fragments after osteotomy is often a real 3D problem. Typical examples are bilateral repositioning of the zygomas or reconstruction of facial symmetry.
- To a patient, it is not only important to predict the post-operative shape of his/her face, but also how this shape will look in combination with his/her natural complexion.

This paper describes the current state of an image based system that is meant to cope with the above requirements. With this system, surgical actions on underlying bony structures are simulated. Their implications on surrounding soft tissue (the shape of the skin) are calculated. The expected result of the surgery is shown to the patient in a convincing and realistic manner.

Section 2 discusses current planning procedures and related research work for maxillofacial surgery including soft tissue implications. In section 3 our developments are explained. Concluding remarks finish the paper in section 4.

2   Background

A maxillofacial intervention is normally planned by means of lateral X-ray images. Using these so-called cephalograms, distances (based on cephalometric landmarks) are measured and compared to their normal values. In this way a surgeon derives a surgical plan while the patient is provided with the expected new contour of the face. This image-on-film based planning has been extended towards 2D image based computer systems, some of them even capable of introducing video images [1]. However, predictability is limited due to the lack to explore 3D movement and its consequences. Planning methods based on 3D images may open new possibilities to handle the requirements mentioned in the previous section.

One 3D attempt is the use of tangible skull models produced by e.g. stereolithograpy [2]. These models make realistic bone surgery simulation possible. However, disadvantages are a large extra cost of the model, a considerable production time and a loss of information concerning soft tissues. Instead of tactile models, 3D software planning systems are another line of work. Ideally, such systems would include capabilities for osteotomy simulation, cephalometric reference data for guidance during repositioning, and finally ways for modelling soft tissue deformation. In practice, no single system integrating these features has been reported on:

1. Osteotomy simulation for craniofacial surgery is surveyed by Vannier et al. [3]. More recent examples are the work of Altobelli et al. [4], Keeve et al. [5] and Bohner et al. [8]. In general this work is restricted to planar cuts.
2. Cutting et al. [21] describe an early method to introduce 3D cephalometric constraints. However, only a limited transfer of well-known cephalometric

landmarks from lateral and frontal 2D X-ray analysis towards 3D image analysis is possible (see also [9]). Altobelli et al. [4] apply interactive repositioning using cephalometric and anthropometric databases. This previous work mentioned the paucity of normative 3D data as a significant obstacle. Mollard et al. [10] recently report on an integration of 3D cephalometry into a simulator for orthognatic surgery.

3. For modelling soft tissue deformation, a number of (intuitive) physics based, models are described in the literature. In all these approaches, the derivation of tissue material properties (e.g. generalised constant of Hooke) from image data is treated harshly. On the other hand, applying such models in a simulation environment usually means to trade-off interactivity against accuracy. *Mass-spring* models represent soft tissue as a collection of point masses connected by (nonlinear) springs in a lattice structure. E.g. in [5] mass-spring modeling of the skin tissue is used resulting in a model that can be updated at interactive speeds, but represents a significant approximation. In *continuum* models, deformation is described as a function of external forces and of the tissue's material properties. When such models are solved by finite element methods (FEM), physically realistic simulations can be provided , however at the expense of loosing interactivity, e.g. [11]. To speed up FEM, several assumptions (and thus reduced flexibility) can be made to perform part of the calculations in a pre-processing step [12, 13]. *Voxel-based methods*, focusing on fast respons time without sacrificing to much realism, are explored by Gibson et al., [6, 7]. Such methods combine a kinematic model (ChainMail) determining the coarse motion of a discretized deformable object to a dynamic model (mass-spring model) to refine the final shape of the object.

3   Methods

3.1   3D environment

Our current simulation system expands on the ideas we have previously described in [14] and applied to other surgical disciplines in [15] and [16]. Basically we adhere to a scene-based approach in which image derived visualizations (MPR, surfaces, volume renderings) and additional 3D structures (external to the medical image volume) are co-presented and manipulated. As an example of the latter – typical for maxillofacial applications –, see figure 1. The underlying graphics environment is OpenInventor [17].

Primarily we employ CT data. It is reasonably easy to segment bone structures and soft tissues of interest from this source. To provide the patient with a realistic view of the natural complexion of his/her face, we also acquire a 3D photograph. Currently we use an "active" 3D system (projecting a pattern on the face and recovering 3D from the deformation of the pattern on the 2D picture), see [18]. The surface thus obtained is registered with the skin surface extracted from the CT using point/surface matching algorithms like ICP [19] or a 3D extension of RPM [20]. A result was shown in figure 1 already.

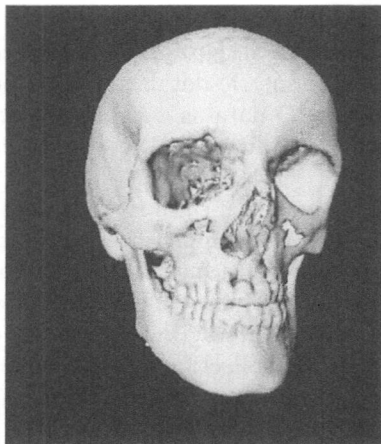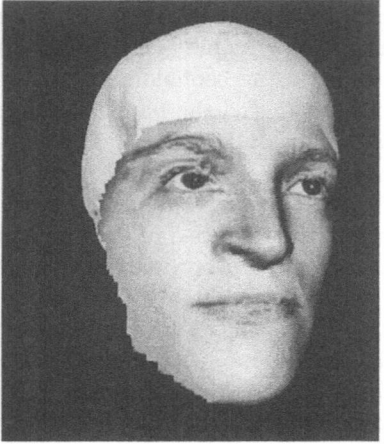

Fig. 1. Our surgical simulation environment presents anatomical objects in a 3D scene. The bony structures derived from CT images, can be co-presented with arbitrarily chosen multiplanar reslices and for example so-callled 3D photographs.

3.2   Osteotomy planning: cutting and repositioning of bone

To simulate osteotomy, first a cutting blade is defined on a surface representation of the bone, then the cutting action is performed, and finally repositioning of the bone fragments is made possible.

The definition of the cutting blade is a two step procedure. First, the surgeon draws a trajectory on the bone surface (using the workstation's mouse). While drawing, this surface can be rotated and translated to have an optimal sight on the structure of interest (figure 2). Real time manipulation is possible due to graphics features such as overlay planes and depth buffers. Second, the surgeon specifies the depth along the cutting trajectory. This depth is edited by means of a manipulator (see figure 2 or by means of a 3D cursor (3D mouse) in combination with stereoviewing (shutter glasses)). Once the trajectory is thus extended into a cutting blade, the actual cutting action is performed on the volume data itself (by labeling voxels adjacent to the blade and recalculating bone surfaces, see figure 3).

Repositioning is the final step in every osteotomy simulation. However it is not sufficient to provide general tools to freely rotate and translate resectioned bone fragments in 3D space. Extra guidance should be introduced. In [15] we have already shown that in this way the repeatability of a planning procedure can be increased and the planning time be decreased. It will be clear that 3D cephalometry is the best provider of medical knowledge in this context. However as pointed out in section 2, no reliable sources are yet to be found, leaving this part of our simulation environment as work in progress.

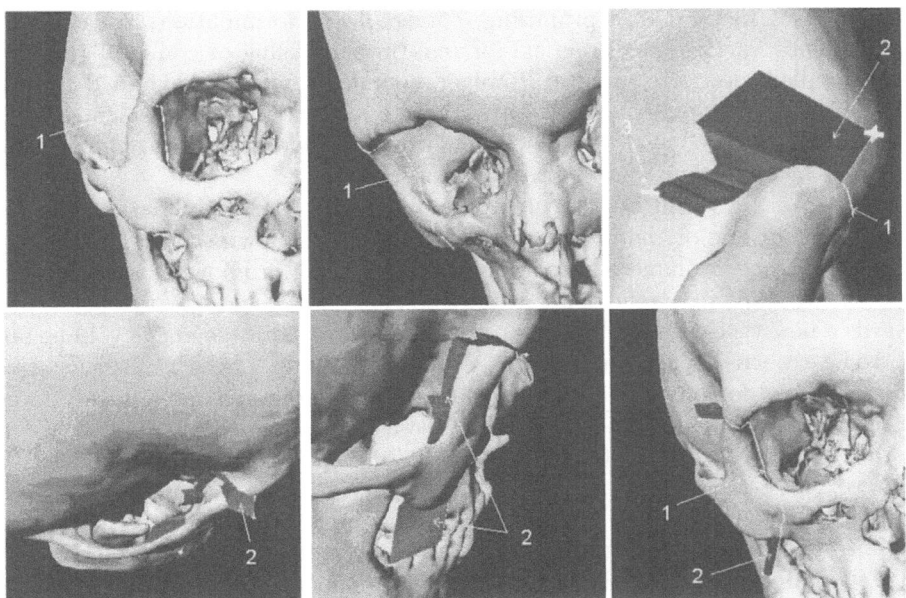

Fig. 2. In this example, an osteotomy trajectory (1) is being drawn on a zygoma. Due to its complex anatomy, the outlined trajectory is a true 3D curve. The cutting blade (2) is specified as shown in the upper right image. The manipulator (3) is used to change the direction and extent of the depth of the blade along the cutting trajectory. The final result is depicted in the bottom row.

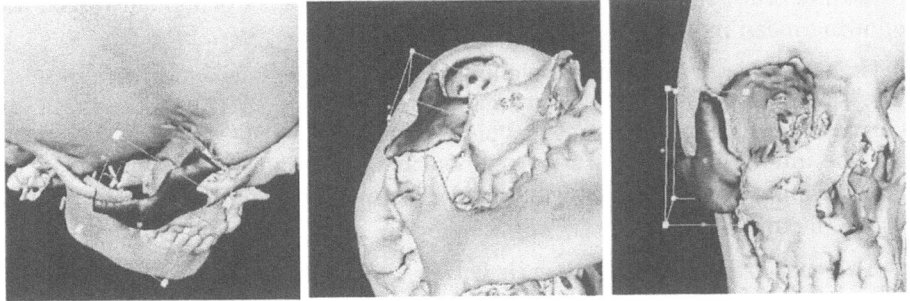

Fig. 3. As a result of applying the cutting blade, the zygoma is resectioned (darker part) from the skull. A manipulator is attached to it in order to allow repositioning.

3.3   Soft tissue modelling

While FEM methods are promising, current FEM formulations and software implementations are not practical for real-time modeling of complex geometry and detailed interior structure. However, complex system behaviour can result from applying simple behaviour patterns to a large number of elements. Based on this observation, we state a new formalism for voxel-based tissue displacement induced by sectioning and repositioning of bone.

Indeed, as a result of our osteotomy and repositioning simulation, the displacement of one or more bone tissue part(s) B is known. Hence, in the pre-operative image volume a displacement vector $\Delta(v)$ is known for every voxel $v \in B$. We want to extend this partially defined displacement vector field Δ towards a new vector field $\overline{\Delta}$ that maps the entire pre-operative image volume into a "to be expected" postoperative image volume. Of course, $\forall v \in B, \overline{\Delta}(v) = \Delta(v)$. Furthermore, for our application of maxillofacial surgery, we are mainly interested in the behaviour of $\overline{\Delta}$ on voxels "between" bone and skin.

So how can $\Delta(v)$ be extended towards $\overline{\Delta}(v)$ on a voxel level? We model $\overline{\Delta}(v)$ in a voxel $v \notin B$ by taking into account three factors (sources of influence). First, suppose $N_v = \{w_1, \cdots, w_n\}$ is a set of voxels neighbouring v. Then it is reasonable to expect that $\overline{\Delta}$ is behaving in v in a way consistent with its behaviour in N_v. Stated otherwise, the displacement in v depends on the displacement of its neigbouring voxels. Second, as v belongs to a given tissue type, also material properties, say $M(v)$ will contribute to the expected displacement. Finally, the way v interacts with its neighbouring voxels ties the previous sources together. We denote this interaction as the function Φ, resulting in the relationship

$$\overline{\Delta}(v) = \Phi(\overline{\Delta}(w_1), \cdots, \overline{\Delta}(w_n), M(v))$$

This equation will generally be used in an iterative way starting from the known values of $\overline{\Delta}$ in the voxels belonging to B. In this way the equation drives a relaxation scheme. Of course a variety of extended displacement fields can be obtained by varying N_v, M and Φ.

To illustrate this approach, assume the three sources of influence have the following meaning:

1. Let N_v the set of six facet neighbours of v.
2. Assume that for a voxel v belonging to soft tissue, $M(v)$ represents a displacement attenuation factor typical for the soft tissue.
3. The interaction of v with its neigbouring voxels is expressed as taking the maximum of the neighbouring displacement vectors and attuenuating it by the factor $M(v)$.

For each iteration and for each voxel v belonging to the soft tissue of interest, $\overline{\Delta}(v)$ is calculated as stated by source 3. Convergence of iteration is assumed when the difference in the displacement field between two iteration steps is smaller than a given ϵ.

A result is shown in figure 4. Initially the zygoma was repositioned according to the expertise of the surgeon. The original 3D photograph has been locally displaced by apptying the extended displacement field to the skin surface.

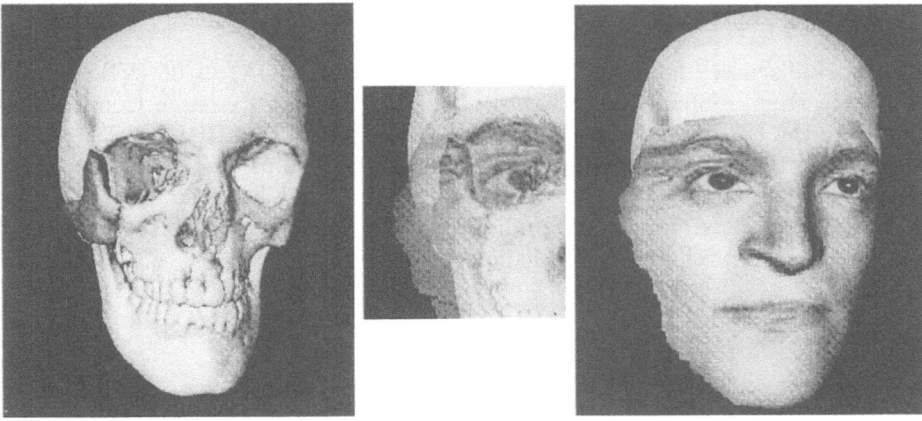

Fig. 4. On the left, a hypoplastic zygoma is repositioned to approximate the ideal sizes of the skull. Using our approach of extending the displacement field known on the bone fragment towards the surrounding soft tissues, the skin surface is locally deformed.

4   Conclusion

This paper describes a 3D environment for simulation and prediction of true 3D problems in maxillofacial surgery. Examples are treating asymmetries, bilateral repositioning of the zygoma's, ... These problems comprise three parts: cutting of the skull, repositioning of the bone fragments and modelling the soft skin tissue to predict the expected face after surgery.

Concerning osteotomies, we are able to cut the bone according to free-hand drawn 3D trajectories and cutting blades. Uptill now, we allow free 3D repositioning of the bone fragments (three dimensions of freedom for rotation and three dimensions of freedom for rotation). Giving the surgeon extra guidance to reposition the bone fragments using 3D cephalometry can be an interesting tool speeding up the simulation process. However, as explained, analysis based on 3D cephalometry needs further investigations.

We introduced a general voxel-based formalism for predicting the face after surgery. We instantiated the formalism in a concrete implementation. Comparing our approach to the voxel-based methods of Gibson [6, 7] it will be clear that the latter requires adaptions and generalisations for the application of maxillo-facial surgery: at least two different kind of tissue need to be introduced and attention needs to given to displacements induced by osteotomy and repositioning. Also the ChainMail's important property of visiting only once needs reconsideration in the case of different types of tissue and the presence of non-convex structures.

The focus of further research will be on refinement of the soft tissue deformation model on incorporation of 3D cephalometric analysis and on validation of this approach towards clinical application.

Acknowledgments

The work discussed here belongs, partly to the grant GOA/99/05 (VHS+ Variability in Human Shape and Speech) of the K.U.Leuven Research Council, and partly to the EU-funded Brite Euram III *PISA* project (nr. BRPR CT97 0378). Partners in the latter are Materialise NV, Belgium; Philips Medical Systems BV, the Netherlands: ICS-AD; DePuy International Ltd, UK; Ceka NV, Belgium; K.U. Leuven, Belgium: ESAT/Radiology & Div. Biomechanics; University of Leeds, UK: Research School of Medicine.

References

1. G. Schultes, Q. Gaggl, H. Kärcher: Accuracy of Cephalometric and Video Imaging Program Dentofacial Planner Plus in Orthognathic Surgical Planning. Computer Aided Surgery, Vol. 3, Nr. 3, p 108–114, 1998
2. J. Kragskov, S. Sindet-Petersen, C. Gyldensted, K.L. Jensen: A comparison of three-dimensional computed tomography scans and stereolithographic models for evaluation of craniofacial anomalies. Journal of Oral and Maxillofacial Surgery, 54:4, p 402–411, April 1996
3. M. Vannier, J. Marsh, A. Tsiaras: Craniofacial Surgical Planning and Evaluation with Computers. Computer Integrated Surgery (eds. Taylor, Lavallee, Burdea, Mosges) MIT press 1996, p 673–678
4. D. Altobelli, R. Kikinis, J. Mulliken, H. Cline, W. Lorensen, F. Jolesz Computer-Assisted Three-Dimensional Planning in Craniofacial Surgery Plastic and Reconstructive Surgery, 1993, vol 92, p 576–585
5. E. Keeve, S. Girod, B. Girod: Craniofacial Surgery Simulation. Proceedings of the 4th International Conference on Visualisation in Biomedical Computing VBC'96, p 541–546
6. S. Gibson 3D Chainmail: a fast algorithm for deforming volumetric objects. Proc. Symposium on Interactive 3D Graphics, ACM SIGGRAPH, p 149–154
7. S. Gibson, C. Fyock, E. Grimson, T. Kanade, R. Kikinis, H. Lauer, N. McKenzie, A. Mor, S. Nakajima, H. Ohkami, R. Osborne, J. Samosky, A. Sawada Volumetric modeling for surgical simulation. Medical Image Analysis, 2(2), p 121–132
8. P. Bohner, C. Holler, S. Hassfeld Operation Planning in Craniomaxillofacial Surgery Computer Aided Surgery, 1997, Vol 2(3/4), p 153–161
9. R. Fuhrmann, H. Feifel, A. Schnappauf, P. Diedrich: Integration of Three-Dimensional Cephalometry and 3D-Skull Models in Combined Orthodontic/Surgical Treatment Planning. Journal of Otofacial Orthopedics, 57:1, p 32–45, February 1996
10. B. Mollard, S. Lavallée, G. Bettega: Computer Assisted Orthognatic Surgery. Proc. MICCAI98, Lect. Notes in Computer Science, 1496, 1998, p 21–28
11. S.D. Kirby, B. Wang, C.W.S. To, H.B. Lampe: Nonlinear, Three-Dimensional Finite-Element Model of Skin Biomechanics Journal of Otolaryngology, 27:3, p 153–160, June 1998
12. Fast finite elements for surgery simulation. Medicine Meets Virtual Reality V, 1997
13. Real-time volumetric deformable models for surgery simulation using finite elements and condensation. Proc. Eurographics, vol. 15, p 57–66, 1996
14. J. Van Cleynenbreugel, K. Verstreken, G. Marchal, P. Suetens: A flexible environment for image guided virtual surgery planning. Proc. VBC96, Lect. Notes in Computer Science, 1131, 1996, p 501–510
15. F. Schutyser, J. Van Cleynenbreugel, V. Vander Poorten, P. Delaere, G. Marchal, P. Suetens: An experimental image guided surgery simulator for hemicricolaryngectomy and reconstrunction by tracheal autotransplantation. Proc. MICCAI98, Lect. Notes in Computer Science, 1496, 1998, p 919–925
16. K. Verstreken, J. Van Cleynenbreugel, K. Martens, G. Marchal, D. van Steenberghe, P. Suetens: An image-guided Planning System for Endosseous Oral Implants. IEEE Transactions on Medical Imaging Vol 17, no 5, pp. 842-852, October 1998
17. J. Werneke: The Inventor Mentor, Programming Object-Oriented 3D Graphics with OpenInventor Addison-Wesley, release 2, 1994
18. ShapeSnatcher, www.eyetronics.com
19. Paul J. Besl and Neil D. McKay: A Method for Registration of 3-D Shapes. IEEE Trans. on Pattern Analysis and Machine Intelligence, 14:2, p 239–256, 1992
20. Anand Rangarajan, Haili Chui, Eric Mjolsness, Suguna Pappu, Lila Davachi, Patricia Goldman-Rakic, James Duncan: A robust point-matching algorithm for autoradiograph alignment. Medical Image Analysis, Vol. 1, Nr. 4, p 379–398, 1997
21. C. Cutting, F. Bookstein, B. Grayson, L. Felligham, J. McCarthy Three-Dimensional Computer-Assisted Design of Craniofacial Surgical Procedures: Optimization and Interaction with Cephalometric and CT-Based Models. Plastic and Reconstructive Surgery, 1986, vol 77, p 877–885

Surgical Forces and Tactile Perception During Retinal Microsurgery

Puneet K. Gupta, Patrick S. Jensen, Eugene de Juan, Jr.[1]

The Microsurgical Advanced Design Laboratory
Wilmer Eye Institute
Johns Hopkins University
721 Maumenee
600 North Wolfe Street
Baltimore, MD 21287
puneet@jhu.edu

Abstract. Purpose: Vitreoretinal surgery involves the manipulation of delicate retinal membranes with a required surgical accuracy often on the order of tens of microns, a scale at or near the limit of human positional ability. In addition, forces imposed by the tissue on the surgical tool are exceedingly small. Here we investigate the magnitude of forces generated during retinal surgery in cadaveric porcine eyes and compare the results with the magnitude of forces discernable by retinal surgeons. This data will be used as a design guideline for robotic surgical augmentation systems currently under development. Methods: The study was performed in two phases. First, retinal surgeons manipulated the retina of porcine cadaver eyes with a calibrated 1-axis force sensing retinal pick while data was simultaneously recorded. In the second phase, blindfolded subjects held the pick and were instructed to press a button whenever an "event" was felt. Events were generated by slowly tapping the end of the pick with varying force while both the magnitudes of forces applied and the responses of the subjects were recorded. The magnitudes of forces generated during retinal surgery were then compared with those that could be discerned by the subjects. Results: Roughly 75% of all forces measured during retinal microsurgery were found to be less than 7.5 mN in magnitude, however, only $19.3 \pm 8.1\%$ (N=492) of events generated at this level could be felt by the subjects. Conclusions: The results of this study indicate that a majority of retinal surgery is probably performed without the surgeon being able to "feel" interactions between retinal tissue and the surgical tool. Prior studies have indicated that relying on visual feedback alone increases the length of manual manipulation tasks and reduces task accuracy. The lack of tactile sensation during retinal surgery similarly could adversely affect surgical outcome.

[1] We gratefully acknowledge the support of the National Science Foundation under grant #IIS9801684.

1. Introduction

Retinal microsurgery is a complex manual manipulation task requiring judgement, microscopic visualization and precision [1,2]. In addition, we feel that the delicate nature of microsurgical procedures probably provides limited tactile sensation to the surgeon about the tissue manipulation being performed. A lack of tactile information during similar manual manipulation tasks has been shown to reduce both speed and accuracy of manipulation [3]. With an end goal of developing microsurgical augmentation devices capable of enhancing positional accuracy and tactile sensation [4], we investigate the threshold of tactile sensation during retinal microsurgery. This study will be used as a design guideline for such augmentation systems.

2. Background

Vitreoretinal ophthalmic microsurgery deals with the vitreous chamber and the associated retina, which covers the inner surface of the eye and is responsible for vision (figure 1). Sometimes the retina becomes diseased such as in diabetic retinopathy [5] where scar tissue forms on the surface of the retina, requiring the gentle peeling off of the thin membrane without compromising vision. Vitreoretinal procedures involve placing instruments through the sclera while observing the visual field through the cornea and lens using a steromicroscope [6].

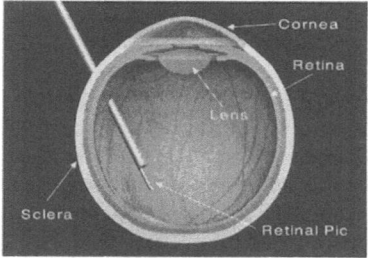

Fig. 1. Basic anatomy of the eye along with sample insertion of surgical pick.

Manipulation of retinal membranes is very delicate and generates forces believed to be below what the surgeon can feel. In studies by Howe et. al. and Patkin [7], the lack of tactile feedback drastically slowed the manipulation and resulted in positional errors possibly as a result of slow visual pathways [8]. Tactile feedback, through touch, pressure, or vibration, results from the stimulation of one or more of four types of mechanoreceptors [3,9]. The minimum threshold for these receptors can be affected by many variables, from such things as age and gender to inhomogeneity of the body surface noted by Weber [10]. Weinstein found the fingers to have a threshold range of 50-100 mg (0.5 - 1 mN) over an area of less than 1 mm^2.

A particular sense can convey more information concerning a particular aspect of an occurrence than another sense could provide [11]. For example, vision is most perceptive to spatial changes, while tactile sensations are sensitive to such things as force/pressure changes. Microsurgery is a manual manipulation task performed primarily using visual feedback. Therefore, in microsurgery, the visual sense predominates followed by touch [12]. However, if these sensory inputs are synergistically integrated, performance could be improved substantially through intersensory integration.

Vitreoretinal surgery is a delicate microsurgical procedure that possibly lacks sufficient tactile feedback. Three interesting topics to investigate in this study are the nature of the forces during retinal microsurgery, the tactile perception thresholds in a simulated microsurgical environment, and the comparison of the two categories to assess the need of enhancing tactile sensation through such robotic platforms as the "steady hand" micromanipulator.

3. Methods

The study was performed in two phases. First, retinal surgeons manipulated the retina of porcine cadaver eyes with a calibrated force sensing retinal pick. In the second phase, blindfolded subjects held the pick and were instructed to press a button whenever a simulated "event" was felt. The magnitudes of forces generated during retinal surgery were then compared with the magnitudes of forces that could be perceived by the subjects.

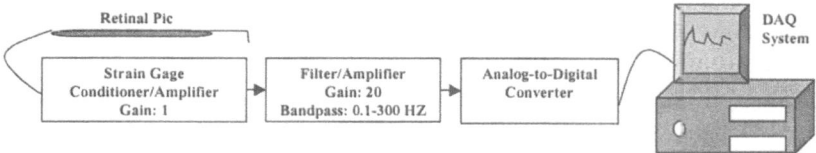

Fig. 2. Block diagram for the experimental setup. Strain gages placed on the retinal pick are conditioned using a strain gage amplifier, filtered prior to A/D conversion at 1 kHz and then stored in data files on a computer.

3.1 Data Acquisition System

The shaft of a retinal pick was flattened and fitted into an ergonomic surgical handle. Foil gages (Measurement Group, Model #EA-06-030LB-120) were affixed with adhesive in a half-bridge configuration and coated with a layer of silicone and shrink wrap tubing. The half-bridge was connected to a strain gage conditioner/amplifier system (Measurements Group, System 2100) with unity gain. The amplifier output was filtered with a bandpass of 0.1-300 Hz and was amplified as a single-ended referenced input with a gain of 20. The signal was digitized at 1 kHz using a PC based (450 MHz Dell computer) analog-to-digital converter (National Instruments, Model PCI 6024E) into files using a custom LabView (National Instruments) application (figure 2). The raw voltage values were converted to forces using a pre-determined calibration curve (R^2 = 0.9995, Rice Lakes Weighing Systems, Model #0F51, Class F).

3.2 Experimental Protocol

Retinal Manipulation Porcine cadaver eyes were used to determine the force range experienced during retinal manipulation (figure 3). An eye was placed in the socket of a model head. The cornea and lens were removed, exposing the anterior chamber and the iris. The calibrated instrumented retinal probe was then inserted through the pupil to the retina. The subject manipulated the retina while observing the procedure through a microscope. The strain resulting from the soft tissue forces on the pick during manipulation was acquired for approximately 2 minutes. Care was taken so that the pick shaft did not come in contact with the iris at the point of insertion to avoid extraneous data. This was repeated with 10 subjects.

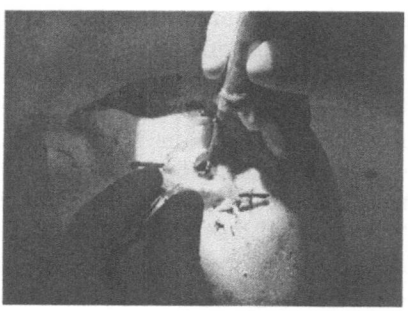

Fig. 3. Ten subjects manipulated the retina of porcine cadaver eyes with a calibrated force sensing retinal pick while force data was continuously recorded.

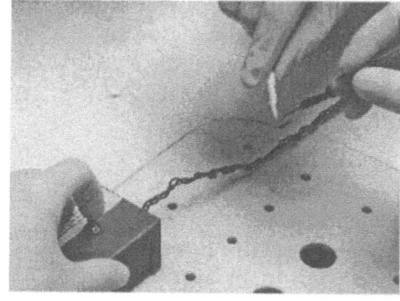

Fig. 4. Blindfolded subjects held the pick and were instructed to press a button whenever an "event" was felt. Events were generated by slowly tapping the end of the pick with varying force.

Threshold Testing of Tactile Perception The threshold values of tactile perception were determined using the same instrumented retinal pick (figure 4). The subject, wearing surgical gloves, held the pick using a wrist rest, mimicking a vitreoretinal surgical procedure. The subject then closed his/her eyes while maintaining the surgical position. A twisted paper towel then was used to create distinct unique events at the tip of the pick. If the event was felt by the subject, the subject would push a button. A time span of at least 1 second passed between events to allow the subject a chance to respond to the stimuli. The events varied in amplitude. Between 40-60 events were produced per subject. The subject was allowed trial runs to become accustomed to the stimuli.

4.   Results

A total of 10 subjects were tested, 6 medical doctors, including residents, fellows, and attending surgeons, all with microsurgical experience and 4 non-experienced personnel without medical degrees. The age range was from 21 to 45 years old. The range of surgical experience amongst those medical doctors was from 1 to 18 years.

4.1 Retinal Manipulation

The force traces from the two most experienced vitreoretinal surgeons of the group were used as indicative measures of the magnitudes and frequencies of forces that are exerted during retinal manipulations.   Figure 5 depicts a typical 30 second force trace during retinal manipulation. The positive values denote lifting of the retina.   Figure 6 is the associated power spectrum for a characteristic manipulation event from the same 30 seconds. Figure 7 shows that roughly 75% of manipulation events (N=181) used less than 7.5 mN of force.

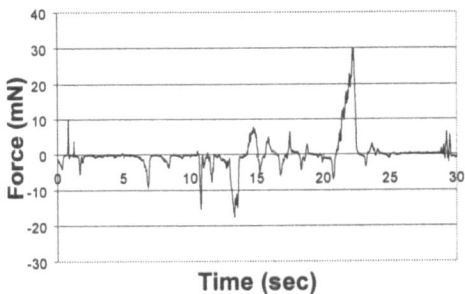

Fig. 5. A sample 30 second force trace during retinal manipulation. The positive values denote lifting of the retina.

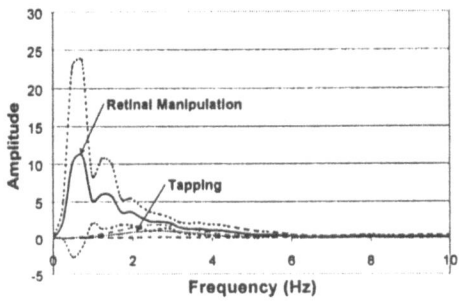

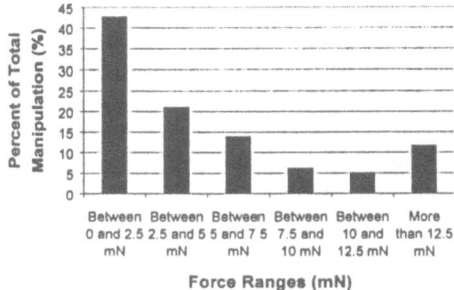

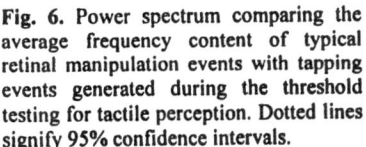

Fig. 6. Power spectrum comparing the average frequency content of typical retinal manipulation events with tapping events generated during the threshold testing for tactile perception. Dotted lines signify 95% confidence intervals.

Fig. 7. Shows the percentage of events that fell within each force range during retinal manipulation. Note that 75% of all manipulations are less than 7.5 mN.

4.2 Threshold testing of tactile perception

Data from all ten subjects were used in the analysis. Figure 8 shows a 20 second sample of the tapping test. The solid black spikes denote an event. The downshift of the lighter grey lines denotes tactile sensation. Figure 6 shows the power spectrum of a characteristic induced event. A total of 492 events were recorded. Since 75% of all manipulations occurred less than 7.5 mN, the data was divided into two groups based on this value. The percent of detection within the two groups was determined (figure 9). Only 19.3 ± 8.1% of events less than 7.5 mN could be detected, while 59.2 ± 28.2% of events greater than 7.5 mN were perceived. This difference was found to be highly significant (p=0.0005) using the F-test.

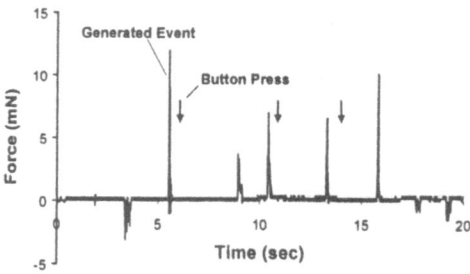

Fig. 8. A 20 second sample demonstrating how the threshold measurements were taken. The solid black spikes denote stimuli. The arrows below the time axis denote tactile sensation.

5. Discussion

It was crucial to obtain both data sets with the same measuring device and under similar operating conditions in order to minimize variables that could alter data correlation. It is important to realize the other variables that can affect the data from one individual to another, such as fatigue, stress, and level of training.

The presented data demonstrates that the majority of retinal surgery is performed without being able to "feel" tool-tissue interactions since most of the manipulative events are below the

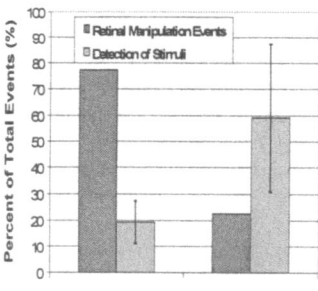

Fig. 9. Only 19.3 ± 8.1% of events less than 7.5 mN, which made up 75% of all retinal manipulations, could be detected, while 59.2 ± 28.2% of events greater than 7.5 mN, which made up only 25% of manipulations, were perceived.

threshold of tactile sensation. This supports the theory that most microsurgery is performed utilizing predominately visual feedback alone, which is slower and not as accurate as when combined with from tactile sensation.

The threshold values obtained in this study are higher than those from Weinstein's study. This is probably attributed to using a blunt instrument handle instead of Weinstein's pointed stimulator [10] since the area of application of the blunt surface is more, and hence a greater force is needed to reach the threshold pressure. In the microsurgical environment, the interfacing surfaces are blunt, thus requiring a higher amount of force to elicit a tactile sensation. There are also other factors that may contribute to the difference, such as wearing surgical latex gloves in addition to sitting in a more stressful position.

In addition to the magnitudes of forces, another interesting parameter to consider is the power spectrum. The frequency content of the events during retinal manipulation was compared to that of the stimuli during the sensitivity test to determine whether or not the events being produced were indicative of those that are actually experienced during vitreoretinal microsurgery (figure 6). The DC component of the frequencies was eliminated by subtracting the mean of the magnitude of the data sets before running a power spectral analysis on them. From the spectrum plot, it can be seen that though the two data sets are predominately composed of low frequencies (less than 20 Hz), the frequency content of the events generated during the threshold testing of tactile perception seems to be higher than that of retinal manipulation. A way of generating events that better follow the power spectrum of retinal manipulation is currently being explored.

Tactile Augmentation With intense training, surgical performance can be further enhanced, though as can be seen by the presented data, much of what is done during retinal surgery cannot be felt. However, via tactile surgical augmentation, enhanced tactile sensation will allow for further increase in performance encompassing accuracy, speed, and safety. One solution incorporates force sensing and tactile feedback into the "steady-hand" micromanipulator, an augmentative approach conceived at Johns Hopkins University [4]. In this system, the forces that exist at the tool tip-tissue interface are monitored by the robot's controller and are used in control system algorithms. The result is force scaling which would enhance tactile sensation by detecting and amplifying the forces described above to a level perceptible by human touch. The end result would be enhanced positional accuracy and augmented tactile sensation during microsurgical procedures such as retinal manipulation.

6. Conclusions

Though modern day microsurgical instruments and procedures have revolutionized ophthalmologic surgery, human performance is still limited. Scientifically exploring these limitations will lead to novel augmentative surgical devices that will remove some of these limitations, such as with tactile sensation. This could potentially lead to new microsurgical techniques that are not currently possible.

7. References

[1] Charles, S. "Dexterity Enhancement for Surgery." *Proc First Int'l Symp Medical Robotics and Computer Assisted Surgery.* 1994, 2: 145-160.

[2] Tamai, S. "History of Microsurgery -- from the beginning until the end of the 1970s." *Microsurgery,* 1993. 14(1): 6.

[3] Howe, R.D., *et. al.* "Tactile Display of Vibratory Information in Teleoperation and Virtual Environments." *Presence,* 1995. 4(4): 387-402.

[4] Taylor, R., *et. al.* "A Steady-Hand Robotic System for Microsurgical Augmentation." Accepted to *the Second International Conference on Medical Image Computing and Computer-Assisted Intervention.*

[5] Michels, R.G. *Vitreous Surgery.* C.V.Mosby: St. Louis, 1981.

[6] Eisner, G. *Eye Surgery.* Springer-Verlay: New York, 1978.

[7] Patkin, M. "Ergonomics Aspects of Surgical Dexterity." *Medical Journal of Australia,* 1967. 2(17): p.775-5.

[8] Patkin, M. "Ergonomics applied to the practice of microsurgery." *Aust NZ J Surg.,* 1977. 47(3): p.320-329.

[9] Kandel, E.R., Schwartz, J.H., Jessell, T.M. *Principles of Neuroscience, 3rd ed.* Elsevier Science: New York, 1991.

[10] Weinstein, S. "Intensive and extensive aspects of tactile sensitivity as a function of body part, sex, and laterality", in *The Skin Senses,* D.R. Kenshalo, Ed. Thomas: Springfield, IL, 1968.

[11] Sage, G.H. *Introduction to Motor Behavior: A Neuropsychological Approach.* Addison-Wesley Publishing: Reading, MA, 1984.

[12] Knudson, D.V., Morrison, C.S. *Qualitative Analysis of Human Movement.* Human Kinetics: Champaign, IL, 1997.

A Novel Technique for Simulating Transcranial Doppler Examinations *In Vitro*

Robin Hart[1], Philip D. Hart[2] and Stuart Bunt[1]

[1] Department of Anatomy and Human Biology, University of Western Australia
[2] The Hart Combination Company Limited, Bath, United Kingdom

Abstract. The left internal carotid artery of a cadaveric head was injected with a methyl methacrylate casting resin. The cast of the vessels of the Circle of Willis was used to construct an artificial arterial system from Tygon R3603 tubing. Sylgard 527 elastomer gel was used to replace the intracranial contents. Sylgard 184 was used to replicate the extracranial tissues. The model was perfused with a fluid consisting of sephadex particles and glycerine, which approximates normal blood characteristics. Physiologically accurate fluid flow was achieved using a custom designed computer controlled syringe pump which could deliver normal or pathological flow profiles as required. Age and sex matched control data were compared with data obtained from the model system using a Transcranial Doppler scanner. The results showed that a close approximation between the artificial and *in vivo* flow patterns could be achieved by manipulation of the flow profile.

1 Introduction

Transcranial Doppler Ultrasound (TCD) is a diagnostic technique used to assess blood flow in the head. This is important in the management of cerebral vasospasm (VSP), a condition commonly seen in survivors of acute subarachnoid haemorrhage. The detection of VSP is most accurately performed using Digital Subtraction Angiographic studies, but such invasive procedures carry high inherent risk, and may be contraindicated. TCD, although less sensitive and specific, poses significantly less risk to the patient [1].

Transcranial Doppler ultrasound suffers two significant limitations:
a. It is a conceptually difficult technique to learn and demonstrate; and
b. Intra-operator variability may lead to high rates of false positive or false negative results [1].

This study aims to construct an artificial system which is able to simulate TCD examinations of both normal and pathologic vascular states. Training in TCD examination technique can then be performed in a controlled environment. This study forms the first part of the development of a system of co-registration between digital subtraction angiography images of vascular anatomy, and physiological data from TCD examinations.

2 Methods

2.1 Preparation of the Cadaveric Model

A 74 year old female cadaver was cannulated through the left internal carotid artery, and the cerebral circulation flushed using normal saline. An injection of 50 mls of green methyl methacrylate casting material ("Vertex" Dentimex Zeist, Holland) was then made using a 12 french arterial catheter, with hand injection from a 50 ml syringe [2]. The arterial catheter was withdrawn, the wound closed, and the body embalmed for three months via cannulation of the femoral artery and infusion of embalming solution (Formalin (7.5%), Glycerin (20%), Phenol (6%), Methylated Spirit (40%), Water (26.5%)).

Specimen Dissection. After removal of the head at the fourth cervical vertebra, a plaster cast impression of the head was taken. The postero-superior part of the skull was then removed at its widest diameter. The extracranial tissues were grossly dissected, and the cervical spine removed.

All brain tissues, including the arachnoid mater, were removed. The Circle of Willis (COW) was left *in situ*, and sectioned to remove all arteries except: the distal internal carotid; anterior , middle and posterior cerebral (ACA, MCA and PCA respectively); anterior (ACoA) and posterior (PCoA) communicating, vertebral (VA), basilar (BA) and cerebellar arteries. The vessel walls were completely dissected to reveal the previously injected Vertex casting medium, which was removed from the skull, and immersed in saturated potassium hydroxide for three days.

Vessel Reconstruction. The vertex cast of the vessels was used as a model from which an artificial circulation was constructed, using direct measurement, from Tygon R3603 tubing (Lab Supplies Australia). This material has some elastic properties, although there was no attempt to closely replicate *in vivo* arterial elasticity. This model was then re-inserted into the skull.

A de-aerated silicone based gel, Sylgard 527 dielectric polymer (Dow Corning), was used to replace the intracranial contents. All air was removed by placement under vacuum of 29 inches of mercury for 30 minutes This material is recognised as possessing physical and ultrasonic properties similar to those of brain tissue [3], [4].

After a seven day delay for cure, a second polymer gel, Sylgard 184 (Dow Corning) was mixed and de-aerated. This was then poured around the skull assembly, previously placed in the facial cast, to form a robust seal, which also recreated the facial features of the cadaver.

2.2 Perfusion

Pump Construction. The pump consists of a 12 ml capacity, 12 mm stroke piston and cylinder assembly, driven by a stepper motor. The cylinder head has an inlet and an outlet ball valve, both being closed by a compression spring. The outlet valve closing spring has a tension adjustment screw to vary the opening and closing pressures. The output of the pump was designed to allow emulation of a typical maximum cerebral supply of 1 litre of perfusate per minute.

The stepper motor was driven by a drive card (GSM5, Greenwich Instruments), controlled by a 300 MHz Pentium® personal computer. With a step angle of 1.8 degrees, the pump has 330 steps in the full travel of the piston.

Software. A program was written in Visual Basic 6° (Microsoft) which allowed digitised data from *in vivo* flow conditions to be delivered to the pump. Up to seven different waveforms may be previously defined, and these may be combined in any order to a maximum of thirteen in any one wave train. This train is self-repeating. Data plots of normal left ventricular volume against time were obtained [5]. These were manually digitised, using graph paper, with sample points at 25 ms intervals. Data points were plotted as percentage of maximal contraction against time. These were converted to the appropriate number of motor steps. This output was delivered to the program at pulse rates of 30 to 180 beats per minute (bpm).

Delivery System. The delivery system was a development of previous work [6], [7], [8], [9]. The pump output was taken from the outlet valve via vinyl laboratory tubing (Nylex, Australia) of 8mm internal diameter. This tube fed into the middle of a capacitance tank holding 1L of perfusate. The outlet from the tank was in the middle of the vessel on the side opposite the inlet. A baffle plate was set vertically from the bottom of the tank dividing the line between the inlet and the outlet to ensure that the smoothing effect of the tank was not eliminated by direct streaming between inlet and outlet. At maximal filling, the additional pressure head provided by the tank was 5cm.

The 8mm outlet from the tank terminated in a four-way flow divider. The output from the divider was taken via 5mm tubing to the inlet ports of the VAs and ICAs of the model. The differential flow through each of these tubes was controlled by a tap. The system was set to deliver 82% through the anterior circulation, and 18% through the posterior circulation. This simulates the typical *in vivo* distributions [10].

2.3 Perfusate

A perfusate with the same effective acoustic reflector surface as blood was developed to provide return echo signals from which doppler data was derived. The perfusion medium was prepared using the following concentrations of materials:

Glycerol: 5%
Sephadex particles (80 µm average particle size)   0.28%
Distilled water   94.72%

The glycerol allows sufficient reduction in surface tension of the water to allow
perfusion of the models. The concentration of sephadex particles allowed the use of
identical gain settings on the TCD scanner for both *in vitro* and *in vivo* examinations.

2.4 Ultrasound Scanning

Model. The model was subjected to a TCD examination of all major arterial
segments accessible from the trans-pterional window: ICA, M1 and M2 MCA
segments, A1 ACA and P1 PCA segments, using an EME Companion (Nicolet
Biomedical, Madison, WI, USA) single channel 2MHz TCD scanner. Trans-orbital
access was used for the ophthalmic artery and carotid artery siphon.   These
examinations were undertaken while the model was perfused with a normal cardiac
output wave. The TCD data (Table 1) were taken from the insonation attempt which
yielded the best signal:noise ratio for each vessel segment. Controls were side-
matched scans of age and sex matched patients, with normal cerebral circulation.
Figures 1 and 3 were obtained from the MCA with the sample volume at a depth of
60mm for both *in vivo* and *in vitro* cases.

Gel Samples. The gels used do not have the identical behaviour when insonated as
the tissues that they replace. A sample of each was prepared to generate correction
factors.   These correction factors take into account the difference in transmission
speed of ultrasound through the gel and tissue, and hence the difference between real
and apparent depth measurements.

A degassed sample of 527 gel was poured into a cylindrical container measuring
75.5mm deep, and 18mm in diameter. Degassed 184 gel was poured into a cuboid
container, 44.5mm deep, 34mm wide and 53mm long. All measurements taken with
vernier calipers. To measure the apparent depth of the gel samples (the TCD system
being unable to produce an image) the sample of both 527 and 184 gel were imaged
with a Toshiba PowerVision ultrasound system. A small quantity of Scan ultrasound
coupling medium (Parker Laboratories Inc., Fairfield, N.J., USA) was used between a
7.5 MHz linear array ultrasound probe and the surface of the gel sample. As speed of
transmission of ultrasound through a given medium is frequency independent, these
results are also comparable to those of a 2 MHz TCD probe. The samples were
insonated from the exposed gel surface at the top of the container, and measurements
taken between this gel surface and the bottom of the container, using the on-screen
cursors supplied as part of the Toshiba ultrasound system software (Table 2). These
are accurate to ± 0.1mm (Toshiba).

3 Results

3.1 Model

The model demonstrated circulatory tubal patency, and successful perfusion at rates of up to 900 mls/min was achieved.

3.2 Waveform Data

Figures 1a and 1b show that the artificial circulation closely mimics actual flow. The waveform shown in Figure 1a was generated using the pump input shown in Figure 2a, applied at a rate of 30 beats per minute. There is, however, considerable angularity of the wave shape, with elements resembling square wave functions seen throughout the profile. In contrast, the *in vivo* waveform demonstrates a smooth profile.

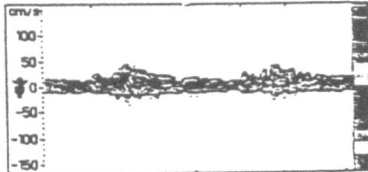   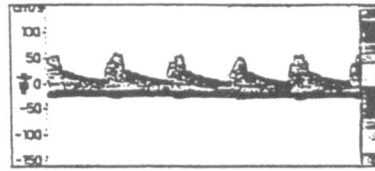

Fig. 1a. Artificial TCD Output   **Fig. 1b.** *In Vivo* TCD Output

Figure 1a shows the TCD output with a sample depth of 60mm. This equates to a real depth of 59.76mm (See Table 2). This is within the sample volume size of 15mm, and hence the error can be ignored. Figure 1b illustrates a normal control graph from a 73 year old female. This waveform represents a heamodynamic state in the same anatomic location[1]

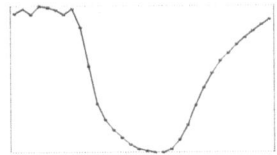
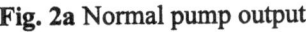   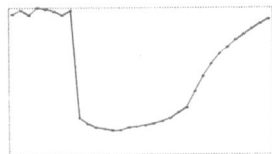

Fig. 2a Normal pump output   **Fig. 2b** Modified pump output

Figure 2 shows input waveforms to the pump, as piston position (% of travel) against time. Figure 2a illustrates a normal left ventricular contraction profile. Figure 2b shows a modified input waveform with the systolic contraction more rapid, and the time at contraction lengthened

---

1 These are exact replicas of the original TCD scanner output

A modification of the wave supplied to the pump (Figure 2b), and an increase in the pump rate to 62 beats per minute, led to the results shown by Figures 3a and 3b.

The altered (non-physiologic) input waveform, when combined with the artificial circulation, yields a hybrid circulation which has the effect of smoothing the TCD output, and hence closely approximating a true *in vivo* TCD output wave profile.

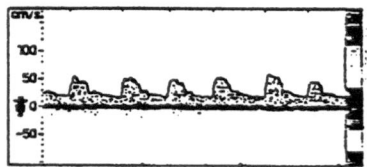   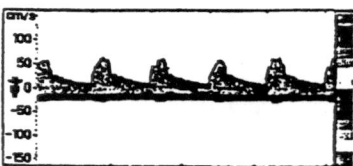

Fig. 3a. Modified artificial TCD Output   **Fig. 3b** *In Vivo* TCD output

Figure 3a illustrates the TCD output using the modified pump waveform, and Figure 3b illustrates the age-matched control at the same depth[1]

Table 1. Data comparing the waveforms shown in Figure 1 and Figure 3

		Mean Velocity	Systolic Velocity	Diastolic Velocity	P.I	R.I
Figure 1	In Vitro (Fig. 1a)	21 cm/s	43 cm/s	10 cm/s	1.43	0.77
	In Vivo (Fig. 1b)	34 cm/s	70 cm/s	18 cm/s	1.49	0.75
Figure 3	In Vitro (Fig. 3a)	22 cm/s	48 cm/s	9 cm/s	1.63	0.81
	In Vivo Fig. 3b)	34 cm/s	70 cm/s	18 cm/s	1.49	0.75

P.I. = Pulsatility Index, R.I. = Resitivity Index

In all cases the blood flow velocity of the *in vitro* circulation is between one half and two thirds of that *in vivo*. This may be due inertial effects of the pump mechanism, and differences in the compliance of the vessels between the pump and model

Table 2. Data showing the derivation of ultrasound depth correction factors for the gels

	Sylgard 527 Gel	Sylgard 184 Gel
Sample depth (mm)	75.5	44.5
Measured depths (mm)	65.4, 66.1, 66.9, 67.3	67.9, 68.0, 67.6, 67.6
= Average (mm)	66.4	67.8
Measured /real depth (%)	88	152

From these data, a table (Table 3) was generated to allow correction of scanning depth errors.

Table 3. Correction table for different skin thicknesses (Sylgard 184) over typical insonation depths

Real Depth (mm)	Skin Thickness (mm)					
	4.00	6.00	8.00	10.00	12.00	14.00
	Error (mm)					
40	-1.66	-0.40	0.86	2.12	3.38	4.64
44	-1.88	-0.62	0.64	1.90	3.16	4.42
48	-2.10	-0.84	0.42	1.68	2.94	4.20
52	-2.32	-1.06	0.20	1.46	2.72	3.98
56	-2.54	-1.28	-0.02	1.24	2.50	3.76
60	-2.76	-1.50	-0.24	1.02	2.28	3.54
66	-4.74	-3.48	-2.22	-0.96	0.30	1.56
70	-5.18	-3.92	-2.66	-1.40	-0.14	1.12
76	-5.84	-4.58	-3.32	-2.06	-0.80	0.46
80	-6.28	-5.02	-3.76	-2.50	-1.24	0.02

4 Discussion

Alteration of both the wave profile and the rate of the pump input has a smoothing effect on the TCD output. The lack of a real circulation (particularly small vessels), the lack of elastic capacitance vessels, and the relatively high inertia of the pump, combine to produce a circulatory system very different from that in the human subject. The use of an artificial pump input is required to emulate a normal output wave. Further refinement of the vessels of the circulation may lead to a closer approximation to the real situation.

There is close correlation between the resistivity (0.77 versus 0.75 = 2.5%) and pulsatility (1.43 versus 1.49 = 4%) indices of the real and artificial waveforms in the input wave shown in Figure 2a. For the modified input waveform shown in Figure 2b, these values are slightly worse: resistivity: 0.81 versus 0.75 = 9%; pulsatility: 1.63 versus 1.49 = 9%. However, this input wave yields a closer output wave shape. This may reflect the artificial nature of the circulation, particularly the lack of peripheral resistance vessels.

This study confirms that Sylgard 527 is a useful tissue analogue for brain. In combination with Sylgard 184, Table 3 demonstrates that sample depth errors lie within the resolution limit of current TCD scanners (typically 2 mm), when imaging through typical tissue thicknesses.

5 Conclusion

This study describes a technique to create anatomically accurate models of the cerebral circulation from cadaveric material. The apparatus described allows these models to be perfused in a way that can simulate *in vivo* flow within the resolution limits of the TCD technique. Future studies will reveal whether the restrictions imposed by the artificial nature of the system can be overcome to allow accurate replication of other *in vivo* flow profiles.

Acknowledgments

This work was in part supported by a grant from the Medical Research Foundation of Royal Perth Hospital; and by the Lotteries Commission of Western Australia. The authors wish to thank Dr Mark Kanghure, Ms Helen Wines, and Mrs Elvie Haluszkiewicz (Royal Perth Hospital Radiology Department); Mr Darryl Kirk, Mr Mark Peterson Mr Brian Peppler and Mr Albert Kalajzich (Department of Anatomy and Human Biology, University of Western Australia).

References

1. Babikian, V.L., Weschler, L.R.: Transcranial Doppler Ultrasonography. Mosby Year Book, St Louis (1993)
2. Kerber, C.W., Heilman, C.B.: Flow Dynamics in the Human Carotid Artery: 1. Preliminary Observations using a Transparent Elastic Model. A.J.N.R. 13 (1992) 173-180
3. Meaney, D.F., Smith, D.H., Shreiber, D.I., Allison, C.B., Miller, R.T., Ross, D.T., Gennarelli, T.A.: Biomechanical Analysis of Experimental Diffuse Axonal Injury J. Neurotrauma 12 4 (1995) 689-694
4. Kerber, C.W., Heilman, C.B., Zanetti, P.H.: Transparent Elastic Models 1: A Brief Technical Note. Biorheology 26 (1989) 1041-1049
5. Anthony, C.P., Thibodeau, G.A., Preszbindowski K.S.: Textbook of Anatomy and Physiology. The C.V. Mosby Company, St Louis (1979)
6. Lutz, R.J., Hsu, L., Menawat, A., Zrubek, J., Edwards, K.: Comparison of Steady and Pulsatile Flow in a Double Branching Arterial Model. J. Biomechanics 16 (1983) 753-766
7. Roach, M.R., Scott, S., Ferguson, G.G.: The Hemodynamic Importance of the Geometry of Bifurcations in the Circle of Willis (Glass Model Studies). Stroke 3 (1972) 255-267
8. Stehbens, W.E.: Turbulence of Blood Flow. Quart. J. Exp. Physiol. 44 (1959) 110-117
9. Cohen, M.I., Wang, D.-M., Tarbell, J.M.: Measurement of Oscillatory Flow Pressure Gradient in an Elastic Artery Model. Biorheology 32 4 (1995) 459-471
10. Boyajian, R.A., Schwend, R.B., Wolfe, M.M., Bickerton, R.E., Otis, S.M.: Measurement of Anterior and Posterior Circulation Flow Contributions to Cerebral Blood Flow: An Ultrasound-Derived Volumetric Flow Analysis. J. Neuroimag. 5 (1995) 1-3

Author Index

Homma, S., 430
Homolka, P., 883
Hoogeveen, R. M., 358
Howe, R. D., 1133
Hu, R., 852
Huber, K., 883
Hug, J., 106
Hughes, A. D., 90
Hurdal, M. K., 279

Inkpen, K. B., 1072
Ionecsu, G., 768

Jackson, A., 524
Jahnke, M., 832
Jakopec, M., 1116
Jaramaz, B., 868, 876
Jenkinson, M., 308
Jensen, P., 1031, 1108, 1218
Jolesz, F. A., 1, 62, 202, 441, 809, 928, 1020

Kainberger, F., 883
Kakinuma, R., 386, 394
Kalvin, A., 820
Kanade, T., 621
Kaneko, M., 386, 394
Kansy, K., 832
Karlik, S., 218
Kasrai, R., 726
Katila, T., 192, 481
Kaus, M. R., 1
Kavoussi, L. R., 1031, 1052
Kawata, Y., 386, 394
Kazanzides, P., 820, 1010
Keen, M. C., 328
Kennedy, F. E., 900
Kerrien, E., 664
Kettenbach, J., 883
Khidhir, B., 441
Khosla, P. K., 1080
Kikinis, R., 1, 62, 202, 271, 441, 809, 928, 1020
Kim, B., 631, 638
Kim, J., 473
King, A. P., 579, 842
Kingdom, F. A. A., 726
Kleinszig, G., 1199
Knisely, J., 567
Ko, J. P., 245

Komarek, P., 973
Korvenoja, A., 481
Krempien, R., 963
Kruggel, F., 52
Kubota, T., 338
Kumar, R., 1010, 1031, 1098, 1108
Kusumoto, M., 386
Kwoh, C. K., 297

LaBarca, R. S., 876
Lacey, A. J., 524
Laine, A., 430
Lapeer, R. J., 1143
Laugier, C., 1156, 1191
Launay, L., 664
Lavallée, S., 138, 768, 1175
Lawrence, P. D., 1062
LeBihan, D., 453
Lethor, J. P., 508
Levison, T. J., 876
Liang, J., 116
Lichtenstein, S., 1088
Liebig, T., 945
Linney, A. D., 998
Lötjönen, J., 192
Lohmann, G., 489
Lohou, C., 98
Loth, F., 368
Lueth, T. C., 1125

Ma, B., 936
Machado, A. M. C., 378
Maciewicz, R. A., 328
Maes, F., 11, 128, 348
Männer, R., 981, 1166
Magnin, I. E., 192
Maier, S. E., 441
Malandain, G., 168, 555
Mangin, J.-F., 453
Mao, Z., 402
Marchal, G., 860, 1210
Martínez-Pérez, M . E., 90
Martel, A. L., 22
Martens, K., 860
Martin, A.J., 910
Mattes, J., 646
Maurer, C. R., 842, 910, 953
Maurincomme, E., 664
McInerney, T., 116
Mei, Q., 1042

Lecture Notes in Computer Science

For information about Vols. 1–1610
please contact your bookseller or Springer-Verlag